Clinical Neurophysiology of Infancy, Childhood, and Adolescence

Clinical Neurophysiology of Infancy, Childhood, and Adolescence

Gregory L. Holmes, M.D.
Professor of Medicine (Neurology) and Pediatrics
Dartmouth Medical School
Chief, Section of Neurology
Dartmouth-Hitchcock Medical Center
Lebanon, New Hampshire

H. Royden Jones, Jr., M.D.
Jaime Ortiz-Patiño Chair in Neurology
Lahey Clinic
Burlington, Massachusetts
Clinical Professor of Neurology
Harvard Medical School
Director, Electromyography Laboratory
Children's Hospital Boston
Boston, Massachusetts

Solomon L. Moshé, M.D.
Professor of Neurology, Neuroscience and Pediatrics
Vice Chair, Department of Neurology
Albert Einstein College of Medicine of
    Yeshiva University
Director, Child Neurology and Clinical Neurophysiology
    at Montefiore
The University Hospital of Albert Einstein
    College of Medicine
    and Jacobi Medical Center
Bronx, New York

BUTTERWORTH
HEINEMANN

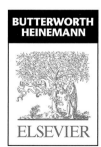

ELSEVIER

BUTTERWORTH
HEINEMANN
ELSEVIER

1600 John F. Kennedy Blvd.
Ste 1800
Philadelphia, PA 19103-2899

Library of Congress Cataloging-in-Publication Data

Clinical neurophysiology of infancy, childhood, and adolescence/Gregory L. Holmes,
    Solomon L. Moshé, H. Royden Jones, Jr.—1st ed.
        p. cm.
    ISBN 0-7506-7251-X
        1. Pediatric neurology.   2. Neurophysiology.   3. Electroencephalography.   4. Evoked potentials (Electrophysiology) I. Holmes, Gregory L. II. Moshé, Solomon L. III. Jones, Jr., H. Royden

    RJ488.C56 2006
    618.92'8—dc22

                                                                    2005042084

Acquisitions Editor: Susan Pioli
Developmental Editor: Kim J. Davis
Publishing Services Manager: Frank Polizzano
Senior Project Manager: Peter Faber
Design Direction: Steven Stave

Printed in the United States of America

Last digit is the print number: 9 8 7 6 5 4 3 2 1

Dedicated to the many children who have passed through our neurophysiology labs.

To my wife Colleen, for her enthusiasm and perseverance.
GLH

To my mentor and father-in-law Dr. Marvin Cornblath (1925–2005), my wife Nancy, my son Jared, and all the children.
SLM

To my mom, a wonderful and vigorous, now 99-year-old, retired school teacher who loves children dearly, our own kids Roy, Kate, Fred and David, and to my wife Mary who is a terrific grandmother for Erik, Kristin, Kendall, Sam, and Natalie.
HRJ

Contributors

P. IAN ANDREWS, MBBS, FRACP
Senior Lecturer, School of Women's and Children's
  Health, University of New South Wales; Paediatric
  Neurologist, Division of Neurology, Sydney Children's
  Hospital, Sydney, Australia
Neuromuscular Transmission Defects

WARREN T. BLUME, MD, FRCPC
Professor of Neurology and Paediatrics, Department of
  Clinical Neurosciences, University of Western Ontario;
  Neurologist, Department of Clinical Neurosciences,
  University Hospital, London, Ontario, Canada
*Normal Development of the Electroencephalogram: Infancy
Through Adolescence*

CHARLES F. BOLTON, MD
Adjunct Professor, Department of Medicine, Division of
  Neurology, Queen's University, Kingston, Ontario,
  Canada
*Neuromuscular Problems of the Critically Ill Neonate, Child,
and Adolescent*

ALEXIS D. BORO, MD
Assistant Professor, Department of Neurology, Albert
  Einstein College of Medicine; Attending Physician,
  Department of Neurology, Montefiore Medical Center,
  Bronx, New York
Basic Principles of Electroencephalography
The Diagnosis of Brain Death

DEBORAH Y. BRADSHAW, MD
Clinical Associate Professor, Department of Neurology,
  Upstate Medical University, Syracuse, New York
Clinical Neurophysiology of Pediatric Polyneuropathies

SAMUEL L. BRIDGERS, MD
Assistant Clinical Professor, Department of Neurology,
  Yale University School of Medicine; Director, EEG
  Laboratory, Hospital of St. Raphael, New Haven,
  Connecticut
Ambulatory Electroencephalography

PHILIP J. BRUNQUELL, MD
Associate Professor of Pediatrics and Neurology,
  University of Connecticut School of Medicine,
  Farmington, Connecticut; Medical Director, Clinical
  Neurophysiology Laboratories, Connecticut Children's
  Medical Center, Hartford, Connecticut
Head Trauma

TED M. BURNS, MD
Assistant Professor, Department of Neurology, University
  of Virginia, Charlottesville, Virginia
Clinical Neurophysiology of Pediatric Polyneuropathies
Autonomic Testing in Childhood
Clinical Neurophysiology of Pediatric Polyneuropathies

EDUARDO M. CASTILLO, PhD
Assistant Professor, Department of Neurosurgery,
  University of Texas at Houston Medical School;
  Faculty, MEG Laboratory, Hermann Hospital,
  Houston, Texas
Magnetoencephalography

THOMAS O. CRAWFORD, MD
Associate Professor of Neurology and Pediatrics,
  Departments of Neurology and Pediatrics, Johns
  Hopkins University; Associate Professor of Neurology
  and Pediatrics, Department of Neurology, Johns
  Hopkins Hospital, Baltimore, Maryland
*Spinal Muscular Atrophies and Other Disorders of the
Anterior Horn Cell*

BASIL T. DARRAS, MD
Professor of Neurology, Department of Neurology, Harvard Medical School; Director, Neuromuscular Program, Department of Neurology, Children's Hospital Boston, Boston, Massachusetts
Neuromuscular Problems of the Critically Ill Neonate, Child, and Adolescent
The Interrelation of DNA Analysis with Clinical Neurophysiology in the Diagnosis of Chronic Neuromuscular Disorder of Childhood

MICHAEL DUCHOWNY, MD
Professor of Clinical Neurology, University of Miami School of Medicine; Director, Comprehensive Epilepsy Program, Miami Children's Hospital, Miami, Florida
Long-Term Electroencephalogram and Video Monitoring

KARIN EDEBOL EEG-OLOFSSON, MD
Associate Professor, University of Uppsala, Institute of Neuroscience; Assistant Professor, Department of Clinical Neurophysiology, Neurocentre, University Hospital, Uppsala, Sweden
Transcranial Magnetic Stimulation: An Overview
Sphincter Dysfunction

ALAN B. ETTINGER, MD
Director, Comprehensive Epilepsy Center and Chief of EEG, Department of Neurology, Long Island Jewish Medical Center, New Hyde Park, New York; Chief of EEG, Department of Neurology, North Shore University Hospital, Manhasset, New York; Chief of EEG and Epilepsy, Department of Neurology, Huntington Hospital, Huntington, New York
Basic Principles of Electroencephalography

KEVIN J. FELICE, DO
Professor of Neurology and Director, Neuromuscular Program and EMG Laboratory, Department of Neurology, University of Connecticut School of Medicine, Farmington, Connecticut
Focal Neuropathies in Children

ROBIN L. GILMORE, MD
Staff Neurologist, Department of Neurology, Neurology Center of Middle Tennessee; Staff Neurologist, Department of Medicine, Maury Regional Hospital, Columbia, Tennessee
Somatosensory Evoked Potentials in Pediatrics—Normal
Somatosensory Evoked Potentials in Pediatrics—Abnormal

WILLIAM D. GOLDIE, MD
Associate Clinical Professor, Departments of Pediatrics and Neurology, University of California—Los Angeles; Associate Clinical Professor, Division of Child Neurology, Children's Hospital—Los Angeles, Los Angeles, California; Director, Child Neurology, and Director, Clinical Neurophysiology, Ventura County Medical Center, Ventura, California
Visual Evoked Potentials in Pediatrics—Normal
Visual Evoked Potentials in Pediatrics—Abnormal

SANDRA L. HELMERS, MD
Associate Professor, Department of Neurology, Emory University School of Medicine; Associate Professor, Department of Neurology, Grady Health System, Atlanta; Associate Professor, Department of Neurology, Children's Healthcare of Atlanta, Atlanta, Georgia
Brainstem Auditory Evoked Potentials in Pediatrics—Normal
Intraoperative Neurophysiologic Monitoring Using Evoked Potentials
Brainstem Auditory Evoked Potentials in Pediatrics—Abnormal

GREGORY L. HOLMES, MD
Professor of Medicine (Neurology) and Pediatrics, Dartmouth Medical School; Chief, Section of Neurology, Dartmouth-Hitchcock Medical Center, Lebanon, New Hampshire
Basic Principles of Electroencephalography
Visual Analysis of the Neonatal Electroencephalogram
Age-Specific Seizure Disorders
Drug Effects on the Human Electroencephalogram

PAUL A. L. S. HWANG, MDCM, MSc, FRCPC
Associate Professor of Neurology, University of Toronto Epilepsy Program; Head of Paediatric Neurology, North York General Hospital, Toronto, Ontario, Canada
Age-Specific Seizure Disorders

PRASANNA JAYAKAR, MD, PhD
Director, Neuroscience Center, Children's Brain Institute, Miami Children's Hospital, Miami, Florida
Long-Term Electroencephalogram and Video Monitoring

H. ROYDEN JONES, JR., MD
Jaime Ortiz-Patiño Chair in Neurology, Lahey Clinic, Burlington, Massachusetts; Clinical Professor of Neurology, Harvard Medical School; Director, Electromyography Laboratory, Children's Hospital Boston, Boston, Massachusetts
The Floppy Infant
Plexopathies and Nerve Root Lesions
Focal Neuropathies in Children

Clinical Neurophysiology of Pediatric Polyneuropathies
Neuromuscular Problems of the Critically Ill Neonate, Child, and Adolescent
The Interrelation of DNA Analysis with Clinical Neurophysiology in the Diagnosis of Chronic Neuromuscular Disorder of Childhood

SUSAN K. KLEIN, MD, PHD
Assistant Professor, Department of Pediatrics, Case Western Reserve University; Child Neurologist, Department of Pediatrics, University Hospitals of Cleveland—Rainbow Babies and Children's Hospital, Cleveland, Ohio
Neurophysiology of Language and Behavioral Disorders in Children

SAMUEL E. KOSZER, MD
Associate Professor of Neurology, Section Head, Epilepsy and Neurophysiology, Department of Neurology, Albany Medical College Hospital, Albany, New York
Visual Analysis of the Neonatal Electroencephalogram
Visual Analysis of the Pediatric Electroencephalogram

SURESH KOTAGAL, MD
Professor, Departments of Neurology and Pediatrics, Mayo Clinic, Rochester, Minnesota
Childhood Sleep-Wake Disorders

EDWARD H. KOVNAR, MD
Attending Physician, Department of Pediatric Neurology, Children's Hospital of Wisconsin, Milwaukee, Wisconsin
Drug Effects on the Human Electroencephalogram
Manifestations of Metabolic, Toxic, and Degenerative Diseases
Infectious Diseases

NANCY L. KUNTZ, MD
Assistant Professor of Neurology and Pediatrics, Department of Neurology, Mayo College of Medicine; Consultant in Child and Adolescent Neurology, Department of Neurology, Mayo Clinic, Rochester, Minnesota
Clinical Neurophysiology of the Motor Unit in Infants and Children
Clinical Neurophysiology of Pediatric Polyneuropathies
Autonomic Testing in Childhood
Muscle Disorders in Children: Neurophysiologic Contributions to Diagnosis and Management

WILLIAM N. MAY, MD, MBA
Associate Professor, Department of Pediatrics and Neurology, University of Tennessee; Chief Medical Officer, Administration Department, Le Bonheur Children's Medical Center, Methodist Healthcare—Memphis Hospitals, Memphis, Tennessee
Electroencephalography and Structural Disease of the Brain

FAYE MCNALL, MED, REEG T
Director of Education, American Society of Electroneurodiagnostic Technologists, Kansas City, Missouri
Drug Effects on the Human Electroencephalogram

THOMAS A. MILLER, MD, FRCPC
Associate Professor, Department of Physical Medicine and Rehabilitation, Schulich School of Medicine; Faculty of Medicine and Dentistry, University of Western Ontario; Director, Electrodiagnostic Laboratory, Co-Director, Peripheral Nerve Clinic, Consultant Physiatrist, Hand and Upper Limb Centre, St. Josephs Health Care, London, Ontario, Canada
Plexopathies and Nerve Root Lesions

SOLOMON L. MOSHÉ, MD
Professor of Neurology, Neuroscience and Pediatrics, Vice Chair, Department of Neurology, Albert Einstein College of Medicine of Yeshiva University; Director, Child Neurology and Clinical Neurophysiology at Montefiore, The University Hospital of Albert Einstein College of Medicine and Jacobi Medical Center, Bronx, New York
Basic Principles of Electroencephalography
Visual Analysis of the Neonatal Electroencephalogram
Visual Analysis of the Pediatric Electroencephalogram
The Diagnosis of Brain Death

HIROSHI OTSUBO, MD
Assistant Professor, Department of Paediatrics, University of Toronto; Director of Operations, Department of Clinical Neurophysiology and Epilepsy Monitoring, Division of Neurology, Hospital for Sick Children, Toronto, Ontario, Canada
Age-Specific Seizure Disorders

ANDREW C. PAPANICOLAOU, PHD
Professor and Director, Division of Clinical Neurosciences, Department of Neurosurgery, University of Texas—Houston Medical School; Director, MEG Center, Memorial-Hermann Hospital; Director, Institute of Rehabilitation and Research; Adjunct Professor, Department of Psychology, University of Houston; Adjunct Professor, Department of Linguistics, Rice University, Houston, Texas
Magnetoencephalography

MATTHEW PITT, MD, FRCP
Attending Physician, Clinical Neurophysiology, Great
    Ormond Street Hospital for Children NHS Trust,
    London, United Kingdom
*Maturational Changes vis-à-vis Neurophysiology Markers
and the Development of Peripheral Nerves*

SUSANA QUIJANO-ROY, MD, PhD
Assistant, Faculty of Medicine, Université de Versailles
    Saint-Quentin-en-Yvelines; Pediatric Neurologist,
    Department of Pediatrics, Intensive Care and Neuro-
    respiratory Rehabilitation Department, Hôpital
    Universitaire Raymond Poncaré, Garches, France;
    Assistant, Pediatric Neurophysiology Unit, Hôpital
    d'Enfants Armand-Trousseau, Paris, France
Facial and Bulbar Weakness

FRANCIS RENAULT, MD
Associate Professor, Université Pierre et Marie Curie;
    Head, Pediatric Neurophysiology Unit, Hôpital
    d'Enfants Armand-Trousseau, Paris, France
Facial and Bulbar Weakness

TREVOR J. RESNICK, MD
Associate Professor and Director, Division of Pediatric
    Neurology, University of Miami School of Medicine;
    Chief, Department of Neurology, Miami Children's
    Hospital, Miami, Florida
Long-Term Electroencephalogram and Video Monitoring

JAMES J. RIVIELLO, JR., MD
Professor of Neurology, Department of Neurology,
    Harvard Medical School; Director, Epilepsy Program,
    Division of Epilepsy and Clinical Neurophysiology,
    Department of Neurology, Children's Hospital Boston,
    Boston, Massachusetts
Age-Specific Seizure Disorders
Drug Effects on the Human Electroencephalogram
Infectious Diseases

MONIQUE M. RYAN, MBBS, M MED, FRACP
Senior Lecturer, Discipline of Paediatrics and Child
    Health, University of Sydney; Paediatric Neurologist,
    T. Y. Nelson Department of Neurology and
    Neurosurgery, Children's Hospital at Westmead,
    Sydney, Australia
Autonomic Testing in Childhood

DONALD B. SANDERS, MD
Professor, Division of Neurology, Duke University
    Medical Center, Durham, North Carolina
Neuromuscular Transmission Defects

MARK S. SCHER, MD
Professor of Pediatrics and Neurology, Department of
    Pediatrics, Case School of Medicine; Division Chief,
    Pediatric Neurology, Director, Pediatric/Epilepsy and
    Fetal/Neonatal Neurology and Programs, Rainbow
    Babies and Children's Hospital, University Hospitals of
    Cleveland, Cleveland, Ohio
Electroencephalography of the Newborn: Normal Features
Neonatal Electroencephalography: Abnormal Features

KATHRYN J. SWOBODA, MD
Associate Professor, Department of Neurology, University
    of Utah School of Medicine; Adjunct Associate
    Professor, Department of Pediatrics, Primary
    Children's Medical Center, Salt Lake City, Utah
The Floppy Infant

ROBERTO TUCHMAN, MD
Associate Professor, Department of Neurology, University
    of Miami, Florida; Director, Autism Program,
    Department of Neurology, Miami Children's Hospital
    Dan Marino Center, Weston, Florida
*Neurophysiology of Language and Behavioral Disorders in
Children*

JAMES W. WHELESS, MD
Professor and Chief of Pediatric Neurology, Le Bonheur
    Chair in Pediatric Neurology, University of Tennessee
    Health Science Center; Director, Pediatric
    Neuroscience Center; Director, Le Bonheur
    Comprehensive Epilepsy Center, Le Bonheur
    Children's Medical Center; Clinical Director and Chief
    of Pediatric Neurology, St. Jude Children's Research
    Hospital, Memphis, Tennessee
Magnetoencephalography (MEG)

ELAINE WYLLIE, MD
Head, Section of Pediatric Neurology and Pediatric
    Epilepsy, Department of Neurology, Cleveland Clinic
    Foundation, Cleveland, Ohio
*Electroencephalography in the Evaluation for Epilepsy
Surgery in Children*

LEON ZACHAROWICZ, MD, MA
Neurologist, Department of Psychiatry, North Shore
    Child and Family Guidance Center, Roslyn Heights,
    New York
Visual Analysis of the Pediatric Electroencephalogram

Preface

Neurophysiologic testing is an important component of the clinical assessment of children with neurologic disorders. Early in the history of clinical neurophysiology, testing primarily involved electroencephalography (EEG), and later on measuring the speed of conduction along peripheral nerves became available. This field has dramatically expanded during the past decades and now additionally includes evoked potentials, electromyography (EMG), magnetoencephalography, and magnetic stimulation.

The physiologic parameters measured in the child's nervous system change rapidly from birth to the teenage years, with age-specific patterns expressed during discrete developmental periods. Clinical neurophysiologists must be aware of the challenges in testing and interpreting neurophysiologic studies in a continuously evolving system. Although many of the clinical neurophysiology techniques in adults can be extrapolated to children, there is a need to have a textbook dedicated solely to the performance and interpretation of these various neurophysiologic testing modalities in infancy and childhood.

The wide diversity of clinical neurophysiologic studies has made it impossible for a single physician to review this entire field in detail. We have been successful in obtaining contributions from a wonderful group of authors with expertise in all aspects of pediatric neurophysiology. All of our contributors have graciously accepted the difficult task of providing a state-of-the-art perspective of the key elements appropriate to the performance and interpretation of clinical neurophysiologic studies in children of all ages.

Neurophysiologic studies provide an important extension to the clinical evaluation and are predicated on a careful neurologic history and examination. These various parameters should never be interpreted in isolation from the neurologic condition for which testing was obtained.

Rather one should strive to make a "clinical correlation" of the neurophysiologic data vis-à-vis the history and examination findings. To this end, we have asked our contributors to provide succinct descriptions of clinical disorders where neurophysiologic testing is a valuable adjunct. Our authors have accepted this challenge and have provided beautiful summaries of clinical features and neurophysiologic findings for both common and rare neurologic disorders. We made every effort to blend the details important to classic electrophysiologic techniques of EEG and EMG studies with the newest techniques such as magnetic stimulation and magnetoencephalography.

Since the era of Hans Berger, who made the first EEG recording at Jena, Germany, in 1924, and Edward Lambert, in Rochester, Minnesota, who brought clinical EMG to the fore in the early 1950s and later became the teacher of more than 50% of North American electromyographers, clinical neurophysiology has attracted talented and prolific investigators. The early contributions in the field remain important and are frequently cited in these chapters. We asked our contributing authors to balance the "classic, old," but pertinent literature with more recent studies. Although it is not possible to cite every paper dealing with childhood clinical neurophysiology, our authors have succeeded in accurately and concisely surveying the neurophysiology literature.

This textbook was designed to be of value to both trainees and established clinicians. While we hope some readers, particularly those in fellowships, will read the book cover to cover, it is likely that other colleagues will find specific chapters of primary interest. By providing a systematic and critical approach to childhood clinical neurophysiologic studies, this volume should serve as a stand-alone reference source of clinical neurophysiology information for professionals working with children who have one of the many neurologic disorders that can be better defined with neurophysiologic testing.

We extend our heartfelt thanks to all of the authors who contributed to this volume. Because of each person's well-deserved reputation in his or her respective fields of expertise, their contributions provide a special strength to this first monograph dedicated to the principles of pediatric clinical neurophysiology. Each clinical neuro-physiologist has provided a special dedication to this project, and for this the editors are most grateful. We know that no first effort is perfect, and we hope our readers will feel free to advise us of any areas of confusion or mistakes that we have inadvertently overlooked. We very much appreciate the alacrity that our authors applied to our ministrations as well as their good humor when we occasionally applied pressure to come to closure. At times one has to state there is enough paint on the canvas and move forward in hopes the next round will provide opportunity to enhance the color. That is often difficult to achieve with such dedicated and conscientious colleagues, who seek perfection in their given fields as they have with their participation in this venture.

We greatly appreciated the efforts of Mr. Dennis Druin for his expertise in producing many of the illustrations in this volume and the wonderful assistance provided by our support staff: Emily R. Clough at Dartmouth Medical School; Ms. Pat Clements, the supervisor of the EEG laboratory at Montefiore Medical Center; and Mrs. Mary Kreconus of the Lahey Clinic.

No project of this sort can come to fruition without the dedication of a top-notch executive publisher. Each of the editors is particularly indebted to Susan Pioli for her faith in this project and her unceasing urging, cajoling, and good humor while asking us to bring this project to conclusion. We also thank her colleague at Elsevier, Kim Davis, a developmental editor who was most helpful as we entered the gun lap for this project.

Lastly, we thank our many neurologic colleagues in our respective institutions who have provided us support and constructive critique over the years. We are proud to have worked with each and every one of you!

Gregory L. Holmes
H. Royden Jones, Jr.
Solomon L. Moshé

Contents

I

Basic Principles and Maturational Change

1

Basic Principles of Electroencephalography

Alan B. Ettinger, Alexis D. Boro, Gregory L. Holmes and Solomon L. Moshé

Successful electroencephalograph (EEG) interpretation and analysis are predicated on a thorough understanding of the basic concepts of electrical neurophysiology. This chapter discusses the physiologic basis of the EEG, the fundamental principles of the electrical circuit, filters, the EEG apparatus, electrodes and their application to the scalp, special electrodes, digital technology, the EEG penwriting apparatus, frequency and voltage considerations, testing the recording system, sources of the EEG, localization of activity, artifacts, electrical safety, and special considerations in performing the EEG in children. Definitions of terms used in the chapter are presented in Appendix I.

PHYSIOLOGIC BASIS OF THE EEG

The human brain contains more than 10^{12} neurons interconnected and communicating with each other via 10^{15} synaptic connections. It is through this communication process, termed *signaling*, that electrical activity is generated, resulting in the human EEG.

The cells of the nervous system can be divided into two major categories: neurons and neuroglial cells. Although neurons come in many shapes and sizes, the major components of most neurons consist of the dendrites (which receive information), the cell body (which processes and integrates the information), and the axon (which conducts signals to other brain regions). Neuroglial cells, often referred to as *glia*, may also be involved. The three major categories of glial cells are (1) the astrocytes (which maintain the correct metabolic milieu for neuronal signaling); (2) the oligodendrocytes (which myelinate neurons); and (3) the microglia (which serve as the brain's macrophages and assist in brain recovery from injury).

Neurons are classified into three broad types on the basis of the shape of the cell body and the patterns of the dendrites and axons. These types are the multipolar, pseudounipolar, and bipolar cells. Multipolar neurons are characterized by multiple dendrites that emerge from the cell body, resulting in a polygonal shape. The cell body of a pseudounipolar neuron is round and gives rise to a single dendritic process that divides close to the cell body into a peripheral and central branch. The peripheral branch transmits incoming sensory information while the central branch relays information onward to its target in the central nervous system. The two processes therefore act as a combined axon and dendrite. An example of a pseudounipolar neuron is the cell that relays information from the periphery into the central nervous system in the dorsal root ganglion. Bipolar neurons have a round or oval-shaped cell body with a large process emanating from each end of the cell body. Bipolar cells occur in the retinal and olfactory epithelium, vestibular ganglion, and auditory ganglion.

Neurons are organized into neuronal ensembles of circuits that process specific kinds of information. Neurons that carry information into the circuit are termed *afferent neurons*, whereas neurons signaling information away from the circuit are referred to as *efferent neurons*. Nerve cells that participate only in the local aspects of a circuit are called *interneurons*. Processing circuits are combined to form systems that serve broader functions such as memory, vision, and hearing.

Clinical neurophysiologic studies are based on the recording of both spontaneous electrical activity, as with the EEG, and stimulated response, such as evoked potentials. It is through the electrical signaling of information within these neuronal circuits that both spontaneous and evoked electrical activity can be measured. This chapter reviews some of the basic concepts of neuronal signaling that are important to the understanding of clinical neurophysiology.

Basis of Brain Electrical Activity

Membrane Polarity

The atom is composed of three basic particles: neutrons, electrons, and protons. The net charge of the three particles is zero. Neutrons are neutral, electrons carry a negative charge, and protons carry a positive charge. Upsetting this electrical balance by separating positive and negatively charged ions results in forces aimed at reinstitution of the electrical equilibrium and thereby a flow of charged ions. Ions may be separated by the application of energy of variable types such as mechanical, electrical, magnetic, or chemical. Electrical or chemical energy can separate charges in nerve cell membranes.[1]

All neurons and glia have lipid bilayer membranes separating the delicate internal machinery of the cell from the external environment. The neuronal membrane is an excellent insulator and separates different concentrations of ions inside the cell from those outside the cell. The activity of ion channels is fundamental to signaling in the nervous system. The movement of ions that carry electrical charge through ion channels results in voltage changes across the membrane.

Electrical potentials are generated across the membranes of neurons because there are differences in the concentration of specific ions across the membrane and the membrane is selectively permeable to ion flow. Movement of ions across the membrane occurs through ion channels that consist of proteins that transverse the neuronal membrane and allow certain ions to cross in the direction of their concentration gradient. Na^+ and Cl^- are more concentrated outside the cell, but K^+ and organic anions (consisting of amino acids and proteins) are more concentrated inside the cell. Na^+ and Cl^- therefore tend to flow into the cell, whereas K^+ tends to flow outward. Because of the large size of the organic anions, flow through ion channels is not possible. However, ion flow is not strictly related to concentration gradients. Because of the selective permeability of ion channels, anions

(negatively charged ions) and cations (positively charged ions) inside the cell are not equal; therefore, there is a potential difference between the inside and outside of the cell—the membrane potential. In most neurons at rest the inside of the membrane is –70 mV compared with the outside (resting membrane potential). Ions are therefore subjected to two forces driving them across the membrane: (1) a chemical driving force that depends on the concentration gradient across the membrane and (2) an electrical driving force that depends on the electrical potential across the membrane. Ions flow from high-concentration areas to low-concentration areas (chemical driving force), and they flow to areas of opposite charge, where like charges repel and unlike charges attract (electrical driving force).

The flux of ions through ion channels is passive and requires no metabolic energy. The kinetic properties of ion permeation are described by the channel's conductance, which is determined by measuring the current (ion flux) that flows through the open channel in response to a given electrochemical driving force. The net electrochemical driving force is determined by the electrical potential difference across the membrane and the concentration gradient of the ions selective for the channel.

To illustrate these physiologic features, the flow of K^+ ions is considered (Fig. 1-1). Because K^+ ions are present at a high concentration inside the cell, they tend to diffuse from inside to outside the cell down their chemical concentration gradient. As a result, the outside of the membrane becomes positively charged compared with the inside of the membrane. Once K^+ diffusion has proceeded to a certain point, a potential develops across the membrane at which the electrical force driving K^+ into the cell exactly balances the chemical force driving K^+ out of the cell; that is, the outward movement of K^+ (driven by its concentration gradient) is equal to the inward movement of K^+ (driven by the electrical potential difference across the membrane). This potential is called the *potassium equilibrium potential* (E_K).

The equilibrium potential for any ion X can be calculated from the Nernst equation,

$$Ex = (RT/zF) \ln ([X]o/[X]i)$$

where R is the gas constant, T is the temperature, z is the valence of the ion, F is the Faraday constant, and X is the concentration of the ion inside (i) and outside (o) the cell. Since RT/F is 25 mV at 25°C and the constant for converting from natural logarithms to base 10 logarithms is 2.3, z is +1 for K^+, and the concentration of free K^+ inside and outside the typical mammalian neuron is around 100 mmol and 3 mmol, respectively, the Nernst equation can be rewritten as

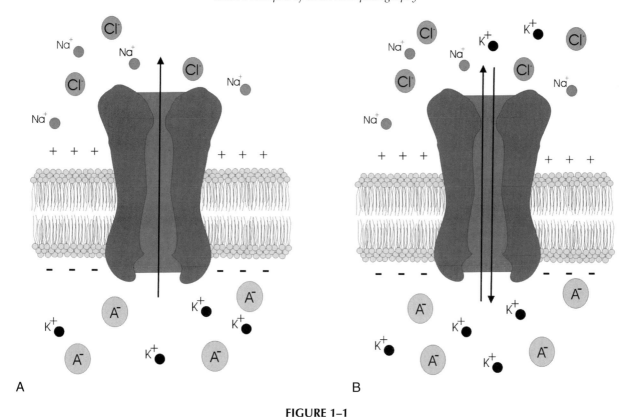

FIGURE 1–1

Passive K⁺ channel. In neurons, K⁺ has a higher concentration inside than outside (A). Because of the concentration differences, K⁺ diffuses from inside the cell to the outside. With K⁺ outflow, the inside of the cell becomes even more negative since the K⁺ ion is carrying a positive charge (B). At some point, an equilibrium is reached in which the electrical and chemical driving forces are equal and opposite and there is a balance between K⁺ entering and leaving the cell.

$$Ex = (58 \text{ mV}/1) \log ([3]/[100]) = -90 \text{ mV}$$

Na⁺ is more common outside the cell than inside; therefore, it tends to flow into the cell down its chemical concentration gradient. The equilibrium potential for Na⁺ is around +60 mV. Therefore, there is also an electrical driving force that drives Na⁺ into the cell by virtue of the negative electrical potential difference across the membrane. However, Na⁺ conductance of membrane at rest is very small (about 10 times smaller) compared with K⁺ conductance, and the influx of Na⁺ depolarizes the cell only slightly from the K⁺ equilibrium potential (–90 mV). Eventually, the resting membrane potential is established at the level at which the outward movement of K⁺ just balances the inward movement of Na⁺. This balance point (–70 mV) is only slightly more positive than the equilibrium potential for K⁺ (–90 mV) since neurons have relatively few Na⁺ channels open at rest and the conductance to Na⁺ is therefore low.

The resting membrane potential (Vm) is not equal to either E_K or E_{Na} but lies between them. As a general rule, when Vm is determined by two or more ions, the influence

of each ion is determined not only by the concentration of the ion inside and outside the cell but also by the relative permeability of the membrane to each ion. The Goldman equation was developed to determine the membrane potential by taking into account the concentrations and permeability for the "big three" ions (in terms of concentration): Na⁺, K⁺, and Cl⁻.

$$Vm = 58 \log \frac{Pk[K]i + PNa[Na]i + PCl[Cl]i}{Pk[K]o + PNa[Na]o + PCl[Cl]o}$$

where P is the permeability of the membrane to each ion.

The Goldman equation is an extension of the Nernst equation that considers the relative permeabilities of the ions involved. Table 1-1 provides the extracellular and intracellular free ion concentrations that can be used in the formula.

Since ion leaks would eventually result in a rundown of Na⁺ and K⁺ gradients, the resting membrane potential would eventually be altered. The Na⁺-K⁺ pump, which moves Na⁺ and K⁺ ions against their net electrochemical gradients, extrudes Na⁺ from the cell while bringing K⁺

TABLE 1–1
Extracellular and Intracellular Ion Concentrations

Ion	Intracellular, mmol	Extracellular, mmol
Potassium	100	3
Sodium	10	110
Chloride	4-30	110
Calcium	0.00001	2

into the cell. The energy to run this pump comes from the hydrolysis of adenosine triphosphate. At the resting membrane potential, the cell is not in equilibrium but rather in a steady state. The continuous passive influx of Na^+ and efflux of K^+ ions is counterbalanced by the Na^+-K^+ pump.

At rest, the total electrical current flow through the membrane is null; therefore, no signal is recorded by an extracellular field potential electrode.

Channel Gating

Thus far we have discussed ion channels that are open in the resting state and are selectively permeable to ions. Resting channels normally are open and are not influenced significantly by extrinsic factors, such as the potential across the membrane. Resting channels are therefore critically important in maintaining the resting potential. There are also gated channels that can exist in several configuration states. The term *gating* is used to describe the transition of a channel between these different states. Most gated channels are closed when the membrane is at rest. Each ion channel has at least one open state and one or two closed states (Fig. 1-2).

The two categories of gated channels are characterized by having an appropriate sensor—either a *voltage type* or a *ligand type* (i.e., the ligand receptor site). In voltage-gated channel function the voltage across the membrane determines whether a conformational change in the channel occurs. In ligand-mediated channels the ligand binds to the channel, either at an extracellular site, as with neurotransmitters such as glutamate or γ-aminobutyric acid (GABA), or at an intracellular site, as in the case of certain cytoplasmic compounds such as Ca^{2+} and nucleotides. Ligands can also activate cellular signaling cascades that can covalently modify a channel through phosphorylation.

Action Potential

For a neuron to transmit information it must generate an electrical signal termed an *action potential*. Development of the action potential requires an electrical or chemical stimulus that alters ion flow into the cell.

The electrical current that flows into and out of the cell is carried by ions, both positively charged (cations) and negatively charged (anions). The direction of current flow is conventionally defined as the direction of net movement of positive charge. Cations move in the direction of the electrical current while anions move in the opposite direction. Whether or not there is a net flow of cations or anions into or out of the cell, the charge separation across the resting membrane is disturbed, altering the polarity of the membrane. A reduction of charge separation resulting in a less negative membrane potential is termed *depolarization,* and an increase in charge separation leading to a more negative membrane potential is called *hyperpolarization.*

When the membrane potential depolarizes to a threshold (which is around –55 to –60 mV), the voltage-gated Na^+ channels open rapidly. The influx of Na^+ inward makes the interior of the cell more positive than before. The increase in depolarization causes still more voltage-gated Na^+ channels to open, resulting in further acceleration of the depolarization. The positive feedback cycle initiates the action potential and is responsible for its all-or-none character. Once initiated, the action potential is independent of the stimulus. The membrane potential approaches, but never reaches, the equilibrium potential for Na^+ (+60 mV) because K^+ efflux continues during the depolarization and there is influx of Cl^-. Depolarization during the action potential is very large but also very brief, lasting only 1 millisecond. These features of the action potential allow neuronal signaling with high fidelity at a very high rate (up to hundreds of action potentials per second). Termination of the action potential is due to rapid inactivation of Na^+ channels and delayed (compared to Na^+ channels) opening of voltage-gated K^+ channels. The delayed increase in K^+ efflux combines with a decrease in Na^+ influx to produce a net efflux of positive charge from the cell, which continues until the cell has repolarized to its resting membrane potential. Figure 1-3 demonstrates the sequential opening of voltage-gated Na^+ and K^+ channels during the action potential.

Thus, during the action potential, Na^+ channels undergo transitions among three different states: resting, activated, or inactivated. On depolarization, the channel goes from the resting (closed) state to the activated (open) state. If the depolarization is brief, the channels go directly back to the resting state on repolarization. If the depolarization is maintained, the channels go from the open to the inactivated closed state. Once the channel is inactivated, it cannot be opened by further depolarization. The inactivation can be reversed only by repolarization of the membrane to its negative resting potential, which allows the channel to switch from the inactivated to the resting state. Each Na^+ channel has two kinds of gates that must be opened simultaneously for the channel to conduct Na^+ ions. An activation gate is closed when the membrane is at its negative resting potential and is rapidly opened by depolarization; an inactivation gate is open at the resting potential and closes slowly in response to depolarization.

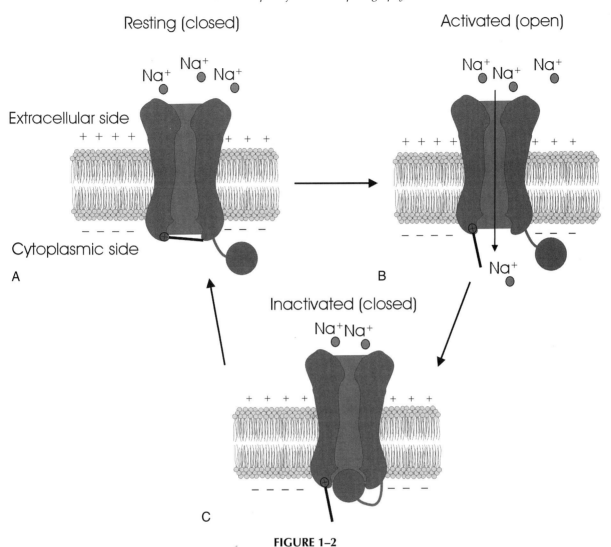

FIGURE 1–2

Voltage-gated Na$^+$ channel. In the resting condition (A) *the activation gate* (black bar) *is closed and the inactivation gate* (ball and chain) *is open. No Na$^+$ flows because of the closed activation gate. With depolarization there is a conformational change of the channel and the activation gate opens* (B). *Na$^+$ flow then occurs. This is followed by inactivation by the inactivation gate, prohibiting the further flow of Na$^+$ ions* (C). *With repolarization of the membrane, the inactivation gate opens and the activation gate closes and the channel is ready for another cycle.*

The channel conducts only for the brief period during a depolarization when both gates are open. Repolarization reverses the two processes, closing the activation gate rapidly and opening the inactivation gate more slowly. After the channel has returned to the resting state, it can again be activated by depolarization.

Following an action potential the Na$^+$ channels are inactivated and the K$^+$ channels are activated. These transitory events make it more difficult for another action potential to be generated quickly. This refractory period limits the number of action potentials that a given nerve cell can produce per unit time. This phenomenon also explains why

action potentials do not reverberate up and down the neuronal membrane.

Extracellular field potential electrodes can detect the action potentials from the individual neurons only if the size of electrode is comparable to the size of the cell (tens of microns) and if the electrode is very close to the cell soma, where the action potential is generated. The amplitude of the extracellularly recorded action potential is small, in the order of tens of microvolts, and the duration is less than a millisecond. With conventional EEG electrodes, the action potentials from individual neurons are too small to be detected. However, when many neurons

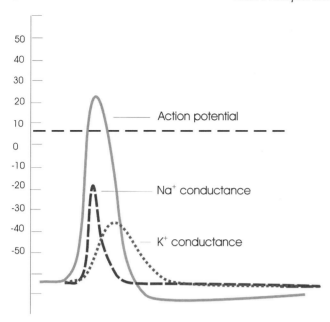

FIGURE 1–3

Generation of the action potential. The sequential opening of voltage-gated Na+ and K+ generates the action potential. Note that the Na+ conductances begin before the K+ conductances. The influx of Na+ makes the interior of the cell more positive than before, increasing the degree of depolarization, which causes still more voltage-gated Na+ channels to open, resulting in further acceleration of the depolarization. With the depolarization there is a greater electrical driving force on the K+ ions and K+ ions flow outward. The increase in K+ efflux combined with a decrease in Na+ influx results in an efflux of positive charge from the cell, which continues until the cell has repolarized.

fire action potentials simultaneously, which can occur, for instance, in patients with epilepsy, their summated action potentials can be detected in EEG recordings as a "population spike."

Transmission of Action Potentials

The action potential can transverse long axonal distances without loss of amplitude despite the fact that neuronal membranes have relatively poor conducting properties. During the generation of the action potential there is some passive flow of current downstream from the action potential. The passive current flow depolarizes the membrane potential in adjacent regions of the axon, opening Na+ channels. The local depolarization results in another action potential that then spreads again in a continuing cycle until the end of the axon is reached.

Signaling Changes

When the postsynaptic membrane is stimulated through either electrical stimulation through gap junctions or at

chemical synapses, there is a change in membrane potential. The change in membrane potential is typically not instantaneous because the membrane has both a resistive and a capacitive component. Neurons have three passive electrical properties that are important to electrical signaling: the resting membrane resistance, the membrane capacitance, and the intracellular axial resistance along the axons and dendrites. These membrane properties are important in determining whether an action potential will be generated.

Current is defined as the amount of charge that flows through a conductor over a given set of time. Current is either direct or alternating in that

1. Direct current represents electricity that flows in one direction only and is exemplified by the electrical current supplied by a routine battery used in common mechanical devices.
2. Alternating current repetitively changes direction between two opposite directions within the same circuit. This source of electricity is used to power mechanical devices that are plugged into home, office, and hospital wall outlets. In the United States, the frequency of alternation is 60 Hz (cycles/sec).

Current is described in units called *amperes*, commonly abbreviated amps (A). Units of charge have been named *coulombs* (Q). By convention, when 1 Q of charge (6×10^{18} electrons) has traveled through a conductor over a period of 1 second, a current of 1 A has been observed. Conversely, a coulomb of charge represents the charge caused by a current of 1 A flowing for 1 second. One coulomb is approximately equal to the charge of 6×10^{18} electrons. This is expressed mathematically as

$$I = Q/T$$

where I is the current, Q is the charge, and T is time.

All cell membranes have a resistance. Resistance is the part of the circuit that "resists" the flow of charges by converting the electrical flow of energy into heat. *Energy* is defined in the term of *joules* (J). One joule of energy is expended when 1 Q is moved across a potential difference of 1 V. The term *impedance* is used to describe the resistance in a circuit that is powered by an alternating current source and includes a device known as a *capacitor*. Quantified units of resistance or impedance have been termed *ohms* (Ω). All circuits always have some degree of resistance.

The input resistance (R_{in}) of the cell determines how much the cell depolarizes in response to a steady current. The magnitude of the depolarization, that is, the change in membrane voltage (ΔV), is given by Ohm's law:

$$\Delta V = I \times R_{in}$$

Of two neurons receiving identical synaptic current inputs, the cell with the higher input resistance will have a greater change in membrane voltage. Input resistance depends on both the density of resting ion channels in the membrane and the size of the cell. The larger the neuron, the greater is its membrane surface area and the lower the input resistance, since there will be more resting channels to conduct.

Membranes also act as capacitors. A capacitor consists of two conducting plates separated by an insulating layer. The fundamental property of a capacitor is its ability to store charges of opposite sign: positive charge on one plate, negative on the other. Voltage across a capacitor is proportional to the charge stored on the capacitor. Capacitors store electrical charge by maintaining a separation between positive and negative electrical charges.[2] Although the plates are relatively close to each other, charges cannot traverse the insulating material to reach the opposite plate when direct current is applied. Ions of similar charge but on opposite plates repel each other, resulting in a further establishment of separated charges. On connecting a capacitor to an energy (voltage) source, the capacitor finally attains a separation in charges (or voltage) equal to that of the voltage source. When connected to a source of voltage where one side remains positive and the other negative as in "direct current," one plate remains positive and the other negative. When alternating current is applied, the voltage source repetitively alternates from positive to negative and therefore the associated connected capacitor plates alternate from positive to negative charge. This, in effect, is comparable to a traversing of the insulating substances by charged ions.[1]

$$V = Q/C$$

where Q is the charge in coulombs and C is the capacitance in farads (F). To alter the voltage, charge must either be added or removed from the capacitor. *Capacitance* is a term indicating the amount of current a capacitor can store. When capacitance is small, it takes very little current to fully charge the capacitor. Figure 1-4 is an example of a circuit that includes a capacitor.

$$\Delta V = \Delta Q/C$$

The change in charge ΔQ is the result of the flow of current across the capacitor (Ic). Since current is the flow of charge per unit time (Ic = $\Delta Q/\Delta t$), the change in voltage across a capacitor can be calculated as a function of current and the time that the current flows.

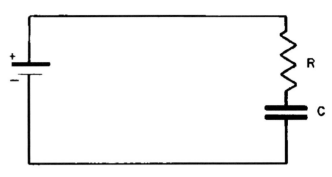

FIGURE 1–4
An example of a circuit that includes a capacitor. R, resister; C, capacitor

$$\Delta V = Ic \times \Delta t/C$$

The magnitude of the change in voltage across a capacitor in response to a current pulse depends on the duration of the current, because time is required to deposit and remove charge on the plates of the capacitor.

Capacitance is directly proportional to the area of the plates of the capacitor. The larger the area of a capacitor, the more charge it will store for a given potential difference. Since all biologic membranes are composed of lipid bilayers with similar insulating properties that provide a similar separation between the two plates (4 nm), the specific capacitance per unit area of all biologic membranes has the same value. The total input capacitance of a spherical cell, Cin, is therefore given by the capacitance per unit area multiplied by the area of the cell,

$$Cin = Cm(4\pi r^2)$$

where r is the radius of the cell. Since capacitance increases with the size of the cell, more charge, and therefore current, is required to produce the same change in membrane potential in a larger neuron than in a smaller one. The capacitance of the membrane has the effect of reducing the rate at which the membrane potential changes in response to a current pulse. If the membrane had only resistive properties, a step pulse of outward current passed across it would change the membrane potential instantaneously. Biologic membranes have both capacitive and resistive properties in parallel.

Cell-to-Cell Communication

The EEG represents a set of field potentials as recorded by multiple electrodes on the surface of the scalp. The electrical activity of the EEG is an attenuated measure of potentials alter the probability that an action potential will be produced in the postsynaptic cell. If there is depolarization of the membrane, the potential is termed an *excitatory postsynaptic potential* (EPSP), whereas if there is hyperpolarization the change in membrane potentials is referred to as an *inhibitory postsynaptic potential* (IPSP). EPSPs bring the membrane potential closer to threshold for action potential generation, whereas IPSPs keep the membrane potential more negative than the threshold potential. In the chemical synapses, whether the event is an EPSP or IPSP is dependent on the neurotransmitter released from the presynaptic neuron and the type or receptor activated in the postsynaptic neuron. In the cerebral cortex, about 90% of neurons (called the *principal neurons*) synthesize and release on their postsynaptic targets neurotransmitter glutamate, which is the principal neurotransmitter of excitation in the cortex. The remaining 10% of neurons (interneurons) synthesize and release the neurotransmitter GABA, which is the principal neurotransmitter of inhibition in the cortex.

Electrical signal transmission from one cell to another occurs through the gap junctions. Gap junctions consist of hexameric complexes formed by the close juxtaposition of pores consisting of proteins called *connexons*, which span the neuronal membrane. The pore of a gap junction is larger than the pores of the voltage-gated ion channel and can therefore transfer much larger substances such as intracellular metabolites between cells. Electrical transmission across gap junctions occurs rapidly since passive current flow across the gap junction is virtually instantaneous. Gap junctions appear to have an important role in the synchronization of neuron firing, in particular in the interneuron networks.

Chemical synapses have a wider spacing between cells, termed the *synaptic cleft*, and operate through release of neurotransmitter stored in vesicles. The neurotransmitter diffuses from the presynaptic membrane to the postsynaptic membrane. Neurotransmitter release occurs when an action potential reaches the terminals and initiates the opening of voltage-gated Ca^{2+} channels. The openings of these channels causes a rapid influx of Ca^{2+} into the presynaptic terminal. Elevation of the intracellular Ca^{2+} permits synaptic vesicles to fuse with the plasma membrane of the presynaptic neuron. Precisely how Ca^{2+} triggers the fusion and release of neurotransmitters is not clear. There are a number of proteins that bind with Ca^{2+} to elicit the cascade of events that lead to release of the transmitter. The fusion of the vesicular and neuronal membranes allows release of the neurotransmitter. Figure 1-5 is a drawing that illustrates the process of neurotransmitter release.

Glutamate is the primary excitatory neurotransmitter in the brain. It has been estimated that more than half of the brain synapses release glutamate. Synaptic transmission is mediated by glutamate, which is released from the principal (granular cells also release glutamate) neurons and depolarizes and excites the target neurons via three types of ionotropic receptors, named after their selective agonists (α-amino-3-hydroxy-5-methylisoxazole-4-proprionic acid [AMPA], kainate [KA], and *N*-methyl-D-aspartate [NMDA]). Although all types of the glutamate receptors respond to glutamate, they have individual characteristics. The AMPA receptor rapidly responds to glutamate with opening of the short-living channel equally permeable to Na^+ and K^+ (the reversal potential ~ 0 mV), and current through the AMPA receptors results in neuronal depolarization. One synapse contains tens of AMPA receptors on the postsynaptic membrane, and summation of the currents through the AMPA receptors results in an EPSP of 0.1 mV. Therefore, to depolarize the postsynaptic neuron to the action potential threshold, simultaneous activation of several excitatory synapses is necessary. KA receptors are similar to AMPA receptors in the ionic selectivity but have slower kinetics. The third type of glutamate ionotropic receptors—NMDA receptor—does not directly participate in the information processing, but it plays the critical role in the synaptic plasticity. The NMDA channel has characteristics of both a neurotransmitter or ligand-activated and voltage-sensitive channel. At resting membrane potential, Mg^{2+} sits in the channel blocking the flow of ions. Only with depolarization of the membrane is Mg^{2+} displaced and Na^+ and Ca^{2+} ions able to cross the channel. The high permeability of NMDA receptor to Ca^{2+} underlies its role in the synaptic plasticity, such as long-term potentiation of the strength of the synaptic transmission, which presumably participates in learning and memory.

GABA is the principal inhibitory transmitter of the brain. Inhibitory synapses made by interneurons and employing GABA as their transmitter use two types of receptors: $GABA_A$ and $GABA_B$. $GABA_A$ receptors are ligand-gated ion channels while $GABA_B$ receptors are metabotropic receptors (see later). $GABA_A$ receptors are inhibitory because their associated channels are permeable to Cl^-. Since the reversal potential for Cl^- is more negative than the threshold for neuronal firing, Cl^- flow prevents action potential generation. Activation of $GABA_B$ receptors results in opening of K^+ channels that also inhibit the postsynaptic cell. In the spinal cord, GABA and glycine act as neuroinhibitors by activating presynaptic autoreceptors.

Physiologic Basis of the EEG

Through either neurotransmitter release at chemical synapses or current flow through gap junctions, the postsynaptic membrane opens ligand-gated or voltage-gated channels and elicits postsynaptic potentials. Postsynaptic

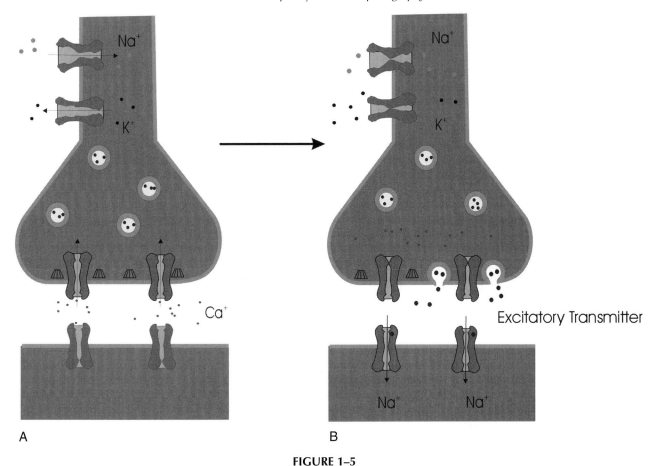

A   B

FIGURE 1–5

Synaptic neurotransmission. An action potential travels down the axon until it reaches the synapse. The depolarization causes voltage-gated Ca^{2+} channels to open. The influx of Ca^{2+} results in high concentrations of Ca^{2+} near the active zone. This triggers fusion of vesicles with neurotransmitter to the presynaptic cell membrane and emptying of the vesicles into the synaptic cleft. The neurotransmitter crosses to the postsynaptic membrane and results in depolarization of the membrane if it is an excitatory neurotransmitter. With glutamate release there is binding of the ligand to postsynaptic receptors (AMPA, NMDA, or KA) with subsequent inflow of Na^+ ions.

the extracellular current flow from the summed activity of many neurons. The surface EEG predominately reflects the activity of cortical neurons close to the EEG electrode. The depth structures such as the hippocampus, thalamus, or brain stem do not contribute directly to the surface EEG. However, transmission of electrical impulses from distant sites has substantial effects on the surface EEG. For example, thalamocortical connections are critical in the synchronization of electrical activity such as sleep spindles. Oscillatory EEG patterns occur because of pacemaker cells where membrane voltage fluctuates spontaneously or because of the reciprocal interaction of excitatory and inhibitory neurons in circuit loops. The human EEG shows activity over the range of 1 to 150 Hz with amplitudes in the range of 20 to 100 µV. Until recently

electroencephalographers have concentrated on activity between 1 and 30 Hz. However, it is now recognized that frequencies in the gamma range are clinically relevant in normal[3,4] and abnormal states.[5]

The waveforms recorded by the surface electrodes depend on the orientation and distance of the electrical source with respect to the recording electrode. To understand how the EEG is recorded it is helpful to use a diagram with a single neuron, although it is recognized that EEG activity is the result of thousands of neurons functioning within neuronal networks. Figure 1-6 shows a single neuron with current flowing into the dendrite at the site of generation of the excitatory postsynaptic potential creating a current sink. Current must complete a loop and therefore creates a source somewhere along the dendrites

Cortical surface

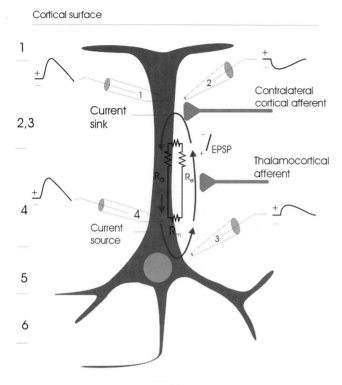

FIGURE 1–6
Current flow in a cortical neuron. See text for discussion.

or cell body. The size of the voltage created by the synaptic current is predicted by Ohm's law ($V = I \times R$). The Rm (membrane resistance) is much larger than the extracellular fluid, and the corresponding voltage recorded by an intracellular electrode is larger and of opposite polarity to an extracellular electrode positioned near the current sink. At the site of generation of an EPSP the extracellular electrode detects current (positive ions) flowing away from the electrode into the cytoplasm as a downward deflection, whereas the intracellular electrode detects a positive signal owing to the influx of Na^+ ions. An extracellular electrode near the source has an opposite deflection. The direction of pen deflection is determined by location in regard to the sink and source. Note the differences in pen deflection depending on whether the extracellular electrode is near the source or sink.

Now consider pen deflection as a function of location of the afferent signal in cortical neurons. In Figure 1-7 there are afferent inputs into either the apical dendrites (Fig. 1-7A) or cell body (Fig. 1-7B). In both cases the afferent stimuli lead to depolarization (sink) with current flow into the cell body. This results in an extracellular negativity. The current flow in Figure 1-7A results in a source in the apical dendrites, whereas in Figure 1-7B the source is

located at the soma. Surface EEG electrodes detect the electrical field generated at the surface, and there is little influence from activity occurring at the cell body. Therefore, the deflection of the pen is opposite in the two conditions.

Origin of EEG Rhythms

Despite numerous advances in the recording of the EEG and its usage in clinical neurology, the origin of the fundamental frequencies of the normal EEG remains surprisingly poorly understood. Even 75 years after Hans Berger's initial characterization of the alpha rhythm,[6] it is only recently that the basic cellular and synaptic mechanisms underlying the EEG have begun to be uncovered. A detailed analysis of the studies (predominantly animal experiments) concerned with generation of EEG rhythms is beyond the scope of this chapter, but the reader is referred to a number of excellent references on this subject.[7-10]

Such studies have led to the speculation that sleep spindles may originate from repetitive burst depolarizations from neurons in the reticular nucleus of the thalamus, which in turn has extensive thalamocortical connections with networks of cortical pyramidal cells. Delta activity associated with deep levels of sleep is also believed to be driven by the thalamus. Focal pathologic irregular delta (and theta) activity has been rigorously correlated with an assortment of deep white matter structural abnormalities[11] and may result in part from loss of synaptic inputs toward cortical neurons, although specific mechanisms of this waveform generation remains unclear.

Extensive work by Andersen and Andersson[12] suggested that the thalamus was also responsible for the alpha rhythm, but more recent work suggests that islands of pyramidal neurons in the occipital cortex may be a more likely source and that large neuronal networks in the cortex have an intrinsic capacity for rhythmicity.[13] The origins of beta activity associated with arousal and theta frequencies of drowsiness remain more obscure.

Large EPSPs involving dendritic connections in more superficial cortical layers may produce major sustained depolarizations with a resultant negativity in extracellular regions. This major depolarization has been termed the *paroxysmal depolarization shift* (PDS)[14] and may explain negative spikes, the hallmark of focal interictal epileptiform activity. It is a relatively slow depolarization that correlates in time and duration with spikes or sharp waves seen in the EEG. PDSs have been demonstrated in many animal models of epilepsy. The hyperpolarization following this PDS may explain the slow wave that often follows spikes or sharp waves seen on the EEG.[15]

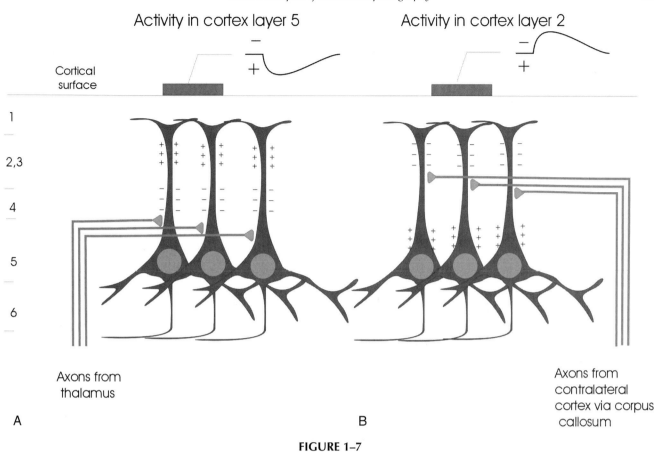

FIGURE 1–7

A and B, Polarity of the surface EEG depends on the location of the synaptic activity within the cortex. See text for discussion.

FUNDAMENTAL PRINCIPLES OF THE ELECTRICAL CIRCUIT

An electrical circuit comprises a conductor through which current flows, a power source that leads to the flow of charges, and a resistor. The power source produces energy that separates charges and thereby leads to the flow of charges in the attempt to re-establish electrical equilibrium. Nerve cell membranes separate charges through chemical diffusion gradients and active transport systems.

Principles known as *Kirchoff's laws* govern the properties of linked electrical circuits. Kirchoff's Law No. 1 states that the voltages around a closed path in a circuit must sum to zero. It can be demonstrated by using Kirchoff's Law No. 1 together with Ohm's law that the total resistance in a circuit is equal to the sum of all component resistances. Kirchoff's Law No. 2 states that the voltage between any two points in a circuit is the same, regardless of the path taken between those points.

A transformer is a device designed to transfer increased or decreased voltages and currents. It is produced by wrapping a wire that is conducting current into a coil formation, which sets up a magnetic field around it. When a second coil of conducting material is placed nearby, the second wire acquires some amount of the voltage and current from the first coil. This is achieved without directly connecting the conducting wires. The number of turns of the coil determines the strength of the voltage and current produced and provided to the second coil. Altering this variable determines whether increased or decreased current is lent to the second coil. Transformers are used to step down the major voltage produced by electrical generators of alternating current to the much reduced voltage levels used for delivery to buildings, allowing the use of common electrical appliances.

Amplifiers are devices that increase, or "amplify," the input signal produced by a voltage source. Amplifiers are designed to leave the input signal (voltage or current) unaltered except for multiplying the signal in magnitude. They use an external power supply to achieve the amplification. The degree of amplification is the ratio of input to output voltage.[1]

The EEG machine can be considered as a series of circuits, including amplifiers. Brain-generated electrical signals are small and are further attenuated by the impedances of brain, skull, and skin. Production of the EEG requires the use of several amplifier circuits. Electrical signals generated by the brain are magnified by a preamplifier. Following this, the signal is modified by additional circuits known as *filters* (explained later), which select out undesired signal information. This final product is magnified once more by another group of amplifiers that produce a signal large enough to drive the pen-writing apparatus of the EEG machine.

The EEG machine uses amplifiers known as differential, or "push-pull," type, as opposed to single-ended amplifiers. The single-ended amplifier magnifies the signal of an input compared to a ground reference potential. For EEG recordings, a single-ended amplifier is problematic, since we are interested in voltage differences between electrode pairs. If two electrodes, each connected to ground, were connected together to compose one channel of EEG recording, a short circuit would occur that would in effect connect the voltages at the first and second electrode, producing no net differential signal. Differential amplifiers, in contrast, amplify only the potential difference between two inputs. A common signal to both electrodes is not amplified. Thus, a "common mode rejection" is achieved (Fig. 1-8). The 60-Hz interference arising from electrostatic effects of wires conducting alternating current as well as from electromagnetic effects of nearby appliances affects two inputs equally and is abolished by common mode rejection. With differential amplifiers, cerebral activity of large magnitude received at similar voltages at two electrodes is not easily seen.

FILTERS

EEG circuitry incorporates devices known as *filters* that attenuate frequencies of little relevance to the interpretation of brain wave activity. The high-frequency filter (HFF) attenuates high frequencies, and the low-frequency filter (LFF) attenuates low-frequency activities.

Cerebral generators of EEG activity can be considered as a battery producing varying voltages at different frequencies, connected to a circuit that includes a capacitor and a resistor. This simple model is displayed in Figure 1-9A. Using a switch, the resistor can be connected to the battery in such a way that three possibilities can be

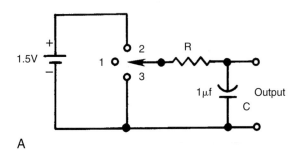

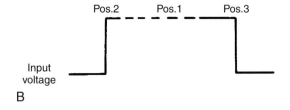

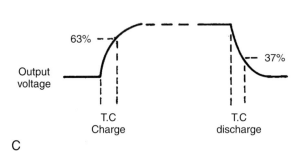

FIGURE 1–9

A, EEG rhythms are composed of rising and falling voltages at a given frequency and are comparable to a battery supplying input voltages that run on and off repetitively, as measured at the site of the capacitor. Diagrammatically this is comparable to the rapid connection and disconnection of a battery from its circuit. B, The actual input voltages produced by the battery. C, Voltages seen at the capacitor. T.C., time constant. (From Tyner F, Knott J, Mayer W. Fundamentals of EEG technology. Basic concepts and methods. New York: Raven Press, 1983, p. 48.)

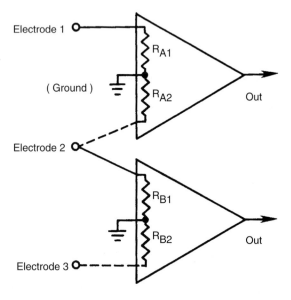

FIGURE 1–8

Use of differential amplifiers to record from a common electrode (electrode 2). (From Tyner F, Knott J, et al. Fundamentals of EEG technology. Basic concepts and methods. New York, Raven Press, p. 58.)

attained depending on the final connection. One possibility would be to complete the circuit and charge the capacitor. A second option would be to leave the circuit disconnected, thereby keeping the capacitor at whatever charge it has acquired. A third possibility would be to connect the resistor to a part of the circuit that does not include the battery. In this case, the capacitor discharges any voltage it has acquired.[16]

EEG rhythms are composed of rising and falling voltages at a given frequency and are comparable to a battery supplying input voltages that run on and off repetitively, as measured at the site of the capacitor. Diagrammatically this is comparable to the rapid connection and disconnection of a battery from its circuit. The EEG signal seen on paper depicts what a voltmeter would detect as changes in the voltage at the capacitor at specific point in time. There is an inherent difference between the actual input voltages produced by the battery and the voltages seen at the capacitor, because it takes time for the capacitor to charge, and because of such factors as impedance in the circuit and properties of the capacitor itself. For example, when the battery is at maximal voltage at a specific point in time, the capacitor has not yet achieved the same voltage as the source. Displayed graphically (Fig. 1-9B, part 2), a line representing the rise of the battery's voltage would be vertical, whereas the capacitor's voltage curve would have a substantial slope, implying that the battery had not achieved its maximal voltage at that point but would theoretically achieve it at a later point in time.

Analog filters can be characterized in terms of the *time constant*, which is the time required to charge or discharge a capacitor to a specified degree. Since the time constant is subject to the properties of capacitance and resistance, the relationship between these variables may be expressed as

$$TC = C \times R$$

where TC is the time constant, R is resistance, and C is capacitance.

Based on exponential properties related to the rate of charge or discharge of a capacitor, the time constant is defined as the amount of time for a 1 μF capacitor to either charge or discharge 63% of maximum charge. For example, if the capacitance is 1 μF and the resistance is 1 megaohm (MΩ), the time constant will equal 1 second, indicating that it requires 1 second for the capacitor to charge or discharge 63% of its initial charge. In the example provided earlier (Fig. 1-10B), the time required for 63% charge of the capacitor is comparable to the time required for voltage decline across the resistor to 37% of the original voltage. This is applicable to both HFFs and LFFs. In EEG terms, however, the time constant usually refers to voltage activity at the resistor and is used synonymously with the LFF (see later).

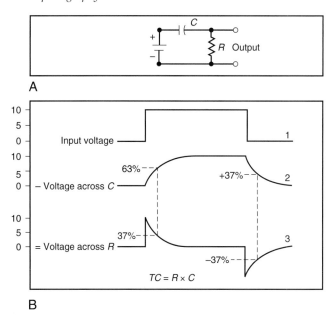

A

B

FIGURE 1–10

Voltage drops in an RC circuit. A, In contrast to Figure 1-9, the low-frequency filter (LFF) is achieved by monitoring the voltage across the resistor rather than across the capacitor. See text. B, (1) Input voltage; (2) Voltage across the capacitor, reflecting the function of the high-frequency filter; (3) Voltage across the resistor, reflecting the function of the LFF. (From Tyner F, Knott J, Mayer W. Fundamentals of EEG technology. Basic concepts and methods. New York: Raven Press, 1983, p. 51.)

High-Frequency Filter

The HFF attenuates waveforms of high frequencies. Moving the switch rapidly between positions 2 and 3 simulates a high-frequency input. As shown in Figure 1-9, with this configuration there is a gradual increase of the recorded voltage. The resultant wave has the appearance of being shifted in time, as if its maximum would be achieved at a later point in time. When there is insufficient time for each wave to reach its maximum, such as when a wave is part of a rapid frequency, the amplitude of the wave experiences a relative attenuation.[16]

The HFF does not abruptly attenuate frequencies at any given setting but rather affects all high-frequency rhythms to varying degrees along a spectrum, with the fastest frequencies most affected and the slower frequencies least affected. The slowest frequencies are unaffected. For example, a 70-Hz filter attenuates frequencies near 70 Hz or higher, and a 35-Hz filter attenuates frequencies near 35 Hz and higher. The principles of the analog HFF are presented in Appendix II.

Low-Frequency Filter

The LFF attenuates low frequencies and can be represented diagrammatically by switching the location of the battery and resistor seen in Figure 1-9 and connecting the circuit at point 2 (Fig. 1-10A). Another term for LFF is *high-pass filter* because it allows high frequencies to pass through.

The LFF is often used synonymously with the time constant. This is because the time constant can be easily measured with a calibration signal, and since there is an inverse relationship between time and frequency, the setting of the LFF can be alternatively expressed as a setting for the time constant. One can select filter frequencies for attenuation of undesired rhythms and signify this in terms of an alteration in the time constant. The relationship is expressed mathematically as

$$f = 1/2\pi TC$$

where f is the frequency selected for the filter and TC is the time constant. The ratio $1/2\pi = 0.16$, so the formula can be easily remembered as

$$f = 0.16/TC$$

For example, if the time constant was set at 0.1 second, the LLF would equal 1.6 Hz. If the time constant was increased to 0.3 second, the filter frequency would equal 0.53 Hz. More details regarding the theory of the LFF are given in Appendix II.

During the performance of an EEG, one of several LFF (or time constant) settings may be selected at a given time. The switch on the EEG panel selects a different capacitive resistance configuration. These configurations may be designed with the same value for resistance but a different capacitance. Alternatively, each configuration may have the same value for capacitance but a different resistance.

As the value of the LFF setting goes up (i.e., from 1 to 5 Hz), attenuation of low-frequency rhythms increases. As higher values for LFF are set, individual slow waves of interest experience decrements in amplitude and phase shifts. The peak appears earlier in time. Using measurements of sine waves of different frequencies against different LFF settings, one can determine the output amplitudes at each LFF setting per given frequency. The amplitudes become progressively smaller at frequencies increasingly below the filter setting.

In a similar fashion to that of the LFF, several different resistance-capacitance configurations may be selected for the input circuit to travel through in the HFF setting. The system may be designed to select circuits with varying capacitors with resistance held constant or varying resistors with the capacitance held constant. A larger capacitance results in an increased attenuation of high frequencies.

Just as in the case of the LFF, sine waves can be used to see the effects of the HFF on different frequencies. As

opposed to the LFF where there is no attenuation when a pure direct current signal without a filter is used, some attenuation of signal occurs with the pen-writing apparatus when increasingly high-frequency sine waves are applied purely because of electromechanical forces that prevent the pen from writing so quickly. This is not an issue with digital EEG, in which the limiting factors for recording fast frequencies are the sample rates and the filters installed by the manufacturers.

Determining the Effect of Filters on the Input Signal

By comparing the absolute amplitude to the output attained, the percentage of output attenuation can be determined. A frequency response curve can be drawn by plotting the percentage of attenuation of the absolute amplitude on the *y* axis with 0 at the top and 100 at the bottom against input frequency on the *x* axis (Fig. 1-11). For any LFF frequency, a curve emerges with a line arising from the lower left corner of the graph and reaching a plateau at the 0% attenuation mark. The LFF not only attenuates frequencies below the filter setting but also attenuates frequencies slightly above the LFF setting. However, most of the attenuation involves frequencies below the LFF setting.

On the frequency response curve, the given number for a filter is called the *cutoff frequency*. At this setting the predetermined frequency is attenuated by 20% to 30% depending on the particular instrument. The cutoff frequency distinguishes between significant and insignificant attenuation, since one might consider attenuation greater than 20% or 30% to be a "significant" attenuation. At frequencies higher than the cutoff frequency, an essentially linear relationship exists between input and output voltage.

When the HFF is applied, attenuation involves frequencies not just at or above the frequency setting value but also to some extent frequencies near but below that

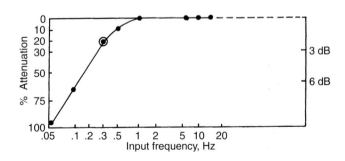

FIGURE 1–11

Frequency response curve with low-frequency filter of 0.3 Hz.

TABLE 1–2

Output Amplitude (mm) at Twelve Input Frequencies at Three HF Filter Settings°

| HF Filter, Hz | Input Frequency (Hz) | | | | | | | | | | | |
	5	**10**	**15**	**20**	**25**	**35**	**40**	**50**	**55**	**60**	**70**	**100**
None	10	10	10	10	10	10	10	10	10	9.5	8	3.5
70	10	10	10	10	10	10	10	10	10	9.5	8	3.5
35	10	10	10	9.5	9	8	7.5	7	6	5	3	2
15	10	9	8	7	6	4.5	3	2.5	2	1.5	1	1

° LF = 0.1 Hz; S = 10 µV/mm; input = 100 µV.
  † No LF in this channel.
  HF, high-frequency; LF, low-frequency; S, sensitivity.
  From Tyner F, Knott J, Mayer W: Fundamentals of EEG Technology: Basic Concepts and Methods. New York, Raven Press, 1983.

frequency setting. A comparison between HFF values against amplitudes produced at different frequencies is shown in Table 1-2. Alternatively, a table comparing HFF values against percentages of amplitude attenuation at different frequencies can be generated.[16] Graphs can also be generated by placing percent attenuation with 0 on top and 100% on bottom of the *y* axis and input frequencies on the *x* axis. Frequency response curves can be generated for each filter setting (Fig. 1-12). The curve typically arises from the top approximately mid-graph and descends toward the right lower hand corner, reaching a frequency of 100 Hz and 100% attenuation. These curves are also influenced by the electromechanical effects of the ink-writing apparatus on analog machines. Similar to that of the LFF, the cutoff frequency for the HFF is that frequency which is attenuated 20% or 30%. Joining the frequency response curves for a given LFF (or time constant) and HFF over a range of low to high frequencies results in bell-shaped curves. An example is shown in Figure 1-13.[16]

The currently recorded EEG consists of frequencies between 0.1 and 100 Hz. The most commonly used filters are 1 Hz (LFF) and 70 Hz (HFF). Frequencies greater than 70 Hz are not considered clinically significant, whereas the percentage of slow frequencies may increase with brain insults. Filters can be considered windows, allowing for better depiction of certain frequencies and

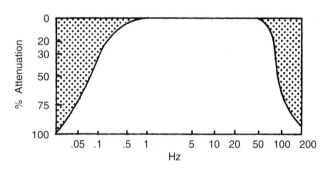

FIGURE 1–13

Joining of the frequency response curves for a low-frequency filter of 0.3 Hz and high-frequency filter of 70 Hz.

attenuation of others. For example, to see slow waves, one method is to change the LFF from 1 Hz to 0.3 Hz. Another strategy would be to reduce the HFF to a lower setting, such as a reduction to 35 Hz, which attenuates faster frequencies that may obscure slower electrographic activity of interest. Frequencies of interest can also be viewed by changing the "paper" speed, which traditionally was 30 mm/sec. For example, changing the paper speed to 15 or 10 mm/sec allows slower rhythms to be readily identified. Digital EEGs have the advantage of changing the paper speed after the test has been performed in contrast with paper EEGs, in which changes must be performed during the data acquisition.

The LFF and HFF are filters that attenuate rhythms at the low or high ends of the EEG spectrum. The "notch" filter attenuates a narrow band of frequencies with a maximum at 60 Hz.[6] This is necessary because the EEG apparatus is in an environment leaving it susceptible to a 60-Hz interference pattern resulting from the commonly used 60-Hz alternating electrical current. Since the filter cannot distinguish between frequencies of cerebral and extracerebral origin, the filter also attenuates cerebral frequencies in the selected range (Fig. 1-14). The use of the 60-Hz filter can be avoided if all electrode impedances are

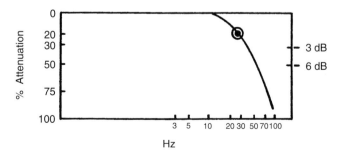

FIGURE 1–12

Frequency response curve with high-frequency filter of 35 Hz.

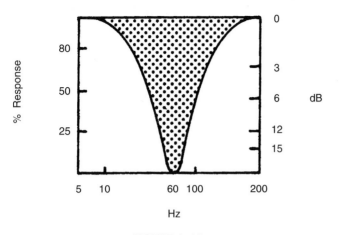

FIGURE 1–14
Frequency response curve of a 60-Hz notch filter.

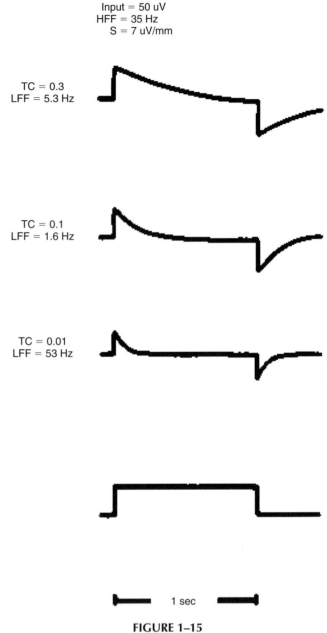

FIGURE 1–15
Changing the morphology of square waves with the use of different low-frequency filters. TC, time constant; HFF, high-frequency filter; S, sensitivity.

equal. In this case, 60 Hz will be rejected by the common mode arrangement.

At the beginning of the EEG recording, a process of calibration is performed involving the display of uniform square wave pulses that allows each channel of recording to be compared for uniformity. Calibration also shows the effects of different filters on such uniform waves. A square wave can be thought of as a complex combination of multiple sine wave components of different frequencies. The use of filters changes the morphology of square waves (Fig. 1-15). Based on the morphology of the altered square waves, the electroencephalographer can deduce an alteration in filter frequency.[16]

As the time constant is progressively decreased (LFF is increased), square wave pulses assume a more narrow morphology, since the fast phase of waves decays more rapidly (see Fig. 1-15). Additionally, square wave amplitudes are also diminished since the square wave is also composed of low-frequency sine wave components attenuated by the increased LFF setting.

The effect of HFF on the square wave calibration pulse can also be demonstrated since the square wave also has high-frequency sine wave components. As the HFF gets a lower value (setting a lower limit for more attenuation), the high-frequency components of the square wave are more affected and contribute a more rounded-off appearance on the square wave. For example, one might see a progression from a narrow peak to a rounded-off upphase. Figure 1-16 demonstrates the combined effects of different HFFs and LFFs on the square pulse.

THE EEG APPARATUS

The complete EEG apparatus is composed of several major components. These include electrodes placed on the head as well as a wire emanating from each electrode that has a terminal pin. Each pin goes into a receptacle known as a "jack" located on an electrode board jackbox. A cable connects the jackbox to the EEG machine. The EEG machine includes master control switches for all amplifiers as well as individual switches for each amplifier. These can select the sensitivity of the recording and the LFF and HFFs. There are also other components including the notch filter, pen-writing devices with paper

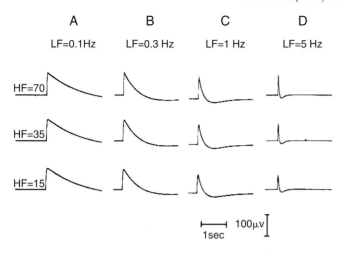

B   C   D

LF=0.1Hz   LF=0.3 Hz   LF=1 Hz   LF=5 Hz

HF=70

HF=35

HF=15

├──┤ 100μv
1sec

FIGURE 1–16

A-D, *Changing the morphology of squares with the use of different low-frequency (LF) and high-frequency (HF) filters. (From Tyner F, Knott J, Mayer W. Fundamentals of EEG technology. Basic concepts and methods. New York: Raven Press, 1983, p. 115.)*

recordings, a device to control paper speed, a calibration device, a device to gauge electrode impedance, and a power supply and cord.[16]

Each electrode is connected to a specific point on the electrode selector. The electrode selector connects any pair of electrodes to a single amplifier and the resulting signal is displayed on the corresponding channel on the EEG. The first channel may represent the voltage at a frontal electrode compared with that at the vertex. A second channel could hypothetically compare voltage at the vertex with that at an occipital electrode. The typical routine EEG comprises multiple channels varying from as few as 8 to as many as 21. The specific order and arrangement of these pairs of electrodes are known as a montage. Multiple montages are used sequentially during each recording to attempt to study activity from all major portions of the cortex. EEG laboratories tend to use uniform mon-

tages among the different patients recorded. A discussion of the referential and bipolar montages is included later in the chapter.

ELECTRODES AND THEIR APPLICATION TO THE SCALP

Resistance and impedance are important considerations in the EEG since the electrical changes comprising EEG signals are affected at multiple sites and are subject to many potential alterations before their final appearance on paper. Sites of resistance include resistance in the brain, skull, and skin-electrode interface; in the conducting wires from the head of the patient to the EEG apparatus; and in the EEG apparatus, including the pen-writing device.

Before electrodes are placed, a process of lightly abrading the skin is performed to remove superficial layers of oils and dead skin that may have some degree of conductivity and could thereby alter the signal delivered to the EEG apparatus. After the electrodes are applied, impedances should be checked, and if they are persistently high, the abrasion process should be repeated as necessary. Subsequently, an electrolyte gel is applied to the electrode as the latter is placed on the scalp. This gel facilitates the direct connection between the electrode and the skin and lowers the impedance at the electrode-skin interface.[16]

Electrodes should be well applied to avoid movement artifact, shown in the EEG as an electrode "pop" (Fig. 1-17), which is a change in electrostatic potential due to movement and loss of common mode rejection. The conductive solution collodion, which requires more time and effort to apply, has the advantage of providing a more secure contact between the electrode and the scalp. This reduces movement artifact and is particularly useful for prolonged recordings.

The typical electrode is a silver chloride (AgCl) electrode. The electrode provides acceptable conductivity and does not irritate the skin of the scalp; it may be immersed

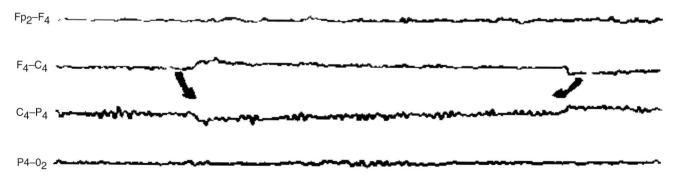

Fp2–F4

F4–C4

C4–P4

P4–02

FIGURE 1–17

Electrode pop artifact (between arrows).

in an electrolyte gel such as sodium chloride (NaCl). This chemical combination promotes a flow of charges that is ultimately received at the amplifier. When a negative charge arises from cortical generators, it causes negative chloride ions to leave the gel immersing the skin. The Cl^- ion combines with the positive silver (Ag^{2+}) ion to yield the product of AgCl and a residual free electron ion that is recorded at the amplifier. The process of ion exchange lends the name *reversible* to this type of electrode. Non-reversible electrodes are considered to be less optimal for EEG use because they are more prone to modifying incoming signals.[1]

A systematic and generally accepted convention for electrode placement over the scalp was developed by Jasper to avoid a haphazard application of electrodes. This convention, known as the *International 10-20 System*,[17] was designed to avoid the errors inherent in a mere visual approximation for the site of electrode placement and to encourage replicability in EEG results among different EEG laboratories and different patients. The International 10-20 System is based on anatomic landmarks and percentages of the distances between them instead of absolute interelectrode distance values. The latter would be problematic since the same absolute distances over a small head would produce a very different localization over a large head.

The convention recommends the use of 21 electrodes for standard conditions of recording and assigns odd numbers to the electrodes on the left and even ones to those on the right. Letters linked to these numbers refer to regions of the head and are shown in Table 1-3. The system also allows for the use of additional electrodes, at intermediate points beyond or between the above mentioned electrodes. For example, Fpz would represent a mid-prefrontal region and Oz a mid-occipital area.

The specific locations of these electrodes are based on four landmarks on the head: the nasion, the inion, and the

left and right preauricular areas. The following is a summary of the locations[16]:

- A mark placed midway between the nasion and inion localizes Cz.
- Points representing 10%, 20%, 20%, 20%, 20%, and 10% of the total distance along the line linking the nasion and inion over the vertex of the head represent the locations of Fpz, Fz, Cz, Pz, and Oz, respectively.
- Points representing 10%, 20%, 20%, 20%, 20%, and 10% of the total distance along the line linking the two preauricular points assign the locations of T3, C3, Cz, C4, and T4, respectively.
- Points representing 10%, 20%, 20%, 20%, 20%, and 10% of the total distance along the line linking Fpz and Oz going through T3 represent the locations of Fp1, F7, T3, T5, and O1, respectively.
- Points representing 10%, 20%, 20%, 20%, 20%, and 10% of the total distance along the line linking Fpz and Oz going through T4 represent the locations of Fp2, F8, T4, T6, and O2, respectively.
- A position midway between Fp1 and C3 represents F3, and a position midway between Fp2 and C4 represents C4.
- A position midway between Fp2 and C4 represents the location of F4.
- A position midway between C3 and O1 localizes P3, and a position midway between C4 and O2 localizes P4.

In 1991 the American Electroencephalographic Society (now called the American Clinical Neurophysiology Society) added nomenclature guidelines that designated specific identifications and locations of 75 electrode positions along 10 anteroposterior planes and 4 coronal chains (Fig. 1-18).[18] Several electrodes have different names in the 10-20 system and the extended nomenclature: The electrodes T3 and T4 in the 10-20 system are referred to as T7 and T8 in the expanded system, and T5 and T6 are referred to as P7 and P8 under the new nomenclature.

Although there is uniformity with localization and naming of electrodes, there is still variation among centers in the type of montages used, that is, the specific configurations of electrode comparisons in a set of channels. Some laboratories employ additional electrodes at intermediate distances between the 21 electrodes already mentioned, with the hope of enhancing the yield and localization of specific EEG activity of interest such as epileptiform abnormalities. Examples of montages are shown in Figures 1-19 to 1-21.

SPECIAL ELECTRODES

Specific clinical situations may warrant the use of special electrodes. However, because of patient comfort and

TABLE 1–3

Electrode Positions

Electrodes	Approximate Region of Brain Coverage
Fp1, Fp2	Anterior frontal
F3, F4	Frontal
F7, F8	Anterior temporal
C3, C4	Posterior frontal (overlying central sulcus)
T3, T4	Mid-temporal
T5, T6	Posterior temporal
A1, A2	Ear
P3, P4	Parietal
O1, O2	Occipital
Fz	Frontal midline
Cz	Posterior frontal midline
Pz	Parietal midline

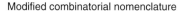

Modified combinatorial nomenclature

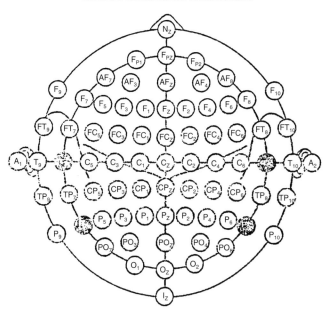

FIGURE 1–18

Modified International 10-20 System nomenclature.

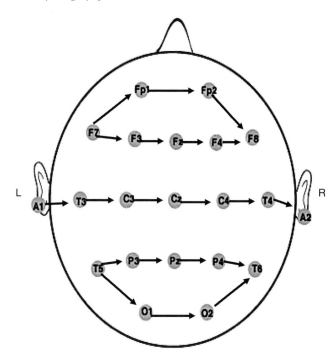

FIGURE 1–20

Transverse montage.

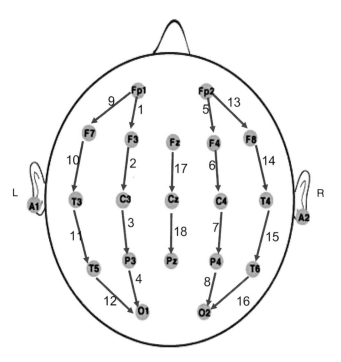

FIGURE 1–19

Bipolar montage (double banana).

reliability, these special electrodes are now rarely used, particularly in children. Nasopharyngeal electrodes are made of small silver spheres attached to long wires. These

are inserted though the nares to lie in the nasopharynx. They are designed to record electrical activity from the anteromesial surfaces of the temporal lobes, regions that are thought to be somewhat less accessible to scalp electrodes. They are usually employed to increase the yield on mesial temporal ictal and interictal epileptiform abnormalities. Nasopharyngeal electrodes are uncomfortable and often are contaminated by artifact. Infrequently used nasoethmoidal electrodes inserted into the nose and through the floor of the ethmoid sinus may be used to better sample EEG activity of the basal frontal lobe.[19]

Sphenoidal electrodes are more invasive electrodes used for even better recording of the mesial temporal area.[10-12] These wires are inserted through a cannula into the inferotemporal fossae with their tips lying in the vicinity of the foramen ovale on each side. Although they sample the same area as nasopharyngeal electrodes, they can be left in place for prolonged recordings (several days to more than a week), are better tolerated by patients after insertion, and provide a recording less compromised by artifacts.[20]

Anterotemporal electrodes (T1/T2) that are placed 1 cm above a point one third of the distance from the external auditory meatus to the outer tragus of the eye may delineate anterior temporal lobe discharges more than conventional electrode placement. There is controversy whether T1/T2 electrodes provide as much information as sphenoidal electrodes. Sphenoidal electrodes can be safely placed in children.[20-22]

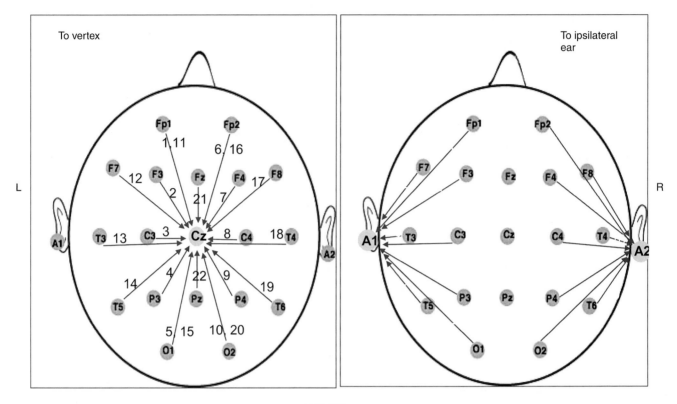

FIGURE 1–21

Reference montage.

DIGITAL TECHNOLOGY

Digital EEG machines record, amplify, and filter the electrical activity generated by the brain in much the same way as the analog machines described earlier in this chapter. In an analog machine, the resulting signal is used to drive a pen-writer. Digital processing, however, begins with conversion of this continuous signal into a series of discreet, regularly spaced data points.

The key component of the digital EEG machine is the analog-to-digital converter (ADC).[23] The signal from a single EEG channel is delivered to the converter, its voltage is measured at regular intervals, and this numerical value is stored in memory. The precision with which the ADC digitizes the input voltage depends on the voltage range of the ADC and the number of "bits" with which it represents the measured voltage, where each bit corresponds to a digit in a binary number. An n-digit binary number can represent 2^n different states. A two-digit binary number, for example, has four possible values: 00, 01, 10, and 11. A 2-bit ADC with an input range of ±100 μV would assign voltages of –75, –25, 25, or 75 μV to each measurement. More generally, if Vr is the voltage range of the ADC and n is the number of bits, the input signal can be resolved in steps of $Vr/2^n$ volts. At a resolution of 2 bits,

digitization would unacceptably distort the original signal. The resolution could be improved by limiting the input range of the ADC, but this would come at the expense of the ADC's dynamic range. Not surprisingly, digital EEG did not gain wide acceptance until 12- and 16-bit ADCs became widely available.[23] A typical ADC on the market today has an input range of ±10 mV and a 22-bit sampling resolution and can resolve voltage differences of $20 \text{ mV}/2^{22}$ = 4.8 nV. For most applications, increasing precision beyond this increases storage requirements without improving clinical utility.

The fidelity with which the analog signal is replicated also depends on the frequency with which it is sampled. The Nyquist theorem states that to unambiguously characterize a signal of a given frequency F, the signal must be sampled at a rate of more than two times F.[23] For example, a 50-Hz signal must be sampled at 100 Hz or more. This procedure prevents "aliasing," the phenomenon in which a signal of a certain frequency is sampled too slowly so that the resulting samples represent a signal with a frequency that is lower than that of the original analog signal. Figure 1-22 illustrates this phenomenon.

The EEG frequencies of clinical interest lie between 0.1 and 70 Hz. This necessitates a sampling rate of at least 140 Hz. To prevent the aliased representation of the higher

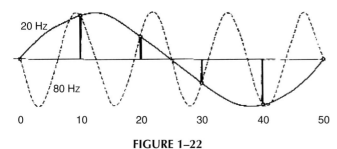

FIGURE 1–22

Digitizing an EEG signal at a frequency that is too low (i.e., using time intervals that are too long). Sampling of a 20-Hz waveform and an 80-Hz waveform end up looking the same.

frequency components of the analog EEG signal from contaminating the digitized signal, the signal is filtered with analog "antialiasing" filters prior to digitization. These are HFFs whose cutoff frequencies are one half or less of the sampling rate. In practice, most EEG machines sample at 200 Hz or more. First, this oversampling permits a smoother representation of the analog waveform. Second, this allows for the fact that the antialiasing filters do not block all the signal energy above their cutoff frequency—by choosing a sampling rate that is greater than twice the highest EEG frequency of interest, one can then choose an antialiasing filter with a cutoff frequency that is significantly less than one half of the sampling rate to prevent aliasing without filtering EEG frequencies of clinical interest. Unfortunately, increasing the sampling rate comes at the cost of increased storage requirements.

Digital Filters

Digital filters offer several advantages over the analog filters discussed earlier. First, analog filters operate on the signal as it is being acquired, prior to its representation on paper or digitization and storage. The information removed by analog filtering is irrevocably lost. By contrast, digital filters operate on the digitized signal. As is the case with other aspects of the visualization of the digitized EEG, post hoc digital filtering does not alter the stored signal and so refiltering with any combination of filters is possible. Second, digital filters can be designed so as not to introduce the phase delay inevitably associated with analog filters. Third, unlike analog filters, which are realized in relatively inflexible circuits of resistors and capacitors, digital filters exist in a program stored in the processor's memory and can therefore be modified without changing the hardware. Finally, analog filters can be sensitive to temperature changes and are subject to drift over time. Digital filters are stable in these respects. A brief introduction to the theory of digital filters is presented in Appendix III.

Visualizing the Digital EEG

The digitally recorded EEG is typically displayed on a computer monitor.[23] Important determinants of how a digital signal will look on a monitor are monitor size and the number of pixels used to demonstrate the EEG signal. Increasing the number of the pixels increases the accuracy and crispness of the visual display. Larger monitors may improve the visualization of tracings and allow space for each channel.

Advantages of Digital EEG

In contrast with analog machines, which record the EEG in the same montage in which it is displayed, digital EEG machines normally record the signal in a fixed referential montage. A common reference electrode or combination of electrodes serves as the second input into the differential amplifier for each channel. Recording the data in this way facilitates its display in any conceivable montage: Fp1-F3 can be obtained by simply subtracting Fp1-reference from F3-reference. Digital EEG therefore allows for both on-line and post hoc reformatting of an EEG segment in different montages. The ability to view a particular discharge or sequence in a variety of montages is one of the key advantages of the digital EEG. This is useful in addressing a host of localization problems.

Similarly, the digitized EEG can be reviewed using a variety of different filters. The EEG signal is normally acquired with "wide-open" analog filters prior to digitization that prevent aliasing and eliminate low-frequency artifact but permit the frequencies of clinical interest to be recorded without attenuation. Specific combinations of digital HFFs and LFFs and notch filters are then applied during review as needed. For example, filtering muscle artifact by reducing the cutoff frequency of the HFF often makes it possible to analyze portions of a record that would otherwise be uninterpretable. The filtered muscle artifact, however, can resemble spikes. By momentarily changing the cutoff frequency of the HFF, this issue can usually be resolved without difficulty. To better appreciate slow waves, one can increase the cutoff frequency of the low filter. Conversely, another strategy would be to reduce the cutoff frequency of the HFF to attenuate faster frequencies that may obscure underlying slow activity.

The voltage and time scales of the displayed EEG can also be changed during review. Compressing the time scale is another strategy to appreciate subtle background slowing that complements the adjustment of the filter parameters. Expanding the time scale can be helpful in determining phase relationships of transients across channels. This can be useful to resolve localization problems and to identify secondary bilateral synchrony. The ability to change the voltage scale during review is often helpful when, for example, the record contains occasional high-voltage discharges. Most of the record can be viewed at a scale appropriate to analyze background abnormalities, while the scale can be compressed (i.e., the sensitivity increased) to evaluate the lateralizing and localizing features of the high-voltage transients.

The ease with which the digital EEG can be reformatted has changed the way it is recorded and interpreted. Prior to the digital era, EEG technicians recorded the EEG in a sequence of montages and carefully monitored the sensitivity at which the signal was displayed. Because post hoc reformatting was impossible, the burden of selecting a nonstandard montage to resolve interpretive questions usually fell to the technician. In many institutions the technician still cycles the default montage in which the EEG appears through the routine montages and monitors the default sensitivity. These decisions are often less crucial than they were in the past because reformatting does not alter the stored data. Digital EEG does not, however, reduce the burden on the technician. No amount of manipulation allows the reader to compensate for a poorly recorded EEG. In particular, a poorly applied reference electrode can render the entire record uninterpretable.

New Applications of Digital EEG

The data-handling capabilities and flexibility of digital EEG have facilitated the development of long-term monitoring. This has revolutionized the use of the EEG for the classification of seizures and the presurgical evaluation in the epilepsy monitoring unit. Correlation of the digitized EEG with digital video is routine. Storing an EEG on a compact disk requires approximately 1000 times less physical space than on paper. Digital technology has also increased the role of the EEG in the neurointensive care unit (NICU), where it is used to detect subclinical seizures and to titrate antiepileptic therapy in status epilepticus. Digital EEG can also be used in the NICU to screen for the development of focal cerebral ischemia and increased intracranial pressure.[24] Ambulatory EEG monitoring, which was difficult to realize in the era of bulky analog machines, is now an expanding application of digital EEG.

Digital technology has also permitted the development of computer-aided quantitative techniques for analyzing the EEG. Spectral analysis and spike and seizure detection algorithms are available and may be useful to prioritize portions of records obtained during long-term EEG monitoring for visual analysis. Automated scoring of sleep studies is approaching clinical utility. Spike modeling and localization techniques are fertile areas of research, and a variety of clinical applications are under development;

registration of spike and seizure foci with imaging studies is emerging as a particularly promising technique.

Finally, since the inception of electroencephalography, clinical attention has focused on a fairly narrow frequency band. The upper end of this band reflects both an inherent limitation of the surface EEG—both lipid membranes and the skull act as HFFs and higher frequency activity overlaps with the scalp EMG—as well as the electromechanical limitations of a pen-writing apparatus. Baseline drift at the scalp-electrode interface and the characteristics of conventional amplifiers and filters have limited recording at very low frequencies. With the advent of intracranial recording with microelectrodes, it is now possible to record fast-field oscillations of 500 Hz and higher. It is now recognized that frequencies in the gamma range are clinically relevant in normal[3,4] and abnormal states.[5] Direct current–stable electrodes and direct current–coupled amplifiers have become increasingly available, which, in combination with digital technology, has greatly simplified the recording and analysis of very low-frequency EEG activity. The exploration of the full bandwidth of the EEG is one of the frontiers of encephalography.

THE EEG PEN-WRITING APPARATUS

Analog EEG machines have a pen-writer that uses simple electromagnetic forces.[17] The pen-writer produces deflections that represent the rhythms and patterns seen on the EEG. A conducting coil is used for receiving the amplified EEG signal, and an electromagnetic field develops around it. In one type of design, the coil is attached on one end to a pivot point, which allows it to rotate. Each coil is placed between the poles of a stable magnet, creating forces of action and repulsion between the coil and the magnetic poles that are constantly changing in accordance with the changing EEG signal. Forces of attraction or repulsion cause the coil to experience a deflection in upward and downward directions corresponding to the alternating voltages of the EEG signal. A pen attached to each coil transcribes the EEG signal onto paper (Fig. 1-23).

An oscillating pen-coil device is susceptible to the problem of extending beyond the intended range of motion (overshooting). Mechanical properties such as inertia and friction can lead to overshooting.[25] Although the initial tendency to begin movement is much less than that of a body already in motion, the weight of the pen contributes to inertia, causing a pen in motion to continue moving and therefore overshoot. An electrical or mechanical system of "damping" is employed to avoid these excessive oscillations. Electrical damping systems work by electrically adjusting the pen positions when they stray from normal positions. Mechanical systems alter the pressure exerted

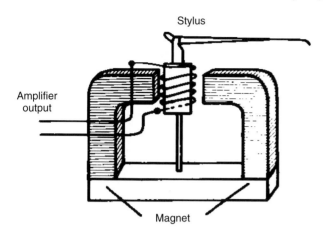

FIGURE 1–23

A pen attached to each coil in an analog EEG, which transcribes the EEG signal onto paper.

by the pen on the paper. However, both damping systems may result in some degree of modification of the frequency response to the EEG signal, especially at the high-frequency end. The pen actually writes the form of an arc instead of a perfectly vertical deflection. This results from the pivot point attachment of the pen. A signal of high amplitude assumes an arc form in a more obvious fashion than does a signal of lower amplitude. In the interpretation of the EEG, this may produce subtle timing errors, with higher amplitude waveforms most affected. The distance between EEG channels is designed to avoid pens hitting each other.[16]

With digital technology the EEG is typically displayed on a computer monitor.[23] Important determinants of how a digital signal will look on a monitor are monitor size and the number of pixels used to demonstrate the EEG signal. The fewer the pixels, the less crisp, the less accurate, and the less detailed will be the visual display. Larger monitors may help better visualize tracings and allow space for each channel.

FREQUENCY AND VOLTAGE CONSIDERATIONS

The EEG paper commonly used in the United States is designed to have each 1-second interval correspond to a 30-mm distance between any two repeating adjacent bold vertical lines, as that paper speed is set at 30 mm/sec. Most recordings use 30 mm/sec as a standard rate. However, many laboratories use a recording speed of 15 mm/sec for neonatal EEGs. When the intention is to better identify rhythms composed of waves of longer duration, slowing down the paper speed to 15 mm/sec results in the consolidation of EEG activities over a smaller amount of

paper and easier recognition of slow-frequency waveforms. In some centers, 15 mm/sec is the standard paper speed used in neonatal recordings. With digital technology, paper speed can be altered as desired and is not restricted to the speed at which the technician recorded.

Gain refers to the ratio of output to input at the amplifier. The *sensitivity* of the recording is the amount of millimeters of pen deflection assigned to each microvolt of output signal amplitude and is expressed as microvolt per millimeter. The sensitivity can be changed during the recording to enhance or diminish the representation of voltages on paper. EEGs often begin with a sensitivity of 7 μV/mm, since most voltages of cerebral origin and of interest to the electroencephalographer are reasonably displayed with this sensitivity.

Since each channel displayed on the EEG represents the comparison of two inputs, a convention has been established for the direction of the pen deflection. When the voltage in the first input is positive (less negative) with respect to the second input, the pen is deflected downward. When the first input is negative (less positive) with respect to the second input, the pen is deflected upward. Alternatively, when the second input is more negative (less positive) with respect to the first input, the pen moves downward. When the second input is more positive (less negative) with respect to the first input, the pen moves upward.[23,26] These variations are displayed in Figure 1-24.

TESTING THE RECORDING SYSTEM

To ensure that the EEG faithfully represents the voltages it receives, the recording system is tested by delivering external cerebral signals of uniform voltage to each

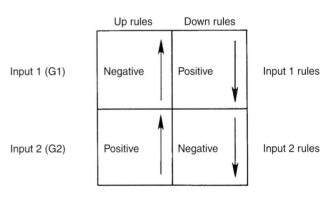

FIGURE 1–24

Established convention for the direction of the pen deflection in response to polarity of the first and second electrode composing the input signal. (From Tyner F, Knott J, Mayer W. Fundamentals of EEG technology. Basic concepts and methods. New York: Raven Press, 1983, p. 146.)

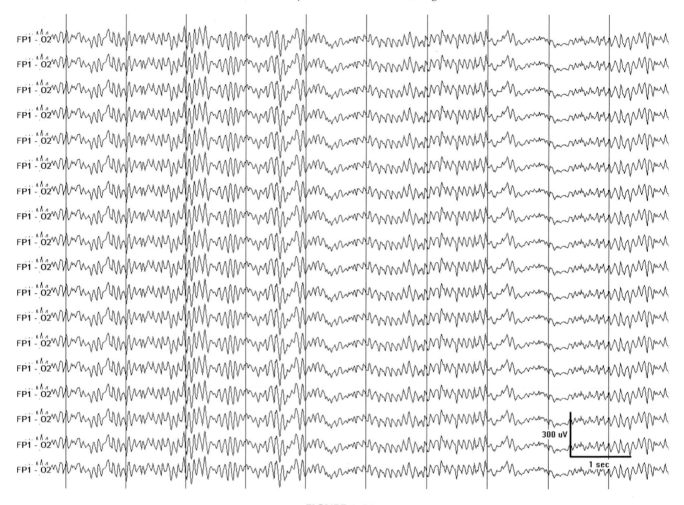

FIGURE 1–25

Biocalibration that uses a frontal-to-occipital derivation.

amplifier and assessing the produced EEG pattern or aberrations in wave morphology. During this calibration process,[25] a consistent current input signal is applied to produce square waves or sinusoidal waves that can be compared among the different channels of recording. It is easier to understand calibration using a square wave, although sinusoidal waves or even brain waves can be used as the calibration signal. The use of brain waves derived from the front and back of the head in the contralateral hemispheres (Fpl-O2) is a longstanding ritual called *biocalibration* and is performed just prior to the actual recordings. This is an opportunity to detect subtle differences in the display of uniform signals of cerebral origin and to correct them before the actual recording of the routine EEG (Fig. 1-25).

At arbitrarily selected sensitivity and filter settings,[16] a calibration button that applies the input signal is pressed. As described in the section explaining filters, the calibration pulse seen on the EEG represents the voltage at the resistor. With a slope of decline governed by the value setting of the LFF (or time constant), the signal undergoes a decay in voltage, ultimately reaching a 0 baseline (see Fig. 1-10*B*). When a manual setting is used, continuing to press the calibration button preserves the input voltage but the voltage across the resistor remains at 0. Immediately on release of the calibration button, the pen deflects in an opposite direction.

At the end of the test recording, filter settings and sensitivity changes used during the actual recording of the patient are applied to the calibration signal to demonstrate proper response by the EEG apparatus.

LOCALIZATION OF ACTIVITY

In the interpretation of the EEG, pattern recognition alone is insufficient for the accurate assessment of normal and abnormal rhythms. Tables 1-4 and 1-5 summarize the

Text continued on p. 31

TABLE 1–4
EEG Abnormalities and Their Clinical Significance

EEG CHARACTERISTICS	SIGNIFICANCE
Background Abnormalities	
Posterior dominant rhythm < 8 Hz (subject ≥ 3 yr of age)	Diffuse disturbance. Nonspecific, but may occur in toxic-metabolic disorders (electrolyte abnormalities, medication effects) and degenerative disorders, including dementia
Generalized background slowing, including or excluding slowing of the posterior rhythm	Diffuse, bilateral polymorphic delta activity and loss of reactivity indicate more severe cerebral dysfunction. Usually reflects a global process such as drug intoxication, uremia, hepatic disease, hypoxia, degenerative disorders, encephalitis, or meningitis. Can be seen with thalamic or midbrain dysfunction on the basis of bilateral structural lesions or herniation
Disorganization	Absence of the anteroposterior frequency and amplitude gradients appropriate for the patient's age and state of arousal. Implies a significant, diffuse disturbance of cerebral function
Excessive or distorted sleep patterns	In the absence of other findings, suggests a mild, diffuse abnormality of cerebral function
Abnormal Slow Waves	
Focal or lateralized slowing	Can represent a transient focal disturbance (consider the postictal state, complicated migraine, or head trauma) or a structural lesion, characteristically involving white matter (consider tumor, vascular, infectious, traumatic, local developmental, and degenerative diseases). A demonstrable structural lesion is more likely if the slowing is continuous, polymorphic, and of delta rather than theta frequency. Structural lesions are often associated with a focal loss of faster frequencies or in some cases with a focal attenuation of all EEG activities
Intermittent rhythmic delta activity (IRDA), generalized	Bisynchronous rhythmic slow waves with a wide distribution. Usually associated with a diffuse encephalopathy. Occasionally occurs in the setting of widespread structural damage involving subcortical and cortical gray matter to a greater extent than white matter and in the setting of circumscribed structural lesions involving mesial frontal, diencephalic, or brain stem structures
Frontally predominant intermittent rhythmic delta activity (FIRDA)	Common presentation of bisynchronous rhythmic slow waves in adults. Significance similar to that of IRDA. Occasionally seen with increased intracranial pressure, deep midline or subcortical lesions
Occipitally predominant intermittent rhythmic delta activity (OIRDA)	More common in children. Significance similar to that of IRDA. Must be differentiated from posterior slow waves of youth and other normal presentations of occipital slow waves
Abnormal Fast Activity	
Generalized excessive fast activity	Most often represents a medication effect (barbiturates or benzodiazepines). Also can occur in hyperthyroidism, acute or chronic anxiety, and as a normal variant
Focal excessive fast activity	Suggests a dysplastic cortical lesion
Periodic Patterns	
Periodic generalized complexes	May be seen in Creutzfeldt-Jacob disease (CJD), subacute sclerosing panencephalitis (SSPE), and phencyclidine intoxication. In both CJD and SSPE, the discharges may be associated with myoclonus. In CJD, the complexes are often stereotyped diphasic or triphasic transients occurring at intervals on the order 1 sec. Also are often triggered by sudden, loud noises. In SSPE, the complexes consist of high-voltage polyspikes, sharp waves, and slow components occurring at intervals of 3-20 sec. The complexes are usually not provoked by stimulation
Triphasic waves	Consist of three phases, each longer than the one before. The second phase is positive in polarity and has the greatest amplitude. Voltage is usually maximal over the anterior head regions. There is often an anterior-to-posterior phase delay. May appear at 0.5- to 1-sec intervals or sporadically. Reflect a metabolic derangement. Classically associated with hepatic encephalopathy but also occur in other conditions such as uremia, hyponatremia, and lithium intoxication. Usually seen in patients with a mild alteration of consciousness rather than stupor or coma

TABLE 1–4
Continued

EEG CHARACTERISTICS	SIGNIFICANCE
Pseudoperiodic lateralized epileptiform discharges (PLEDs)	Pseudoperiodic, sharply contoured waveforms with lateralized fields. Typically involve large areas of one hemisphere and may involve the homologous regions of the other. Bilaterally independent discharges (BiPLEDs) occur. If the pseudoperiodic discharges are localized to a region, e.g., anterior temporal lobe (as with herpes encephalitis), the term *pseudoperiodic focal epileptiform discharges* (PFEDs) may be more appropriate. PLEDs are associated with relatively acute structural lesions including those caused by encephalitis, infarction, hemorrhage, tumor, or abscess. Sometimes appear in the setting of an acute toxic or metabolic insult in a patient with a preexisting lesion. Can also represent an ictal or postictal pattern and a consequence of anoxia
Burst-suppression pattern	Pseudoperiodic complexes variably composed of polyspikes, sharp waves, and slow components separated by periods of background attenuation. Seen with severe diffuse disturbances such as anoxia, hypothermia, and high doses of central nervous system depressant medications
Coma Patterns	
Beta, alpha, and theta coma patterns	Generalized, invariant, monorhythmic activity in the beta, alpha, or theta frequency ranges. In beta coma, the activities are widespread and are usually of high amplitude. In alpha and theta coma, the expected anterior-to-posterior amplitude and frequency gradients are absent. The beta coma pattern often occurs in coma caused or complicated by benzodiazepines or barbiturates and in this setting is associated with a good outcome. The alpha and theta coma patterns are of less prognostic significance than the presence or absence of reactivity and spontaneous variability
Spindle coma pattern	Repetitive sleep spindles and sometimes vertex waves resembling stage II sleep in a comatose patient. Depending on the underlying etiology, this pattern is often associated with a good prognosis
Voltage suppression, generalized	Defined as the absence of electrical brain activity > 10 μV. Consistent with severe encephalopathy. This pattern should be considered abnormal only in the setting of impaired consciousness because some normal individuals have brain activity that does not exceed this threshold
Electrocerebral inactivity	Defined as the absence of electrical brain activity > 3 μV. In the appropriate clinical scenario, a technically adequate EEG demonstrating this pattern supports the diagnosis of brain death. This pattern can be seen in potentially reversible conditions such as benzodiazepine overdose
Epileptiform Abnormalities	
Spike	Sharply contoured waveform standing out from the background with a duration of 20-70 msec. The major deflection is most often surface negative. Indicates a focal area of epileptogenic potential. Rarely seen in individuals who have no history of seizures
Sharp wave	Sharply contoured waveform standing out from the background with a duration of 70-200 msec. Similar significance to that of spikes
Polyspikes	Repetitive spikes without intervening background. Rarely seen in individuals who have no history of seizures. Their detailed interpretation depends on their distribution and other features of the EEG
Centrotemporal spikes	Stereotyped spikes located in the central and temporal regions. May have a slightly shifting distribution. Unilateral in about 70% of routine records. Individual spikes characteristically have the field distribution of horizontal dipoles, such that a positive phase reversal over the anterior head regions and a negative phase reversal over the central and temporal regions is seen in longitudinal bipolar recordings. These spikes often dramatically increase in frequency. In the appropriate clinical setting, these discharges support the diagnosis of childhood epilepsy with centrotemporal spikes
Spike-wave complex	A spike followed by a slow wave. Most often the major deflections have the same polarity

TABLE 1–4
Continued

EEG CHARACTERISTICS	SIGNIFICANCE
Rapid spike-wave complexes	Rhythmic runs of bisynchronous spike-wave complexes with a repetition rate > 3 Hz. Indicative of generalized seizure disorder, usually of the genetically determined type
3-Hz spike-wave complexes	Indicative of generalized seizure disorder. Classically seen in absence seizures, although this pattern also occurs in other genetically determined epilepsy syndromes
Slow spike-wave complexes	Rhythmic runs of bisynchronous spike-wave complexes with a repetition rate < 3 Hz. Indicative of a generalized seizure disorder. Often seen in the symptomatic and cryptogenic epileptic syndromes such as Lennox-Gastaut syndrome. Prolonged runs of these complexes, in the absence of evolution of their frequency or morphology and clinical manifestations, often represent an interictal phenomenon
Polyspike-wave complex	Two or more spikes occurring in sequence followed by a slow wave. The major deflections of each component usually have the same polarity. These are indicative of a generalized seizure disorder. Their detailed interpretation depends on their repetition rate
Photoparoxysmal response	Bisynchronous polyspike or polyspike-wave discharges appearing during photic stimulation that are not synchronized with the flash rate. Indicative of a predisposition to photogenic seizures. Seen in a subset of patients with genetically determined generalized and occipital epilepsies and rarely in patients with other epilepsy syndromes
Hypsarrhythmia	High-amplitude (>200 μV), disorganized and slow background with multifocal spikes. This pattern is usually present interictally in patients with infantile spasms
EEG seizure patterns	Repetitive, rhythmic waveforms evolving in frequency and morphology that usually begin abruptly and interrupt the patient's background activities. These sequences may consist of waveforms similar to the patient's interictal epileptiform abnormalities or entirely distinct patterns
	Sudden attenuation of amplitude preceded by a frontally maximal or generalized paroxysmal complex composed of a high-amplitude slow wave with or without superimposed sharp components. The most common ictal pattern associated with infantile spasms. Also seen with atonic seizures

Data from References 32-38.

TABLE 1–5
Pseudoepileptiform Patterns (benign EEG variants)

Pattern	Morphology	Distribution	Context	Comment
14- and 6-Hz positive bursts	Negative arciform deflection alternates with sharply contoured positive component. Discharges occur in <3-sec bursts at 13-17 Hz or less frequently at 6-7 Hz. Isolated electropositive transients occasionally occur	Maximal over posterior temporal regions. Bisynchronous with shifting emphasis or bilaterally independent. Best seen in widely spaced bipolar or referential montages	Drowsiness and light sleep	Seen in 10-60% of normal population, most often in adolescents
Frontal arousal pattern	Trains of sinusoidal discharges. Superimposed rhythms may produce a notched or spiky appearance. $\approx$ 20-sec duration, 7-20 Hz	Predominantly frontal	Occurs on arousal from sleep. Disappears when fully awake	Occurs in children
Lambda waves	Bilaterally synchronous diphasic or triphasic transients. Maximal deflection usually positive. <20 μV, 100-200 msec	Maximal in occipital regions. Field may extend to parietal and temporal regions	Evoked by scanning patterned images. Eliminated by darkening room, staring at blank field	Seen in 50% of normal EEGs

TABLE 1–5

Continued

Pattern	Morphology	Distribution	Context	Comment
Rhythmic temporal theta bursts of drowsiness (also known as psychomotor variant)	Sharply contoured, often notched discharges. Occur in bursts or runs without evolution. 5-7 Hz	Maximal over the temporal regions. Bisynchronous with shifting emphasis or bilaterally independent	Occurs in quiet wakefulness or drowsiness	Overall incidence of 0.5-2%. Most often seen in adolescents and young adults
Positive occipital sharp transients of sleep (POSTS); also known as lambdoid waves	Sharply contoured monophasic or, less often, biphasic transients. The initial deflection is positive. Occur singly or in irregular 4- to 5-Hz bursts	Bioccipital. Always synchronous, but may have considerable amplitude asymmetry	Drowsiness and light sleep	Most often seen in adolescents and adults
Posterior slow waves of youth	Slow wave interrupting alpha rhythm, often abruptly. Superimposed alpha waves then become increasingly distinct during latter part of slow wave	Same distribution as alpha rhythm	Same reactivity as alpha rhythm	Uncommon before 2 yr of age. Maximal from 8-14 yr of age. Incidence 15% in adolescents. Rare after 21 yr of age
6-Hz spike and wave; also known as phantom spike-wave	Bursts or trains of 5- to 7-Hz spike-wave complexes. The spike tends to be of lower amplitude than the associated slow wave. High amplitude (<5 Hz) patterns more likely to be associated with seizures	Usually bisynchronous with a widespread field. Infrequently asymmetrical. Frontally maximal patterns more likely to be associated with seizures	Occurs in relaxed wakefulness and drowsiness. In contrast with more epileptogenic patterns, these discharges disappear during sleep	Seen in 2.5% of the population, most often in adolescents and adults
Small sharp spikes; also known as benign sporadic sleep spikes and benign epileptiform transients of sleep	Low-voltage (≤50 μV), short duration (≤50 msec) monophasic or diphasic transients with steep ascending and steeper descending limbs. May have an after-coming slow wave, but there is no disruption of the background or focal slowing	Very widespread fields, maximal over temporal regions. Bilateral independent or bisynchronous	Occur in drowsiness and light sleep	Seen in 20-25% of adults
Subclinical rhythmic electrographic discharges of adults (SREDA)	Rhythmic, prolonged sequences (often ≈ 40 sec) typically evolving from irregular, sharply contoured, low-frequency discharges to a faster (5-7 Hz) sinusoidal pattern	Often maximal over parietal or temporal regions. Bisynchronous or unilateral	Usually seen in quiet wakefulness. Occasionally in sleep. Sometimes provoked by hyperventilation	Rare. Seen in adults. Discharges are asymptomatic
Wicket spikes	Positive arciform deflection alternates with sharply contoured negative component. Isolated discharges or in trains. Emerges out of background. 6-11 Hz, 60-200 μV	Occur maximally over the temporal regions, either synchronously or independently	Occur in drowsiness and light sleep	Overall incidence of 1%. Seen most often in adults

Data from References 32, 33, 35, 37, and 39.

classification of EEG abnormalities and pseudoepileptiform patterns of no clinical significance.

Identification of rhythm types requires the assessment of localization of activity. Although the EEG is actually only a two-dimensional recording, the EEG is derived from a three-dimensional brain that conducts electrical currents. In accordance with volume conduction theory, current flows in a direction of the shortest path between two points. However, even portions of this conducting volume that are distant from the site of maximal current may be affected to some degree by this current. Considering the case of a single point of charge helps elucidate this concept (Fig. 1-26).

Around any single point of positive or negative charge, a surrounding field of activity of similar charge is present. The potential close to the point of charge is greater than a potential distant from it. The rate of drop of the potential further away from the point of maximal charge is contingent on the conducting qualities of the medium the charge exists in. The potential decrements can be displayed as concentric circles with a point along each circle being isopotential to all other points on that circle.[26] This

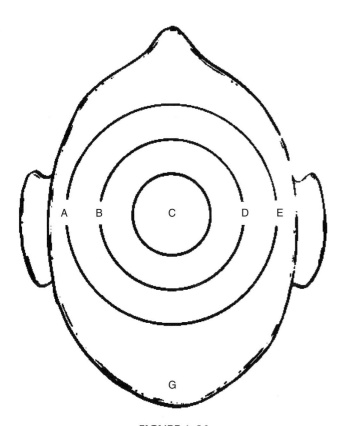

FIGURE 1–26

Field surrounding any single point of positive or negative charge. The center of the activity is in C and is represented by the smallest concentric circle.

diagrammatic display could be thought of as comparable to the concentric ripples a stone produces when thrown in water.

In the case of a dipole, positive and negative charges are separated in space and the concentric fields are now elliptical in shape. A flat plane of zero isopotential charge runs perpendicularly halfway between a hypothetical line connecting positive and negative charges. When simultaneous positive and negative charges are recorded by separate scalp electrodes, a horizontal dipole is observed. When dipoles are uniformly aligned perpendicular to the cortical surface, the recording electrodes see only the potentials of the dipole aspect closest to it.

For the interpretation of the EEG a model has been adopted that assumes that dipoles are aligned perfectly perpendicular to the cortical surface. In fact, the surface of the cortex is marked by multiple convolutions that would distort this idealized arrangement. Additionally, the principles discussed apply to only one moment in time even though the EEG is a dynamic process.

To assess the localization of potentials, two methods of recording are used. The first is known as the *bipolar mode* and the second as the *referential derivation*.[26] Bipolar montages are composed of chains of several adjacent electrodes, and the recorded activity represents the comparison of voltages at two different electrodes.[27] Each channel depicts the potential differences of consecutive pairs of electrodes. In the referential montage, potentials at each electrode are compared to the same voltage at one site arbitrarily designated as the "reference" potential. Ideally, this reference is not in the field of the activity of interest (Fig. 1-27).

The following exemplifies how different types of activity may appear in bipolar and referential montages. As mentioned earlier, convention dictates a downward pen deflection when voltage at the first input is relatively positive compared to the second input and upward when the first input is relatively negative compared to the second.[16,26] To assess sites of minimal and maximal activity, the electroencephalographer uses amplitudes as well as the direction and relationships of deflections of the activities of interest. Deflections among a series of channels that follow the same direction are "in-phase"; those involving activity that varies in direction are "out-of-phase." Two adjacent opposing deflections demonstrate a "phase reversal." In a bipolar montage (but not in a referential montage), the phase reversal signifies the site of maximum voltage.

Figure 1-27 demonstrates one example of a series of potentials seen in a referential montage. All deflections are in-phase, and the point of maximal amplitude corresponds to the site of maximal potential (electrode A). The reference electrode C is at the lowest potential among the series and is relatively uninvolved in the activity. The site

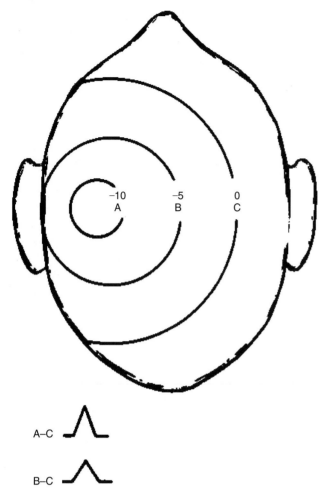

A–C

B–C

FIGURE 1–27

In the referential montage, potentials at each electrode are compared with the same voltage at one site designated as the "reference" potential, in this case electrode C.

minimum. If C were the minimum, this would produce highly unusual fields of activity. The field shown in Figure 1-28 would be a much more likely possibility.

The same activity is displayed in Figure 1-29 in a bipolar montage. In the bipolar montage, reversal in phases is seen at two adjacent channels. The channels involved in this phase reversal have a common electrode C, which is the electrode of maximum potential. In the bipolar montage, therefore, the electrode common to any two channels that exhibit a phase reversal is the site of maximum voltage. In a referential montage, however, the phase reversal does not relate to the point of maximal activity, as demonstrated in Figure 1-30. In this montage, a phase reversal indicates that activity is not completely in-phase and therefore the reference is neither the maximum nor minimum of activity.

In Figure 1-30, the maximum of activity exists at the end of a chain of electrodes. In the bipolar montage, all deflections are in-phase with each other. In the referential montage deflections are out-of-phase, indicating that the reference electrode is neither the maximum nor minimum of activity. Although electrode E was the maximum for that particular array of electrodes, it is quite possible that E would not be the maximum for a broader array of electrodes, as shown in Figure 1-31.

There are merits and disadvantages to the bipolar or referential mode.[27] For this reason, most laboratories use a combination of assorted bipolar and referential montages to provide varying views of the patient's EEG activity. A disadvantage of the bipolar montage is the inability to directly infer absolute amplitudes of activity, which can be done more readily in the referential montage. Another problem in the bipolar montage concerns "in-phase cancellation": Any activity similar in amplitude in both inputs to the amplifier of a given channel is canceled out. This results in deflections that are nearly flat for that specific activity. During the interpretation of the EEG, these apparent very low amplitudes can deceptively suggest the absence of activity despite the actual presence of substantial voltage in that area. In the referential montage, this activity would be more readily seen in each channel. Figure 1-32 exemplifies this point. In this case, the difference in voltage between

of maximal activity, however, does not always correspond to the electrode with the highest recorded amplitude. In Figure 1-28, potentials at electrodes A, B, D, and E are compared with that of the selected reference electrode C. These two examples demonstrate the rules for the localization of activity in the referential montage shown in Box 1-1. When evaluating EEG activity that is completely in-phase among all channels considered, two possibilities exist for that field of activity: one in which the reference is minimal in activity and one in which it is maximal. The decision about which possibility applies to the particular recording can be deduced by drawing the fields that correspond to each possibility. The possibility that produces a more reasonable field of activity is the more likely one. In the example provided, the series of in-phase deflections leads to two possibilities for fields of activity: one with the reference electrode C as the maximum and one with C as

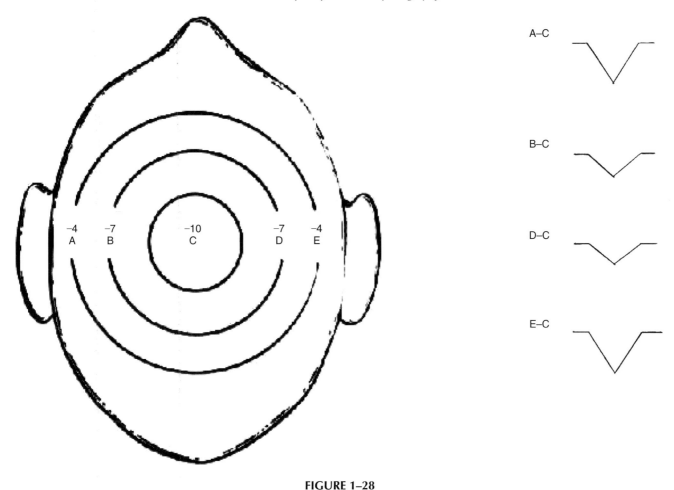

FIGURE 1–28
In this referential montage, the reference electrode C is at the maximum of the activity. All EEG activity is in-phase.

sequential electrodes comprising each channel of recording is minimal. The activity is much more difficult to appreciate in the bipolar montage. The same activity represented in the referential montage is more easily seen since the amplitude differences are more substantial when comparing each electrode to the reference electrode. To avoid the problems inherent in recording from adjacent electrodes that are exposed to very similar voltages in the bipolar montage, pairing electrodes that have larger electrode distances may show this activity better. This concept is employed, for example, in neonates and brain death recordings.

A caveat in the use of the bipolar montage is to avoid, when possible, the use of nonlinear arrays of electrodes in any one chain of sequential channels (Fig. 1-33). In this example, electrical fields of activity are unusual and difficult to interpret.

The referential montage is actually a modified bipolar montage since it compares the voltages at two different electrodes in each channel. However, the second input is always the same for each hemisphere and is called the

reference. Ideally one would like to have "active" electrodes over the area of interest and a standard reference with minimal involvement. This would make the interpretation of the EEG simple, since fields would be represented exactly by amplitudes, with the highest amplitude reflecting the site of maximal voltage in every case. Unfortunately, the reference is rarely completely uninvolved. Placing the reference off the scalp, such as on the ear or on the face, does not prevent volume conduction from the cerebral cortex, and these areas are especially susceptible to noncerebral electrical potentials. Placing the reference on the body makes it vulnerable to electrocardiogram potentials, whose amplitudes are usually much larger than cerebral activity. Potentials arising from these "contaminants" of the reference usually are seen in all channels that include the reference, although at varying amplitudes. When the ipsilateral ear is used as a reference, the electrocardiogram signal may be of opposite polarity.

Analysis of the referential montage assumes an electrical field distribution that is unipolar, as would be attained by

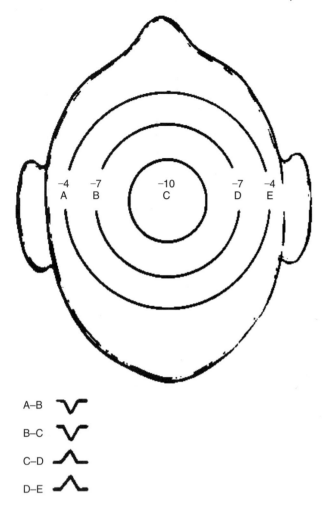

FIGURE 1–29.

The same activity seen in Figure 1-28 is now represented in a bipolar montage. Phase reversals demonstrate maximum activity at electrode C.

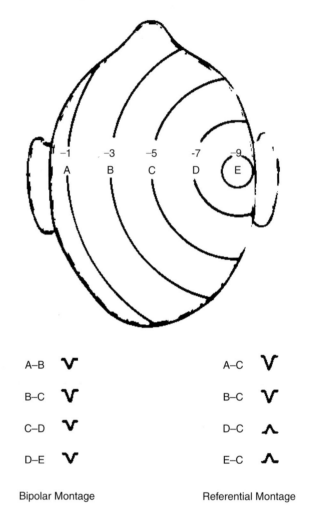

Bipolar Montage   Referential Montage

FIGURE 1–30

In this example, the maximum of activity is at the end of an electrode chain. In a bipolar montage there is no phase reversal. When C is used as the reference, a phase reversal occurs and does not relate to the point of maximal activity. In this case, the phase reversal indicates that the reference is located within the field.

sampling only one side of the dipoles produced by pyramidal cells perpendicular to the cortical surface. This assumption is not always true as in the case when these dipoles are aligned in horizontal or diagonal orientations to the recording surface (Fig. 1-34). Since voltage differences tend to be larger in the referential montage, the sensitivity of recording often needs to be reduced to avoid blocking of pens undergoing wide deflections. This reduction in sensitivity may diminish the prominence of more subtle lower amplitude activity intermixed with the higher voltage type, making the former more difficult to appreciate.

One special kind of referential montage employed by some EEG laboratories is the "average montage." This is a referential montage in which the voltage in every electrode is compared with that of one reference. The value of the reference is achieved by taking the average of the voltages of all electrodes selected. With the notion of the random-

ness of relationships among potentials in the selected electrodes, it is hoped that the average would approximate a value of zero and in this way become a very good reference. When this happens, the recording produced may accentuate the activities of interest, making them readily apparent to the electroencephalographer. Unfortunately, this reference may not achieve its intended value. As the number of electrodes connected to the average reference point is increased, the activity of any one electrode has a proportionately smaller effect on the other channels, thereby encouraging the incorporation of many electrodes in the formulation of the average reference. However, when activity of interest is widespread and involves mul-

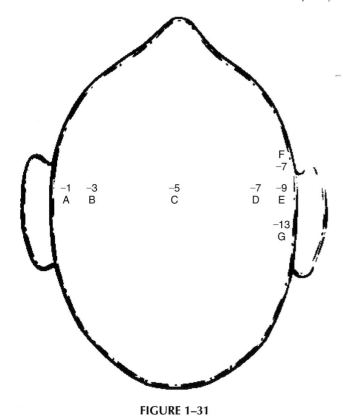

FIGURE 1–31

The same activity shown in Figure 1-30 is now shown with additional electrodes outside the linear array of Figure 1-30. This shows that although electrode E was the maximum for the initial array of electrodes, it is not the maximum for a broader array of electrodes. The field maximum is now at electrode G.

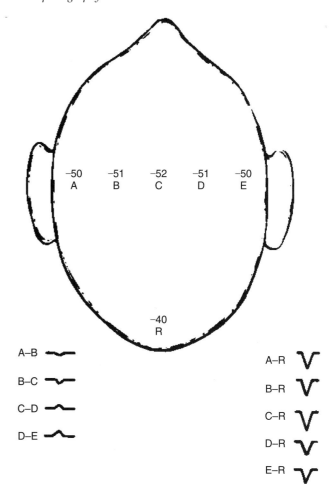

FIGURE 1–32

Similar voltages at each adjacent electrode result in relative attenuation of activity in the bipolar montage. EEG activity in each channel is more clearly seen in the referential montage.

tiple electrodes, a greater amount of electrodes involved in a given activity will skew the potential of the average reference to a large degree. The problem here is that the potential of activity of interest as the first input to the amplifier will be compared to a very similar potential value in the average, resulting in a relative cancellation. Conversely, when an area not involved in the activity is compared with the average, an inverted signal will be seen at that electrode. An example of the normal waking EEG background in the average montage is displayed in Figure 1-35.

The average montage is superior for displaying focal activity involving a minimal number of electrodes. In this case, the differences in potential between the electrodes of interest and the average reference are substantial and the visualization of localization is enhanced. The average montage is particularly vulnerable to obfuscation caused by artifactual activity such as that seen with eye blink artifact. Many average montages are set up to specifically exclude the most frontal electrodes in the summation of the average with the hope of partially avoiding this contamination of the average reference. Selected electrodes in areas of

focal abnormalities may be excluded from the average so that these areas will be accentuated when comparing them with an uncontaminated average potential.

There is a limit to the number of electrodes that can be excluded since removing an electrode diminishes the total number of electrodes participating in the average and thereby makes this potential less of a true "average." At least 10 electrodes should be included in the average.

ARTIFACTS

The EEG often contains activity of extracerebral origin that may resemble cerebral activity. These artifacts can be quite subtle and need to be recognized to avoid an inaccurate interpretation of the EEG. Although vigorous use of the LFFs and HFFs may substantially reduce the

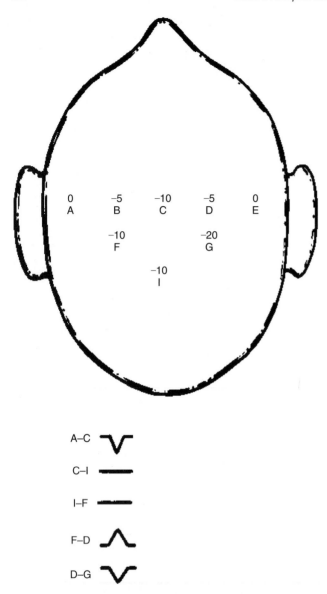

FIGURE 1–33

A caveat in the use of the bipolar montage is to avoid when possible the use of nonlinear arrays of electrodes in any one chain of sequential channels. Here, electrical fields of activity are unusual and difficult to interpret.

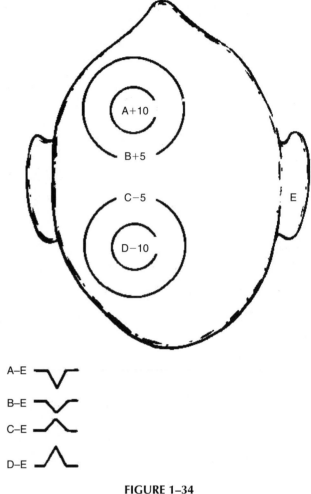

FIGURE 1–34

Electrical field distribution associated with a horizontally oriented dipole.

appearance of many types of artifacts on the recording, this may often compromise the interpretation of normal background activity. Therefore, it is desirable to correct the source of artifact.

The wide range of artifacts may be conveniently divided into *physiologic* and *nonphysiologic*.[28] The former refers to those artifacts arising from a part of the patient's body other than the brain. The latter refers to artifacts created by influences outside the patient. Physiologic types include artifact secondary to muscle activity, electrocardiogram,

pulse, eye movements, movements of the tongue (glossokinetic potential), respiration, tremor, and perspiration. Nonphysiologic types[17] include artifacts related to faulty junctions between the electrodes and the scalp, 60-Hz electrical interference, "noise" inherent in amplifiers composing the EEG apparatus, movements in the recording environment, intravenous drip artifact, electromagnetic radiation emanating from nearby devices, electrostatic potentials from clothing, and even the ringing of a nearby telephone. Several examples are displayed in Figures 1-36 (pulse artifact), 1-37 (electrode pop artifact), and 1-38 (artifact from patting an infant).

ELECTRICAL SAFETY

Principles of electrical safety must be carefully applied to avoid danger to the patient. Patient exposure to

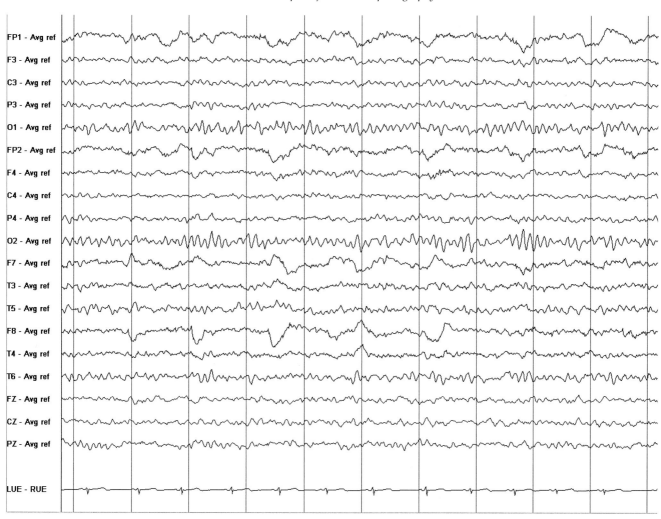

| FP1 - Avg ref |
| F3 - Avg ref |
| C3 - Avg ref |
| P3 - Avg ref |
| O1 - Avg ref |
| FP2 - Avg ref |
| F4 - Avg ref |
| C4 - Avg ref |
| P4 - Avg ref |
| O2 - Avg ref |
| F7 - Avg ref |
| T3 - Avg ref |
| T5 - Avg ref |
| F8 - Avg ref |
| T4 - Avg ref |
| T6 - Avg ref |
| FZ - Avg ref |
| CZ - Avg ref |
| PZ - Avg ref |
| LUE - RUE |

FIGURE 1–35

Normal waking recording in an 8-year-old child.

electrical current can cause a wide spectrum of serious adverse effects depending on the region of the body involved, the amount of voltage, and the electrical resistance in that area. Based on experimental animal data involving threshold currents for the production of ventricular fibrillation and burns, it has been estimated that patients with surface electrodes connected to electrical devices such as the EEG machine can tolerate only 100 µA of current safely. Patients with direct connections to the heart such as the Swan-Ganz catheter can tolerate only 10 µA of current before the risk of serious morbidity.[1,29] The major potential cause of electrical problems for the patient is exposure to "leakage" current. This is current that strays from its intended pathway. Older buildings using two-wire delivery systems for alternating current to power electrical devices were vulnerable to short circuiting of current to a part of the apparatus itself. Coming into contact with that part

of the apparatus led to connecting the patient to this unintended additional circuit.

Modern hospitals and other buildings commonly use three-wire outlet systems that are composed of a wire that delivers the alternating current, a "neutral" (for return of current to complete the circuit), and an additional ground connection that receives a ground wire connected to the chassis of the apparatus and channels stray current from the chassis to ground. Another safety device is the "circuit breaker," which represents a conducting material placed along important circuits. The circuit breaker is designed to open and thereby disconnect the circuit immediately when current exceeds safe levels.

Improper ground protection may result in a broken ground wire in the power cord or poor connections of the building ground to the earth ground. A patient should not be connected to multiple electrical devices with separate

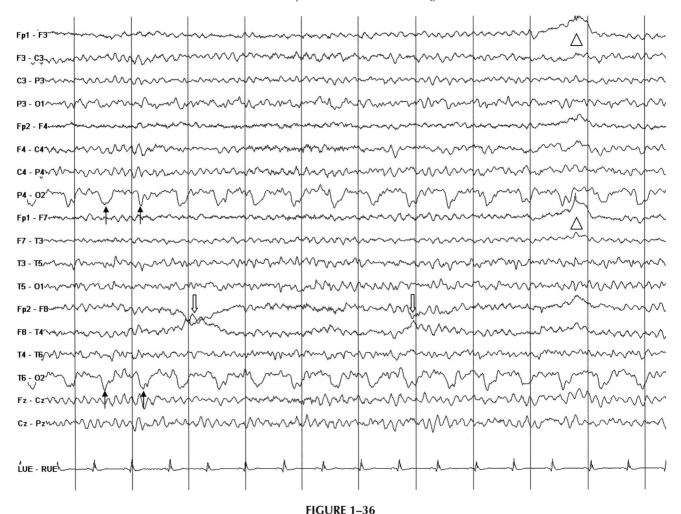

FIGURE 1–36

Pulse artifact at O2 (solid arrows). This artifact occurs when an electrode is placed over a superficial artery. Note the primarily leftward eye movements in the 3rd and 4th as well as in the 7th and 8th seconds, best seen at F8 (open arrows). F8 becomes relatively negative as a result of the cornea moving away from the right temporal area. An eye movement predominantly in the downward direction occurs in the 10th second (arrowheads).

grounds because an electrical current can be established flowing from a properly grounded instrument through the patient into the apparatus with a faulty ground. Such a circuit has been termed a *ground loop*. All devices used should be connected to the same power strip leading to a unified outlet.

Short circuits are not the only cause of leakage current. Other causes include "stray capacitance," which occurs among long power lines such as extension cords that have wires running parallel to each other separated by an insulating material.[27] Extension cords should therefore be avoided. "Stray inductance" can also create electrical current outside of its intended pathway since any current going through a conducting wire creates an electromagnetic field. An easily avoidable dangerous situation is the "power

surge," which is a transient, uncontrolled elevation in current that occurs when a device is turned on or off. It can be avoided by turning equipment on before connecting the patient and by disconnecting the patient before the EEG machine is shut off.[16]

SPECIAL CONSIDERATIONS IN PERFORMING THE EEG IN CHILDREN

Difficulties in performing the EEG may arise in the pediatric population because of fear, hyperactivity, or limitations in the ability to cooperate with the procedure. Sedation is employed when clinical features of the patient make a technically satisfactory recording unlikely to be

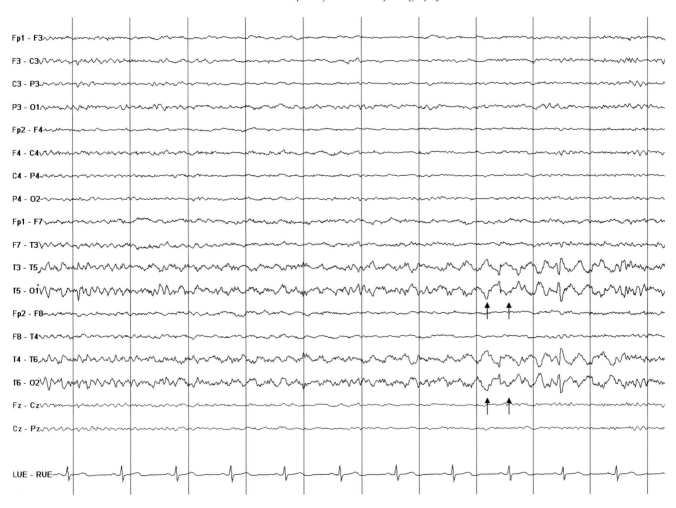

FIGURE 1–37

Electrode artifact at T5 and T6. These rhythmic, evolving discharges have some of the characteristics of an electrographic seizure pattern (arrows). *They were created when the subject rubbed his temples.*

obtained or when attention is focused on abnormalities better elicited in sleep. In our opinion, however, sedation should not be routinely performed on neonates, infants, or children because of the risks associated with medications and limitations on the ability to assess background abnormalities in wakefulness. In neonates, alternatives to sedation include bundling, postfeeding recordings, and other means of pacification. (For specific suggestions on how to perform neonatal EEG, see Chapter 2.) In older infants and children, sleep deprivation may facilitate sleep recordings and may have an independent activating effect on epileptiform abnormalities. When indicated, sedation may be effected with the use of chloral hydrate administered orally or per rectum. In our laboratory, suggested oral doses range from 50 mg/kg for routine sedation to 100 mg/kg for

patients who are very difficult to sedate. Potential adverse effects include irritability, paradoxical hyperactivity, prolonged sedation, or gastric upset. Other agents such as pentobarbital (5 or 6 mg/kg per rectum 30 to 45 minutes prior to the EEG) may be administered to children who fail or are intolerant to chloral hydrate. Associated potential risks include effects on the respiratory, cardiovascular, and central nervous systems. Patients should be restricted to clear liquids up to 3 hours prior to the administration of any sedative agent.

Acknowledgments

We also acknowledge Dr. Aristea Galanopoulou for providing the EEG montage figures.

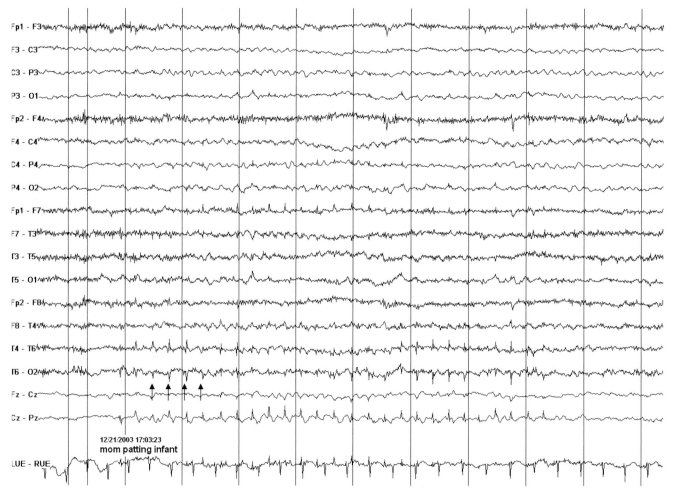

FIGURE 1–38

Electrode artifact at multiple electrodes. This EEG of a 4-month-old child was recorded with the child sitting in the mother's lap. The sharply contoured discharges were created when the mother patted the child's back (arrows). *Note the coincident electrocardiogram artifact.*

Appendix I Definitions

Action potential A depolarization of sufficient magnitude to cause a spreading wave of depolarization along the neuronal membrane

Ampere (amp) (A) Unit of current. By convention, when 1 coulomb of charge has traveled through a conductor over a period of 1 second, a current of 1 A has been observed.

Amplifier A device that increases, or "amplifies," the input signal produced by a voltage source

Atom A fundamental unit of matter composed of three basic particles: neutrons, electrons, and protons

Calibration The display of uniform square wave pulses on the EEG that allows each channel of recording to be compared for uniformity

Capacitance The amount of current a capacitor can store

Capacitor A device that stores electrical charge by maintaining a separation between positive and negative electrical charges. It is composed of two metal plates separated by a relatively nonconducting (i. e., insulating) substance.

Circuit An electrical pathway composed of a conductor through which current flows, a power source that leads to the flow of charges, and a resistor

Circuit breaker A conducting material placed along important circuits, designed to open and thereby disconnect the circuit immediately when current exceeds safe levels

Conductor   The substance through which ions flow

Coulombs (Q)   Units of charge. A coulomb of charge represents the charge lent by a current of 1 A flowing for 1 second.

Current   The flow of charges

Depolarization   A reduction in the negativity of the resting potential

Dipole   A uniform separation of negative and positive extracellular charges along neuronal membranes

Electrons   One of three basic particles comprising the atom. Electrons have a negative charge.

Filter   A device used to attenuate specified frequencies on the EEG. The high-frequency filter (HFF) attenuates high frequencies and the low-frequency filter (LFF) attenuates low-frequency activities.

Gain   The ratio of output to input at the amplifier

Glossokinetic potential   An artifact on the EEG created by movements of the tongue

Ground connection   The wire that diverts stray current from the chassis of the EEG apparatus to ground

Hyperpolarization   An increase in the negativity of the resting potential

Impedance   The resistance in a circuit that is powered by an alternating current source and includes a device known as a capacitor

Montage   A configuration of sequential electrode voltage comparisons designed to attempt to study activity from all major portions of the cortex. Montages are bipolar or referential.

Neutrons   One of three basic particles comprising the atom. Neutrons are neutral in charge.

"Notch" filter   A filter that attenuates a narrow band of frequencies with a maximum at 60 Hz

Ohm (Ω)   Quantified unit of resistance or impedance

Ohm's law   Voltage = Current × Resistance ($V = iR$)

Paroxysmal depolarization shift (PDS)   A relatively slow major depolarization across neuronal membranes believed to be associated with spikes or sharp waves seen in the EEG

Phase reversal   EEG activity with opposite directions of deflection

"Pop" electrode   A change in electrostatic potential seen on the EEG that is due to movement and loss of common mode rejection

Postsynaptic potentials   Small changes in potential along the neuronal membrane resulting from neurotransmitter release. Inhibitory postsynaptic potentials (IPSPs) are associated with hyperpolarization and excitatory postsynaptic potentials (EPSPs) are associated with depolarization.

Protons   One of the basic particles comprising the atom. Protons have positive charge.

Resistance   The part of the circuit that "resists" the flow of charges by converting the electrical flow of energy into heat

Resting potential   The voltage difference between the inside and outside of the cell

Sensitivity   The amount of millimeters of pen deflection assigned to each microvolt of output signal amplitude

Transformer   A device designed to transform either increased or decreased voltages and currents

Voltage   The disparity in electrical potential between two sites that leads to a flow of current

Appendix II Quantitative Analysis of Analog Filters

THE HIGH-FREQUENCY FILTER

The high-frequency filter (HFF) attenuates waveforms of high frequencies. In Figure 1-9, moving the switch rapidly between positions 2 and 3 simulates a high-frequency input. With this configuration there is a gradual increase of the recorded voltage. If there is sufficient time for the capacitor to achieve its full charge, the graph displaying voltages at the capacitor shows the waves reaching maximal voltage. Input voltages that are delivered slowly, as in a slow-frequency rhythm of rising and falling voltages, would allow complete charging and discharging of the capacitor. This circuit allows low-frequency rhythms to pass unaltered in amplitude and therefore is a "low-pass" situation. Hence the HFF is also known as a low-pass filter. Conversely, an input frequency could be delivered that is too fast for the capacitor to fully charge and discharge. By the time an input voltage has gone up and begins its descent, the voltage at the capacitor is still on its way up.

When the input voltage begins to drop, the capacitor does not continue to charge but also begins to drop in voltage. This produces a wave at the capacitor that has a smaller amplitude than that of the input. At the point in time that the input voltage has dropped to its maximal depression, the capacitor voltage is still on its way down and does not have the time to drop to the same extent as the input. Since the input voltage now goes up again, the voltage at the capacitor does not have time to drop further and it begins to rise also. The faster the input frequency, the more the attenuation of the waves at the capacitor, since a faster frequency leaves increasingly less time for the charging or discharging of the capacitor.

The time required for charging or discharging a capacitor is a function not only of the capacitance but also of the impedance in the circuit. The greater the circuit impedance, the greater the amount of time required for charging or discharging the capacitor. Based on these properties, the HFF filter can attenuate high frequencies by altering capacitance or impedance characteristics. A lower HFF setting implies that more frequencies at the faster spectrum will be attenuated. The lower the setting of the HFF, the longer it takes to charge or discharge a capacitor and therefore the greater the attenuation of fast frequencies.

THE LOW-FREQUENCY FILTER

The low-frequency filter (LFF) represents the voltage output across the resistors. Since the resistor and capacitor are connected in series, the input voltage must equal the voltage across the capacitor plus the voltage across the resistor.

Expressed mathematically, this is written as

$$Vb = Vc + Vr$$

where Vb is the battery voltage, Vc is the voltage across the capacitor, and Vr is the voltage across the resistor.

Because the LFF corresponds to the voltage across the resistor,

$$Vr = Vb - Vc$$

Consider the following hypothetical scenario of one square pulse of input as is seen in the typical calibration of the EEG machine (see Fig. 1-10B). At point 0 in time, the input voltage suddenly shoots up to 10. At point 0, therefore, Vb = 10, Vc = 0 (because it has not charged up yet), and since Vr = Vb – Vc, Vr = 10.

In the EEG calibration mode, the signal is recorded as a sudden upward motion. At theoretical point 1 second in time, the battery voltage remains at 10 V; that is, Vb = 10 V. By this point, the capacitor has been theoretically charged up to 7 V. Again, because R = Vb – Vc, Vr = 3 V. Therefore, on the EEG machine, the signal is seen as a downslope. At theoretical point 2 seconds, Vb remains at 10, Vc has fully charged to 10 V, and therefore Vr must equal 0. This value of 0 at the resistor represented by a flat line at the baseline persists until the voltage input is released (not delivered anymore). At theoretical point 3 seconds, the battery is suddenly disconnected; that is, the square pulse signal is no longer sustained. At this point, Vb now equals 0 V. Vc is still 10 V (it has not begun to discharge yet), and since Vr = Vb – Vc, Vr now equals –10 V. This is represented on the EEG as an inverted signal down to 10 V. Notice that even though the EEG displays a negative signal, this corresponds to a voltage of

0 in the battery, not a negative voltage. At theoretical point 4 seconds, Vb remains at 0 V and the capacitor has discharged theoretically down to a voltage of 3. Since Vr = Vc – Vb, Vr equals –3 V. Therefore, on the EEG, the signal is below the 0 V baseline but is a little higher and closer to the 0 V baseline. At theoretical point 5 seconds, Vb remains at 0 V, the capacitor has fully discharged, and therefore Vc = 0. Since Vr = Vb – Vc, Vr equals 0 now. If very fast frequencies for input were applied, the signal seen at the resistor would correspond to the frequency of input and would be relatively unaltered. Only the slow frequencies in this model are altered.

The LFF and HFF are both components of the circuits comprising the EEG apparatus. Voltages across the capacitor (HFF) reflect low-frequency components of a signal and attenuate high frequencies. The voltages across the resistor (LFF) reflect high-frequency components and attenuate lower frequencies. For EEG purposes the LFF affects frequencies less than 10 Hz, whereas the HFF affects frequencies higher than 10 Hz.

Appendix III The Theory of Digital EEG Filters

We only briefly introduce the theory of digital filters. Interested readers are referred to References 23, 30, and 31. Digital filters can be conceptualized in either the frequency domain or in the time domain.[31] The time domain representation of the EEG is the familiar one, where the amplitude of the signal voltage is graphed as a function of time. In the frequency domain, a section of the EEG is approximated by a sum of a series of sine waves of increasing frequencies, where the amplitudes of the contributing sine waves are graphed as a function of their frequency. In Figure 1-39, for example, a sine wave composed of a high-amplitude 3-Hz sine wave and a lower amplitude 17-Hz sine wave are shown in the time and frequency domains. In practice, the frequency components of the EEG are usually found with the Fourier transform. To filter the EEG in the frequency domain, one computes the Fourier transform of the digitized signal, sets the amplitudes of the frequencies to be filtered out to 0, and then computes the inverse Fourier transform of the remaining sine waves. In the example described earlier, a perfect HFF with a cutoff frequency less than 17 Hz would set the amplitude of the 17-Hz component of the composite wave to 0 (see Fig. 1-39).

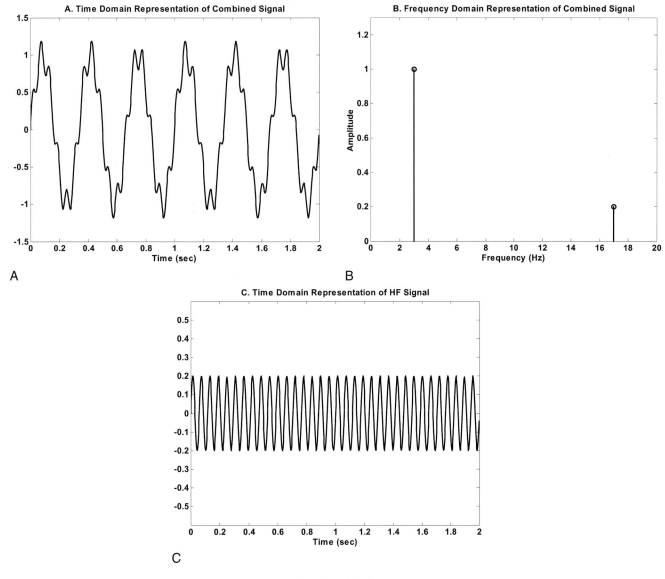

FIGURE 1–39

Time and frequency domain representations of signals. A, A time domain representation of a signal composed of 3-Hz and 17-Hz sine waves. B, A representation of this signal transformed into the frequency domain. It is evident that the 17-Hz component of the signal is of much lower amplitude. Conceptually, a high-pass frequency domain filter with a cutoff frequency greater than 3 Hz would operate on the frequency domain representation of this signal by setting the amplitude of the 3-Hz component to 0 and then transforming the signal back into the time domain. This would result in a 17-Hz sine wave represented in the time domain (C). HF, high frequency.

Digital filtering in the time domain can be conceptualized in terms of a moving average, where each digitized value is replaced by a weighted sum of several adjacent values. A highly efficient HFF—one that attenuated frequencies just above its cutoff frequency to a great extent and had little effect on frequencies just below its cutoff frequency—would require a large number of values to contribute to this sum. The "order" of such a filter would be large. In practice, filter orders from as low as 3 to more than 100 are used. The general form for a kth order finite impulse response (FIR) filter is given by

$$y(t) = \sum_{i=0}^{t=k-1} x(t-i)a(i)$$

where y(t) is the value of the filtered signal at time t, x(t) is the value of the unfiltered signal at time t, and a(i) is the ith coefficient of the filter. For example, consider the signal composed of the 3-Hz and 17-Hz sine waves discussed earlier. The first four values of this signal are 0, 0.1195, 0.2324, and 0.3328. A third order FIR filter could have filter coefficients 1/3, 1/3, 1/3. In this case, each output of the filter is simply the mean of three successive inputs. The third and fourth outputs of the FIR filter with these filter coefficients are

$$y(3) = 0(1/3) + 0.1195(1/3) + 0.2324(1/3)$$

and

$$y(4) = 0.1195(1/3) + 0.2324(1/3) + 0.3328(1/3)$$

The first two outputs are undefined because there are not yet enough inputs to form the sum specified by the first equation. The effect of passing a composite 3-Hz and 17-Hz signal through a 20th order filter of this type is shown in Figure 1-40. This filter is an HFF. The contribution of the 17-Hz sine wave to the original signal has been effectively removed. In addition, the filter introduces a phase shift; the peaks of the filtered data are delayed with respect to the input data. FIR filters can be designed so as not to introduce phase shift.

The equation for an infinite impulse response (IIR) of order k is

$$y(t) = \sum_{j=1}^{j=k} y(t-j)b(j) + \sum_{i=0}^{t=k-1} x(t-i)a(i)$$

where y(t) and x(t) are defined as in the first equation. Here a(i) represents filter coefficients that operate on input samples and b(j) represents filter coefficients that operate on output samples. Unlike FIR filters, which depend only on past input samples, IIR filters depend on both previous input samples and previous output samples. IIR filters are computationally more efficient than FIR filters. They require a lower filter order owing to the fact that they feed their outputs back into subsequent steps of the calculation. As compared with FIR filters, the design and analysis of IIR filters are more complex. Unlike FIR filters, IIR filters necessarily introduce phase distortion into the filtered time series. This can be dealt with if the filtering is done post hoc: The data can be filtered in both the forward and reverse directions to cancel the phase distortion.

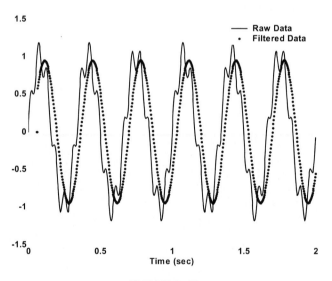

FIGURE 1–40
Filtering a signal composed of 17-Hz and 3-Hz sine waves with a 20th order finite impulse response (FIR) filter with filter coefficients all equal to 1/20. This is a high-frequency filter. The contribution of the 17-Hz sine wave to the original signal has been effectively removed. In addition, this filter introduces a phase shift: the peaks of the filtered data are delayed with respect to those of the input data. FIR filters can be designed so as not to introduce phase shift.

REFERENCES

1. Misulis K: Electronics for clinical neurophysiology. J Clin Neurophysiol 1989;6:41-74.
2. Kooih K, Tucker R, Marshall R: Instrumentation and Signal Analysis: Fundamentals of Electroencephalography, 2nd ed. New York, Harper & Row, 1978, pp 9-11.
3. Sederberg PB, Kahana MJ, Howard MW, et al: Theta and gamma oscillations during encoding predict subsequent recall. J Neurosci 2003;23:10809-10814.
4. Uchida S, Maehara T, Hirai N, et al: Cortical oscillations in human medial temporal lobe during wakefulness and all-night sleep. Brain Res 2001;89:7-19.
5. Park SA, Lim SR, Kim GS, et al: Ictal electrocorticographic findings related with surgical outcomes in nonlesional neocortical epilepsy. Epilepsy Res 2002;48:199-206.
6. Berger H: Über das Elektrenkephalogramm des Menschen. Arch Psych Nervenkrankheiten 1929;87:527-570.
7. Buzsaki G, Traub RD: Physiologic basis of EEG activity. *In* Engel JJ, Pedley TA (eds): Epilepsy: A Comprehensive Textbook. Philadelphia, Lippincott-Raven, 1997, pp 819-830.
8. Steriades M: Cellular substrates of brain rhythms. *In* Niedermeyer E, Da Silva FL (eds): Electroencephalography: Basic Principles, Clinical Applications, and Related Fields, 4th ed. Philadelphia, Williams & Wilkins, 1999, pp 28-75.
9. Speckmann E-J, Elger CE, Altrup U: Neurophysiologic basis of the electroencephalogram. *In* Wyllie E (ed): The Treatment of Epilepsy: Principles and Practice, 3rd ed. New York, Lippincott Williams & Wilkins, 2001, pp 149-163.
10. Buzsaki G, Traub RD, Pedley TA: The cellular basis of EEG activity. *In* Ebersole JS, Pedley TA (eds):

Current Practice of Electroencephalography, 3rd ed. Philadelphia, Lippincott Williams & Wilkins, 2002, pp 1-11.

11. Schaul N, Green L, Peyster R, Gotman J: Structural determinants of electroencephalographic findings in acute hemispheric lesions. Ann Neurol 1986;20:703-711.

12. Andersen P, Andersson SA: Physiologic Basis of the Alpha Rhythm. New York, Appleton-Century-Crofts, 1968.

13. Lopes de Silva FH, Sotrm van Leewan W: The cortical source of the alpha rhythm. Neurosci Lett 1977;6:237-241.

14. Matsumoto H, Ajmone-Marsan C: Cortical cellular phenomena in experimental epilepsy: Interictal manifestations. Exp Neurol 1964;9:286-304.

15. Engel J Jr: Seizures and Epilepsy. Philadelphia, FA Davis, 1989.

16. Tyner F, Knott J, Mayer W: Fundamentals of EEG Technology: Basic Concepts and Methods. New York, Raven Press, 1983.

17. Cooper R, Osselton J, Shaw J: EEG Technology. Boston, Butterworth, 1980.

18. Society AE: Guidelines for standard electrode position nomenclature. J Clin Neurophysiol 1991;8:200-202.

19. Quesney L, Katsarkas A, Gloor P, Andermann F: Contribution of naso-ethmoidal electrode recording in the electrographic exploration of frontal and temporal lobe epilepsy. *In* Dam M, Gram L, Penry J (eds): Advances in Epileptology: XIIth Epilepsy International Symposium. New York, Raven Press, 1981, pp 293-304.

20. Wyllie E, Wyllie R, Kotagal P, et al: Comfortable insertion of sphenoidal electrodes in children. Epilepsia 1990;31:521-523.

21. Septien L, Gras P, Girourd M, Dumas R: Sphenoidal electrode insertion under local analgesia in children. Child Nerv Syst 1992;8:129-132.

22. Welsh FA, Sims RE, Harris VA: Mild hypothermia prevents ischemic injury in gerbil hippocampus. J Cereb Blood Flow Metab 1990;10:557-563.

23. Litt B, Caranstoun SD: Engineering principles. *In* Ebersole JS, Pedley TA (eds): Current Practice of Clinical Electroencephalography. Philadelphia, Lippincott Williams & Wilkins, 2003, pp 32-71.

24. Claassen J, Mayer SA: Continuous electroencephalographic monitoring in neurocritical care. Curr Neurol Neurosci Rep 2002;2:534-540.

25. Niedermeyer E, Lopes da Silva F: Electro-Encephalography Basic Principles, Clinical Applications, and Related Fields. Baltimore, Urban & Schwarzenberg, 1983.

26. Maulsby R: Polarity convention, principles of localization, and electrical fields. *In* Klass D, Daly D (eds): Current Practice of Clinical Electroencephalography. New York, Raven Press, 1979, pp 27-36.

27. Kiloh L, McComas A, Osselton J: Clinical Electroencephalography. London, Butterworth, 1972.

28. Saunders M: Artifacts: Activity of noncerebral origin in the EEG. *In* Klass D, Daly D (eds): Current Practice of Clinical Electroencephalography. New York, Raven Press, 1979, pp 37-67.

29. Hill D, Dolan A: Intensive Care Instrumentation. New York, Academic Press, 1976.

30. Lyons R: Understanding Digital Signal Processing. Englewood Cliffs, NJ, Prentice Hall, 2001.

31. Gotman J: The use of computers in analysis and display of EEG and evoked potentials. *In* Daly D, Pedley T (eds): Current Practice of Clinical Electroencephalography, 2nd ed. New York, Raven Press, 1990, pp 51-83.

32. Blume WT, Kaibara M, Young GB: Atlas of Adult Electroencephalography. Philadelphia, Lippincott Williams & Wilkins, 2002.

33. Blume WT, Kaibara M: Atlas of Pediatric Electroencephalography. Philadelphia, Lippincott-Raven, 1999.

34. Chatrian GE, Turella GS: Electrophysiological evaluation of coma, other states of diminished responsiveness, and brain death. *In* Ebersole JS, Pedley TA (eds): Current Practice of Clinical Electroencephalography. Philadelphia, Lippincott Williams & Wilkins, 2003, pp 405-462.

35. Fisch BJ: Fisch and Spehlman's EEG Primer. Amsterdam, Elsevier, 1999.

36. Ikeda A, Klem GH, Luders HO: Organic brain syndromes and dementias. *In* Ebersole JS, Pedley TA (eds): Current Practice of Clinical Electroencephalography. Philadelphia, Lippincott Williams & Wilkins, 2003, pp 348-377.

37. Kellaway P: Orderly approach to the visual analysis: Characteristics of the normal EEG of adults and children. *In* Ebersole JS, Pedley TA (eds): Current Practice of Clinical Electroencephalography. Philadelphia, Lippincott Williams & Wilkins, 2003, pp 100-159.

38. Zifkin BG, Cracco RQ: An orderly approach to the abnormal electroencephalogram. *In* Ebersole JS, Pedley TA (eds): Current Practice of Clinical Electroencephalography. Philadelphia, Lippincott Williams & Wilkins, 2003, pp 288-302.

39. Westmoreland BF: An orderly approach to the abnormal electroencephalogram. *In* Ebersole JS, Pedley TA (eds): Current Practice of Clinical Electroencephalography. Philadelphia, Lippincott Williams & Wilkins, 2003, pp 235-245.

2

Electroencephalography of the Newborn: Normal Features

MARK S. SCHER

Advances in neonatal intensive care have led to improved survival for high-risk infants. Concomitant with these improvements has been an increasing awareness of two groups of at-risk neonates. One group, manifesting a "new morbidity," comprises acutely ill neonates who have survived neonatal disease because of sophisticated neonatal intensive care unit (NICU) management. These children remain subsequently at risk for sequelae.1 Despite marked improvements in neonatal care, long-term follow-up studies of these infants have indicated that a substantial number will manifest variable degrees of long-term neurodevelopmental sequelae.2-5

Although many infants at risk for neurologic sequelae can be identified as high risk by epidemiologic or clinical factors, the second group of at risk neonates lacks such markers and appear neurologically intact based on their limited clinical repertoire during the neonatal period. There is, therefore, a need for more sensitive diagnostic evaluation of the central nervous system (CNS) to supplement clinical observations.

STRUCTURAL AND FUNCTIONAL ASSESSMENT OF THE NEONATAL BRAIN

Brain imaging techniques developed over the last several decades have revolutionized the diagnosis of major structural disorders of the neonatal brain. Cranial ultrasonography, cranial computed tomography, magnetic resonance imaging, and positron emission tomography extend the clinician's ability to detect specific areas of the brain with either acquired or congenital structural disorders.

Newborn brain abnormalities, however, may also be expressed in functional terms, with or without demonstrable structural correlates. Neurophysiologic studies provide continuous documentation of CNS function. The diagnostic evaluation of the neonatal patient, therefore, would benefit from neurophysiologic studies that complement structural studies. Recent advances in the neurophysiologic assessment of newborn brain function offer unique opportunities for the coordinated evaluation of the dysfunctional nervous system. This chapter and a subsequent one (see Chapter 13) elucidate how electroencephalography can assess both healthy neonates and those with suspected CNS dysfunction.

Implementation of innovative methods to assess brain structure and function should always complement and extend clinical observations. Reliable and rapid identification of infants at risk by these methods may allow the neonatologist the opportunity to offer cerebral resuscitation at a time when such injury is potentially reversible, as well as provide a therapeutic avenue for early intervention to improve outcome.

GENERAL CONSIDERATIONS

Together with the establishment of present-day tertiary-level NICU care, technical improvements in the recording apparatus as well as standardization of recording procedures assist the neurologic consultant in making sophisticated neurophysiologic assessments. Proper instrumentation and technique yield reliable neonatal EEG studies that can be used to evaluate CNS functioning.

Several basic tenets assist in understanding the principal applications of neonatal electroencephalographic (EEG) interpretation (Box 2-1). The electroencephalographer needs to be aware of the gestational age of the infant which is the duration of the pregnancy, whereas conceptional age (CA) is the age of the child from the time of conception and is the gestational age plus the chronological age of the child. There are expected changes in scalp-generated EEG patterns of neonates at different gestational ages. A trained interpreter of a neonatal EEG can approximate the electrical maturity of the neonatal brain within 2 weeks of the gestational age for preterm (PT) infants and within 1 week for fullterm (FT) infants.[6,7] Evolving electrical patterns reflect the CA age of the infant independent of his or her birthweight. Concordance between electrographic

Of paramount importance in the assessment of the neonatal EEG is knowledge of the age and state of the neonatal patient.[7-9] Close communication between the electroneurodiagnostic technologist performing the study and the electroencephalographer is also required since technical aspects of recording may affect the interpretation of the study.

INSTRUMENTATION AND RECORDING TECHNIQUES

At least 10 electrodes are required as the minimum number for adequate EEG recordings.[10] A greater area of cerebral activity can certainly be monitored using more channels of EEG. However, this must be weighed against the more limited ability to visualize electrographic activity, given the smaller potential differences between adjacent electrodes due to the smaller head size of the neonate. The 10-20 International System of Electrode Placement is the standard method of application of scalp electrodes, but specific electrodes (i.e., parietal, anterior, or posterior temporal) may need to be eliminated to increase interelectrode distance. Specific locations such as the occipital, temporal, midline, and frontal regions should always be included for monitoring because of the abundant activity occurring in these brain regions. Other technical aspects are stressed in Box 2-2.

BOX 2-1
GUIDELINES FOR INTERPRETATION OF THE NORMAL NEONATAL EEG

1. EEG features reflect gestational or conceptional age rather than birthweight.
2. Estimates of electrical maturity should be within 2 weeks for a preterm neonate's stated estimated gestational age (EGA) and 1 week for a fullterm neonate's EGA.
3. Knowledge of neonatal behavioral state during the recording is essential.
4. Serial EEG studies more accurately document ontogeny of rhythms than do single studies.
5. Attention to both temporal and spatial characteristics of the EEG record should be explicitly stated in the electrographic interpretation (e.g., occipital theta, delta brushes, synchrony, sleep cycles).
6. Concordance between electrographic and polygraphic components of EEG sleep begins as early as 30 weeks EGA and is complete after 36 weeks EGA.
7. Antepartum, intrapartum, and neonatal medical facts must be applied to formulate a clinical correlation that accurately interprets either electrographic evidence of acute or chronic encephalopathic abnormalities.

BOX 2-2
TECHNICAL ASPECTS OF NEONATAL EEG RECORDINGS

A. Recording environment
1. Maintain a positive working relationship with the medical staff. Coordinate EEG studies with other testing procedures. Position monitoring equipment in a way that least affects working conditions.
2. Recognize potential sources of artifact.
3. Recordings in an open bed warmer vs. an incubator require different concerns with respect to artifacts.
4. The technologist should recognize situations when additional help is needed to place equipment or reposition the patient.
5. Anticipate a 1.5- to 2-hour time commitment.
B. Recording equipment
1. Devices should be properly shielded to minimize artifact from other monitoring equipment.
2. The technologist should be proficient in operating evoked potential and synchronized EEG monitoring equipment.

---

and polygraphic signals marks the maturation of the CNS as reflected in EEG sleep development. Serial studies more accurately document normal ontogeny or the evolution of encephalopathic changes than do single recordings.

Continued

BOX 2-2
TECHNICAL ASPECTS OF NEONATAL
EEG RECORDINGS—cont'd

3. Care and attention should be directed to patient and electrical safety guidelines.
   a. Communication with clinical engineering of the hospital to maintain Joint Commission on Accreditation of Healthcare Organizations guidelines for hospital equipment safety.
   b. Maintain infection control standards (e.g., pay close attention to hand washing and electrode cleaning).
C. Instrumentation—electrode application
   1. Use of collodion or paste: Either technique is acceptable, but collodion is less desirable within the incubator owing to inadequate ventilation.
   2. Use of neonatal electrode sizes is strongly suggested.
   3. Use hypoallergenic skin tape to minimize skin irritation.
   4. Use a minimum of 10 scalp electrodes.
   5. Fp1 and Fp2 are often displaced to Fp3 and Fp4 owing to smaller frontal brain regions.
   6. Select one or two montages for best assessment of sleep state changes.
   7. Use 15 mm/sec paper to depict state changes, synchrony, and periodic discharges.
   8. Use long time constant to assess slow activity.
   9. Pay attention to cardiorespiratory, electromyographic, and electro-oculographic monitoring during the recordings.
D. Technologist notations
   1. The occipitofrontal circumference should be accurate. Be alert to skull deformities that might affect this measurement (e.g., molding of the cranium and scalp edema).
   2. Review the chart for documentation of gestational maturity. Be alert for discrepancies between estimations of gestational age based on obstetric vs. clinical information. Note the infant who is either large or small for gestational age.
   3. Assist the electroencephalographer by identifying which medical personnel (nurse *or* physician) has the most information with respect to questionable seizure activity or clinical status.
   4. Document areas of scalp edema, cephalhematomas, extraventricular drains, and so forth.
   5. Record blood studies obtained during or around the recording session, including blood gases, antiepileptic drug levels, and other metabolic values.

6. Record ventilatory status, including ventilator rate changes.
7. Frequent notations during recording are of paramount importance, especially head position, respiratory excursions, suspicious clinical activity, and personnel around the recording equipment.
8. Note the start and finish times of recordings, medication administrations, and clinical changes (e.g., bradycardia, apnea).
9. Actively attempt to identify and correct sources of artifact.

Silver chloride electrodes are most commonly used, and their application to the scalp can be achieved with either paste or collodion. Needle electrodes are no longer recommended. The electrode arrays or montages can be either bipolar or referential, although the former montage choice is preferable given the importance of regional localization. A variety of montages may be used depending on the specific needs for the study, but a single bipolar or combined bipolar-tangential montage allows the technologist and the electroencephalographer to more readily observe changes in EEG sleep state without interruption.

Instrumental control settings can be similar to those obtained for the older child and adult. However, adjustments in sensitivity, paper speed, and filter settings may help facilitate the electrographic interpretation. With digital technology this is not quite as easy. Sensitivity settings should begin with the standard 7 μV/mm but may need to be periodically adjusted throughout the record. Both high- and low-frequency filters should be correctly chosen to allow accurate representation of an appropriate range of frequencies of cerebral origin. Overzealous use of filter settings may eliminate brain-generated activities while attempts are made to minimize undesirable noncerebral artifactual signals. For the newborn patient, lower frequency filter settings, commonly referred to as *time constants*, should preferably remain at 0.25 to 0.5 Hz rather than 0.1 Hz to avoid the elimination of commonly occurring slow-frequency waveforms. Fifteen rather than the conventional 30 mm/sec paper speed may be advantageous. Slower paper speeds permit easier visualization of slowly recurring or periodic cerebral activity. With digital EEG recordings the control settings used to record the EEG are less important since the electroencephalographer can change paper speed, montages, filters, and sensitivity at the time of the interpretation. However, improper settings at the time of the recording may cause the technologist to miss critical findings.

Important information can be derived from recording motility, cardiorespiratory, and eye movement data. Such monitors assist in the identification of specific segments of the EEG sleep cycle. Noncerebral physiologic observations may have relevance to the clinical problem that prompted the request for the EEG study. Important sources of artifact can be identified more readily or eliminated by using noncerebral monitors. As with adults, physiologic and nonphysiologic artifacts must be properly identified in neonatal recordings because they may interfere with the interpretation of cerebral activity. Three basic forms of artifacts—instrumental, external, and physiologic—all may occur in the neonate. Accurate descriptions by the technologist assist the neurologist in the diagnosis of a neurologic disorder in the neonate. The technologist should not only try to identify the source of the artifact but eliminate such artifacts during the recording. Figures 2-1 through 2-4 illustrate some of the artifacts encountered during neonatal EEG recordings.

Both skill and speed are required to obtain a quality recording within a busy NICU. Ample time should be allowed for proper electrode application because of the special challenges of recordings of sick PT neonates confined to an incubator. Information from the medical record should include the child's gestational age and conceptional age as well as the state of arousal of the neonate. The physician who ordered the study should be identified so that a clearly written request for the EEG study will state the clinical concerns. Many patients may have been administered medications, and each of these drugs should be listed by the technologist. Skull defects, vital signs, pertinent laboratory studies, and medications all should be described since they may affect the electrographic and clinical impressions of the recording.

Frequent and accurate annotations by the technologist throughout the study must corroborate changes in state of the neonatal patient. Eye opening and closing as well as repositioning of the patient's head are some examples of annotations that are essential for proper interpretation. Consensual validation of suspicious cerebral activity between the electroencephalographer and technologist is always a high priority at the time of the review of the record.

ASSESSMENT OF CENTRAL NERVOUS SYSTEM MATURATION

Specific features of the EEG in the asymptomatic neonate relate to the gestational age of the neonate. It is generally accepted that a combination of intrahemispheric as well as interhemispheric electrical features correlates with CNS maturation within 2 weeks of the clinically derived gestational age.

Current methods for assessing CNS maturation include the gestational age calculation from the mother's last menstrual period, fetal ultrasonographic changes in head and body size, and a variety of obstetric signs that correlate with overall fetal maturation. Clinical examination of the neonate at birth also offers an estimation of CNS maturation. A variety of clinical scoring techniques emphasize neurologic parameters of tone and postural reflexes.[11-13] However, these standard methods are inaccurate for the early premature infant as well as misleading in specific clinical situations. In these circumstances, electrographic estimation of CNS maturation can be especially useful to verify clinical estimates of gestational age. Detailed electroanatomic correlations with changes in sulcation and gyral development have been compared with electrical patterns and clinical information pertaining to gestational maturity.[14] Ninety-two percent of PT infants demonstrated an agreement within 2 weeks between electrical maturity and gyral measurements of the inferior frontal, superior temporal, and calcarine gyri as well as the cytoarchitecture of various brain regions. This compared more favorably than the 70% agreement among last menstrual periods, fetal sonography, and clinical examination findings with these gyral measurements. Examples of corresponding EEG patterns and anatomic features are illustrated in Figures 2-5 and 2-6.

ONTOGENY OF EEG FEATURES

The description of evolving EEG sleep patterns in the asymptomatic, presumably healthy neonate has been the subject of many excellent reviews.[6,7,9,15] Improvements in neonatal intensive care, however, require periodic revisions to include more premature neonates.[16-18] This is particularly relevant for early premature infants of less than 32 weeks' gestation for whom tremendous improvements in survival rates have occurred over the last decade. It is always important to verify EEG sleep patterns as normal *after* systematic neurodevelopmental assessment of such children.

Regional and hemispheric EEG patterns for PT and FT neonates are described in the following sections, designated arbitrarily by specific gestational age ranges. Temporal, spatial, and state organization of the EEG recordings that comprise the cerebral activity during each age range are highlighted with appropriate illustrations.

Gestational Age of Less than 28 Weeks

Neonates with a gestational age of less than 25 weeks may fall below the limits of viability and, therefore, may not survive long enough to receive even one EEG recording. However, useful information is now available to characterize the neurophysiologic profile of these very premature neonates. There are no distinctive features noted between waking and sleep portions. The record is largely discontinuous, with short periods of continuous EEG activity that may last for as long as 1 minute. Patterns of motility alternate between segmental myoclonic movements of the face

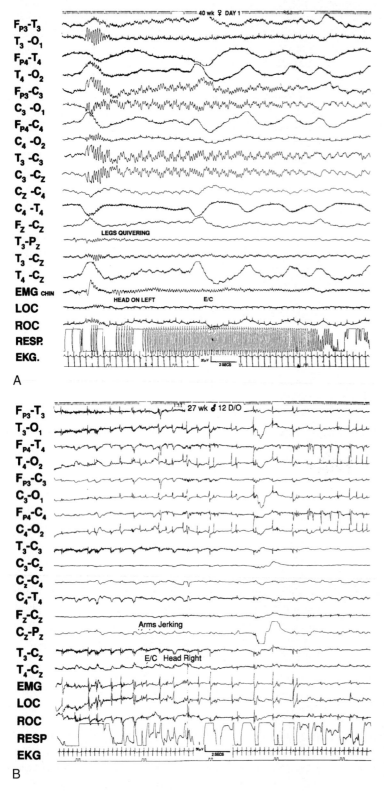

FIGURE 2–1

A, *Physiologic artifact secondary to clonus of the legs in a 40-week, 1-day-old girl after a severe hypoxic-ischemic episode at delivery. Electrodes in contact with the mattress generate a rhythmic signal secondary to movement of the head during tremulous episodes.* B, *Physiologic artifact consisting of myogenic potentials seen on multiple channels of a recording of a 27-week, 12-day-old infant with herpes encephalitis. Although the background is markedly abnormal because of severe suppression of background activity, the muscle-generated artifacts are not of cerebral origin, despite a "spikelike" morphology.*

or body to more generalized myoclonic and tonic posturing either in an axial or appendicular distribution.

A pattern of alternating active and sleep periods in PT infants is characterized as discontinuity or tracé discontinu.[9,19,20] Anderson and associates[16] found that 60% of EEG recordings consisted of discontinuity. These same authors found that the average interburst interval during this age range was between 8 and 16 seconds, with the

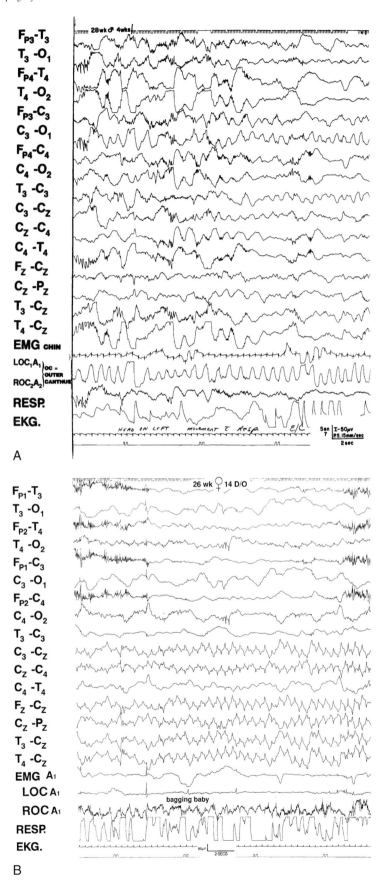

FIGURE 2–2

A, *Ventilatory artifact noted in the left central region on an EEG recording of a 32-week conceptional age boy synchronized to the respiratory excursions.*
B, *Physiologic artifacts created during ventilatory assistance using an ambu bag by a neonatal nurse. Unusual waveforms are noted at the midline and in the parasagittal regions.*

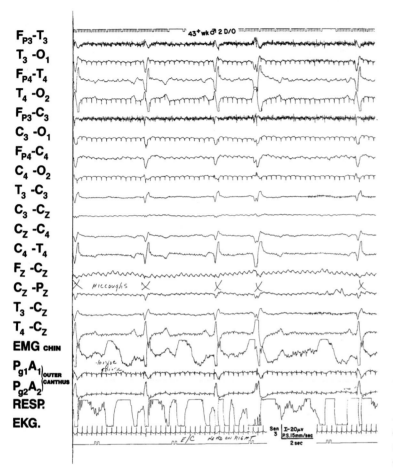

FIGURE 2–3

Hiccoughing artifact in a 43-week, 2-day-old boy creating diffuse, repetitive sharp-wave discharges. (Note that the "X" marks indicate the occurrence of each hiccough.)

longest interburst intervals being between 15 and 88 seconds. Similar ranges for the duration of interburst intervals have been found by other authors, as listed in Table 2-1.[21-25] This is sharp contrast to earlier descriptions of interburst intervals as long as 2 minutes in duration.[7] This difference may be, in part, based on the medical condition of the neonate at the time of the recording and/or the lack of information concerning long-term follow-up.

Activity predominates in the vertex, central, and occipital regions. Bitemporal attenuation is common and may reflect intrahemispheric asynchrony.[14] Underdevelopment of the inferior frontal and superior temporal gyri may also help explain the relative quiescence of activity in this brain region.

EEG activity consists of mixed frequencies, predominated by delta activity in the parasagittal and occipital regions. Occipital delta activity is either isolated to one or two waveforms and is rarely longer than 5 or 6 seconds or of a rhythmic nature. Faster frequencies in the theta, alpha, and beta ranges are also intermixed in multiple head regions. Diffuse theta bursts (see Fig. 2-5) are commonly seen during either continuous or discontinuous periods.

TABLE 2–1

Interburst Intervals (IBIs) in Very Preterm Neonates

Reference	Gestational Age, wk	Mean IBI	Maximum IBI
Anderson et al[16]	27	12	48
	29	9	36
	31	7	20
Connell et al[22]	27	12-14	40-75
	29	11-15	35-65
	31	7-16	20-70
Eyre et al[23]	26	26	—
	28	24	—
	30	12	—
Hughes et al[24]	26	5-6	7-19
	28	5-6	4-32
	30	4.5-5	2-6
Benda et al[21]	25-29	—	≤30
	30-35	—	≤30

Beta-delta complexes are transient patterns that identify premature neonates of varying conceptional ages. Such a pattern is the principal landmark regional electrographic

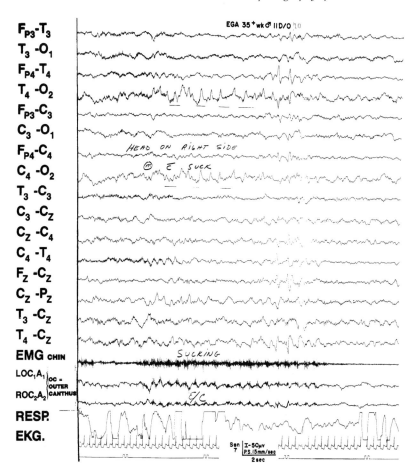

FIGURE 2–4

Buccolingual artifact from sucking in a 35-week, 11-day-old boy resulting in sharp-wave discharges in the right occipital area.

feature of the PT infant. Random or briefly rhythmic 0.3- to 1.5-Hz delta activity of 50 to 250 μV have superimposed bursts of low-to moderate-amplitude faster frequencies with a frequency range of 10 to 20 Hz. The amplitude of such activity on bipolar recordings rarely exceeds 60 to 75 μV. Historically, various terms such as *spindle delta bursts*, *brushes*, *spindle-like fast waves*, and *ripples of prematurity* have been applied to these complexes, which can be readily seen as early as 24 to 26 weeks, largely in the central and midline regions as well as the occipital regions (Fig. 2-7A and *B*).

Runs of monorhythmic alpha and/or theta activity are seen independent of delta brushes principally in the occipital regions in the neonate of less than 28 weeks' gestation (Fig. 2-7B and *C*). This transient pattern has been described in more detail and can last 6 to 10 seconds in either an asynchronous or asymmetrical manner.[26] Such activity should be distinguished from the more diffuse bursts of moderate-to high-amplitude theta, which commonly are noted at this degree of prematurity (see Fig. 2-5).

Intrahemispheric and interhemispheric synchrony have been variably described by different authors. Lombroso

described synchronous bursts as morphologically similar bursts of activity appearing within 1.5 seconds.[7,9] He described asynchrony periods from 50% at 31 and 32 weeks to 100% at 40 to 43 weeks CA with a midpoint of 70% to 85% at 35 to 36 weeks CA. This is in sharp contrast to the observation of Anderson and associates[16] that interhemispheric synchrony has a mean of 93% for 1-minute epochs at 27 weeks CA with a mean of 94% at 29 to 32 weeks CA.

The methodology for defining synchrony can vary between authors, but one must consider that a high degree of intrahemispheric synchrony does exist even in very PT infants. However, it should be accepted that greater asynchrony may occur as the distance from the midline increases with rapid brain growth beyond 30 weeks CA. Rapid growth of temporal and parietal structures may contribute to more frequent episodes of asynchrony.[6] Measures of asynchrony must include not only information about CA but also state changes. Definitions of asynchrony should involve all background rhythms rather than only bursts during discontinuous epochs.

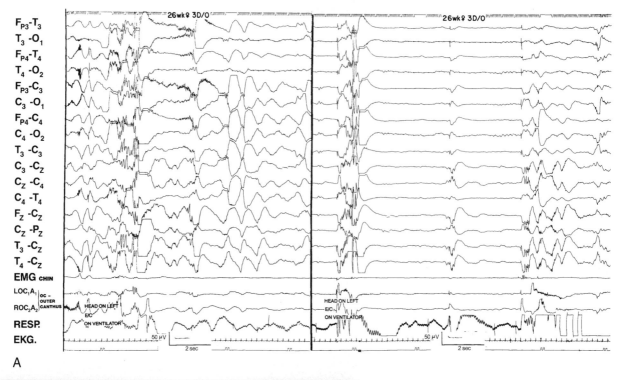

A

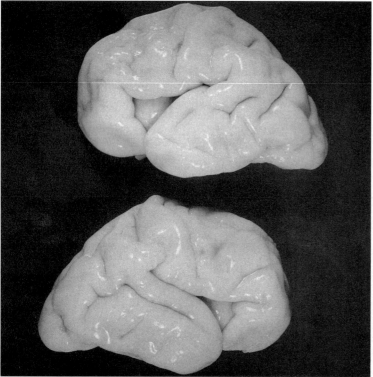

B

FIGURE 2–5

A, Two EEG tracings for a 26-week, 3-day-old girl. The first frame demonstrates generalized theta and delta slowing with prominent vertex central slow activity. Note the bitemporal attenuation. In the second frame, synchronous interburst intervals of less than 30 seconds are noted. Note the prominent delta brush patterns in the vertex region. B, Lateral view of the brain for the same patient in A. Underdeveloped frontal and temporal lobes with a clearly visible insula are shown. There is an immature sulcation pattern, especially involving the rolandic, calcarine, and superior temporal sulci.

Gestational Age of 28 to 31 Weeks

In the period of 28 to 31 weeks gestational age, cyclic organization of states remains undifferentiated. However, periods of body and eye movements are more distinctively associated with irregular respirations during continuous periods of EEG.

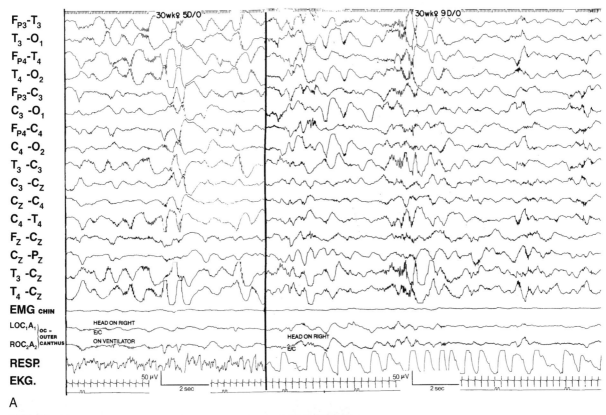

F_{P3}-T_3
T_3 -O_1
F_{P4}-T_4
T_4 -O_2
F_{P3}-C_3
C_3 -O_1
F_{P4}-C_4
C_4 -O_2
T_3 -C_3
C_3 -C_Z
C_Z -C_4
C_4 -T_4
F_Z -C_Z
C_Z -P_Z
T_3 -C_Z
T_4 -C_Z
EMG CHIN
LOC_1A_1 | OC = OUTER CANTHUS
ROC_2A_2 |
RESP.
EKG.

A

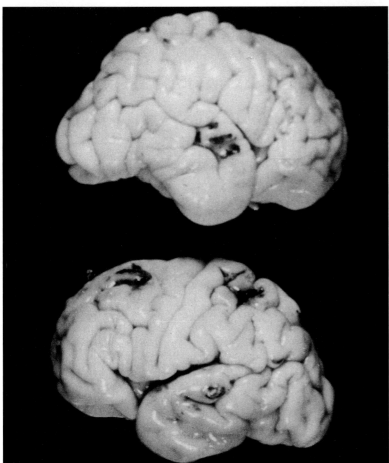

B

FIGURE 2–6

A, Two EEG tracings for a 30-week, 5-day-old girl. In the first frame, continuous EEG activity with prominent temporal delta brush and delta patterns is noted. In the second frame, occipital delta and theta brush patterns are recorded. B, Lateral view of the brain for the patient in A, showing a greater degree of sulcation evident than in Figure 2-5B. Note the more complete elaboration of the rolandic, superior temporal, and calcarine sulci. There is shortening of the anteroposterior brain length and a persistently visible insula, both of which reflect dysmaturity of the brain.

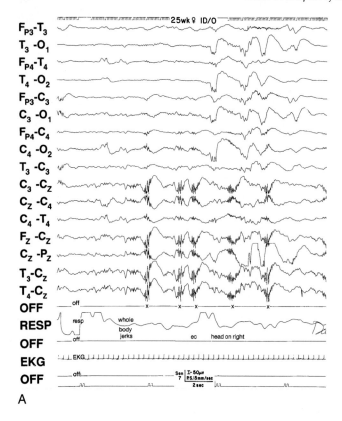

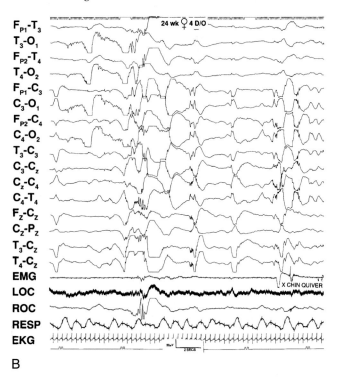

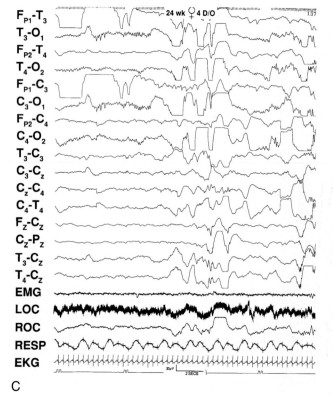

FIGURE 2–7

A, *EEG tracing of a 25-week, 1-day-old girl depicting prominent vertex delta brushes as well as occipital theta and delta brushes. Briefly rhythmic occipital delta are noted as well as myoclonic movements ("X" marks) that appear coincident with the delta brush patterns. B, EEG tracings of a 24-week, 4-day-old girl demonstrating features characteristic of this gestational age (i.e., <28 weeks estimated gestational age). Isolated occipital delta with theta-alpha bursts are noted. Bitemporal attenuation and parasagittal delta brushes are also recorded. C, An EEG tracing of a 24-week, 4-day-old infant with a more prolonged period of occipital theta-alpha brushes that are asymmetrical in amplitude. Shifting asymmetries of such features are common.*

Discontinuous epochs still predominate but decrease in duration as compared to the very premature neonate of less than 28 weeks CA. Interbursts become progressively briefer with a dramatic increase in low- to moderate-amplitude faster rhythms primarily in the theta range (Fig. 2-8A).

By 32 weeks, the degree of discontinuity has decreased to 45% of the record.[16] Dreyfus-Brisac[27] found an alternating pattern in 24% of records at 32 to 34 weeks' gestation. The average interburst intervals at 29 to 31 weeks CA ranged between 5 and 14 and 4 and 11 seconds, respectively, with means of 9 and 7 seconds, whereas the longest interburst periods for these two CA groups were found to be between 16 and 57 and 6 to 41 seconds with means of 36 and 20 seconds, respectively (see Table 2-1).

Monorhythmic occipital delta is now quite abundant at 28 to 31 weeks with durations that are greater than 30 seconds (Fig. 2-8B).

Delta brush patterns continue to be abundant involving not only the vertex and central regions but also the occipital and temporal regions.[28] It may, at times, be difficult to differentiate superimposed delta brushes in the temporal region particularly because of the abundance of temporal theta bursts (see Fig. 2-8 and later discussion).

Another useful developmental marker is the appearance of rhythmic 4.5- to 6-Hz activity occurring independently as well as synchronously in each mid-temporal region (see Fig. 2-8B). Although this activity is noted at less than 28 weeks CA, it is expressed maximally between 28 and 32 weeks CA. Historically, this feature has been described as *temporal sawtooth waves*.[29] Amplitudes range from roughly 20 to 200 μV, and with maturation these bursts may reach the alpha frequency. In a study of 436 infants a parabolic polynomial function has described the age incidence of this temporal theta activity, strongly reflecting the pattern as a maturational landmark.[30] Temporal theta can obtain a maximum incidence of 36% at 29 to 30 weeks, after which it diminishes rapidly. At 32 weeks, only 12% of the record persists in this pattern.[16] This rhythmic theta activity should be distinguished from repetitive sharp activity in the theta range seen at near-FT and FT ages in the midline and rolandic regions, particularly during the quiet sleep segment.

The clinical significance of sharp wave transients in healthy PT infants has been poorly documented at these early PT ages. Regional patterns associated with maturation as discussed earlier must be considered before assigning independent spike- or sharp-wave criteria to a transient waveform. Sharply contoured delta brushes, temporal, or occipital theta bursts may appear epileptiform without clearly satisfying morphologic criteria for a spike or sharp wave (Fig. 2-9A). (Also see Table 13-4 in Chapter 13).

Sporadic and multifocal spikes and sharp waves can be seen at any age in newborns, but few studies include PT infants less than 32 weeks estimated gestational age (EGA) (see Box 2-1)[13,29]

Anderson and associates[16] studied the incidence and location of spikes and sharp waves in 33 PT infants, 27 to 32 weeks EGA (Fig. 2-9B). Both features were infrequent, with spikes less common than sharp waves. Both morphologies were most abundant in frontal and temporal regions, with frontal and temporal sharp waves increasing in incidence from 27 to 32 weeks EGA. Central sharp waves decreased in number over time, whereas occipital and vertex discharges had the lowest incidence. Unfortunately, only 555 of infants were verified as normal on follow-up at 6 to 8 months of age. Larger PT populations with longer periods of neurodevelopment follow-up are needed before assigning clinical significance to sharp waves in asymptomatic PT infants.

Gestational Age of 32 to 34 Weeks

Body and eye movement take on a more phasic rather than tonic pattern with a better differentiation of cycles between continuous sleep associated with active sleep and quiet or non-rapid eye movement (-REM) sleep segments that remain without movements, except for mouth and tongue movements and occasional myoclonic jerks.[31] Variable respirations persist, but short periods of regular respirations are present in the context of discontinuous portions of the recording.

EEG background is more continuous with cyclic periods of tracé discontinue (Fig. 2-10A and B). Synchronous delta frequencies of varying amplitude still predominate, interrupted by random inactive periods. Faster frequencies, also of variable amplitudes, are also present represented by the faster component of a delta brush pattern. Regional patterns (i.e., brushes, theta bursts) are prominent in the rolandic and occipital regions as well as the temporal and midline regions (Fig. 2-10C).

The most characteristic feature at this age range is the notable increase in multifocal sharp waves (see later section) as well as the appearance of reactivity to stimulation, characterized by transient periods of attenuation independent of discontinuity.

Sharply contoured activity predominates in the temporal and central regions, where positive temporal sharp waves are frequently seen in synchronous or independently occurring runs (Fig. 2-11). The sharp activity in the central regions is more likely negative in polarity and should be carefully distinguished from physiologic artifacts that can occur owing to fontanelle pulsation or ventilatory excursions. Positive temporal sharp waves need to be differentiated from pathologic rolandic and vertex positive sharp waves that are seen in the sick neonate with either intraventricular hemorrhage or periventricular leukomalacia (see Chapter 13).

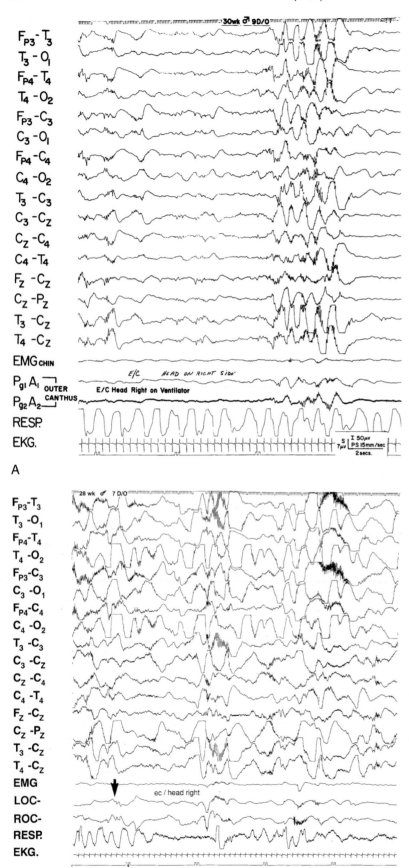

A

B

FIGURE 2–8

A, EEG tracing of a 30-week, 9-day-old boy illustrating a discontinuous background with comparatively shorter interburst intervals than those seen at more immature ages. Prominent delta brushes in the temporal region as well as central and midline locations are noted. More abundant temporal activity is characteristic at this gestational age range. B, EEG tracing of a 28-week, 7-day-old boy showing continuous activity comprising prominent rhythmic occipital delta lasting greater than 20 seconds. Prominent temporal sawtooth waves are noted, as are horizontal eye movements (arrows). Rapid eye movements (REMs) commonly occur during continuous EEG tracing of the premature neonate.

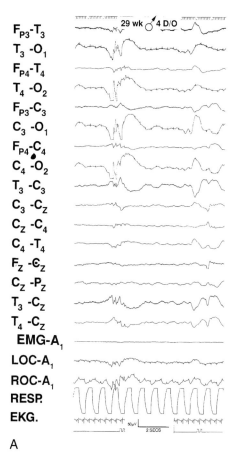

A

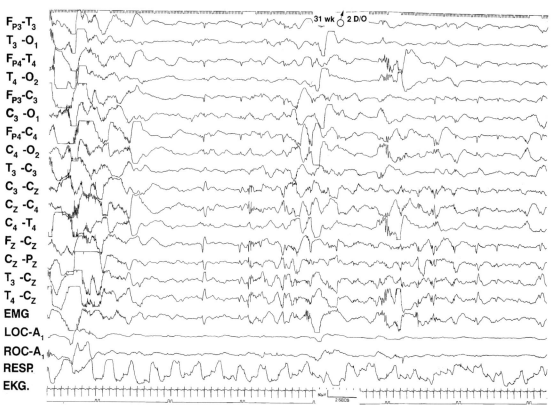

B

FIGURE 2–9

A, EEG tracing for a 29-week, 4-day-old boy with sharply contoured occipital theta giving the appearance of pathologic sharp activity. Superimposed waveforms may appear sharp and must be clearly distinguished from abnormal epileptiform discharges in this young age group. B, EEG tracing of a 31-week, 2-day-old boy demonstrating prominent frontal and central sharp activity intermixed with delta brush and other intermixed frequencies characteristic for the age. Note the prominent frontal parasagittal and midline sharp waves in this healthy asymptomatic premature infant.

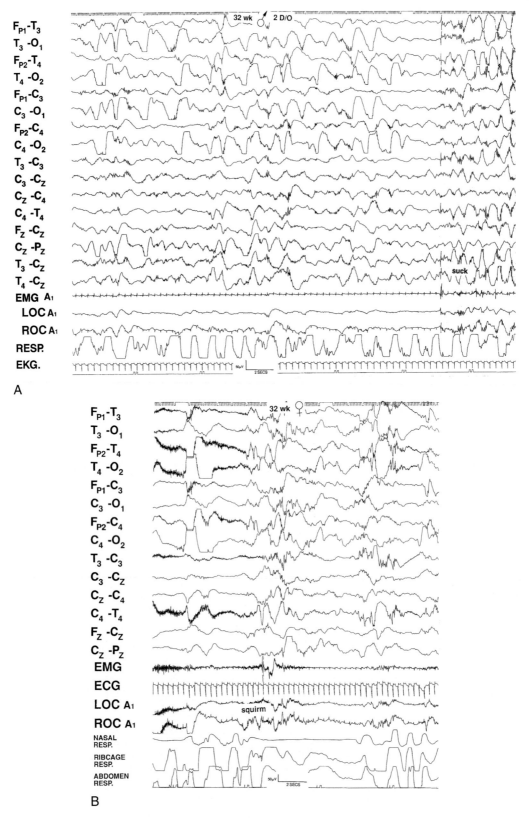

FIGURE 2–10

A, *EEG tracing of a 32-week-old infant demonstrating a continuous background of fast and slow frequencies.* B, *Discontinuous EEG segment of the same infant as in A demonstrating reactivity.*

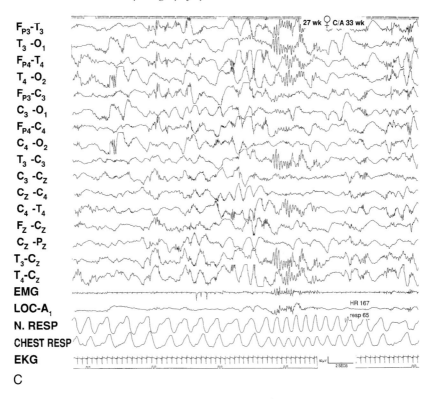

FIGURE 2–10—cont'd

C, An EEG tracing for a 33-week-old girl demonstrating an abundance of regional patterns characteristic at this gestational age, including temporal theta and brushes. Frontal sharp activity and frontal brushes, occipital theta, and occipital brushes are also noted in the context of a continuous EEG background.

Reactivity to stimulation appears in this gestational age range. Nonspecific EEG changes are induced by tactile or painful stimulation, usually with an abrupt attenuation or desynchronization of background (see Fig. 2-10*B*). This can be difficult to distinguish from low-amplitude quiescent periods but becomes more obvious with maturation, allowing a better distinction between active and quiet sleep. Uncommonly, bursts of higher amplitude delta activity may also characterize this reactivity. It is unknown whether these are the precursors of more discrete arousal patterns such as K complexes and hypersynchronous delta that are seen at older ages.

Reactivity to photic stimulation has been studied more systematically.[16] Responses to photic stimulation clearly are seen in the EEG of the early premature infant.[32] Responses to isolated flashes have a prominent negative wave component. Ellingson[33] described the later positive component occurring with maturation, with decreasing latency in proportion to increasing CA. In contrast with isolated flashes, repetitive flashes or photic driving have also been investigated by several authors, but such responses are difficult to detect in the EEG of the neonate.[33] Only between 4% and 5% of premature and FT infants exhibit photic driving with a wide range of flicker frequencies. Anderson and associates[16] found that even early premature infants between 27 and 32 weeks exhibited driving in 64% of 34 neonates when the frequencies were limited to 2 to 10 flashes per second.

Responses to other forms of sensory stimulation such as auditory or painful stimulation have been the object of less attention in either the premature or FT neonate. Monod and Garma[34,35] investigated behavioral and physiologic responses to auditory clicks in the premature neonate. These authors found vertex spikes in response to auditory clicks readily noted in neonates at 32 to 34 weeks CA. This is in contrast with a less distinctive response with more mature ages. Sudden, loud auditory stimuli more effectively produce EEG than do visual or tactile stimuli. Such periods of desynchronization have been postulated to be associated with the psychophysiologic property of habituation and may represent electrographic representation of perceptual memory and discriminatory functions of the neonate.[16]

Gestational Age 34 to 37 Weeks

Cyclic alterations between wakefulness and sleep as well as longer periods of continuous periods of EEG predominate

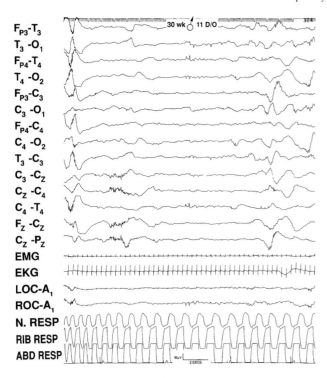

FIGURE 2–11

An EEG tracing for a 30-week, 11-day-old boy with briefly repetitive positive temporal sharp waves in this healthy asymptomatic neonate. Normal neurodevelopment has been documented at 1 year of age.

during the age range of gestational age 34 to 37 weeks CA. More concordant segments between cerebral and noncerebral signals resemble active and quiet sleep of the FT infant. For instance, motility patterns take on a distinctive phasic quality that predominates during active sleep. An absence of motility except for generalized myoclonic and facial movements is seen during quiet sleep. Myogenic activity measured at the chin characteristically remains low during the periods of active sleep while it is higher and more phasic during quiet sleep. The cyclic nature of the active and quiet sleep periods still lacks the well-defined 30- to 70-minute cycle seen in the FT infant.

Electrographic components of the EEG sleep cycle in this gestational age range show a predominance of continuous EEG activity comprising mixed delta and theta wave activity usually lower in amplitude (20 to 100 µV) than at younger gestational ages. Low-amplitude faster rhythms of alpha and beta activity are also present, with delta brushes persisting primarily over the temporal and occipital regions. Brushes also more commonly appear during quiet sleep than during active sleep.

Frontal sharp transients of 50 to 150 µV are predominantly noted at 34 to 35 weeks' gestation (250 µV) but may

have been seen at earlier gestational ages (Fig. 2-12).[36,37] Historically, these waveforms were termed *encoches frontales* and were popularly identified as *frontal sharp transients* as well as *pointes lents diphasiques frontales*. These sharp waves usually have an initial surface-positive component followed by a negative component but are also associated with rhythmic sharply contoured frontal delta activity and can occasionally be high amplitude (250 µV).[38]

In contrast, fewer multifocal sharp transients occur, and as with more PT neonates are sometimes difficult to distinguish from the intermixed background theta or beta frequencies.

The discontinuous quality of the EEG sleep tracing during this CA range indicates the appearance of a tracé alternant (TA) pattern rather than a tracé discontinu pattern noted for younger premature infants. The quiescent periods now consist of activity that may exceed 15 µV/mm with a greater mixture of low-amplitude faster rhythms noted.

Gestational Age 38 to 42 Weeks

Electrographic and polygraphic patterns are fully elaborated at this age range. Alternating periods of wakefulness and sleep as well as cyclic changes between four segments of sleep state can be identified. Two active sleep and quiet EEG patterns comprise this cycle (Fig. 2-13), with a length varying from 30 to 70 minutes, associated with the presence or absence of REMs, body movements, autonomic signs, and arousal episodes.

Although conventional wisdom dictates that only FT and near-FT infants possess such an organized EEG sleep cycle, concordance among specific EEG and polygraphic parameters has been described in the PT infant as early as 30 weeks' gestation. A developmental match between cerebral and noncerebral physiologic parameters fundamentally reflects the coordination of specific neural systems within the maturing system. There indeed may be a more established order of state in the premature infant that cannot be readily recognized by visual analysis techniques. A more rudimentary cycle may be detected in the premature neonate by more quantitative techniques.[39]

The EEG sleep organization of the FT neonate has traditionally been considered to be similar for a premature infant who has matured to a FT age as compared to the appropriate-for-gestational-age FT neonate. Two active sleep segments occupy 50% of the sleep time of the FT infant and comprise the mixed-frequency pattern (M) and low-voltage irregular (LVI) pattern that begin and end the sleep cycle. Quiet sleep segments consist of high-voltage slow (HVS) and TA segments and make up 10% to 15% of the cycle. The mixed-frequency active sleep pattern comprises moderate-amplitude delta and lower amplitude theta, alpha, and beta range activities (Fig. 2-14A). The low-voltage EEG pattern

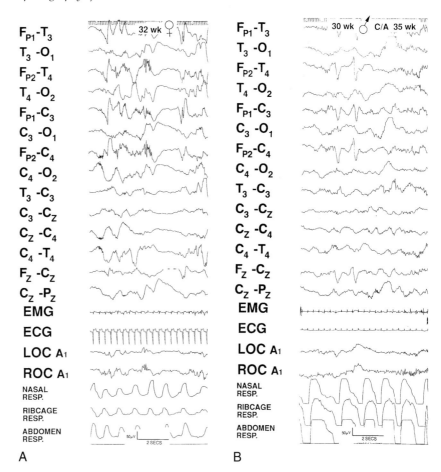

FIGURE 2–12

A, *EEG tracing of a 32-week-old boy with frontal sharp waves.* B, *EEG tracing of a 35-week old-boy with frontal sharp waves.*

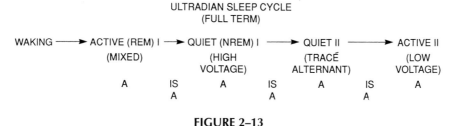

ULTRADIAN SLEEP CYCLE (FULL TERM)

WAKING ⟶ ACTIVE (REM) I ⟶ QUIET (NREM) I ⟶ QUIET II ⟶ ACTIVE II

	(MIXED)		(HIGH VOLTAGE)		(TRACÉ ALTERNANT)		(LOW VOLTAGE)
	A	IS A	A	IS A	A	IS A	A

FIGURE 2–13

Ultradian sleep cycle of a fullterm neonate indicating the four-segment sleep cycle beginning and ending with an active sleep period with two intervening quiet sleep periods. Arousals (A) occur as periods of reactivity either within or between sleep segments, which can be on either a spontaneous or an evoked basis. Transitional or interdeterminate sleep (IS) periods punctuate changes in sleep state segments. REM, rapid eye movement; NREM, non-REM.

consists of lower amplitude activity (Fig. 2-14B). This EEG background can also be seen during the awake state. Considerable amounts of alpha activity are intermixed both posteriorly and anteriorly. This pattern can be seen either during wakefulness or active sleep.

Two quiet sleep segments, HVS and TA (Fig. 2-14C and D), occupy the second and third positions in this idealized EEG sleep cycle. The HSV pattern comprises diffuse, continuous high-amplitude 50 to 150 µV delta activity, inter-

mixed with theta and beta range activity of lower amplitude. The HVS segment is quite brief (4% to 6% of the cycle) and is rapidly replaced by the TA pattern. The TA segment comprises a discontinuous tracing of high-amplitude bursts of slow activity in the delta and theta range alternating with lower amplitude faster frequencies in sharp waves seen synchronously over both hemispheres.

Frontal sharp waves may be abundant especially during quiet sleep. These waveforms are bilateral and synchronous

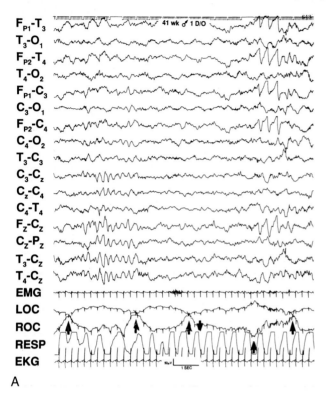

A

FIGURE 2–14

A, *Example of a mixed-frequency active sleep state in a 41-week, 1-day-old boy. Note the rhythmic theta activity in the midline and the frontal sharp waves during a transition to indeterminate sleep. (Arrows indicate the horizontal eye movements characteristic of rapid eye movements of sleep.) B, EEG tracing of a 40-week, 2-day-old girl depicting the low-voltage irregular active sleep segment. Rapid eye movements are prominent during this portion of the sleep cycle with frontopolar sharp waves reflecting eye movement-induced artifact. C, High-voltage EEG tracing in a healthy fullterm (41-week, 1-day-old) boy, characteristic of a quiet sleep segment with absence of movements and regular respiratory and cardiac rhythms. D, EEG tracing of a 38-week, 1-day-old boy depicting a tracé alternant quiet sleep segment. Note the occasional brush patterns as well as sharp transients that can be seen in various head regions in the sleep segment, particularly in the right hemisphere.*

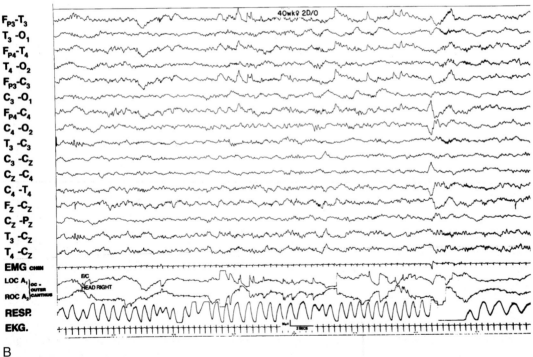

B

but also can be asymmetrical. Frontal sharp waves are seen less often during active and indeterminate sleep segments and are least likely to be noted during LVI active sleep.[40] During sleep, frontal sharp transients are noted until the beginning of the second month of life.[29]

As with PT infants, the clinical significance of spikes and sharp waves in asymptomatic FT neonatal populations remains controversial. Most groups do not have adequate follow-up data or were selected based on clinical problems. Clancy and Spitzer[41] identified 69 healthy

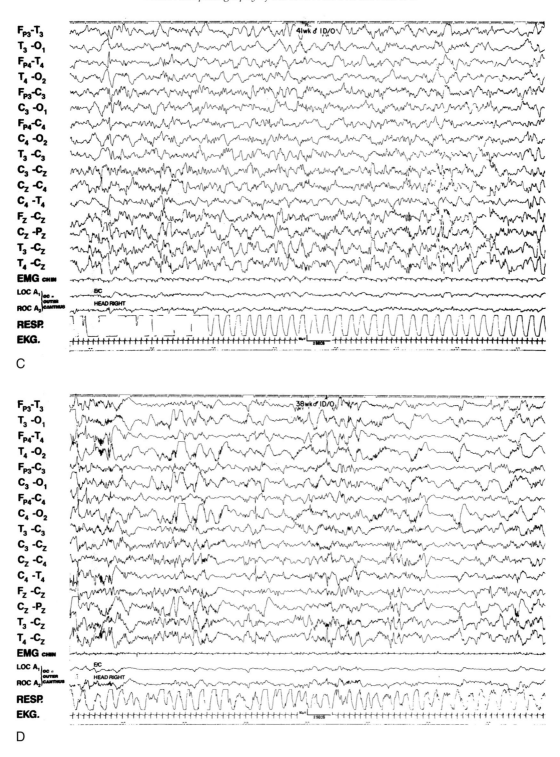

C

D

infants who had an acute life-threatening event (e.g., near-miss sudden infant death syndrome). Analyses of 10 minute of active sleep documented more frequent sharp waves in near-FT than in FT infants. Temporal sharp waves were more abundant than centrally located dis-

charges, persisting until 50 weeks CA and disappearing by 30 weeks CA.

Karbowski and Nencka[42] studied 1-hour sleep recordings in 82 FT healthy newborns without subsequent follow-up. Eighty-one percent had predominately right centrotemporal

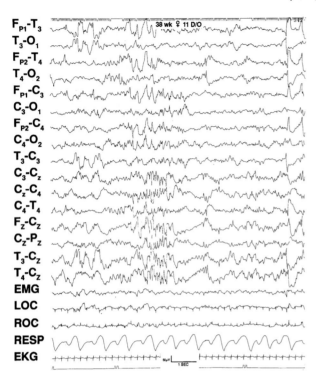

F_P1-T_3
T_3-O_1
F_P2-T_4
T_4-O_2
F_P1-C_3
C_3-O_1
F_P2-C_4
C_4-O_2
T_3-C_3
C_3-C_z
C_z-C_4
C_4-T_4
F_z-C_z
C_z-P_z
T_3-C_z
T_4-C_z
EMG
LOC
ROC
RESP
EKG

38 wk ♀ 11 D/O

FIGURE 2–15

EEG tracing of a 38-week, 11-day-old girl with sharply contoured midline and parasagittal sharply contoured theta. Also note the isolated sharp waves seen in the right temporal region. Both patterns can be seen in healthy patients and have no prognostic significance.

sharp waves with an average interval of 3 minutes and 47 seconds (Fig. 2-15). Only 12% had predominately left central waves with an average interval of 15 minutes. All discharges were noted primarily in indeterminate sleep.

As a final illustration, Statz and colleagues[40] followed 24 FT healthy infants to 9 to 12 months of age after obtaining a neonatal sleep recording. They noted sporadic, multifocal, nonrepetitive discharges during quiet sleep in all infants, whereas only 25% of infants had discharges during active sleep. The parietal region had the most abundant discharges with an interval between 38 seconds and 25 minutes.

Clearly, the clinical significance of spikes and sharp waves in both PT and FT infants needs more investigation. As recently emphasized, sporadic sharp waves may be either normal or abnormal, depending on the clinical context, EEG background activity, location, morphology, and CA. Unless discharges are repetitive, periodic, or positive in polarity, pathologic significance should not be definitively assigned.

Central sharp wave transients and rhythmic sharply contoured theta seen in the parasagittal and vertex regions are also seen. This midline pattern is rhythmic and has a

spindle-like appearance (see Fig. 2-15).[43] It is unknown whether this rhythmic activity is rudimentary sleep spindle activity that is seen at 2 to 3 months of age.

Delta brush patterns are occasionally noted during the quiet sleep segment but are rare and isolated primarily to the temporal and central regions.

As described earlier, synchrony should be 100% during sleep of the FT neonate. Transient asymmetries, mainly in the temporal regions, can be observed, particularly during the initial minutes of quiet sleep.[44]

Ontogeny of EEG sleep by the end of the neonatal period (i.e., 28 days following a FT birth) has been systematically investigated by only several researchers.[45,46] Gradual disappearance of TA by 3 to 6 weeks following an FT birth has been described as well as a change of REM and active sleep onset to quiet sleep onset. Sleep spindles commonly noted at 2 to 4 months of age may be seen as early as 4 to 6 weeks of age, and frontal sharp waves are normally noted 3 to 4 weeks following birth.

Although no significant differences can be distinguished between the maturational criteria at 1 month in PT as compared with FT infants, some differences have been noted. These differences comprise elements of sleep architecture. Longer bursts during TA, early sleep spindle appearance, more immature patterns, better phase stability, and specific frequency bands are described.[47] Behavioral criteria of sleep are also different between the two groups, suggesting that sleep organization of the PT neonate to FT and beyond is not entirely equivalent to the FT newborn.[48]

NEONATAL EEG SLEEP AS AN ULTRADIAN RHYTHM

During the last several decades, extensive information has been published with respect to the existence and functional significance of ultradian rhythms in humans. Durations of ultradian rhythms between 30 minutes and 24 hours may represent an important portion of the entire spectrum of human biologic rhythms. The human sleep cycle fits into a longer ultradian period, whereas individual EEG frequencies that comprise EEG activity represent markedly shorter periods.

The neonatal ultradian EEG sleep cycle has been approximated between 30 and 70 minutes.[29,49] The sleep architecture that comprises this cycle includes two active and two quiet sleep segments, usually beginning as sleep-onset active sleep portion. Transitional sleep segments within and between active sleep segments are commonly termed *indeterminate sleep segments*. Reactivity or arousal periods also punctuate within and between sleep segments. Indeterminate sleep and arousal phenomena represent the measure of sleep continuity.

Mathematical relationships among sleep components better define the development of this ultradian neonatal sleep cycle in the infant.[50] Sleep parameters including EEG sleep state, motility, REMs, and arousal can be better expressed quantitatively in terms of period length, amplitude, and phase. For a particular gestational age, specific period phase and amplitude relationships may better define the ontogeny of the EEG sleep cycle. With maturation of the CNS, relationships solidify among these parameters.

Longitudinal studies of the EEG sleep cycles as an ultradian rhythm in premature neonates maturing to FT under extrauterine conditions explore developing relationships that emerge as a function of CNS maturation. Comparisons of premature neonate sleep cycles at corrected FT age with FT infants can better assess the degree to which premature neonates must adapt to this extrauterine environment. What is more, such studies may then be compared with fetal state patterns. Differences between groups reflect differences in CNS maturation, in part due to maternal circadian influence on fetal development that is lacking in the children prematurely born.

Specific studies of PT EEG sleep parameters involving quantitative techniques have not yet been compared with those of the FT infant. There may be interesting relationships among EEG sleep, REM, and motility patterns in either single studies or with maturation across different gestational ages. Although circadian influence may not be established until sometime after birth, important periodic phasic and amplitude relationships may exist as ultradian rhythms during the premature neonatal or fetal periods.

A brief discussion of the noncerebral components of the EEG sleep rhythm highlights the importance of correlating such parameters with the EEG portion of the sleep rhythm during maturation.

REMs represent one of the main identifying features of active sleep. Active sleep constitutes most of the neonatal sleep cycle. REMs appear to be time locked to continuous EEG activity as early as 31 to 32 weeks' gestation.[51] However, REM activity is not a random rhythm and may have predictable intervals of occurrence.[52] Different classes of REM at different times of the sleep cycle may exist, and the numbers and types of REM increase with maturation.[53] This feature also can be measured during fetal life and is associated with continuous EEG activity in PT neonates as early as 30 weeks EGA. Closer identification of REM occurrence as well as quantification during different EEG states is needed to better understand this important developing ultradian rhythm. REM occurrence during active sleep segments constitutes an important maturational milestone of the immature brain and may have significance as a biologic marker for a variety of biologically relevant events.

Motility patterns are also an integral part of the neonatal sleep cycle. Different motility patterns appear at successively older neonatal ages up to FT infancy. Their ontogenic patterns are seen in both extrauterine-reared neonates as well as fetuses.[54-58] Myoclonic and whole-body movements predominate in the PT infant, whereas smaller, slower body movements are seen in the FT neonate. Attention to specific segments of the EEG sleep cycle of the neonate is important since motility patterns may differ during different segments of the cycle.[43,58,59] Similar motility patterns reflect in utero maturational changes detected by fetal ultrasonography.[54,57]

SUMMARY

Neonatal electroencephalography can accurately document the ontogeny of both regional and hemispheric electrographic patterns by visual analyses of paper records as well as ultradian EEG sleep rhythms by automated analyses of digitized records. Such patterns can serve as templates for normal extrauterine brain development. Furthermore, comparisons with physiologic profiles of fetal state behavior obtained by abdominal sonographic studies can follow intrauterine brain maturation. Such strategies ultimately will improve our diagnostic skills for the successful care of the high-risk fetus as well as the neonate.

Electroencephalography remains the only neurodiagnostic procedure that provides a continuous record of cerebral function over long periods. Although other advanced methods of anatomic or functional inquiry provide detailed but brief "snapshots" into cerebral pathophysiology, electroencephalography provides the important aspect of its evolution and structure in time. Knowledge of the temporal dimensions of developmental changes or pathologic processes is essential to acquiring an understanding of both the significance of normal ontogeny as well as deviations from these biologically programmed processes in pathologic conditions.

REFERENCES

1. Scher MS, Painter MJ, Guthrie RD: Cerebral neurophysiologic assessment of the high-risk neonate. *In* Guthrie RD (ed): Recent Advances in Neonatal Care. New York, Churchill Livingstone, 1987.
2. Davis DW: Cognitive outcomes in school-age children born prematurely. Neonatal Netw 2003;22:27-38.
3. Lorenz JM: The outcome of extreme prematurity. Semin Perinatol 2001;25:348-359.
4. Perlman JM: Cognitive and behavioral deficits in premature graduates of intensive care. Clin Perinatol 2002;29:779-797.

5. Sweet MP, Hodgman JE, Pena I, et al: Two-year outcome of infants weighing 600 grams or less at birth and born 1994 through 1998. Obstet Gynecol 2003;101:18-23.

6. Hrachovy RA, Mizrahi EM, Kellaway P: Electroencephalography of the newborn. *In* Daly DD, Pedley TA (eds): Current Practice of Clinical Electroencephalography. New York, Raven Press, 1990, p 201.

7. Lombroso CT: Neonatal polygraphy in full-term and premature infants: A review of normal and abnormal findings. J Clin Neurophysiol 1985;2:105-153.

8. Lombroso CT: Normal and abnormal EEGs in neonates. *In* Henry CE (ed): Current Clinical Neurophysiology: Update on EEG and Evoked Potentials. Amsterdam, Elsevier, 1980, p 83.

9. Lombroso CT: Neonatal electro-encephalography. *In* Niedermeyer E, Lopes da Silva F (eds): Electro-Encephalography Basic Principles, Clinical Applications, and Related Fields. Baltimore, Urban & Schwarzenberg, 1982, p 599.

10. Anders T, Emde R, Parmelee AH: A Manual of Standardized Terminology, Techniques, and Criteria for Scoring of States of Sleep and Wakefulness in Newborn Infants. Los Angeles, UCLA Information Service. NIDS Neurological Information Network, 1971.

11. Ballard JL, Novak KK, Driver M: A simplified score for assessment of fetal maturation of newly born infants. J Pediatr 1979;95:769-774.

12. Dubowitz LM, Dubowitz V, Goldberg C: Clinical assessment of gestational age in the newborn infant. J Pediatr 1970;77:1-10.

13. Dubowitz LM, Dubowitz V, Goldberg C, Keith I: Rapid assessment of gestational age at birth. Arch Dis Child 1976;51:986-987.

14. Scher MS, Barmada MA: Estimation of gestational age by electrographic, clinical, and anatomic criteria. Pediatr Neurol 1987;3:256-262.

15. Torres F, Anderson C: The normal EEG of the human newborn. J Clin Neurophysiol 1985;2:89-103.

16. Anderson CM, Torres F, Faoro A: The EEG of the early premature. Electroencephalogr Clin Neurophysiol 1985;60:95-105.

17. Sofue A, Okumura A, Hayakawa F, Watanabe K: Sharp waves in preterm infants with periventricular leukomalacia. Pediatr Neurol 2003;29:214-217.

18. Olischar M, Klebermass K, Kuhle S, et al: Reference values for amplitude-integrated electroencephalographic activity in preterm infants younger than 30 weeks gestational age. Pediatrics 2004;113:e61-e66.

19. Dreyfus-Brisac C: The electroencephalogram of the premature and full-term newborn: Normal and abnormal development of waking and sleeping patterns. *In* Kellaway P, Petersén I (eds): Neurological and Electroencephalographic Correlative Studies in Infants. New York, Grune & Stratton, 1964, p 186.

20. Hahn JS, Monyer H, Tharp BR: Interburst interval measurements in the EEGs of premature infants with normal neurological outcome. Electroencephalogr Clin Neurophysiol 1989;73:410-418.

21. Benda GI, Engel RC, Zhang YP: Prolonged inactive phases during the discontinuous pattern of prematurity in the electroencephalogram of very-low-birthweight infants. Electroencephalogr Clin Neurophysiol 1989;72:189-197.

22. Connell JA, Oozeer R, Dubowitz V: Continuous four-channel EEG monitoring: A guide to interpretation, with normal values, in preterm infants. Neuropediatrics 1987;18:138-145.

23. Eyre JA, Nanei S, Wilkinson AR: Quantification of changes in normal neonatal EEGs with gestation from continuous five-day recordings. Dev Med Child Neurol 1988;30:599-607.

24. Hughes JR, Fino J, Gagnon L: Periods of activity and quiescence in the premature EEG. Neuropediatrics 1983;14:66-72.

25. Vecchierini MF, D'Allest AM, Verpillat P: EEG patterns in 10 extreme premature neonates with normal neurological outcome: Qualitative and quantitative data. Brain Dev 2003;25:330-337.

26. Hughes JR, Miller JK, Fino JJ, Hughes CA: The sharp theta rhythm on the occipital areas of prematures (STOP): A newly described waveform. Clin Electroencephalogr 1990;21:77-87.

27. Dreyfus-Brisac C: Ontogenesis of sleep in human prematures after 32 weeks of conceptional age. Dev Psychobiol 1970;3:91-121.

28. Watanabe K, Iwase K: Spindle-like fast rhythms in the EEGs of low-birthweight infants. Dev Med Child Neurol 1972;14:373-381.

29. Stockard-Pope JE, Werner SS, Bickford RG: Atlas of Neonatal Electroencephalography, 2nd ed. New York, Raven Press, 1992.

30. Hughes JR, Fino JJ, Hart LA: Premature temporal theta (PT theta). Electroencephalogr Clin Neurophysiol 1987;67:7-15.

31. Curzi-Dascalova L, Peirano P, Morel-Kahn F: Development of sleep states in normal premature and full-term newborns. Dev Psychobiol 1988;21:431-444.

32. Ellingson RJ: Electroencephalograms of normal, full-term newborns immediately after birth with observations on arousal and visual evoked responses. Electroencephalogr Clin Neurophysiol 1958;10:31-50.

33. Ellingson RJ: Cortical electrical responses to visual stimulation in the human infant. Electroencephalogr Clin Neurophysiol 1960;12:663-677.

34. Monod N, Garma L: Auditory reactivity during sleep in the premature human. Electroencephalogr Clin Neurophysiol 1970;29:535.

35. Monod N, Garma L: Auditory responsivity in the human premature. Biol Neonate 1971;17:292-316.

36. Hughes JR, Kuhlman DT, Hughes CA: Electro-clinical correlations of positive and negative sharp waves on the temporal and central areas in premature infants. Clin Electroencephalogr 1991;22:30-39.

37. Okumura A, Hayakawa F, Kato T, et al: Abnormal sharp transients on electroencephalograms in preterm infants with periventricular leukomalacia. J Pediatr 2003;143:26-30.

38. Goldie L, Svedson-Rhodes V, Easton J, Robertson NRC: The development of innate sleep rhythms in short gestation infants. Dev Med Child Neurol 1971;13:40-51.

39. Scher MS, Sun M, Hatzilabrou GM, et al: Computer analyses of EEG-sleep in the neonate: Methodological considerations. J Clin Neurophysiol 1990;7:417-441.

40. Statz A, Dumermuth G, Mieth D, Duc G: Transient EEG patterns during sleep in healthy newborns. Neuropediatrics 1982;13:115-122.

41. Clancy RR, Spitzer AR: Cerebral cortical function in infants at risk for sudden infant death syndrome. Ann Neurol 1985;18:41-47.

42. Karbowski K, Nencka A: Right mid-temporal sharp EEG transients in healthy newborns. Electroencephalogr Clin Neurophysiol 1980;48:461-469.

43. Hayakawa F, Watanabe K, Hakamada S, et al: Fz theta/ alpha bursts: A transient EEG pattern in healthy newborns. Electroencephalogr Clin Neurophysiol 1987;67:27-31.

44. O'Brien MJ, Lems YL, Prechtl HF: Transient flattenings in the EEG of newborns—a benign variation. Electroencephalogr Clin Neurophysiol 1987;67:16-26.

45. Ellingson RJ, Peters JF: Development of EEG and daytime sleep patterns in normal full-term infant during the first 3 months of life: Longitudinal observations. Electroencephalogr Clin Neurophysiol 1980;49:112-124.

46. Lombroso CT, Matsumiya Y: Stability in waking-sleep states in neonates as a predictor of long-term neurologic outcome. Pediatrics 1985;76:52-63.

47. Joseph JP, Lesevre N, Dreyfus-Brisac C: Spatio-temporal organization of EEG in premature infants and full-term newborns. Electroencephalogr Clin Neurophysiol 1976;40:153-168.

48. Watt JE, Strongman KT: The organization and stability of sleep states in fullterm, preterm, and small-for-gestational-age infants: A comparative study. Dev Psychobiol 1985;18:151-162.

49. Parmelee AH, Akiyama Y, Stern E, Harris HA: A periodic cerebral rhythm in newborn infants. Exp Neurol 1969;25:575-584.

50. Harper RM, Leake B, Miyahara L, et al: Development of ultradian periodicity and coalescence at one cycle per hour in electroencephalographic activity. Exp Neurol 1981;73:127-143.

51. Haas GH, Prechtl HF: Normal and abnormal EEG maturation in newborn infants. Early Hum Dev 1977;1:69-90.

52. Andrade JP, Cardete-Leite A, Madeira MD, Paula-Barbosa MM: Long-term low-protein diet reduces the number of hippocampal mossy fiber synapses. Exp Neurol 1991;112:119-124.

53. Lynch JA, Aserinsky E: Developmental changes of oculomotor characteristics in infants when awake and in the "active state of sleep." Behav Brain Res 1986;20:175-183.

54. Robertson SS: Intrinsic temporal patterning in the spontaneous movement of awake neonates. Child Dev 1982;53:1016-1021.

55. Robertson SS: Human cyclic motility: Fetal-newborn continuities and newborn state differences. Dev Psychobiol 1987;20:425-442.

56. Robertson SS: Cyclic motor activity in the human fetus after midgestation. Dev Psychobiol 1985;18:411-419.

57. Robertson SS, Dierker LJ, Sorokin Y, Rosen MG: Human fetal movement: Spontaneous oscillations near one cycle per minute. Science 1982;218:1327-1330.

58. Fukumoto M, Mochizuki N, Takeishi M, et al: Studies of body movements during night sleep in infancy. Brain Dev 1981;3:37-43.

59. Prechtl HFR, Theorell K, Blair AW: Behavioural state cycles in abnormal infants. Dev Med Child Neurol 1973;15:606-615.

3

Visual Analysis of the Neonatal Electroencephalogram*

SAMUEL E. KOSZER, SOLOMON L. MOSHÉ, AND GREGORY L. HOLMES

INTRODUCTION

The electroencephalogram (EEG) provides useful information that reflects the function of the neonatal brain. The EEG may assist in determining brain maturation and identifying focal or generalized abnormalities, existence of potentially epileptogenic foci, or ongoing seizures. It is useful in assessing prognosis for neonates at risk for neurological sequelae. Basic guidelines for visual analysis and techniques of recording and interpretation of the EEG in infants younger than 44 weeks are discussed in this chapter.

TECHNIQUE

While the principles of electroencephalography are the same in neonates as in older children and adults, successfully recording and interpreting neonatal EEGs require additional skills. Considerable experience and patience are required to obtain technically satisfactory EEGs from neonates in a busy intensive care nursery. Sick neonates often have multiple organs being monitored by a variety of devices that can lead to unusual artifacts and may make reaching the infant's head difficult.

The number of electrodes used in recording the neonatal EEG is reduced owing to the small head circumference of the newborn. A standard 10-20 system is used with a single combined longitudinal and transverse montage. The frontal-temporal, frontal-central, temporal-occipital, and central-occipital longitudinal measurements are double distance-recordings. Instead of each interelectrode distance being 20% of the diameter of the head, they are 40%. Transverse and midcentral interelectrode distances are the standard 20% distances (Fig. 3-1).

Additional physiological leads that consist of two eye-movement monitors, electromyogram (EMG), and ECG and respiratory monitor electrodes (chest wall and/or nasal airflow) are placed to aid in determination of state. One eye electrode is placed 0.5 cm below the outer canthus and the other electrode is placed 0.5 cm above the outer canthus of the other eye. Differential field effects of the retina-to-cornea dipoles recorded in these opposing electrodes provide data on the types of eye movements. EMG electrodes are useful in differentiating subcortical or peripheral myoclonus from movements associated with epileptiform activity recorded at the surface of the brain.

Recording settings are chosen to acquire the necessary spectrum of data and to eliminate artifact. A time constant of 0.3 seconds typically is chosen to record the slower frequencies present in the neonatal EEG. A low-pass filter of 70 Hz is recommended. Filtering of high-frequency muscle artifact with 35 Hz (or other low-pass filter) is not recommended because EEG activity can be distorted and may be

*The chapter (including text and tables and figures) is from the article entitled "Visual Analysis of Neonatal EEG" by Drs. Koszer, Moshé, and Holmes, published on *www.emedicine.com/neuro/topic493.htm*. ©Copyright 2005, eMedicine, Inc.

Electrode configuration

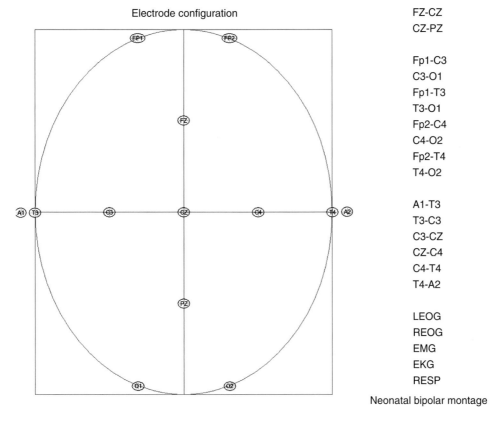

FZ-CZ
CZ-PZ

Fp1-C3
C3-O1
Fp1-T3
T3-O1
Fp2-C4
C4-O2
Fp2-T4
T4-O2

A1-T3
T3-C3
C3-CZ
CZ-C4
C4-T4
T4-A2

LEOG
REOG
EMG
EKG
RESP

Neonatal bipolar montage

FIGURE 3–1

Electrode map and montage.

misinterpreted as sharp activity. Sensitivity typically is set at 7 μV/mm and adjusted, if necessary. ECG, EMG, and eye electrodes are set at sensitivities of 50 μV/mm, 50 μV/mm, and 7 μV/mm, respectively, and adjusted as necessary.

The EEG test typically is run for 60 minutes or more to ensure the recording of at least one change in sleep state (a full sleep cycle in the neonate is typically 50 to 60 minutes).

Traditionally, neonatal EEGs were performed on paper EEG writers and a consensus regarding paper speed was not established. Recording speed often was chosen to be half the speed of the typical adult record (i.e., 15 mm/sec instead of 30 mm/sec).

Detection of asymmetries or asynchronies may be enhanced by slow speed. This becomes less of an issue as digital EEG acquisition and review allows for postrecording change of the time base of the recording. Review at different speeds is available, when necessary. Unfortunately, waveform morphology is different in records that are recorded at different paper speeds. At 15 mm/sec, sharp waves and spikes are half the width in the EEG record and "look sharper." Sharp waves and spikes must stand out from the background, be sharply contoured, and be 70 to 200 milliseconds and 20 to 70 milliseconds in duration, respectively.

VISUAL ANALYSIS

A five-step process should be performed when analyzing a neonatal EEG. The five steps comprise the following:

1. Knowledge of the post conceptional age and topography of the infant's head
2. Identification of artifacts in the EEG
3. Identification of sleep and wake states
4. Feature extraction
5. Classification of the record as normal or abnormal and clinical correlation provided to clinician

Post Conceptional Age and Topography

An accurate estimate of post conceptional age is required because features in the EEG will vary with the age of the newborn. *Post Conceptional age* is defined as gestational age (in weeks) plus the number of weeks since birth. Gestational age is the number of weeks/months the child was in the womb. Legal age is the age of the child since birth. *Prematurity* (PT) is defined as birth at a gestational age of less than 38 weeks; *fullterm* (FT) is defined as birth at a gestational age of 38 to 42 weeks.

As in the adult, a description of skull and scalp topography is necessary. Scalp swelling and other forms of trauma can increase interelectrode resistance and attenuate the recording. Meningocele or subdural or epidural fluid collections can alter interelectrode resistance as well. Skull fractures provide a low-resistance pathway for electric fields and result in increased voltage. Distorted cranial vaults (common after birth trauma) also alter the topography of the EEG.

Artifact Rejection

As with the older child, all artifacts must be identified before a visual analysis of the EEG can begin, so that they are not considered part of the background or paroxysmal activity. The neonate should lie still with the head in the midline position to minimize artifacts. The technician must try to determine the nature of artifacts at the time they occur, because once the child is disconnected from the EEG, identification of artifacts is difficult (Table 3-1 and Figs. 3-2 and 3-3).

Identification of Sleep and Wake States

Observation of the infant's movements, by the technician description of the infant's behavior, and analysis of the data in the noncerebral electrodes determine the neonate's state. Table 3-2 describes types of activity expected for each state. Lateral eye movements, ventilatory rate, and ECG and EMG patterns do not become reliable indicators of state, however, until 34 to 36 weeks CA.

TABLE 3–1. COMMON ARTIFACTS SEEN ON NEONATAL EEG

Cardiac	ECG and pulse (see Fig. 3-2)
	Ballistocardiographic (movement of the head with heartbeat)
Body	Respiratory, twitches, and tremor (see Fig. 3-3)
Head	Vertical, horizontal, and rotatory head movements
	Electrode "pops" and fontanelle-related pulsations
Face	Sucking glossokinesthetic, eye movements and blinks, frontotemporal muscle contraction
Other	60-Hz electrical
	Electromechanical devices (e.g., ventilators, IV drips) (see Fig. 3-2)

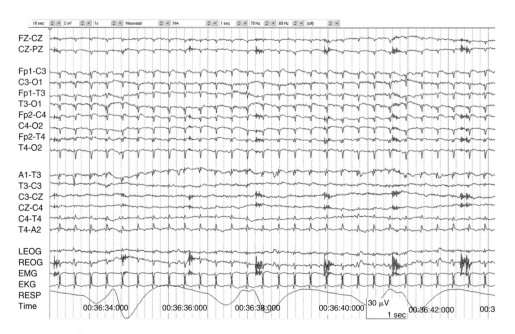

FIGURE 3–2

Artifacts and a low-voltage record: A full-term infant at day 4 of life with anoxia at birth and seizures. No spontaneous respirations occur. The record is low voltage with no activity of cerebral origin greater than 2 μV. All other activity can be accounted for by physiologic or nonphysiologic artifacts. ECG artifacts are diffuse. Pulse artifact is time locked to the ECG. An IV artifact occurs in multiple electrodes every 1 75 seconds and is most prominent in the right electro-oculogram (REOG). The RESP channel demonstrates mechanical ventilation artifact.

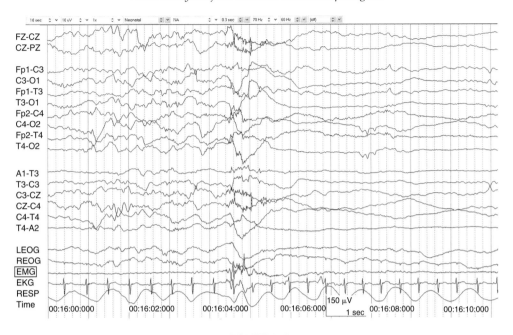

FIGURE 3–3

Twitching artifact: A full-term, 3-day-old infant with anoxic encephalopathy and episodes of generalized twitching lasting 1 to 2 seconds at a time. Muscle artifacts are seen in multiple electrodes and are particularly prominent in the EMG channel. After the twitch the background attenuates and appears to be a state change rather than an electrographic seizure correlate.

TABLE 3–2. STATE-RELATED POLYGRAPHIC CHANGES IN THE NEONATE

Physiological Measure	Awake/Sleep State		
	Awake	Active Sleep	Quiet Sleep
EMG (chin)	Phasic and tonic	Phasic	Tonic
Respiration	Irregular	Irregular	Regular
Eye movements	Random or pursuits	Rapid eye movements	Absent
Body movements	Facial, limbs, and body	Sucking and irregular limb movements	None

EEG is a useful test in providing reliable clues for assessing postconceptional age. Quantification of various sleep states from the newborn period to adulthood show that FT infants spend more time in rapid eye movement (REM) sleep than any other age group. Furthermore, as a PT baby approaches FT, the amount of non-rapid eye movement (NREM) sleep increases while REM sleep decreases. *Quiet sleep* is analogous to NREM sleep, and *active sleep* is analogous to REM sleep in the adult. Quiet sleep is characterized by an absence of lateral eye movements and increased chin EMG activity with regular respirations and ECG (Fig. 3-4).

Neonates often enter active sleep at onset of sleep. Low-to-moderate voltage; continuous EEG pattern with REMs; irregular respirations and cardiac rate; decreased chin EMG activity; and quick irregular movements of the fingers, hand, or face characterize active sleep. By term, two patterns of REM may be seen if the recording continues long enough. In the first REM cycle, the EEG shows fairly continuous mixed frequencies in the delta, theta, and alpha ranges with a paucity of faster activity, and the voltages range from 40 to 100 μV. In the second REM cycle, which occurs after a period of NREM sleep, the background is more continuous, voltage is lower (20 to 50 μV), and frequencies are faster than in the first REM period (Fig. 3-5).

Delta brushes are present in the premature infant beginning at 26 weeks postconceptional age. Delta brushes are analogous to K-complexes in the adult; however, they typically occur asynchronously in the neonate. Delta brushes consist of a mixture of medium- to high-voltage delta activity inter-mixed with low- to medium-voltage fast activity, commonly with 18- to 22-Hz maximum in the central region. Delta brushes are a prominent feature in active sleep by 29 to 33 weeks postconceptional age, and by 33 to 38 weeks postconceptional age they are expressed maximally in quiet sleep.

Prior to 28 to 30 weeks postconceptional age the record is discontinuous, with interbursts of low voltage or inactivity alternating with higher amplitude and mixed-frequency activity, a pattern termed *tracé discontinu* (TD) (Fig. 3-6).

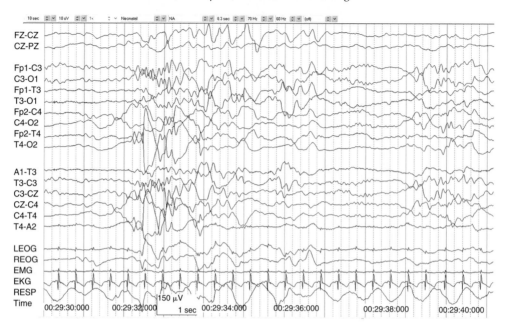

FIGURE 3–4

Quiet sleep and tracé alternant (TA): An infant of 39 weeks' postconceptional age with hydrocephalus and possible seizures. During quiet sleep, respirations are regular, EMG activity is low-voltage tonic with no phasic activity, and no spontaneous eye movements occur. TA is seen with medium- to high-voltage mixed frequencies alternating with periods of relative voltage attenuation.

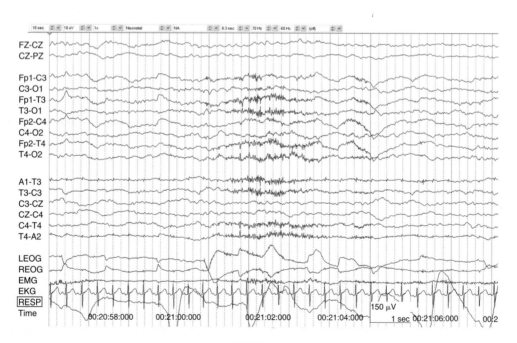

FIGURE 3–5

Active sleep: An otherwise healthy infant of 41 weeks' postconceptional age with episodes of arm and leg extension without EEG correlates. This segment of normal active sleep shows irregular respirations; frequent eye movements on electro-oculogram (EOG); and a mixed pattern of delta, theta, and alpha frequency activity.

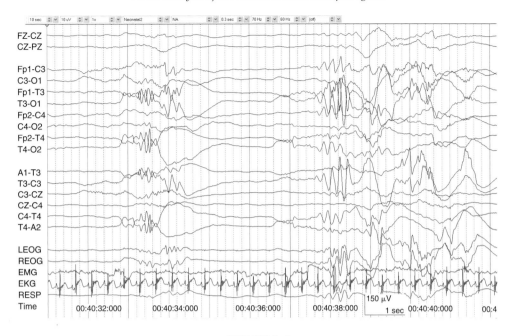

FIGURE 3–6

Tracé discontinu (TD) An infant of 24 weeks' gestational age at 4 weeks with an intraventricular hemorrhage and left shoulder twitching. Periods of alternating high-voltage mixed frequencies and periods of voltage suppression are normal findings before 28 to 30 weeks' postconceptional age.

Beginning at 28 to 30 weeks postconceptional age, some sleep-state differentiation occurs, with active sleep having more continuous patterns than quiet sleep. However, sleep-state differentiation may be difficult until 32 to 34 weeks CA. As the infant matures, the interburst durations decrease, and the amplitude and morphologies of the interburst activity change. Beginning at approximately 34 to 35 weeks postconceptional age, other physiological features become increasingly helpful in determining sleep state.

Tracé alternant (TA) is defined as the discontinuous pattern of NREM sleep in which bursts of prevalent slow activity (1 to 4 Hz) alternate with random faster transients at 50 to 200 μV. The bursts appear roughly every 4 or 5 seconds and last 2 to 4 seconds. The interburst consists of low-voltage continuous, somewhat rhythmic activity with a dominant frequency in the theta range and voltages between 20 and 50 μV. TA usually emerges by 36 to 38 weeks CA (Fig. 3-7).

By term, the infant often has a slow wave sleep pattern (SWS) of NREM state, which consists of prominent diffuse delta with some theta rhythms. Although some brief periods of SWS can occur as early as 36 weeks postconceptional age, the amount of SWS gradually increases until 44 to 48 weeks postconceptional age when it almost completely replaces the TA pattern.

FEATURE EXTRACTION

The process of feature extraction is performed for each state that is identified in the EEG record. The types of features to be identified include amplitude, continuity of background activity, frequency, symmetry, reactivity, synchrony, and maturational and paroxysmal patterns.

I. *Amplitude*: The spectrum of abnormalities of background varies from the ominous pattern of electrocerebral inactivity to the more benign finding of low-amplitude activity during discontinuous sleep. Note that caput succedaneum, scalp edema, and subdural effusions or hematomas may affect the apparent amplitude of the EEG.

A. The most extreme abnormality in amplitude consists of electrocerebral inactivity (isoelectric/inactive) (see Fig. 3-2). This is a record in which no cerebral electrical activity is present. Before concluding that this pattern is present, the electroencephalographer must be certain the test was performed satisfactorily and for a long enough time to include potential sleep cycling. Increased sensitivities, long time constants, and long interelectrode distances are used. Artifacts are identified and eliminated, when possible. The technician always performs various stimulations (auditory and nociceptive) to establish lack of reactivity. This EEG pattern carries a grave prognosis in both PT and FT infants if not due to postictal state, hypothermia, acute hypoxia, or drug intoxication. Most infants with persistent electrocerebral inactivity either die or have severe neurological sequelae.

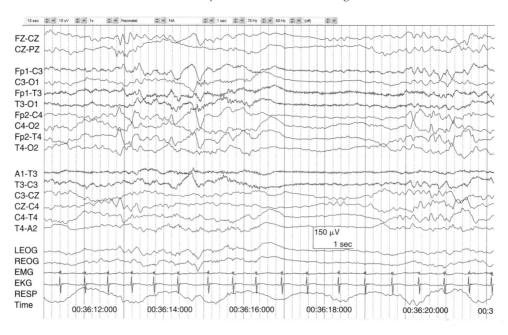

FIGURE 3–7

Tracé alternant: An infant of 42 weeks' postconceptional age delivered via cesarean birth, with Apgar scores of 4/4/4 and left arm and leg jerking movements. TA occurs with regular respirations, low-voltage tonic EMG, and minimal eye movements. Periods of relative voltage attenuation may occur periodically during quiet sleep.

B. A second abnormality of amplitude occurs when the low-voltage undifferentiated pattern consists of background activity between 5 and 15 μV in all states. Distinct state changes typically do not occur. This background pattern is easier to recognize in PT infants because discontinuity and high-voltage bursts are normal, and a decrease or absence of delta brushes, which should be quite prominent at this age, is common. The low-voltage undifferentiated pattern is associated with poor outcomes, particularly when the pattern persists beyond the first weeks of life. Low-voltage records can be observed in a variety of neonatal encephalopathies, including hypoxia-ischemia, congenital hydrocephalus, and severe intracranial hemorrhages such as large subdural hematomas. They also may occur in various toxic or metabolic disturbances. A low-voltage record shortly after a hypoxic or ischemic event is less concerning than one obtained days after the event.

II. *Continuity*: One of the most striking features of the neonatal EEG is its discontinuity (i.e., periods of higher voltage activities followed by periods of lower ones that occur during portions of the recording). Degrees and morphologies of discontinuity vary significantly in healthy neonates according to their postconceptional age (most dramatic in young PT and almost nonexistent in healthy FT infants reaching 3 to 4 weeks of postnatal life). These features also vary according to the newborn's states.

A. No absolute criteria currently exist that can be used to determine whether records are excessively discontinuous. However, recent studies do provide some guidance. Hahn et al studied interburst intervals (IBIs).[1] Conservatively stated, the maximum IBI duration should be less than 40 seconds in infants younger than 30 weeks postconceptional age; by term, the IBIs should be less than 6 seconds in duration.

B. The most obvious abnormality of continuity is burst-suppression (BS). This pattern consists of bursts of high-voltage activity lasting 1 to 10 seconds. BS is composed of various features (e.g., spikes, sharp waves, theta, delta), which are followed by periods of marked background attenuation (voltage < 5 μV). The bursts (highly synchronous between hemispheres) contain no age-appropriate activity. In the most austere form, this pattern is invariant, minimally altered by stimuli, and persistent throughout awake and sleep states. This pattern is easy to differentiate from the discontinuous features normally seen during NREM sleep in infants older than 34 to 36 weeks postconceptional age when TA begins to emerge clearly (Fig. 3-8).

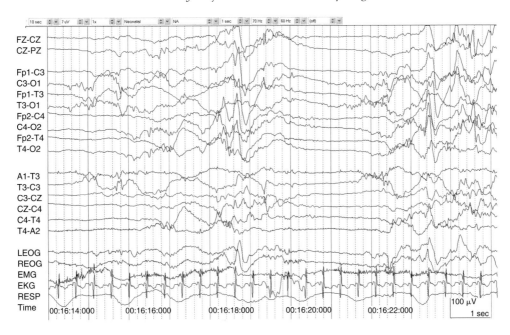

FIGURE 3–8

Burst-suppression: An infant of 42 weeks' postconceptional age with asphyxia. An alternating pattern of high-voltage mixed-frequency activity and voltage attenuation in a term infant indicates severe diffuse cerebral dysfunction. Compare this with tracé discontinu in Figure 3-6 where similar activity may be considered normal prior to 30 weeks gestational age.

C. The discontinuous EEG pattern of TA is distinguished from BS by the presence of higher amplitude interburst activity, reactiveness to stimulation, and containment of EEG features normal for postconceptional age (i.e., delta brushes, temporal theta, or frontal sharp transients). Most importantly, cycling of the discontinuous pattern of TA with the continuous pattern of REM sleep is prevalent.

D. Problems may arise in young PT infants (34 weeks postconceptional age and younger) owing to discontinuous periods of practically absent activities between bursts, which are typical at this age. Unlike the normal discontinuous pattern of TD, BS usually is invariant and not associated with other features characteristic of the EEGs of neonates of various postconceptional age. Testing for reactivity, usually but not invariably absent in BS, is also helpful. In young PT infants, serial recordings are advisable before reaching the dire prognosis generally attached to BS. However, the most reliable clue to distinguish the pathological pattern of BS from the ontogenetically normal TD is an accurate postconceptional age of the infant.

III. *Frequency*: Records that are excessively slow or fast are unusual in neonates. Rarely, a neonatal record consists of diffuse delta activity in both waking and sleep states, minimal theta or faster frequencies, and poor reactivity. When these conditions persist longer than 2 weeks in FT neonates, the prognosis is poor.

IV. *Symmetry*: Neonatal records with voltage asymmetries of 25% or more are abnormal. Noncerebral hemisphere abnormalities should be excluded when evaluating records for amplitude abnormalities. These noncerebral hemisphere abnormalities include unilateral cephalhematomas, subgaleal or scalp edema, and technical faults (e.g., asymmetric placement of electrodes, sweating, smearing of electrode paste). Because of the nature of their lesions, neonates exhibiting this pattern often develop seizures. Ictal EEG discharges can be seen over the depressed side and sustained focal discharges superimposed on this abnormal background represent the rare occurrence of focal ictal events in direct proximity with underlying anatomical lesions.

A. Transient interhemispheric asymmetry is likely a normal variant. A sudden markedly exaggerated TA pattern approaching a BS pattern involving only one hemisphere while the other hemisphere maintains normal features is seen occasionally. This finding may be indicative of a focal lesion.

B. Persistent attenuation of voltage involving only one scalp region can be associated with focal or

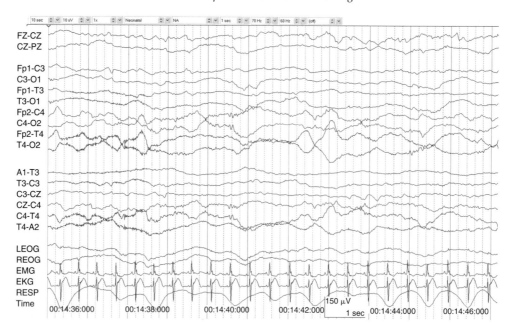

FIGURE 3–9

Voltage attenuation—focal: An infant of 40 weeks' postconceptional age with a left middle cerebral artery infarction and intermittent posturing and hyperextension of the neck. Background activity demonstrates attenuation of delta, and fast activity on the left is indicative of a structural lesion on the left.

lateralized neuropathological lesions. The technician must be aware that improper placement of electrodes or localized scalp edema can result in an EEG pattern that resembles focal attenuation (Fig. 3-9).

V. *Synchrony*: Synchronous activity is defined as simultaneous EEG activity in homologous regions of each hemisphere. Synchrony is assessed during TA and NREM sleep. In well-established TA in healthy FT infants, the bursting activities between hemispheres occur almost simultaneously. In younger infants (32 to 38 weeks postconceptional age) these bursts occur with less synchrony. In even younger PT infants (27 to 28 weeks postconceptional age), the bursts of TD are synchronous between hemispheres.

VI. *Sleep-state transitions*: While observation of sleep-state changes provides the electroencephalographer with a considerable amount of information regarding the status of the infant's brain, those interpreting neonatal EEGs must be cautioned that considerable variation occurs during a routine 1-hour EEG, not only in different neonates but also in the same infant when tested at intervals of a few days. These marked individual fluctuations often overlap with those observed in impaired newborns. Care must be taken in interpreting an abnormal record solely based on sleep features. As with other

abnormalities, persistence of the abnormality on serial records adds to the strength of the predictive value of the EEG.

A. Records in which no recognizable sleep states exist, despite lengthy recordings, are abnormal. In infants older than 30 weeks postconceptional age the lack of sleep-state differentiation usually is readily apparent (continuous activity typically appears in active sleep by 30 weeks postconceptional age). In addition to lack of cyclical states, the EEGs often contain other abnormalities such as persistent low voltage or excessive discontinuity, monotonous moderate theta or alpha range frequencies, and even interictal or ictal discharges. Disruption in the ability to develop cyclic states often is observed in infants in a coma state due to a variety of causes. In these patients, the following factors should be ruled out: reversible toxic factors, hypothermia, and use of drugs for controlling seizures or minimizing brain damage due to anoxic-ischemic insults. Lack of distinct sleep states is associated with poor outcomes.

B. Transitional or indeterminate sleep is used by some to indicate periods of sleep in which lack of concordance between criteria does not allow their classification as either REM or NREM. An excessive amount of transient sleep is considered abnormal. A similar pattern, excessive labile sleep states, refers to rapid changes of sleep state, with the infant spending only a few minutes or even seconds in one sleep state before entering into another state.

C. Both excessive transient sleep state and excessive labile sleep state have been observed in infants born to mothers on drugs such as alcohol.

VII. *Maturation*: EEG maturation from PT to FT and beyond occurs in a predictable time-linked fashion. The observation that the maturation of the EEG is primarily dependent on the postconceptional age renders the EEG a valuable tool in assessing central nervous system physiological maturation.

A. A number of indices are used in determining whether the EEG is appropriate for the infant's postconceptional age. These indices include the percentages of interhemispheric synchrony during TA, amount of delta brushes in both REM and NREM states, and sleep-state transitions including concordance between EEG and other bioelectric and behavioral parameters.

B. The neonatal record is considered to have a pattern of dysmaturity when the background patterns lag behind postconceptional age by at least 2 weeks. Dysmaturity may be either transient or persistent.

C. A constellation of electroencephalographic and physiological information goes into determining whether a record is mature or not. The following criteria may be helpful in determining when an EEG is maturationally delayed:

1. By 32 to 34 weeks postconceptional age the background activity should have some periods of continuous activity as periods of better organized REM and NREM states begin to emerge. The average interburst interval should be less than 20 seconds. The range of interhemispheric synchrony between bursts of the emerging TD varies between 50% and 70%. Delta brushes still abound, tending to localize more over rolandic and occipital areas. The high-voltage temporal theta of younger PT infants is less frequent, while lower voltage, multifocal, sharp transients occur between bursts. In the absence of an isoelectric reading, distinguishing immature records in this age group from those with more severe disturbances of background activity may be difficult.

2. By 34 to 36 weeks postconceptional age, clear EEG distinction between REM and NREM states should be observed. REM should consist of a continuous pattern with mixed delta and theta waves of variable voltage (usually 30 to 100 μV). Delta brushes are present more frequently in NREM than in REM sleep. Interhemispheric synchrony

of bursts of NREM TD ranges from 70% to 85%.

3. By 36 to 38 weeks TD prevails in NREM sleep, and activity greater than 20 μV is present during most of the interburst interval. Brief periods (<3 seconds) of lower voltage activity still can be seen during the interburst interval. During REM sleep abundant clusters of rapid eye movements, frequent body movements, decreased muscle tone, and irregular respiration are present. In NREM sleep only rare eye movement, general body quiescence, increased muscle tone, and regular respirations (in the absence of pulmonary disease) are present. Interhemispheric synchrony of bursts in TD ranges from 85% to 95%. Delta brushes still occur, but are diminished during NREM sleep, with an average of approximately 20 during every 5 minutes of REM sleep.

4. By 38 to 40 weeks postconceptional age, the infant should cycle through clear sleep states. TA occurs during NREM sleep. Bursts are 90% to 100% synchronous (< 2 seconds difference in time of onset). Bursts and interburst intervals are of similar duration. Occurrence of delta brushes decreases, with only 1 or 2 during every 5 minutes of REM sleep.

5. By 40 to 42 weeks no delta brushes are present. If present, delta brushes occur only during NREM sleep, at most four per 5-minute epoch. Complete interhemispheric synchrony between bursts of TA is observed. The infant should cycle through clear sleep states.

6. By 44 weeks continuous slow-wave pattern should be predominant during NREM sleep.

7. By 48 weeks TA should be minimal with NREM sleep dominated by high-voltage slow-wave activity. Some sleep spindles also should emerge.

VIII. *Paroxysmal patterns*: These include interictal discharges (positive rolandic sharp waves, frontal and temporal sharp transients), ictal discharges (focal spikes and sharp waves, pseudo delta, theta, alpha and beta), and low-frequency discharge patterns.

A. Interictal patterns

1. While *spikes or sharp waves* are defined the same way in neonates, older children, and adults, their significance may be different. In many cases, spikes and sharp waves are normal features, especially in PT infants. Spikes and sharp waves are common during the bursting phase of TD or TA and may be observed over the temporal region during the inactive phase.

2. In healthy FT neonates, sporadic spikes predominate over frontal areas (usually synchronously) and are incorporated within the bursts of TA. They often coexist with rhythmic slow waves, misnamed "anterior slow dysrhythmia." These transients may shift between hemispheres; they begin to appear clearly at approximately 34 to 35 weeks postconceptional age, persisting with diminished frequency into the beginning of the early infancy period. Because these spikes and sharp waves can be ontogenetically normal in spite of their epileptiform morphology, they have been labeled *frontal sharp transients* to defuse implications of an epileptiform signature.

3. *Positive rolandic sharp waves* are surface-positive, broad-based, sharp transients with duration up to 500 milliseconds, localized over the rolandic areas (C3-C4). In spite of their paroxysmal features that might suggest an epileptiform signature, positive rolandic spikes do not correlate with ictal phenomena. Although these waves can be observed in the context of intracerebral hemorrhages, the present consensus is that they are associated more directly with pathologies that induce deep white matter lesions. Their underlying generator remains obscure, especially since explaining them simply based on white matter necrosis is difficult.

4. *Positive temporal sharp waves* are EEG transients with morphology and polarity similar to the positive rolandic sharp waves; however, they occur over the mid-temporal areas. They occur in neonates with intracranial hemorrhages or a history of perinatal asphyxia (Fig. 3-10).

5. A clear differentiation between normality and abnormality for spikes and sharp waves may be difficult, because the boundaries still are not distinct and are a matter of controversy. Spikes and sharp waves that occur over frontal, rolandic, and temporal areas are abnormal if they are excessively frequent for the postconceptional age, appear in short runs, are consistently unilateral, occur frequently during the attenuated phase of TA, or persist during the more continuous patterns of REM sleep or wakefulness (Fig. 3-11).

6. The significance of excessive numbers of spikes and sharp waves is not clear. While excessive numbers of spikes and sharp waves are more common in neonates with seizures than in neonates without them, the correlation is tenuous. Many neonates with electroencephalographic and/or behavioral

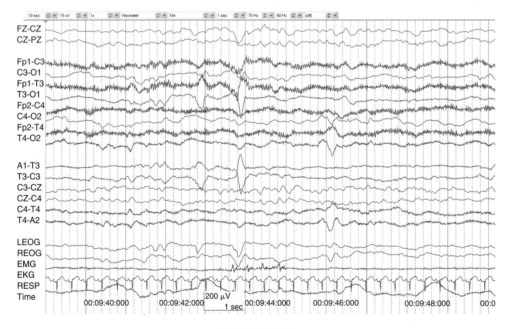

FIGURE 3–10

Positive temporal sharps: An infant of 41 weeks' postconceptional age with a fever of 102°F and three episodes of right arm and leg jerking with eye deviation lasting 5 to 10 seconds each. Left positive temporal sharps are seen in the 4th and 5th seconds at T3 and independently at T4 during the 8th second.

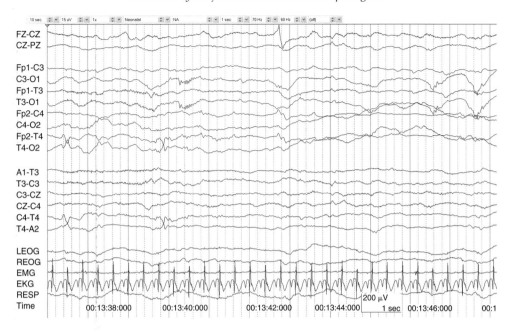

FIGURE 3–11

Excessive sharp transients: An infant of 36 weeks' postconceptional age with hypoxic-ischemic encephalopathy and seizures on days 2 and 3 of life. Sharp transients are seen in the 1st and 3rd seconds at T4.

seizures may have few interictal spikes or sharp waves. Conversely, the presence of excessive spikes or sharp waves can be seen in neonates without a history of seizures.

B. Ictal patterns

1. A generally accepted definition of what constitutes an ictal discharge has not been established. Some authors classify a discharge as ictal if it lasts at least 10 seconds, while other authors require duration of at least 20 seconds. However, documented clinical and electrical seizures long have been described as lasting only a few seconds. With increasing age electrical seizure activity becomes more frequent and longer in duration. Some have proposed that any rhythmic discharge accompanied by clinical changes be considered an ictal event, while rhythmic discharges lasting 10 seconds or longer be considered EEG events, regardless of whether behavioral changes occur.

2. *Electrographic seizure discharges* typically consist of rhythmic theta, alpha, delta or beta waves, or sharp waves or spikes that are focal or multifocal and vary in frequency and amplitude as the seizure progresses. The electroencephalographer must be aware that a variety of artifacts may resemble EEG seizures. Changing location, waveform morphology, or frequency suggests that the rhythmic activity is cerebral. The cerebral hemispheres in the neonate function relatively autonomously, so that even when seizures spread they may not spread to the other hemisphere. In cases when seizures do spread to the opposite hemisphere, the discharges often alternate from side to side (Figs. 3-12 to 3-16).

3. Focal spikes or sharp wave discharges consist of trains of rhythmic spikes or sharp waves that erupt focally out of the background activity, usually abruptly. While initially the amplitude may be low, it often increases as frequency decreases. Frequency of discharge varies most commonly in the delta to alpha bands (from 4 to 10 Hz), with the most frequent location in the rolandic areas. Discharge may spread to the adjacent cortex but usually at a much slower pace in neonates than in older patients. The discharge may appear in homotopic areas of the other hemisphere. In general, these types of focal patterns correlate well with the clinical manifestations of seizures that are usually clonic.

4. Ictal focal EEG discharges do not necessarily indicate an underlying lesion because they often occur in the context of transient metabolic disorders following a mild hypoxic-ischemic event or a

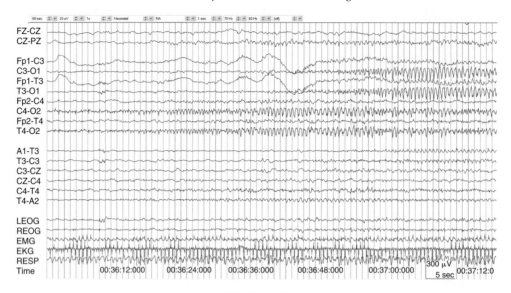

FIGURE 3–12

Alternating seizure 1: An infant of 32 weeks' gestational age at 40 weeks' conception with serratia meningoencephalitis. Surgery for drainage and dural repair was performed. This seizure begins at 00:36:12 in the right posterior quadrant with sharply contoured rhythmic delta at 1.5 to 2 Hz. Note the compressed nature of the time base with each gradation representing 1 second. By 00:36:50 the spread to the left posterior quadrant is evident. The seizure continues in Figure 3-13.

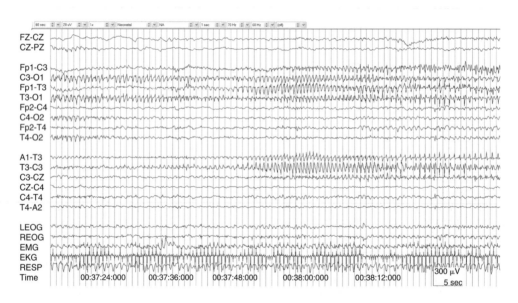

FIGURE 3–13

Alternating seizure 2: In the first 10 seconds of the page, the electrographic seizure pattern in the right posterior quadrant attenuates is leaving behind the ongoing left posterior quadrant discharge. By 00:37:32 spread to T3 is evident. Seizures in neonates often alternate, or "ping pong," from one side to the other.

subarachnoid hemorrhage. In these situations the background activities and state organizations usually are normal, and prognosis is good. Similar focal ictal discharges also may occur in the presence of acquired or congenital brain lesions. In these infants the EEG often exhibits abnormalities of background, such as interhemispheric amplitude asymmetry and focal attenuation.

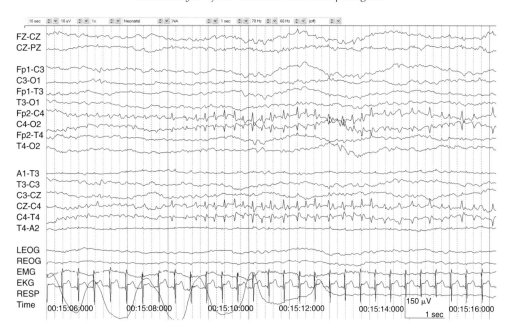

FIGURE 3–14

Electrographic seizure, surface positive: An infant of 40 weeks' postconceptional age with partial seizures and hypocalcemia. An asymptomatic surface-positive electrographic seizure occurs at C4 with rhythmic spikes at 4 Hz.

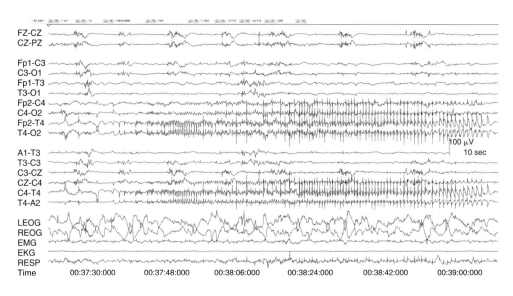

FIGURE 3–15

Electrographic seizure, focal 1: An infant of 40 weeks' postconceptional age with meningitis. This page contains 2 minutes of compressed EEG to demonstrate the entire extent of the seizure. At 00:37:32, repetitive T4 spikes begin and over the next 10 seconds become rhythmic spikes. This spreads centrally; by 00:39:05 the discharge begins to end with slow spike discharges at T4 and then attenuates completely.

5. *Pseudo-delta, -theta, -alpha, and -beta activity* consists of runs of rhythmic monomorphic waves ranging from 0.5 to 15 Hz, therefore resembling normal background activities. Their amplitude varies from a low of 20 to 30 μV to a high of 200 μV, generally being higher for the slower frequencies. They may occur with a generalized or a focal distribution. They can appear in all states, but as they often occur

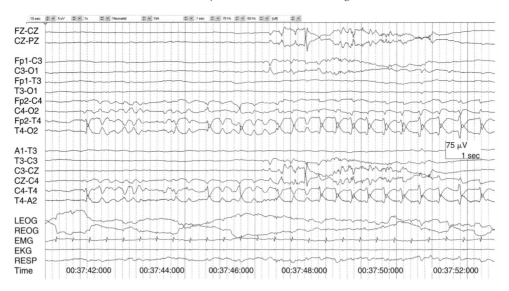

FIGURE 3–16

Electrographic seizure focal 2: Expanded time base of seizure onset from Figure 3-15. In the 2nd second, a clear rhythmic spike onset is seen in the right temporal region.

in severely compromised neonates, state organization may be disrupted, and background activities undifferentiated. These discharges can be seen (1) after severe hypoxic-ischemic insults, (2) after intraventricular hemorrhages, (3) in neonates with inborn metabolic defects, or (4) in infants with various chromosomal and dysgenetic brain abnormalities (Fig. 3-17).

C. Low-frequency discharge patterns
    1. Low-frequency discharge patterns are stereotyped, repetitive, rhythmic, or "quasi-rhythmic" paroxysmal discharges consisting of sharp, broad-based waves occurring at low frequencies (around 0.5 to 1Hz). These discharges may involve focal or multifocal areas or involve an entire hemisphere. This pattern is similar to the periodic lateralized epileptiform discharges (PLEDs) seen in older children.
    2. To fit the definition of PLEDS, these discharges cannot exhibit evolution in morphology, frequency, or field and cannot be associated with ictal manifestations. Almost invariably these discharges occur in the context of abnormal backgrounds, usually of invariant, inactive, or low-voltage patterns.

Computerized seizure detection in newborns recently has been described with seizure detection rates at greater than 70% accuracy, with a false detection rate of 1.7/hr. A confirmatory study revealed similar findings. This may be a helpful tool in long-term monitoring of the newborn.

CLASSIFICATION AND IMPRESSION

Classification of the record as normal or abnormal is the most important step in interpreting a neonatal record. If the record is abnormal, a list of abnormal features is reported.

Impression takes into account the classification made, abnormal features, and patient's history (including use of medications and findings prior to EEG testing). Even in neonates, barbiturates and benzodiazepines may cause diffuse beta activity and should not be interpreted as a seizure or abnormal record.

Follow-up examinations may be suggested if the examination is technically difficult or technically unsatisfactory, maturation of the neonate is inconsistent with the EEG findings, or results of therapeutic interventions are analyzed (Table 3-3).

ANALYZING A NEONATAL EEG—FIVE-STEP APPROACH

I. Postconceptional age and topography
    A. Determination of postconceptional age
    B. Topography
        1. Confirm head position
        2. Confirm the location of scars or intravenous lines
        3. Confirm any edema
II. Artifacts

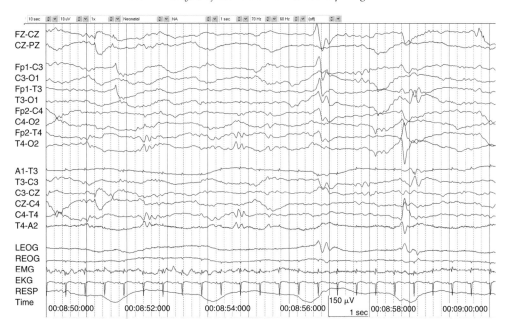

FIGURE 3–17

Pseudo-theta: An infant of 35 weeks' gestational age at 3 days of life. Patient is having alternating jerking movements of all four extremities. Focal monorhythmic theta at 7 Hz is seen in the right temporal and left central regions, independently.

TABLE 3–3. INTERPRETATION OF THE NEONATAL EEG

Classification of Features	Impression
Normal features	Normal for gestational age
Immature pattern	Cerebral dysfunction or gestational age not calculated correctly
Multifocal abnormalities	Multifocal or diffuse cerebral dysfunction
Background abnormalities	Multifocal or diffuse cerebral dysfunction
Focal abnormalities	Focal cerebral dysfunction
Electrographic seizures	Focal or multifocal epileptogenic regions

    A. Locate

    B. Describe

  III. Identification of sleep and wake states

    A. Determine cycling through awake, quiet, and active sleep states

    B. Analyze the distinctness of the changes in sleep state

    C. Determine and evaluate the duration of each sleep state

    D. Determine the presence of a quiet sleep pattern, tracé discontinu, tracé alternant, or high-voltage slow wave

      1. Evaluate noncerebral physiological patterns and determine whether they are consistent with quiet sleep

      2. Determine whether the EEG pattern is appropriate for postconceptional age

    E. Determine whether REM sleep is continuous

      1. Determine whether noncerebral physiological patterns are concordant with quiet sleep

      2. Determine whether the pattern is appropriate for postconceptional age

  IV. Feature extraction

    A. Determine whether abnormalities in quiet sleep, active, sleep or wakefulness are present

    B. Determine amplitude

    C. Determine continuity

    D. Determine frequency

    E. Determine synchrony

    F. Determine maturation

    G. Note any paroxysmal abnormalities

      1. Interictal

      2. Ictal

  V. Classification of the record

    A. Determine whether normal or abnormal

    B. Determine the clinical correlation

    C. Determine the need for follow-up

REFERENCE

1. Hahn JS, Monyer H, Tharp BR: Interburst interval measurements in EEGs of premature infants with normal neurologic outcome. Electroencephalogr Clin Neurophysiol 1989;73:410-418.

SUGGESTED READING

Gotman J, Flanagan D, Zhang J, Rosenblatt B: Automatic seizure detection in the newborn: Methods and initial evaluation. Electroencephalogr Clin Neurophysiol 1997;103:356-362.

Gotman J, Flanagan D, Rosenblatt B, et al: Evaluation of an automatic seizure detection method for the newborn EEG. Electroencephalogr Clin Neurophysiol 1997;103:363-369.

Hrachovy RA, Mizrahi EM, Kellaway P: Electroencephalography of the newborn. *In* Daley DD, Pedley TA (eds): Current Practice of Clinical EEG. New York, Raven Press, 1990, pp 201-242.

Mizrahi EM, Kellaway P: Characterization and classification. *In* Diagnosis and Management of Neonatal Seizures. Philadelphia, Lippincott-Raven, 1998, pp 15-34.

Stockard-Pope JE, Werner SS, Bickford RG: Atlas of Neonatal Electroencephalography. NY, Raven Press, 1992.

Tharp BR, Cukier F, Monod N: The prognostic value of the electroencephalogram in premature infants. Electroencephalogr Clin Neurophysiol 1981;51:219-236.

Volpe JJ: Neonatal seizures: Current concepts and revised classification. Pediatrics 1989;84:422-428.

4

Normal Development of the Electroencephalogram: Infancy Through Adolescence

WARREN T. BLUME

Accurate and confident interpretations of pediatric electroencephalograms are afforded by optimal technique and by a full appreciation of normative values. Avoiding the pitfalls of pediatric electroencephalogram (EEG) interpretation includes the recognition of normal patterns during wakefulness and sleep.[1] Because pediatric electroencephalography differs in certain ways from both adult and neonatal EEGs in each of these respects, this chapter covers both topics, particularly the latter.

TECHNIQUE

Certain modifications of preparation and recording are needed to accommodate the needs and particularities of the infant and child.

Personnel

An experienced pediatric EEG technologist generally obtains a higher quality recording than a novice for several reasons. First, a confident approach relaxes the child. An experienced technologist generally is more able to handle the difficult child and to apply electrodes and obtain valuable data from a recalcitrant patient.

Knowledge of the sign posts of wakefulness, drowsiness, and sleep as well as the occasionally different morphology of recorded seizures helps the experienced technologist to adjust the recording according to its initial findings and also according to the question posed by the clinician. Thus, the technologist should also be familiar with pediatric neurologic conditions in which diagnosis and management can be clarified by EEG.

However, it has been my experience that the quality of the EEG recording relates more closely to the overall competence of the technologist more than any specific quantity of experience with children. Highly qualified technologists can record patients competently at any age. (Therefore, our laboratory has long maintained the policy that all its technologists should be competent in performing children's EEGs.)

The technologist should make every effort to present him or herself to the patient and relatives in a clean, and positive manner. As with adults, a child can recognize a poor, incompetent approach and will deal with it directly and accordingly.

Recording Room

If practical conditions and patient volume permit, devotion of one or two rooms of a general EEG laboratory to the pediatric EEG is useful. The clean and well-organized room should be large enough to contain an EEG, a sink, a small table for electrodes, a large mattress-covered surface such as an examining table, and a comfortable chair. Oversized and under-sized rooms have disadvantages and frighten young patients. All equipment required for the recording should be ready and accessible beforehand because continuity of preparation increases the infant's and child's confidence and cooperation.

Appointments

At any age, the quality of recording is improved if patient discomfort is kept to a minimum. For infants and young children, this means that they should be fed, dry, and warm. Thus, for children in the first year of life an appointment shortly after feeding is optimal. Young children are best recorded early in the afternoon to coincide with a nap so that both a sleep and an awake recording can be accomplished. So that the child does not sense that the technologist is rushing the procedure, appointment intervals of at least 90 minutes are necessary.

Parents and Guardians

A frequently asked question is whether a parent or guardian should remain in the room during the electrode placement and recording. During the initial history taking, the technologist can assess a parent's attitude toward his or her child and to the concept of having an EEG. A parent with a relatively positive attitude helps the child behave during the procedure, whereas a parent who feels that the test is an imposition generally hinders the child's cooperation. At times, a well-intentioned parent will impair the child's cooperation. In such negative circumstances, the technologist can explain to the parent that the procedure will proceed more fluidly if limited to the technologist and the child.

Electrode Application

As stated earlier, all necessary equipment required to apply the electrodes should be organized beforehand so that interruptions do not occur. Electrodes applied with collodion are generally preferred to other means because movement creates less artifact and is less likely to dislodge an electrode. Because gross movements are less likely to occur in patients younger than 1 year of age, disk electrodes with electrolyte paste can be satisfactorily used.

Between ages 3 months to 18 months, electrodes are applied with the patient placed in a supine position. The infant is partially bundled up to reduce movements and is usually being fed during electrode application.

The most difficult age to apply electrodes is between 18 months and 6 years. Electrodes are usually applied with the patient seated. After a general explanation of the procedure, each step is explained as it is carried out. Close technologist-patient relationship during the 20 minutes or

more required for electrode application is essential. Beyond age 6 years cooperation usually spontaneously improves and becomes similar to that of an adult. Children with cognitive impairment may present with cooperation difficulties at any age. However, a calm and reassuring attitude with the mentally impaired child makes the application of electrodes much less difficult.

The EEG Recording

Montages, Electrode Positions, and Settings

For infants less than 3 months old, FP1/2, C3/C4, O1/2, T3/4, and Cz positions suffice in our laboratory. However, other pediatric laboratories choose to use a full complement of electrodes in patients of all ages except the very preterm infant. A full complement of positions can be used at later ages unless the head is small.

Straight longitudinal anteroposterior and coronal montages are the simplest to interpret and best resist movement and other artifact. An ear reference montage may follow, particularly to identify morphology of some diffuse waveforms. Additional montages are rarely required in my experience.

For infants younger than 3 months of age, a single bipolar anteroposterior montage and a coronal chain through Cz will record all electrode positions adequately and no additional montage is required. At this age, recording the extraocular movements, respiration, and heart rate is a useful guide to state.

EEG voltages are usually higher in children than in adults and therefore the usual initial sensitivity setting is 10 to 15 μV/mm. Because quantity of delta activity is important to assess, a time constant of 0.3 second is preferred. Higher frequencies are usually not filtered unless uncorrected muscle artifact obscures the tracing, but this occurs rarely.

However, recording situations differ widely, particularly in children. General recording principles will guide the technologist to more appropriate settings. When using paper EEGs, technologists should avoid frequent changes of montages, sensitivity, filters, and paper speed since this hinders the electroencephalographer from assessing changes of EEG with state, and this is an important component in EEG interpretation of children. This is much less of an issue with digital technology.

Although digital recording permits offline frequency response, sensitivity adjustments, and montage selection; the technologist should employ optimal settings to address the purpose of the EEG and its findings en route.

For a detailed review of recording techniques, the reader should refer to Chapter 1.

Age-Related Procedures

Between ages 3 and 18 months, wrapping the child in a blanket keeps him or her sufficiently warm and limits movements, thus encouraging sleep. Sleep is also encouraged by a monotonous sound such as tap water, a darkened room, and soft whispering by the technologist. Avoid rocking because it may create artifactual delta activity. At this age it is particularly important to have the EEG close to the patient so that behavioral changes can be observed. Because the electrode application procedure usually fatigues a child at this age (and the technologist!), the child usually falls asleep for the initial part of the tracing. Following arousal, some portion of awake recording can be obtained, including use of passive eye closure. To accomplish this maneuver, which reveals the basic alpha rhythm not otherwise seen, a technologist blows gently on the eyes to elicit closure and then holds the eyes lightly closed for a few seconds.

Between the ages of 18 months and 6 years, the child is also recorded supine, but bundling the child is less often required unless movements are excessive. Spontaneous sleep usually occurs in the younger children of this age group during the initial part of the recording and therefore the awake portion can be reserved for the latter half of the procedure. Passive eye closure is important when the child is alert and can be accomplished as described earlier. Older children may close their eyes spontaneously if requested. Again, the EEG should be close to the child so that behavioral observations can be easily viewed.

Between ages 6 and 16 years children can be recorded supine or seated. Most of the recording time is taken up by wakefulness. Cooperative children usually close and open their eyes on request in this age group. Sleep could be obtained spontaneously by placing a blanket over the child and creating a monotonously quiet room.

The technologist should reassure the child who arouses during the recording because the environment is a strange one for most patients. It is important to continue recording during arousal because abnormalities may appear only during this phase.

Hyperventilation

Hyperventilation is obtained in older children and adolescents in the usual fashion as adults. Younger children can be encouraged to blow on a plastic windmill or a handkerchief. As at other ages, hyperventilation may elicit focal or epileptiform abnormalities and therefore is a valuable component of the recording.

Photic Stimulation

Because a photoparoxysmal response is often indicative of an ongoing seizure tendency in children with febrile seizures and may be markedly present in patients with progressive myoclonic encephalopathies, it should not be omitted in pediatric EEG recordings. The procedure does not differ from that used in adults.

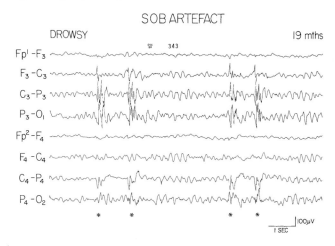

FIGURE 4–1

Example of sob artifact.

Annotation

Surprisingly, one of the aspects that most clearly distinguishes experienced technologists from novices is the quality, appropriateness, and legibility of annotation. Because changes of state occur more readily in pediatric patients, a notation of the apparent clinical state enables the electroencephalographer to judge whether the clinical EEG correlation is normal for age. Moreover, annotation of movement, sucking, rocking, and other potentially artifact-producing phenomena helps the electroencephalographer distinguish such events from cerebral potentials (Fig. 4-1). On occasion the lack of any movement or other event should be annotated if an EEG phenomenon usually associated with a clinical change appears.

Sedation

Sedation may augment both theta and beta activity, slow the background rhythms, and even impair the development of deep sleep. Therefore, a more accurate recording is obtained when it is sedation free. Only about 1% of pediatric patients require sedation for electroencephalography, and these are usually cognitively impaired patients or those with major behavior disorders. A technologist who realizes that sedation is not an alternative develops techniques to elicit adequate patient cooperation.

THE NORMAL EEG

Introduction

As compared with normal EEGs in adults, those of normal infants and children contain a greater variety of waveforms of usually higher voltage. The resulting superimposition of rhythms at various frequencies creates complex, often sharply contoured and bizarre waveforms that can confuse the inexperienced reader. Conservative interpretation is advisable. By answering the following five questions and by memorizing some reasonably consistent facts, the complexities can be unraveled:

1. In what state is the patient? A greater percentage of children's recordings is carried out in drowsiness and sleep and the corresponding modifications are generally more pronounced and peculiar to the pediatric age group.
2. Is the electrical maturation for this state adequate?
3. Are there any consistent, marked, nonartifactual asymmetries that are not usually accepted for the waveform in question?
4. Are there any spikes? Remember that these must be clearly distinguished from sharply contoured waveforms created by combinations of frequencies.
5. Is there any focal or diffuse excess delta activity for age and state?

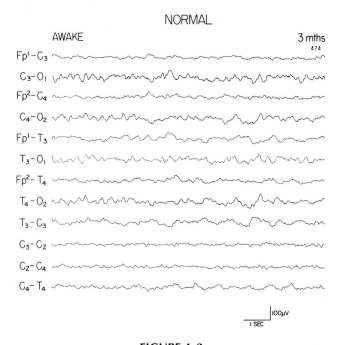

FIGURE 4–2
Normal awake EEG in a 3-month-old child.

Wakefulness

Delta and Theta

Except for older children and adolescents, the reader will initially be faced with a mixture of delta and theta activity in awake tracings with the eyes open. With age, the proportion of theta activity gradually increases in comparison with delta activity.

Studies using frequency analysis suggest that delta activity dominates during the first 12 months of life[2,3]; theta and delta appear in approximately equal quantity to visual analysis in the first year with the eyes open (Fig. 4-2). Although the absolute quantity of delta increases even to the fifth year, this increase is less than that for theta and therefore the theta-to-delta ratio increases with age. Delta may be transiently asymmetrical, and a slight predominance on one side should not be given any clinical significance. A prolonged portion of the record should be carefully examined, and the possibility of an artifact component should be carefully excluded before concluding that delta activity was significantly more prominent on one side. Scrutiny of recordings in older children and even to adolescence reveals the continuing presence of some delta activity, principally when the eyes open to attenuate alpha.

The quantity of theta increases during the first few years of life to reach a peak of about 5 to 6 years and then declines.[4,5] Theta involved in "posterior slow of youth" may, however, become more prominent in later ages. With eyes open or closed, theta is the most prominent activity in recordings of the 2- to 5-year-old age group. Because eye closure elicits alpha activity, the total quantity of theta is

about equal to alpha at age 5 to 6 years, after which alpha gradually becomes the more prominent waveform. Because the absolute quantity of theta varies considerably among normal children, assessment of theta quantity is not among the five questions suggested earlier.

However, there are two instances in which prominent diffuse theta is clearly abnormal. Theta may be the only rhythm in globally impaired children who have a static encephalopathy. In this instance, it is the lack of other rhythms that constitutes the abnormality. Second, bursts of 3- to 4-Hz waves during definite wakefulness may occasionally herald the later presence of spike waves. Rhythmic theta may be the more obvious component of such complexes.

"Background" Frequencies

Among his many other accurate observations on the EEG of humans, Berger[6] was the first to recognize that the frequency of background activity in childhood increased with age. Such frequencies are best appreciated by passive eye closure, which can be accomplished as early as 3 months of age.[7-9] No discernible dominant occipital activity appears until age 3 months, when a 3- to 4-Hz rhythm can be seen.[10,11] This rhythm increases to about 5 Hz by age 5 months, to 6 to 7 Hz at age 12 months, and to about 7 to 8 Hz in the third year of life (Fig. 4-3).[12,13] By age 3 years, an 8-Hz posterior rhythm appears, usually of higher voltage than in adolescents. Petersen and Eeg-Olofsson[9] found a 9-Hz rhythm to be the mean at age

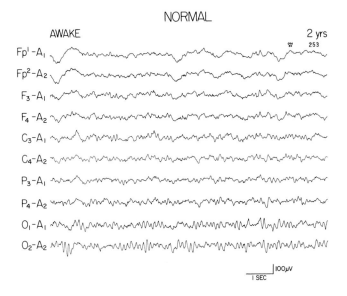

FIGURE 4–3
Normal awake recording in a 2-year-old child.

7 years and a 10-Hz rhythm by age 15 years. These authors found an 8- to 12-Hz background in middle to late adolescence, usually higher on the right than left.

In assessing the normality of background rhythms, a conservative approach is suggested. There remain wider ranges of normality in this and other respects in pediatric electroencephalography. Drowsiness, sometimes difficult to clinically appreciate by the technologist, can slow the background rhythm by 1 to 2 Hz. A more confident decision of abnormality would be justified if the background rhythm, in a definitely awake child whose eyes were actively or passively closed, was 2 or more Hz lower than the values listed earlier.

Although many studies have shown background activity to be higher in the right hemisphere, normal shifts of prominence can appear during a recording and between bipolar and referential montages. No convincing relationship between higher background amplitude and handedness has been demonstrated.

Posterior Rhythms

A prominent feature confounding interpreters of children's EEGs is the wide variety of waves that normally appear in the posterior head. Because most of these appear with eyes closed, they become superimposed on the background activity, creating sharply contoured and other bizarre waveforms. These can be distinguished from occipital spikes by the even sharper configuration of the latter with prominent aftercoming slow waves. Moreover, at least some patients with occipital spikes have abnormal background activities such as a lack of background over the side of the spikes.

The various forms of posterior slow of youth were studied by Aird and Gastaut[14] and by Petersen and Eeg-Olofsson.[9] Each of these varieties is described below.

Polyphasic Potentials

Two- to 4-Hz (250 to 500 millisecond) single or multiple waves can be seen inserted between alpha waves whose amplitudes are suddenly larger than usual. This combination of a larger alpha and such rhythmic slow waves may superficially resemble spike waves. The distinction is made by assessing the morphology of the associated alpha wave, which differs little from that of other alpha waves (Fig. 4-4). These preceding alpha waves and others that may be superimposed on the slower wave create the polyphasic morphology of the phenomenon and hence its name. Curiously, such polyphasic potentials are usually moderately more prominent on the right posterior temporal area (T6) than the left. Petersen and Eeg-Olofsson[9] found such phenomena in almost all normal controls. The quantity of this activity increases gradually in the first 10 years of life, becoming most prominent in very early adolescence. Residual amounts of such activity can be seen far beyond the pediatric age group.

Slow Posterior Rhythms or Posterior Rhythmic Waves

Rhythmic or sinusoidal 3- to 4-Hz waves may appear in groups or prolonged runs posteriorly in 25% of normal subjects (Fig. 4-5).[9] Eye closure may precipitate such rhythms for 1 to 3 seconds. Prolonged runs of such rhythmic waves may gradually merge into posteriorly situated spike waves.[10,15] In such situations, hyperventilation or photic stimulation may elicit such spike-wave paroxysms.

Slow Alpha Variant

Not infrequently, the background rhythm with the eyes closed may simply be a semirhythmic or notched 4- to 5-Hz series of waves either unilaterally or bilaterally. This may simply represent drowsiness and/or the "slow alpha variant," which is an approximate halving of the usual background rhythm.

Lambda Waves

In contrast with the three previously described posterior phenomena that appear with the eyes closed, lambda waves occur exclusively with eyes open. Although the most constant and prominent phase is surface positive, a negative phase may also appear. Blinking or saccadic eye movements may elicit such phenomena whose sharply contoured appearance may resemble occipital spikes. However, occipital spikes appear almost exclusively with the eyes closed, are virtually always electronegative, are often less

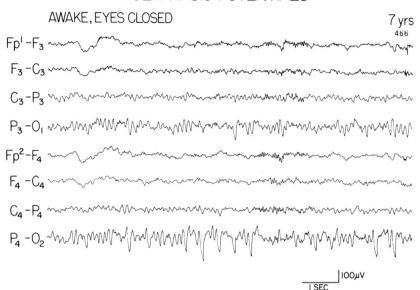

FIGURE 4–4

Polyphasic activity in the posterior head region of a 7-year-old child. Note the mixture of alpha and delta range frequencies.

confined to the O1-2 electrodes, and are usually followed by an aftercoming slow wave. There is a strong correlation between the presence of lambda waves and photic driving.[16]

Contamination of the EEG by the electrocardiogram (ECG) may occasionally produce potentials resembling lambda. An ECG monitor and the regularly repetitive nature of such potentials would distinguish them from lambda. Lambda waves are usually bilaterally symmetrical, but I am unaware of any study in children that ascribes an abnormality to unilateral or predominantly unilateral lambda.

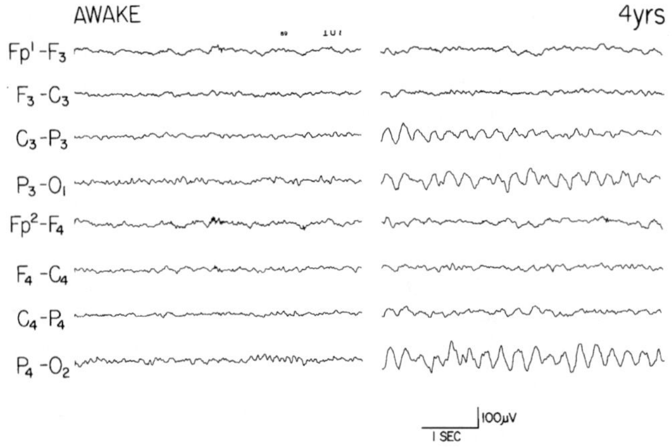

Finally, blinking may evoke high voltage (100 to 200 μV) electronegative, sharply contoured occipital waves with preceding and following electropositive waves. This phenomenon is unique to children, occurring from ages 6 months to about 10 years. Because they can be associated with scanning objects that also produce lambda, these phenomena may share its physiologic mechanism.

Central Rhythms

Sustained activity develops earlier in the rolandic regions (C3, C4) than other areas.[2] A 6- to 7-Hz rolandic rhythm may appear before age 3 months and its frequency may increase to 8 to 10 Hz after 3 months.[8,15] The most prominent EEG rhythm in an awake 1- to 5-year-old child with his or her eyes open is this central rhythm that can wax and wane on either side. The transient presence of moderate asymmetries of such rhythms may therefore be within normal limits. There may be a close resemblance of the frequently sharply contoured normal central rhythms with rolandic spikes.[17] The field of rolandic spikes is more widespread than that of the central rhythm, and a referential recording may demonstrate a dipole.[10]

Frontal Activity

Because there is normally a relative paucity of frontal rhythms during wakefulness in children, any high-voltage activity in that region can result from either disconnection of electrodes or a marked frontal abnormality. Abnormal attenuation frontally would be most difficult to establish in children unless the sensitivity settings were increased considerably.

FIGURE 4–5

Posterior rhythmic waves induced by eye closure (right panel) in a 4-year-old child.

Symmetrical Activity

As already emphasized, many features of the child's EEG may be at least transiently asymmetrical. These include alpha, varieties of posterior slow of youth, central rhythms, and a left hemisphere-predominant theta.

Abnormal asymmetries can be identified more confidently if they persist and if other associated rhythms are also asymmetrical. Thus, a persistently lower posterior slow of youth with a lower alpha rhythm, each less than 50% of the homologous side likely represents an underlying abnormality. Fortunately, most abnormalities in pediatric EEG are sufficiently marked as to be identified with confidence (Figs. 4-6 and 4-7).

"ACTIVATING" PROCEDURES

Hyperventilation

When not present in the "resting record," hyperventilation can be useful in eliciting generalized spike-and-wave discharges, focal spikes, or even nonspecific focal activity

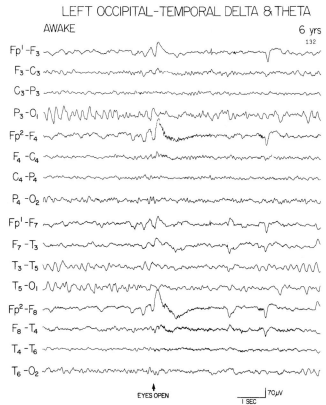

LEFT OCCIPITAL-TEMPORAL DELTA & THETA

FIGURE 4–7

Abnormal asymmetry with left occipital-temporal delta and theta activity in a 6-year-old child. Note the change of background with eye opening.

such as theta and delta. This principle applies to both children and adults. As compared with adults, the response to hyperventilation is usually greater: Alpha, theta and rhythmic delta amplitudes all augment markedly, particularly the latter. Such rhythmic delta activity initially appears posteriorly in patients younger than 8 to 10 years of age (Fig. 4-8); with continued hyperventilation it becomes diffuse. Because hyperventilation often creates high-voltage waveforms, these may appear sharply contoured. Moreover, the superimposition of ongoing background activity (not attenuated by hyperventilation) with such rhythmic waves may create a spike-and-wave–like appearance. Neither of such responses should be identified as epileptiform, "sharpish," or "spikey" because the receiver of the report may falsely identify such normal potentials as epileptogenic. Among a parade of errors commonly made in interpreting children's EEGs, this is among the more usual. The morphology of a true spike-and-wave discharge differs significantly from ongoing background activity and is seen synchronously in three or more channels in a bipolar recording.

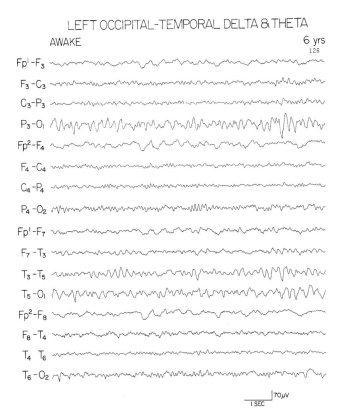

FIGURE 4–6

Abnormal asymmetry with left occipital-temporal delta and theta activity in a 6-year-old child.

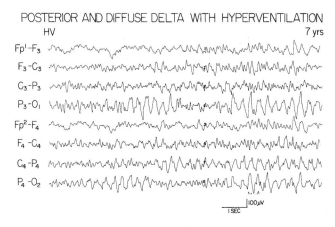

FIGURE 4–8

Posterior and diffuse delta elicited by hyperventilation in a 7-year-old child.

The quantity of slow waves elicited by hyperventilation depends on the age of the patient, effort in hyperventilating, and any hypoglycemia. Therefore, the quantity of such "build-up" cannot be assessed as normal or abnormal. The quantity of response to hyperventilation gradually decreases throughout adolescence to reach adult proportions in the late teenage years.

The effect of hyperventilation should subside by about 1 or 2 minutes after its cessation. However, the technologist should ensure that the child has indeed stopped over-breathing when requested to do so.

Photic Stimulation

The main role of photic stimulation is to elicit generalized spike-and-wave complexes in children who are suspected of having seizure disorders.

The photic following and driving response is usually maximum at lower flash rates among young children and the flash rate eliciting the maximum driving response increases in rough parallel with age.[11] The driving response can occasionally be normally notched resembling a spike-and-wave discharge. Distinction from an abnormal spike-and-wave discharge derives from the following: (1) the former, normal response is time locked to the flash rate and (2) it ceases immediately on cessation of flash rate. This low-amplitude spike-and-wave–like response has no clinical significance.

In contradistinction, photically induced spike and waves repeat at a frequency independent of the flash rate and often outlast its cessation. In contrast with normal photic driving, the field of such spike and waves extends considerably beyond the occipital region and may usually be frontally dominant in a bisynchronous fashion.

Although most patients with photically induced spike-and-wave discharges that outlast the flash rate have a generalized seizure disorder,[18] such a response may appear in persons who will not have a seizure disorder, particularly in siblings of patients with photic-sensitive generalized seizures.[19]

The most sensitive method of photic stimulation in eliciting spike-and-wave complexes is flash rates of 10 to 16 Hz with eye closure. To avoid precipitation of a grand mal seizure in extremely photic-sensitive patients, commencing photic stimulation with the eyes open and at low flash rates is advised.

Photic stimulation, searching for spike and waves, may be useful in evaluating patients suspected of having one of the progressive myoclonic epilepsies.[20] Neuronal ceroid lipofuscinosis may also produce very large bilateral occipital potentials to low flash rates.[21]

DROWSINESS AND SLEEP

Fatigued from the trip to the hospital, the preparation process, and a feed, infants and young children spend most of a routine recording in sleep. Older children commonly show episodes of drowsiness and light sleep. Patterns occur in normal drowsiness, sleep, and arousal that do not appear in adults, and the morphology of other universally appearing patterns differs in some respects from those produced by the more mature nervous system. For all these reasons, a thorough appreciation of such phenomena substantially helps the electroencephalographer read pediatric EEGs. Having become familiar with such patterns, they then serve as sign posts indicating state of the patient. Such indicators are often not present among the elderly, for example.

Drowsiness Patterns

Because the EEG signs of drowsiness usually begin while the child still appears awake, the recording could be falsely interpreted as containing excessively slow activity for age. Thus, in a young child, drowsiness may appear before sleep, following a prolonged sleep, and after crying.

Reflecting the greater tendency for rapid eye movement (REM) sleep in younger ages, the drowsy pattern in the first few months consists of low-voltage theta and beta activity diffusely without major regional preponderance. The most common drowsy pattern in older children is diffuse rhythmic to sinusoidal theta appearing maximally centrally, more posteriorly, or frontocentrally. This pattern is first seen at about age 3 months and becomes more prominent over the ensuing months, then becoming less evident after age 5 to 6 years (Fig. 4-9). Initially, the

THETA WITH DROWSINESS

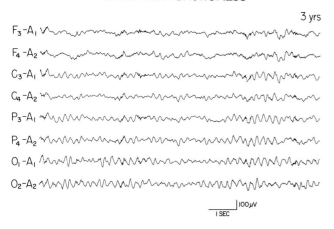

FIGURE 4–9
Theta activity during drowsiness in a 3-year-old child.

predominant rhythm is 3 to 5 Hz in the first year of life, increasing to 4 to 6 Hz by 4 to 5 years. Although the delta activity of normal wakefulness may augment slightly in drowsiness, this increase is far less than that of theta in infants and young children. Therefore, a marked delta increase with light drowsiness would represent a diffuse abnormality.

Less common are bursts of 2 to 5 Hz, rhythmic to sinusoidal, bilaterally synchronous waves whose amplitude may attain 350 μV (Fig. 4-10). Although these are usually

NORMAL DROWSINESS & SPIKE-WAVE

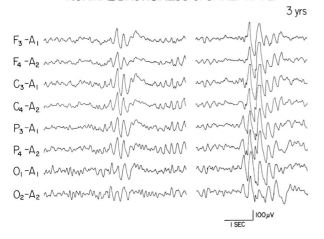

FIGURE 4–10
Comparison of a normal drowsy burst of slow activity (left panel) *versus spike-wave discharge* (right panel). *In the right panel, note the clear sequence of spike followed by slow wave and the widespread distribution of the discharge.*

maximum in the frontal central regions, they may appear principally in the posterior head regions in the first year. Although this phenomenon may first appear at 4 to 6 months of age, it is most common from 14 months to 5 years and may normally appear in rudimentary form to age 10 years. The superimposition of background rhythms, particularly those in the central head regions, may create a notch in the waveform and therefore could superficially resemble a spike-and-wave discharge. However, the sharply contoured component more closely resembles higher frequency central rhythms than any spike, and the distribution of this sharply contoured form is less widespread than that seen in a spike-and-wave discharge. Coronal bipolar and ipsilateral ear reference montages are the best in distinguishing these two phenomena (see Fig. 4-10). Fortunately, such bursts do not normally appear in light and moderate sleep, whereas spike-and-waves would continue to do so.

From 3 to 5 years of age onward, rhythmic 6- to 7-Hz frontally predominant but diffuse waves appear in drowsiness, with less tendency to burst. At the onset of drowsiness, this pattern may become superimposed on normal elements of wakefulness such as normal alpha rhythm. Subsequently, the alpha rhythm slows 1 to 2 Hz and any "posterior slow of youth" phenomenon increases. The slowing of alpha may merge with the continuous theta rhythms described earlier.

Even in children who are not taking medication, beta activity at 20 to 30 Hz may become more prominent in drowsiness from age 5 to 6 months. This activity may be diffusely distributed or may appear with an anterior or posterior maximum. Lateralizing asymmetries may normally appear, shifting from side to side. As with adults, such beta may appear in bursts and therefore distinction from bursts of polyspikes may be difficult.

A small percentage of children adopt an "adult" form of drowsiness: a diffuse reduction of electrical activity occurs such that low-voltage beta and theta are the principal drowsy components. After age 13 years, this feature becomes more common.

Sleep Patterns

Although REM sleep occupies 50% of total sleep time at birth, its quantity descends to 40% at 3 to 5 months and to about 30% at 12 to 24 months.[11] Therefore, this discussion covers primarily non-REM patterns.

V Waves

Rudiments of vertex waves can be detected at age 3 to 4 months, but well-developed V waves first appear at 5 months. Their maximum expression is attained at about 4 to 5 years and then gradually declines. Their higher voltage and briefer duration in children create a very sharply contoured morphology resembling spikes. V waves may be principally negative, positive, or diphasic. In children they may appear in 1- to 3-wave/sec sequences, lasting 5 to 10 seconds, giving an astonishingly spikelike allure to the tracing (Figs. 4-11 and 4-12). V waves are not as sharply contoured as most spikes, however, and any aftercoming slow wave is usually opposite in polarity to the major V-wave component, whereas the spike and wave have the same polarity. The V-wave field may be asymmetrical both in voltage and extent; usually these features shift from side to side. Therefore, in a coronal bipolar run, V waves may "phase reverse" alternately at C3 and C4. The extent of their field may also vary, creating a false impression of a higher voltage on the more peaked hemisphere in anteroposterior bipolar montages. Possibly because of the shifting nature of such asymmetries, V-wave asymmetry provides no guide to lesion lateralization.

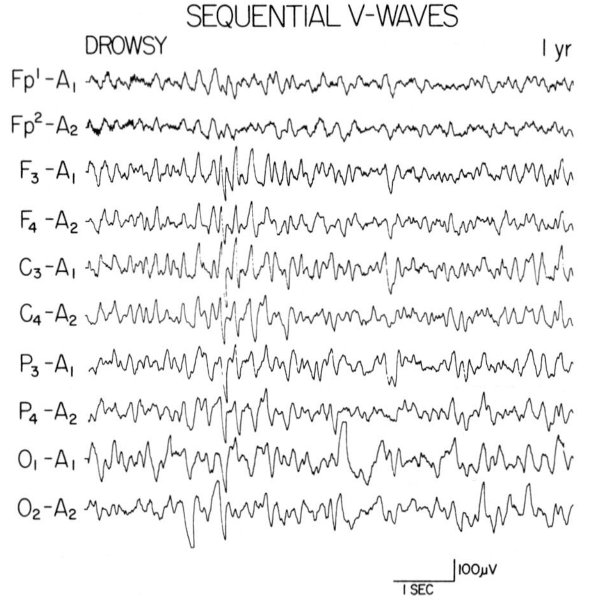

Spindles

Sequences of rhythmic 13- to 14-Hz waves may appear in light sleep in the first few days after term in infants. These may evolve to 14-Hz spindle-like activity by 1 to 3 months. More clearly defined spindles are normally present by 3 to 4 months of age. In the first year of life spindles are seen maximally in the central and parietal regions and frequently exhibit shifting asymmetries. Their morphology is often comb shaped and therefore resembles somewhat the mu rhythm of older ages (Fig. 4-13).

Total number of spindles and their length increase to a maximum at age 3 to 6 months and then decline.[22,23] Therefore, spindles are almost always present in non-REM sleep of normal children between ages 3 and 9 months.[24] The only exception would be a child who fell very rapidly into very deep sleep, deeper than the usual spindle range. Because such deep sleep may occur more prominently in the second year of life and the spindle quantity normally decreases in this period, the absence of spindles should not be considered a definite abnormality at that age.

Spindle rhythmicity is usually at 14 Hz with a mean of 12 to 15 Hz in infants and young children but such may slow to 10 to 12 Hz in deep sleep after age 3-5 years.

FIGURE 4–11

Example of vertex sharp waves during drowsiness in a 1-year-old child.

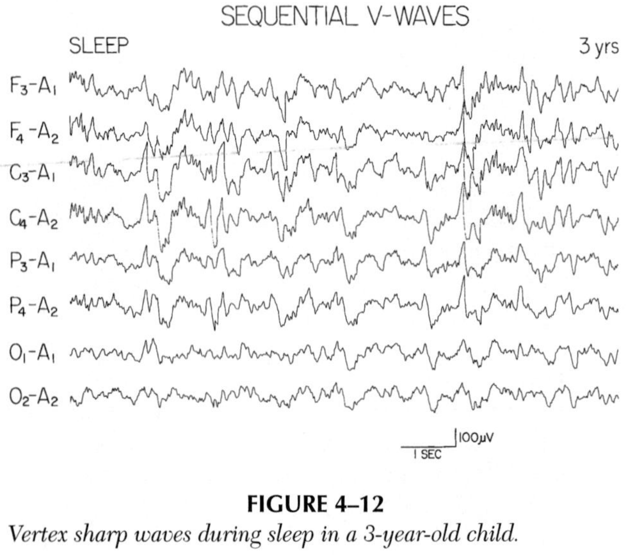

FIGURE 4–12

Vertex sharp waves during sleep in a 3-year-old child.

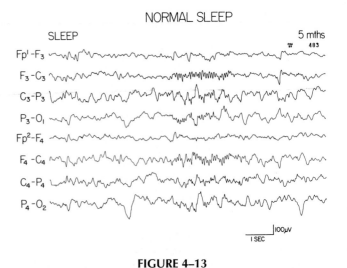

FIGURE 4–13

Bilateral sleep spindles in the central region in a 5-month-old child.

As stated earlier, spindle asynchrony or shifting asymmetry is common in the first year of life but spindles usually become more bilaterally synchronous and symmetrical in children 12 to 36 months of age. A consistent spindle asymmetry may reflect a lesion on the lower side. To ensure oneself of this, the aforementioned shifting asymmetry and a breach rhythm should be excluded. Bilateral anteroposterior and ipsilaeral ear reference montages best serve this evaluation.

Delta and Theta in Sleep

As non-REM sleep deepens, the quantity of 1- to 3-Hz waves increases whereas that of 4 to 6 Hz relatively decreases. Such delta activity almost always appears principally over the occipital regions in children younger than 4 years of age (see Fig. 4-13). In fact, Slater and Torres[25] found that the lack of such posterior-accentuated delta activity in sleep at this age constituted an abnormality.

Positive Occipital Sharp Transients of Sleep (Lambdoid Waves)

Positive occipital sharp transients of sleep appear moderately well developed in light sleep at ages 3 to 5 years but are less commonly present than among adolescents and adults.[15] These and the occasionally sharply contoured posterior delta of deep sleep can create sharply contoured waves posteriorly that are not spikes.

Fourteen and Six Per Second Positive Spikes and "Rhythmic Mid-Temporal Discharges"

The term *14 and 6* refers to an overpublicized drowsiness or light sleep phenomenon consisting of a 60- to 70-μV comb-shaped burst whose sharp components repeat at about 14 Hz and/or about 6 to 7 Hz and that last usually less than 1 second. As with other clinically innocent sharply contoured waveforms, the 14-and-6 field is widely distributed in the involved hemisphere even though its maximum voltage is relatively low. Montages with long interelectrode distances would best disclose their presence. Occasionally, distinction from sleep-activated posterior polyspikes can be difficult, but this can be usually achieved by recognizing three properties of such abnormal spikes: (1) the multiple-spike field is more restricted to the occipital posterior temporal region(s); (2) its frequency exceeds 14 Hz; and (3) they persist in moderately deep sleep.

Because neither Schwartz and Lombroso,[26] Lombroso and associates,[27] nor Eeg-Olofsson[28] found any correlation between the presence of such waveforms and any personality type or neurologic abnormality, they can be considered clearly normal phenomena. Indeed, Schwartz and Lombroso[26] found these in 55% of control subjects who were adolescents and young adults.

The psychomotor variant pattern is seen most commonly in adolescents and young adults and consists of a prolonged sequence of sawtoothed waves of 5 to 7 Hz appearing over one or both of the temporal regions in drowsiness. The lack of any further evolution of this pattern would distinguish it from a complex partial seizure of temporal lobe origin.[10] Although there have been rare associations of this pattern with underlying structural pathology,[29] in most patients this pattern can be considered a normal phenomenon.[8]

Arousal

From 0 to 2 months of age, arousal is associated with a simple attenuation of voltage of the EEG. By age 3 months, a low-amplitude diphasic slow wave may be evoked by afferent stimuli that would arouse the patient. By age 5 to 6 months, this diphasic wave may merge into a series of delta waves. By age 7 months, 4- to 8-Hz rhythmic waves may appear diffusely, maximum frontal-centrally for several seconds. This phenomenon becomes most prominent at age 13 months to 3 years and gradually declines.

Occurring simultaneously or directly after the aforementioned rhythmic 4- to 8-Hz theta is diffuse 1- to 3-Hz high-voltage delta activity that may initially appear maximally anteriorly but actually can persist longer posteriorly. This rhythm itself gradually increases in hertz to become diffuse theta.

This entire prolonged sequence is maximally expressed at 12 to 18 months of age and gradually declines to minimal after 4 to 5 years. Therefore, a pronounced delta pattern in arousal after age 4 to 5 years likely represents a diffuse encephalopathy.

Arousal attains the instantaneous adult form after approximately 7 years of age.

Acknowledgments

Mrs. Maria Raffa carefully typed the manuscript. The author offers special thanks to Mrs. Masako Kaibara for help with the illustrations and Mrs. Cathy Johnson for advice on the technology section.

REFERENCES

1. Mizrahi EM: Avoiding the pitfalls of EEG interpretation in childhood epilepsy. Epilepsia 1996;37(Suppl 1):S41-S51.
2. Hagne I, Peersson J, Magnusson R, Petersen I: Spectral analysis via fast Fourier transform of waking EEG in normal infants. *In* Kellaway P, Petersen I (eds): Automation of Clinical Electroencephalography. New York, Raven Press, 1973, p 103.
3. Walter WG: Normal rhythms—their development, distribution and significance. *In* Hill JDN, Parr G (eds): Electroencephalography. London, McDonald, 1950.
4. Corbin HPF, Bickford RG: Studies on the electroencephalogram of normal children: Comparison of

visual and automatic frequency analyses. Electroencephalogr Clin Neurophysiol 1955;7:15-28.

5. Hagne I: Development of the waking EEG in normal infants during the first year of life. *In* Kellaway P, Petersen I (eds): Clinical Electroencephalography of Children. New York, Grune & Stratton, 1968, p 97.

6. Berger H: On the electroencephalogram of man: Fifth report. Electroencephalogr Clin Neurophysiol 1969;(Suppl 28):151-171.

7. Pampiglione G: Development of rhythmic EEG activities in infancy: Waking states. Rev Electroenceph Neurophys Clin 1977;7:327.

8. Pampiglione G: Some criteria of maturation in the EEG of children up to the age of 3 years. Electroencephalogr Clin Neurophysiol 1972;32:463.

9. Petersen I, Eeg-Olofsson O: The development of the electroencephalogram in normal children from the age of 1 through 15 years: Non-paroxysmal activity. Neuropadiatrie 1971;2:247-304.

10. Blume WT, Kaibara M: Atlas of Pediatric Electroencephalography, 2nd ed. Philadelphia, Lippincott Williams & Wilkins, 1999.

11. Niedermeyer E, Lopes da Silva F: Maturation of the EEG: Development of waking and asleep patterns. *In* Niedermeyer E, Lopes da Silva F (eds): Electro-Encephalography. Basic Principles, Clinical Applications, and Related Fields, 2nd ed. Baltimore, Urban & Schwarzenberg, 1987, p 133.

12. Stroganova TA, Orekhova EV, Posikera IN: EEG alpha rhythm in infants. Clin Neurophysiol 1999;110:997-1012.

13. Marshall PJ, Bar-Haim Y, Fox NA: Development of the EEG from 5 months to 4 years of age. Clin Neurophysiol 2002;113:1199-1208.

14. Aird RB, Gastaut Y: Occipital and posterior electroencephalographic rhythms. Electroencephalogr Clin Neurophysiol 1959;11:637-656.

15. Niedermeyer E: Maturation of the EEG: Development of waking and sleep patterns. *In* Niedermeyer E, Lopes da Silva F (eds): Electro-Encephalography Basic Principles, Clinical Applications, and Related Fields. Baltimore, Urban & Schwarzenberg, 1982, p 133.

16. Shih JJ, Thompson SW: Lambda waves: Incidence and relationship to photic driving. Brain Topogr 1998; 10:265-272.

17. Beaumanoir A, Ballis T, Varfis G, Ansari K: Benign epilepsy of childhood with rolandic spikes: A clinical, electroencephalographic, and telencephalographic study. Epilepsia 1974;15:301-315.

18. Reilly EL, Peters JF: Relationship of some varieties of electroencephalographic photosensitivity to clinical convulsive disorders. Neurology 1973;23:1050-1057.

19. Doose H, Gerken H, Hien-Völpel KF, Völzke E: Genetics of photosensitive epilepsy. Neuropädiatrie 1969;1:56-73.

20. Berkovic SF, Andermann F, Carpenter S, Wolfe LS: Progressive myoclonus epilepsies: Specific causes and diagnosis. N Engl J Med 1986;315:296-305.

21. Pampiglione E, Harden A: So-called neuronal ceroid lipofuscinosis: Neurophysiological studies in 60 children. J Neurol Neurosurg Psychiatry 1977;40:323-330.

22. Lenard HG: The development of sleep spindles in the EEG during the first two years of life. Neuropädiatrie 1970;1:264-276.

23. Tanguay PE, Ornitz EM, Kaplan A, Bozzo ES: Evolution of sleep spindles in childhood. Electroencephalogr Clin Neurophysiol 1975;38:175-181.

24. Dreyfus-Brisac C, Curzi-Dascalova L: The EEG during the first year of life. *In* Leiry G (ed): Handbook of Electroencephalography and Clinical Neurophysiology, Vol 6-B. Amsterdam, Elsevier, 1975, p 24.

25. Slater GE, Torres F: Frequency-amplitude gradient: A new parameter for interpreting pediatric sleep EEGs. Arch Neurol 1979;36:465-470.

26. Schwartz IH, Lombroso CT: 14 and 6/second positive spiking (ctenoids) in the electroencephalogram of primary school pupils. J Pediatr 1968;72:678-682.

27. Lombroso CT, Schwartz IH, Clark DM, et al: Ctenoids in healthy youths: Controlled study of 14- and 6-per-second positive spiking. Neurology 1966;16:1152-1158.

28. Eeg-Olofsson O: The development of the electroencephalogram in normal children from the age of 1 through 15 years: 14 and 6 Hz positive spike phenomenon. Neuropädiatrie 1971;2:405-427.

29. Hennessy MJ, Koutroumanidis M, Hughes E, Binnie CD: Psychomotor EEG variant of Gibbs: An association with underlying structural pathology. Clin Neurophysiol 2001;112:686-687.

5

Visual Analysis of the Pediatric Electroencephalogram

Samuel E. Koszer, Leon Zacharowicz, and Solomon L. Moshé

Performing, analyzing, and interpreting the electroencephalogram (EEG) of a child may be an arduous task if one does not take into account special considerations. Some children lack insight into the need for such an examination and may work hard to thwart many attempts made by the technician to adequately record the EEG. During analysis the electroencephalographer may find that pediatric EEG patterns differ from those of the adult. Many features are age dependent, the EEG features may change dramatically with changes in state, there are a wide variety of intermixed waveform, and transient interhemispheric asymmetries are common. Certain patterns occur normally only in the pediatric EEG, and this must be considered when interpreting the examination.

As a practical guide to the analysis of the pediatric EEG, the goal of this chapter is to visually analyze the EEG, correlating patterns with age, state, and clinical context, and to arrive at the best possible description, classification, and interpretation of the EEG.

TECHNIQUE

In most children a technologist should be able to perform an EEG without the aid of sedation. When necessary, chloral hydrate is preferred to benzodiazepines because it produces less prominent beta activity (Fig. 5–1).[1] However, this can only be performed under supervision. In our laboratory, we currently do not sedate children, preferring to obtain natural sleep. This may be taxing for the technician and family because the child and the family may have to stay for a longer period. Whenever possible, a sleep-deprived EEG is obtained. Hyperventilation should be attempted. Photic stimulation is always included. Frequent, accurate, and legible notation by the technologist is important and helps the electroencephalographer to exclude artifacts and make electroclinical correlations.

PREREQUISITE INFORMATION

The technologist should provide information as discussed in the following sections.

Age. Since the EEG changes dramatically with maturity, knowing the age of the child is critical in determining whether patterns are normal or abnormal. In newborns the technician must note the conceptional and gestational age in weeks. During the first 3 years, the age in months should be provided; thereafter, the age in years is sufficient.

State. Waveforms may be normal or abnormal, depending on the state of the child. For example, a vertex spike may be a normal finding during sleep but would be abnormal during the awake state. The technologist should note whether the patient is awake, drowsy, or asleep. When necessary (e.g., coma), reactivity should be assessed by auditory, tactile, and/or noxious stimulation.

In addition to observing the child, the technician and electroencephalographer may obtain some clues about state

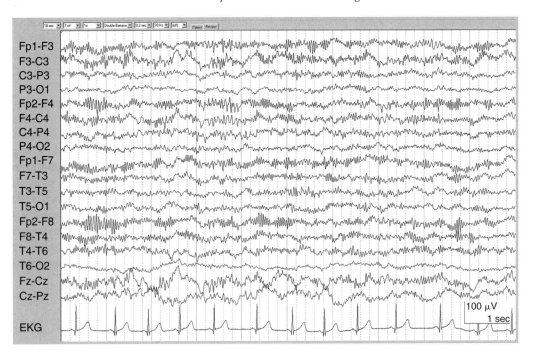

FIGURE 5–1

A 7½-year-old child was given chloral hydrate prior to the EEG administration. Diffuse fast activity is more prominent in the frontocentral regions.

by EEG findings. Artifacts such as muscle or eye blinks (Fig. 5–2) would suggest that the child is awake, whereas rolling eye movement (Fig. 5–3) or an increase in beta activity would suggest drowsiness (Fig. 5–4). Hypnogogic hypersynchrony in younger children would also suggest drowsiness.

Skull Defects. It is important for the technician to search for and note any skull defects. The intact skull and dura dampen the amplitude of cerebral activity by a factor of 10 to 1000 (as compared to the electrocorticogram). Skull defects may alter the scalp EEG with a breach rhythm (increased local voltage) due to increased current flow through the defect (Fig. 5–5). Skull defects can result in asymmetries in voltage and accentuated sharp activity on the side with a skull breach. Failure to recognize a skull defect can result in errors in the interpretation of the EEG.

Calibration. On pen-writing mechanical machines, the technologist and electroencephalographer should check the calibration carefully to be certain that the pen deflections occur synchronously, with the same amplitude and the same time constant. The alignment, height of the pen deflections, and slope of the curve as the pens return to baseline should be the same in each channel. Calibration errors may complicate the visual analysis of the EEG. If there is a defect in one or more pens, a number of errors can occur: if pen deflections are not accurate, errors will occur in determining the maximum amplitude of a discharge; if pen alignment is

faulty errors will occur in determining the area of onset of focal epileptiform discharges.

On digital EEG machines, calibration of the amplifiers is done automatically at the beginning of acquisition of data. To ensure that this is consistently being done accurately by the computer, a short examination of a calibration run is recommended at the beginning of the record.

Clinical History. Some electroencephalographers prefer to interpret the EEG with prior knowledge of the clinical context to expeditiously search for supportive or contradictory findings. Others perform the visual analysis (description) without prior knowledge of the clinical history, so that the analysis is not biased. Regardless of the personal style of the electroencephalographer, in approaching an EEG, there is a basic "formula":

EEG visual analysis + clinical history → clinical interpretation

The history is crucial for proper interpretation. It behooves the technician to obtain a brief history, in particular, why the EEG was requested. For children, a birth and developmental history may be helpful. Although this should be noted on the referral form, in reality many referring physicians provide insufficient information. Current medications taken and results of prior neuroimaging studies should be documented. Any family history of seizures should be

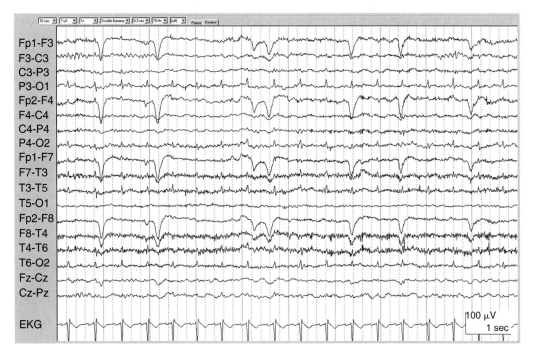

FIGURE 5–2

A 17-year-old child with psychosis. Bilateral temporal high-frequency muscle artifacts (35 to 40 Hz) are present along with seven prominent eye blinks. Note the downward deflections of eye closure followed by smaller upward deflections due to eye opening.

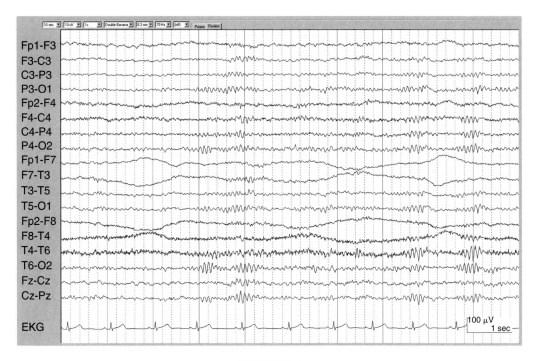

FIGURE 5–3

A 13-year-old child with impulsive behavior. Eye rolling is seen with 0.3-Hz slow waves occurring in the anterior-temporal areas bilaterally. Activity at F8 is 180 degrees out of phase with activity at F7.

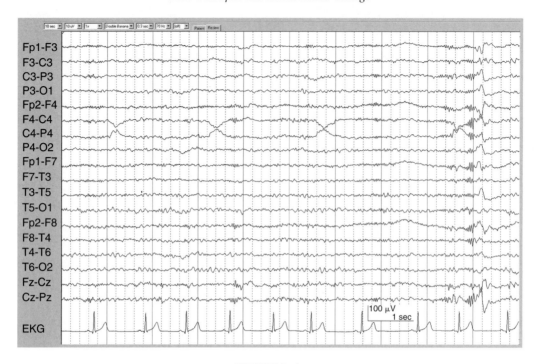

FIGURE 5–4

A drowsy 18-year-old with diffuse low-voltage beta that becomes more prominent in the 9th second just before a vertex wave.

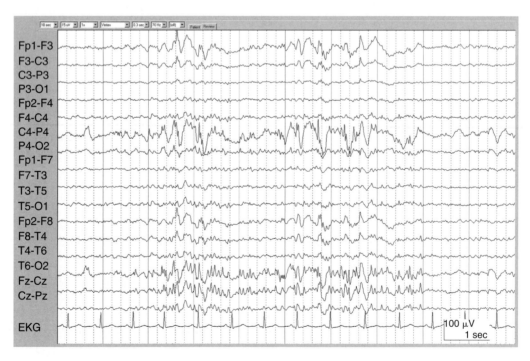

FIGURE 5–5

Mental retardation, seizures, and a breach in the right temporal region. Sharp, high-voltage, 20-to 25-Hz fast activity occurs in the right frontotemporal region.

mentioned. The time of the last and first seizure should be noted.

FEATURE EXTRACTION

Artifacts

The main aim of the electroencephalographer is the analysis and interpretation of features that are of cerebral origin. The EEG often contains activity of extracerebral origin that may resemble cerebral activity. These artifacts can be quite subtle and need to be recognized to avoid the inaccurate interpretation of the EEG. Artifacts in children are similar to the types seen in adults but may occur more frequently in a restless child. A fundamental concept in assisting the electroencephalographer in the differentiation of artifact from activity of electrocerebral origin is the *field*. The electrical fields produced by the dipoles of the cortex decrease in intensity proportional to the distance from their source. The greater the distance an electrode is from the source, the weaker the voltage field measured. This is visualized on the EEG by gradually diminished waveform amplitudes on at least one other adjacent channel and indicates greater distances from the source. Extracerebral activity such as movements or electrode "pops" does not produce a field (Fig. 5–6). Be aware, however, that strong external electromagnetic fields or cardiac-generated fields can show up on multiple or all recording electrodes. The stereotypic nature of these fields is usually sufficient to determine that they are not of electrocerebral origin.

The wide range of artifacts is divided into physiologic and nonphysiologic types. *Nonphysiologic artifact* refers to activity created by influences outside patients themselves. *Physiologic artifact* refers to activities generating electrical fields arising from a part of the patient's body other than the brain. Physiologic artifacts include muscle activity, the electrocardiogram (Fig. 5–7), pulse, eye movements (Fig. 5–8), movements of the tongue (glossokinetic potential) (Fig. 5–9), respiration, tremor, and perspiration (Fig. 5–10).

Although appropriate use of the high- and low-frequency filters may reduce the appearance of many types of artifacts on the recording, this may often compromise the interpretation of normal background activity. Therefore, it is more desirable to correct the source of artifact. Even if the artifact cannot be corrected, it is important for the technologist to try to determine the nature of artifacts at the time they occur. It may be difficult for the electroencephalographer to identify the cause of the artifacts after they have occurred.

In some cases, the electroencephalographer may initially be unsure whether a particular pattern is an artifact or cerebral in origin. Examination of subsequent pages and various montages may help in this determination.

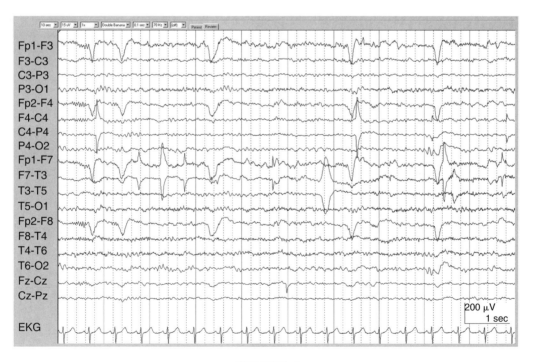

FIGURE 5–6

An 11-year-old boy with seizures. Three electrode pops are seen as mirror image artifacts in the 2nd and 3rd seconds at F7. An electrode pop occurs in T3 during the 6th second. A C4 pop is seen in the 7th second.

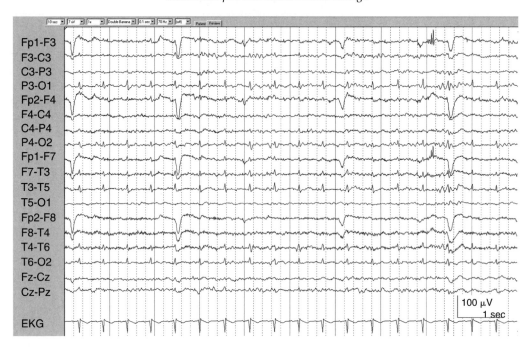

FIGURE 5–7

A 17-year-old child with psychosis. Left and right temporal occipital artifacts occur each 600 milliseconds coincident with the QRS complexes in the accompanying electrocardiogram seen at the bottom of the record.

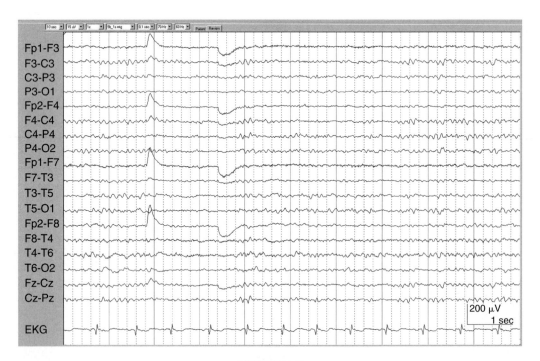

FIGURE 5–8

An 8-year-old boy with partial seizures. At the end of the 2nd second, there is an upward (negative) deflection in the frontal leads with eye opening. Note that the posterior background attenuates. In the middle of the 4th second there is a small frontal downward deflection with eye closure.

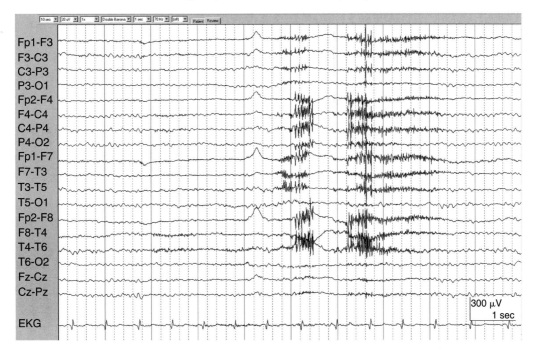

FIGURE 5–9

Glossokinetic potentials. In the 6th second, tongue movements with swallowing cause a temporal surface negativity and simultaneous frontal surface positivity.

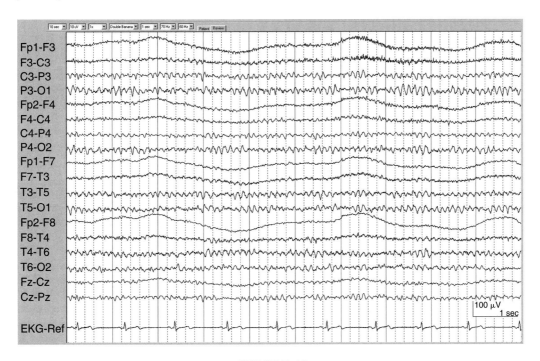

FIGURE 5–10

Very low-frequency frontal activity due to the presence of sweat.

Nonphysiologic Artifacts

All nonphysiologic artifacts need to be identified and excluded from further analysis. Most of the artifacts have no field or a limited field confined to one electrode or may appear as double-phase reversals (Fig. 5–11).

Some of the common artifacts are as follows:

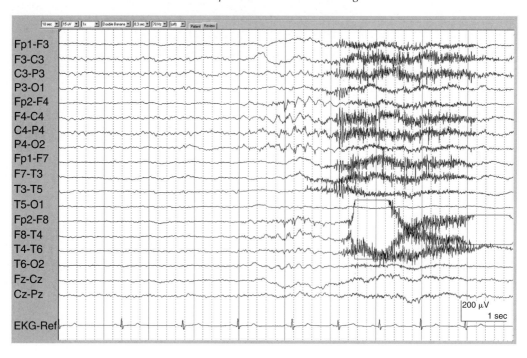

FIGURE 5–11

An adolescent with a right central rhythmic movement artifact. There are clear double-phase reversals seen at the 6th second in the right parasagittal chain.

1. *Electrode pops* are mirror-like activities involving only one electrode. These occur when the electrode-to-skull interface impedance varies. This is usually due to improperly applied electrodes or unequal impedances (see Fig. 5–6).

2. *60-Hz electrical interference* can occur when alternating voltage sources from nearby electrical devices emit a field strong enough to be picked up by the EEG machine. Poorly grounded EEG machines are also susceptible to 60-Hz artifact (Fig. 5–12).

3. *Amplifier "noise"* refers to noise inherent in amplifiers composing the EEG apparatus. With properly functioning amplifiers, this should be very low voltage.

4. *Movements in the recording environment* induce voltages when there are movements of conducting materials (in the external environment or from the patient) through ambient electromagnetic fields.

Physiologic Artifacts

Some of the physiologic artifacts are the following:

1. *Lateral and vertical eye movements*—Eye blink artifacts are of greatest amplitude in the anterior leads, and they need to be differentiated at times from frontal intermittent rhythmic delta activity (FIRDA) and other activities of cerebral origin. An eye montage may help

in this differentiation. The electrophysiologic model of the eye is a dipole with a negativity at the retina and a positivity at the cornea. On looking upward, which is also what occurs when the eyes are closed (Bell's phenomenon), the corneal positivity gets closer to Fp1 and Fp2 and causes a downward deflection in the channels that include the frontal electrodes in horizontal bipolar or standard reference montages. On opening the eyes or looking upward, the corneal positivity moves away from the frontal electrodes creating a change in voltage that is a relative negativity in the frontopolar regions. This appears as an upward deflection in horizontal or standard reference montages. Combinations of these vertical eye movements commonly occur with an eye blink, a downward deflection with a quick eye closure followed by a smaller upward deflection on opening (Fig. 5–13).

Lateral eye movements are more complex in their interpretation. A quick gaze to the right results in a surface-positive field from the right cornea to be seen in the right frontal and right temporal electrodes. Simultaneously, the left cornea moves *away* from the left temporal electrodes, creating a surface negativity in the left temporal region. Therefore, lateral eye movements to the right may be interpreted when a surface positivity appears in the right temporal region and a surface negativity occurs simultaneously in the left

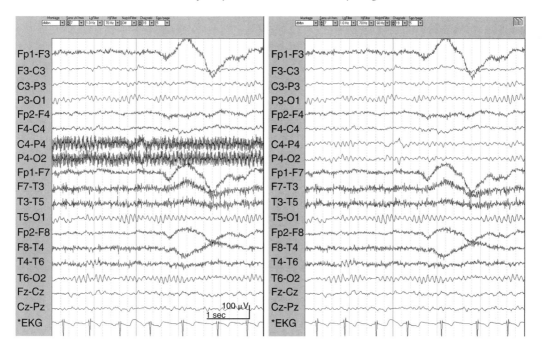

FIGURE 5–12

An 8-year-old boy with prominent P4 60-Hz electrical artifact. The left-sided EEG is one without a notch filter. The EEG on the right has a notch filter applied, demonstrating an underlying alpha rhythm on the right.

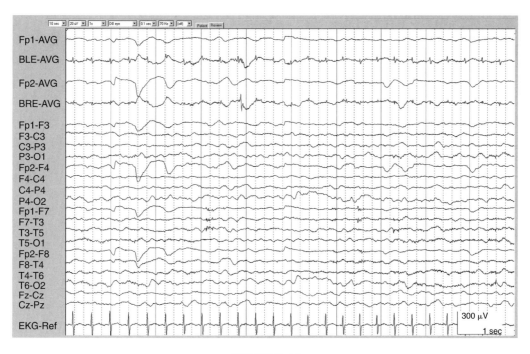

FIGURE 5–13

Adolescent with an eye blink in the 2nd second. This shows downward positive deflections in the frontal eye leads. Confirmation that these are eye movements rather than of cerebral origins is accomplished with the use of eye leads BLE (below left eye) and BRE (below right eye) and the use of an "eye montage."

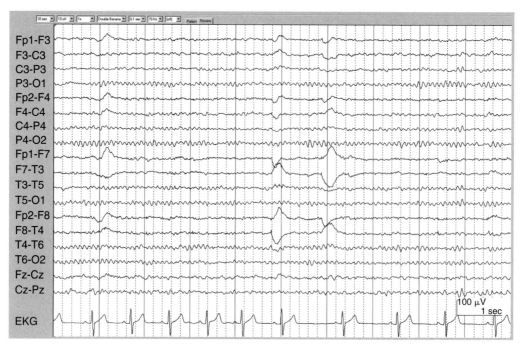

FIGURE 5–14

A 13-year-old child with inattentiveness and possible seizures. Lateral eye movements occur with characteristic surface positivity in the right anterior temporal area (F8) at the end of the 5th second and surface negativity in the left anterior temporal area (F7). The reverse polarity occurs in the 6th second when the patient looks to the left.

temporal region. A gaze to the left results in the reverse. Keep in mind that oblique eye movements have field characteristics with components of both vertical and lateral eye movements (Fig. 5–14).

2. *Electrocardiographic artifacts*—The heart generates an electrical field that is measured on the surface of the body with a magnitude of 1 mV. The high sensitivity of the EEG machine (measuring in microvolts) often detects distant electrocardiographic activity, especially in the temporal and ear leads (see Fig. 5–7).

3. *Movement artifact*—These appear as slow waves without an electrocerebral field due to changes in electrostatic potentials leading to voltage differences in an electrode pair (Fig. 5–15).

4. *Motor unit artifact*—Using a high-frequency filter of 70 Hz these are very sharp, fast, not followed by slow wave, and are elicited when the electrodes are placed on top of the belly of the muscle.

5. *Glossokinetic artifacts (tongue movements)*—These are rhythmic or semirhythmic potentials elicited by tongue movements. The back of the tongue dipole is positive with respect to the tip. When the tongue is thrust forward, the frontocerebral regions become surface negative and the temporal regions become surface positive (see Fig. 5–9).

6. *Pulse artifacts*—This is a synchronous artifact due to electrode location on or adjacent to a pulsating artery or fontanelle.

7. *Ballistocardiographic artifacts*—Caused by head movements with each heartbeat.

8. *Sweat artifacts*—Perspiration may cause a change in the impedance of the interface region between the electrode and the scalp. This change often causes medium-voltage slow waves that are often less than 1.0 Hz (see Fig. 5–10).

BACKGROUND ACTIVITY

After exclusion of artifacts, the next task is the recognition and classification of normal and abnormal cerebral activity. The EEG should be analyzed for age-dependent normal and abnormal features in both the awake and sleep states. In neonatal and infant EEGs, the patterns in each state should be checked to see if the maturation for each state is adequate (see Chapter 3 and eMedicine.com [http://www.emedicine.com/neuro/topic493.htm]).

A good starting point is the sequential examination of features in the posterior, central, and anterior head regions. The dominant background activity should be assessed when the child is alert and relaxed and the eyes are closed. Even in children as young as 3 to 6 months, a dominant rhythm

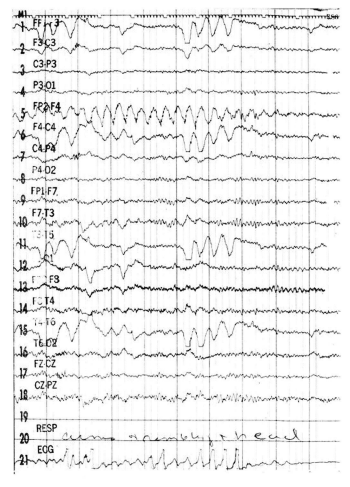

FIGURE 5–15
Movement artifacts of the arms and head trembling. Note the high-voltage, low-frequency artifacts in the ECG electrodes as well as the bilateral frontal and temporal rhythmic artifacts.

can be assessed if the technician gently closes the eyes. Alertness can be assessed by the technician asking the patient to count or perform some calculations before closing the eyes. The drowsy patient can have a posterior background rhythm 1 or 2 Hz slower than when alert. The predominant frequency and amplitude should be recorded.

Frequency

As the infant matures, the record contains faster rhythms with a decrease in the amount of slow activity. However, delta and theta activity are common during the first few years of life.

Posterior Activity

From 3 to 12 months, the background activity consists of delta and theta waves (generalized, arrhythmic, and rhythmic) more prominent over the occipital areas, which

TABLE 5–1
Age-Related Changes in Posterior Background Frequency

Age	Frequency (Hz)
3 mo	3–4
5 mo	5
12 mo	6–7
2 yr	7–8
3 yr	8
7 yr	9
15 yr	10–11

may be synchronous over wide areas of both hemispheres. An occipital rhythm can be distinguished from the background at 3 months. This activity, which occurs at a frequency of 3 or 4 Hz, is partially attenuated by eye opening. The frequency of posterior background activity increases with age. By age 5 months, rhythmic occipital activity usually increases in frequency to about 5 Hz. Table 5–1 lists the background rhythms as a function of age. A posterior background rhythm slower than the values listed, by 1 Hz or more, is abnormal if the child were clearly awake with eyes closed. By 2 to 3 years of age the posterior background evolves into an *alpha rhythm*. This rhythm consists of sinusoidal waves occurring at 8 to 13 Hz that appears during relaxed wakefulness, usually while the eyes are closed. Alpha rhythm is blocked or clearly attenuated by eye opening, sleep, drowsiness, attention to a task, and mental effort. The amplitude is greatest over the posterior head regions but may extend forward to the central regions and beyond. Just after eye closure it is common to see an increase in the frequency of the alpha rhythm lasting 1 to 2 seconds. This phenomenon is called the *alpha squeak*. It has no known clinical significance (Fig. 5–16).

Rhythmic theta may be present in the posterior region and prominent in temporal and posterior regions until adolescence. Until 4 years of age, posterior theta may be more prominent than posterior alpha activity. By 5 to 6 years of age, theta and alpha are equally prominent. Intermixed random theta and delta waveforms are commonly present over the posterior regions during childhood and adolescence; they may be seen in more than 5% of normal subjects up to 30 years of age. Normal posterior slow waves should rarely exceed the voltage of the alpha rhythm by 1.5 times. Asymmetries of slow waves should conform to asymmetries of the alpha rhythm. Slow waves should have the same topographic distribution as alpha. Like alpha activity, posterior slow waves should attenuate during alerting.

A wide variety of waveforms peculiar to children are present in the posterior quadrant; most are present only with the eyes closed. A few of these waveforms are described.

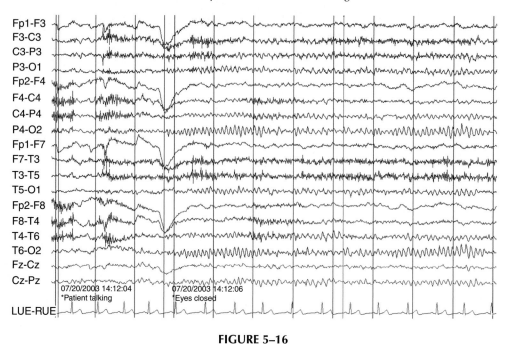

FIGURE 5–16

Alpha squeak. Alpha activity in the 5th second with eye closure is at 10.5 Hz, whereas by the 6th second the alpha rhythm has slowed to its stable rate of 9.5 Hz.

Posterior Slow Waves of Youth (Polyphasic Potentials). This activity consists of 2- to 4-Hz waves lasting 250 to 500 milliseconds. The activity occurs as single or multiple waves. It is interposed between alpha waves, causing a "polyphasic" morphology. This activity gradually increases in quantity during the first decade of life, becoming maximal early in adolescence. This activity has the same reactivity as the alpha rhythm[2] (Fig. 5–17).

Slow Alpha Variant. This pattern consists of semirhythmic, 4- to 5-Hz theta activity that has a morphology, distribution, and reactivity similar to alpha, hence the term *alpha variant*. The activity occurs either unilaterally or bilaterally. When bilateral, the waveforms are usually synchronous. In children this appears to be a rare pattern.[3]

Lambda Waves. These waveforms are primarily elicited by saccadic eye movements while the child scans a visual field of interest. They consist of a surface-negative or surface-positive, sharply contoured, broad waveform. These biphasic or triphasic potentials occur less than three or four times per second and are synchronous in the occipital regions of both hemispheres.[4] At times electrocardiogram artifact and lambda waves may resemble one another.

Central Activity

Sustained rhythmic activity appears earlier in the central than in other regions. Central rhythm may be the most prominent rhythm in children aged 1 to 5 years. As the child gets older, central activity is up to 2 Hz slower than the alpha rhythm. A normal variant pattern may be present in the central region called the *mu rhythm*. This activity is in the theta or alpha frequency bandwidths at 9 ± 2 Hz. The activity characteristically has sharp surface-negative and rounded surface-positive phases. The spatial distribution is in the precentral to postcentral region, although spread into parietal leads is not uncommon. Mu rhythm may occur unilaterally or bilaterally. The activity is attenuated with movement, or the thought of movement, of the contralateral arm or hand (Fig. 5–18).

Anterior Activity

During wakefulness, frontal activity is usually of lower voltage than central or posterior activity. Normal records often demonstrate low-voltage beta activity (18 to 24 Hz or even faster) in the anterior quadrants. Beta should not exceed 25 µV in amplitude. Beta occurs only rarely in children and adolescents during wakefulness. It should be cautioned that amplitude of the beta activity may be artifactually increased adjacent to a skull defect (breach effect). Excessive beta activity, especially in the 18- to 25-Hz range, is an abnormality that is frequently due to a medication effect (e.g., benzodiazepines, barbiturates) (see Fig. 5–1).

The amplitude of beta over the two hemispheres should be compared. We consider an interhemispheric difference of greater than 35% as abnormal with the reduced beta amplitude typically over the pathologic hemisphere. Absence of beta frequencies in one hemisphere (which, if

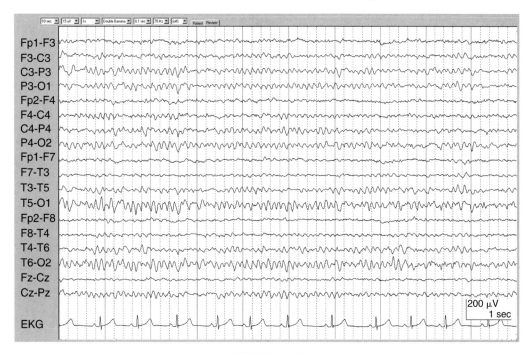

FIGURE 5–17

Posterior slow waves of youth in a 9-year-old girl with seizures. These occur in the first 3 seconds of the record.

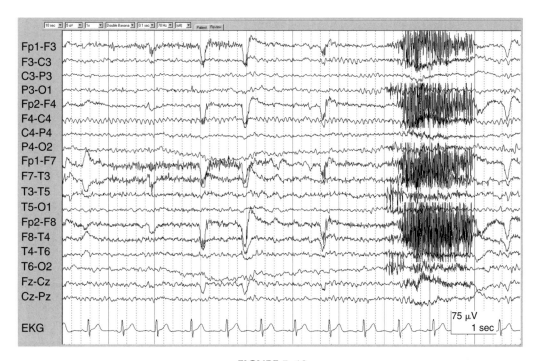

FIGURE 5–18

A boy with a 10.5-Hz central or mu rhythm on the right.

severe, is called "balding") may indicate a structural abnormality in that hemisphere.

Rhythmic theta waves are present in frontocentral regions in 15% to 20% of normal children 8 to 16 years old.

The presence of 5- to 7-Hz frontal or frontocentral theta in runs lasting several seconds is normal. Frontocentral theta may normally occur through early adulthood. High-voltage frontal activity in the delta range is abnormal. Anterior dominant (or generalized) slowing may occur for a variety of reasons suggesting bilateral cerebral dysfunction. The etiologies may include head injury, central nervous system infection, and toxic/metabolic encephalopathies.

Abnormalities of Background Frequencies

Posterior dominant slowing or diffuse slowing occur frequently as a nonspecific response to a variety of diffuse conditions, including head injury, central nervous system infection, and toxic/metabolic encephalopathies. EEGs that cycle through distinct states and have normal sleep features such as spindles and vertex sharp waves clearly differ from records that are monotonous and have no normal sleep features. Any patient with a slow record should be stimulated with a variety of stimuli (sound, tactile, noxious) to determine if there is reactivity. Slow records that are not reactive to stimuli are associated with a poor prognosis, regardless of etiology. When confronted with a slow record, the electroencephalographer should determine if the slowing is continuous or intermittent. The final step is to determine if there are other abnormal features such as asymmetries or epileptiform discharges.

Continuous slowing may be focal, lateralized, or diffuse (generalized). Slow waves may be characterized as polymorphic (arrhythmic) or rhythmic. Slowing in the delta range is usually indicative of a greater degree of dysfunction than waveforms in the theta range. Likewise, high-amplitude slow waves are usually more pathologic than medium- or low-amplitude slow waves. The absence of beta (14 to 25 Hz) activity often implies a superficial cortical lesion.

Continuous rhythmic slowing indicates gray matter dysfunction. This may involve the cerebral cortex, deep structures (thalamus or midbrain), or both. Rhythmic slowing may be due to a structural lesion or the result of a diffuse insult such as encephalitis or a metabolic disturbance.

Continuous focal polymorphic arrhythmic slowing is generally indicative of a structural abnormality involving the white matter; exceptions include slowing concurrent or subsequent to migraine headaches and slowing following seizures.

The surface location of the slowing may not perfectly correlate with the location of the structural abnormality. For example, a parasagittal frontal structural abnormality may demonstrate temporal slowing; in such a case, the temporal surface leads are said to act as a "broadcaster" of dysfunction from adjacent lobes.

Focal Intermittent Slowing. Intermittent rhythmic delta activity (IRDA) may be frontal (FIRDA), occipital (OIRDA), or limited to other regions. If these activities occur during the awake state, they may be indicative of dysfunction affecting cortical and subcortical white matter (Figs. 5–19 and 5–20). In the presence of normal background rhythms, they may be indicative of increased intracranial pressure; otherwise, they may be indicative of a metabolic or diffuse dysfunction.

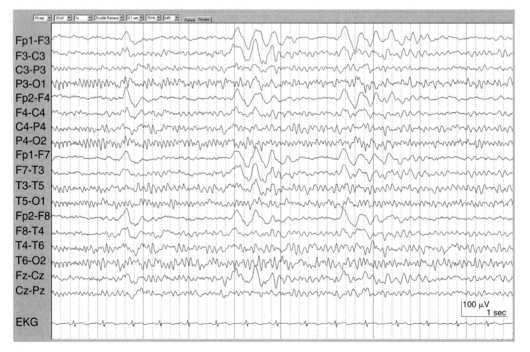

FIGURE 5–19

Frontal intermittent rhythmic delta activity in a 13-year-old child with a closed head injury. This is a nonspecific finding of diffuse dysfunction that can be seen with various etiologies.

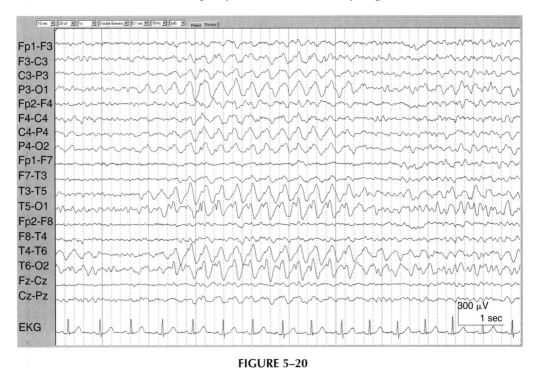

FIGURE 5–20

Occipital intermittent rhythmic delta activity in an 8-year-old girl with absence seizures.

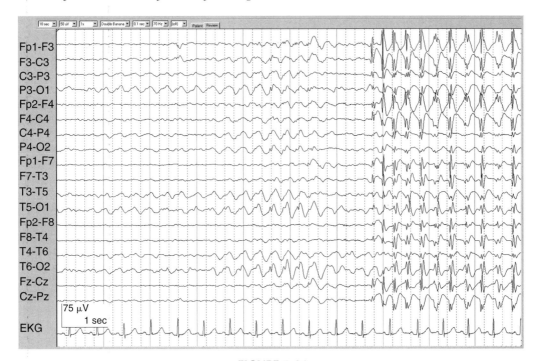

FIGURE 5–21

Occipital intermittent rhythmic delta activity (OIRDA) and generalized spike wave (GSW): OIRDA and 3-Hz generalized spike wave often occur within the same record in those with absence epilepsy syndrome.

Fifteen percent of children with 3-Hz spike-and-wave activity on EEG and absence seizures may have short bursts of OIRDA without overlapping spike components. Activation of 3-Hz spike-and-wave activity by hyperventilation is more common when OIRDA coexists (Fig. 5–21).[5]

Amplitude

There is an inverse relationship between amplitude and frequency. Although the frequency of background activity increases with maturation, amplitude decreases with age. EEGs rarely are abnormal because of generalized amplitude abnormalities alone. Occasionally children have low-voltage EEGs. In the absence of any other abnormality, this may represent a normal variant. When there is no reactivity, background activity of less than 30 µV in all states is a poor prognostic sign. A focal or lateralized amplitude asymmetry is abnormal.

The voltage of the posterior dominant rhythm on the right side is normally greater on the right than on the left (possibly due to skull thickness asymmetry); hence, a voltage (amplitude) of the left posterior dominant rhythm greater by more than 35% than the right posterior dominant rhythm is an abnormal finding, whereas the right posterior dominant rhythm voltage must be more than 50% greater than the left posterior dominant rhythm to be an abnormal finding. In general, the side with the lower voltage posterior dominant rhythm is the abnormal side. In addition, shifting asymmetries of alpha rhythms are common during recording, especially in bipolar montages. An asymmetry of frequency of greater than 1 Hz usually indicates an abnormality on the slower side.

Abnormalities of Symmetry

In a normal EEG, right and left homologous regions should demonstrate symmetrical activity during all three states (awake, drowsy, and asleep). Although transient asymmetries may occur, particularly during state transitions, a persistent asymmetry is abnormal. In patients with persistent abnormalities, the side with the attenuated activity is usually the most severely affected area.

Asymmetries of voltage of posterior dominant rhythms are common. As discussed earlier, the amplitude of posterior dominant rhythms over the left hemisphere is typically lower than over the right hemisphere. An asymmetry may be short lived (e.g., postictal or migraine) or long-standing (e.g., mass lesion, infarction). Repeating the EEG usually differentiates the two conditions.

Other Types of Background Abnormalities

Subacute Sclerosing Panencephalitis (SSPE). A diagnostic EEG pattern occurs with a chronic measles virus infection of childhood characterized by bilateral, usually synchronous and symmetrical bursts of very high amplitude (>500 µV) delta waves that occur every 4 to 7 seconds. The bursts of delta activity have a variable relationship with myoclonic jerks (Fig. 5–22).

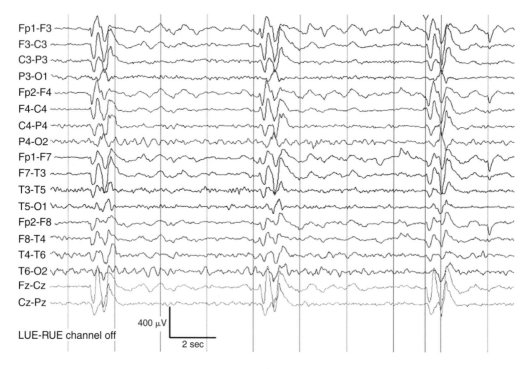

FIGURE 5–22

High-amplitude periodic generalized delta waves in a child with subacute sclerosing panencephalitis.

Theta, Alpha, and Beta Coma. These are patterns in which one frequency is predominant in a comatose patient. The patterns have a widespread distribution and a monotonous monorhythmic appearance that do not react to stimuli. The best known, alpha coma, consists of alpha frequency patterns that are widespread. Unlike alpha rhythm, this pattern is not primarily occipital and is not altered by eye movements. Beta coma may be seen in patients with drug intoxication. Clinically, the patient is comatose (Fig. 5–23).

Spindle Coma. Spindle-like activity is the predominant waveform morphology in this pattern that may occur in comatose patients. This type of pattern may have a somewhat better prognosis than other coma patterns (Fig. 5–24).

Triphasic Waves. These are high-voltage generalized delta waves seen intermittently or rhythmically. Triphasic waves are bilaterally synchronous and frontally predominant. They typically occur at 1.5 to 3.0 Hz with a small, sharp, surface-negative component followed by a large, sharp surface-positive component and then a negative slow wave. The waveform often has an anterior-to-posterior lag (Fig. 5–25). Triphasic waves are often seen in metabolic encephalopathies (including hepatic and uremic), toxic encephalopathies, and diffuse structural abnormalities.

Periodic Lateralized Epileptiform Discharges (PLEDs). PLEDs may take on the form of spikes, sharp waves, or slow waves that, as the name implies, occur periodically. They most often repeat once per second, but the period may vary from 0.5 to 3 seconds (Fig. 5–26). PLEDs indicate a lateralized acute or subacute structural lesion or may be a residue of status epilepticus.

Burst-Suppression Pattern. This consists of synchronous or asynchronous bursts of cerebral activity, lasting 0.5 to 10 seconds, followed by periods of a generalized isoelectric background lasting from 2 to more than 10 seconds. The record is invariant and unreactive (Fig. 5–27). Be aware that the preterm infants may normally have a similar pattern. In the absence of a clinical explanation (e.g., barbiturate intoxication, accidental or deliberate), after the 28 weeks' gestation, a nonreactive burst-suppression pattern is indicative of bilateral cerebral dysfunction. A burst-suppression pattern with complete asynchrony may suggest agenesis of the corpus callosum and in females this may occur in Aicardi's syndrome.

Electrocerebral Silence (Electrocerebral Inactivity, Isoelectric Pattern). For discussion, see Chapter 20.

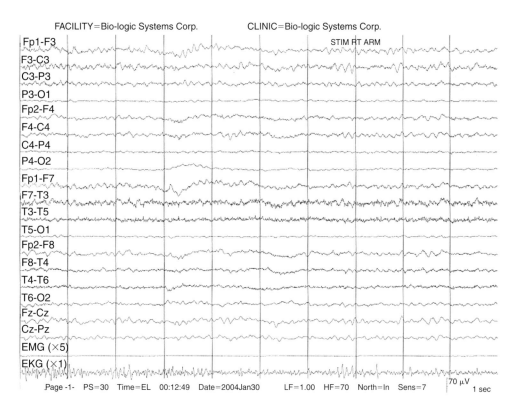

FIGURE 5–23

Alpha theta coma: diffuse 7- to 8-Hz activity more prominent frontally in a comatose child. This activity is invariant to noxious stimuli delivered to the right arm.

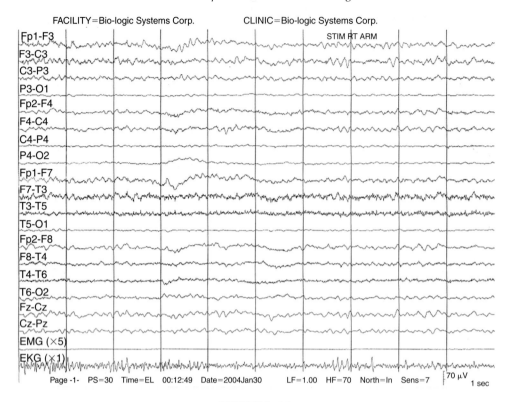

FIGURE 5–24

Spindle coma: diffuse 14-Hz spindle activity in a comatose child.

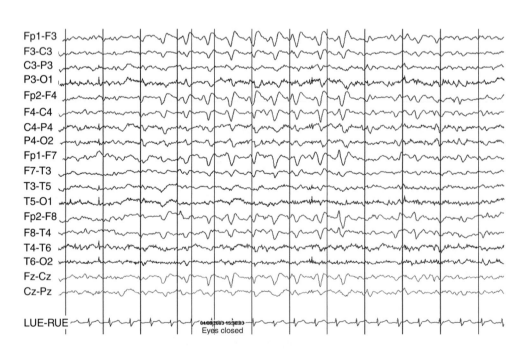

FIGURE 5–25

Triphasic waves in an encephalopathic child.

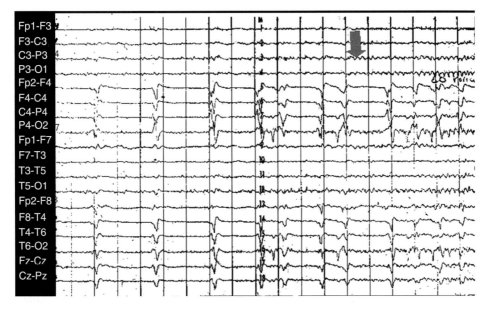

FIGURE 5–26

Periodic lateralized epileptiform discharges (PLEDs) occur once every 1 to 2.5 seconds in the right hemisphere.

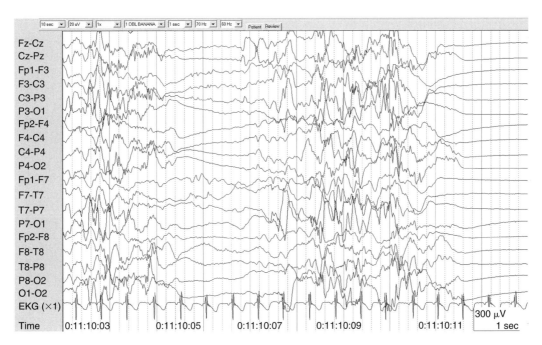

FIGURE 5–27

Burst-suppression: a 13-month-old infant with seizures receiving oxygen.

ORGANIZATION

A record is said to be organized with an adequate "anterior-to-posterior voltage gradient" when there is a steadily increasing amplitude of waveforms demonstrable from anterior to posterior regions. A disorganized record lacks an age-appropriate, anterior-to-posterior voltage gradient. The term *disorganization* can be applied to one hemisphere or be used to reflect bilateral disruption of the voltage gradient. A disorganized record is an abnormal but nonspecific finding.

STATE-RELATED CHANGES

In routine pediatric and adolescent EEGs, there are often three states: awake, drowsy (stage I sleep), and sleep (stage II). Stages III and IV are deep stages of sleep that are uncommonly seen in the routine EEG recording due to the short nature of the examination. Likewise, recording of rapid eye movement (REM) sleep during electroencephalography is rare unless the patient has narcolepsy.

Drowsiness and Sleep

An infant or child may clinically appear awake and yet have EEG signs of drowsiness. EEG features of drowsiness in older children and adults include diffuse slowing, slowing of the posterior background rhythm, attenuation of the dominant posterior background rhythm, rolling lateral eye movements, and mild to moderate increased low-voltage beta activity.

Beta activity (20 to 30 Hz, especially 20 to 25 Hz) increases in drowsiness from age 5 to 6 months to 2 years. In younger children this beta activity occurs diffusely or is maximal over central and posterior regions. In older children, beta activity is most prominent in frontocentral regions (Fig. 5–28).

Hypnagogic hypersynchrony, which consists of rhythmic widely distributed bisynchronous waves of high amplitude (75 to 200 μV), occurs frequently during the first few years

of life. The pattern can occur intermittently or continuously for up to several minutes at the beginning of sleep (hypnagogic) and end of sleep (hypnopompic). Between 3 months to 6 years the frequency is 3 to 5 Hz. It increases to 4 to 6 Hz by 5 years of age. Thereafter, this activity gradually declines and disappears by age 10 years.

At 10 years of age, adult patterns of drowsiness are common. As the child enters stage II of sleep, the background consists of a mixture of beta and theta frequencies. Vertex sharp waves, K-complexes, and sleep spindles are prominent.

Vertex (V) waves appear by age 5 to 6 months. Vertex waves can be very sharply contoured and usually have negative polarity, but they can have positive, negative, or diphasic polarity with voltages of up to 250 milliseconds. The duration is less than 200 milliseconds but can occur in sequences lasting 5 to 10 seconds. The following slow wave is opposite in polarity to the major vertex wave deflection. The fields may shift slightly from side to side, appearing asymmetrical at times. These waveforms may be present in short bursts or repetitive runs. They become maximally expressed at 4 to 5 years of age. In some infants, these can be distinguished in rudimentary form during the neonatal period.

Spindles are distinct waveforms that first appear at 2 months of age in term infants. They consist of rhythmic, sinusoidal 12- to 14-Hz or 14- to 16-Hz waves appearing in the central and frontal regions during non-REM sleep (Fig. 5–29). Until 3 to 4 months the spindles may be

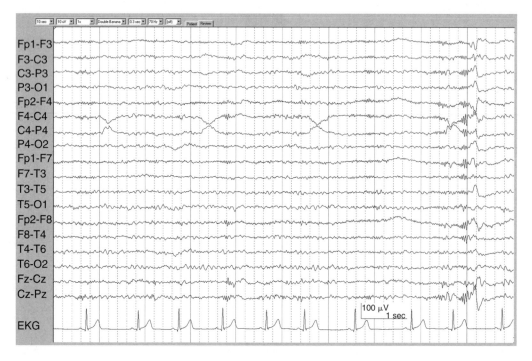

FIGURE 5–28

Beta activity with drowsiness in an 18-year-old.

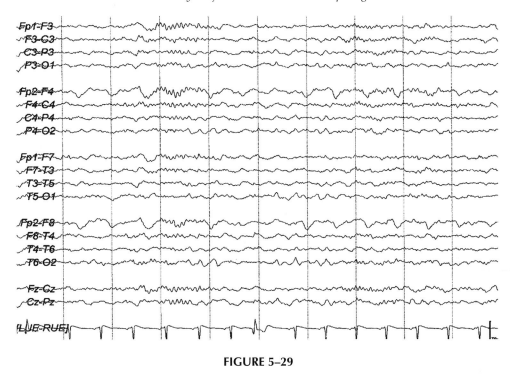

FIGURE 5–29

Sleep spindles.

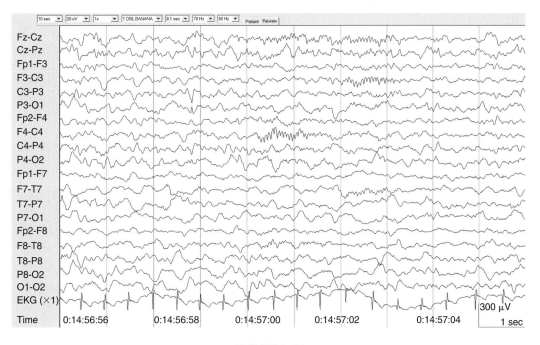

FIGURE 5–30

Asynchronous sleep spindles in a 1-year-old infant with staring, stiffening, and shaking events.

fragmentary and difficult to clearly distinguish. After 3 to 4 months spindles are prominent and often occur in runs lasting 5 to 6 seconds. During the first 2 years of life the spindles are often asynchronous (Fig. 5–30).

K-complexes are sharp, negative high-voltage waves (>200 μV), followed by moderate- to high-voltage positive waves of longer duration (>0.5 seconds), and can occur spontaneously during non-REM sleep. They can also be elicited during sleep by sensory stimulation, especially auditory, with a positive component occurring 0.75 second after a stimulus and may or may not be followed by a 1- to 2-second run of sleep spindles.[6]

Differentiating abnormal midline or parasagittal spikes and sharp waves from normal vertex activity can be quite difficult in children. Midline spikes during the awake and alert state are always abnormal. However, occasionally patients have vertex sharp waves during the very early stages of drowsiness. Abnormal spikes and sharp waves can sometimes be differentiated from normal vertex activity by the presence of an asymmetrical field, the presence of multiple spikes, or concurrent slowing. Many patients with midline lesions may have both midline spikes and normal vertex activity.

Positive occipital sharp transients of sleep (POSTS) or lambdoid waves are cone-shaped waveforms occurring in runs of four or five waves at a time. They are common in light sleep during childhood and are a normal finding. They may be superimposed on posterior delta to give sharply contoured posterior waveforms in non-REM sleep (Fig. 5–31).

Small sharp spikes (SSS, benign epileptiform transients of sleep [BETS]) are low-amplitude spikes with a duration of less than 50 milliseconds that occur during drowsiness.

The distribution is in the mid- and anterior temporal region and they typically shift in location. They can be unilateral, or bilateral, occurring independently or bisynchronously. They are rare in young children but can be seen in adolescents. BETS are a normal finding (Fig. 5–32).

Wicket Spikes. These are repetitive spikes that have an appearance of a series of arches, lasting a few seconds. They are distributed in the anterior and mid-temporal region during wakefulness and, more commonly, during drowsiness and light sleep. These waveforms are unusual in children. Despite their sharp appearance, this pattern is not associated with epileptic disorders.

Six-Hertz Spike-and-Slow Wave (SW) (Phantom Spike and Wave). This pattern consists of miniature spike and wave activity occurring at a frequency of 4 to 7 Hz. The typical duration is less than 1 second. The distribution is generalized, often with a maximum voltage predominance. The pattern is seen in adolescents and young adults and occurs primarily during drowsiness, but it can also be seen in the awake state. Some authors make a distinction between frontal and occipital accentuation. Hughes and Fino[7] described the acronyms WHAM (*w*aking, *h*igh amplitude, *a*nterior, *m*ales) and FOLD (*f*emales, *o*ccipital, *l*ow amplitude, *d*rowsy). The frontal type has been associated with epileptic seizures, whereas the occipital type

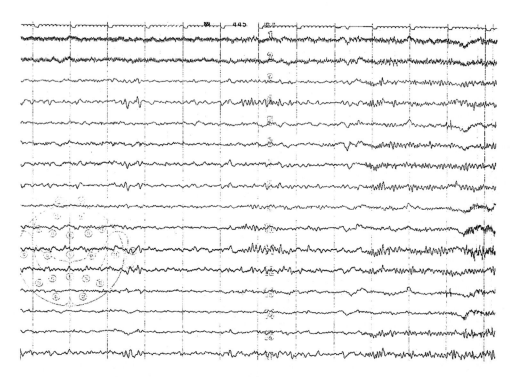

FIGURE 5–31

Positive occipital sharp transients in sleep. Surface-positive left occipital sharp waves are seen in the 3rd second. Montage is the double-banana without a central chain.

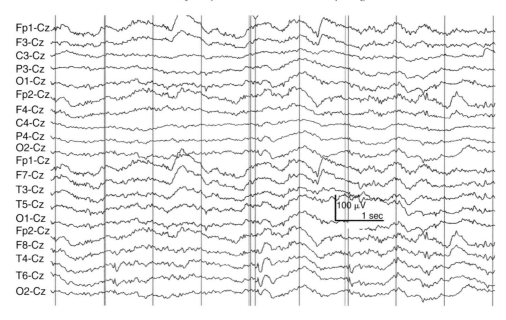

FIGURE 5–32

Small sharp spikes. Right temporal small sharp spikes are seen in the 3rd and 6th seconds.

is found predominantly in patients without evidence of seizures.

Fourteen- and Six-Hertz Positive Spikes. This pattern consists of repetitive surface-positive spikes, lasting 1 to 2 seconds, that have a distinct comblike appearance and occur during drowsiness or stage II of sleep. The typical voltage is 60 to 70 µV and occurs at a frequency of approximately 14 Hz, 6 Hz, or both. The location is in the posterior temporal/parietal region and can occur unilaterally or bilaterally (either independently or synchronously). They can be seen in children but are most common in adolescents. These are considered normal variants (Fig. 5–33).

Mittens. This is an unusual waveform that is confined to sleep. This waveform is seen in the prefrontal, frontal, and central regions and consists of anterior delta wave with interspersed minor sharp transients. The sharp component is the thumb portion, whereas the slow component represents the hand section. This normal variant is seen primarily in stage III of sleep.

Rhythmical Mid-temporal Discharge (Psychomotor Variant). This normal variant is a common pattern consisting of 4- to 7-Hz theta activity with notched negative sharp waves followed by rounded notched or flat positive phases. These discharges last for a few seconds and occur in the mid-temporal region. They can be unilateral or bilateral. When bilateral they can occur independently or bisynchronously. They typically occur during drowsiness and are more common in adults than children.

TABLE 5–2

Age-Specific Differences in Arousal Patterns

Age	Arousal Pattern
0–2 mo	Voltage attenuation
2–3 mo	Low-amplitude diphasic wave
4–6 mo	Delta waves
7–13 mo	4–8 Hz rhythmic waves, diffusely and frontocentrally for several seconds
13 mo-3 yr	Prominent theta waves (disappearing after 5 yr of age)
12–18 mo	Prolonged sequence of theta, delta, and then theta
By 7 yr	Arousal patterns are similar to those of an adult

Activations

Reactivity. In a routine light sleep recording, the EEG should be reactive to auditory, tactile, or noxious stimulation with vertex waves, increased theta activity, and/or global attenuation.

Arousal from sleep is usually characterized by marked and prolonged activity of high-voltage slow wave activity in all brain areas with some intermixed slower frequencies.

There are age specific differences and they are listed in Table 5–2.

Hyperventilation. Even children as young as 2 years of age may participate in hyperventilation. Asking the child to blow on a pin-wheel or other toy frequently produces the desired results. The typical EEG response consists of

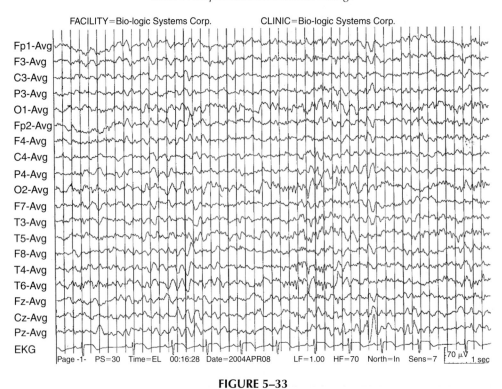

FIGURE 5–33

Fourteen- and 6-Hz positive spikes seen in a drowsy child during the 6th and 7th seconds in the right posterior temporal region.

slowing of the background frequencies. In children older than 6 years of age, the slowing may start over the posterior regions and gradually move forward. The degree of slowing is age dependent. Younger children (<6 years) typically develop a slower pattern than that of adolescents.

The primary purpose of hyperventilation is to activate epileptiform activity. Although generalized abnormalities, such as the 3-Hz spike-and-wave in absence epilepsy (see "Paroxysmal Features") is particularly sensitive to hyperventilation, focal abnormalities, including focal asymmetries, may also be seen. In children with a considerable amount of beta activity on the EEG, it is important for the electroencephalographer to be able to distinguish between the random occurrence of beta at the beginning of a slow wave from true epileptiform activity (Fig. 5–34).

Protracted slowing, occurring either as continuous delta-theta activity or bursts of rhythmic delta, following hyperventilation suggests the child is either continuing to hyperventilate or has some degree of hypoglycemia.

Photic Stimulation. Photic driving can be seen in newborns, usually at frequencies lower than 5 Hz. As the child matures, there is a greater response to faster frequencies. From 6 years on the maximum driving responses are in the range of 6 to 16 Hz.

The primary purpose of photic stimulation is to activate epileptiform activity. A photoconvulsive or photoparoxysmal response consists of spike-and-wave or multiple spike-and-wave complexes that are bilaterally synchronous and symmetrical and that may or may not outlast the stimulus by a few seconds. Spikes that are time linked to the photic stimulus are not considered a photoconvulsive response. Photoconvulsive responses (Fig. 5–35) are most frequently induced by 15-Hz stimulation with eyes closed and by 20-Hz stimulation with eyes closed. A photomyoclonic response can also occur that consists of rapid synchronous eye blinking in response to flashing. The significance of this response is unclear (Fig. 5–36).

PAROXYSMAL FEATURES

Spikes

These are sharply contoured, transient waveforms (monophasic, diphasic, or polyphasic) with at least one of the prominent phases lasting 20 to 70 milliseconds and visually are differentiated from the background activity. The waveform should have an electrical field and be followed by a slow wave (Fig. 5–37). The electroencephalographer should determine their morphology and degree of stereotypy, location, field extension, and relative frequency and whether they occur spontaneously or in

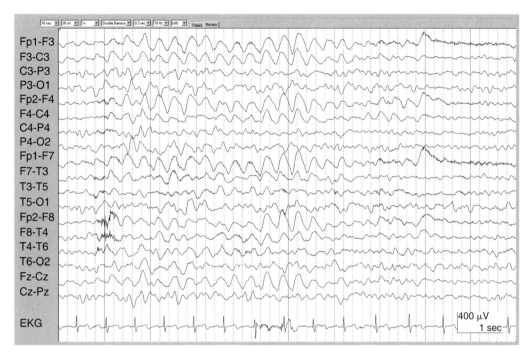

FIGURE 5–34

Rhythmic, high-voltage, frontally predominant delta with hyperventilation.

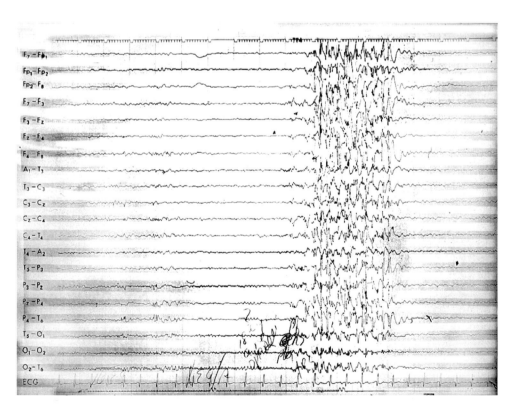

FIGURE 5–35

A photoconvulsive response of irregular generalized spike wave occurring during 17- to 18-Hz photic stimulation. Note the convulsive responsive persists after the end of the photic stimulation.

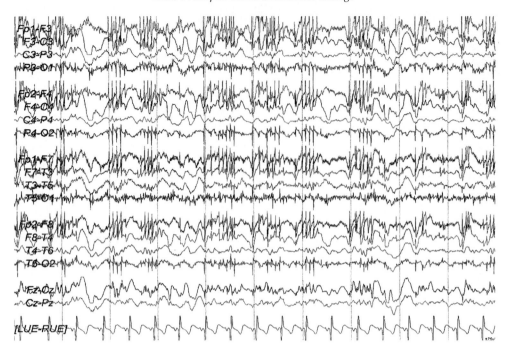

FIGURE 5–36

Photomyoclonic response. Blinking in response to photic stimulation. This is not epileptiform in nature. Eyeblink and muscle artifacts are prominent frontally.

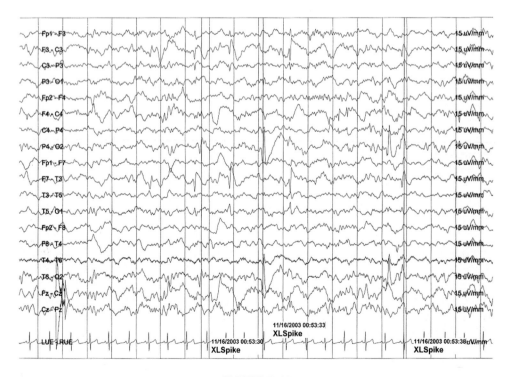

FIGURE 5–37

Spikes: left temporal spikes in the 8th, 9th, 12th, and at the end of the 16th seconds. These spikes are maximum at T3 = T5. Note the field that extends to the central region on the left.

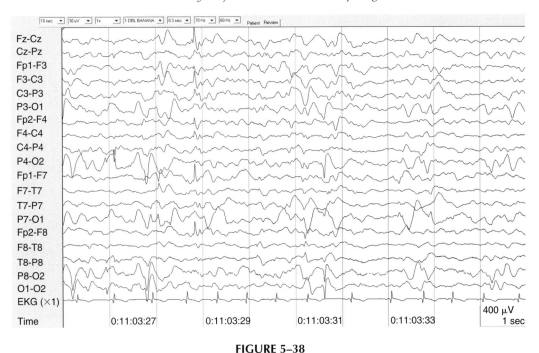

FIGURE 5–38

Multifocal spikes seen in a 13-month-old infant with seizures. Spikes are seen independently at F7 and Fp2 in the 3rd second and at F8 in the 6th second. Right occipital spikes are also seen in the 2nd and 6th seconds.

association with a particular state or activation procedure. If spikes occur in more than one electrode location, the electroencephalographer needs to determine whether they are coming from one or more foci. Spikes occurring in three separate locations, separated by at least two electrodes and occurring in both hemispheres, are called *multifocal spikes* (Fig. 5–38).

Sharp Waves

Sharp waves are sharply contoured, transient waveform (monophasic, diphasic, or polyphasic) lasting 70 to 200 milliseconds and visually are differentiated from the background activity. The waveform should have an electrical field and be followed by a slow wave. Their characterization and significance are similar to spikes.

Spike-and-Slow-Wave Patterns

As stated previously, slow waves follow nearly all focal or generalized spikes and sharp waves. A regular, repetitive sequence of high-voltage SW complexes may occur with a bilateral onset and termination. Specific patterns of generalized seizures occur such as the 3-Hz SW pattern seen in childhood absence epilepsy (Fig. 5–39), the 4- to 6-Hz (rapid) SW in juvenile myoclonic epilepsy (JME) (Fig. 5–40), and the 2-Hz (slow) SW (Fig. 5–41) often associated with Lennox-Gastaut syndrome. It is important

to measure the frequency of the discharge in the middle of the paroxysm because the frequencies may be somewhat faster at the start and slower at the end.[8] Hyperventilation activates 3-Hz SW in 50% to 80% of patients with absence epilepsy,[5] and similar results have been found with other primarily generalized epilepsies.[9] The rapid SW in JME frequently has polyspikes associated with it, and sleep often accentuates slow SW in Lennox-Gastaut syndrome. At times a generalized paroxysm may not perfectly fit a typical syndrome's characteristics, and the syndrome is often referred to as *atypical* (e.g., atypical absence).

Documentation of alterations in the level of consciousness or the presence of automatisms during paroxysms is essential. The use of responsive button pushing in the "clicker" test or simply counting or reading out loud may assist in demonstrating lapses in the level of consciousness.

A secondary bilateral synchrony or rapid generalization of an epileptic focus may occur resulting in a generalized burst of SW that may be electrographically indistinguishable from the SW of the absence epilepsy. This rare occurrence has been termed *frontal absence* and has been localized to a unilateral mesial frontal lobe lesion causing 3-Hz generalized SW.[10]

Seizure Patterns

Depending on whether clinical seizure manifestations (e.g., clonic motor activity, automatisms, or altered mental

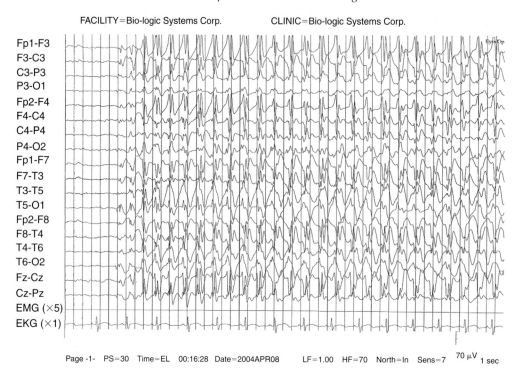

FACILITY=Bio-logic Systems Corp.   CLINIC=Bio-logic Systems Corp.

FIGURE 5–39

Three-Hertz generalized spike wave in childhood absence epilepsy.

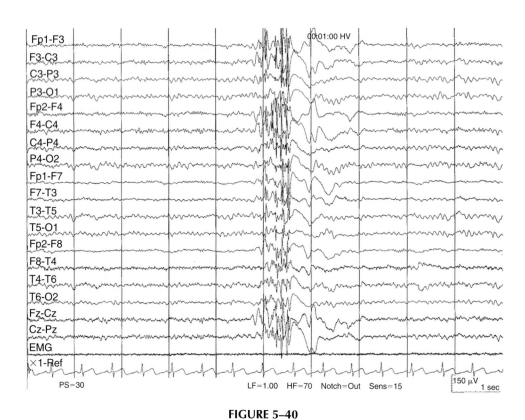

FIGURE 5–40

Rapid, generalized spike wave with intermixed polyspikes occurring during hyperventilation.

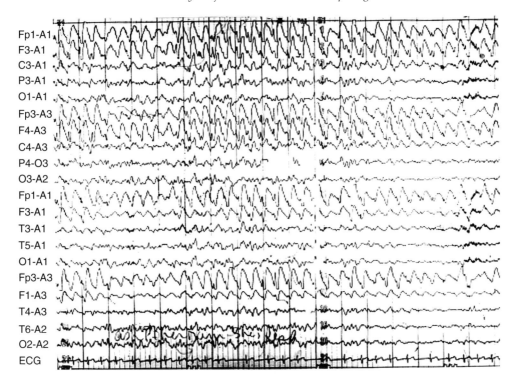

FIGURE 5–41
Slow spike wave at 2 Hz seen in a patient with Lennox-Gastaut syndrome.

status) are absent or present, a seizure pattern may be classified as electrographic or electroclinical, respectively.

Electrographic Seizures

It is well known that electrographic seizures may be generalized, lateralized, or focal in onset, evolution, and/or conclusion; however, there are surprisingly few studies that describe how often each of these patterns occur.[11] There are no studies that specifically address how often specific seizure patterns occur in children. The hallmark feature of an electrographic seizure pattern is an evolution as it progresses. This evolution may include a change in frequency, a change in amplitude, or a change from rhythmic activity to repetitive spiking or vice versa. The duration of an electrographic seizure may vary from less than 1 second to more than 30 minutes in status epilepticus.

Seizures may consist of any of the following paroxysmal abnormalities: global voltage attenuation; focal or diffuse fast activity; rhythmic slow waves or sharp waves that evolve (change in frequency, amplitude, and distribution); runs of spikes followed by rhythmic activity or vice versa; and mixed spike and rhythmic activity.[12] A decrease in interictal spiking may also be seen prior to seizure onset.[13] In infantile spasms, one may see an electrodecremental response characterized by a high-voltage generalized delta wave followed by global voltage attenuation (Fig. 5–42).[14]

The technologist and the electroencephalographer must look for any evidence suggestive of laterality or focality prior to, during, and following the ictal event.

Electroclinical Seizure Determination

An electroclinical seizure consists of an electrographic seizure pattern correlated with abnormal clinical behavior or alteration in consciousness. The technician's notations may describe impaired clinical reactivity, as demonstrated by the patient's inability to respond to cues during a clicker test. Recording simultaneous video can greatly assist in this task and is becoming increasingly available for the use in routine studies as well as with long term monitoring. The electroencephalographer can observe characteristic muscle artifacts on EEG and video of seizure induced movements such as tonic, clonic, tonic/clonic and atonic activity. Spasms in the infant, automatisms in temporal lobe, frontal lobe, and generalized epilepsies and complex motor behaviors in seizures involving the frontal lobes should be distinguished.

CLASSIFICATION

Depending on the findings, the EEG is classified as follows:

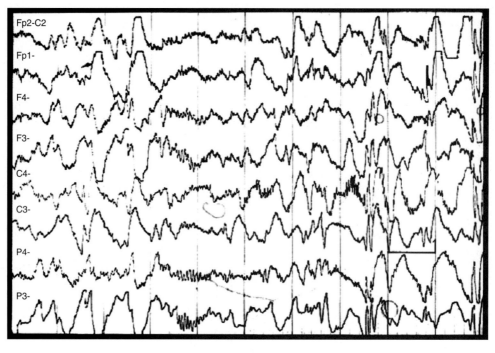

FIGURE 5–42

An electrodecremental response in an infant with attenuation of high-voltage delta and a 1-second burst of low- to medium-voltage beta activity. This is followed by return of baseline chaotic delta activity and generalized spikes.

1. Normal—a statement of states obtained should also be mentioned (e.g., awake, drowsy, and asleep)
2. Abnormal—with a listing of each abnormality including, when appropriate, lateralization, location, and how often they occur
3. Technically difficult—an EEG limited by factors outside the control of the technician, such as lack of cooperation by the patient or an unfriendly electrical environment. A repeat examination may be suggested if clinically indicated.
4. Technically unsatisfactory—"technically unsatisfactory" refers to an EEG limited by factors within the control of the technician, such as failure to try to eliminate electrode artifacts. A repeat examination should be performed.

INTERPRETATION

The electroencephalographer should use the interpretation section to make concise statements tying together the description, classification, and clinical context in a meaningful way. For example, the reader might state that "continuous polymorphic slowing in the left frontal region in the clinical context of a 4-week history of right hemiparesis is indicative of a structural lesion in the left frontal area." Medications and metabolic and toxic factors also play a significant role in how the record is interpreted. Drug effects are numerous and may suggest reasons for some diffuse abnormalities, but they would be highly unusual as the sole explanation for lateralized or focal abnormalities.

The EEG may confirm or argue against the referring physician's clinical impression. If it argues against, the referring physician will use this information to focus on other possible diagnostic testing. The electroencephalographer may suggest other EEG-related tests (with the caveat "if clinically warranted" mentioned), such as a sleep-deprived EEG, ambulatory or prolonged video-EEG monitoring study.

Don't forget to sign and date your reports!

REFERENCES

1. Glaze DG: Drug effects. *In* Daley DD, Pedley TA (eds): Current Practice of Clinical Electroencephalography, 2nd ed. New York, Raven Press, 1990, pp 490–493.
2. Petersen I, Eeg-Olofsson O: The development of the electroencephalogram in normal children from the age of 1 through 15 years: Non-paroxysmal activity. Neuropaediatrie 1971;2:247–304.

3. Aird RB, Gastaut Y: Occipital and posterior electroencephalographic rhythms. Electroencephalogr Clin Neurophysiol 1959;11:637–656.

4. Laget P, Salbreux R: Atlas of EEG in the Child. Paris, Masson, 1982.

5. Sato S, Dreifuss FE, Penry JK, et al: Long-term follow-up of absence seizures. Neurology 1983;33:1590–1595.

6. Loomis AL, Harvey EN, Hobart G: Distribution of disturbance patterns in the human electroencephalogram with special reference to sleep. J Neurophysiol 1938;1:413–430.

7. Hughes JR, Fino JJ: Changes in reactivity during 6/second spike and wave complex. Clin Electroencephalogr 1992;23:31–36.

8. Gibbs FA, Gibbs EL: Atlas of Encephalography III, 2nd ed. Reading, MA, Addison-Wesley Press, 1964.

9. Janz D: Epilepsy with impulsive petit mal (juvenile myoclonic epilepsy). Acta Neurol Scand 1985;72:449–459.

10. Bancaud J, Talairach J: Clinical semiology of frontal lobe seizures. Adv Neurol 1992;57:3–58.

11. Anziska B, Cracco RQ: Changes in frequency and amplitude in electrographic seizure discharges. Clin Electroencephalogr 1977;8:206–210.

12. Goldensohn ES, Legatt AD, Koszer S, Wolf SM: EEG patterns associated with clinical seizures. *In* Goldensohn's EEG Interpretation, 2nd ed. Armonk, NY, Futura, 1999, pp 331–372.

13. Geiger LR, Harner RN: EEG patterns at the time of focal seizure onset. Arch Neurol 1978;35:276–286.

14. Kellaway P, Hrachovy RA, Frost JD Jr, Zion T: Precise characterization and quantification of infantile spasms. Ann Neurol 1979;6:214–218.

6

Clinical Neurophysiology of the Motor Unit in Infants and Children

Nancy L. Kuntz

The motor unit (Fig. 6-1) includes the lower motor neuron, spinal roots, peripheral nerves, neuromuscular junction, and muscle. Neurophysiologic tests can elucidate the ongoing physiology of this functional unit and contribute significantly to differential diagnosis. This section of the book describes neurophysiologic techniques and their application to diagnosing and treating neuromuscular disorders in infants, children, and adolescents. This chapter briefly describes commonly used neurophysiologic techniques, reviews relevant physiology, and discusses technical issues relating to testing infants and children. Optimum understanding of the information derived from commonly used neurophysiologic tests requires an understanding of the involved physiology of generation of action potentials, volume conduction, saltatory conduction, neuromuscular transmission, and muscle contraction. In depth review of these principles is beyond the scope of this chapter, and the reader is referred to recently published comprehensive reviews.[1,2]

The neurophysiologic techniques described in this chapter include motor nerve conduction studies (MNCS), sensory nerve conduction studies (SNCS), F-wave latencies, H reflexes, blink reflexes, repetitive stimulation of motor nerves, and needle electromyography (EMG). All these techniques are well established and have well-accepted normative data for use with adult patients.[1,3-5] Application of these techniques to infants and children was initiated several decades ago[6,7] and has proved to be a critically valuable adjunct to neuromuscular diagnosis in children.[8] Performing neurophysiologic testing on infants, children,

and adolescents requires special attention to technical issues related to small and variable size and to the unique psychosocial needs of these patients. Chapter 7, written by Dr. Matthew Pitt, explores in greater depth the developmental changes in nerve conduction and motor unit potentials throughout childhood.

Virtually all the disorders of the motor unit encountered in adults also occur in infants, children, and adolescents. However, one must also be prepared to evaluate and diagnose other congenital or acquired disorders that present somewhat selectively in younger patients. Disorders such as congenital myasthenic syndromes, dysmyelinating neuropathies, congenital myopathies, congenital muscular dystrophies, and hypoplasias of various portions of the motor unit are relatively unique to children. An acquired disorder such as infantile botulism has a distinct pathophysiology that causes it to selectively present in young infants. There are several excellent references that provide overviews of technical issues as well as address these unique differential diagnoses.[8-10]

REVIEW OF PHYSIOLOGY

Generation of Action Potentials

Action potentials are an "all-or-none" response. In human muscle or nerve cells, when the resting membrane potential depolarizes by about 15 to 25 mV, a critical threshold is

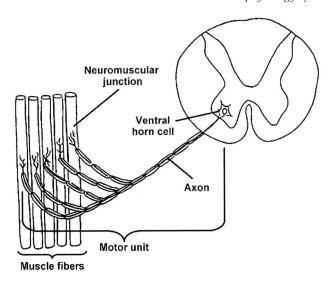

FIGURE 6–1

Motor unit anatomy.

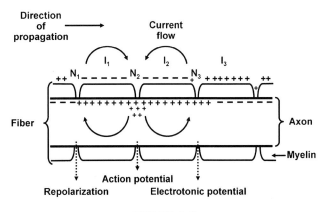

FIGURE 6–2

Saltatory Conduction.

reached and an action potential is generated. This is an energy-dependent process. Generated action potentials cause sodium channels in the membrane to open, which gives rise to a 500-fold increase in permeability to sodium ions. Increased potassium conductance and inactivation of sodium conductance are responsible for rapid recovery of the cell membrane from depolarization.[11]

Volume Conduction

In clinical diagnostic settings, recording electrodes are rarely placed directly on the nerve or muscle. Rather, they are placed on the surface of the extremity and the underlying, variably deep nerve or muscle generates potentials in a "volume conductor." Current flow decreases in proportion to the square of the distance from its source. Therefore, the amount of current required for stimulation and the amplitude of evoked responses depend on the depth of the target of stimulation and source of generated action potential.

Nerve Conduction

Nerve fibers of varying diameter possessing myelin sheaths of different thicknesses conduct impulses within the human peripheral nervous system. Unmyelinated nerve fibers conduct action potentials along the entire length of their cell membrane with predictably slow conduction velocity (1 to 2 m/sec). These fibers serve autonomic and some somatic pain pathways. Myelinated fibers conduct at a faster velocity due to larger fiber diameters with lower axoplasmic resistance to current flow and to saltatory

conduction. The latter refers to the rapid "jumping" of depolarization from the gap at the end of myelin produced by one Schwann cell (node of Ranvier) to the next node (Fig. 6-2). This produces conduction velocities between 20 and 60 m/sec. The largest myelinated fibers function in motor nerves and vibratory and proprioceptive sensory pathways.

Physiology of Nerve Injury

Neuropraxia describes a type of nerve injury in which there is a proportionate decrease in amplitude (conduction block) with stimulation proximal to the site of a lesion (Fig. 6-3). This is a physiologic or functional loss of conduction without structural injury to the axon. With another type of injury involving transection of the axon, stimuli applied distal to the site of the lesion continue to be conducted for up to 5 to 7 days, after which wallerian degeneration disrupts function. *Axonotmesis* refers to disruption of continuity of axons with immediate failure of conduction across the lesion and subsequent wallerian degeneration of the portion of axon disconnected from its cell body. *Neuronotmesis* describes a situation in which the nerve injury causes discontinuity of both axon and associated connective tissue structures. Physiologic studies cannot differentiate this from axonotmesis. However, the prognosis for nerve regeneration is poorer with neuronotmesis due to a higher incidence of failed or misdirected axonal regrowth. Nerve conduction studies (NCS) performed a week after nerve injury can differentiate axonal loss from conduction block. In the case of a complete brachial plexus lesion that has been present since birth, NCS performed at 5 to 10 days of age have prognostic value. Nerve stimulation distal to the spinal root or plexus site of injury produces preserved amplitude of motor response with neuropraxia but produces proportionately decreased amplitudes with

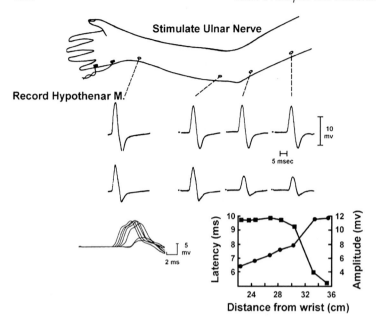

FIGURE 6–3

Conduction Block.

axonal degeneration. These data provide important physiologic and prognostic information to practitioner and family.

Neuromuscular Transmission

Action potentials reach the nerve terminals of motor nerves and activate a physiologic cascade of events that carries the impulse across the synaptic cleft and generates an action potential in muscle fibers if stimulation threshold is reached (Fig. 6-4). The physiology of this process is discussed in more detail in Chapter 25. Clinical neurophysiologic techniques including repetitive stimulation of motor nerves, standard needle electromyography, and single-fiber electromyography can be used to assess neuromuscular transmission in infants and children. Maturational issues regarding neuromuscular transmission are discussed in Chapter 7.

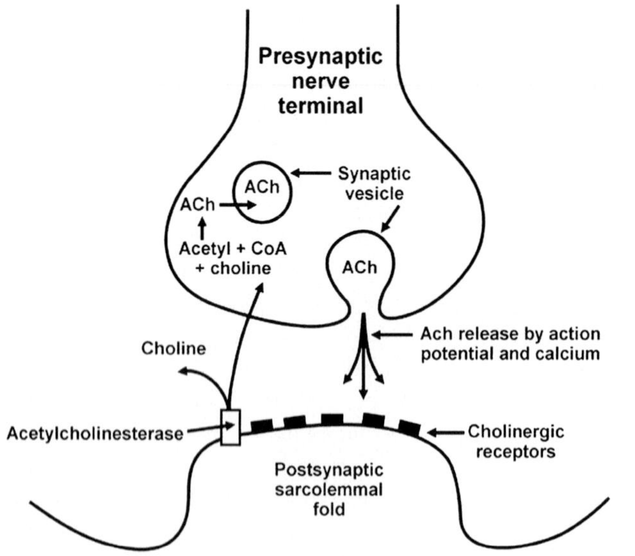

Muscle Contraction

Contraction of muscle fibers begins when action potentials cause calcium to be released into the sarcoplasmic reticulum and transverse tubules. This disinhibits troponin and leads to unmasking of active binding sites by tropomyosin. At this point, development of cross-bridges between actin and myosin filaments generates contraction of the fiber. Force is generated by the summated contraction of multiple muscle fibers pulling against the point of tendinous insertion into bone. Motor unit potentials recorded during needle electromyography are the electrical summation of activation of all the muscle fibers innervated by a single motor neuron that are within the reach of a recording probe.

DEVELOPMENTAL CONSIDERATIONS IN NEUROPHYSIOLOGIC EXAMINATION

Cooperation and Tolerance for Testing

Most clinical neurophysiologic techniques evaluating the motor unit include stimuli that can be described as

FIGURE 6–4

Neuromuscular Junction. ACh, acetylcholine; CoA, coenzyme A.

annoying, mildly painful, or frightening. In fact, a survey of physicians performing neurophysiologic testing of the motor unit on infants and children was conducted with respondents reporting that 35% of children undergoing study experienced extreme behavioral distress (screaming, needing additional restraint, or attempting to leave the examining table).[12] The electromyographer needs to consider the developmental status of the patient and, with those issues in mind, work with the family to coordinate the examination from pretest information and consent through the completion of the study. The primary decision is whether the study should be performed under sedation or carefully orchestrated in a nonsedated child. In an older child, it is also reasonable to perform the examination in multiple, shorter sessions organized to minimize discomfort and development of anxiety toward future testing.

The most important factors to be considered during this decision are the probability of completing a nonsedated examination without unacceptable emotional trauma to the child and consideration of the potential medical risks of sedation in a given child. Hays, in 1992, correlated behavioral distress during electrodiagnostic procedures with a younger age, a history of being uncooperative with previous painful procedures, having had previous negative medical or dental experiences, or having parents who reported greater fear and anxiety about undergoing EMG or NCS. Potential medical risks of sedation relate primarily to underlying medical status with hypotonia or underlying cardiopulmonary disease increasing the risk of airway collapse or respiratory depression. Sedation for outpatient procedures cannot be performed as informally as in years past. Joint Commission on the Accreditation of Healthcare Organizations regulations require written procedures and monitoring by licensed personnel until effects of sedation are documented to have worn off. Heightened attention to safety concerns has transformed conscious sedation for outpatient medical procedures from a casual procedure using less than a dollar's worth of medication administered by laboratory personnel to a formal protocol with charges of several hundred dollars.

Children who can be successfully studied without sedation tend to be very young infants as well as older children and young adults. Newborn and very young infants can sleep through NCS if the stimulation is administered slowly—allowing 10 to 60 seconds rather than a fraction of a second between stimuli. With careful attention to the system and preparation for the examination, older children or young adults can tolerate these studies without sedation.

The family and the patient (if he or she is old enough) need to be provided with information about the proposed study. However, the referring physician has the opportunity to play an important role in the success of the study by carefully phrasing his or her description of the study.

Graphic descriptions of shocks and needles provided for the sake of informed consent tend to become magnified into nightmares over the days or weeks between referral and testing. A simple explanation provided by the referring physician for the parent or older child is preferable. It is much more reassuring to compare the shock to being similar to what one experiences with a simple static discharge in the winter months. Similarly when discussing the use of needles to the parent these are best compared with the size of an acupuncture tool. If the parents have continued concerns prior to the EMG they should be encouraged to speak with the electromyographer per se to lessen their anxieties. We instruct our laboratory appointment team to feel free to tell the parent we will be pleased to personally speak with them prior to the study. This often adds greatly to the rapport at the time of the procedure.

Later at the time of the procedure, it is important for the performing electromyographer to provide a detailed discussion to the parent and older child. He or she should carefully explain the two primary techniques before the EMG is performed.

Finally, it is most important to assure the parents that they will have control over continuation of the examination. Parenthetically, however, some electromyographers find that on some occasions the parents may wish to continue the study when the physician feels it is best to discontinue and have the child return to have the procedure under conscious sedation as described later. It is reasonable to consider providing special instruction in visualization techniques, guided imagery, and/or self-hypnosis for appropriate older children. A calm manner and positive approach by the electromyographer produce much greater tolerance of the procedure by the patient and parent. Assuring the parents that the physician is empathetic and often has children of his or her own is also reassuring.

Since 1998, a significant number of infants and children have had NCS and EMG performed under conscious sedation in a cooperative effort by the Mayo Clinic Clinical Electromyography Laboratory and pediatric anesthesiologists. Oral midazolam for sedation, and a topical mixture of prilocaine and lidocaine creams to prepare the intravenous site, are administered while the child is with parents in the waiting room, prior to entering the outpatient surgery room. Additional medication, including inhaled nitrous oxide and/or intravenous midazolam, propofol, or ketamine, are used to provide necessary sedation and amnesia. Fentanyl is also frequently used to provide analgesia. Patient and family satisfaction has been very high. The only observed side effect has been a small number of markedly weak or hypotonic infants or young children who developed transient atelectasis after sedation and required more prolonged observation. These sedative medications have little effect on peripheral NCS. However, central conduction may be altered by these medications, with the effect more marked at cortical than subcortical levels. F-wave responses are suppressed proportionate to the degree of clinical sedation. Clinical experience suggests that propofol suppresses the frequency of F-wave responses more than other agents used for conscious sedation.

Size Issues

Infants and young children have shorter extremities, proportionately thicker subcutaneous fat layers, and greater surface areas than older children. The short extremities and small hands and feet make electrode separation more difficult and increase potential for artifact owing to spread of the electrical stimulus. Also, short distances magnify the effect of small errors in measurement. For example, in an 8-month-old infant, a measurement error of only 2 mm creates a 2% difference in conduction velocity, whereas a 1-cm error can create an 8% to 12% difference. Finally, the greater surface area in infants and children makes them more susceptible to cooling of extremities and slowing of nerve conduction (at 2 m/sec per degree centigrade temperature loss). Lower temperatures also affect neuromuscular transmission and the appearance of motor unit potentials. These technical issues are compounded when studies are done portably in intensive care units where electronic equipment increases likelihood of electrical interference.

Nerve Conduction Studies

The procedure for NCS should be explained to the parent(s) to obtain informed consent. When appropriate, assent should be obtained from older children. As necessary, reassurances should be given regarding issues that are worrisome to children: The fact that the adhesive tape and the application of recording electrodes are not painful, that the stimulus is produced by the machine and is not electricity from a wall socket, and that it is normal for the stimulus to cause involuntary movement.

Most children tolerate the NCS portion quite well when the electromyographer recognizes that the peripheral nerves of children are close to the surface and require a relatively low stimulus intensity in comparison with the adult patient. Furthermore, enlisting the interest of older children by having them watch the waveform develop on the screen as they "build mountains," so to speak, is a useful technique.

Parents, who have spent much time keeping their children away from electric sockets in the home, are quite reassured to hear that the electrical stimuli used are not the same as "electricity" or household current. It helps to emphasize that the stimulus is of short duration (demonstrated by a click of the tongue) and that the sensation does not linger. Occasionally gaining the help of Mom or Dad is sometimes very useful, as one may perform a brief sensory NCS on them to gain their understanding of the relatively benign sensation that their child will experience with the NCS. If the patient wants more information, the stimulus can be likened to and demonstrated as the fast, sharp flick of finger against the skin of the electromyographer's extremity. When older children or youth are awake during NCS, it is useful to warn them of the arrival of each stimulus using a cue such as a tongue click. This frequently helps children retain a sense of control during a stressful experience.

Pediatric NCS are best accomplished by an experienced team consisting of an electromyographer and an EMG resident or technician. A large examination room is needed because a parent or extra personnel to monitor sedation are required in addition to standard equipment and personnel. Room lights that dim are helpful to promote patient relaxation and sedation. Extra time must be allotted for pediatric cases to allow for the slower pace and/or the administration of sedation. Pediatric cases can take nearly twice as long as a similar examination in a cooperative adult.

Several features unique to infants and children create technical problems for the electromyographer. In newborn infants, a significant layer of subcutaneous baby fat provides an energy reserve to provide for future growth. For example, muscle contributes to less than 60% of the cross-sectional diameter of the calf in newborn infants, whereas the proportion of muscle is greater than 80% in school-age children. Cutaneous nerves are relatively superficial; however, most major nerve trunks are contained in neurovascular bundles deep to baby fat. This requires the distance between anode and cathode to be greater than otherwise might be estimated necessary in these short limbs. Baby fat also tends to obscure palpable bony landmarks in infants and toddlers.

The ease with which sensory nerves are studied in children varies. For example, sural SNCS can be technically challenging in infants with proportionately large layers of baby fat. Alternatively, medial plantar NCS are technically easier. In children younger than 10 years of age, sensory potentials can be frequently recorded at the ankle and the knee with stimulation of the medial plantar sensory fibers in the foot. This allows calculation of sensory nerve conduction velocity along a proximal segment.

Increases in height and extremity length are dramatic throughout childhood. A simple rule of thumb is that length/ height and arm span double between birth and 2 years of age and double again by adulthood. Short distances between electrodes increase the potential for shock artifact due to spread of current, paste bridges, and so forth. Special stimulating electrodes need to be used in infants and toddlers to provide shorter and variable interelectrode distances. Factors that help alleviate shock artifact include careful cleansing of the skin prior to electrode application, careful physical separation of lead wires, prevention of paste bridges, use of the largest ground electrode possible, and use of paper or cloth towels to immobilize or manipulate the extremity. Constant current stimulators and near-nerve needle stimulating electrodes are used in some laboratories and have certain technical advantages.[7,9]

Two prospective studies on normal children demonstrated that nerve conduction measurements obtained in a given child were highly reproducible. In one study with infants,[6] motor nerve conduction velocities performed on different days in 15 infants demonstrated a mean difference of 1.6 m/sec. In another study,[13] the difference in sensory nerve conduction velocities performed on different days in several adolescent patients was less than 2 m/sec.

Needle Electromyography

Infants and children frequently experience a degree of difficulty tolerating the needle examination owing both to the discomfort of the needle insertion and probing as well as to psychological issues relating to fear of mutilation, body penetration, or loss of control. Children should be considered for conscious sedation if they present with a history of poorly tolerating painful medical or dental procedures or if they are believed, on a developmental basis, to be unlikely to tolerate the examination.

Parents are told that we expect the children to be partially alert and possibly object when the needle examination is started since there is some discomfort. We emphasize that no medication is being injected through the needle, so the child will not experience delayed soreness as with immunizations. When describing or discussing needle EMG, it is useful to call the needle electrode an "electrode" or "wire" and to assiduously avoid showing it to the patient. Some experienced electromyographers find that children respond well when they refer to the EMG needle as a "microphone that listens to the muscle".[14] The children are told they will feel a small pinch in the skin—"like a mosquito"—preceding the placement of the electrode in the muscle. Once the motor units are activated, the children are asked if they knew that their muscle could make such funny noises or what this response sounds like. The electromyographer may be surprised sometimes by the varied responses of children; in fact, their answer often creates a laugh, bringing some relaxation to the procedure per se.

Simultaneous tape-recording of the needle EMG for later detailed assessment or quantitation is frequently useful. Positioning and repositioning the extremity (particularly with the muscle at its shortest length) can aid in attaining a silent background for examination of insertional or spontaneous activity. Observation of voluntarily activated motor unit potentials can be more difficult if the patient is deeply sedated. With experience, pediatric anesthesiologists can titrate the degree of conscious sedation to allow controlled amounts of spontaneous movement. In infants or children unable or unwilling to contract the muscle voluntarily, motor unit activity initiated by repeated passive movements, tactile stimulation, or activation of infantile or protective reflexes can be used. The quality of motor unit potential activation can be improved by use of analgesic medication to decrease ongoing discomfort and midazolam to create amnesia for most of the experience.

As discussed earlier, infants and toddlers have a thick layer of body fat. One of the most important technical considerations is to use a needle electrode that is long enough to reach the muscle being studied. Use of standard concentric needle electrodes (37 to 42 mm in length, 26 gauge) has been most satisfactory. Experience has shown that the "child and facial" needles with a length of 20 mm are not long enough to reach limb muscles in many infants and children. Although monopolar needles are preferred by some clinicians, in my experience the minimal decrease in discomfort with insertion and manipulation of these needles is outweighed by the increase in background noise from the reference electrode in active limbs.

Certain muscles are easier to study in children of different ages. Therefore, if the process is diffuse and does not need to be "mapped out," the technically easiest muscles should be studied. Tibialis anterior, gluteus medius, iliopsoas, abductor digiti minimi, biceps brachii, and deltoid are muscles that can be immobilized and/or activated easily for study. The triceps is frequently activated voluntarily if the child's hand is gently placed over the eyes or nasal bridge. Infants and children usually receive immunizations in the anterior thigh rather than the deltoid. For this reason, the anterior thigh muscles should generally be avoided on needle examination.

CLINICAL NEUROPHYSIOLOGIC TECHNIQUES

Nerve Conduction Studies

Nerve conduction studies can help differentiate among many similarly presenting disorders of the motor unit. Findings can outline the following:

1. Types of nerve fibers involved, such as motor versus sensory, large- versus small-diameter fibers
2. Pattern of involvement, such as diffuse versus focal or multifocal, proximal versus distal

3. Type and degree of the physiologic insult, such as conduction block versus axonal injury

Knowledge of whether the axons have been partially or totally severed can determine the prognosis for and time course of recovery and whether surgical intervention may be useful. Nerve conduction techniques involve the application of brief, low-current, electrical square-wave pulses to peripheral nerves while recording the desired response over nerve or muscle. The amount of current used is adequate to stimulate the nerve fibers of interest (usually large myelinated motor or sensory fibers) but is subthreshold for the unmyelinated pain fibers. Therefore, the stimulus is usually described as a tapping, thumping, or stinging sensation. If motor fibers are activated, an involuntary brief contraction or twitch of the muscles innervated by those fibers distal to the site of stimulation occurs. Most commonly, tin disks can be taped or applied to the skin for both stimulation and recording. On occasion, subcutaneous needle electrodes must be employed to stimulate or record selectively from deeply placed nerves. Surface electrodes are obviously better tolerated by infants and children. The usefulness of the neurophysiologic information provided by NCSs is being increasingly demonstrated in pediatric medicine. Developmental changes in normative values for each of the techniques is discussed in detail in Chapter 7.

Motor Nerve Conduction Studies

MNCSs are performed by stimulating motor or mixed nerves and recording over the endplate region of a muscle innervated by those fibers. The summated electrical response of all the muscle fibers appears as the M wave, or compound muscle action potential (CMAP), whose onset latency, amplitude, and shape provide physiologic information. Stimulation at multiple points along the nerve produces CMAPs at different latencies. The difference in latency divided by the distance separating the points of stimulation calculates the conduction velocity of the fastest conducting fibers (Fig. 6-5). Any muscle whose nerve supply is superficial enough to be stimulated and whose endplate region is superficial enough and geometrically suited to producing a summated response can have motor nerve conduction recorded. Therefore, in addition to the commonly tested nerves in the forearms and legs, the phrenic nerve can be stimulated in the neck with the diaphragmatic CMAP recorded over the lower chest wall.[15] Another clinical application of NCS would be early in the course of idiopathic facial nerve palsy when evaluation of the CMAP amplitude and distal latency evoked by facial nerve stimulation accurately predicts the clinical outcome.[16] NCS have been used in countries with endemic outbreaks of poliomyelitis as a cost-effective, quick, and easy way to distinguish

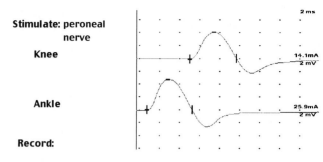

FIGURE 6–5

Motor Nerve Conduction Study

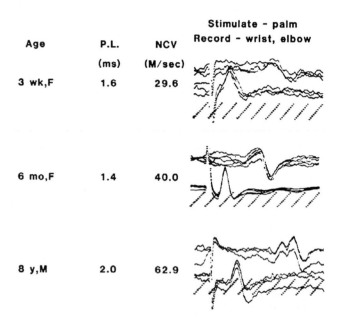

FIGURE 6–6

Sensory Nerve Conduction Studies: ulnar sensory nerve action potentials. F, female; M, male; PL, peak latency; NCV, nerve conduction velocity.

poliomyelitis from other motor nerve disorders such as Guillain-Barré syndrome.[17]

Sensory Nerve Conduction Studies

Sensory nerve action potentials (SNAPs) (Fig. 6-6) provide sensitive and specific information regarding the status of the peripheral sensory nerve fibers. As volume-conducted direct nerve action potentials, the amplitude of sensory potentials is low compared with motor responses, arising from the muscles per se (microvolts rather than millivolts). This makes it important to manage technical issues such as

TABLE 6–1

Methods of Performing Sensory Nerve Conduction Studies

Stimulation Site	Recording Site
Cutaneous sensory nerve	Same cutaneous sensory nerve fibers at a distance
	Mixed nerve containing same cutaneous sensory fibers
Mixed nerve	Cutaneous sensory nerve containing sensory fibers from mixed nerve

background noise and shock artifact. The shorter distances between stimulating and recording electrodes in infants and small children and the greater surface area in infants, which promotes extremity cooling, create potential challenges to high-quality SNCS in infants and children. SNCS are performed by stimulating and recording directly over sensory fibers. This can be accomplished in several manners as shown in Table 6-1.

In the peripheral nervous system, sensory neurons are located in the dorsal root, in ganglia extrinsic to the spinal cord—the dorsal root ganglia. Therefore, disorders or injury to the spinal cord or anterior spinal roots may occur without disrupting the connection between a dorsal root ganglion and its peripheral sensory processes. As long as that connection is preserved, the peripheral sensory potentials remain intact. For example, spinal nerve root avulsion from severe trauma can be associated with significant motor and sensory deficit with a complete disconnection of spinal motor neurons from their anterior roots and central sensory processes from their dorsal root ganglion. In this circumstance, despite dense clinical sensory loss, the SNAPs remain intact—the lesion having occurred proximal to the dorsal root ganglion. SNCS are valuable diagnostically because they are both

sensitive indicators of injury to peripheral nerves and useful in localizing disorders of the motor unit to *preganglionic* (proximal to dorsal root) and *postganglionic* (at or distal to the dorsal root ganglia).

F-Wave Latencies

F-wave latencies are late responses recorded over muscle and occur when retrograde conduction along motor axons stimulates anterograde impulses from a portion of the pool of anterior horn cells reached by the initial stimulus (Fig. 6-7). The F-wave latency includes conduction along the proximal portion of the motor axon that is not evaluated in standard peripheral MNCS. Because this response is an absolute latency, the value reflects both the conduction velocity as well as the distance traveled along the limb. Normal F-wave latencies cannot, therefore, be directly extrapolated from motor nerve conduction velocities but also need to account for limb length.[9,18]

H Reflexes

H reflexes are a motor response elicited via activation of the same monosynaptic reflex arc that is responsible for the clinically activated muscle stretch reflex. They are produced by activation of sensory fibers by a stimulation that submaximally activates motor fibers. The name (*H reflex*) reflects that the initial recordings were made in hand muscles. H reflexes are more easily elicited in infants than in older children and adults. Advantages of recording H reflexes lie in the low stimulation intensity required to elicit them and in their ability to convey information about the proximal sensory and motor pathways. Normal values have been published for H reflexes recorded in hand and calf muscles (Fig. 6-8).[19] Changes in H reflexes have been used to titrate optimum dosage of intrathecal baclofen in spastic children.[20]

Individual Responses

Superimposed Responses

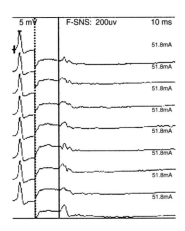

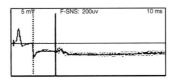

FIGURE 6–7

F-wave Latencies: tibial nerve.
SNS, sensivity or gain.

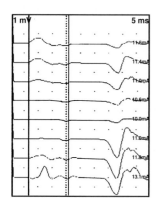

M wave   **H reflex**

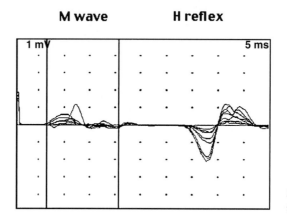

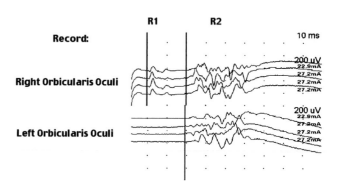

FIGURE 6–8
H Reflex: stimulate tibial nerve and record soleus muscle.

Blink Reflexes

Blink reflex study consists of early and late electrical responses recorded over bilateral orbicularis oculi muscles with low-intensity electrical stimulation of the supraorbital branch of the trigeminal nerve. This is a reflex arc with afferent impulses through the trigeminal nerve, multiple synapses in the pons, and an efferent limb through the facial nerve. Responses in term infants are less consistent and occur with longer latencies than those in adults. Normative data have been published for infants and children (Fig. 6-9).[21]

Repetitive Motor Nerve Stimulation

Neuromuscular transmission can be tested with pairs of stimuli or with trains of stimuli (repetitive stimulation). Disease states frequently lower the safety margin of neuromuscular transmission such that repeated stimuli in quick succession are followed by failure of the postsynaptic membrane to generate an action potential. With repetitive stimulation, the amplitude and area of serially generated responses are compared. Repetitive stimulation at 2 to 3 Hz (Fig. 6-10) is used to evaluate postsynaptic disorders of neuromuscular transmission, including acquired autoimmune myasthenia gravis and most forms of congenital myasthenic syndrome. Rapid, repetitive stimulation at 20

FIGURE 6–9
Blink Reflex: stimulate right supraorbital nerve.

to 50 Hz (Fig. 6-11) is needed to test for the facilitation or increment in amplitude characteristic of infantile botulism and other presynaptic disorders of neuromuscular transmission.

Rapid, repetitive motor nerve stimulation is uncomfortable and can be technically difficult to perform in infants and children because voluntary movement of the extremity produces artifact. Normal infants younger than 6 months of age can demonstrate decrements in CMAP amplitude

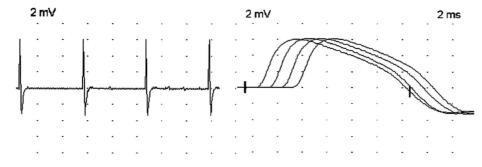

Sequential responses   **Superimposed responses**

FIGURE 6–10
Slow Repetitive Stimulation: stimulate spinal accessory nerve and record trapezius muscle.

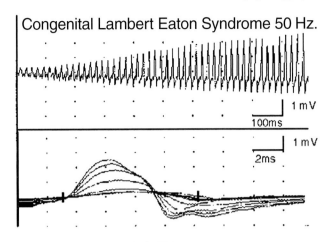

FIGURE 6–11
Rapid Repetitive Stimulation. LES, Lambert Eaton syndrome; stimulate femoral nerve, record rectus femoris muscle.

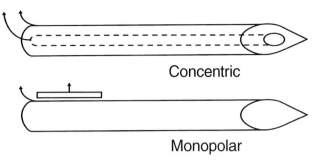

FIGURE 6–12
Electrodes for Needle Electromyography: concentric needle/monopolar.

of up to 50% in response to 20- to 50-Hz repetitive stimulation.[22] Repetitive stimulation has been useful in differentiating the pathophysiologic causes of prolonged respiratory paralysis following critical illness in children. For example, polyneuropathy of critical illness and persistent neuromuscular blockade secondary to prolonged pharmacologic neuromuscular blockade can be differentiated by NCS including repetitive stimulation.[23] More detailed descriptions of applying these techniques to neuromuscular disorders common to infants and children are contained in Chapter 27.

Motor Unit Number Estimation

Motor unit number estimation is a neurophysiologic method to estimate the number of motor units (and, therefore, lower motor neurons) innervating a specific muscle. There are several different techniques (all-or-none incremental, spike-triggered averaging, and the statistical method) that have been developed to obtain such estimates, and these are not reviewed in detail here.[24,25] The multiple-point stimulation technique is based on electrical activation of single motor axons in an all-or-none fashion. A sample of single motor unit potentials can be obtained by moving the stimulating electrode to multiple points along a nerve. Motor unit number estimation values are calculated from the ratio of the maximal CMAP to the average single motor unit potential. This technique can be applied easily to the ulnar nerve–hypothenar muscle group in infants and young children with reproducible results. A modified multiple-point stimulation technique for monitoring the loss of motor neurons in infants and young children with spinal muscular atrophy has shown promise in documenting the natural course of disease progression in these patients.[26]

EMG

Needle Electromyography

Needle electromyography is the technique most frequently used to provide qualitative and quantitative descriptions of voluntary motor units. Standard EMG is performed with a specialized recording electrode with a thickness equivalent to a 26-gauge needle and a length adequate to reach the muscle (Fig. 6-12). The electrode is inserted into a muscle, pausing at a number of sites for evaluation of the electrical response to needle insertion. Spontaneously occurring electrical activity is noted.

Concomitantly, one needs to assess the voluntarily activated motor unit potentials. However, in contrast with the adolescent and the adult patient, one needs to examine the motor unit potentials when they are activated, often involuntarily, in the infant and toddler. One attempts to observe both the recruitment pattern and details of individual motor unit potentials (amplitude, duration, number of phases, stability over time). As discussed later, there are a number of different methods to quantitate the character of voluntary motor unit potentials; however, an audiovisual semiqualitative assessment is most frequently used. Standard needle EMG can reliably differentiate neurogenic processes from other motor problems in infants and children. Needle EMG can provide important information about the pathophysiology of the disease process—for example, the presence or absence of ongoing reinnervation.

Most muscles in the body can be studied by EMG. The muscles that are most superficial and distinct from vascular structures and other muscles are the most easily studied. However, hooked-wire electrodes have been inserted into posterior cricoarytenoid and thyroarytenoid muscles to differentiate between vocal cord fixation and paralysis[27,28] and into the diaphragm for evaluation of that muscle. Surface EMG recordings of diaphragm and intercostal muscles have been shown to correlate with the forced expiratory volume in one second in children with asthma.[29] Cranial nerve-innervated muscles can be monitored by intramuscular wire electrodes as part of intraoperative monitoring.

For example, EMG activity in lateral rectus and facial muscles during resection of fourth ventricular tumors was shown to correlate with postoperative facial weakness.[30]

The more complete and specific the differential diagnosis and physiologic questions to be answered, the better able the electromyographer is to select and prioritize the muscles to be studied. If a muscle biopsy is planned, the electromyographer should be informed so that that particular muscle will not be examined because needle insertion can produce artifacts difficult to differentiate from pathologic change. Patients with bleeding tendencies should be evaluated individually with consideration given to the magnitude of the clotting disorder as well as the location of the muscles to be examined. Examination of superficial muscles can usually be safely performed in patients with mild clotting problems.

The findings on needle examination are somewhat different in infants and children than in adults. Frequent motor endplate regions are encountered, especially in children younger than 1 year of age or with significant central nervous system immaturity.[31] Initially positive, low-amplitude, short-duration "preinnervation infantile activity" has been described in premature infants and in children with developmental disorders such as myelomeningocele when innervation has not naturally occurred.[32] There is no evidence that typical fibrillation potentials occur in fullterm or older infants unless there is an abnormality in the peripheral nervous system.

The time frame for appearance of positive sharp waves and fibrillation potentials as EMG evidence of denervation may well be shorter in infants than in adults. In adults, extremity muscles frequently do not demonstrate denervation for up to 21 days after spinal root injury. Fibrillation potentials may appear after a shorter interval after denervation in infants and young children. A well-documented case report of a 4030-gm infant delivered vaginally with clinical shoulder dystocia and subsequent flaccid, areflexic paralysis of the right arm demonstrated increased insertional activity with continuous runs of positive sharp waves in right shoulder and proximal forearm muscles during the first EMG on the fourth day of life. Similar changes were seen in right hand muscles on the fifth day but had not been present on the fourth day. Although an intrauterine injury was not completely excluded, the root avulsion seen on a magnetic resonance imaging study, the pattern of soft tissue injury, and the clinical history were strongly suggestive of an intrapartum insult.[33]

Motor unit potential recruitment does not differ significantly between children and adults. To obtain maximum information from needle EMG, it is important to characterize motor unit potential recruitment separately from evaluation of individual motor unit potential size. This is even more critical in infants and young children, in whom

congenital malformations (such as hypoplasia of muscle) can produce findings not commonly seen in adults.

During standard needle EMG, judgments about motor unit potential characteristics are made by visually estimating measurements on 20 to 40 motor unit potentials individually isolated during mild to moderate contractions. The motor unit potentials recorded during standard needle EMG represent a summation of the potentials from individual muscle fibers that are innervated by a single anterior horn cell and that are within several millimeters of the recording electrode (Fig. 6-13).[34] The exact number of fibers that contribute to a motor unit potential depends on the characteristics of the recording electrode (the pickup area) and its relationship to the patchy distribution of individual fibers in a given motor unit.

Motor unit potentials in infants and young children are characterized by simpler configuration, shorter duration, and lower amplitude.[35] In premature infants, motor unit potentials are described as monophasic or biphasic, less than 100 μV in amplitude and 1 to 4 milliseconds in duration.[36] Shorter duration motor unit potentials are seen in all muscles in infants.[37] The rate at which duration increases with age varies between muscles. At 20 weeks' gestation, the range of muscle fiber diameter is 5 to 12 μm. This increases to 7 to 12 μm in fullterm infants. The muscle fiber diameter increases slowly until it reaches the adult range of 45 to 64 μm by 12 years of age. Concomitantly, the width of the endplate zone increases. In the biceps, this distance is 6 mm in fullterm infants and increases to 25 mm in adults. The increasing muscle fiber diameter means that there is more spatial dispersion of the different fibers whose action potentials summate to form the motor unit potential.

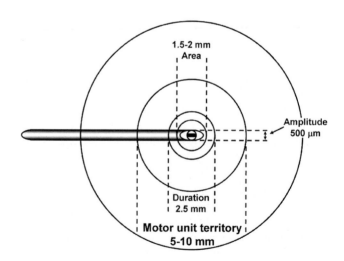

FIGURE 6–13
Contribution to Motor Unit Potential Recordings with Concentric Needle Electrode.

Willison and Smythe have described a method of motor unit potential quantitation that produces a mean ratio of amplitude per turns per second.[38] Further quantitative refinement has been proposed for turns analysis of the EMG interference pattern. These include "upper centile amplitude" (which defines the upper limit of the maximum peak-to-peak amplitude of the motor unit action potentials) and "number of small segments" (which is a reflection of the polyphasicity of the component motor unit action potentials).[39] These techniques have evolved into development of "clouds" of turns and amplitude measurements on 500-millisecond epochs of interference pattern that vary with the force of voluntary contraction.[40] This and other methods of motor unit quantitation, including motor unit number estimation, remain to be standardized in infants and children.

However, individual motor unit potential characteristics in infants are different from those in adults. In infants, motor unit potentials are simpler in configuration, shorter in duration (≈ 70% adult values), and lower in amplitude (≈ 20% to 50% of adult values).[35] Motor unit potential changes with aging are therefore greater with respect to amplitude (a twofold to fivefold increase) as compared to duration (an increase of only one third).

Quantitative methods increase the sensitivity to minor degrees of abnormality. These may vary from manual graphic measurements to computer-generated measurements of individual motor units to theoretically derived computer programs for quantitating motor units or motor unit populations from partial interference patterns (a more moderate contraction with multiple motor units firing simultaneously).[41] The latter methods are appealing for potential application to pediatric patients because they require less voluntary cooperation and are increasingly available as part of commercial EMG systems. Surface electrode recordings of interference patterns (motor unit potentials produced by a strong enough voluntary contraction to make it difficult to isolate individual potentials) have been studied quantitatively (mean ratio of amplitude per turns per second) in babies and young children.[38] Reports of extensive experience with quantitative EMG methods in infants and children have not yet been published. Serum muscle enzymes should be drawn before needle EMG because the repeated needle insertions involved in most studies can produce a transient elevation of muscle enzymes that may confound the diagnostic effort.

Disease processes that primarily involve abnormalities of the contractile mechanism of the muscle fiber tend to cause milder changes in the characteristics of the individual motor unit potentials: a tendency toward lower amplitude, briefer duration, and increased percentage of polyphasic motor unit potentials (Fig. 6-14). There is a change in motor unit potential recruitment proportional to the degree of reduced-strength–recruitment of greater numbers of motor unit potentials firing more rapidly and producing relatively less strength of contraction—but this cannot be quantified with standard EMG laboratory equipment. Therefore, it is understandable that NCS and EMG results produced changes characteristic of a myopathy in only 10% to 40% of biopsy-proven myopathies.[42,43] Motor unit potentials and recruitment patterns can be difficult to differentiate from normal in some myopathic processes, including carrier states or subclinical phases of muscular dystrophies and congenital structurally distinct myopathies. Further discussion of neurophysiologic changes noted in myopathic processes is noted in Chapter 26.

Disease processes that involve loss of innervation to the muscle fibers are initially characterized by decreased numbers of motor unit potentials that can be voluntarily

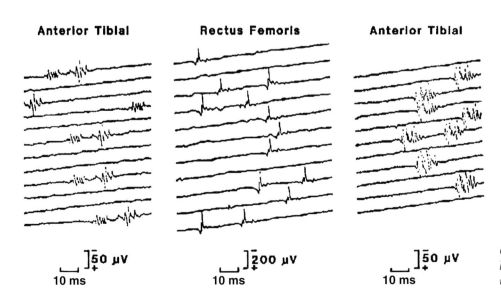

Anterior Tibial   **Rectus Femoris**   **Anterior Tibial**

]50 µV   ]200 µV   ]50 µV

10 ms   10 ms   10 ms

FIGURE 6–14

Congenital Myotonic Dystrophy: low amplitude, polyphasic motor unit potentials.

Anterior Tibial

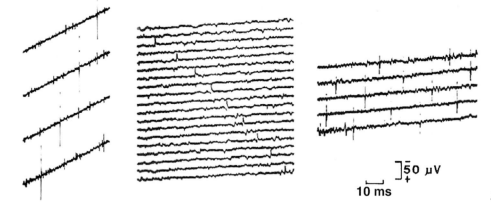

50 µV

10 ms

FIGURE 6–15
Congenital Myotonic Dystrophy: fibrillation potentials.

recruited. If the denervation persists, fibrillation potentials occur spontaneously and signal the presence of denervated muscle fibers (Fig. 6-15). As reinnervation occurs, there are usually fewer but larger (higher amplitude, longer duration) motor unit potentials (Fig. 6-16). Many disease states involve variable degrees of both muscle fiber involvement and nerve fiber loss. In such cases, the concept of "myopathic" and "neurogenic" motor unit potentials is too simplistic and can be misleading. Characterization of distinct motor unit populations is useful in understanding the pathophysiology of the disease process. For example, a population of low-amplitude, polyphasic-varying motor unit potentials with decreased recruitment suggests a chronic neurogenic process with a component of ongoing reinnervation.

Single-Fiber EMG

Single-fiber EMG (Fig. 6-17) is a technique that selectively records from a single or pair of muscle fibers from the same motor unit. This technique provides physiologic information about neuromuscular transmission, which can be affected by primary pathologic change in the neuromuscular junction or secondarily by denervation and reinnervation. Single-fiber EMG is particularly valuable in infants and children because of the wide range of disorders of neuromuscular transmission that occur in this age group. Collated norms for single-fiber EMG jitter and fiber density have been published in older children.[44] Standard single-fiber EMG requires patient cooperation and sustained control of voluntary activation of motor unit potentials. This

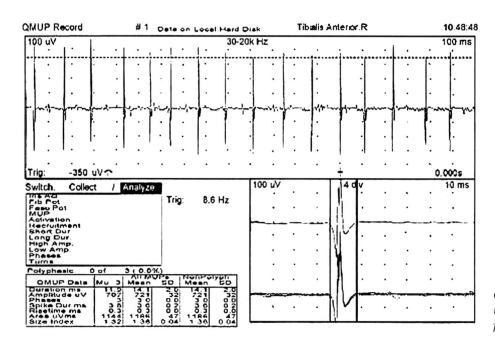

FIGURE 6–16
Chronic Reinnervation: decreased numbers of large motor unit potentials.

Pair 1

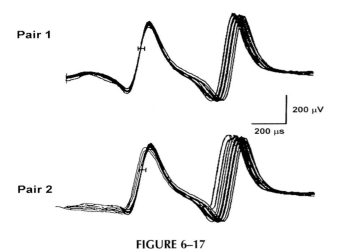

200 μV

200 μs

Pair 2

FIGURE 6–17
Single-fiber electromyography.

is extremely difficult to achieve in infants or younger children. A technique using electrical stimulation of the axon to produce the motor unit potentials to record by single-fiber EMG electrode has been described.[45] This technique does not require sustained voluntary contraction and, therefore, can be used in the pediatric age group. Stimulated single-fiber EMG can be performed with the infant or child under conscious sedation. This technique has been used to facilitate evaluation of infants with botulism[46] and congenital myasthenic syndromes[47] and to promote an improved understanding of the pathophysiology of childhood neuromuscular disorders such as Schwartz-Jampel syndrome.[48]

SUMMARY

With careful attention to technical details and constant awareness of the continuous process of maturation, NCS and EMG are powerful diagnostic tools for evaluating infants and children. Despite the increasing array of molecular genetics tests available for diagnosing neuromuscular disorders in infants and children, NCS and EMG remain a necessary and valuable component of our pediatric neuromuscular practice.[49] NCS and EMG are useful in developing differential diagnoses, establishing prognosis, and monitoring the course of disease during surgical intervention or ongoing treatment trials.

NCS and EMG continue to play an important role in the diagnosis of neuromuscular disorders. These physiologic techniques are not performed in all children with neuromuscular symptoms. For example, infants and children who present with likely diagnoses of dystrophin-deficient muscular dystrophy or spinal muscular atrophy are likely to undergo initial molecular genetics testing in an attempt to establish a definitive diagnosis. However, NCS and EMG

remain important diagnostic techniques in infants and children with less stereotyped clinical presentations (e.g., floppy infants) or unusual clinical problems such as vocal cord paralysis[28] or acute poliomyelitis.[17] NCS and EMG are also valuable when disorders of neuromuscular transmission or peripheral nerve are suspected or when initial molecular genetics testing is unrevealing. NCS and EMG play a particularly important diagnostic role in the evaluation of infants and children with acute onset of weakness seen in critical care settings.[23,50,51]

NCS and EMG delineate the physiologic changes in many disorders and can thereby give important clues about prognosis. For example, by differentiating among acute inflammatory demyelinating polyradiculopathy, acute motor and sensory axonal neuropathy, acute motor axonal neuropathy, and inexcitable nerves in clinical Guillain-Barré syndrome, the likelihood and timeline of clinical recovery can be projected.[52-54] Similarly, prognosis in focal neuropathies (including facial neuropathies) can be projected from physiologic information obtained from NCS and EMG.[16] Other studies have shown that CMAP amplitude and findings on needle electromyography can supplement clinical findings to develop a prognosis for infants and children presenting with spinal muscular atrophy.[55]

NCS, EMG, and evoked potentials are increasingly being used during surgical intervention to monitor neurophysiology and minimize morbidity. These techniques are particularly useful in monitoring posterior fossa surgery,[30] spinal cord surgery, and surgical dissections of the anterior neck.[56] NCSs, including repetitive stimulation, have been used in randomized clinical trials to assess effectiveness of new anesthetic agents[57] and to monitor prolonged therapeutic paralysis.[58] Surface EMG has been used to evaluate movement disorders in children.[59] EMG-guided botulinum toxin injections are used to treat disorders of motor control.[60] Surface EMG is also used as an integral component of biofeedback training in children with voiding dysfunction unresponsive to other therapies.[61,62]

In summary, clinical neurophysiologic techniques can be used to characterize the neurophysiology of the motor unit. Application of these techniques allows one to define disorders affecting the anterior horn cell, spinal nerve roots, peripheral nerves, nerve terminals, neuromuscular junction, and/or muscle. Technical problems relating to small size, decreased voluntary cooperation, rapid change of normal values during maturation, and less well-defined normal values make the application of these techniques in infants and children more challenging. Nevertheless, with collaboration between the referring physician, parent, patient, and electromyographer, exacting pathophysiologic information can be obtained that may not be available by any other means. The potential exists to use these techniques not only for diagnostic purposes but also for prognostic purposes and for following the course of disease during clinical treatment trials.

REFERENCES

1. Brown WF, Bolton CF, Aminoff MJ: Neuromuscular Function and Disease: Basic, Clinical, and Electrodiagnostic Aspects, Vol 2. Philadelphia, WB Saunders, 2002, Sections I (pp 1-102), IV (pp 247-400), V (pp 401-432).

2. Daube JR (ed): Clinical Neurophysiology, 2nd ed. Oxford, Oxford University Press, 2002.

3. Sorenson EJ: Nerve action potentials. *In* Daube JR (ed): Clinical Neurophysiology, 2nd ed. Oxford, Oxford University Press, 2002, pp 169-180.

4. Daube JR: Compound muscle action potentials. *In* Daube JR (ed): Clinical Neurophysiology, 2nd ed. Oxford, Oxford University Press, 2002, pp 237-267.

5. Hermann RJ Jr: Assessing the neuromuscular junction with repetitive stimulation studies. *In* Daube JR (ed): Clinical Neurophysiology, 2nd ed. Oxford, Oxford University Press, 2002, pp 268-281.

6. Thomas JE, Lambert EH: Ulnar nerve conduction velocity and H reflex in infants and children. J Appl Physiol 1960;15:1-9.

7. Wagner AL, Buchthal F: Motor and sensory conduction in infancy and childhood: Reappraisal. Dev Med Child Neurol 1972;14:189-216.

8. Jones HR Jr, Bolton CF, Harper CM Jr: Pediatric Clinical Electromyography. Philadelphia, Lippincott-Raven, 1996.

9. Miller RG, Kuntz NL: Nerve conduction studies in infants and children. J Child Neurol 1986;1:19-26.

10. Garcia A, Calleja J, Antolin FM, Berciano J: Peripheral motor and sensory nerve conduction studies in normal infants and children. Clin Neurophysiol 2000;111:513-520.

11. Kimura J: Electrodiagnosis in Disease of Nerve and Muscle: Principles and Practice. Philadelphia, FA Davis, 1983.

12. Hays RM, Hackworth SR, Speltz ML, Weinstein P: Physicians' practice patterns in pediatric electrodiagnosis. Arch Phys Med Rehabil 1992;74:494-496.

13. Kuntz NL: Childhood sensory nerve conduction studies. Unpublished data, 1983.

14. Jones HR Jr and Darras BT: Pediatric Electromyography. *In* Brown WF, Bolton CF, and Aminoff MJ (eds): Clinical Indications and Methodology in Neuromuscular Functional Disease: Basic, Clinical and Electrodiagnostic Aspects Vol 2. WB Saunders, Philadelphia, 2002;pp 1539-1551.

15. Moosa AL: Phrenic nerve conduction in children. Dev Med Child Neurol 1981;23:434-448.

16. Danielides V, Skevas A, Kastanioudakis I, Assimakopoulos D: Comparative study of evoked electromyography and facial nerve latency test in the prognosis of idiopathic facial nerve palsy in childhood. Childs Nerv Syst 1994;10:122-125.

17. Agboatwalla M, Kirmani SR, Sonawalla A, Akram DS: Nerve conduction studies and its importance in diagnosis of acute poliomyelitis. Indian J Pediatr 1993;60:265-268.

18. Parano E, Uncini A, DeVivo DC, Lovelace RE: Electrophysiologic correlates of peripheral nervous system maturation in infancy and childhood. J Child Neurol 1993;8:336-338.

19. Mayer RF, Mosser RS: Excitability of motoneurons in infants. Neurology 1969;19:932-945.

20. Dachy B, Dan B: Electrophysiological assessment of the effect of intrathecal baclofen in spastic children. Clin Neurophysiol 2002;113:336-340.

21. Kimura J, Bodensteiner J, Yamada T: Electrically elicited blink reflex in normal neonates. Arch Neurol 1977;34:246-249.

22. Churchill-Davidson HC, Wise RP: Neuromuscular transmission in the newborn infant. Anesthesiology 1963;24:271-278.

23. Heckmatt JZ, Pitt MC, Kirkham F: Peripheral neuropathy and neuromuscular blockade presenting as prolonged respiratory paralysis following critical illness. Neuropediatrics 1993;24:123-125.

24. Daube JR, Gooch C, Shefner J, et al: Motor unit number estimation (MUNE) with nerve conduction studies. Clin Neurophysiol 2000;53(Suppl):112-115.

25. Daube JR: Estimating the number of motor units in a muscle. *In* Clinical Neurophysiology, 2nd ed. Oxford, Oxford University Press, 2002, pp 358-371.

26. Bromberg MB, Swoboda KJ: Motor unit number estimation in infants and children with spinal muscular atrophy. Muscle Nerve 2002;25:445-447.

27. Jacobs IN, Finkel RS: Laryngeal electromyography in the management of vocal cord mobility problems in children. Laryngoscope 2002;112:1243-1248.

28. Gartian MG, Peterson KL, Hoffman HT, et al: Bipolar hooked-wire electromyographic technique in the evaluation of pediatric vocal cord paralysis. Ann Otol Rhinol Laryngol 1993;102:695-700.

29. Maarsingh EJ, van Eykern LA, deHaan RJ, et al: Airflow limitation in asthmatic children assessed with a noninvasive EMG technique. Respir Physiol Neurobiol 2002;133:89-97.

30. Grabb PA, Albright AL, Sclabassi RJ, Pollack IF: Continuous intraoperative electromyographic monitoring of cranial nerves during resection of fourth ventricular tumors in children. J Neurosurg 1997;86:1-4.

31. Turk MA: Pediatric electrodiagnosis. Phys Med Rehabil 1989;3:791-808.

32. Inberg HO, Johnson EW: Electromyographic evaluation of infants with lumbar meningomyelocele. Arch Phys Med Rehabil 1963;44:86-92.

33. Mancias P, Slopis JM, Veakley JW, Vriesendrop FJ: Combined brachial plexus injury and root avulsion after complicated delivery. Muscle Nerve 1994;17:1237-1238.

34. Stalberg E, Nandedkar SD, Sanders DB, Falck B: Quantitative motor unit potential analysis. J Clin Neurophysiol 1996;13:401-422.

35. Sacco G, Buchthal F, Rosenfalck P: Motor unit potentials at different ages. Arch Neurol 1962;6:366-373.

36. Marinacci A: Dynamics of neuromuscular diseases. Arch Neurol 1959;6:243-257.

37. Buchthal F: Introduction to Electromyography. Copenhagen, Scandinavian University Books, 1957.

38. Willison RG, Smythe DPL: Quantitative electromyography in babies and young children with no evidence of neuromuscular disease. J Neurol Sci 1982;56:209-217.

39. Nandedkar SD, Sanders DB, Stalberg EV: Automatic analysis of the electromyographic interference pattern: I. Development of quantitative features. Muscle Nerve 1986;9:431-439.

40. Nandedkar SD, Sanders DB, Stalberg EV: On the shape of the normal turns-amplitude cloud. Muscle Nerve 1991;14:8-13.

41. Hermann RJ Jr: Quantitative electromyography. *In* Daube JR (ed): Clinical Neurophysiology, 2nd ed. Oxford, Oxford University Press, 2002, pp 324-342.

42. Russell JW, Afifi AK, Ross MA: Predictive value of electromyography in diagnosis and prognosis of the hypotonic infant. J Child Neurol 1992;7:387-391.

43. Davis WS, Jones HR Jr: Electromyography and biopsy correlation with suggested protocol for evaluation of the floppy infant. Muscle Nerve 1994;17:424-431.

44. Bromberg MB, Scott DM, and the ad hoc committee of the AAEM Single-Fiber Special Interest Group: Single-Fiber EMG reference values: Reformatted in tabular form. Muscle Nerve 1994;17:820-821.

45. Trontelj JV, Stalberg E, Mihelin M, Khuraibet A: Jitter of the stimulated motor axon. Muscle Nerve 1992;15:449-454.

46. Chaudry V, Crawford TO: Stimulated single-fiber EMG in infantile botulism. Muscle Nerve 1999;22:1698-1703.

47. Harper CM: Neuromuscular transmission disorders in childhood. *In* Pediatric Clinical Electromyography. Philadelphia, Lippincott-Raven, 1996, pp 353-385.

48. Jablecki C, Schultz P: Single muscle fiber recordings in the Schwartz-Jampel syndrome. Muscle Nerve 1982;5: S64-S69.

49. Darras BT, Jones HR Jr: Diagnosis of pediatric neuromuscular disorders in the era of DNA analysis. Pediatr Neurol 2000;23:289-300.

50. Jones HR Jr, Darras BT: Acute care pediatric electromyography. Muscle Nerve 2000;999:S53-S62.

51. Chetaille P, Paut O, Fraisse A, et al: Acute myopathy of intensive care in a child after heart transplantation. Can J Anaesth 2000;47:342-346.

52. Bradshaw DY, Jones HR Jr: Guillain-Barré syndrome in children: Clinical course, electrodiagnosis, and prognosis. Muscle Nerve 1992;15:500-506.

53. Phillips JP, Kincaid JC, Garg BP: Acute motor axonal neuropathy in childhood: Clinical and MRI findings. Pediatr Neurol 1997;16:152-155.

54. Massaro ME, Rodriguez EC, Pociecha J, et al: Nerve biopsy in children with severe Guillain-Barré syndrome and inexcitable motor nerves. Neurology 1998;51:394-398.

55. Kuntz NL, Gomez MR, Daube JR: Prognosis in childhood proximal spinal muscular atrophy. Neurology 1980;30:378.

56. Horn D, Rotzscher VM: Intraoperative electromyogram monitoring of the recurrent laryngeal nerve: Experience with an intralaryngeal surface electrode—a method to reduce the risk of recurrent laryngeal nerve injury during thyroid surgery. Langenbecks Arch Surg 1999;384:392-395.

57. Kenaan CA, Estacio RL, Bikhazi GB: Pharmacodynamics and intubating conditions of cisatracurium in children during halothane and opioid anesthesia. J Clin Anesth 2000;12:173-176.

58. Brandom BW, Yellon RF, Lloyd ME, et al: Recovery from doxacurium infusion administered to produce immobility for more than four days in pediatric patients in the intensive care unit. Anesth Analg 1997;84:307-314.

59. Oguro K, Kobayashi J, Aiba H, et al: Electrophysiological study of myoclonus in pediatric practice. Electromyogr Clin Neurophysiol 1998;38:207-221.

60. Heinen F, Wissel J, Philipsen A, et al: Interventional neuropediatrics: Treatment of dystonic and spastic muscular hyperactivity with botulinum toxin A. Neuropediatrics 1997;28:307-313.

61. McKenna PH, Herndon CD, Connery S, Ferrer FA: Pelvic floor muscle retraining for pediatric voiding dysfunction using interactive computer games. J Urol 1999;162:1056-1062.

62. Yamanishi T, Yasuda K, Murayama N, et al: Biofeedback training for detrusor overactivity in children. J Urol 2000;164:1686-1690.

7

Maturational Changes vis-à-vis Neurophysiology Markers and the Development of Peripheral Nerves

MATTHEW PITT

PERIPHERAL NERVES

Embryology

In early embryonic life cells migrate from the ependymal layer of the primitive spinal cord to the mantle layer and become differentiated into neuroblasts (Figs. 7-1 and 7-2). Those in the anterior and lateral parts of the mantle layer produce the fibers of the ventral roots and enter the myotomes of the mesodermal somites, ultimately becoming the alpha and gamma efferents of the ventral nerve roots (Fig. 7-3). The fibers of the dorsal roots develop from the spinal ganglia, which develop from the proliferating cells in the neural crest. The ventral and dorsal roots combine to produce the spinal nerves.

Peripheral nerve myelination begins about the 15th week of gestation[1] and continues throughout the first 2 to 5 years of life (Figs. 7-4 and 7-5).[2,3] A direct relationship exists between the diameter of the axon and the thickness of the myelin sheath. Conduction velocity (CV) increases in proportion to the diameter of the nerve fibers, the ratio being about 6:1.[4] Rexed[3] reported that the diameter of the seventh cervical ventral root in the newborn is 3 to 5 μm and increases to 8 to 11 μm at 2 to 5 years. The diameters of peripheral nerves range from 1 to 3 μm in the newborn and between 1 and 7 μm in children 4 years of age.[2] The nodes of Ranvier are remodeled during maturation with

the maximum internodal distances occurring at 5 years,[5] and there is a linear relationship between diameter and internode difference, as in adults.

Motor Nerve Studies

Studies in premature infants show the expected increase in motor conduction velocity (MCV) with age, although many of the studies suffer from the problem of small numbers of subjects. At the beginning of the third trimester, the median MCV may be as low as 9 to 11 m/sec, about a third of the values expected at birth.[6] In a group below 34 weeks the mean median MCV was 15.6 m/sec.[7] The mean ulnar nerve MCV in a group between 33 and 41 weeks was 20.2 m/sec,[8] similar to the mean peroneal MCV of 19.1 m/sec. Bahtia and associates[7] reported a velocity of around 27 m/sec for the median at birth.

The effects of growth retardation on this maturation have been studied and the results have been inconsistent. Using the weight of the baby as an indicator of maturity, Cerra and Johnson,[8] in their study of babies between 33 and 41 weeks of age, found that CV could be correlated with birthweight, a conclusion not supported by Cruz-Martinez and colleagues[6] studying similar-aged infants. Weight alone may be a sufficiently sensitive measure of maturity in babies only if there is severe intrauterine growth retardation. Bahatia and Prakash,[9] comparing premature babies (mean gestational

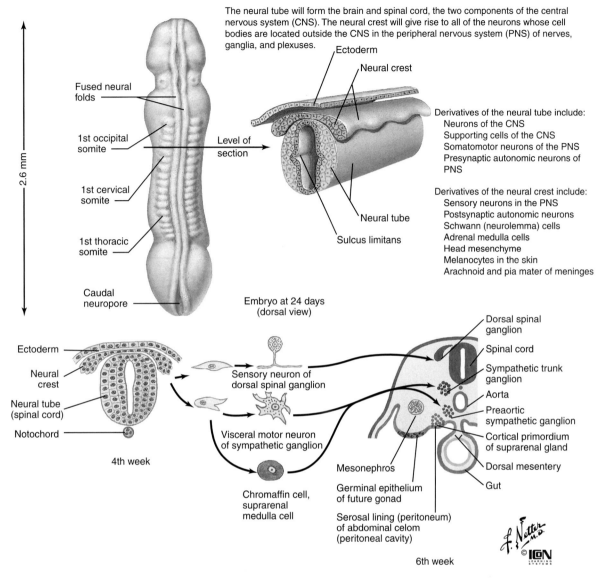

The neural tube will form the brain and spinal cord, the two components of the central nervous system (CNS). The neural crest will give rise to all of the neurons whose cell bodies are located outside the CNS in the peripheral nervous system (PNS) of nerves, ganglia, and plexuses.

Derivatives of the neural tube include:
Neurons of the CNS
Supporting cells of the CNS
Somatomotor neurons of the PNS
Presynaptic autonomic neurons of PNS

Derivatives of the neural crest include:
Sensory neurons in the PNS
Postsynaptic autonomic neurons
Schwann (neurolemma) cells
Adrenal medulla cells
Head mesenchyme
Melanocytes in the skin
Arachnoid and pia mater of meninges

FIGURE 7–1

Neural tube development. (Courtesy of Icon Learning Systems. Copyright©, Icon Learning Systems, LLC. A subsidiary of MediMedia, USA, Inc. All rights reserved.)

age [GA] 34.6 weeks) to fullterm babies (mean GA 38.1 weeks), found the expected differences, mean MNCV 18 m/sec versus mean MNCV 21 m/sec, when birthweights in the two groups were between 1801 and 2100 gm. When the two groups' birthweights were between 1500 and 1800 gm, a more severe intrauterine growth retardation, there was a greater effect on the fullterm group, whose mean motor nerve conduction velocity (MNCV) was 19 m/sec while the premature group remained at 18 m/sec. Bhatia and coworkers[7] analyzed their results for the influence of other factors and crown-heel length and maternal serum albumin were found to be significant independent variables with MNCV

values being lower in those with lower values of these two variables. Skin-fold thickness is another parameter that might be a better measure of the adequacy of fetal nutrition than weight. Robinson and Robertson [10] found a significant correlation between this and nerve CV when studying 27 babies born around term. Schulte and associates[11] found a wide variation in the velocities in small-for-date babies, which suggests that the contributions of myelination and nutrition vary widely in these children.

There are other differences between nerves of newborns and those of adults. The MCVs of the median, ulnar, and peroneal nerves are similar (average 27 m/sec) at birth,

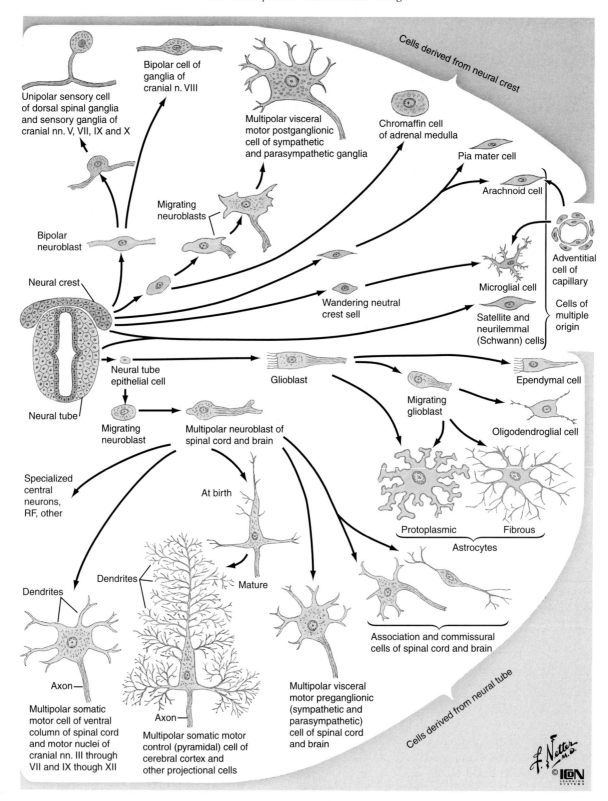

Unipolar sensory cell of dorsal spinal ganglia and sensory ganglia of cranial nn. V, VII, IX and X

Bipolar cell of ganglia of cranial n. VIII

Multipolar visceral motor postganglionic cell of sympathetic and parasympathetic ganglia

Chromaffin cell of adrenal medulla

Cells derived from neural crest

Pia mater cell

Arachnoid cell

Migrating neuroblasts

Bipolar neuroblast

Adventitial cell of capillary

Cells of multiple origin

Neural crest

Microglial cell

Wandering neutral crest sell

Satellite and neurilemmal (Schwann) cells

Neural tube epithelial cell

Glioblast

Neural tube

Ependymal cell

Migrating neuroblast

Migrating glioblast

Oligodendroglial cell

Multipolar neuroblast of spinal cord and brain

Specialized central neurons, RF, other

At birth

Protoplasmic   Fibrous

Astrocytes

Dendrites

Dendrites

Mature

Dendrites

Axon

Association and commissural cells of spinal cord and brain

Multipolar somatic motor cell of ventral column of spinal cord and motor nuclei of cranial nn. III through VII and IX though XII

Axon

Multipolar somatic motor control (pyramidal) cell of cerebral cortex and other projectional cells

Multipolar visceral motor preganglionic (sympathetic and parasympathetic) cell of spinal cord and brain

Cells derived from neural tube

FIGURE 7–2

Neural crest formation. (Courtesy of Icon Learning Systems. Copyright©, Icon Learning Systems, LLC. A subsidiary of MediMedia, USA, Inc. All rights reserved.)

Differentiation and Growth of Neurons at 26 Days

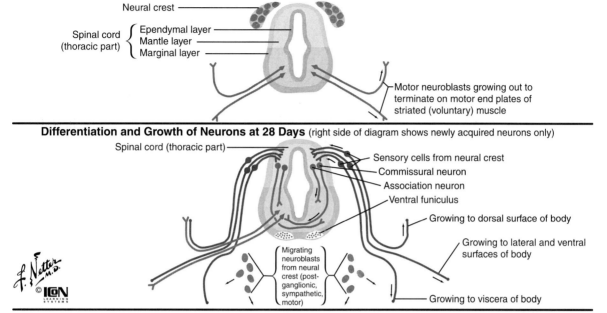

Differentiation and Growth of Neurons at 28 Days (right side of diagram shows newly acquired neurons only)

Differentiation and Growth of Neurons at 5 to 7 Weeks (right side o diagram shows neurons acquired since 28th day only)

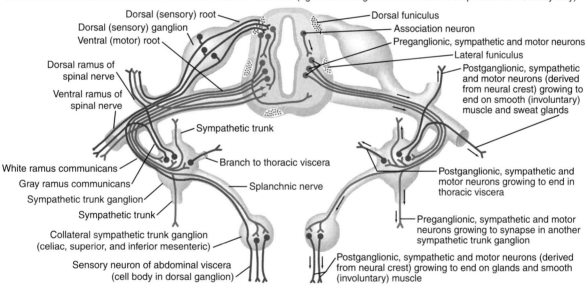

FIGURE 7–3

Development of peripheral nerves. (Courtesy of Icon Learning Systems. Copyright©, Icon Learning Systems, LLC. A subsidiary of MediMedia, USA, Inc. All rights reserved.)

unlike in adults where the leg MCVs are about 10 m/sec slower.[12,13] The exact reverse of the adult situation has even been reported, with a 5-week-old infant reported in whom the peroneal MCV was greater than those of both the median and ulnar MCVs.[14]

Differences also exist between the specific nerves in how they reach the adult distribution of CVs. The myelination of *ulnar* and *peroneal nerves* occurs concomitantly at a similar

rate, allowing for a gradually increased speed of conduction through infancy. This is especially true during the first 6 months of life. In contrast, the *median nerve* lags in maturation. Therefore, its MCV does not increase significantly until the child reaches approximately 1 to 3 years of age.[14] Within just 3 years of age, ulnar MCV values have achieved the lower adult range.[12] The modest early difference between ulnar and median MCV gradually disappears in

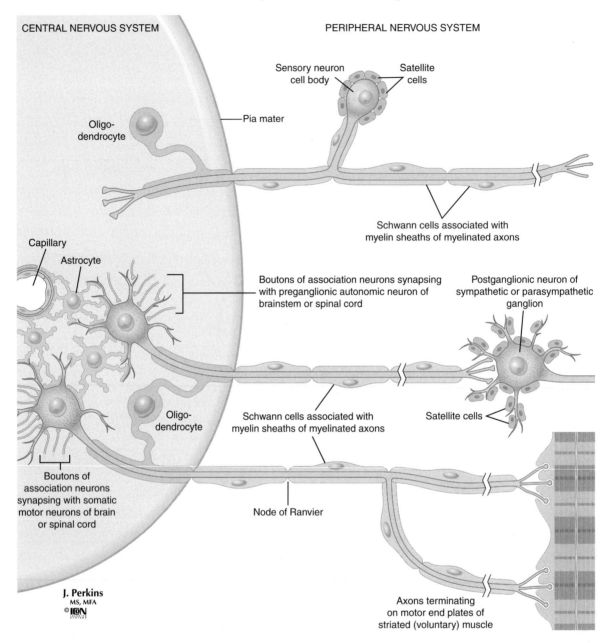

CENTRAL NERVOUS SYSTEM

PERIPHERAL NERVOUS SYSTEM

Sensory neuron cell body

Satellite cells

Pia mater

Oligo-dendrocyte

Schwann cells associated with myelin sheaths of myelinated axons

Capillary

Astrocyte

Boutons of association neurons synapsing with preganglionic autonomic neuron of brainstem or spinal cord

Postganglionic neuron of sympathetic or parasympathetic ganglion

Oligo-dendrocyte

Schwann cells associated with myelin sheaths of myelinated axons

Satellite cells

Boutons of association neurons synapsing with somatic motor neurons of brain or spinal cord

Node of Ranvier

Axons terminating on motor end plates of striated (voluntary) muscle

J. Perkins
MS, MFA
©IGN

FIGURE 7–4

Myelination of central nervous system and peripheral nerves. (Courtesy of Icon Learning Systems. Copyright©, Icon Learning Systems, LLC. A subsidiary of MediMedia, USA, Inc. All rights reserved.)

children by 4 or 5 years of age. Further disparities occur in middle childhood: while the MCVs of the ulnar and median nerves continue to increase, those of the peroneal nerve do not. The process of peripheral nerve maturation is reflected not only by increasing MCVs but also the values for distal latencies and compound muscle action potential (CMAP) amplitudes. As the child matures, CMAPs triple in size for the upper extremity and double in amplitude for the lower extremity (Tables 7-1 through 7-11).[12-14]

Sensory Conduction Studies

Maturational changes for orthodromic sensory conductions are similar to those for motor fibers. With proximal sensory stimulation in infants, two distinct peaks occur in the sensory nerve action potential (SNAP). This bifid response may first appear at 3 months of age[15] and persist until 4 to 6 years of age.[16] These findings are attributed to differences in maturation of two groups of sensory fibers.

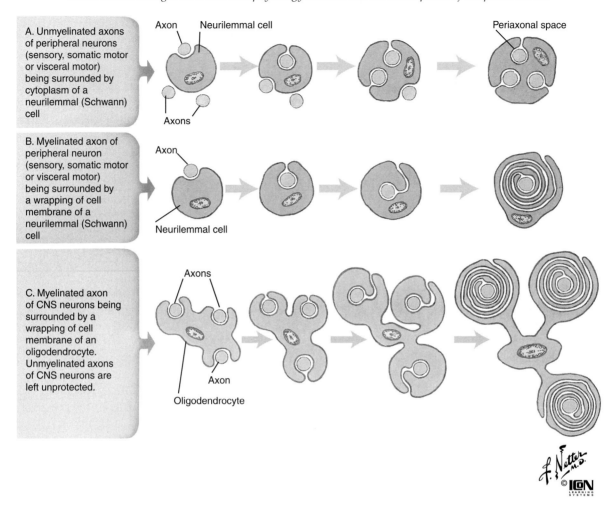

A. Unmyelinated axons of peripheral neurons (sensory, somatic motor or visceral motor) being surrounded by cytoplasm of a neurilemmal (Schwann) cell

Axon   Neurilemmal cell   Periaxonal space

Axons

B. Myelinated axon of peripheral neuron (sensory, somatic motor or visceral motor) being surrounded by a wrapping of cell membrane of a neurilemmal (Schwann) cell

Axon

Neurilemmal cell

C. Myelinated axon of CNS neurons being surrounded by a wrapping of cell membrane of an oligodendrocyte. Unmyelinated axons of CNS neurons are left unprotected.

Axons

Axon

Oligodendrocyte

FIGURE 7–5

Development of myelination and axonal ensheathments. (Courtesy of Icon Learning Systems. Copyright©, Icon Learning Systems, LLC. A subsidiary of MediMedia, USA, Inc. All rights reserved.)

In the fullterm infant, sensory nerve conduction velocity (SNCV) is 50% that of the adult and it gradually increases to the adult SNCV value by 4 years of age. By 12 months, the figures approach 75% of adult values.[15,17,18] SNAP amplitudes in the newborn, using surface electrodes, are slightly below those of the adult for the median and ulnar nerves. These amplitudes attain adult values by 6 to 12 months of age and surpass them by 1 to 6 years.[16] At the end of this chapter, Tables 7-12 through 7-15 provide normal values for sensory NCS for children 0 to 5 years of age.[19] The values for mixed NCS and pure sensory conduction are similar.

The sensory nerve fiber populations differ significantly in myelination and diameter and consequently show marked variation in their velocity. This means that there is considerable phase cancellation of nerve action potentials and the compound SNAP amplitude measurements correlate only

with the number of axons in the population of the faster conducting fibers. Details of the smaller diameter fibers' function can be obtained from needle recording electrodes. This is not an easy option in children and therefore only the largest diameter myelinated fibers can be tested routinely.

Proximal Measures of Nerve Conduction

H Reflexes

The H reflex is carried over group 1A afferent fibers, which are the fastest conducting peripheral fibers. These nerves have the lowest threshold to submaximal stimuli. An ulnar nerve H reflex was identified in 34 of 39 fullterm infants.[12] By 1 year of age it had disappeared (see Tables 7-6 and 7-11). The CV of afferent fibers of the H reflex between wrist and elbow segments in newborns was 10% faster than that of motor fibers of the ulnar nerves. The presence of the H reflex in the upper extremities most likely represents incomplete central nervous system myelination similar to that accounting for the presence of Babinski's sign in the newborn and young infant. H reflexes are also identified in the median nerves in children (see Table 7-3)[9,20-22] and tibia[23,24] up to age 1 year including premature and fullterm infants.[20]

The latency of the H reflex, recorded from the intrinsic muscles of the hand, correlates with the child's body length until 1 year of age.[15] Only the tibial H reflex can be consistently obtained in adults. With the opposing influences of progressive axonal myelination and increasing limb length, H reflex and F wave latencies initially decrease and later increase with age when recorded from the triceps surae[23] and the abductor pollicis brevis[25] muscles, respectively.

F Waves

Some studies have defined the normal spectrum of F wave latencies from newborns and young infants.[15,17,25,26] These are shown in Tables 7-2, 7-5, 7-8, and 7-10 as in neuromuscular disorders of infancy and so forth. Some of these studies reported the length of the limb, but no attempt has been made to correct for this as well as age. There is a broad measure of agreement between the studies, and attempts to make corrections for height are likely to make the calculations extremely complex and require prohibitively large numbers of controls to allow them. As discussed, there is an initial decrease before the values increase with age.

Phrenic Nerve Studies

Phrenic nerve studies present another circumstance where the increased distance between stimulus and recording site is interlinked to the effects of myelination so that there is an initial decrease in the absolute latency before the steady increase up to adult levels. Moosa's study[27] of 94 children used the technique of Newsom-Davis.[28] The results are shown in Table 7-16.

Use of Nerve Conduction Velocity to Predict Gestational Age

Before the advent of other technical advances in obstetrics, particularly the use of ultrasonography, there was an argument that the variation in nerve CVs might lead to a breakthrough in the solution of the difficult problem of the estimation of gestational age.[29] Blom and Finnsstrom[30] identified that there was a variation among fullterm infants outside the experimental error that resulted when measuring the distances and the latencies of the responses and consequently the interpretation of the results may be insufficiently precise to allow its routine use.

Despite this caveat, Schulte and colleagues[11] concluded that when babies of similar weight were compared, the *light-for-date babies* would have faster CVs than the premature babies. They were able to produce a rule stating that if a low-birthweight baby has an ulnar CV greater than 30 m/sec or a tibial nerve CV greater than 26 m/sec, it was likely that the baby is at or near term. Wagner and Buchthal[31] found equivalent maturation of myelinated nerve fibers whether the child had been delivered at term or was born prematurely but was otherwise healthy.

Rather than look at the absolute measurements of CV, Ruppert and coworkers[32] reported that the truly premature babies had a much more rapid increase in nerve CVs over the first 3 months of life and that this would allow differentiation of intrauterine growth retardation from true prematurity. Dubowitz and associates[33] found that the increase in MCV was greater after birth than in utero. In contrast, Smit and colleagues[34] found a quite different result when they looked at a cohort of 100 very preterm babies. They found that there was a significant delay in extrauterine maturation of the ulnar nerve as compared to intrauterine. Suggestions as to why it should be slower include the effects of concomitant illness, such as hyaline membrane disease and hypothyroxinemia, which is more common in the premature infant. No such delay was found in the tibial nerve studies. They did not find that any confounding variables such as weight, twin pregnancy, or intrauterine growth retardation influenced the findings.

NEUROMUSCULAR TRANSMISSION

The neuromuscular junction is not fully matured at birth. Unfortunately, there are only a few control studies reported of normal infants. One of the most detailed was the evaluation of 17 newborns, including 6 premature infants with GAs between 34 and 42 weeks, by Koenigsberger and coworkers.[35] Continuous stimulation at rates of 1, 2, 5, 10, 20, and 50 impulses per second (IPS) was carried out for 15 seconds. In their study group no change in CMAP amplitude was observed at a rate of 1 to 2 IPS. When the stimulus was increased to between 5 and 10 IPS, 5 and 8 infants, respectively, showed at least a 10% facilitation. At 20 IPS, 12 of 17 showed decremental changes that averaged 24%. The degree of decrement was greatest in the most premature infants studied, who were born at 34 weeks' gestation. The neuromuscular junction of the newborn was most sensitive to 50 IPS stimulation; all 17 infants studied demonstrated a decrement averaging 51%. The results at 20 and 50 IPS as shown in their paper are plotted in Figures 7-6 and 7-7.

In summary their findings indicated that newborns exhibit less neuromuscular reserve than do older children

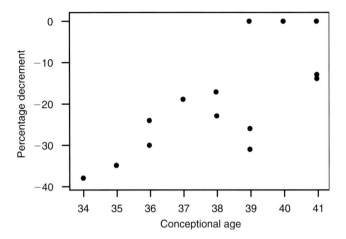

FIGURE 7–6

Plot of the percentage decrement of the thenar compound motor nerve action potential during 20 impulses per second stimulation. (From Koenigsberger MR, Patten B, Lovelace RE: Studies of neuromuscular function in the newborn: A comparison of myoneural function in the fullterm and premature infant. Neuropediatrics 1973;4:350-361.)

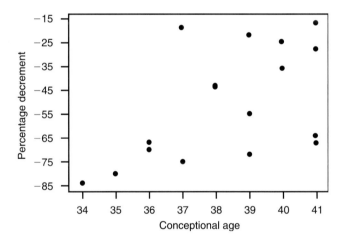

FIGURE 7–7

Plot of the percentage decrement of the thenar compound motor nerve action potential during 50 impulses per second stimulation. (From Koenigsberger MR, Patten B, Lovelace RE: Studies of neuromuscular function in the newborn: A comparison of myoneural function in the fullterm and premature infant. Neuropediatrics 1973;4:350-361.)

and that premature infants have less neuromuscular junction reserve than do fullterm infants. Therefore, the rapid and most uncomfortable forms of repetitive stimulation are not as helpful in evaluating postsynaptic infantile neu-

romuscular transmission defect because of the poor safety factor present in the immature neuromuscular junction.

On a practical note, C. Michel Harper, speaking from experience at the Mayo Clinic (personal communication, 1999), expressed the belief that the use of 3/sec stimulation is most probably without difficulties in interpretation when screening premature babies for a neuromuscular transmission defect but rates of 10/sec and above should not be used for babies less than 3 months post-term. Cornblath[36] stated that decremental changes of greater than 10% at the rates of 2 to 5 Hz and facilitatory changes of greater than 23% at 20 to 50 Hz are significant for the diagnosis of the most common infantile presynaptic neuromuscular junction disorder, namely infantile botulism.

DEVELOPMENT OF MUSCLES

At 6 weeks' gestation the myoblasts begin to elongate. At 10 weeks nerve fibers reach the muscle cells and create the neuromuscular junctions. Only after this has occurred is it possible to see the fiber type develop following a specific sequence of changes.[37] Up to 19 weeks most fibers have properties that would conform to the type IIc (fast twitch), and these are larger in diameter and greater in number than the type I fibers that are present. Through weeks 10 to 20 the nuclei become peripheral but the type II remain the larger fibers. There is a progressive increase in the diameter of type I fibers, particularly in the 15- to 20-week period.

During the last 3 months of pregnancy there is a decrease in the number of type IIc and the appearance of type IIa and IIb fibers. Fibers with type IIb characteristics are seen at about 30 weeks and type IIa appear at around 35 weeks. Others have indicated that the adult anatomic configuration of the motor unit is achieved by as early as 20 weeks.[38] There are some mild reported differences between limb and trunk muscles.[39] The percentage of type I fibers increases to around 50% in the psoas (a trunk muscle), whereas quadriceps (a limb muscle) may only reach 23%.

The differentiation is not complete at birth. A significant percentage (15% to 20%) of all the fibers may not be differentiated at this time. Gradually there is an increase in types I, IIa, and IIb fibers.[40] By this time type IIc fibers are usually absent from the muscle of infants older than 1 or 2 weeks.

Additionally there are changes in the diameter of the fibers with development. At birth, the average diameter of the type I and II fibers in quadriceps is 10 to 15 μm. Growth continues during postnatal development up until puberty, when the fibers reach their final diameter of 60 to 65 μm.[41] At birth the fibers have a rounded polygonal shape and are all closely apposed without evidence of endomysial connective tissue. This shape is in contrast with the angular polygonal profiles found in older children and adults.

NERVE CONDUCTION AND ELECTROMYOGRAPHIC CORRELATIONS WITH MOTOR UNIT MATURATION

Background

When performing electromyographic (EMG) procedures in infants and young children, it is important to relate the known anatomic changes to the likely changes that will be seen on EMG. The interference pattern is determined by the interactions of the compound motor action potentials from the motor units, which are within the range of pick-up for the needle in use. In adults the biceps muscle has been studied extensively and the muscle fibers are distributed within a 6-mm oval, which may be shared with between 5 and 10 different motor units. The length of an individual terminal axonal after division from the point of division from the motor nerve may be as much as 30 mm.[42] The same motor unit generates a different action potential depending on where the needle enters this oval.

The major tools that have elucidated the extent of the motor unit in vivo have been either the scanning EMG needle[43] or the macro EMG.[44] Both procedures are painful and it is therefore no surprise to discover that this information on the motor unit territory is scanty in children, with reliance placed on the anatomic studies, such as they are.

Reference values produced by the Laboratory of Clinical Neurophysiology, Righospitalet, Copenhagen, give the mean duration of the motor unit potentials for a large number of muscles. These show increasing duration of the motor unit potentials with age (Fig. 7-8). Some muscles such as orbicu-laris oris and genioglossus show a rapid increase over the first 10 to 20 years followed by a little increase over the rest of adulthood. Most other muscles do not show the same rapid increase over the first 2 decades of life.

The increase in duration is thought to be due to an increase in the width of the endplate zone with growth and to the higher fiber density obtained by a closer packing of the subunits.[45] Unfortunately, for the most part, the invaluable information held in this reference manual cannot be used by most pediatric neurophysiologists practicing today because the needle diameters are different. The values were obtained using a concentric needle diameter of 0.64 mm, a core diameter of 0.15 mm, and a recording area of 0.07 mm^2.

To be most humane, we use the thinnest needle that has a diameter of 0.3 mm and the recording area is 0.03 mm^2. It is unlikely that it will be possible to produce a conversion factor. A very limited analysis has been done using the smaller needles. Sacco and associates[45] (Tables 7-17 and 7-18) used needles with an external diameter of 0.65 mm and the leading-off surface of the platinum core was 0.03 mm^2. Only 4 of the 38 subjects studied were infants and the next group began at 16 years, so *there is no information over the whole age range of childhood*. This study does confirm that the values in infancy are reduced to the same order as indicated by the studies using more conventional needle electrodes. This gives more impetus to use the multi-motor unit action potential automatic analysis[46] now available on many EMG machines.

Motor Unit Number Estimation

The mean duration of the motor unit potentials gives an indication of the size and density of the motor units being increased in situations where reinnervation has taken place. For the reasons discussed it is not possible to use the macroelectrodes or other similar techniques in children. Motor unit number estimation (MUNE) does not require needles and can be defined by incremental nerve stimulation. These MUNE values are calculated from the ratio of the maximal CMAP to the average single motor unit potential. It is therefore a technique that is suitable for use in children of any age and gives further information about the motor unit.

Bromberg and Swoboda[47] described its use in patients with spinal muscular atrophy where the number of motor units is reduced. They used the multiple-point stimulation technique[48] and refined it for use in children. With such a recent application the data available over the whole range of childhood are limited. These authors confirmed that the values obtained are in line with the anatomic studies done by Feinstein and colleagues.[49] This was a study on 12 cadavers ranging from 22 to 54 years and as yet maturational changes have not been identified.

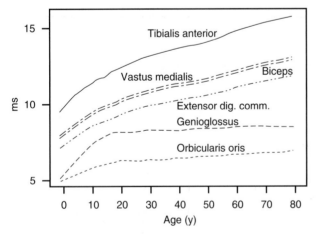

FIGURE 7–8

Plots of mean duration of the motor unit potentials against age. Findings are in normal subjects at the Laboratory of Clinical Neurophysiology, Righospitalet, Copenhagen.

CONCLUSION

It is not easy in pediatrics to relate the anatomic and pathologic studies directly to findings on the EMG because of ethical considerations. For example, we cannot use the scanning EMG needle to accurately determine the electrical characteristics of motor units.

That said, there is a great deal that is known about the maturational changes and how they affect our interpretation of results. The study of the changes in nerve CVs provides one such example. On a practical note, it is easy to make more of the differences in values obtained by different laboratories

of nerve CVs than is justified. There are undoubtedly differences, but a cautious pediatric electromyographer should be wary of overinterpreting minor deviations from normal unless corroboration is found from other aspects of the examination such as the clear demonstration of neurogenic potentials by needle EMG in a child with borderline slow MCVs.

With increasing interest in the diagnosis of the infantile myasthenic syndromes, the work done on normal premature infants and neonates is invaluable. With knowledge of the maturational effects on the neuromuscular system, the examinations in pediatric groups can be as accurate as those in the adult population.

TABLE 7–1. MEDIAN MOTOR NERVE CONDUCTION STUDY REFERENCE VALUES

Table 7–1A. Values Obtained Using Surface Electrodes*

Age	No.	Amplitude, mV	Distal Latency, msec	Distance, cm	MNC, m/sec
Neonate	4	2.6-5.9	2.0-2.9	1.9-3.0	22.4-27.1
1-6 mo	6	3.5-6.9	1.6-2.2	2.1-4.1	37.0-47.7
7-12 mo	13	2.3-8.6	1.5-2.8	1.9-4.3	33.3-46.3
13-24 mo	16	3.7-11.6	1.8-2.8	2.2-4.3	39.2-50.5

MNC, motor nerve conduction.
   Data are presented as mean ± SD or as normative ranges.
   * Data from Miller RG, Kuntz NL: Nerve conduction studies in infants and children. J Child Neurol 1986;1:19.

Table 7–1B. Values Obtained Using Surface Stimulating and Recording Electrodes*,†

Age	No.	Amplitude, mV	Distal Latency, msec	MNCV, m/sec
7 days-1 mo	20	3.00 ± 0.312.23 ± 0.29	25.43 ± 3.84	
1-6 mo	23	7.37 ± 3.242.21 ± 0.34	34.35 ± 6.61	
6-12 mo	25	7.67 ± 4.452.13 ± 0.19	43.57 ± 4.78	
1-2 yr	24	8.90 ± 3.612.04 ± 0.18		48.23 ± 4.58
2-4 yr	22	9.55 ± 4.342.18 ± 0.43		53.59 ± 5.29
4-6 yr	20	10.37 ± 3.662.27 ± 0.45	56.26 ± 4.61	
6-14 yr	21	12.37 ± 4.792.73 ± 0.44	57.32 ± 3.35	

MNCV, motor nerve conduction velocity.
   Data are presented as mean ± SD or as normative ranges.
   * Data from Parano E, Uncini A, De Vivo DC, Lovelace RE: Electrophysiologic correlates of peripheral nervous system maturation in infancy and childhood. J Child Neurol 1993;8:336.
   † Stimulating anode and cathode are 15 mm apart, with stimulation at the wrist and elbow (cubital fossa). Recording electrodes are over the abductor pollicis brevis.

Table 7–1C. Values Obtained Using Surface Electrodes for Stimulation and Recording*,†

Age	Mean (range) Amplitude, mV	Distal Latency, msec	MNCV, m/sec
Premature (mean gestation 35.8 wk)		2.8 ± 0.46	22.4 ± 2.60
Newborn (38-42 wk gestation)		2.5 ± 0.31	26.9 ± 2.60
0-1 mo	4 (2-7)	2.60 ± 0.26	28.5 ± 2.04
1-3 mo		2.30 ± 0.31	30.8 ± 2.61
3-6 mo		2.10 ± 0.26	39.4 ± 3.64
6-12 mo		2.12 ± 0.34	42.5 ± 4.65
1-2 yr		2.0 ± 0.23	47.0 ± 2.89
2-4 yr		2.17 ± 0.14	53.4 ± 3.84
4-6 yr		2.23 ± 0.20	56.4 ± 4.22
6-11 yr	14.1 (6-20)	2.50 ± 0.20	59.5 ± 2.71

MNCV, motor nerve conduction velocity.
   Data are presented as mean ± SD or as normative ranges.
   * Data from Cruz-Martinez A, Ferrer MT, Perez-Conde ML, Bernacer M: Motor conduction velocity and H-reflex in infancy and childhood: Intra and extrauterine maturation of the nerve fibers: Development of the peripheral nerve from 1 month to 11 years of age. Electromyogr Clin Neurophysiol 1978;18:11-27; and Cruz-Martinez A, Perez-Conde ML, Ferrer MT: Motor conduction velocity and H-reflex in infancy and childhood: I. Study in newborns, twins, and small-for-dates. Electromyogr Clin Neurophysiol 1977;17:493-505.
   † Stimulating anode and cathode are 15 mm apart with stimulation at the wrist and proximal to the elbow; stimulus duration is 0.1-0.5 milliseconds. Recording electrodes are placed on the belly of the thenar eminence and the proximal phalanx of the first finger of the hand. Compound muscle action potential amplitude is measured peak to peak. Skin temperature is measured and warmed when necessary using an infrared lamp.

(Continued)

TABLE 7–1. Cont'd

Table 7–1*D.* Values Obtained Using Surface Electrodes for Stimulation and Recording[*],[†]

Average Age	No.	Mean MNCV, m/sec
5 wk	12	33.1
18 wk	11	35.8
34 wk	12	41.8
56 wk	12	40.4
88 wk	12	47.5
140 wk	12	49.4
210 wk	12	54.9
4-16 yr		57.2 ± 8.2

MNCV, motor nerve conduction velocity.

Data are presented as mean ± SD or as normative ranges.

[*] Data from Baer RD, Johnson EW: Motor nerve conduction velocities in normal children. Arch Phys Med Rehabil 1965;46:698-704.

[†] Stimulating anode and cathode are 15 mm apart with stimulation at the elbow medial to the biceps tendon and at the wrist lateral to the palmaris longus tendon; stimulation duration is 0.1 milliseconds. Recording electrodes are placed over the opponens pollicis (active) and over the distal phalanx of the thumb (reference).

Table 7–1*E.* Recording from Abductor Pollicis Brevis[*]

Age	No.	MNCV, m/sec
<3 mo	3	27 ± 9.1
4 mo-2 yr	11	49 ± 12
3-5 yr	5	55 ± 3.5
6-10 yr	6	56 ± 4.9
11-16 yr	16	59 ± 5.1

MNCV, motor nerve conduction velocity.

Data are presented as mean ± SD or as normative ranges.

[*] Data from Shahani BT, Young RR: Clinical significance of late response studies in infants and children [Abstract]. Neurology 1981;31:66.

Table 7–1*F.* Stimulating at the Wrist and Elbow[*]

Age	No.	Amplitude, mV	Distal Latency, msec	MNCV, m/sec
1-28 days	20	2.25 ± 1.29	2.12 ± 0.28	25.19 ± 2.52
1 mo-1 yr	20	2.39 ± 2.24	2.07 ± 0.32	34.44 ± 6.01

MNCV, motor nerve conduction velocity.

Data are presented as mean ± SD or as normative ranges.

[*] Data from Misra UK, Tiwari S, Shukla N, et al: F-response studies in neonates, infants, and children. Electromyogr Clin Neurophysiol 1989;29:251-254.

Table 7–1*G.* Using Surface Electrodes and Recording from the Right Abductor Pollicis Brevis on Right Median Nerve Stimulation*

Age/Subject Type	Gestation, wk	No.	MNCV, m/sec
Fullterm newborn normal (37-41 wk) appropriate for gestational age (birthweight 10th-90th percentiles of local standards)	39.14 ± 0.77	14	26.56 ± 3.95
Fullterm newborn (37-41 wk), intrauterine growth retarded with weight			
1500-1800 gm	38.6 ± 1.8	5	18.5 ± 2.21
1801-2100 gm	38.1 ± 1.2	15	21.3 ± 2.36
Preterm newborn appropriate for gestational age (as defined above) with gestation of			
≤34 wk	32.0 ± 1.73	5	15.56 ± 5.34
>34 wk	35.5 ± 0.54	6	19.40 ± 3.41
or with weight			
1500-1800 gm	33.2 ± 1.6	5	17.5 ± 1.84
1800-2100 gm	34.6 ± 0.9	8	17.5 ± 3.2

MNCV, motor nerve conduction velocity.

Data are presented as mean ± SD or as normative ranges.

[*] Data from Bhatia BD, Prakash U, Singh MN, et al: Electrophysiological studies in newborns with reference to gestation and anthropometry. Electromyogr Clin Neurophysiol 1991;31:55-59; and Bhatia BD, Prakash U: Electrophysiological studies in preterm and growth retarded low birth weight babies. Electromyogr Clin Neurophysiol 1993;33:507-509.

TABLE 7–2. MEDIAN MOTOR NERVE F WAVE REFERENCE VALUES

Table 7–2A. According to Miller and Kuntz[°]

Age	No.	Latency, msec	Distance, cm
7-12 mo	3	13-16	23-30
13-24 mo	4	14-18	22-27

Data are presented as mean ± SD or as normative ranges.
[°] Data from Miller RG, Kuntz NL: Nerve conduction studies in infants and children. J Child Neurol 1986;1:19-26.

Table 7–2B. According to Shahani and Young[°]

Age	No.	Minimal Latency, msec
<3 mo	3	16 ± 1.4
4 mo-2 yr	11	14.4 ± 1.6
3-5 yr	5	17.1 ± 0.6
6-10 yr	6	19.4 ± 1.5
11-16 yr	16	25.3 ± 2.3

Data are presented as mean ± SD or as normative ranges.
[°] Data from Shahani BT, Young RR: Clinical significance of late response studies in infants and children [Abstract]. Neurology 1981;31:66.

Table 7–2C. According to Parano and Associates[°]

Age	No.	Latency, msec
7 days-1 mo	20	16.12 ± 1.5
1-6 mo	23	16.89 ± 1.65
6-12 mo	25	17.31 ± 1.77
1-2 yr	24	17.44 ± 1.29
2-4 yr	22	17.91 ± 1.11
4-6 yr	20	19.44 ± 1.51
6-14 yr	21	23.23 ± 2.57

Data are presented as mean ± SD or as normative ranges.
[°] Data from Parano E, Uncini A, De Vivo DC, Lovelace RE: Electrophysiologic correlates of peripheral nervous system maturation in infancy and childhood. J Child Neurol 1993;8:336-338.

Table 7–2D. Stimulating the Median Nerve at the Wrist with the Cathode Proximal, Recording from Abductor Pollicis Brevis, and Measuring Latency from the Stimulus Artifact to the First Deflection from the Base Line[°],[†]

Age	No.	Minimum Latency, msec	Amplitude, mV	Duration, msec	Minimal-Maximal Latency Difference, msec
1-28 days	20	16.95 ± 1.30	1.06 ± 0.45	8.46 ± 1.45	1.89 ± 1.01
1 mo-1 yr	20	14.93 ± 1.50	0.24 ± 0.14	7.41 ± 2.68	2.01 ± 0.89

Data are presented as mean ± SD or as normative ranges.
[°] Data from Misra UK, Tiwari S, Shukla N, et al: F-response studies in neonates, infants and children. Electromyogr Clin Neurophysiol 1989;29:251-254.
[†] 10 F waves were recorded.

Table 7–2E. Using Surface Electrodes for Supramaximal Stimulation of the Median Nerve at the Wrist and a Concentric Needle Electrode for Recording from Abductor Pollicis Brevis[°],[†]

Age, yr	No.	Minimum Latency, msec	Minimal-Maximal Latency Difference, msec
0-1.5	20	15.4 ± 0.9	203.0 ± 1.1
1.5-3	14	15.3 ± 0.7	122.9 ± 1.1
3-5	23	17.0 ± 1.1	233.6 ± 1.4
5-7	13	18.2 ± 1.0	134.1 ± 1.4
7-12	20	19.5 ± 1.1	173.8 ± 1.2

Data are presented as mean ± SD or as normative ranges.
[°] Data from Kwast O, Krajewska G, Kozlowski K: Analysis of F-wave parameters in median and ulnar nerves in healthy infants and children: Age-related changes. Electromyogr Clin Neurophysiol 1984;24:439-456.
[†] 20-100 F waves were recorded.

TABLE 7–3. MEDIAN NERVE H REFLEX REFERENCE VALUES

Table 7–3A. According to Bhatia and Associates*

Age/Subject Type	Gestation, wk	No.	Latency, msec
Full-term newborn (37-41 wk: birthweight 10th-90th percentile)	39.14 ± 0.77	14	17.11 ± 1.25
Full-term newborn (37-41 wk), intrauterine retarded			
1500-1800 gm	38.6 ± 1.8	5	18.8 ± 1.68
1801-2100 gm	38.1 ± 1.2	15	17.0 ± 1.73
Preterm newborn appropriate for gestational age			
≤34 wk	32.0 ± 1.73	5	20.10 ± 1.55
>34 wk	35.5 ± 0.54	6	19.16 ± 2.09
or with weight			
1500-1800 gm	33.2 ± 1.6	5	20.1 ± 1.24
1801-2100 gm	34.6 ± 0.9	8	19.1 ± 1.24

* Data from Bhatia BD, Prakash U, Singh MN, et al: Electrophysiological studies in newborns with reference to gestation and anthropometry. Electromyogr Clin Neurophysiol 1991;31:55-59; and Bhatia BD, Prakash U: Electrophysiological studies in preterm and growth-retarded low birth weight babies. Electromyogr Clin Neurophysiol 1993;33:507-509.

Table 7–3B. Using Submaximal Stimulation of the Median Nerve at the Wrist and Recording from the Abductor Pollicis Brevis*

Age	No.	Latency, msec
1-28 days	20	17.86 ± 1.60
1 mo-1 yr	20	15.69 ± 1.67

* Data from Misra UK, Tiwari S, Shukla N, et al: F-response studies in neonates, infants, and children. Electromyogr Clin Neurophysiol 1989;29:251-254.

TABLE 7–4. ULNAR MOTOR NERVE CONDUCTION REFERENCE VALUES

Table 7–4A. Using Surface Electrodes and Recording over the Belly of the Hypothenar Muscles and the Proximal Phalanx of the Fifth Finger, Stimulating at the Wrist and Proximal to the Elbow with the Elbow Straight*,†

Age	No.	MNCV, m/sec
Premature (studied 1-46 days after birth)		618.1-22.2 (20.7 ± 1.83)
Fullterm newborn	42	20.8-33.3 (27.9 ± 3.08)
6 mo		−35-45
12 mo		−40-60

Data are presented as mean ± SD or as normative ranges.

  * Data from Thomas JE, Lambert EH: Ulnar nerve conduction velocity and H-reflex in infants and children. J Appl Physiol 1960;15:1-9.

  † Stimulation is at the elbow medial to the olecranon and at the wrist lateral and superior to the styloid process, and the active recording electrode is over the abductor digiti minimi (manus), and the reference recording electrode is over the proximal phalanx of the little finger.

Table 7–4B. According to Miller and Kuntz*

Age	No.	Amplitude, mV	MNCV, m/sec	Distal Latency, msec	Distance, cm
Neonate	56	1.6-7.0	20.0-36.1	1.3-2.9	1.0-3.4
1-6 mo	22	2.5-7.4	33.3-50.0	1.1-3.2	1.7-4.4
7-12 mo	28	3.2-10.0	35.0-58.2	0.8-2.2	1.9-4.6
13-24 mo	53	2.6-9.7	41.3-63.5	1.1-2.2	2.4-4.8

MNCV, motor nerve conduction velocity.

  Data are presented as mean ± SD or as normative ranges.

  * Data from Miller RG, Kuntz NL: Nerve conduction studies in infants and children. J Child Neurol 1986;1:19-26.

(Continued)

TABLE 7–4 Cont'd

Table 7–4C. According to Baer and Johnson*

Average Age	No.	Mean MNCV, m/sec
5 wk	11	34.5
18 wk	12	35.4
34 wk	12	46.1
56 wk	10	46.7
88 wk	12	51.6
140 wk	12	52.4
210 wk	12	56.1
4-16 yr		58.2 ± 9.7

MNCV, motor nerve conduction velocity.
Data are presented as mean ± SD or as normative ranges.
° Data from Baer RD, Johnson EW: Motor nerve conduction velocities in normal children. Arch Phys Med Rehabil 1965;46:698-704.

TABLE 7–5. ULNAR MOTOR NERVE F WAVE REFERENCE VALUES

Table 7–5A. According to Miller and Kuntz*

Age	No.	Latency, msec	Distance, cm
1-6 mo	1	17	21
7-12 mo	6	13-16	21-30
13-24 mo	10	14-17	25-39

Data are presented as mean ± SD or as normative ranges.
° Data from Miller RG, Kuntz NL: Nerve conduction studies in infants and children. J Child Neurol 1986;1:19-26.

Table 7–5B. According to Kwast and Associates*,†

Age, yr	No.	Minimum Latency, msec	No.	Minimal-Maximal Latency Difference, msec
0-1.5	19	14.6 ± 0.7	18	2.5 ± 0.9
1.5-3	12	14.7 ± 0.4	10	3.6 ± 1.3
3-5	25	15.9 ± 0.8	25	3.1 ± 1.0
5-7	15	17.6 ± 0.9	15	3.6 ± 1.2
7-12	15	19.1 ± 1.0	15	3.6 ± 1.5

Data are presented as mean ± SD or as normative ranges.
° Data from Kwast O, Krajewska G, Kozlowski K: Analysis of F-wave parameters in median and ulnar nerves in healthy infants and children: Age related changes. Electromyogr Clin Neurophysiol 1984;24:439-456.
† Stimulation is at the wrist for the ulnar nerve with recordings from abductor digiti quinti.

TABLE 7–6. ULNAR NERVE H REFLEX REFERENCE VALUES*

Age	No.	Latency, msec (mean)
1-3 days	6	16.0-19.0 (17.3)
6-12 mo	5	14.0-17.0 (15.8)

Data are presented as normative ranges, using surface electrodes for stimulation and recording.
° Data from Mayer RF, Mooser RS: Excitability of motoneurons in infants. Neurology 1969;19:932-945.

TABLE 7–7. PERONEAL MOTOR NERVE CONDUCTION REFERENCE VALUES

Table 7–7A. According to Miller and Kuntz°

Age	No.	Amplitude, mV	MNCV, m/sec	Distal Latency, msec	Distance, cm
Neonate	4	1.8-4.0	21.0-26.7	2.1-3.1	1.9-3.8
1-6 mo	10	1.6-8.0	32.4-47.7	1.7-2.4	2.5-4.1
7-12 mo	19	2.3-6.0	38.8-56.0	1.4-3.2	2.2-5.5
13-24 mo	36	1.7-6.5	39.2-54.3	1.6-3.5	2.2-5.8

MNCV, motor nerve conduction velocity.
° Data from Miller RG, Kuntz NL: Nerve conduction studies in infants and children. J Child Neurol 1986;1:19-26.

Table 7–7B. According to Parano and Associates°

Age	No.	Amplitude, mV	MNCV, m/sec	Distal Latency, msec
7 days-1 mo	20	3.06 ± 1.26	22.43 ± 1.22	2.43 ± 0.48
1-6 mo	23	5.23 ± 2.37	35.18 ± 3.96	2.25 ± 0.48
6-12 mo	25	5.41 ± 2.01	43.55 ± 3.77	2.31 ± 0.62
1-2 yr	24	5.80 ± 2.48	51.42 ± 3.02	2.29 ± 0.43
2-4 yr	22	6.10 ± 2.99	55.73 ± 4.45	2.62 ± 0.75
4-6 yr	20	7.10 ± 4.76	56.14 ± 4.96	3.01 ± 0.43
6-14 yr	21	8.15 ± 4.19	57.05 ± 4.54	3.25 ± 0.51

MCNV, motor nerve conduction velocity.
° Data from Parano E, Uncini A, De Vivo DC, Lovelace RE: Electrophysiologic correlates of peripheral nervous system maturation in infancy and childhood. J Child Neurol 1993;8:336-338.

Table 7–7C. According to Baer and Johnson*

Age	Amplitude, mV	MNCV, m/sec
5 wk	6	37.2
18 wk	12	39.1
34 wk	12	44.1
56 wk	12	46.7
88 wk	12	49.5
140 wk	11	44.2
210 wk	12	52.2
4-16 yr		53.0 ± 9.6

MCNV, motor nerve conduction velocity.
° Data from Baer RD, Johnson EW: Motor nerve conduction velocities in normal children. Arch Phys Med Rehabil 1965;46:698-704.

TABLE 7–8. PERONEAL MOTOR NERVE F WAVE REFERENCE VALUES

Table 7–8A. According to Miller and Kuntz*

Age	No.	Latency, msec	Distance, cm
1-6 mo	2	22-25	35-36
7-12 mo	3	19-23	20-47
13-24 mo	10	21-26	30-53

Data are presented as mean ± SD or as normative ranges.
° Data from Miller RG, Kuntz NL: Nerve conduction studies in infants and children. J Child Neurol 1986;1:19-26.

Table 7–8B. According to Parano and Associates*

Age	No.	Latency, msec
7 days-1 mo	20	22.07 ± 1.46
1-6 mo	23	23.11 ± 1.89
6-12 mo	25	25.86 ± 1.35
1-2 yr	24	25.98 ± 1.95
2-4 yr	22	29.52 ± 2.15
4-6 yr	20	29.98 ± 2.68
6-14 yr	21	34.27 ± 4.29

Data are presented as mean ± SD or as normative ranges.
° Data from Parano E, Uncini A, De Vivo DC, Lovelace RE: Electrophysiologic correlates of peripheral nervous system maturation in infancy and childhood. J Child Neurol 1993;8:336-338.

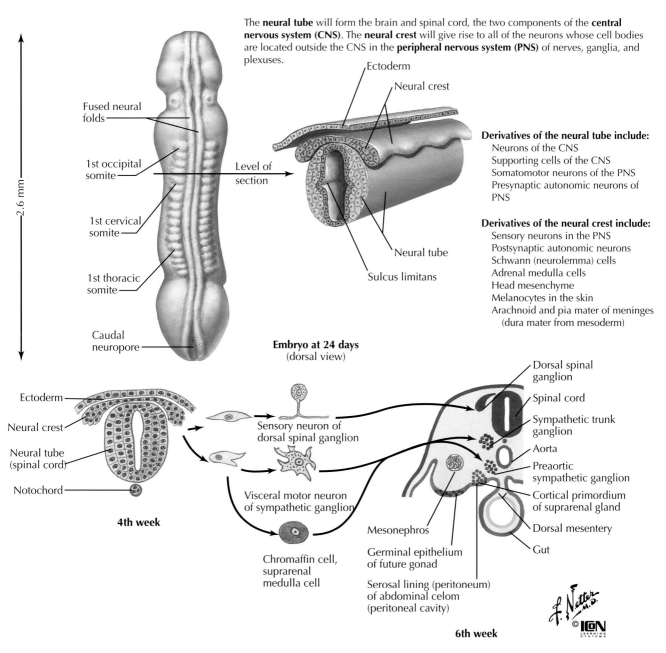

The **neural tube** will form the brain and spinal cord, the two components of the **central nervous system (CNS)**. The **neural crest** will give rise to all of the neurons whose cell bodies are located outside the CNS in the **peripheral nervous system (PNS)** of nerves, ganglia, and plexuses.

Ectoderm
Neural crest

Derivatives of the neural tube include:
Neurons of the CNS
Supporting cells of the CNS
Somatomotor neurons of the PNS
Presynaptic autonomic neurons of PNS

Derivatives of the neural crest include:
Sensory neurons in the PNS
Postsynaptic autonomic neurons
Schwann (neurolemma) cells
Adrenal medulla cells
Head mesenchyme
Melanocytes in the skin
Arachnoid and pia mater of meninges
(dura mater from mesoderm)

Fused neural folds

1st occipital somite

Level of section

1st cervical somite

Neural tube

1st thoracic somite

Sulcus limitans

Caudal neuropore

Embryo at 24 days
(dorsal view)

2.6 mm

Ectoderm
Neural crest
Neural tube (spinal cord)
Notochord

4th week

Sensory neuron of dorsal spinal ganglion

Visceral motor neuron of sympathetic ganglion

Chromaffin cell, suprarenal medulla cell

Dorsal spinal ganglion
Spinal cord
Sympathetic trunk ganglion
Aorta
Preaortic sympathetic ganglion
Cortical primordium of suprarenal gland
Dorsal mesentery
Gut

Mesonephros
Germinal epithelium of future gonad
Serosal lining (peritoneum) of abdominal celom (peritoneal cavity)

6th week

FIGURE 7–1

Neural tube development. (Courtesy of Icon Learning Systems. Copyright©, Icon Learning Systems, LLC. A subsidiary of MediMedia, USA, Inc. All rights reserved.)

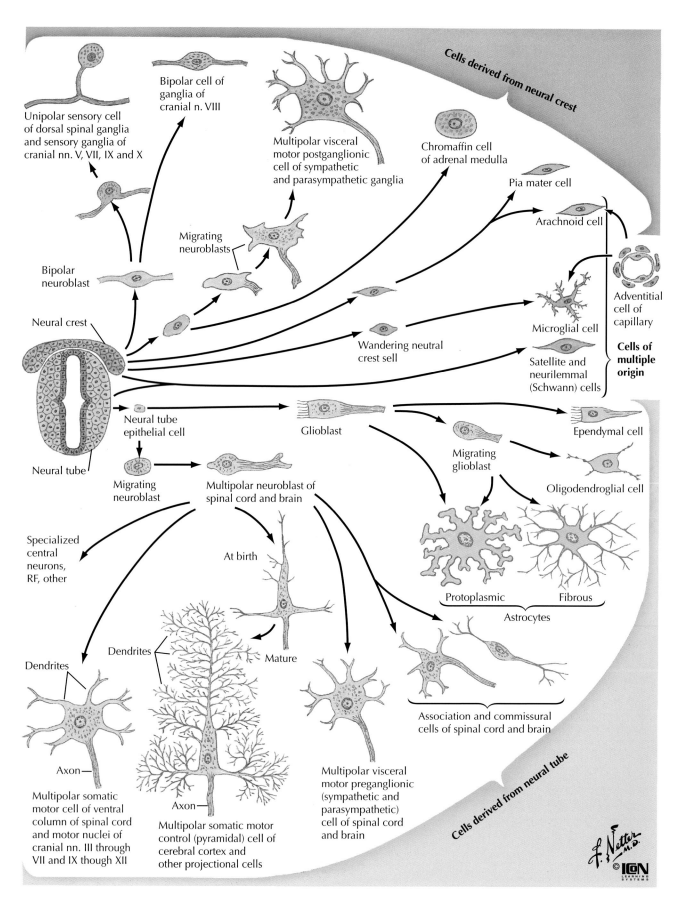

Unipolar sensory cell of dorsal spinal ganglia and sensory ganglia of cranial nn. V, VII, IX and X

Bipolar cell of ganglia of cranial n. VIII

Multipolar visceral motor postganglionic cell of sympathetic and parasympathetic ganglia

Chromaffin cell of adrenal medulla

Pia mater cell

Arachnoid cell

Migrating neuroblasts

Bipolar neuroblast

Neural crest

Adventitial cell of capillary

Cells of multiple origin

Microglial cell

Wandering neutral crest sell

Satellite and neurilemmal (Schwann) cells

Neural tube epithelial cell

Glioblast

Migrating glioblast

Ependymal cell

Neural tube

Migrating neuroblast

Multipolar neuroblast of spinal cord and brain

Oligodendroglial cell

Specialized central neurons, RF, other

At birth

Protoplasmic   Fibrous

Astrocytes

Dendrites

Dendrites

Mature

Dendrites

Axon

Association and commissural cells of spinal cord and brain

Multipolar somatic motor cell of ventral column of spinal cord and motor nuclei of cranial nn. III through VII and IX though XII

Axon

Multipolar somatic motor control (pyramidal) cell of cerebral cortex and other projectional cells

Multipolar visceral motor preganglionic (sympathetic and parasympathetic) cell of spinal cord and brain

Cells derived from neural crest

Cells derived from neural tube

F. Netter m.d.

© ICON LEARNING SYSTEMS

FIGURE 7–2

Neural crest formation. (Courtesy of Icon Learning Systems. Copyright©, Icon Learning Systems, LLC. A subsidiary of MediMedia, USA, Inc. All rights reserved.)

Differentiation and Growth of Neurons at 26 Days

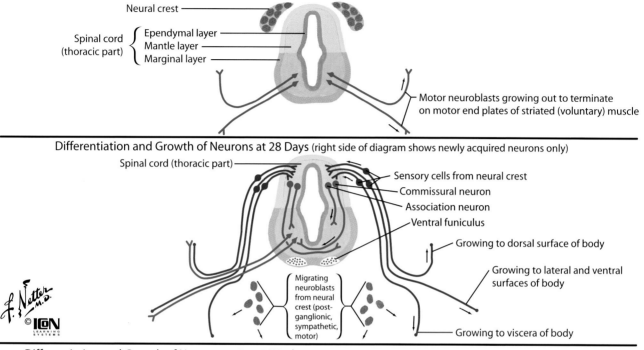

Neural crest

Spinal cord (thoracic part)
- Ependymal layer
- Mantle layer
- Marginal layer

Motor neuroblasts growing out to terminate on motor end plates of striated (voluntary) muscle

Differentiation and Growth of Neurons at 28 Days (right side of diagram shows newly acquired neurons only)

Spinal cord (thoracic part)

Sensory cells from neural crest
Commissural neuron
Association neuron
Ventral funiculus

Growing to dorsal surface of body

Growing to lateral and ventral surfaces of body

Migrating neuroblasts from neural crest (post-ganglionic, sympathetic, motor)

Growing to viscera of body

Differentiation and Growth of Neurons at 5 to 7 Weeks (right side of diagram shows neurons acquired since 28th day only)

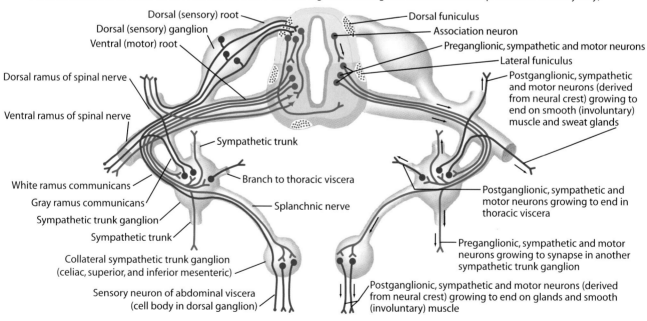

Dorsal (sensory) root
Dorsal (sensory) ganglion
Ventral (motor) root

Dorsal ramus of spinal nerve

Ventral ramus of spinal nerve

White ramus communicans
Gray ramus communicans
Sympathetic trunk ganglion
Sympathetic trunk

Collateral sympathetic trunk ganglion (celiac, superior, and inferior mesenteric)

Sensory neuron of abdominal viscera (cell body in dorsal ganglion)

Sympathetic trunk
Branch to thoracic viscera
Splanchnic nerve

Dorsal funiculus
Association neuron
Preganglionic, sympathetic and motor neurons
Lateral funiculus
Postganglionic, sympathetic and motor neurons (derived from neural crest) growing to end on smooth (involuntary) muscle and sweat glands

Postganglionic, sympathetic and motor neurons growing to end in thoracic viscera

Preganglionic, sympathetic and motor neurons growing to synapse in another sympathetic trunk ganglion

Postganglionic, sympathetic and motor neurons (derived from neural crest) growing to end on glands and smooth (involuntary) muscle

FIGURE 7–3

Development of peripheral nerves. (Courtesy of Icon Learning Systems. Copyright©, Icon Learning Systems, LLC. A subsidiary of MediMedia, USA, Inc. All rights reserved.)

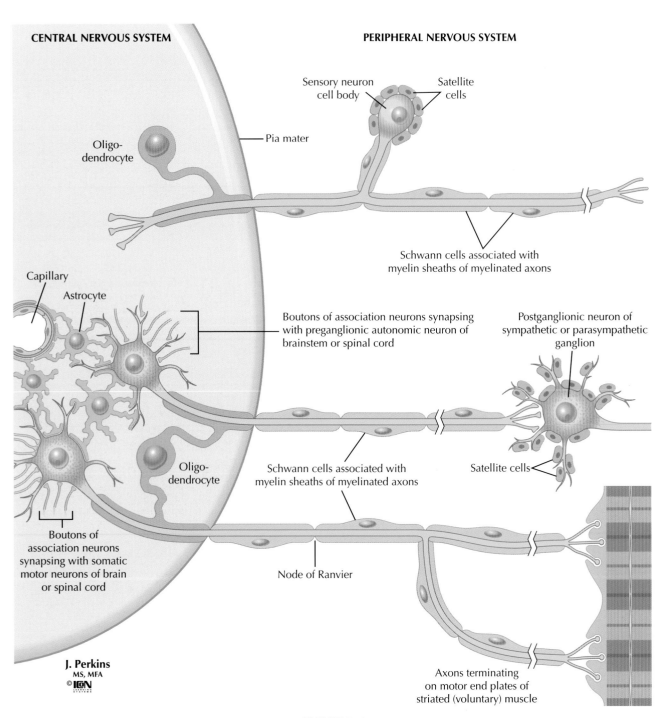

CENTRAL NERVOUS SYSTEM

PERIPHERAL NERVOUS SYSTEM

Oligo-dendrocyte

Pia mater

Sensory neuron cell body

Satellite cells

Schwann cells associated with myelin sheaths of myelinated axons

Capillary

Astrocyte

Boutons of association neurons synapsing with preganglionic autonomic neuron of brainstem or spinal cord

Postganglionic neuron of sympathetic or parasympathetic ganglion

Satellite cells

Oligo-dendrocyte

Schwann cells associated with myelin sheaths of myelinated axons

Boutons of association neurons synapsing with somatic motor neurons of brain or spinal cord

Node of Ranvier

Axons terminating on motor end plates of striated (voluntary) muscle

J. Perkins
MS, MFA
© ICON
LEARNING
SYSTEMS

FIGURE 7–4

Myelination of central nervous system and peripheral nerves. (Courtesy of Icon Learning Systems. Copyright©, Icon Learning Systems, LLC. A subsidiary of MediMedia, USA, Inc. All rights reserved.)

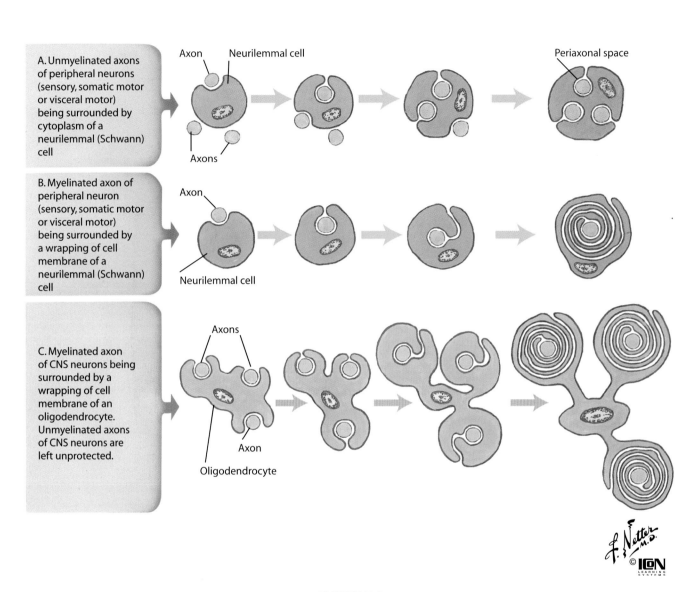

A. Unmyelinated axons of peripheral neurons (sensory, somatic motor or visceral motor) being surrounded by cytoplasm of a neurilemmal (Schwann) cell

Axon   Neurilemmal cell   Periaxonal space

Axons

B. Myelinated axon of peripheral neuron (sensory, somatic motor or visceral motor) being surrounded by a wrapping of cell membrane of a neurilemmal (Schwann) cell

Axon

Neurilemmal cell

C. Myelinated axon of CNS neurons being surrounded by a wrapping of cell membrane of an oligodendrocyte. Unmyelinated axons of CNS neurons are left unprotected.

Axons

Axon

Oligodendrocyte

FIGURE 7–5

Development of myelination and axonal ensheathments. (Courtesy of Icon Learning Systems. Copyright©, Icon Learning Systems, LLC. A subsidiary of MediMedia, USA, Inc. All rights reserved.)

TABLE 7–9. TIBIAL MOTOR NERVE CONDUCTION REFERENCE VALUES

Table 7–9A. According to Cruz-Martinez and Associates*,†

Age	Mean (range) Amplitude, mV	MNCV, m/sec	Distal Latency, msec
Premature (mean gestation, 35.8 wk)		19.0 ± 2.73	3.6 ± 0.53
Newborn (38-42 wk gestation)		24.5 ± 2.35	3.35 ± 0.41
0-1 mo	(5-8)	25.3 ± 1.96	3.20 ± 0.61
1-3 mo		27.8 ± 3.89	2.86 ± 0.45
3-6 mo		36.3 ± 4.98	2.20 ± 0.24
6-12 mo		39.9 ± 3.89	2.46 ± 0.34
1-2 yr		42.6 ± 3.80	2.40 ± 0.27
2-4 yr		49.8 ± 5.79	2.81 ± 0.47
4-6 yr		50.0 ± 4.26	3.20 ± 0.56
6-11 yr	12 (5-20)	52.4 ± 4.19	3.60 ± 0.67

MNCV, motor nerve conduction velocity.
   Data are presented as mean ± SD or as normative ranges.
   ° Data from Cruz-Martinez A, Ferrer MT, Perez-Conde ML, Bernacer M: Motor conduction velocity and H-reflex in infancy and childhood: Intra and extrauterine maturation of the nerve fibers: Development of the peripheral nerve from 1 month to 11 years of age. Electromyogr Clin Neurophysiol 1978;18:11-27; and Cruz-Martinez A, Perez-Conde ML, Ferrer MT: Motor conduction velocity and H-reflex in infancy and childhood: I. Study in newborns, twins, and small-for-dates. Electromyogr Clin Neurophysiol 1977;17:493-505.
   † Stimulation is at the popliteal fossa and close medial malleolus, and the recording electrodes are on the intrinsic muscles of the fifth toe.

Table 7–9B. According to Baer and Johnson*, †

Average Age	No.	Mean MNCV, m/sec
5 wk	11	34.3
18 wk	11	32.7
34 wk	12	38.3
56 wk	12	39.8
88 wk	12	44.5
140 wk	10	43.1
210 wk	12	48.4
4-16 yr		47.9 ± 9.2

MNCV, motor nerve conduction velocity.
   Data are presented as mean ± SD or as normative ranges.
   ° Data from Baer RD, Johnson EW: Motor nerve conduction velocities in normal children. Arch Phys Med Rehabil 1965;46:698-704.
   † Stimulation is in the upper mid-popliteal fossa and just proximal to the medial malleolus, and the active recording electrode is over the abductor digiti quinti (pedis) and the reference recording electrode over the lateral aspect of the little toe.

TABLE 7–10. TIBIAL MOTOR NERVE F WAVE REFERENCE VALUES*

Age, mo	No.	Latency, msec	Distance, cm
7-12	2	19-24	43-48
13-24	9	22-26	42-52

Data are presented as normative ranges.
   ° Data from Miller RG, Kuntz NL: Nerve conduction studies in infants and children. J Child Neurol 1986;1:19-26.

TABLE 7–11. TIBIAL NERVE H REFLEX REFERENCE VALUES

Table 7–11A. According to Mayer and Mooser[°],[†],[‡]

Age	No.	Latency, msec (mean)
1-3 days	25	13-17 (15.7)
4-30 days	9	13-17 (14.8)
1-5 mo	13	14-15 (14.3)
6-12 mo	17	13.5-16.5 (14.9)
1-3 yr	10	14.0-18.5 (15.8)
3-7 yr	5	16.0-19.5 (17.7)
1-3 days	7	22.0-25.0 (23.7)
6-12 mo	5	17.0-21.0 (18.4)

Data are presented as mean ± SD or as normative ranges, using surface recording electrodes.

[°] Data from Mayer RF, Mooser RS: Excitability of motoneurons in infants. Neurology 1969;19:932-945.

[†] Stimulation with the 7.5-mm diameter silver disk cathode is at the popliteal fossa and the large silver plate anode 12 cm proximally over the buttock, and with the 7.5-mm diameter silver disk active recording electrode on the surface of the distal edge of the calf muscle at a point where the three components of the triceps surae are close together and the 7.5-mm diameter silver disk reference recording electrode is on the Achilles tendon.

[‡] Recordings were also made with the active recording electrode over the center of the plantar foot muscle and the reference recording electrode on the great toe, 2.5 cm distally.

Table 7–11B. According to Bryant and Eng[°],[†]

Conceptional Age (gestational age plus age from birth), wk	No.	Latency, msec
31-34	30	19.19 ± 2.16
35-39	26	16.67 ± 1.49
40-45	27	15.95 ± 1.45

Data are presented as mean ± SD or as normative ranges, using surface recording electrodes.

[°] Data from Bryant PR, Eng GD: Normal values for the soleus H-reflex in newborn infants 31-45 weeks post conceptual age. Arch Phys Med Rehabil 1991;72:28-30.

[†] Stimulation is applied to the nerve in the popliteal fossa with the cathode proximal to the anode; stimulus duration is 0.1 msec and intensity subthreshold to the motor response. The ground electrode is between the stimulating and recording electrodes. The 5-mm diameter silver cup active recording electrode is over the gastrocnemius muscle midpoint and the reference recording electrode on the Achilles tendon.

TABLE 7–12. MEDIAN SENSORY AND MIXED NERVE CONDUCTION REFERENCE VALUES

Table 7–12A. According to Miller and Kuntz[°],[†]

Age	No.	Amplitude, μV		SNCV, m/sec	Distal Latency, msec	Distance, cm
		Antidromic SNAP	Orthodromic SNAP			
Neonate	10	7-15	8-17	25.1-31.9	2.1-3.0	3.8-5.4
1-6 mo	11	13-52	9-26	36.3-41.9	1.5-2.3	4.3-6.3
7-12 mo	15	14-64	11-36	39.1-60.0	1.6-2.4	5.5-6.8
13-24 mo	29	14-82	7-36	46.5-57.9	1.7-3.0	5.7-9.1

SNCV, sensory nerve conduction velocity; SNAP, sensory nerve action potential.

Data are presented as mean ± SD or as normative ranges.

[°] Data from Miller RG, Kuntz NL: Nerve conduction studies in infants and children. J Child Neurol 1986;1:19-26.

[†] Stimulation is on the index finger using ring electrodes; recording electrodes are over the median nerve at the wrist; and up to 30 responses are averaged.

(Continued)

TABLE 7–12. Cont'd

Table 7–12*B.* According to Parano and Associates[*],[†]

Age	No.	SNCV, m/sec	Amplitude, μV
7 days-1 mo	20	22.31 ± 2.16	6.22 ± 1.30
1-6 mo	23	35.52 ± 6.59	15.86 ± 5.18
6-12 mo	25	40.31 ± 5.23	16.00 ± 5.18
1-2 yr	24	46.93 ± 5.03	24.00 ± 7.36
2-4 yr	22	49.51 ± 3.34	24.28 ± 5.49
4-6 yr	20	51.71 ± 5.16	25.12 ± 5.22
6-14 yr	21	53.84 ± 3.26	26.72 ± 9.43

SNCV, sensory nerve conduction velocity.

   Data are presented as mean ± SD or as normative ranges.

   [*] Data from Parano E, Uncini A, De Vivo DC, Lovelace RE: Electrophysiologic correlates of peripheral nervous system maturation in infancy and childhood. J Child Neurol 1993;8:336-338.

   [†] Stimulation is with metal ring electrodes on digits I, II, and III; stimulus duration is 0.1 milliseconds. Bipolar recordings with interelectrode distance of 20 mm are made at the wrist for stimulation of each of the three digits and at the elbow for stimulation of digit III for determination of the wrist-elbow segment data.

Table 7–12*C.* According to Cruz-Martinez and Associates, 1978[*],[†]

Age	Digit I Amplitude		Digit II Amplitude		Digit III Amplitude	
	NCV, m/sec	μV	NVC, m/sec	μV	NCV, m/sec	μV
Newborn	19.4 ± 2.03	10.3 ± 4.38	19.7 ± 3.3	7.0 ± 2.6	20.8 ± 2.17	7.2 ± 2.1
1-3 mo	21.2 ± 2.3	16.2 ± 3.56	26.7 ± 5.21	12.4 ± 4.77	29.0 ± 5.24	12.2 ± 4.71
3-6 mo	29.2 ± 4.92	23.8 ± 4.19	34.9 ± 4.6	17.8 ± 5.1	37.1 ± 4.68	17.7 ± 3.75
6-12 mo	31.8 ± 4.4	27.3 ± 7.8	36.5 ± 3.79	16.7 ± 6.0	38.7 ± 4.47	18.0 ± 7.19
1-2 yr	35.5 ± 5.8	35.2 ± 10.2	43.3 ± 7.36	22.6 ± 3.8	44.0 ± 6.27	2.1 ± 4.22
2-4 yr	38.8 ± 5.27	38.3 ± 8.64	46.4 ± 4.6	22.8 ± 4.22	47.5 ± 4.33	22.0 ± 3.08
4-6 yr	38.9 ± 3.52	36.6 ± 6.41	46.1 ± 4.36	19.2 ± 5.37	46.5 ± 4.79	19.2 ± 6.59
6-14 yr	42.9 ± 3.78	36.1 ± 8.82	49.3 ± 4.65	16.8 ± 4.6	48.9 ± 4.21	19.0 ± 4.65
	NCV, m/sec	Component 1	Component 2			
Newborn	30.6 ± 2.93	2.9 ± 1.02				
1-3 mo	31.4 ± 0.98	2.22 ± 1.29				
3-6 mo	44.9 ± 4.92	3.5 ± 1.5	5.2 ± 1.83			
6-12 mo	51.4 ± 6.85	2.78 ± 1.5	6.7 ± 1.77			
1-2 yr	57.1 ± 5.72	3.37 ± 1.4	8.1 ± 1.73			
2-4 yr	61.7 ± 4.95	2.6 ± 0.69	5.9 ± 1.8			
4-6 yr	63.1 ± 6.26	2.7 ± 0.94	4.75 ± 1.51			
6-14 yr	64.9 ± 15.39	1.71 ± 0.77	3.1 ± 1.35			

Using surface stimulating and recording electrodes.

   NCV, nerve conduction velocity; SNAP, sensory nerve action potential.

   Data are presented as mean ± SD or as normative ranges.

   [*] Data from Cruz-Martinez A, Perez-Conde MC, del Campo F, et al: Sensory and mixed conduction velocity in infancy and childhood: I. Normal parameters in median, ulnar, and sural nerves. Electromyogr Clin Neurophysiol 1978;18:487-504.

   [†] The stimulating pipe-cleaner cathode is wrapped around the index (second) finger at the metacarpophalangeal joint with the 6-15-mm wide copper strip anode around the tip of the finger; stimulus duration is 0.05-0.1 milliseconds. Recording electrodes are over the nerve at the wrist. Distance is measured from the pipe cleaner to the distal recording electrode. Latency is from the start of the stimulus to the peak of the SNAP response, with approximate conduction velocity calculated by dividing distance by latency.

Table 7–12*D.* According to Cruz-Martinez, 1977[*],[†]

Age	NCV, m/sec	Amplitude, μV
Newborn	30.6 ± 3.82	7.75 ± 3.12
1-3 mo	34.0 ± 4.56	10.8 ± 6.27
3-6 mo	47.6 ± 7.2	21.6 ± 4.22
6-12 mo	54.9 ± 9.6	37.9 ± 16.2
1-2 yr	59.7 ± 6.13	43.5 ± 18.5
2-4 yr	66.4 ± 5.0	44.1 ± 14.16
4-6 yr	63.4 ± 4.18	33.4 ± 12.4
6-14 yr	66.2 ± 3.89	32.2 ± 13.3

Data are presented as mean ± SD or as normative ranges.

   NCV, nerve conduction velocity.

   [*] Data from Cruz-Martinez A, Perez-Conde ML, Ferrer MT: Motor conduction velocity and H-reflex in infancy and childhood: I. Study in newborns, twins, and small-for-dates. Electromyogr Clin Neurophysiol 1977;17:493-505.

   [†] Stimulation is at the wrist percutaneously, with recording of the action potential at the elbow.

TABLE 7–13. ULNAR SENSORY AND MIXED NERVE CONDUCTION REFERENCE VALUES

Table 7–13A. According to Cruz-Martinez and Associates°

| | Digit V-Wrist Segment | | Wrist-Elbow Segment Amplitude, mV | | |
Age	NCV, m/sec	Amplitude, μV	NCV, m/sec	Component 1	Component 2
Newborn	18.4 ± 3.97	5.5 ± 3.1	25.2 ± 3.64	2.2 ± 0.88	
1-3 mo	27.7 ± 6.37	9.4 ± 3.2	28.9 ± 1.45	2.62 ± 0.94	
3-6 mo	37.1 ± 5.25	13.2 ± 3.23	41.9 ± 3.03	3.1 ± 1.5	4.5 ± 1.0
6-12 mo	40.0 ± 5.13	13.0 ± 5.6	51.6 ± 6.6	2.8 ± 1.12	6.0 ± 1.65
1-2 yr	44.2 ± 7.79	16.3 ± 2.44	55.0 ± 6.15	3.5 ± 1.41	6.8 ± 1.19
2-4 yr	48.81 ± 3.01	16.0 ± 3.6	60.3 ± 5.25	3.0 ± 1.3	6.2 ± 1.15
4-6 yr	47.7 ± 6.75	14.2 ± 2.72	58.4 ± 2.59	2.9 ± 0.98	4.1 ± 1.17
6-14 yr	46.6 ± 5.6	13.4 ± 4.2	60.5 ± 5.38	2.4 ± 1.15	4.7 ± 1.53

NCV, nerve conduction velocity.

Data are presented as mean ± SD or as normative ranges.

° Data from Cruz-Martinez A, Perez-Conde MC, del Campo F, et al: Sensory and mixed conduction velocity in infancy and childhood: I. Normal parameters in median, ulnar and sural nerves. Electromyogr Clin Neurophysiol 1978;18:487-504.

† Digit V is stimulated, with recordings at the wrist and elbow.

‡ Stimulation is on the little (fifth) finger, with recording from the wrist.

§ Stimulation is at the wrist percutaneously, with recording of the action potential at the elbow.

Table 7–13B. According to Cruz-Martinez and Associates*

Age	NCV, m/sec	Amplitude, μV
Newborn	30.5 ± 2.29	7.4 ± 2.22
1-3 mo	37.1 ± 3.72	11.3 ± 4.96
3-6 mo	45.3 ± 6.36	23.4 ± 7.73
6-12 mo	56.2 ± 4.13	31.0 ± 13.7
1-2 yr	60.0 ± 7.67	48.6 ± 13.7
2-4 yr	62.5 ± 3.51	41.8 ± 15.4
4-6 yr	62.3 ± 2.56	40.3 ± 19.5
6-14 yr	62.7 ± 4.61	45.8 ± 16.7

NCV, nerve conduction velocity.

Data are presented as mean ± SD or as normative ranges.

° Data from Cruz-Martinez A, Perez-Conde MC, del Campo F, et al: Sensory and mixed conduction velocity in infancy and childhood: I. Normal parameters in median, ulnar and sural nerves. Electromyogr Clin Neurophysiol 1978;18:487-504.

TABLE 7–14. SURAL SENSORY NERVE CONDUCTION REFERENCE VALUES

Table 7–14A. According to Miller and Kuntz°,†

Age	No.	Amplitude, μV	NCV, m/sec	Distal Latency, msec	Distance, cm
Neonate	1	8		3.3	5.5
1-6 mo	2	9-10		1.7-2.3	5.8
7-12 mo	5	10-28	40.6	1.7-2.5	5.8-7.6
13-24 mo	9	8-30		1.4-2.8	4.5-8.6

NCV, nerve conduction velocity.

Data are presented as mean ± SD or as normative ranges.

° Data from Miller RG, Kuntz NL: Nerve conduction studies in infants and children. J Child Neurol 1986;1:19-26.

† Stimulation is below and distal to the lateral malleolus; recording electrodes are over the sural nerve 4-10 cm above the ankle; and up to 30 responses are averaged.

Table 7–14B. According to Parano and Associates°

Age	No.	SNCV, m/sec	Amplitude, μV
7 days-1 mo	20	20.26 ± 1.55	9.12 ± 3.02
1-6 mo	23	34.63 ± 5.43	11.66 ± 3.57
6-12 mo	25	38.18 ± 5.00	15.10 ± 8.02
1-2 yr	24	49.73 ± 5.53	15.41 ± 9.98
2-4 yr	22	52.63 ± 2.96	23.27 ± 6.84
4-6 yr	20	53.83 ± 4.34	22.66 ± 5.42
6-14 yr	21	53.85 ± 4.19	26.75 ± 6.59

SNCV, sensory nerve conduction velocity.

Data are presented as mean ± SD or as normative ranges.

° Data from Parano E, Uncini A, De Vivo DC, Lovelace RE: Electrophysiologic correlates of peripheral nervous system maturation in infancy and childhood. J Child Neurol 1993;8:336-338.

TABLE 7–15. MEDIAL PLANTAR SENSORY NERVE CONDUCTION REFERENCE VALUES*

Age	No.	Amplitude, μV	NCV, m/sec	Distal Latency, msec	Distance, cm
Neonate	3	10-40		2.1-3.3	4.5-5.8
1-6 mo	2	17-26	35.4-35.7	1.5-1.9	4.5-5.5
7-12 mo	6	15-38	39.4-40.3	1.9-2.7	6.5-7.9
13-24 mo	12	15-60	42.6-57.3	1.8-2.5	6.1-9.3

NCV, nerve conduction velocity.
  Data are presented as normative ranges.
  ° Data from Miller RG, Kuntz NL: Nerve conduction studies in infants and children. J Child Neurol 1986;1:19-26.

TABLE 7–16. PHRENIC MOTOR NERVE CONDUCTION REFERENCE VALUES USING SURFACE RECORDING ELECTRODES°,†

Age	No.	Latency, msec	Stimulus-Response Distance, cm
Preterm (<37 wk)	20	2.6 ± 0.3	7.7 ± 0.7
Fullterm	10	2.5 ± 0.4	9.2 ± 1.4
0-5 mo	24	2.2 ± 0.4	10.4 ± 1.1
6-11 mo	18	2.6 ± 0.7	12.5 ± 0.9
12-23 mo	16	2.8 ± 0.7	13.2 ± 0.7
2-5 yr	13	2.9 ± 0.5	13.8 ± 1.1
5-11 yr	24	4.2 ± 0.7	16.8 ± 1.4

Data are presented as means ± SD or as normative ranges.
  Eng[51] has commented that the latencies of the recordings by Moosa[27] may not be from the diaphragm after phrenic nerve stimulation. Using surface electrodes, preliminary latencies (in young infants with brachial plexopathies) were about 5-6 milliseconds.[52]
  ° Date from Moosa A: Phrenic nerve conduction in children. Dev Med Child Neurol 1981;23:434-448.
  † Subcutaneous stimulation with a hand-held bipolar electrode is at the posterior border of the sternomastoid muscle at the level of the upper border of the thyroid cartilage with the anode over the manubrium sterni; stimulus duration is 0.2 milliseconds. Silver cup recording electrodes are placed at the 5th or 6th intercostal space approximately 2 cm apart with the anterior electrode along the anterior axillary line.

TABLE 7–17. MOTOR UNIT POTENTIAL PARAMETER REFERENCE VALUES

Muscle	Amplitude, μV°				Duration, msec°			
	Mean	SEM	SD	Range	Mean	SEM	SD	Range
Quadriceps femoris, newborn[53]	507	29	290	100-1600	6.27	0.15	1.51	2-10
Tibialis anterior, newborn[53]	498	28	283	100-1500	5.67	0.16	1.65	2.5-10.5
Biceps brachii[44]								
3 mo	96	7			7.7	0.3		
16-23 yr	175	20			10.3	0.2		
Abductor digiti quinti[45]								
3 mo	78	12			5.8	0.1		
16-23 yr	360	20			9.4	0.25		
	Amplitude (μV)†				**Duration (msec)†**			
	Initially 300-500[45]				Initially 2-3[45]			
	Range, 200-2000[45]				Range, 1-5[45]			
	Range, 150-3000[45]				Range, 2-5[45]			

° For muscles of pediatric patients at different ages using concentric needle electrodes with 0.04 mm[15,56] or 0.03 mm[15,49] core surface area.
† For infants, using monopolar needle electrodes.

TABLE 7–18. NORMATIVE VALUES FOR DIFFERENT EMG MUSCLE PARAMETERS FOR DIFFERENT PEDIATRIC AGE GROUPS*,†

Muscle	Age, yr	Fiber Density, 00	Mean MCD	Jitter (>2 of 20 Potentials)
Frontalis	5	1.67	33.6	49.7
	10	1.67	33.6	49.7
	15	1.67	33.7	49.9
	20	1.67	33.9	50.1
Orbicularis oculi	5		39.8	54.6
	10		39.8	54.6
	15		39.8	54.6
	20		39.8	54.7
Orbicularis oris	5		34.6	52.5
	10		34.7	52.5
	15		34.7	52.6
	20		34.7	52.7
Deltoid	5	1.56	32.9	44.4
	10	1.56	32.9	44.4
	15	1.56	32.9	44.5
	20	1.56	32.9	44.5
Biceps	5	1.52	29.5	45.1
	10	1.52	29.5	45.2
	15	1.52	29.5	45.2
	20	1.52	29.6	45.2
Extensor digitorum communis	5	1.77	34.9	50.0
	10	1.77	34.9	50.0
	15	1.77	34.9	50.1
	20	1.78	34.9	50.1
Quadriceps	5	1.93	35.8	47.9
	10	1.93	35.9	47.9
	15	1.93	35.9	48.0
	20	1.94	36.0	48.0
Tibialis anterior	5	1.94	49.4	80.0
	10	1.94	49.4	80.0
	15	1.94	49.4	79.9
	20	1.94	49.3	79.8
Soleus	5	1.56		
	10	1.56		
	15	1.56		
	20	1.56		

MCD, mean consecutive difference.

* Data from Stålberg E, Trontelj JV: The study of normal and abnormal neuromuscular transmission with single fibre electromyography. J Neurosci Methods 1997;74:145-154.

† At 95% upper normal limits.

REFERENCES

1. Gamble HJ, Breathnach AS: An electron-microscope study of human foetal peripheral nerves. J Anat 1965;99:573-584.
2. Cottrell L: Histologic variations with age in apparently normal peripheral nerve trunks. Arch Neurol 1940;43:1138-1150.
3. Rexed B: Contribution to knowledge of postnatal development of peripheral nervous system in man: Study of bases and scope of systematic investigations into fibre size in peripheral nerves. Acta Psychiatry Neurol Scand 1944;Suppl 33:1-206.
4. Carpenter FG, Bergland RM: Excitation and conduction in immature nerve fibers of the developing chick. Am J Physiol 1957;190:371-376.
5. Gutrecht JA, Dyck PJ: Quantitative teased-fiber and histologic studies of human sural nerve during postnatal development. J Comp Neurol 1970;138:117-130.
6. Cruz-Martinez A, Ferrer MT, Martin MJ: Motor conduction velocity and H-reflex in prematures with very short gestational age. Electromyogr Clin Neurophysiol 1983;23:13-19.
7. Bhatia BD, Prakash U, Singh MN, et al: Electrophysiological studies in newborns with reference to gestation and anthropometry. Electromyogr Clin Neurophysiol 1991;31:55-59.
8. Cerra D, Johnson E: Motor nerve conduction velocity in premature infants. Arch Phys Med Rehabil 1962;43:60-164.
9. Bhatia BD, Prakash U: Electrophysiological studies in preterm and growth retarded low birth weight babies. Electromyogr Clin Neurophysiol 1993;33:507-509.
10. Robinson RO, Robertson WC Jr: Fetal nutrition and peripheral nerve conduction velocity. Neurology 1981;31:327-329.
11. Schulte FJ, Michaelis R, Linke L, Notle R: Motor nerve conduction velocity in term, preterm, and small-for-date newborn infants. Pediatrics 1968;42:17-26.

12. Thomas JE, Lambert EH: Ulnar nerve conduction velocity and H-reflex in infants and children. J Appl Physiol 1960;15:1-9.

13. Gamstorp I: Normal conduction velocity of ulnar, median and peroneal nerves in infancy, childhood, and adolescence. Acta Paediatr Scand 1965;54:309-313.

14. Baer RD, Johnson EW: Motor nerve conduction velocities in normal children. Arch Phys Med Rehabil 1965;46:698-704.

15. Miller RG, Kuntz NL: Nerve conduction studies in infants and children. J Child Neurol 1986;1:19-26.

16. Oh SJ: Clinical Electromyography: Nerve Conduction Studies. Baltimore, University Park Press, 1984, pp 115-139.

17. Parano E, Uncini A, De Vivo DC, Lovelace RE: Electrophysiologic correlates of peripheral nervous system maturation in infancy and childhood. J Child Neurol 1993;8:336-338.

18. Cruz-Martinez A, Perez-Conde MC, del Campo F, et al: Sensory and mixed conduction velocity in infancy and childhood: Normal parameters in median, ulnar, and sural nerves. Electromyogr Clin Neurophysiol 1978;18:487-504.

19. Harmon RL, Eichman PL, Rodriguez AA: Laboratory Manual of Pediatric Electromyography. Madison, WI, University of Wisconsin Board of Regents, 1992, pp 1-66.

20. Cruz-Martinez A, Perez-Conde ML, Ferrer MT: Motor conduction velocity and H-reflex in infancy and childhood: I. Study in newborns, twins, and small-for-dates. Electromyogr Clin Neurophysiol 1977;17:493-505.

21. Misra UK, Tiwari S, Shukla N, et al: F-response studies in neonates, infants and children. Electromyogr Clin Neurophysiol 1989;29:251-254.

22. Bhatia BD, Prakash U, Gupka SK, et al: Motor nerve conductor velocity and Hoffman's reflex latency in newborns. Indian J Ped Res 1993;98:227–231.

23. Mayer RF, Mooser RS: Excitability of motoneurons in infants. Neurology 1969;19:932-945.

24. Bryant PR, Eng GD: Normal values for the soleus H-reflex in newborn infants 31-45 weeks postconceptual age. Arch Phys Med Rehabil 1991;72:28-30.

25. Shahani BT, Young RR: Clinical significance of late response studies in infants and children [Abstract]. Neurology 1981;31:66.

26. Kwast O, Krajewska G, Kozlowski K: Analysis of F-wave parameters in median and ulnar nerves in healthy infants and children: Age-related changes. Electromyogr Clin Neurophysiol 1984;24:439-456.

27. Moosa A: Phrenic nerve conduction in children. Dev Med Child Neurol 1981;23:434-448.

28. Newsom-Davis J: Phrenic nerve conduction in man. J Neurol Neurosurg Psychiatry 1967;30:420-426.

29. Dubowitz V, Whittaker GF, Brown BH, Robinson A: Nerve conduction velocity: An index of neurological maturity of the newborn infant. Dev Med Child Neurol 1968;10:741-749.

30. Blom S, Finnstrom O: Motor conduction velocities in newborn infants of various gestational ages. Acta Paediatr Scand 1968;57:377-384.

31. Wagner AL, Buchthal F: Motor and sensory conduction in infancy and childhood: Reappraisal. Dev Med Child Neurol 1972;14:189-216.

32. Ruppert ES, Robertson AF, Johnson EW: Motor nerve conduction velocities in infants of low birth weight. J Pediatr 1967;70:693-694.

33. Dubowitz V: Nerve conduction velocities in premature and full-term infants. Dev Med Child Neurol 1965;7:426-427.

34. Smit BJ, Koh JH, De Vries LS, et al: Motor Nerve Conductors Velocity in Very Preterm Infants. Muscle Nerve 1999;22:372–377.

35. Koenigsberger MR, Patten B, Lovelace RE: Studies of neuromuscular function in the newborn: A comparison of myoneural function in the full term and premature infant. Neuropediatrics 1973;4:350-361.

36. Cornblath DR: Disorders of neuromuscular transmission in infants and children. Muscle Nerve 1986;9:606-611.

37. Farkas-Bargeton E, Diebler MF, Arsenio-Nunes ML, et al: [Histochemical, quantitative and ultrastructural maturation of human fetal muscle]. J Neurol Sci 1977:31:245-259.

38. Fenichel GM: A histochemical study of developing human skeletal muscle. Neurology 1996;16:741-745.

39. Kumagai T, Hakamada S, Hara K, et al: Development of human fetal muscles: A comparative histochemical analysis of the psoas and the quadriceps muscles. Neuropediatrics 1984;15:198-202.

40. Colling-Saltin AS: Some quantitative biochemical evaluations of developing skeletal muscles in the human foetus. J Neurol Sci 1978;39:187-198.

41. Barbet JP, Butler-Browne GS, Labbe S, et al: Quantification of the diameter of muscular fibres in the course of the development of the quadriceps. Bull Assoc Anat (Nancy) 1991;75:25-29.

42. Dumitru D: Electrodiagnostic Medicine. Philadelphia, Hanley & Belfus, 1994.

43. Buchthal F, Guld C, Rosenfalck P: Multielectrode study of the territory of a motor unit. Acta Physiol Scand 1957;39:83-104.

44. Stalberg E, Macro EMG: Muscle Nerve 1983;6:619-630.

45. Sacco G, Buchthal F, Rosenfalck P: Motor unit potentials at different ages. Arch Neurol 1962;6:366-373.

46. Bischoff C, Stalberg E, Falck B, Edebol Eeg-Olofsson K: Reference values of motor unit action potentials obtained with multi-MUAP analysis. Muscle Nerve 1994;17:642-851.

47. Bromberg MB, Swoboda KJ: Motor unit estimation (MUNE) in infants and children with spinal muscular atrophy (SMA). Muscle Nerve 2002;25:445-447.

48. Doherty T, Brown W: The estimated numbers and relative sizes of thenar units as selected by multiple point stimulation in young and older adults. Muscle Nerve 1993;16:355-366.

49. Feinstein B, Lindegard B, Nyman E, Wolhart G: Morphologic studies of motor units in normal human muscles. Acta Anat (Basel) 1955;23:127-142.

50. Kimura J, Bodensteiner J, Yamada T: Electrically elicited blink reflex in normal neonates. Arch Neurol 1977;37:246-249.

51. Eng G: Personal communication to Harmon RL, February 26, 1992.

52. Clay SA, Ramseyer JC: The orbicularis oculi reflex in infancy and childhood. Neurology 1976;26:521-524.

53. de Carmo RJ: Motor unit action potential parameters in human newborn infants. Arch Neurol 1960;3:136-140.

8

Somatosensory Evoked Potentials in Pediatrics—Normal

Robin L. Gilmore

Somatosensory evoked potentials (SSEPs) provide the means to safely and noninvasively study segments of the peripheral and central nervous systems. Physical examination of the infant and young child, especially that of sensory systems, is frequently difficult. In infants and nonverbal children, SSEPs can provide information about the functioning of these systems not assessed by other means. SSEPs may be a valuable diagnostic aid to the clinician. The median nerve (MN)-SSEP[1-5] has been more thoroughly investigated in children than the posterior tibial nerve (PTN)-SSEP.[6-8] In this chapter we examine the generator sources and methodologies of short-latency SSEPs after MN-SSEP and PTN-SSEP stimulation. Effects of maturation—both growth and development—and effects of sleep also are reviewed.

NEUROANATOMY OF SSEPs

Evoked potentials recorded from the body's surface are either near field or far field in nature. That is, the generator source is close or distant to the site of recording. The generators may be in gray matter or white matter. White matter generates compound action potentials (APs) that are propagated through fiber tracts. The latencies of the propagated APs increase proportionate to the distance from the point of stimulation and hence are dependent on recording electrode position. These are recorded only in relative close proximity to the fiber tract itself and thus are

termed *near-field potentials* (NFPs). NFPs have a specific distribution (topographic specificity), latencies that vary according to recording electrode placement, amplitudes greater than 1 V, and generally negative polarity. *Far-field potentials* (FFPs) may be recorded at long distances from the point of propagation and are generated when a traveling impulse (signal) passes through a certain anatomic site or fixed point along the nerve. FFPs have a diffuse distribution, fixed latencies, amplitudes less than 1 V, and polarity that likely reflects volume-conducted positivity.

Potentials are labeled according to the polarity and mean latency of a component derived from a sample of the normal population. As expected, latencies change with body growth and nervous system maturation. Thus, nomenclature differs between children and adults. Although this text is devoted to pediatric clinical neurophysiology, for purposes of discussing generator sources adult terminology is used because this is prevalent in the literature. Neural generators of MN-SSEPs and PTN-SSEPs that have been delineated in adults are reviewed in the following sections and are likely applicable to children. The presumed generators of MN-SSEPs and PTN-SSEPs are summarized in Tables 8-1 and 8-2, respectively.

Median Nerve SSEPs

When SSEPs are recorded from the scalp with a noncephalic reference (shoulder), three (and sometimes four)

TABLE 8–1
Presumed Generators of MN-SSEPs

Component*	Origin
P9 (P7)	FFP of brachial plexus
N9	Brachial plexus
P11 (P8)	FFP of dorsal root entry zone
P13-P14 (P9)	Brainstem lemniscal pathways composite of cervical dorsal horn synaptic activity and brainstem lemniscal pathways
N20 (N16)	Subcortical region and sensory cortex
P23 (P20)	Sensory cortex

* Notations in parentheses are designations for children 1-8 years of age.
  MN-SSEP, median nerve somatosensory evoked potential; FFP, far-field potential.

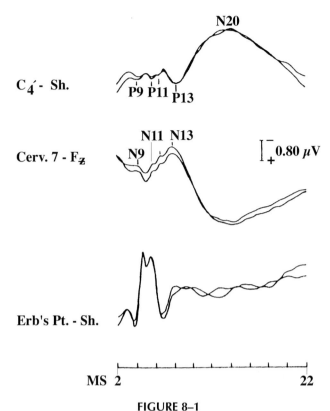

FIGURE 8–1
Somatosensory evoked potential to left median nerve stimulation in a 2-year-old child. Note that the Erb's point, P11, and N11 potentials are bilobed and that the N20 is broader in this young child than in the adult (see Fig. 8-2). (From Cracco JB, Cracco RQ: Spinal, brainstem, and cerebral SEP in the pediatric age group. In Bodis-Wollner I [ed]: Evoked Potentials. New York, Alan R. Liss, 1986, p 471.)

positive potentials are obtained: P9, P11, and P13, regardless of recording site (Fig. 8-1, Channel 1). Since they have fixed latencies, these are FFPs. Two later components are also recorded, the N20 (also called N19) and P23. The P9 is the FFP of the N9 that arises from the distal portion of the brachial plexus.[9,10] Because the N11 has a shorter refractory period than the subsequent N13, it is believed to be generated presynaptically from the dorsal root entry zone.[11,12] The P13 component arises in structures caudal to the thalamus, probably in the brainstem lemniscal pathways.[13] Desmedt and Cheron[14] recorded the P13 from an anterior neck recording and proposed a horizontally oriented dipole arising from the postsynaptic potentials (PSPs) in the interneurons of the dorsal horn.

When recorded from the neck with scalp reference derivation (Cerv 7-Fz in Channel 2 of Fig. 8-1), P9 becomes an upgoing peak, the N9, owing to greater positivity at the scalp than at the neck. Hence, N9 in this channel is an inverted P9. Although it is related to the potential seen in Channel 3 of Figure 8-1, it is not the NFP of Erb's point. The N13 is the major negative peak in this channel. It is a combination of N13 (NFP)[15,16] from the cervical generator and P13 (FFP) from the scalp (Fz). Generator sources proposed for cervical N13 include high cervical cord,[17-19] or mid-cervical dorsal column[12,20] or a site at the foramen magnum.[21] An origin at the cuneate nucleus has also been

TABLE 8–2
Presumed Generators of PTN-SSEPs

Component*	Origin
N8 (N5)	Tibial nerve action potential
N19 (N11)	Cauda equina
N22 (N14)	Lumbar cord gray matter
N29 (N20)	Gracile nucleus
P37 (P28)	Mesial sensory cortex
N45 (N41)	Cortex (association?)

* Notations in parentheses are designations for children 1-8 years of age.
  PTN-SSEP, posterior tibial nerve somatosensory evoked potential.

proposed. The N11 is inconsistently registered as a small notch and is not always recorded. It is a small wavelet "riding on" the ascending limb of N13. The N11 appears to have the same generator as the P11, the dorsal root entry zone.[11] The P11 in Channel 1 and the N11 in Channel 2 may represent the same dipole, vertically oriented.[10]

The N20 generator source is not precisely understood. Some have suggested that it is thalamic in origin,[2,17,21] whereas others have supported a thalamocortical or cortical source.[11,22-25] Yamada[26] has summarized the generators of the several components of the scalp-recorded MN-SSEP. These components show a progressive latency delay from frontal to parietal electrodes over the hemisphere contralateral to the side of stimulation: these include the N17-P20-N29 at the frontal site; the N19-P23-N32 at the central site, and N20-P26-N34 at parietal electrodes. The N20 of this last complex is the same as the N20 in Figure 8-1 and referred to previously. The out-of-phase relationship between frontal P20 and parietal N20 led to the hypothesis that they were the two ends of a dipole oriented across the central sulcus.[27] The central and parietal peaks are recorded only over the contralateral hemisphere, whereas frontal peaks are distributed bilaterally. Because of diffuse distribution the first of the frontal components, the N17, is believed to arise from subcortical structures, possibly from the thalamus[19,28] or just caudal to the thalamus.[29] The P23 appears to arise from somatosensory cortex.[9,30] MN-SSEPs in a 2-year-old child and a 20-year-old man are provided in Figures 8-1 and 8-2, respectively.

Posterior Tibial Nerve SSEPs

Designations for the evoked potential (EP) component of PTN-SSEPs are less consistent than for MN-SSEPs. For purposes of discussion of generators of PTN-SSEPS, adult terminology is used with the child or infant notation following in parentheses. Following PTN stimulation, electrodes over the popliteal fossa record the electronegative peripheral nerve AP N8 (N5 in the child) (Figs. 8-3 to 8-5). Electrodes over the lower spine record two electronegative potentials: the N19 (N11) and the N22 (NI4). The N19 (N11) represents the afferent volley in the cauda equina. The N22 (N20) is a stationary potential and probably

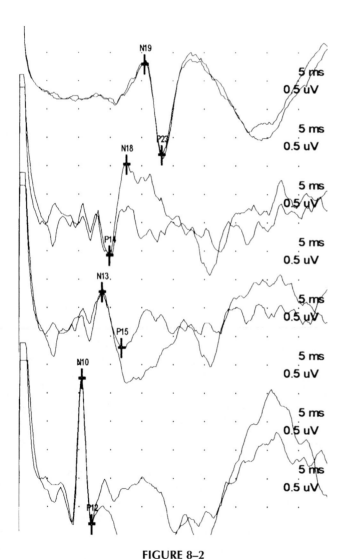

FIGURE 8–2
Somatosensory evoked potential to left median nerve stimulation in a 20-year-old man. Montage, top to bottom: CPc-CPi, CPi-EPc, C5s-EPc, EPi-EPc.

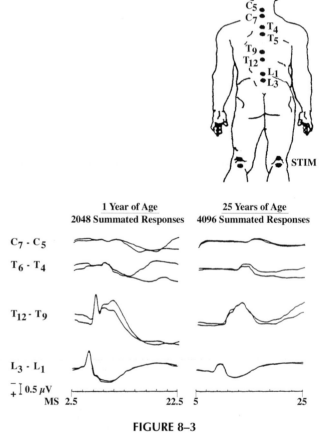

FIGURE 8–3
Comparison of bipolar recordings of the spinal response to peroneal nerve stimulation in a 1-year-old infant and an adult. Over the cauda equina (L1-L3 spine), the response in both the infant and the adult consists of triphasic potentials with poorly defined initial positive phases. In the infant, the response over caudal spinal cord (T12 spine) consists of a positive-negative diphasic potential followed by a broad negative-positive diphasic potential. In the adult it consists of a broad negative potential with two or three inflections. The response over rostral spinal cord in both the infant and adult consists of small initially positive triphasic potentials with poorly defined positive phases. STIM, stimulator. (From Cracco JB, Cracco RQ: Spinal somatosensory evoked potentials: Maturational and clinical studies. Ann N Y Acad Sci 1982;388:526-537.)

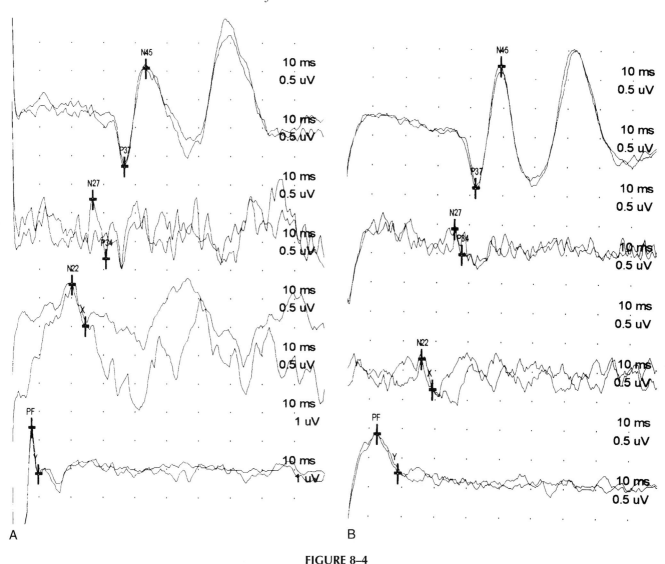

FIGURE 8–4

A, Somatosensory evoked potential (SSEP) to bilateral posterior tibial nerve stimulation in a 20-year-old man. B, SSEP to bilateral posterior tibial nerve stimulation in a 45-year-old woman. Montage, top to bottom: CPz-FPz, C5s-FPz, T12-IC, PF-REF.

reflects postsynaptic activity of internuncial neurons in the gray matter of the spinal cord.[31] Electrodes over the cervical spine record another later stationary potential: N27 (N20). This component may reflect postsynaptic activity in the gracile nucleus.[29] The P37 (P28) is the first major localized scalp recorded component. It reflects the ipsilaterally oriented cortical surface electropositivity while the electronegative end of the dipole may be recorded contralaterally.[32,33] There is a great deal of intersubject variability in the topography of the P37 (P28) in adults[34] and especially in children.[7] This is probably related to known anatomic differences in the location of primary sensory area for the leg.[35] When the leg area is located at the superior edge of the interhemispheric fissure, the cortical generator for P37 (P28) is vertically oriented and its amplitude is maximal

close to the vertex. When the leg area is located more deeply in the fissure, the cortical generator is more horizontally turned and the P37 (P28) projects ipsilaterally.[33] The N45 (N41) is the first large negative recorded at the scalp.

METHODOLOGIES

Stimulation

An SSEP may be generated by physiologic (touch or muscle stretch) or by nonphysiologic stimuli such as electrical stimulation. Because the electrical stimulation is the most easily controlled stimulus and produces EPs of the

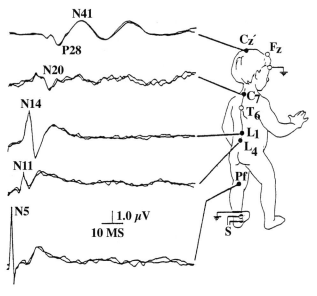

FIGURE 8–5

Somatosensory evoked potential (SSEP) after tibial nerve stimulation at the ankle recorded at various sites simultaneously. Labeling was based on surface polarity and mean peak latency observed in 32 normal young subjects (age = 1 to 8 years, height = 82 to 130 cm). Electrodes were placed at the popliteal fossa (PF), fourth lumbar (L4), first lumbar (L1,) sixth thoracic (T6), and seventh cervical (C7) spinous processes of vertebrae, Cz′ (2 cm behind Cz) and Fz (10-20 System). Fz was the reference for Cz′ and C7 and T6 was the reference for L and pF. Current pulses of 200-second duration were delivered at 5/sec. Two independent averages of 1000 to 2000 responses were superimposed to show intertrial replicability. (From Gilmore RL, Bass NH, Wright EA, et al: Development assessment of spinal cord and cortical evoked potentials after tibial nerve stimulation: Effects of age and stature on normative data during childhood. Electroencephalogr Clin Neurophysiol 1985;62:241-251.)

largest amplitude, electrical stimulation is most commonly used in clinical practice. Stimulation rates are laboratory dependent and should be the same as the rate at which the normative data for the laboratory was acquired. Rates much higher than 5/sec may be associated with degradation of the EP and hence are not recommended. In tibial nerve SSEPs, a rate of 5/sec may be too high and a rate of 2/sec may result in a more clearly defined EP. Even for the MN-SSEP, lower stimulus rates may result in better delineated SSEPs.[36] For children older than 1 year of age, a stimulus duration of 200 milliseconds, the same as used in the adult, is appropriate. For infants, especially preterm newborns, a shorter stimulus duration of 130 to 150 milliseconds may be used.

Stimulus intensity should be adjusted so that there is a consistent, rhythmic movement. It is not sufficient to see the movement only at the beginning of the test, since it is quite possible that it will disappear at borderline low levels of intensity. If that happens, trials during which an EP was recorded will be "averaged out" by subsequent trials during which no potential is evoked or there will be prolongation of the latencies of the EP components. For the older child, stimulus intensity will be approximately 7 to 15 mA.

For small infants, the standard saddle stimulating electrodes are inadequate. Electrodes with smaller surface areas and smaller interelectrode distances are necessary. A typical stimulating electrode surface area is 0.19 cm,[27] and a typical cathode-anode distance is 1 cm.[7] Stimulating intensity of 12 to 14 mA is usually sufficient. Because of a small electrode surface area, there is a high current density, and one should be careful to use a low stimulus rate to avoid superficial burns.

For MN-SSEP, unilateral stimulation is recommended. For tibial nerve EPs, unilateral stimulation is recommended for children older than 1 year of age. For infants, bilateral simultaneous stimulation is usually necessary to record PTN-SSEPs.[7]

Recording

Several methods have been suggested for recording MN-SSEPs in infants and children,[13,36-41] and four are summarized in Table 8-3. The American Electroencephalographic Society guidelines[40] recommend the following as a minimal montage:

- Channel 4: Cc—Ci
- Channel 3: Ci—noncephalic reference
- Channel 2: spC5—noncephalic reference
- Channel 1: Epi—noncephalic reference

Standard electroencephalographic disk electrodes are used for recording, and contact impedance should be less than 5 KΩs. The analysis time should be 30 to 40 milliseconds for MN-SSEP and 50 to 60 milliseconds for PTN-SSEP. The number of trials to be averaged depends on the amount of noise present and the size of the signal of interest. It ranges between 1000 and 2000. Replication is essential to verify that recorded waveforms are time-locked signals and not background noise. Filter bandpass is generally 30 to 3000 Hz (–6 dB/octave). Polarity conventions are indicated in Table 8-3.

For PTN-SSEP, stimulating electrodes are applied at the popliteal fossa (Pf), and over the spinous processes of the first lumbar, sixth thoracic and seventh cervical vertebrae (spL1, spT6, and spC7, respectively). The spL4 electrode may substitute for spC7. Scalp electrodes are placed at Cz′ (2 cm behind Cz [International 10-20 System]; 1 cm behind Cz in the preterm newborn) and Fz. The spT6 electrode was used as the reference for the Pf and spL1 and spL4 electrodes; Fz is the reference for Cz′ and spC7. Proposed American EEG Guidelines suggest the following:

TABLE 8–3

Summary of Four Methods of MN-SSEP Recording in Infants and Children °

Channels	Recording Site	Components Recorded
Cracco Method[13]		
1	C'c-Nc (may be EPc or Shc)	P9, P11, P13-14, N20, P23
2	C'c-Ac	P13-14, N20, P23
3	spC₂-Cz or spC₅-Fz	N9, N11, N13, N14
4	Epi-Epc or Shc	EP potential
Goldie Method[37]		
1	EPc-C'c	P9, P11, P13-14, N20, P23
2	Fpz-C'c	N20
3	Fpz-spC₇	B complex, second negative peak
4	Fpz-EPi	EP potential
Willis Method[36]		
1	C'c-Fz	N1, P1, N2
2	spC₂-Fz	C2
3	Epi-Fz	EP
Taylor Method[38,39,59]		
1	EPi-Fpz	N9
2	spC₇-Fpz	N12, N13
3	C'c-Fpz	P14, P16, N18, N20, P22

° C'c is either C3'c, or C4'c, and is contralateral (c) to the side of stimulation. C3' or C4' is 2 cm behind the standard placement of C3 or C4 of the International 10-20 System. EPc is Erb's point. EPi is ipsilateral to stimulation. EPc is contralateral to stimulation. Ai and Ac are ears ipsilateral and contralateral to stimulation. Notations of spC2, spC5, and spC7 refer to cervical spine at the C2, C5, and C7 levels, respectively. NC is noncephalic reference. It may be the dorsum of the contralateral hand, EPc, or contralateral shoulder, Shc.

MN-SSEP, median nerve somatosensory evoked potential.

- Channel 4: Ci'—Fpz
- Channel 3: Cz'—Fpz
- Channel 2: Fpz'—spC5
- Channel 1: spT12—noncephalic reference

We have found it useful to record whenever possible in the waking state since cortical components are affected by sleep. However, many times this is not possible and it may, in fact, be necessary to sedate the child (see "Effects of Sleep").

The EP can be recorded 1 cm above the axilla rather than at Erb's point.[41] In infants, and especially in newborns, this allows more reliable recording of the potential. Methods for PTN-SSEPs have been less frequently reported in children than have MN-SSEPs but are similar to those for adults.[8] One may use height and, as necessary, age-corrected normative data for latencies of peaks, or one may calculate conduction ("propagation") velocities over

the peripheral nerves and central fibers.[42] The American EEG Society guidelines have recommended the use of velocity calculations.[40] However, there are legitimate objections to this method since there is a potential for error in the measurement of distance as a requisite for the calculation.[43-45] We have preferred using height-based normative data.[7,8,46]

EFFECTS OF MATURATION

Postnatal development of the somatosensory system is complex because of coincident nonparallel changes in parameters of maturation such as (1) the length of the pathway; (2) varying rates of myelination of portions of the pathway; and (3) increasing numbers of synapses in the pathway. These developmental sequences are relatively simple compared with the maturation of brain, which includes the process of synaptogenesis as well as lengthening and myelination of the complex polysynaptic pathways of the thalamocortical system.

Maturation of the Peripheral Nerve

In the developing human infant, the peripheral nerve diameter increases in close association with increasing myelination.[47] There is a close correlation between fiber size and functional properties in developing peripheral nerve. The length of the nerve increases as well, probably parallel to increasing leg length.[48] In newborns, the conduction velocity of peripheral nerve increases linearly with postconceptional age (PCA) from approximately 20 m/sec at 33 weeks PCA to 33 m/sec at 44 weeks PCA.[49-51] The conduction velocity of peripheral nerve has been shown to increase with age, reaching maximal values at 18 to 27 postnatal months for sural nerve.[52] Up until this time the N5 of the PTN-SSEP changes little in latency. This reflects synchronous increases in peripheral nerve conduction velocity (CV) and leg length (distance [D]). The expression of

$$Latency = D/CV$$

would predict latency to be constant if both D and CV change equally. After this time, the latencies of the peripheral components, the EP potential of MN-SSEP and the N5 of PTN-SSEP, parallel increasing height and/or limb length (Fig. 8-6).

Maturation of the Spinal Cord

Myelinogenesis of the spinal cord begins early during prenatal life (Fig. 8-7). Sensory roots start to undergo myelina-

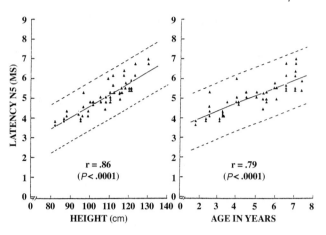

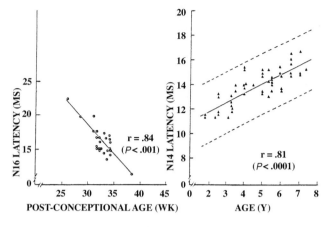

FIGURE 8–6

Left, *Relationship between stature and absolute latency of N5 in children with height ranging from 82 to 130 cm: x = –1.021 + 0.056 (height).* Right, *Relationship between age and absolute latency of N5 in children aged 1 to 8 years: x = 3.23 + 0.38 (age). Based on these functions and those seen in Figures 8-3 and 8-4, absolute latency of N5, N14, and N20 may be provided with reasonable accuracy. In this and other figures, solid line, line of regression; dotted lines ± 3 SD. (Left and Right, From Gilmore RL, Bass NH, Wright EA, et al: Development assessment of spinal cord and cortical evoked potentials after tibial nerve stimulation: Effects of age and stature on normative data during childhood. Electroencephalogr Clin Neurophysiol 1985;62:241-251.)*

FIGURE 8–8

Left, *Relationship between postconceptional age (PCA) and absolute latency of N16 in preterm newborns with PCA ranging from 26 to 38.2 weeks.* Right, *Relationship between age and absolute latency of N14 in children aged 1 to 8 years: x = 10.26 + 0.74 (age). (Left and Right, From Gilmore RL, Bass NH, Wright EA, et al: Development assessment of spinal cord and cortical evoked potentials after tibial nerve stimulation: Effects of age and stature on normative data during childhood. Electroencephalogr Clin Neurophysiol 1985;62:241-251.)*

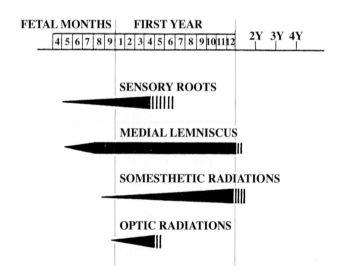

FIGURE 8–7

Myelogenetic cycles of selected somatosensory pathways. Optic radiations data provided for comparison. Point at left indicates when myelin starts to appear and point at right indicates when myelination is believed complete. (From Yakovlev P, Lecours A: The myelogenetic cycles of regional maturation of the brain. In Minkowski A [ed]: Regional Development of the Brain in Early Life. Philadelphia, FA Davis, 1967, p 3.)

tion at 24 weeks PCA and are fully myelinated by 6 months post-term.[53] The fasciculus cuneatus and fasciculus gracilis first appear at 8 weeks PCA.[54] Myelin first appears in the fasciculus cuneatus at 14 weeks PCA and in the fasciculus gracilis at 22 to 24 weeks PCA in the human. In contrast, in the developing kitten the fasciculus gracilis has an increasing fiber diameter that approaches that of the adult cat by 3 postnatal months. There is a parallel increase in central conduction velocity.[55] Presumably, in humans the increased conduction velocity of spinal cord exceeds elongation of the spinal cord in early infancy[7] since latency of the lumbar potential (N16 in newborn) and cervical potential (N27) decreases with increasing PCA in the newborn (Fig. 8-8).

Different portions of the spinal cord may have different conduction velocities. Cracco and colleagues[42] partitioned the spinal cord into several segments and calculated conduction velocities over these segments using surface distance measurements. They found that conduction velocity over rostral segments was faster than over caudal segments and that conduction velocity along the spinal cord progressively increased with age (Fig. 8-9).[42] It is likely that in children the increase in conduction velocity parallels the increase in spinal cord length.[48] The N14 latency of the PTN-SSEP increases with increasing age after 1 year of age (see Fig. 8-8). The N11 latency of the MN-SSEP remains stable over time until 2 to 3 years of age (Fig. 8-10).[42]

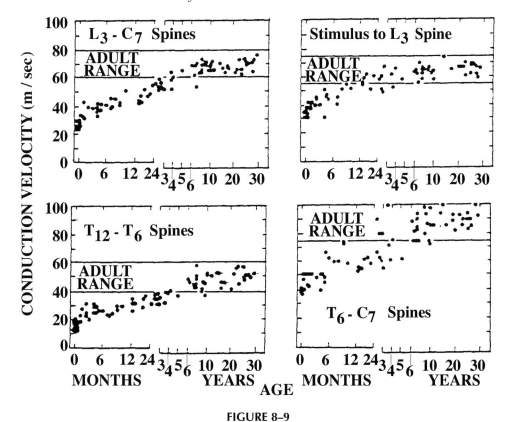

FIGURE 8–9

Relationship between age and overall conduction velocity (L3-C7 spines) and segmental conduction velocities over peroneal nerve and cauda equina (stimulus to L3 spine), caudal spinal cord (T2-T6 spines), and rostral spinal cord (T6-C7 spines). Note the change in age scale (from months to years) on the abscissa. Infants from –1 to 0 months were premature. All conduction velocities progressively increase with age. The overall velocities are in the adult range by 5 years of age. Velocities over peroneal nerve and cauda equina increase rapidly during the first year of life, and most values are in the adult range by 3 years. However, velocities over both caudal and rostral spinal cord are not in the adult range until 5 to 6 years of age. (From Cracco JB, Cracco RQ: Stolove R: Spinal evoked potentials in man: A maturational study. Electroencephalogr Clin Neurophysiol 1979;46:58-64.

Maturation of the Brainstem and Cerebral Hemispheres

The medial lemniscus starts to myelinate at approximately 23 to 25 weeks PCA, proceeds in a caudal-rostral order, and probably concludes myelination approximately 12 months post-term.[53] The functional development of transmission capacities and neuronal responsiveness requires, at the level of the nucleus cuneatus, a period of 2 to 3 months postnatally within the central pathways of the kitten,[56] approximately equivalent to 24 human months post-term. At higher levels than the nucleus cuneatus, in the kitten, the acquisition of mature transmission capacities probably occurs even later.[44]

Because the thalamus is a critical element in cerebral transmission of peripheral signals, one might anticipate that the development of cortical EPs would be closely related to thalamic maturation and myelination. Prior to 32 weeks

PCA, the thalamus has no myelin. By 34 weeks PCA, myelin in the thalamus occurs in less than 20% of the infants; by 36 weeks PCA, some myelin in the thalamus is seen in approximately 70% of brains. By term, 87% of brains contain thalamic myelin.[56] However, there is considerable variability in the sequencing of myelination not only in the thalamus but in other sites.[57] The thalamocortical fibers begin to myelinate at approximately 40 weeks PCA and are thought to be completely myelinated by approximately 12 to 18 months post-term.[53] The wide ranges of time over which the thalamus and subcortical radiations are myelinated undoubtedly play a role in the variable latencies of scalp recorded potentials in preterm newborns.

Because of these maturational changes in infancy affecting generators and pathways of SSEPS, not all components are recorded at term. The time at which various components can be reliably recorded is important. Waveforms may be absent because of a pathologic process or because

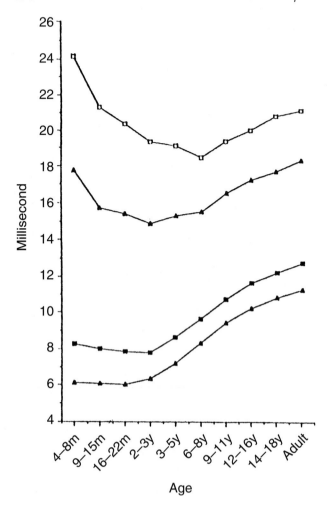

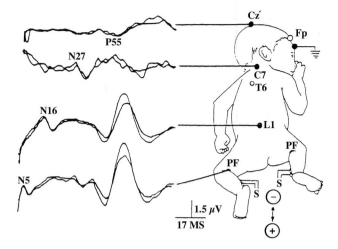

FIGURE 8–11

Somatosensory evoked potential after bilateral simultaneous tibial nerve stimulation at the ankles recorded at various sites simultaneously from a 35-week-old (postconceptional age) infant. Label was based on surface polarity and mean peak latency observed in 29 preterm newborns (gestational age, 26 to 38 weeks; length, 22.5 to 44 cm). Electrodes were placed at the popliteal fossa (PF), first lumbar (L1), sixth thoracic (T6), and seventh cervical (C7) spinous processes (sp) of vertebrae. Cz' (1 cm behind Cz) and Fpz (10-20 System). Cz' and spC7 were referred to Fpz. The reference for SpL1 and PF was spT6. Constant current pulses of 130- to 150-second duration were delivered at 5/sec. Two independent averages of 1000 to 2000 responses were superimposed to show intertrial replicability.

FIGURE 8–10

Developmental changes in latencies of the peripheral (N12 and N13) and cortical (N20, P22) components of median nerve somatosensory evoked potentials demonstrating the different maturational patterns from different aspects of the sensory system. Despite increases in physical size, N12 latency is stable until after 16 to 22 months, N13 decreases slightly in latency until 2 to 3 years of age, N20 decreases more markedly until 2 to 3 years of age, and P22 decreases until 6 to 8 years of age, after which age, all the latencies increase toward adult values, respectively. Open squares, P22; closed triangles, N20; solid squares, N13; solid triangles, N12. (From Fagan ER, Taylor M, Logan WJ: Somatosensory evoked potentials: I. A review of neural generators and special considerations in pediatrics. Pediatr Neurol 1987;3:189-196.)

the necessary central nervous system structures necessary for production of the waveforms have not matured to the point of generating or transmitting the potential.

The cortical EP has been recorded by various authors from 6 to 12 weeks post-term.[36,37,41] Gilmore and coworkers[7] have reported that while the scalp-recorded potential of the

PTN-SSEP was not seen in infants whose PCA was less than 31 weeks, it was not invariably present in infants more than 31 weeks. Approximately 50% have the scalp-recorded component close to term (Fig. 8-11).

Variability of the presence, distribution, and latency of cortical PTN-SSEP components has been found in older infants as well. Georgesco and associates[6] reported PTN-SSEPs in 26 fullterm infants aged 1 day to 3 months. In six infants, no scalp-recorded PTN-SSEP was observed. In the other 20 infants, an electropositive scalp-recorded PTN-SSEP was seen approximately 36 milliseconds (probably P28) after stimulation. Weight, physiologic state of arousal, and intensity of stimulation were not correlated with distribution or latency of the component. Surprisingly, even age failed to correlate with latency or anatomic distribution. In fact, the oldest infant, approximately 3 months post-term, did not have a P28.[6] The appearance or absence of cortical EP as well as the wide range of cortical EP latency may parallel the wide time range over which myelin appears at specific sites within the immature spinal cord and brain.

Age and Height Effects on Latencies of Brain-Generated EP and Central Conduction Time

The short-latency scalp-recorded MN-SSEP of preterm newborns may change morphology and latency with increasing PCA (Fig. 8-12). After 4 years of age, the latencies of the various components change predictably with age. There are several reasons for this. As reviewed earlier, the presence of functional changes that accompany maturation of the nervous system alters the latencies. Other factors are changes in the length of the pathways over which SSEPs are transmitted. This is most important with PTN-SSEPs, but it is also true for MN-SSEPS. In general, the latency of the N20 component of the MN-SSEP decreases from early infancy to 2 to 3 years and then starts to increase (see Fig. 8-10).[42] The increase in latency is correlated with body length and arm lengths.[58] The latencies of N13 are similar in newborns and older infants,[41] probably remaining stable until 2 to

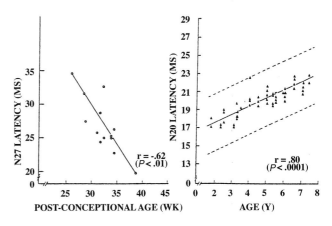

FIGURE 8–13

Left, *Relationship between stature and absolute latency of N27 in children with height ranging from 82 to 130 cm: x = 4.60 + 0.14 (height).* Right, *Relationship between age and absolute latency of N20 in children aged 1 to 8 years: x = 15.51 + 0.95 (age). (From Gilmore RL, Bass NH, Wright EA, Greathouse D, Stanback K, Norvell E: Development assessment of spinal cord and cortical evoked potentials after tibial nerve stimulation: Effects of age and stature on normative data during childhood. Electroencephalogr Clin Neurophysiol 1985;62:241-251.)*

3 years of age, when their latencies start to prolong,[59] reaching adult values by approximately ages 14 to 18 years.[42]

The central conduction time (CCT) for MN-SSEP has been defined as the latency of the N20 minus the latency of the B wave (CCT = N20 – B).[37] The B wave is the N13. After log transformation of CCT, there is a high inverse correlation (r = –.85) between age and CCT; that is, as the infant grows, CCT decreases.

The latency of the N20 (Fig. 8-13) component of the PTN-SSEP increases with increasing age or height in children 1 to 8 years old.[8] The N27 potential of the PTN-SSEP in the preterm newborn is equivalent to the N20 in the older child and decreases with increasing PCA. The latency of the scalp-recorded potential P28 is much more variable in children than adults and correlates only modestly with height (Fig. 8-14).

Table 8-4 demonstrates the use of height-based (measured in centimeters) regression equations in predicting the latency of certain components of both MN-SSEP and PTN-SSEP in children 1 to 8 years old who are awake.[46]

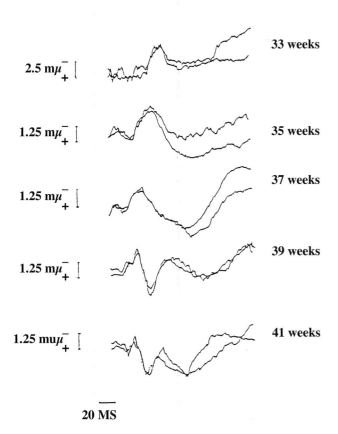

20 MS

FIGURE 8–12

Examples of cortical components of median nerve somatosensory evoked potentials at different postconceptional ages. (From Gallai V: Maturation of SEPs in pre-term and full-term neonates. In Gallai V [ed]: Maturation of the CNS and Evoked Potentials. Amsterdam, Elsevier, 1987, p 95.)

EFFECTS OF SLEEP

The effect of sleep on the short-latency MN-SSEPs has been well studied.[5,60-62] Differences in latency between quiet sleep and active sleep have been reported, whereas no differences between active sleep and wakefulness have been seen.

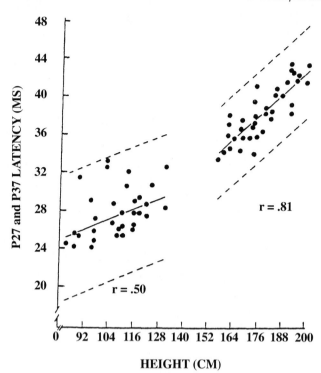

FIGURE 8–14

Effect on height on the cortical evoked potential (P27 in children and P37 in adults). Left, During growth and development (1 to 8 years old). Right, During adulthood (18 to 40 years old). (From Gilmore RL, Bass NH, Wright EA, Greathouse D, Stanback K, Norvell E: Development assessment of spinal cord and cortical evoked potentials after tibial nerve stimulation: Effects of age and stature on normative data during childhood. Electroencephalogr Clin Neurophysiol 1985; 62:241-251.

TABLE 8–4

Regression Equations to Predict Expected Latencies for SSEP

Component	Equation	r	P	Mean Latency ± SD
Median Nerve				
P10	0.41 + 0.059 (ht)	.67	<0.05	6.88 ± 0.74
P13	4.70 + 0.042 (ht)	.76	<0.01	9.28 ± 0.45
N19	13.24 + 0.025 (ht)	.45	<0.01	16.03 ± 0.46
P13-P10	0.32 + 0.018 (ht)	.50	<0.05	2.55 ± 0.77
N19-P13	8.50 + 0.016 (ht)	.56	<0.01	6.57 ± 0.61
Tibial Nerve				
N8	–1.17+0.057 (ht)	.86	<0.001	4.95 ± 0.69
N22	–1.92+0.110 (ht)	.90	<0.001	13.70 ± 1.33
P37	13.71+0.087 (ht)	.50	<0.01	27.74 ± 3.17
N22-N8	2.70+0.059 (ht)	.88	<0.001	
P37-N22	Independent of height			

SSEP, somatosensory evoked potential; ht, height.

The effects of sedating drugs have also been studied.[58,62] One systematic report of sedative effects in children examined MN-SSEPs in 83 children and 7 adults.[58] Components comparable to the adult N20 remained stable during sleep, whereas P22 demonstrated an increase in peak latency during deep sleep but not during REM sleep. It has also been reported that pentobarbital prolongs scalp latencies and attenuates scalp potentials.[59]

Near-field EPs with PTN-SSEPs are not altered with spleen.[63] However, the effect of sleep on the scalp recorded P55 of infants and P28 of children of the PTN-SSEP is even more marked and complicated. In some preterm infants natural sleep actually enhances the appearance of the P55. In older infants and children the effect of sleep is to attenuate the voltage of a component and/or prolong its latency. These effects are most marked in children younger than 48 months of age (Figs. 8-15 and 8-16).

We prefer not to sedate infants younger than 3 months of age. We sedate older infants and children as necessary, recognizing that this attenuates and frequently delays the scalp-recorded components of the MN-SSEP and of the PTN-SSEP. We have used oral chloral hydrate, recognizing, as have others, that barbiturates have an even more marked effect on cortical potentials than chloral hydrate.[64] If the study is abnormal, we will attempt to repeat the study in the waking state. This can be a problem in a busy laboratory, but it must be done to avoid the possibility of false-positive results.

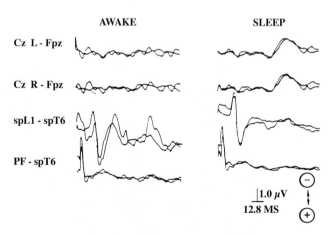

FIGURE 8–15

Posterior tibial nerve somatosensory evoked potential in the awake (left) and sleep (right) states. Note the appearance of the scalp recorded component during sleep. (Left and Right, From Gilmore RL, Brock J, Hermansen MC, Baumann R. Development of lumbar spinal cord and cortical evoked potentials after tibial nerve stimulation in the pre-term newborns: Effects of gestational age and other factors. Electroencephalogr Clin Neurophysiol 1987;68:28-39.)

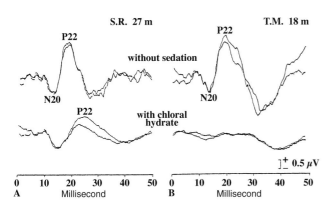

FIGURE 8–16

Median nerve somatosensory evoked potential in two children with and without sedation revealing latency prolongation and diminution in amplitude in one patient (S.R.) and loss of recognizable cortical components in the other patient (T.M.). (From Fagan ER, Taylor M, Logan WJ: Somatosensory evoked potentials: I. A review of neural generators and special considerations in pediatrics. Pediatr Neurol 1987;3:189-196.)

Compared with those in adults, SSEPs in the pediatric population present technical and interpretive challenges that may be met with an understanding of the factors that affect normative data in infants and children.

REFERENCES

1. Allison T, Hume AL, Wood CC, Goff WR: Developmental and aging changes in somatosensory, auditory, and visual evoked potentials. Electroencephalogr Clin Neurophysiol 1984;58:14-24.
2. Chiappa KH, Choi SK, Yount RP: Short-latency somatosensory evoked potentials following median nerve stimulation in patients with neurological lesions. *In* Desmedt JE (ed): Clinical Uses of Cerebral, Brainstem, and Spinal Somatosensory Evoked Potentials, Vol 7. Basel, Karger, 1980.
3. Cullity P, Franks CI, Duckworth T, et al: Somatosensory evoked cortical responses in normal infants. Dev Med Child Neurol 1976;18:11-18.
4. Desmedt JE, Brunko E, Debecker J: Maturation of the somatosensory evoked potentials in normal infants and children with special reference to the early N1 component. Electroencephalogr Clin Neurophysiol 1976;40:43-58.
5. Hrbek A, Karlberg P, Olsson T: Development of visual and somatosensory evoked responses in pre-term newborn infants. Electroencephalogr Clin Neurophysiol 1973;34:225-232.
6. Georgesco M, Radiere M, Seror P, et al: Les potentiels cerebraux somesthesiques evoques a partir du membre inferieur chez le nouveau-ne le nourrisson. Rev Electroencephalogr Neurophysiol Clin 1982;12:123-128.
7. Gilmore RL, Brock J, Hermansen MC, Baumann R: Development of lumbar spinal cord and cortical evoked potentials after tibial nerve stimulation in the pre-term newborns: Effects of gestational age and other factors. Electroencephalogr Clin Neurophysiol 1987;68:28-39.
8. Gilmore RL, Bass NH, Wright EA, et al: Development assessment of spinal cord and cortical evoked potentials after tibial nerve stimulation: Effects of age and stature on normative data during childhood. Electroencephalogr Clin Neurophysiol 1985;62:241-251.
9. Anziska B, Cracco RQ: Short-latency SEPs to median nerve stimulation: Comparison of recording methods and origin of components. Electroencephalogr Clin Neurophysiol 1981;52:531-539.
10. Yamada T, Kimura J, Nitz DM: Short-latency somatosensory evoked potentials following median nerve stimulation. Electroencephalogr Clin Neurophysiol 1980;48:367-376.
11. Leuders H, Kesser RP, Hahn J, et al: Subcortical somatosensory evoked potentials to median nerve stimulation. Brain 1983;106:341-372.
12. Yamada T, Kimura J, Wilkinson JT, Kayamori R: Short- and long-latency median somatosensory evoked potentials: Findings in patients with localized neurological lesions. Arch Neurol 1983;40:215-220.
13. Cracco JB, Cracco RQ: Spinal, brainstem, and cerebral SEP in the pediatric age group. *In* Bodis-Wollner I (ed): Evoked Potentials. New York, Alan R. Liss, 1986, p 471.
14. Desmedt JE, Cheron G: Prevertebral (oesophageal) recording of subcortical somatosensory evoked potentials in man: The spinal P13 component and the dual nature of the spinal generators. Electroencephalogr Clin Neurophysiol 1981;52:257-275.
15. Emerson RG, Pedley TA: Generator sources of median somatosensory evoked potentials. J Clin Neurophysiol 1984;1:203-218.
16. Kimura J, Yamada T, Kawamura H: Central latencies of somatosensory cerebral evoked potentials. Arch Neurol 1978;35:683-688.
17. Chiappa K: Short-latency interpretation somatosensory evoked potentials: Methodology. *In* Chiappa K (ed): Evoked Potentials in Clinical Medicine. New York, Raven Press, 1990, p 307.
18. Lesser RP, Lueders H, Hahn J, Klem G: Early somatosensory potentials evoked by median nerve stimulation: Intraoperative monitoring. Neurology 1981;31:1519-1523.
19. Tsuji S, Shibasaki H, Kato M, et al: Subcortical, thalamic, and cortical somatosensory evoked potentials to median nerve stimulation. Electroencephalogr Clin Neurophysiol 1984;59:465-476.
20. Yamada T, Kameyama S, Fuchigami Y, et al: Changes of short-latency somatosensory evoked potential in sleep. Electroencephalogr Clin Neurophysiol 1988;70:126-136.
21. Goldie WD, Chiappa KH, Young RR, Brooks EB: Brainstem auditory and short-latency somatosensory evoked responses in brain death. Neurology 1981;31:248-256.

22. Desmedt JE, Cheron G: Central somatosensory conduction in man: Neural generators and interpeak latencies of the far-field components recorded from neck and right or left scalp and earlobes. Electroencephalogr Clin Neurophysiol 1980;50:382-403.

23. Allison T: Scalp and cortical recordings of initial somatosensory cortex activity to median nerve stimulation in man. Ann N Y Acad Sci 1982;288:671-678.

24. Hume AL, Cant BR: Conduction time in central somatosensory pathway in man. Electroencephalogr Clin Neurophysiol 1978;45:361-375.

25. Yamada T, Kayamori R, Kamura J, Beck DO: Topography of somatosensory evoked potentials after stimulation of the median nerve. Electroencephalogr Clin Neurophysiol 1984;59:29-43.

26. Yamada T: Anatomic and physiologic basis of median somatosensory evoked potentials. Neurol Clin 1988;6:705.

27. Allison T, Goff WR, Williamson PD, et al: On the neural origin of early components of the human somatosensory evoked potentials. *In* Desmedt JE (ed): Clinical Uses of Cerebral, Brainstem, and Spinal Somatosensory Evoked Potentials, Vol 7. Basel, Karger, 1980, p 51.

28. Desmedt JE, Cheron G: Non-cephalic reference of early somatosensory potentials to finger stimulation in adult or aging normal man: Differentiation of widespread N18 and contralateral N20 from the prerolandic P22 and N30 components. Electroencephalogr Clin Neurophysiol 1981;52:553-570.

29. Mauguiere F, Desmedt JE, Courjon J: Neural generators of N18 and P14 far-field somatosensory evoked potentials studied in patients with lesion of thalamic or thalamocortical radiations. Electroencephalogr Clin Neurophysiol 1983;49:493-499.

30. Dinner DS, Lüders H, Lesser RP, Morris HH: Cortical generators of somatosensory evoked potentials to median nerve stimulation. Neurology 1987;37:1141-1145.

31. Seyal M, Gabor AJ: The human posterior tibial somatosensory evoked potential: Synapse-dependent and synapse-independent spinal components. Electroencephalogr Clin Neurophysiol 1985;62:323-331.

32. Cruse R, Klem G, Lesser RP, Lueders H: Paradoxical lateralization of cortical potentials evoked by stimulation of posterior tibial nerve. Arch Neurol 1982;39:222-225.

33. Seyal M, Emerson RG, Pedley TA: Spinal and early scalp-recorded components of the somatosensory evoked potential following stimulation of the posterior tibial nerve. Electroencephalogr Clin Neurophysiol 1983;55:320-330.

34. Emerson RG: The anatomic and physiologic basis of posterior tibial nerve somatosensory evoked potentials. Neurol Clin 1988;6:705-733.

35. Penfield W, Rasmussen T: The Cerebral Cortex of Man: A Clinical Study of Localization of Function. New York, MacMillan, 1950.

36. Willis J, Seales D, Farazier E: Short-latency somatosensory evoked potentials in infants. Electroencephalogr Clin Neurophysiol 1984;59:366-373.

37. Goldie WD, Spydell JD: Somatosensory evoked potentials following median nerve stimulation in infants: Normative and clinical studies. *In* The American EEG Society Workshop: EPs in Children, 1987.

38. Fagan ER, Taylor M, Logan WJ: Somatosensory evoked potentials: II. A review of the clinical applications in pediatric neurology. Pediatr Neurol 1987;3:249-255.

39. Taylor MJ, Fagan ER: SEPs to median nerve stimulation: Normative data for paediatrics. Electroencephalogr Clin Neurophysiol 1988;71:323-330.

40. American Electroencephalographic Society: Guidelines for clinical evoked potential studies. J Clin Neurophysiol 1984;1:3-53.

41. Cracco JB, Cracco RQ, Stolove R: Spinal evoked potentials in man: a maturational study. Electroencephalogr Clin Neurophysiol 1979;46:58-64.

42. Cracco JB, Cracco RQ, Stolove R: Spinal evoked potentials in man: A maturational study. Electroencephalogr Clin Neurophysiol 1979;46:58-64.

43. Lastimosa ACB, Bass NH, Stanback K, Norvell EE: Lumbar spinal cord and early evoked potentials after tibial nerve stimulation: Effects of stature on normative data. Electroencephalogr Clin Neurophysiol 1982;54:499-507.

44. Simpson JA: Fact and fallacy in measurement of conduction velocity in motor nerves. J Neurol Neurosurg Psychiatry 1964;27:381-385.

45. Young RR, Shahani BT: Clinical value and limitations of F-wave determination. Muscle Nerve 1978;1:248-250.

46. Gilmore RL, Nelson KR: SSEP and F-wave studies in acute inflammatory demyelinating polyradiculoneuropathy. Muscle Nerve 1989;12:538-543.

47. Ouvrier RA, McLeod JG, Conchin T: Morphometric studies of sural nerve in childhood. Muscle Nerve 1987;10:47-53.

48. Merlob P, Sivan Y, Reisner SH: Lower limb standards in newborns. Am J Dis Child 1984;138:140-142.

49. Dubowitz V, Whittaker GF, Brown BH, et al: Nerve conduction velocity: An index of neurological maturity of the newborn infant. Dev Med Child Neurol 1968;10:741-749.

50. Schulte FJ, Michaelis R, Linke I, et al: Motor nerve conduction velocity for term, preterm, and small-for-dates newborn infants. Pediatrics 1968;42:17-26.

51. Wagner AL, Buchthal F: Motor and sensory conduction in infancy and childhood: Reappraisal. Dev Med Child Neurol 1972;14:189-216.

52. Buchthal F, Rosenfalck A, Behse F: Sensory potentials of normal and diseased nerves. *In* Dyck PJ, Thomas PK, Lambert EH (eds): Peripheral Neuropathy. Philadelphia, WB Saunders, 1975, p 442.

53. Yakovlev P, Lecours A: The myelogenetic cycles of regional maturation of the brain. *In* Minkowski A (ed): Regional Development of the Brain in Early Life. Philadelphia, FA Davis, 1967, p 3.

54. Hughes AF: The development of the dorsal funiculus in the human spinal cord. J Anat 1976;122:169-175.

55. Hildebrand C, Skoglund S: Caliber spectra of some fiber tracts in the feline central nervous system during postnatal development. Acta Physiol Scand 1971;364:5-41.

56. Rorke LB, Riggs HE: Myelination of the Brain in the Newborn. Philadelphia, Lippincott, 1969.

57. Gilles FH, Shankle EC, Dooling EC: Myelinated tracts: Growth patterns. *In* Gilles FH, Leviton A, Dooling EC (eds): The Developing Human Brain. Boston, John Wright, 1983, p 117.

58. Hashimoto T, Tayama M, Hiura K, et al: Short-latency somatosensory evoked potentials in children. Brain Dev 1983;4:390-396.

59. Fagan ER, Taylor M, Logan WJ: Somatosensory evoked potentials: I. A review of neural generators and special considerations in pediatrics. Pediatr Neurol 1987;3:189-196.

60. Desmedt JE, Manil J: Somatosensory evoked potentials of the normal human neonate in REM sleep, in slow wave sleep, and in waking. Electroencephalogr Clin Neurophysiol 1970;29:113-126.

61. Hrbek A, Hrbkova M, Lenard H-G: Somatosensory, auditory, and visual evoked responses in newborn infants during sleep and wakefulness. Electroencephalogr Clin Neurophysiol 1969;26:597-603.

62. Boor R, Goebel B, Taylor MJ: Subcortical somatosensory evoked potentials after median nerve stimulation in children. Eur J Paediatr Neurol 1998b;2:137-143.

63. Boor R, Goebel B, Doepp M, Taylor MJ: Somatosensory evoked potentials after posterior tibial nerve stimulation-normative data in children. Eur J Paediatr Neurol 1998a;2:145-152.

64. Roy MW, Gilmore R, Walsh JW: Somatosensory evoked potentials in tethered cord syndrome. Electroencephalogr Clin Neurophysiol 1986;64:42P.

9

Brainstem Auditory Evoked Potentials in Pediatrics—Normal

SANDRA L. HELMERS

The short-latency brainstem auditory evoked potential (BAEP), also commonly known as the *auditory brainstem response* (ABR) or *brainstem auditory evoked response* (BAER), is the auditory system's electrical response to an acoustic stimulus. By definition, the short-latency auditory evoked potential occurs within the first 10 to 15 milliseconds following an acoustic stimulation. The response is generated by the auditory nerve, brainstem, and possibly subcortical structures and can be obtained at almost any age. These features make the BAEP a quite useful test in the evaluation of the peripheral and central brainstem auditory systems at any age. In addition to the evaluation of the peripheral auditory system in assessment of hearing and language development, the central brainstem can be assessed in lesions such as tumors and neurodegenerative diseases. The use of BAERs has also become practical in the operating room to monitor brainstem neurophysiologic function during certain surgical procedures involving the region of the posterior fossa.

ANATOMY OF THE AUDITORY SYSTEM

The vestibulocochlear system performs two functions: the first is audition, and the second is vestibular sense (balance). The external ear consists of the auricle and external auditory meatus or canal. It ends at the tympanic membrane. The canal is angled medially and in an anteroinferior direction. The outer third of the canal is composed of cartilage; the medial two thirds is actually a bony canal in the temporal bone. The external meatus is lined with skin, hair, and sweat glands that produce cerumen. The tympanic membrane or ear drum separates the external auditory canal from the middle ear (Fig. 9-1). The middle ear is lined with a mucous membrane that is continuous with the eustachian tube and mastoid air cells. There are three ear bones (ossicles) arranged in a manner so as to transmit sound vibrations from the tympanic membrane to the inner ear. These bones are the malleus, incus, and stapes (Fig. 9-2).

The inner ear lies in the temporal bone and consists of the cochlea (audition) and the semicircular canals (vestibula). The cochlea can be divided into two parts: the bony spiral or helix and the attached membranes (basilar and vestibular) that subdivide the spiral canals. If the cochlea were cut in half transversely, one would see that the canal is subdivided into three sections by two membranes: the vestibular membrane and the basilar membrane (Fig. 9-3A). The three sections are labeled *scala vestibuli, cochlear duct,* and *scala tympani.* Each scala is filled with a fluid called *perilymph,* whereas the cochlear duct is filled with the fluid endolymph (Fig. 9-3B).

The basilar membrane helps form the cochlear duct, actually forming the "floor" of the duct. On the basilar membrane lies the spiral organ or organ of Corti, which runs the entire length of the cochlea. The spiral organ is composed of a row of inner hair cells and a row of outer hair cells, both of which are direct extensions of cranial nerve VIII. In addition to the hair cells, there is a membrane that

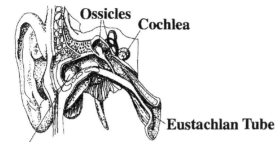

FIGURE 9–1
Anatomy of the external, middle, and internal ear.

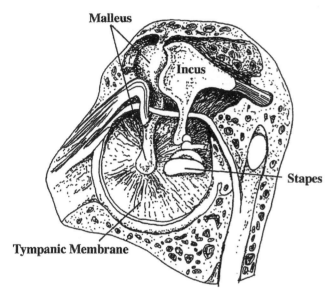

FIGURE 9–2
Anatomy of the middle ear.

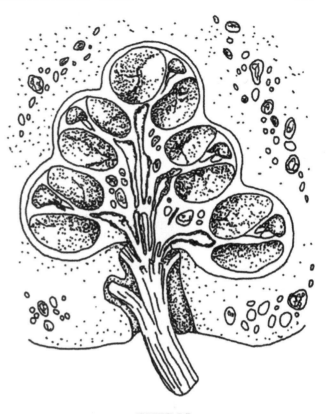

VIII Nerve

A

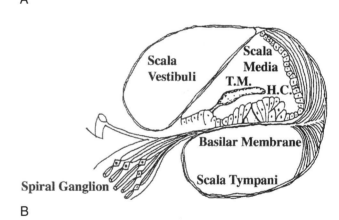

B

FIGURE 9–3
A, *Transverse view of the cochlea.* B, *Transverse view of the cochlear duct. Tectorial membrane (T.M.) and hair cells (H.C.) are demonstrated.*

projects over the hair cells called the *tectorial membrane.* The cochlea is shaped as a spiral and plays a role in sound separation, with the base of the cochlea being involved with higher frequencies and the tip of the cochlea being involved with the lower frequencies. This is due to the basilar membrane being longer near the top and shorter near the base.

From the hair cells, the sound impulse is transmitted to the spiral ganglion, which is the origin of the cochlear nerve. The cochlear nerve enters the dorsolateral brainstem at the level of the inferior cerebellar peduncle in the medulla. The cochlear nerve terminates and synapses in the ventral and dorsal cochlear nuclei. After forming a synapse in the nuclei, the secondary auditory pathways cross to the contralateral brainstem, through the trapezoid body or reticular formation. Once the secondary fibers have crossed, they

form synapses in the superior olivary nucleus, which then projects tertiary fibers into the lateral lemniscus (Fig. 9-4).

The lateral lemniscus ascends along the dorsolateral brainstem to the level of the midbrain. In the midbrain most of the fibers terminate in the inferior colliculus. Following a synapse in the colliculus, some fibers may cross back over in

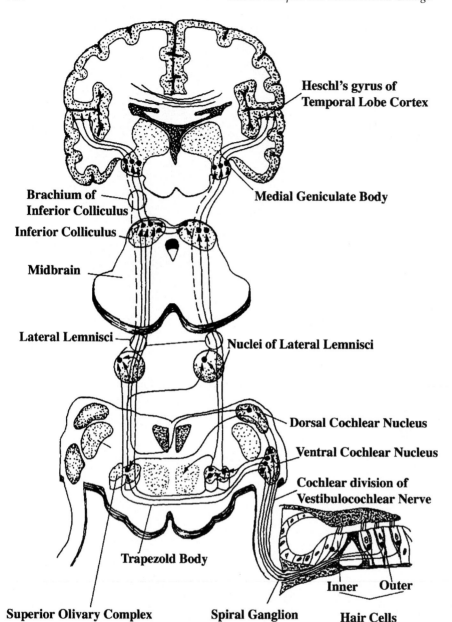

Heschl's gyrus of Temporal Lobe Cortex

Brachium of Inferior Colliculus

Medial Geniculate Body

Inferior Colliculus

Midbrain

Lateral Lemnisci

Nuclei of Lateral Lemnisci

Dorsal Cochlear Nucleus

Ventral Cochlear Nucleus

Cochlear division of Vestibulocochlear Nerve

Trapezold Body

Inner   Outer

Superior Olivary Complex   **Spiral Ganglion**   **Hair Cells**

FIGURE 9–4
Anatomy of the brainstem auditory pathways.

the commissure of the inferior colliculus. The fibers then project to the medial geniculate body of the thalamus, where they synapse once again. The next step is the projection of fibers to the superior gyrus (Heschl's gyrus) of the temporal lobe via the auditory radiations. The last pathway involves projections to the association cortex of the temporoparietal region (Fig. 9-5).

WAVEFORM GENERATORS

Short-latency BAEPs are subcortical, far-field electrical potentials occurring within the first 10 to 15 milliseconds following a stimulus. There are five waveforms of interest, recorded most commonly from the scalp.

Wave I

The first waveform, wave I, is recorded from the ear being stimulated and has a negative polarity (Fig. 9-6). From intraoperative recordings and animal and human clinicopathologic studies, it has been shown that wave I is generated from action potential volleys in cranial nerve VIII near the cochlea.[1-3] It is necessary to obtain wave I to be able to calculate the central auditory brainstem conduction time.

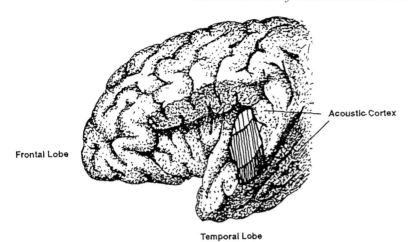

Frontal Lobe

Acoustic Cortex

Temporal Lobe

FIGURE 9–5

Anatomy of the auditory cortex.

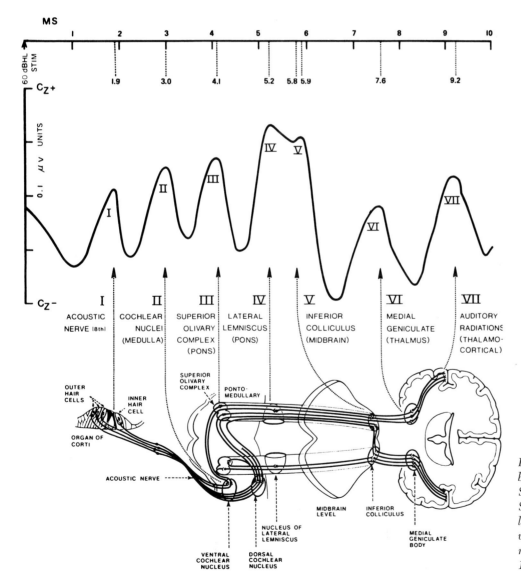

FIGURE 9–6

Far-field recording of auditory brainstem responses. (From Stockard JJ, Stockard JE, Sharbrough FW: Detection and localization of occult lesions with brainstem auditory responses. Mayo Clin Proc 1977;52:761-769.)

Wave II

Wave II is generated from either the intracranial portion of cranial nerve VIII as it enters the lateral medulla, or the cochlear nucleus. Moller and associates[1] recorded simultaneously from the earlobe and directly from the intracranial portion of the eighth cranial nerve in patients undergoing a microvascular decompression. They demonstrated that the latencies of the waveforms from the earlobe recording and the responses recorded from the eighth cranial nerve were almost identical, concluding that wave II is a manifestation of the proximal, intracranial portion of the eighth cranial nerve.

Garg and colleagues[4] studied patients with hereditary motor-sensory neuropathy type I. They demonstrated an abnormally wide separation of the I-II interpeak latency (IPL) with a normal III-V IPL. Since hereditary motor-sensory neuropathy type I affects only the peripheral nerve, this finding demonstrates that the intracranial, extramedullary portion of the eighth nerve generates wave II. Stockard and Rossiter[3] studied patients with infarcts of the pontomedullary junction with destruction of the caudal pons and cochlear nuclei. They were able to record only wave I and concluded that the cochlear nuclei were responsible for generating wave II.

Wave III

The superior olivary complex in the caudal pons is thought to be the primary generator of wave III with some contribution from the medial nucleus of the trapezoid body. Moller and Burgess[5] recorded from near the superior olivary complex and demonstrated a wave that corresponded to wave III. Studying patients with infarctions or hemorrhages in the caudal pontine tegmentum involving the area of the superior olivary nuclei, Stockard and Rossiter[3] recorded normal waves I and II but a prolonged wave III.

Waves IV and V

Wave IV appears to be generated by the nuclei of the lateral lemniscus in the upper pons. The inferior colliculus is postulated to be the origin of wave V. Hashimoto[6] recorded from patients undergoing neurosurgical procedures. He used surface electrodes overlying the eighth nerve, pons, midbrain, and thalamus. Wave IV was maximally recorded from the pons and wave V maximally from the inferior colliculus. Buchwald and Huang[7] lesioned the auditory pathway in cats. When transverse sections were made bilaterally through the ventral nuclear region of the lateral lemniscus, potential 4 was almost abolished, suggesting that wave IV requires an intact ventral nucleus

of the lateral lemniscus. When they aspirated the inferior colliculus, potential 5 was absent and concluded that an intact inferior colliculus was required for wave V. Recording from the lateral lemniscus and inferior colliculus of rhesus monkeys, Moller and associates[1,5] suggested that the principal generator of wave IV was the lateral lemniscus and the inferior colliculus was the origin of wave V.

Starr and Hamilton[2] and Stockard and Rossiter[3] studied patients with tumors, infarcts, or hemorrhages of the mid to rostral pons and midbrain. Using surface recordings and correlating their results with BAEPs, they concluded that wave IV originated in the rostral pons and wave V from the inferior colliculus.

From the previous information it is reasonable to conclude that the origin of wave IV is in the region of the upper pons (lateral lemniscus). Wave V appears to originate in the area of the midbrain (inferior colliculus).

Waves VI and VII

There is little information on the generators of later waves. Wave VI is thought to originate from the area of the brachium of the inferior colliculus and medial geniculate body. Hashimoto,[6] in recordings from patients undergoing neurosurgical procedures, found that wave VI was maximal within the medial geniculate body.

Two patients with tumors were studied by Stockard and Rossiter,[3] one with a rostral midbrain tumor and the other with a caudal thalamic mass. Both patients had selective abnormalities of wave VI only, with normal waves I through V. On pathologic examination, the first lesion was at the level of the brachium of the inferior colliculus, and the second mass involved the medial geniculate body. Stockard and Rossiter[3] also studied a patient with bilateral, deep hemispheric lesions who was completely unresponsive to sound. Waves I through VI were normal, but the latency of wave VII was prolonged. These findings suggest that the neural origin of wave VII is rostral to the thalamus, probably in the region of the auditory radiations.

In summary, and for the purpose of clinical interpretation, wave I is generated by the distal eighth nerve near the cochlea. Wave II is attributed to the extramedullary, intracranial eighth nerve or the cochlear nucleus in the lateral medulla. The superior olivary complex and nuclei of the trapezoid body in the lower pons are the generators for wave III. Waves IV and V are generated in the region of the lateral lemniscus and inferior colliculus, which are in the upper pons and lower midbrain. The last two waveforms, waves VI and VII, are more variable and less helpful clinically. It is suggested that their origins are from the medial geniculate body of the thalamus and the auditory radiations, respectively.

PHYSIOLOGY

Frequency Threshold

The human auditory system is able to perceive a wide range of frequencies, from about 50 Hz to greater than 10,000 Hz. The ear is most sensitive to the frequencies between 2 to 4 kHz, meaning the ear is able to most easily hear this frequency range with the lowest intensity. Outside of this range, the sound has to be louder for the ear to perceive it. In everyday circumstances, most frequencies lie between 100 and 8000 Hz (Fig. 9-7).[8]

Mechanism of Hearing

As sound travels through the air it reaches the external ear, which consists of the auricle and external auditory meatus. It is suggested that the auricle, with its irregular shape and convolutions, may cause delays in the sound, helping in sound localization.

Once the sound has reached the external meatus, it is directed toward the external auditory canal (Fig. 9-8). The canal is cone shaped and ends at the tympanic membrane. The ear drum separates the outer ear from the middle ear, and on the inner side of the membrane is one of the ossicles, the malleus. Attached to the malleus is the incus, which is attached to the stapes. The stapes is attached by its foot-plate to the membrane covering the oval window. The sound entering the external canal causes a vibration that is transmitted to the tympanic membrane, which in

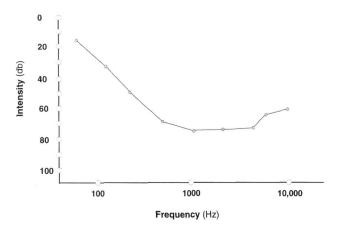

FIGURE 9–7

Range of frequencies with varying stimulus intensities that can be detected by the normal human auditory system. (Adapted from Eyzaguirre C, Fidone SJ: Physiology of the Nervous System. Chicago, Year Book, 1969.)

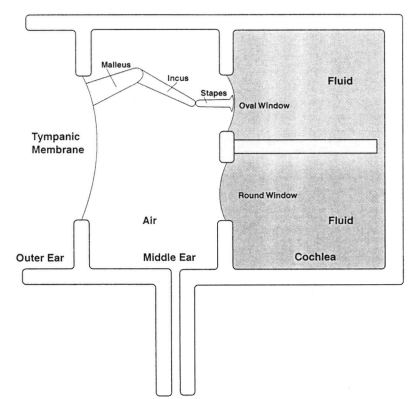

FIGURE 9–8

Schematic showing sound transmission from the external auditory canal, through the middle ear to the cochlea. (Adapted from Eyzaguirre C, Fidone SJ: Physiology of the Nervous System. Chicago, Year Book, 1969.)

turn is transmitted through the ossicles to the oval window of the cochlea. The middle ear acts to match the impedance of the energy from the external ear to the inner ear, since the outer ear transmits through air and the cochlea transmits through fluid.

From the membrane of the oval window, the sound vibrations are transmitted through the perilymph in the scala vestibuli and scala tympani, and with the bulge of the oval window inward, the round window bulges outward. The sound vibrations are passed through the vestibular membrane into the cochlear duct, which is filled with endolymph. It is through this membrane that the vibrations in the cochlear duct deform the hair cells, giving rise to generator-like potentials. These potentials can give rise to action potentials in the auditory nerve if they are of sufficient amplitude.

There are a number of potentials that have been recorded from the cochlea (Fig. 9-9). The endocochlear potential can be recorded from the scala media and is +160 to 180 mV with respect to the scala tympani. The second potential is the cochlear microphonic (CM), which is recorded near the round window. It is generated by the surface of the hair cells. It is a complex waveform with the first wavelet, m, generated by the CM. The successive wavelets n1 and n2, are thought to be due to synchronized action potentials from the auditory nerve. These last waves are variable and therefore are not present all the time.

Once the hair cells generate action potentials, the impulses are transmitted through the auditory nerve to the cochlear nucleus. The cochlear nucleus is the termination of all fibers of the auditory nerve. The cochlear nucleus is organized so that certain neurons respond to specific auditory stimuli. This processing adds to the fine-tuning of the sound. From the cochlear nucleus the secondary fibers project to the superior olivary complex by traversing the trapezoid body. The fibers synapse in the superior olivary nuclei with the tonotopic organization maintained. It is at this level that binaural convergence on single neurons takes place, which is important in directional localization of a sound.

From the superior olivary complex, tertiary fibers join to form the lateral lemniscus and travel to the inferior colliculus and medial geniculate nucleus. These last two nuclear groups act as relays and further fine-tuning takes place. The impulses are then transmitted to the auditory cortex of the temporal lobe via the auditory radiations.

DEVELOPMENTAL CHANGES

Maturation of the Auditory System

In the human, the earliest evidence of the auditory system is seen by 3 weeks postconceptional age (PCA) as the auditory placode, which is a thickening of the ectodermal floor (Fig. 9-10).[9] Complete anatomic development of the cochlea is attained by 25 weeks. Myelination of the auditory nerve begins by the 24th week.[9,10] At 38 to 40 weeks PCA, most peripheral structures are well myelinated with complete anatomic and physiologic maturation by the first few weeks after birth. Myelination of the central auditory components (cochlear nuclei, superior olivary complex, and inferior colliculi) begins between 26 and 30 weeks.[11,12] Central myelination and synaptogenesis has been thought to continue up to 18 to 36 months based on neurophysiologic studies.[13-15] From all of these studies, there appears to be a caudal-to-rostral maturational pattern that parallels the neurophysiologic changes seen with BAEPs.

Maturational changes of the various BAER parameters in the pediatric population have been described in much detail. It has been well documented that absolute and IPLs of the waveforms decrease and amplitudes in general increase with age.[9,10,16-19]

The earliest age at which an evoked response, both ipsilateral and contralateral to the stimulus, can be recorded has been variously reported from 25 to 32 weeks postconception.[10-12,19-22] It has been shown that infants older than 29 weeks conceptional age respond to a sound of 110 dB sound pressure level (SPL) applied transabdominally, whereas in infants younger than 24 weeks conceptional age a response is not generated. Postpartum studies

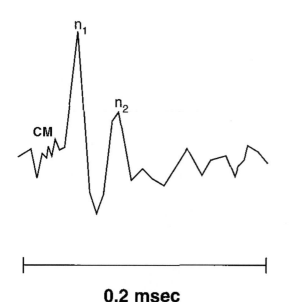

0.2 msec

FIGURE 9–9

Recording of an auditory nerve response to a click stimulation. Cochlear microphonic (CM), nerve responses (n¹ and n²). (Adapted from Eyzaguirre C, Fidone SJ: Physiology of the Nervous System. Chicago, Year Book, 1969.)

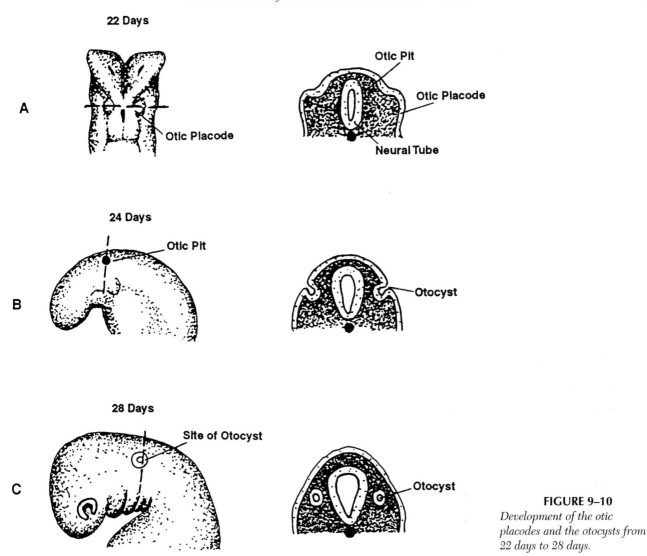

22 Days

Otic Pit
Otic Placode
Otic Placode
Neural Tube

A

24 Days

Otic Pit
Otocyst

B

28 Days

Site of Otocyst
Otocyst

C

FIGURE 9–10
Development of the otic placodes and the otocysts from 22 days to 28 days.

by Starr and coworkers[23] showed recordable brainstem potentials in a small number of infants, 25 to 28 weeks conceptional age, using a stimulus intensity of 75 dB sensation threshold (SL) and a sweep time of greater than 15 milliseconds. They concluded that auditory evoked brainstem responses could be obtained from preterm infants as young as 25 weeks, if the stimulus intensity was great enough and the acquisition time long enough. Krumholz and associates[24] used a stimulus intensity of 65 dB hearing level (HL) and found inconsistently reproducible waveforms in three infants between 25 and 27 weeks conceptional age, recognizable and more consistent responses in three of five infants between 27 and 29 weeks, and consistently recognizable and reproducible waveforms after 30 weeks. Therefore, with so much variability in the waveforms prior to about 30 weeks, interpretation of BAEPs in this age group should be conservative. With increasing age of the infant the reproducibility of the waveforms improves, the latencies decrease, and the amplitudes increase (Fig. 9-11).[15]

Contralateral BAEP waveforms can begin to be recorded by about 31 to 34 weeks. There appears to be a rostral-to-caudal progression in terms of the emergence and stability of the contralateral waveforms III and V.[25]

Specific Change of Waveforms with Age

Latency

After the first appearance of BAEPs at around 25 to 27 weeks, there is a consistent shortening of waves I, III, and V absolute latency and IPL. The most rapid changes in latencies occur between the ages of 28 and 34 weeks conceptional age. Then there appears to be a divergence in the maturational changes between the peripheral and central

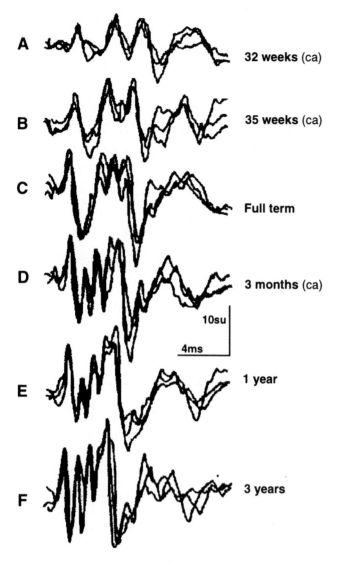

FIGURE 9–11

Maturational changes in BAEP morphology, from 32 weeks (CA) to 3 years. Each trace represents a different individual in the following age groups: A, Preterm, 32 weeks. B, Preterm, 35 weeks. C, Fullterm. D, 3 months. E, 3 years. (A to E, From Salamy A: Maturation of the auditory brainstem response from birth through early childhood. J Clin Neurophysiol 1984;1:293-329.)

auditory systems. The development of the peripheral apparatus, as shown by wave I, levels off and approaches adult values by term. The central components, as reflected by waves III and V, continue to show a decrease in absolute latency, reaching adult values by 18 to 36 months.

These changes in latency can be seen in Table 9-1. The latency of wave I decreases by about 1 millisecond during the conceptional ages of 25 to 34 weeks, from 4.33 (0.49 SD) to 3.15 millisecond (0.65 SD). From 36 to 41 weeks there is a further decrease of about 0.5 millisecond.

This is approximately 0.09 millisecond (0.03 SD) per week according to Krumholz and coworkers.[24] By term, wave I latency has reached the latencies seen in the adult.

The absolute latency of wave III decreases by about 1.5 to 1.8 millisecond during the conceptional ages of 25 to 34 weeks. In Table 9-1 the absolute latency decreases from 7.80 (0.36 SD) to 6.14 (0.81 SD) millisecond. From 36 to 41 weeks the latency shortens further by about 0.5 millisecond. This is a decrease of about 0.16 millisecond (0.03 SD) per week.[24]

The absolute latency of wave V decreases during the conceptional ages of 25 to 34 weeks, from 11.50 msec (0.78 SD) to 8.40 (0.75 SD) millisecond. A further shortening of about 0.75 millisecond is seen from 36 to 41 weeks. This is a change of about 0.17 millisecond (0.03 SD) per week.[24,26]

Waves II and IV are less consistently found. They also show a decrease in absolute latency with maturation.

The IPLs reflect the same changes seen with the absolute latencies.[24] The greatest change occurs during the 28- to 34-week conceptional age period, with a smaller decrease from 36 to 40 weeks. In Table 9-2 one can see that the I-III IPL shortens by about 0.3 millisecond during the conceptional ages of 25 to 34 weeks and about 0.15 millisecond from 36 to 41 weeks. This is about 0.07 millisecond (0.03 SD) per week. The III-V IPL decreases by about 1 millisecond from 25 to 36 weeks conceptional age, with a further decrease of about 0.2 millisecond during the period of 36 to 41 weeks, or about 0.06 millisecond (0.02 SD) per week. The I-V IPL decreases weekly by about 0.09 millisecond (0.02 SD) per week. During the conceptional ages of 25 to 34 weeks, there is a decrease of about 1.5 millisecond, with a further decrease of about 0.5 millisecond from 36 to 41 weeks.

The decrease in absolute latency and IPL continues until about the age of 18 to 36 months. Table 9-3 shows the change in latency of each of the major waves, from term to young adult.[15,27-31] In the first 2 days (0 to 58 hours) there is a small decrease in all of the waves. During the first 3 months the absolute latency of wave I decreases from about 2.0 milliseconds to about 1.5 to 1.8 milliseconds, with only slight changes after that. Wave I reaches adult latencies by approximately 1 to 3 months of age. The absolute latencies of waves III and V continue to decrease significantly over the ages of 18 to 36 months, reaching the adult mean latencies of about 3.8 milliseconds for wave III and about 5.6 milliseconds for wave V. There are no significant changes beyond 3 to 4 years of age.[17]

In summary, the decrease in the absolute latency of wave I is estimated to be about 0.07 to 0.09 millisecond per week up to term. Beyond about 1 month there is very little change.[19] The absolute latency of wave III decreases by approximately 0.06 millisecond per week, up to the age of 18 to 36 months, beyond which there is little change. Up to the age of 4 months the absolute latency of wave V decreases by about 0.1 to 0.65 millisecond per week. The decrease in latency continues at a rate of about 0.01 to 0.02 millisecond per week up to the age of 18 to 36 months, after which there is little change. This is graphically depicted in Figure 9-12.[32]

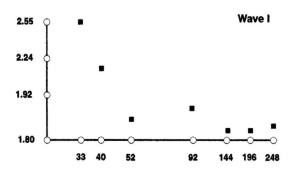

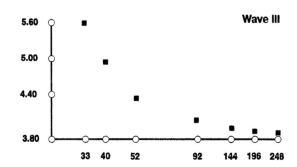

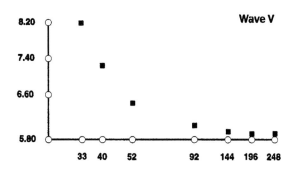

Log postconceptional age (wk)

FIGURE 9–12

Changes in BAEP waveform latencies as a function of age. (From Salamy A: Maturation of the auditory brainstem response from birth through early childhood. J Clin Neurophysiol 1984;1:293-329.)

The change in latency of each of the major waves (I, III, V) from term to young adult is summarized as follows:

1. First 2 days of life (0 to 58 hours)—There is a small decrease in all the waves.
2. First month—The absolute latency of wave I decreases from about 2.0 milliseconds to about 1.5 to 1.8 milliseconds, with only slight changes thereafter.
3. First 36 months—Waves III and V continue to decrease significantly, reaching adult mean latencies of about 3.8 milliseconds for wave III and about 5.6 milliseconds for wave V.

As with the continued decreases in the absolute latencies, the IPLs shorten due to maturation. Table 9-4 shows that the IPLs are approaching adult values by 18 months of age with little change beyond this age. The I-III IPL decreases by about 0.07 millisecond per week for the first 2 to 3 months and continues to decrease by approximately 0.009 millisecond per week up to about 18 months. The III-V IPL shortens by about 0.06 millisecond per week over the first 2 to 3 months with a further change of 0.001 millisecond per week up to 18 months. The I-V IPL decreases by about 0.09 to 0.1 millisecond per week up to 18 months, from about 5 milliseconds at term to about 4.0 milliseconds at about 18 months. There is little change in the IPLs beyond 18 to 36 months.[11,12,18,24]

Thus, from the BAEPs, it would appear that the peripheral components of the auditory system mature sooner than the central auditory components. This can also be inferred from anatomic studies. It has been reported in the human that the earliest anatomic differentiation of hair cells is in the middle of the basal turn and progresses toward the base and the apex. Sufficient development of the cochlea to support auditory function occurs before term, thus antedating the central auditory structures.[33] The earlier decrease in the absolute latency of wave I is thought to be due to the disappearance of mesenchymal tissue in the middle ear, which causes a conductive hearing loss. An increase in signal transduction between hair cells and the dendrites of the VIII nerve also contributes to a decrease in latency.[34] Finally, the latency decreases as maturation of the cochlea is completed.[30]

Additional mechanisms are thought to play a role in the changes of the rostral waveforms and central conduction time. Myelination of the central auditory system with increased synaptic density, efficiency, and synchrony are the principal processes thought to account for changes in the rostral waveforms and central conduction time.[30] There also appears to be a differential maturation of the central auditory system, with most of the change occurring in the pontomedullary area, with a lesser change in the pon-

TABLE 9–1

Mean Absolute Latency of Waves I, II, III, V: Preterm to Term →

Age, wk	I						II			
	Salamy	Krumholz	Rotteveel	Eggermont	Mochizuki	Picton	Rotteveel	Mochizuki	Salamy	Krumholz
25-27			4.33 (0.49)				6.05 (0.21)			
28-29		3.10 (0.38)	4.16 (0.69)				5.04 (0.50)			6.95 (1.36)
30-31	2.90 (0.70)	2.76 (0.56)	3.61 (0.63)				4.85 (0.82)		5.97 (1.12)	5.84 (0.95)
32-33	2.55 (0.47)	2.29 (0.51)	3.25 (0.60)	2.57 (0.54)			4.44 (0.79)		5.73 (0.55)	5.40 (0.64)
34-38		2.25 (0.52)	3.15 (0.65)			2.10 (0.25)	4.13 (0.66)			5.11 (0.62)
36-37	2.43 (1.40)	2.19 (0.46)	3.00 (0.54)	2.41 (0.38)	1.62 (0.13)		4.02 (0.52)	2.96 (0.51)	5.32 (0.44)	5.09 (0.49)
38-41	2.07 (0.36)	1.86 (0.18)	2.74 (0.38)	2.00 (0.31)	1.58 (0.15)	1.95 (0.26)	3.74 (0.49)	2.68 (0.27)	4.84 (0.46)	4.62 (0.26)

Data are shown in milliseconds, followed by the standard deviation in parentheses.

TABLE 9–2

Interpeak Latencies I-III, III-V, I-V: Preterm to Term

Age, wk	I-III			III-V			I-V			
	Rotteveel	Eggermont	Krumholz	Rotteveel	Eggermont	Krumholz	Rotteveel	Eggermont	Mochizuki	Krumholz
25-27	3.20			3.20			7.07 (1.19)			
28-29	3.49 (0.49)		3.43 (1.14)	3.12 (0.50)		3.60 (0.74)	6.52 (0.30)			7.69 (1.23)
30-31	3.30 (0.46)		3.07 (0.97)	2.57 (0.45)		2.97 (0.93)	5.83 (0.47)			6.05 (0.93)
32-33	3.07 (0.34)	3.13 (0.56)		2.41 (0.44)	2.53 (0.48)	2.61 (0.37)	5.50 (0.48)	5.64 (0.70)		5.60 (0.35)
34-35	2.99 (0.50)			2.29 (0.44)		2.50 (0.31)	5.29 (0.42)			5.36 (0.48)
36-37	2.78 (0.32)	2.93 (0.45)		2.23 (0.24)	2.47 (0.46)	2.28 (0.25)	5.01 (0.31)	5.43 (0.55)	5.42 (0.33)	5.10 (0.42)
38-40	2.82 (0.40)	2.80 (0.38)		2.09 (0.40)	2.31 (0.44)	2.18 (0.27)	4.91 (0.31)	5.14 (0.40)	5.18 (0.26)	4.92 (0.29)

Data are shown in milliseconds, followed by the standard deviation in parentheses.

TABLE 9–3

Mean Absolute Latency of Waves I, II, III, V: Term to Adult →

Age	I							II				
	Salamy	Picton	Rotteveel	Eggermont	Mochizuki	Maurizi	Chiappa	Rotteveel	Mochizuki	Chiappa	Salamy	Picton
Term	2.07 (0.36)	1.95 (0.26)	2.74 (0.38)	2.00 (0.31)	1.58 (0.15)						4.84 (0.46)	4.61 (0.33)
0-9 hr						3.0 (1.1)						
10-30 hr						2.2 (0.9)						
31-50 hr						2.2 (0.9)						
3 wk	1.85 (0.25)			1.80 (0.24)							4.61 (0.39)	
4 wk		1.89 (0.24)			1.59 (0.14)				2.74 (0.34)			
6 wk	1.70 (0.22)			1.68 (0.19)							4.40 (0.28)	
8 wk					1.47 (0.07)				2.45 (0.11)			
12 wk	1.70 (0.27)		2.31 (0.39)	1.69 (0.22)	1.49 (0.12)			3.35 (0.53)	2.45 (0.14)		4.23 (0.25)	
4 mo		1.76 (0.19)										4.31 (0.36)
6 mo	1.75 (0.22)			1.70 (0.17)	1.49 (0.09)				2.42 (0.12)		4.09 (0.26)	
9 mo					1.48 (0.14)				2.53 (0.32)			
12 mo	1.75 (0.29)			1.82 (0.30)	1.47 (0.09)				2.56 (0.25)		3.99 (0.32)	
18 mo					1.41 (0.08)				2.54 (0.26)			
2 yr				1.66 (0.12)	1.51 (0.11)				2.60 (0.24)			
3 yr	1.70 (0.16)			1.66 (0.11)	1.42 (0.06)				2.74 (0.14)		3.80 (0.21)	
4 yr				1.67 (0.15)	1.42 (0.06)				2.69 (0.15)			
5-8 yr				1.66 (0.09)	1.42 (0.08)				2.67 (0.14)			
10-20 yr					1.37 (0.06)				2.67 (0.13)			
Adult	1.59 (0.15)			1.70 (0.16)			1.7 (0.15)			2.8 (0.17)	3.72 (0.15)	

Data are shown in milliseconds, followed by the standard deviation in parentheses.

III				V					
Rotteveel	**Eggermont**	**Mochizuki**	**Picton**	**Salamy**	**Krumholz**	**Rotteveel**	**Eggermont**	**Mochizuki**	**Picton**
7.80 (–)						11.50 (0.78)			
7.39 (0.67)					10.11 (2.05)	10.70 (0.86)			
6.94 (0.77)				7.91 (1.22)	8.94 (1.30)	9.45 (0.89)			
6.35 (0.79)	5.68 (0.75)			8.22 (0.54)	7.81 (0.78)	8.76 (0.85)	8.21 (0.79)		
6.14 (0.81)			4.99 (0.36)		7.46 (0.46)	8.40 (0.75)			7.39 (0.40)
5.79 (0.56)	5.35 (0.49)	4.57 (0.27)		7.84 (0.49)	7.24 (0.41)	8.05 (0.52)	7.83 (0.59)	7.04 (0.29)	
5.56 (0.57)	4.82 (0.44)	4.35 (0.19)	4.74 (0.33)	7.16 (0.44)	6.80 (0.28)	7.65 (0.42)	7.14 (0.43)	6.76 (0.25)	7.01 (0.37)

tomesencephalic area of the brainstem.[18,19,34,35] This is reflected by the difference in the rate of change in the I-III and III-V IPLs, with a greater change in the I-III IPL than the III-V IPL. Finally, studies of humans show myelination of the trapezoid body and lateral lemniscus in the pons, detectable by 28 weeks' gestation. Myelination of the cochlear nuclei, olivary complex, lateral lemniscus, and trapezoid body is complete in the neonate, with the tracts of the inferior colliculus being incompletely myelinated at this age.[18,36] This seems to be contrary to the generally held hypothesis of a caudal-to-rostral maturational gradient. Further studies are needed.

Amplitude

There is little in the way of studies on the amplitudes of each waveform with regard to age. From the few studies it appears that the amplitude of waves I, III, and V increase through the first 2 to 4 years. This is demonstrated graphically in Figure 9-13. The graphs depicting each wave, from 33 weeks conceptional age to 4 years show a gradual increase in amplitude up to about 2 to 4 years of age. The amplitudes of waves I and III have been reported to reach adult values by 6 to 12 months, peaking at around 3 years and decreasing thereafter. The amplitude of wave V peaks somewhat later, around 3.5 to 4 years, decreasing thereafter.[35,37] Table 9-5 gives amplitude values for waves I, III, and V from 25 weeks conceptional age to adulthood. There are many factors contributing to this amplitude increase. Some of the variables include a change in thickness of the scalp/skull and dipole orientation and perhaps improving synchrony and efficiency of the auditory system.

Another way of using amplitudes is the V/I amplitude ratio. The ratio is dependent on the stimulus intensity being sufficient for stimulation in the individual with a normal

III					V						
Rotteveel	**Eggermont**	**Mochizuki**	**Maurizi**	**Chiappa**	**Salamy**	**Picton**	**Rotteveel**	**Eggermont**	**Mochizuki**	**Maurizi**	**Chiappa**
5.56 (0.57)	4.82 (0.44)	4.35 (0.19)			7.16 (0.44)						
			5.1 (0.8)							7.2 (0.3)	
			4.5 (0.4)							6.9 (0.4)	
			4.6 (0.3)							6.7 (0.2)	
	4.50 (0.46)				6.90 (0.44)			6.93 (0.37)			
		4.40 (0.22)				6.38 (0.26)			6.87 (0.33)		
	4.32 (0.19)				6.60 (0.29)			6.64 (0.26)			
		4.26 (0.24)							6.61 (0.27)		
4.88 (0.48)	4.12 (0.34)	4.12 (0.14)			6.45 (0.33)		7.03 (0.51)	6.40 (0.22)	6.46 (0.23)		
	4.03 (0.21)	4.05 (0.18)			6.22 (0.24)			6.15 (0.23)	6.37 (0.20)		
		3.93 (0.19)							6.16 (0.27)		
	3.99 (0.49)	3.88 (0.19)			6.03 (0.33)			6.15 (0.22)	6.06 (0.26)		
		3.76 (0.15)							5.90 (0.21)		
	3.84 (0.16)	3.80 (0.13)						5.86 (0.19)	5.86 (0.23)		
	3.81 (0.15)	3.81 (0.13)			5.71 (0.23)			5.81 (0.32)	5.83 (0.23)		
	3.83 (0.22)	3.68 (0.14)						5.80 (0.25)	5.72 (0.62)		
	3.85 (0.17)	3.62 (0.14)						5.60 (0.21)	5.53 (0.19)		
		3.59 (0.14)							5.51 (0.21)		
	3.72 (0.15)		3.9 (0.19)		5.66 (0.23)			5.66 (0.23)			5.7 (0.25)

TABLE 9–4

Interpeak Latencies I-III, III-V, I-V: Term to Adult

Age	I-III		III-V		I-V		
	Eggermont	**Chiappa**	**Eggermont**	**Chiappa**	**Eggermont**	**Mochizuki**	**Chiappa**
Term	2.80 (0.38)		2.31 (0.44)		5.14 (0.40)	5.18 (0.26)	
3 wk	2.73 (0.36)		2.35 (0.45)		5.13 (0.36)		
4 wk						5.27 (0.28)	
6 wk	2.70 (0.28)		2.24 (0.24)		4.96 (0.27)		
8 wk						5.15 (0.27)	
12 wk	2.49 (0.44)		2.22 (0.42)		4.71 (0.27)	4.96 (0.20)	
4 mo							
6 mo	2.36 (0.19)		2.10 (0.23)		4.45 (0.21)	4.87 (0.18)	
9 mo						4.68 (0.23)	
12 mo	2.18 (0.37		2.16 (0.45)		4.33 (0.50)	4.58 (0.24)	
18 mo						4.49 (0.17)	
2 yr	2.19 (0.17)		2.02 (0.16)		4.21 (0.21)	4.35 (0.23)	
3 yr	2.14 (0.16		2.00 (0.31)		4.16 (0.29)	4.31 (0.20)	
4 yr	2.15 (0.17)		1.97 (0.15)		4.14 (0.21)	4.30 (0.19)	
5-8 yr	2.19 (0.21)		1.83 (0.24)		4.02 (0.16)	4.12 (0.18)	
10-20 yr						4.14 (0.18)	
Adult	2.13 (0.21)	2.1 (0.15)	1.83 (0.24)	1.9 (0.24)	4.08 (0.25)		4.0 (0.23)

Data are shown in milliseconds, followed by the standard deviation in parentheses.

hearing threshold. This ratio has been reported to be smaller in neonates than adults, with the change in the ratio being similar to the change in the absolute amplitude of wave V, as seen in Table 9-5. The amplitude ratio is a relative value; therefore, some investigators have argued that it is less variable and perhaps a more sensitive indicator of abnormality than absolute amplitudes. Others have reported a greater variability in the ratio, especially in infants; therefore, the V/I amplitude ratio must be interpreted conservatively. The same factors affecting absolute amplitudes of the waves also must be taken into consideration with the amplitude ratio.

Threshold determinations have also shown a decrease with increasing age. In preterm infants of 28 to 34 weeks

TABLE 9–5

Amplitude (μV) of Waves I, III, V: Preterm to Adult   ⟶

Age	I				III			
	Salamy	**Rotteveel**	**Picton**	**Chiappa**	**Salamy**	**Rotteveel**	**Picton**	**Chiappa**
Preterm, wk								
25-27		0.07 (0.04)				−0.01		
28-29		0.14 (0.07)				0.08 (0.05)		
30-31	0.08 (0.03)	0.14 (0.10)			0.05 (0.02)	0.06 (0.07)		
32-33	0.13 (0.06)	0.16 (0.06)	0.30 (0.11)		0.10 (0.05)	0.07 (0.06)	0.17 (0.08)	
34-35		0.16 (0.07)				0.08 (0.06)		
36-37	0.14 (0.05)	0.17 (0.07)	0.36 (0.12)		0.09 (0.05)	0.08 (0.05)	0.19 (0.10)	
38-41	0.15 (0.60)	0.18 (0.07)	0.37 (0.13)		0.09 (0.04)	0.09 (0.06)	0.20 (0.09)	
Term								
3 wk	0.16 (0.06)				0.09 (0.05)			
6 wk	0.17 (0.06)				0.12 (0.06)			
12 wk	0.21 (0.11)	0.20 (0.09)			0.15 (0.07)	0.09 (0.08)		
4 mo			0.43 (0.15)					
6 mo	0.20 (0.01)				0.18 (0.12)			
12 mo	0.27 (0.15)				0.21 (0.12)			
3 yr	0.19 (0.08)				0.17 (0.10)			
5-6 yr								
Adult	0.19 (0.10)		0.28 (0.15)		0.16 (0.09)			0.23 (0.12)

conceptional age, the threshold has been reported to be about 40 dB HL, 30 dB HL at 35 to 38 weeks, and at or below 20 dB HL at term.[14,19,21] The threshold continues to decrease up to 12 to 15 months.

TEST PROCEDURES

The amplitude of BAEPs lies in the submicrovolt range, which is much smaller than the background electrocerebral activity, ambient environmental noise, and muscle activity. Therefore, recording an evoked potential requires good technique, proper filtering, amplification, and computer averaging of a response that is time locked to the stimulus.[38]

Electrode Application

The routine for performing BAEPs begins with the application of surface disc electrodes. Collodion or standard electrode paste is used after careful skin preparation has been done, as is done in routine electroencephalographic testing. Needle recording electrodes may rarely be necessary due to skin problems such as in burn patients. Impedances of the needle electrodes may differ from the surface electrodes, but waveforms should be able to be recorded. The recording electrodes are placed at the vertex (Cz) as described in the International 10-20 System and at both earlobes or mastoid processes. A ground electrode may be placed anywhere on the body but is most conveniently placed at the FPz position of the International 10-20 System (Fig. 9-14). Electrode impedances must be less than 5 kΩ.

The patient is placed in a supine position to promote maximum relaxation and to decrease muscle artifact. It is helpful to feed and diaper infants right before the start of the test and ensure personal comfort (warmth, comfortable position, dimly lit and quiet room) to relax the infant and allow the infant to fall asleep. In uncooperative patients, sedation may be necessary.

Stimulus

A mixed-frequency or broadband (100 to 8000 Hz) click using acoustic energy over a wide range of audio frequencies is recommended for neurologic evaluations. A single monophasic square-wave click stimulus with a duration of 100 microseconds is used. There are a number of other stimulus types such as pure tone pips that can be used for testing specific frequencies in audiologic testing. The stimulus is delivered monaurally through earphones or intercanalicular inserts.

Stimulus calibration is done with a sound pressure meter used with an artificial ear to simulate as close as possible the actual testing situation. It is recommended that the stimulus intensity be calibrated every 6 months. Click intensity is calibrated in decibels peak-equivalent sound pressure level (dB peSPL). The sound pressure measurement uses a reference level of 0 dB or 20 μPa, which is equal to 0.0002 dyne/cm.[2,39]

The stimulus intensity used in testing can be expressed as decibels above the hearing level, which is defined as decibels above the average hearing threshold of a group of normal young adults tested by the laboratory using identical testing conditions. Intensity also can be expressed as

V				V/I			
Salamy	**Rotteveel**	**Picton**	**Chiappa**	**Eggermont**	**Krumholz**	**Rotteveel**	**Chiappa**
	0.05 (0.06)						
	0.08 (0.04)				1.05 (0.66)		
0.11 (0.04)	0.09 (0.05)				1.36 (0.59)	0.7 (1.3)	
0.12 (0.05)	0.12 (0.07)	0.44 (0.14)		1.3 (1.13)	1.20 (0.62)	0.8 (0.5)	
	0.13 (0.05)				1.34 (0.73)	0.9 (0.6)	
0.17 (0.07)	0.16 (0.06)	0.49 (0.15)		1.29 (0.58)	1.50 (0.55)	1.1 (0.6)	
0.17 (0.06)	0.19 (0.07)	0.52 (0.16)		1.31 (0.86)	1.89 (0.82)	1.1 (0.5)	
0.21 (0.09)				2.35 (0.45)			
0.22 (0.07)				1.30 (0.63)			
0.27 (0.11)	0.20 (0.09)			1.43 (0.75)		1.2 (0.6)	
		0.61 (0.17)					
0.34 (0.20)				1.78 (1.22)			
0.45 (0.21)				2.03 (1.06)			
0.46 (0.13)				2.63 (2.35)			
				1.91 (0.58			
0.35 (0.13)			0.43 (0.16)	2.13 (1.26)	2.14 (0.80)		0.73 (0.48)

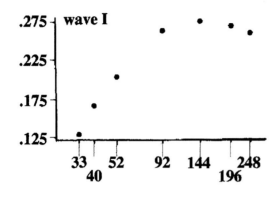

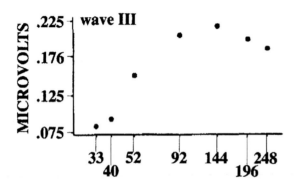

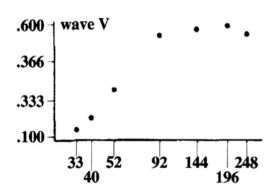

Log postconceptional age (weeks)

FIGURE 9–13
*Changes in BAEP waveform amplitudes as a function of age.
(From Salamy A: Maturation of the auditory brainstem
response from birth through early childhood. J Clin
Neurophysiol 1984;1:293-329.)*

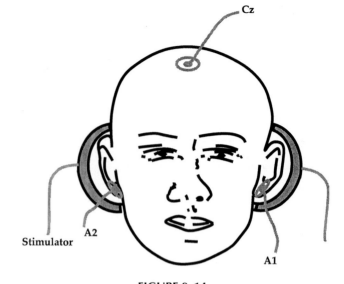

FIGURE 9–14
Electrode placement for BAEP testing.

decibels above sensation threshold, defined as decibels
above the individual's hearing threshold in the ear being
tested. It is recommended that a stimulus intensity of
60 dB above the sensation threshold of the patient be
used. Patients with significant peripheral auditory defects
may require higher stimulus intensities. If the sensation
threshold cannot be obtained because the patient is too

young to cooperate or the patient is comatose and uncooperative, a stimulus intensity of 85 dB HL should ensure
an adequate stimulus intensity in most infants.

To eliminate bone-conducted responses or a crossover
response in the contralateral ear, a masking noise is used.
The masking noise is composed of white noise with an
intensity of 60 dB SPL.

Stimulus Polarity

When using a mixed-frequency click there are three
stimulus polarities that determine the type of pressure applied to the tympanic membrane. Rarefaction click
polarity produces negative pressure and displaces the
tympanic membrane outwardly. Condensation click polarity
produces a positive pressure and displaces the tympanic
membrane inwardly. Alternating polarity alternates
between negative and positive pressure and displaces the
tympanic membrane outwardly and inwardly. For pure-
tone stimuli used in audiologic testing, the polarity
conventions are not used.

For optimal recording and resolution of wave I, rarefaction polarity is best. The amplitude of wave I is maximum.
For this reason, many laboratories select rarefaction polarity initially. If responses are poorly formed, condensation
polarity may improve waveform resolution. Rarely is alternating polarity used due to the "cancellation" effect of the
waveforms and significant latency changes in the responses
in some diseases.

Stimulus Rate

The stimulation rate can vary from 5 to 200 clicks/sec
depending on the type of testing being done. For optimal

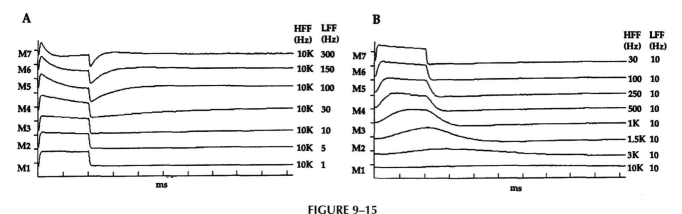

FIGURE 9–15

Effect of changes in the frequency filter upon the BAEP latency and waveform morphology. A, *Low-frequency filter (LFF) changes.* B, *High-frequency filter (HFF) changes.*

resolution of short-latency BAEPs, rates of 10 to 20/sec are best. Using high-frequency stimulation rates can reduce the amplitude of the short-latency responses.

Recording Montages

Only one channel is absolutely necessary for recording BAEPs. The recommended montage for such a recording is vertex-ipsilateral earlobe or mastoid (Cz-Ai or Mi). A two-channel recording is recommended and includes the contralateral ear. The two-channel montage is as follows:

- Channel 1: Vertex-ipsilateral earlobe or mastoid (Cz-Ai or Mi)
- Channel 2: Vertex-contralateral earlobe or mastoid (Cz-Ac or Mc)

In some subjects, the wave IV-V complex can be fused. The contralateral recording can show the separation of waves IV and V better than the ipsilateral, which is helpful in the waveform identifications.

Three- and four-channel recordings can be done, again to help in waveform identification. These montages are as follows:

- Channel 3: Contralateral-ipsilateral earlobe or mastoid (Ac-Ai or Mc-Mi)
- Channel 4: Vertex-Inion (Cz-Inion)

Recording Parameters

The responses are time locked to the stimulus and are recorded over the first 10 to 15 milliseconds following the stimulus. In the premature infant and neonate the sweep time may need to be lengthened to 15 to 20 milliseconds,

but usually no more than this. This is due to the fact that the absolute latencies of the waveforms are longer secondary to the lack of maturation.

The recommended system bandpass for the short-latency BAEP is 10 to 30 Hz and 2500 to 3000 Hz. The low-frequency cutoff can be raised to 100 to 200 Hz if muscle artifact is problematic. In children and infants, raising the low-frequency cutoff is not recommended owing to the substantial effect on the latency and waveform morphology (Fig. 9-15).

To optimally resolve the waveforms, between 1000 and 2000 responses should be averaged during each trial, and at least two trials are acquired from each ear. If waveform resolution remains poor, the number of averages can be increased up to 4000.

Troubleshooting

If waveforms are not well resolved, there are a few things that can be tried to improve waveform morphology. The stimulus intensity can be increased if wave I is not seen or is poorly formed. Special recording electrodes such as external auditory canal needle electrodes may also be of some help. The needle electrodes are not recommended in infants and small children. In the older child their use should be individualized. If there is a problem with stimulus artifact, the stimulus intensity can be decreased. The stimulus polarity may be changed to the opposite polarity or to alternating polarity. The number of stimulus repetitions and trials can be increased.

Waveform Identification

Wave V

The next step is identifying and labeling the responses. The most prominent wave form in the normal individual

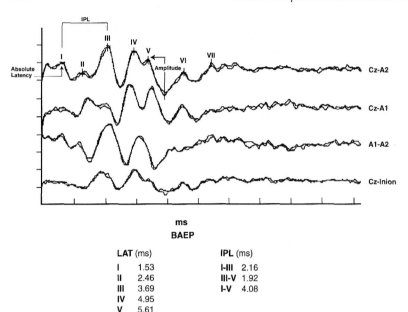

ms
BAEP

LAT (ms)		IPL (ms)	
I	1.53	I-III	2.16
II	2.46	III-V	1.92
III	3.69	I-V	4.08
IV	4.95		
V	5.61		
VI	7.32		
VII	8.67		

FIGURE 9–16

BAEP waveform identification and measurement of parameters. Absolute latency of wave I along with the peak-to-trough amplitude of wave V is shown by the arrows. The absolute latencies (P-LAT) of waves I-VII and interpeak latencies (IP-LAT) are given at the bottom.

is usually the wave IV-V complex (Fig. 9-16). It appears shortly after 5.5 milliseconds in an adult and up to about 10 to 12 milliseconds in a premature infant. Waves IV and V can be fused normally. The IV-V complex has at least six normal patterns that should be recognized when interpreting the test.[40] To distinguish them, one can use the contralateral ear recording that tends to separate the two waves. Another way to better resolve wave V is to decrease the stimulus intensity, and wave V will be the last wave-form to disappear.

Wave I

The next wave to be identified in the normal subject is I, usually occurring at least 1.5 milliseconds following the stimulus. The CM may sometimes be confused with wave I. To differentiate between the two responses, stimulus polarity can be changed, which changes the polarity of the CM but not of wave I. Wave I is also absent in the contralateral ear recording, which may help in identifying this response. If wave I is not able to be recorded using earlobe recording electrodes, special external auditory canal needle recording electrodes can be used. As mentioned previously, they are not recommended in infants and small children but can safely be used in older children who can cooperate with the insertion.

Wave III

Wave III usually occurs equidistant between waves I and V. Wave III may also have more than one appearance. Sometimes it may have a bifid pattern, making it difficult to identify.

The other waveforms—II, IV, VI, and VII—have variable latencies and amplitudes and are not useful clinically.

Latency Measurements

The absolute latencies are measured from the stimulus onset to the peak of each waveform. Difficulties in measuring absolute latencies occur when the peaks are poorly defined. When this happens, several trials superimposed on each other may allow one to estimate where the latency should be measured. IPLs are calculated from the absolute latencies (I-III, I-V, III-V).

Amplitude Measurements

Absolute amplitudes can be measured from the baseline to the peak or from the peak to the following trough. Whichever method is chosen, all waves should be measured the same way. Absolute amplitudes can be so variable, which makes their use clinically difficult to use in the neurologic patient.

NONPATHOLOGIC FACTORS AFFECTING BAEPS

There are a number of factors that need to be taken into consideration when performing and interpreting BAEPs. These include patient and technical factors.

Patient Factors

Age

In pediatrics, one of the most important parameters to consider is the patient age. As was previously stated, BAEPs can be recorded as early as 25 to 27 weeks conceptional age. The waveforms at this early age have much longer absolute latency and IPL, and the waveforms are lower in amplitude, more variable, and less reproducible. With increasing age there is a maturation of the response (Fig. 9-17). The latencies shorten, amplitudes increase, and the waveforms are more reproducible, with an adult configuration being seen by about 3 to 6 months. The absolute latency of wave I reaches adult values usually within the first month of age. This is a decrease of about 0.07 to 0.09 millisecond per week up to term with little change thereafter. Wave V absolute latency does not reach the normal adult range until 18 to 36 months. Wave III maturation lies somewhere in between, with a latency decrease of about 0.06 millisecond per week up to the age of 18 to 36 months, beyond which there is little change.

As with the absolute latency changes, there are significant changes in the IPLs. The I-V IPL decreases by approximately 0.09 to 0.1 millisecond per week up to 18 to 36 months with no clinically significant change beyond this age. The I-III and III-V IPLs shorten by about 0.07 and 0.06 millisecond per week respectively, up to 2 to 3 months, with a much slower rate of change up to 18 to 36 months.

Amplitude changes are more variable. There is an increase in the amplitudes of all the waveforms up to about 3 to 4 years. This is followed by a slow decrease in amplitude through adulthood.

Gender Effects

There have been many studies on the differences in the BAEPs of males and females. It has been shown in adults and children that the absolute latency and IPL are significantly shorter in females.[41-43] Absolute amplitudes are also greater in females.[16,41,44-46]

Most authors attribute the differences to head circumference, body and brain size, shorter anatomic pathways, or perhaps faster maturation in females. Others have suggested that a higher core body temperature might explain the shorter latencies, except that males have a slightly higher temperature than females. Hormonal changes have also been thought to be related to the latency differences, although this would not explain the differences seen in infancy and early childhood. A supposition is that there may be cochlear mechanisms underlying this gender difference.[41] Despite all of these suppositions, nothing has been directly related to the latency and amplitude intersex differences.

Birthweight Influences

Paludetti and associates[47] studied a group of preterm and fullterm, appropriate (ACA) and small (SCA) for conceptional age infants. In their study, BAEP peaks were absent in all preterm SCA infants using 70 dB nHL clicks at birth. Responses were able to be recorded in follow-up testing. In the fullterm SCA newborns, there was also a reduced occurrence of BAEPs, whereas in ACA preterm and fullterm newborns, the responses were normal. Jiang[48] again found that there was no significant difference between preterm low ACA infants and fullterm infants in any BAEP waveforms. It was concluded that birthweight in relation to conceptional age represented a major factor in BAEPs[49] and should be taken into consideration when interpreting results from SCA infants, preterm or fullterm. This factor is most likely due to the stage of maturation of the auditory pathway at the time of testing.

Body Temperature

With progressively decreasing body temperature, there is an increase in the absolute latency and IPL. On average, Picton and colleagues[50] found a 0.17-millisecond increase in the absolute latency of wave V with every 1°C decrease in body temperature. Stockard and coworkers[51] found that temperature-induced alterations of human BAEPs began

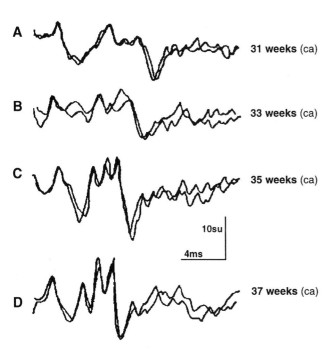

FIGURE 9–17

Changes in BAEP waveform morphology in a single preterm infant, from 31 weeks (CA) to 37 weeks (CA). (From Salamy A: Maturation of the auditory brainstem response from birth through early childhood. J Clin Neurophysiol 1984;1:293-329.)

A   31 weeks (ca)

B   33 weeks (ca)

C   35 weeks (ca)

10su

4ms

D   37 weeks (ca)

around 34.5°C (94.1°F) with abnormal central conduction times occurring at temperatures around 32.5°C (90.5°F). In another study of patients undergoing controlled hypothermic surgery, Stockard and coworkers[51] found that the latencies of waves I to V increased linearly in direct proportion to temperature decreases, from 37°C to 27°C and BAEPs could not be elicited below 27°C. The temperature effect is not so important in the clinical laboratory setting but is a very important factor in intraoperative monitoring.

Pharmacologic Effects

The effects of aminoglycosides on human BAEPs have been studied by Guerit and associates.[52] With rapid intravenous injection of gentamicin, there was a loss of amplitude followed in minutes by an increase in the latency of wave I. These changes returned to the preinjection baseline within 4 hours. Slower injection rates resulted in minor and reversible changes, also in wave I. With long-term aminoglycoside therapy, there is a varying sensorineural hearing loss, with normalization of the BAEPs after the aminoglycoside is stopped.

From animal studies, there appears to be a critical period when exposure to aminoglycosides may obliterate the brainstem auditory response. This critical period is during the time of greatest development in the auditory system, around the 11th to the 15th day after birth in rats. This effect does not occur if the aminoglycoside is given earlier or later than this critical period. Schwent and colleagues[53] used guinea pigs and found considerable variability in the action of kanamycin. Most guinea pigs treated with this aminoglycoside showed no changes on the BAEP. A small number of guinea pigs did show changes, ranging from complete absence shortly after kanamycin administration to absence of the BAEP with low-stimulus intensity only. In a study on rats, using kanamycin during the period of greatest development of auditory function (from the 11th to the 15th day after birth), Osako and coworkers[54] saw complete obliteration of the BAEPs within 10 days of beginning treatment. This did not occur if the kanamycin was given earlier or later than this critical period.

General anesthetics and barbiturates, in doses up to twice that required to produce electrocerebral silence, do not affect the short latency BAEP.[55,56] This allows the BAEP to be used in monitoring intraoperatively and in the evaluation of coma and brain death.

Antiepileptic drugs have also been studied with respect to their effects on BAEPs. Hirose and coworkers[57] reported a case of phenytoin intoxication. The blood level of phenytoin was 54.4 µg/mL when the BAEPs were first performed. Only waves I and V were present with a prolonged I-V IPL. The BAEPs returned to normal with a therapeutic phenytoin level. Green and associates[58] found small changes in BAEP latencies with phenytoin used in con-

junction with other anticonvulsants. In contrast, Stockard and colleagues[56] reported no changes in the BAEPs with chronic or acute phenytoin toxicity despite serum levels greater than 50 µg/mL. They reported no changes with therapeutic levels of phenobarbital and ethosuximide.

Baclofen has little effect on wave I but suppresses waves II, IV, and V.[59]

Sleep

There are no clinically significant effects on the BAEP waveforms with natural or sedated sleep.[60] This is particularly important when performing studies on infants and young children who may need to be recorded during sleep.

Intrasubject Variability

In normal adults, there is little change in the BAEP over time. Chiappa and colleagues[40] tested a number of subjects on two different occasions with a mean interval of 4.8 months. They found no statistically significant difference in latency or amplitude. When BAEPs were continuously recorded over an 8-hour period by Amadeo and Shagass,[60] there was little change. In infants, this consistency is absent due to the latency and amplitude changes occurring with maturation of the auditory system. In older children and adults, this consistency allows the BAEPs to be used to monitor the auditory brainstem system over long periods.

Technical Factors

Click Intensity

Most studies looking at the effect of stimulus intensity on BAEP latencies have been done in adults. As the intensity is decreased, the absolute latency of waves I, III, and V increases and amplitudes are decreased. The increase in latency is fairly linear with an increase in the absolute latency of all the waveforms of about 0.03 millisecond per decibel decrease. The latencies of waves I, III, and V increase roughly by the same amount; therefore, the I-III and I-V IPLs change very little.

In the pediatric population, signal intensity also has a significant effect on the latency of the waveforms. With decreasing stimulus intensity, the absolute latencies increase. Hecox and Burkard[35] reported that the slope of the latency-intensity function shows a small age dependency, with the rate of change in the neonate being approximately 0.7 msec/dB slower than in the adult. Picton and coworkers[50] also found that the latency of wave I may increase slightly less with decreasing stimulus intensity than wave V. This was particularly noted over the middle intensity range.

A particular consideration when performing BAEPs in neonates is that one must be careful in applying the stimulus correctly because the neonatal external auditory canal is a soft cartilage that is easily collapsible. One must be careful with placement of the ear phones so as not to collapse the external auditory canal and cause an artificial conductive defect. Therefore, a false-positive interpretation can be avoided with understanding of neonatal anatomy of the external auditory canal and careful placement of the stimulator.

Stimulus Frequency Spectrum

An effective stimulus is important in standardizing testing of the BAEPs. Many variables can alter the stimulus and must therefore be considered. The usual click stimulus is a 100-μsecond square wave. The click encompasses a broadband of frequencies usually spread over the range of 100 to 8000 Hz. To assume that the stimulus frequency remains constant, these factors must remain unchanged. Filtering the click, mixing specific frequencies of white noise with the click, or using tone pips of a specific frequency shifts the waveform latencies. This is due to stimulating different areas of the cochlea. The frequency of the broadband click at the usual stimulus intensity generates a response from the mid-cochlea, or 2000- to 4000-Hz region. With specific stimulus frequencies, specific regions of the cochlea can be stimulated, that is, low frequencies from the apical region and high frequencies from the basilar area.

Click Polarity

The polarity of the click stimulus, either rarefaction, condensation, or alternating, can also affect the BAEP waveforms and latencies,[61] particularly in subjects with a peripheral auditory defect. Wave V tends to stay at the same latency whereas the latencies of the other waves, especially wave IV, tend to decrease with rarefaction and increase with condensation clicks. IPLs may differ by as much as 0.3 millisecond in a normal subject, only as a function of changing click polarity.

Using rarefaction clicks, Maurer and associates[62] found shorter absolute latencies of wave I and more distinct waves I and IV with larger amplitudes. With condensation clicks the I-III IPL is slightly shorter and there is a better separation of waves IV and V. The latency change in wave I is thought to be due to the possibility that it is phase locked to the outward movement of the tympanic membrane with rarefaction clicks. They state that in cases with marked latency shifts between rarefaction and condensation clicks, there may be a summating process that will obscure the peaks of the waves and diminish their amplitudes, allowing for misinterpretation.

Stockard and associates[34] found that wave I had an earlier latency with rarefaction polarity and that wave V was least affected by a change in polarity. Wave I was best resolved with the largest amplitude using rarefaction

clicks. Wave V was enhanced by the use of condensation clicks. Chan and colleagues[44] found that the latency shifts related to the change in click polarity were independent of sex and race. Emerson and coworkers[63] described a polarity-dependent disappearance of wave V. In summary, wave I has an earlier latency with rarefaction polarity and wave V is least affected by a change in polarity. Wave I is best resolved using rarefaction clicks. Wave V is enhanced by the use of condensation clicks.

In the pediatric age groups the same latency shifts are seen. The latency of wave I is generally shorter and the amplitude greater using rarefaction clicks. Rarefaction clicks also produce longer IPLs. The latency shift with the change in the click polarity is enhanced in the newborn.[34]

Rate of Stimulation

With increases in the stimulation rate, there is an increase in the absolute latency and IPL and a decrease in the absolute amplitudes.[63] Stockard and associates,[34,64] using rarefaction clicks, found that as the stimulus rate was increased from 10 to 80 clicks per second, the latencies of all BAEP components increased, as did the IPLs. The latency of wave V seems to be the most sensitive BAEP component,[29,65] whereas wave I is the most resistant.

This effect from increased stimulation rates on the latencies is more pronounced in newborns.[66,67] Stockard and associates[34] reported a mean adult change in the adult IPL of 0.45 millisecond, while the mean newborn change was 0.89 millisecond going from a stimulation rate of 10 to 80/sec. Jacobson[45] states that wave V exhibits the largest latency change, increasing by 0.006 msec/Hz. This is not a completely linear relationship, because Picton and colleagues[50] noted that the effect is more marked at the shorter interstimulus intervals.

The mechanisms responsible for this latency-rate relationship are unclear. Some have suggested that fatigue of the nerve may play a part. Others hypothesize that adaptation and recovery processes of the synapses, reduced efficiency of the central synapses, or different areas of generation along the basilar membrane are factors.[20,35] Because wave V is affected differently than wave I, it appears that they are generated through different pathways. Some investigators have gone on to suggest that with increasing stimulus rates, you can increase the yield of pathologic findings by stressing the auditory brainstem system.[35]

Monaural Versus Binaural Stimulation

Clicks delivered to both ears simultaneously produce responses that are the sum of the responses obtained from each ear stimulated separately. In human studies there are small and insignificant differences in the latencies of the waveforms from binaural stimulation and the summed monaural waveforms. This difference in waveform or binaural interaction waveform is thought to be due to acoustic cross-talk.[27,50] This waveform is not clinically useful in neurologic testing and therefore stimulation should be done monaurally because an abnormal response from one ear may be masked by normal responses from the good ear. The reason for not using binaural stimulation is that an abnormal response from one ear may be masked by normal responses from the good ear.[68] Levine and McGaffigan[69] used monaural stimulation in normal subjects and found some amplitude asymmetries but no latency differences.

When stimulating monaurally, it is recommended to use a masking white noise in the contralateral ear. This is to prevent bone conduction of the stimulus in the contralateral ear. Masking of the contralateral ear has been shown to have no or little effect on the ipsilateral responses.[70,71]

Filters

Changes in filter bandpasses can affect the waveforms by changing the latency and amplitude of the responses. The frequency spectra that holds most of the energy of the BAEP response is between 15 and 2000 Hz, with about 50% of the energy falling in the range below 200 Hz.[72,73] Underlying the BAEP responses is a slow wave with a frequency of 15 to 80 Hz and a duration of about 4 milliseconds, which can be seen by selecting out the higher frequencies setting the low-pass filter to 150 to 200 Hz. This waveform is clinically important in audiologic testing of thresholds but has not been found useful in neurologic testing at the present.

Since there are few frequencies of interest above 1500 Hz, changing the low-pass filter from 3000 to 1500 Hz does not significantly change the response.[74] In contrast, Chiappa and colleagues[40] found that changing the high-pass filter from 100 to 300 Hz resulted in a 20% loss of amplitude of wave V, and there was no improvement in the resolution of waves, which is also true in children.[75,76] Therefore, in neurologic testing the usual filter settings are 10 to 30 Hz for the high-pass filter and 2500 to 3000 Hz for the low-pass filter to allow the best resolution of the waveforms of interest. Effect of changes in the low- and high-frequency filter settings on waveform morphology and latency is illustrated in Figure 9-15.

The type of filters also may have an effect on the waveform morphology. Analog filters may cause a phase shift of the absolute latency.[77]

INTERPRETATION OF RESULTS

Technical factors are important when performing BAEPs. This is particularly relevant in children who may not be cooperative. Also in the pediatric age group, you must be aware of the developmental changes that occur when interpreting results; the younger the patient, the longer the latencies and the more variable the responses.

The clinical use of BAEPs is in assessment of the peripheral hearing apparatus and the brainstem auditory system. In pediatrics, BAEPs are extremely useful and in some cases, the only way to test hearing. We are now able to assess hearing in patients we were unable to 10 to 15 years ago such as infants, uncooperative patients, and patients in coma.

It is suggested that normal values be defined as the mean plus 2.5 or 3 SDs above the mean. In addition, when interpreting studies from infants, a conservative approach should be taken due to the number of changes that take place developmentally.

Latency Abnormalities

The primary generator of wave I is the distal eighth nerve near the cochlea. Therefore, wave I is affected by pathology of the peripheral auditory apparatus, at or distal to this part of the nerve. This includes not only the nerve but the spiral ganglion, middle ear, and external auditory canal. When all waveforms are clearly seen but there is a prolongation of waves I, III, and V absolute latencies with normal IPLs, a peripheral hearing defect is present with normal central conduction from the peripheral eighth nerve to the midbrain. A shorter than normal I-V IPL with prolongation of all absolute latencies has also been described in high-frequency hearing loss. This is most likely due to a differential response of the cochlea (apical vs. basal) due to the hearing loss, therefore changing the absolute latency of wave I to a greater extent. If wave I is absent with a normal III-V IPL, this is usually due to a peripheral deficit also. The conduction of the click stimulus is normal from the lower pons to the midbrain, but the conduction from the peripheral eighth nerve to the lower pons cannot be determined. Complete absence of responses from one or both ears is rare. If this occurs and is not due to technical difficulties, it suggests a severe high-frequency hearing loss most commonly, or desynchronization of the conducting pathways that may take place in multiple sclerosis. The conduction of the click stimulus from the peripheral eighth nerve through the brainstem cannot be determined.

When the I-III IPL is abnormally prolonged, this suggests a conduction defect in the brainstem auditory system between the distal eighth nerve and the lower pons. When an abnormal increase in the III-V IPL is seen, this suggests a conduction defect in the brainstem auditory system between the lower pons and midbrain.

With monaural stimulation, the responses from each ear should always be compared. If the latencies from both ears are normal, but there is an abnormal asymmetry between the sides, this also suggests a conduction defect from the ear that has the relative prolongation as discussed earlier.

Amplitude Abnormalities

Absolute amplitudes are not a reliable indicator of abnormality owing to the large amount of variability. The V/I amplitude ratio is helpful but should be interpreted conservatively, especially in the pediatric population. It also can vary with the stimulus intensity and shape of the audiogram, so the V/I amplitude ratio can be used only when the hearing threshold is normal. Wave V is usually about twice the size of wave I. With a significant amplitude loss or absence of wave V, this suggests a conduction defect in the brainstem auditory system rostral to the lower pons.

Lateralization

With monaural stimulation, the brainstem pathology is most commonly ipsilateral to the ear showing the most abnormality. This is based on both pathologic and neuroradiologic studies.

REFERENCES

1. Moller AR, Jannetta PJ, Sekar LN: Contributions from the auditory nerve to the brainstem auditory evoked potentials (BAEPs): Results of intracranial recording in man. Electroencephalogr Clin Neurophysiol 1988;71:198-211.
2. Starr A, Hamilton AE: Correlation between confirmed sites of neurological lesions and abnormalities of far-field auditory brainstem responses. Electroencephalogr Clin Neurophysiol 1976;41:595-608.
3. Stockard JJ, Rossiter VS: Clinical and pathologic correlates of brain stem auditory response abnormalities. Neurology 1977;27:316-325.
4. Garg BP, Markand ON, Bustion PF: Brainstem auditory evoked responses in hereditary motor-sensory neuropathy: Site of origin of wave II. Neurology 1982;32:1017-1019.
5. Moller AR, Burgess J: Neural generators of the brain-stem auditory evoked potentials (BAEPs) in the rhesus monkey. Electroencephalogr Clin Neurophysiol 1986;65:361-372.
6. Hashimoto I: Auditory evoked potentials recorded directly from the human VIIIth nerve and brain stem: Origins of their fast and slow components. *In* Buser PA, Cobb WA, Okuma T (eds): The Kyoto Symposia: Electroencephalography and Clinical Neurophysiology, Supplement 36. Amsterdam, Elsevier, 1982, p 305.
7. Buchwald JS, Huang C-M: Far-field acoustic response: Origins in the cat. Science 1975;189:382-384.
8. Eyzaguirre C, Fidone SJ: Physiology of the Nervous System. Chicago, Year Book, 1969.
9. Eggermont JJ: Evoked potentials as indicators of auditory maturation. Acta Otolaryngol 1985;412 (Suppl):41-47.
10. Eggermont JJ: Evoked potentials as indicators of the maturation of the auditory system. *In* Gallai V (ed): Maturation of the CNS and Evoked Potentials. Amsterdam, Elsevier, 1986.
11. Rotteveel JJ, Colon EJ, Stegeman DF, Visco YM: The maturation of the central auditory conduction in preterm infants until three months post term: I. Composite group averages of brainstem (ABR) and middle latency (MLR) auditory evoked responses. Hear Res 1987;26:11-20.
12. Rotteveel JJ, de Graaf R, Colon EJ, et al: The maturation of the central auditory conduction in preterm infants until three months post term: II. The auditory brainstem responses (ABRs). Hear Res 1987;26:21-35.
13. Madonia TH, Serra A, Vancheri M, Lamantia I: Physiological anatomy and maturation of the central auditory pathways. *In* Gallai V (ed): Maturation of the CNS and Evoked Potentials. Amsterdam, Elsevier, 1986, p 154.
14. Salamy A, Eldredge L, Wakeley A: Maturation of contralateral brain-stem responses in preterm infants. Electroencephalogr Clin Neurophysiol 1985;62:117-123.
15. Salamy A: Brainstem ontogenesis in healthy and high risk infants. *In* Gallai V (ed): Maturation of the CNS and Evoked Potentials. Amsterdam, Elsevier, 1986, p 166.
16. Allison T, Hume AL, Wood CC, Goff WR: Developmental and aging changes in somatosensory, auditory, and visual evoked potentials. Electroencephalogr Clin Neurophysiol 1984;58:14-24.
17. Allison TA, Wood CC, Goff WR: Brain stem auditory, pattern-reversal visual, and short-latency somatosensory evoked potentials: latencies in relation to age, sex, and brain and body size. Electroencephalogr Clin Neurophysiol 1983;55:619-636.
18. Beiser M, Himelfarb FZ, Gold S, Shanon E: Maturation of auditory brainstem potentials in neonates and infants. Int J Pediatr Otorhinolaryngol 1985;9:69-76.
19. Cox C, Hack M, Metz D: Brainstem-evoked response audiometry: Normative data from the preterm infant. Audiology 1981;20:53-64.
20. Ken-Dror A, Pratt H, Zeltzer M, et al: Auditory brain-stem evoked potentials to clicks at different presentation rates: Estimating maturation of pre-term and full-term neonates. Electroencephalogr Clin Neurophysiol 1987;68:209-218.
21. Murray AD: Newborn auditory brainstem evoked responses (ABRs): Longitudinal correlates in the first year. Child Dev 1988;59:1542-1554.
22. Murray AD: Newborn auditory brainstem evoked responses (ABRs): Prenatal and contemporary correlates. Child Dev 1988;59:571-588.
23. Starr A, Amlie RN, Martin WH, Sanders S: Development of auditory function in newborn infants revealed by auditory brainstem potentials. Pediatrics 1977;60:831-839.
24. Krumholz A, Felix JK, Goldsstein PJ, McKenzie E: Maturation of the brain-stem auditory evoked potential in premature infants. Electroencephalogr Clin Neurophysiol 1984;59:411-419.
25. Ichiyama T, Hayashi T, Furukawa S: Developmental changes of contralateral brainstem auditory evoked potentials: Evaluation of brainstem maturation. Brain Dev 1995;17:49-51.
26. Eggermont JJ: Development of auditory evoked potentials. Acta Otolaryngol 1992;112:197-200.

27. Chiappa KH: Brain stem auditory evoked potentials: Methodology. In Chiappa KH (ed): Evoked Potentials in Clinical Medicine. New York, Raven Press, 1990, p 173.

28. Eggermont JJ, Don M: Analysis of the click-evoked brainstem potentials in humans using high-pass noise masking: II. Effect of click intensity. J Acoust Soc Am 1980;68:1671-1675.

29. Lasky RE: A developmental study of the effects of stimulus rate on the auditory evoked brain-stem response. Electroencephalogr Clin Neurophysiol 1984;59:411-419.

30. Maurizi M, Almadori G, Cagini L, et al: Auditory brainstem responses in the full-term newborn: Changes in the first 58 hours of life. Audiology 1986;25:239-247.

31. Picton TW, Taylor MJ, Durieux-Smith A, Edwards CG: Brainstem auditory evoked potentials in pediatrics. *In* Aminoff MJ (ed): Electrodiagnosis in Clinical Neurology. New York, Churchill Livingstone, 1986, p 505.

32. Salamy A, McKean CM, Pettett G, Mendelson T: Auditory brainstem recovery processes from birth to adulthood. Psychophysiology 1978;15:214-220.

33. Warren MP: The auditory brainstem response in pediatrics. Otolaryngol Clin North Am 1989;22:473-500.

34. Stockard JE, Stockard JJ, Westmoreland BF, Corfits JL: Brainstem auditory-evoked responses: Normal variation as a function of stimulus and subject characteristics. Arch Neurol 1979;36:823-831.

35. Hecox K, Burkard R: Developmental dependencies of the human brainstem auditory evoked response. Ann N Y Acad Sci 1982;388:538-556.

36. Hosford-Dunn H, Runge CA, Hillel A, Johnson SJ: Auditory brain stem response testing in infants with collapsed ear canals. Ear Hear 1983;4:258-260.

37. Jiang ZD, Zhang L, Wu YY, Liu XY: Brainstem auditory evoked responses from birth to adulthood: Development of wave amplitude. Hear Res 1993;68:35-41.

38. American Electroencephalographic Society: Guidelines for clinical evoked potential studies. J Clin Neurophysiol 1984;1:3-53.

39. Chatrian GE, Wirch AL, Lettich K, et al: Click-evoked human electrocochleogram: Noninvasive recording method, origin, and physiologic significance. Am J Technol 1982;22:151-174.

40. Chiappa KH, Gladstone KJ, Young RR: Brain stem auditory evoked responses: Studies of waveform variations in 50 normal human subjects. Arch Neurol 1979;36:81-87.

41. Don M, Ponton CW, Eggermont JJ, Masuda A: Gender differences in cochlear response time: An explanation for gender amplitude differences in the unmasked auditory brain-stem response. J Acoust Soc Am 1993;94:2135-2148.

42. Maurizi M, Ottaviani F, Paludetti G, et al: Effects of sex on auditory brainstem responses in infancy and early childhood. Scand Audiol 1988;17:143-146.

43. Mochizuki Y, Go T, Ohkubo H, Motomura T: Development of human brainstem auditory evoked potentials and gender difference from infants to young adults. Prog Neurobiol 1983;20:273-285.

44. Chan YW, Woo EKW, Hammond SR, et al: The interaction between sex and click polarity in brain-stem auditory

potentials evoked from control subjects of oriental and caucasian origin. Electroencephalogr Clin Neurophysiol 1988;71:77-80.

45. Jacobson JT: Normative aspects of the pediatric auditory brainstem response. J Otolaryngol 1985;14(Suppl):7-11.

46. O'Donovan CA, Beagley HA, Shaw M: Latency of brainstem response in children. Br J Audiol 1980;14:23-29.

47. Paludetti G, Ottaviani F, Almadori G, et al: Influences of birthweight upon brainstem maturation as reflected by auditory brainstem response (ABR) evaluation. Int J Pediatr Otorhinolaryngol 1987;13:77-84.

48. Jiang ZD: Maturation of the auditory brainstem in low risk preterm infants: A comparison with age-matched fullterm infants up to 6 years. Early Hum Dev 1995;42:49-65.

49. Soares I, Collet L, Deseux V, Morgon A: Differential maturation of brainstem auditory evoked potentials in preterm infants according to birthweight. Int J Neurosci 1992;64:259-266.

50. Picton TW, Stapells DR, Campbell KB: Auditory evoked potentials from the human cochlea and brainstem. J Otolaryngol 1981;10(Suppl 9):1-41.

51. Stockard JJ, Sharbrough FW, Tinker JA: Effects of hypothermia on the human brainstem auditory response. Ann Neurol 1978;3:368-370.

52. Guerit J-M, Mahieu P, Houben-Giurgea S, Herbay S: The influence of ototoxic drugs on brainstem auditory evoked potentials in man. Arch Otorhinolaryngol 1981;233:189-199.

53. Schwent VL, Williston JS, Jewett DL: The effects of ototoxicity on the auditory brain stem response and the scalp-recorded cochlear microphonic in guinea pigs. Laryngoscope 1980;90:1350-1359.

54. Osako S, Tokimoto T, Matsuura S: Effects of kanamycin on the auditory evoked responses during postnatal development of the hearing of the rat. Acta Otolaryngol 1979;88:359-368.

55. Drummond JC, Todd MM, U HS: The effect of high dose sodium thiopental on brain stem auditory and evoked median nerve somatosensory evoked responses in humans. Anesthesiology 1985;63:249-254.

56. Stockard JJ, Rossiter VS, Jones TA, Sharbrough FW: Effects of centrally acting drugs on brainstem auditory responses. Electroencephalogr Clin Neurophysiol 1977;43:550-551.

57. Hirose G, Kitagawa Y, Chujo T, et al: Acute effects of phenytoin on brainstem auditory evoked potentials: Clinical and experimental study. Neurology 1986;36:1521-1524.

58. Green JB, Walcoff M, Lucke JF: Phenytoin prolongs far-field somatosensory and auditory evoked potential interpeak latencies. Neurology 1982;32:85-88.

59. Martin MR: Baclofen and the brain stem auditory evoked potential. Exp Neurol 1982;76:675-680.

60. Amadeo M, Shagass C: Brief latency click-evoked potentials during waking and sleep in man. Psychophysiology 1973;10:244-250.

61. Orlando MS, Folsom RC: The effects of reversing the polarity of frequency-limited single-cycle stimuli on the

human auditory brain stem response. Ear Hear 1995;16:311-320.

62. Maurer K, Schäfer E, Leitner H: The effects of varying stimulus polarity (rarefaction vs. condensation) on early auditory evoked potentials (BAEPs). Electroencephalogr Clin Neurophysiol 1980;50:332-334.

63. Emerson RG, Brooks EB, Parker SW, Chiappa KH: Effects of click polarity on brainstem auditory evoked potentials in normal subjects and patients: Unexpected sensitivity of wave V. Ann N Y Acad Sci 1982;388:710-721.

64. Stockard JJ, Stockard JE, Sharbrough FW: Nonpathologic factors influencing brainstem auditory evoked potentials. Am J EEG Technol 1978;18:177-209.

65. Lina-Granade G, Collet L, Morgon A, Salle B: Maturation and effect of stimulus rate in brainstem auditory evoked potentials. Brain Dev 1993;15:263-269.

66. Teas DC, Klein AJ, Kramer SJ: An analysis of auditory brainstem responses in infants. Hear Res 1982;7:19-54.

67. Salamy A: Maturation of the auditory brainstem response from birth through early childhood. J Clin Neurophysiol 1984;1:293-329.

68. Prasher DK, Gibson WPR: Brain stem auditory evoked potentials: A comparative study of monaural versus binaural stimulation in the detection of multiple sclerosis. Electroencephalogr Clin Neurophysiol 1980;50:247-253.

69. Levine RA, McGaffigan PM: Right-left asymmetries in the human brain stem: Auditory evoked potentials. Electroencephalogr Clin Neurophysiol 1983;55:532-537.

70. Boezeman EHJF, Kapteyn TS, Visser SL, Snel AM: Effect of contralateral and ipsilateral masking of acoustic stimulation on the latencies of auditory evoked potentials from cochlea and brain stem. Electroencephalogr Clin Neurophysiol 1983;55:710-723.

71. Galambos R, Hecox KE: Clinical applications of the auditory brain stem response. Otolaryngol Clin North Am 1978;11:709-722.

72. Elbering C: Auditory electrophysiology: Spectral analysis of cochlear and brain stem evoked potentials. A comment on Kevanishvili and Aphonchenko: "Frequency composition of brain stem auditory evoked potentials." Scand Audiol 1979;8:57-64.

73. Kevanishvili ZS, Aphonchenko V: Frequency composition of brain stem auditory evoked potentials. Scand Audiol 1979;8:51-55.

74. Cacace AT, Shy M, Satya-Murti S: Brainstem auditory evoked potentials: A comparison of two high-frequency filter settings. Neurology 1980;30:765-767.

75. Dorfman LJ, Britt RH, Silverberg GD: Human brainstem auditory evoked potentials controlled hypothermia and total circulatory arrest. Neurology 1981;31:88-89.

76. Fabiani M, Sohmer H, Trait C, et al: A functional measure of brain activity: Brain stem transmission time. Electroencephalogr Clin Neurophysiol 1979;47:483-491.

77. Drift JFC, Brocaar MP, Zanten GA: Brainstem response audiometry: I. Its use in distinguishing between conductive and cochlear hearing loss. Audiology 1988;27:260-270.

78. Stockard JJ, Stockard JE, Sharbrough FW: Detection and localization of occult lesions with brainstem auditory responses. Mayo Clin Proc 1977;52:761-769.

10

Visual Evoked Potentials in Pediatrics—Normal

WILLIAM D. GOLDIE

The visual evoked potential (VEP) is a graphic illustration of the cerebral electrical potentials evoked by a defined visual stimulus (Fig. 10-1). The VEP is elicited by discreet visual stimulation of the eye with subsequent recording of the electrical potentials from the scalp produced by the passage of neural impulses from the eye to the occipital lobe. The VEP elicited in adults has been carefully standardized and evaluated,[1] but the potentials elicited from infants and young children differ from adults and deserve special consideration.[2-4]

In this chapter the reader is introduced to visual pathways from a developmental point of view. The physiologic changes associated with development are reviewed for anatomic sites of the visual pathway and their relationship to the VEP discussed. Various techniques that have been used to elicit the VEP from the infant and child are described, and the advantages and disadvantages of each technique are considered. Finally, techniques that can be used to investigate particular aspects of the developmental physiology of the immature visual system are reviewed.

ANATOMY AND PHYSIOLOGY OF THE VISUAL PATHWAYS, WITH ATTENTION TO DEVELOPMENT DURING INFANCY AND CHILDHOOD

Receptor cells of the retina are arranged in a single layer of cells that are shaped like rods and cones (Fig. 10-2).

Cones respond to bright light and are responsible for color and form vision, whereas the rods respond mainly to low-level light and movement.[5,6] The macula is the area of the retina with high visual sensitivity. In the macula the receptor cells are almost exclusively cones, and the relationship of receptor to ganglion cell is close to one-to-one. The macula is about 5 mm in diameter but accounts for about 50% of the nerve fibers in the optic nerve (see review by Hubel[7]). In the peripheral retina the receptor cells are primarily rods. There are 20 times more rods than cones in the retina.

Rods and cones contain disk-like layers of receptor pigment protein that absorb photon energy from the incident light relative to the color sensitivity of the specific protein. This energy absorption causes a summation potential to be generated that accumulates at the cell body. This summated potential propagates along a neural network consisting of a hierarchy of connections to the *ganglion cells*. *Bipolar cells* modulate and process the input from receptor cells on their way to the ganglion cell. These impulses are modified and modulated in turn by intermediate *horizontal* and *amacrine cells*. There are no action potentials during this passage, and the impulse develops as a graded electrical response with field potentials. At the ganglion cell a nerve action potential is generated. There are estimated to be about 125 million receptor cells that feed into about 1 million ganglion cells. The ganglion cells have a one-to-one relationship to the nerve fibers in the optic nerve. Axons travel across the retina to the optic nerve and continue on to the next synaptic station at the lateral geniculate (Fig. 10-3).

The optic nerves are fairly well myelinated at birth,[8] but the efficiency of their conduction is much less than it will be later on in life. The fibers are small, and the efficiency of the saltatory conduction is probably less than in the adult, so the conduction times are longer.

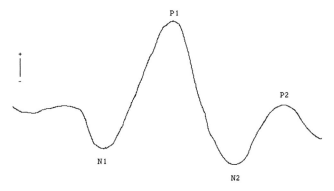

FIGURE 10–1

This demonstrates the ideal waveform of the visual evoked potential obtained with patterned stimulation. With the pattern shift technique, the P1 latency is usually very close to 100 milliseconds and is often referred to as the P100 waveform.

As the ganglion cells send out their axons, they travel back toward the brain in a manner that is topographic with the retina (see Fig. 10-3). As they approach the *optic chiasm*, the more medial fibers cross to the contralateral hemisphere while the more lateral remain ipsilateral. Some fibers cross early, whereas others actually initially follow the tract, reverse direction, and cross to the contralateral side. Approximately 55% of the fibers cross over at the chiasm. This is programmed during development, and it is not subject to maturation or development. As the axonal fibers assemble into the *optic tracts*, some fibers descend into the brainstem. Some of these mediate pupillary constriction to light, eye blinking, and probably even the "bright light sneeze."

The *lateral geniculate*, a remarkably complex structure, is organized topographically, and organizes input from each eye separately into layers that alternate in a predictable manner. The first two layers consist of large cells (*magnocellular*) that respond to low contrast, whereas the other four layers consist of smaller cells (*parvocellular*) that respond to high contrast. The lateral geniculate is the first synaptic junction for axons that are coming from the geniculate cells of the retina. The lateral geniculate appears to

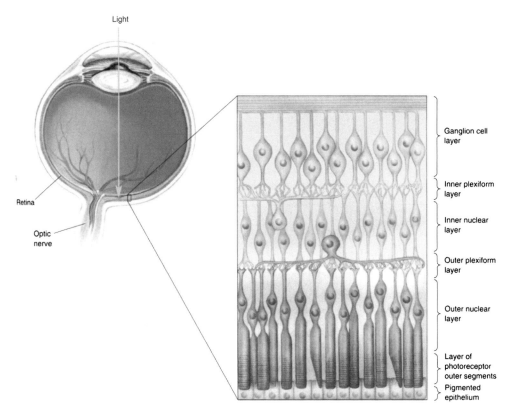

FIGURE 10–2

The laminar organization of the retina. (From Bear MF, Connors BW, Paradiso MA: Neuroscience: Exploring the Brain, 2nd ed. Philadelphia, Lippincott Williams & Wilkins, 2001.)

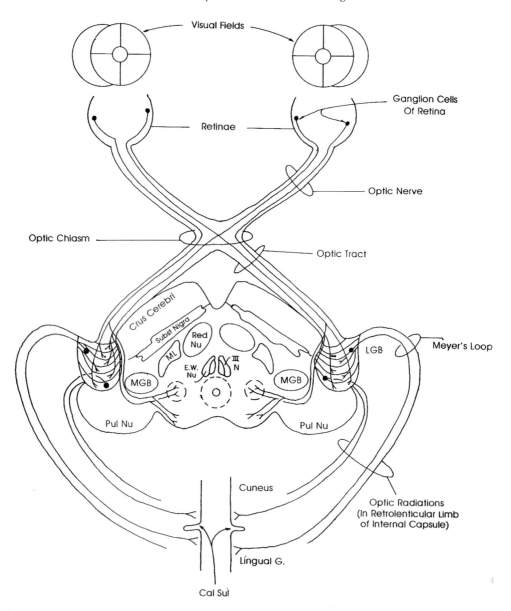

FIGURE 10–3

This drawing illustrates the visual pathways from the retina through the chiasm to the lateral geniculate and to the occipital cortex. Note the complexity of crossings and the portion of the pathways that goes to the brainstem. LGB, lateral geniculate body; MGB, medial geniculate body; ML, medial lemniscus.

provide a "way station" with a booster effect on transmission and may provide a degree of processing that allows for more efficient input to the cortical structures.[9] It is known that the lateral geniculate receives feedback fibers from the occipital lobe and brainstem structures and has a population of cells that responds differently to monocular or binocular stimulation.[10,11] The architecture of the lateral geniculate is well defined even at birth.[8,12]

The components of the visual system subject to the greatest postnatal developmental change are the *optic radiations*. The radiations consist of myelinated axons extending from

the cell bodies of the lateral geniculate while traveling through the posterior aspects of the corona radiata as they reach toward the visual cortex. There is a remarkable linear growth of these fibers during the first several months of development. In addition to linear growth, the fibers also increase in diameter and become myelinated. Conduction along these pathways is initially slow, but as the pathways lengthen they become more efficient and conduct faster. In the very immature brain there is a rather straight pathway between the lateral geniculate and the cortex. With growth of the brain, the distance not only gets longer but the pathway becomes stretched and distorted by other structures, including the ventricles, pulvinar, internal capsule, and corpus callosum. Some of the optic radiation fibers also pass into the temporal lobe as Meyer's loop.

The *occipital cortex* consists of six well-defined cortical layers. The occipital cortex is separated into columns and has a structure that resembles the striping of a tiger.[13] The columns are structured to represent line orientation; the stripes represent binocular integration, and the entire array is oriented in a topographic distribution relative to the retina (see review by Hubel[7]). The fibers of the optic radiations arrive consistently at layer 4. It is this layer that has the myelinated fibers of the radiations and appears as the *line of Gennari*. The vertical orientation of the cellular columns, the alternating linear arrays of the cortical stripes, and electrophysiologic dipole effect that this architecture creates all are present at birth. However, the surface dynamics of the cortical layers, including the folding of the gyri and sulci, become much more complex with maturation.

The latency of the VEP at 1 month of age (44 weeks conceptional age) is about 260 milliseconds. The retina processing can be evaluated by the pattern electroretinogram, which shows that this processing takes up about 100 milliseconds (Fig. 10-4). Over the first few months of age, there is a dramatic decrease in the VEP latency, with only moderate improvement in retinal processing (Fig. 10-5).[4] Physiologic changes are responsible for these decreases in latency. There is improvement in the efficiency of conduc-

tion secondary to myelination, maturation of neurotransmitter receptor sites, and enlargement of the nerve fibers. Authors have estimated that the visual pathways mature within 5 to 8 months after birth.[8,14] Other evidence suggests that there is continuing improvement in the myelination and maturation of receptors up to 2 to 3 years of age.[4,15] By 6 months of age there is already sophisticated visual discrimination, and by 12 months of age most color and form perception is complete.[16,17]

VARIOUS TECHNIQUES FOR STUDYING THE VISUAL PATHWAYS

The VEP can be elicited in a variety of ways by using different techniques for presenting a visual stimulus. Each technique has advantages and disadvantages that are examined in the subsequent sections.

It is preferable to have a specific examination room that is used for all tests. Even in a busy neonatal nursery, there is usually a procedure room that can be used on a periodic basis for the performing of the VEP examination. The ambient light in the room should be kept low and at a constant level across all patients. Infants should be studied just following a feeding, when they are quiet and calm. The tests should be performed quickly and efficiently with as little manipulation of the child as possible. Electrodes should be placed in a standard manner that is held constant across all patients and controls. In our laboratory

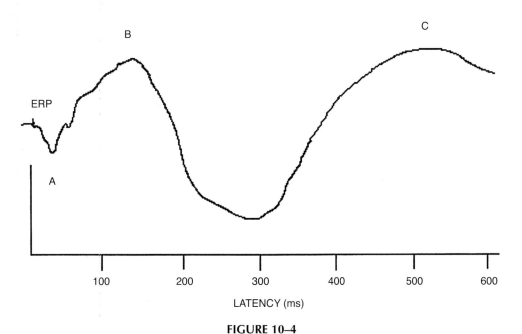

FIGURE 10–4

This drawing illustrates the ideal formation of the electroretinogram (ERG) of the mature eye. It incorporates photopic and scotopic elements all in one figure.

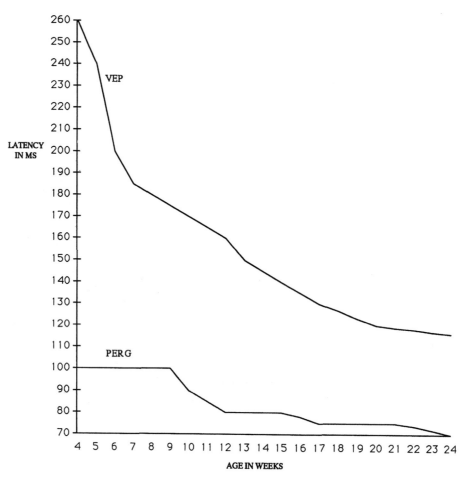

FIGURE 10–5

This graph illustrates a compilation of data that have measured visual evoked potential (VEP) and pattern electroretinogram (PERG) latency data in normal infants of different ages. (Data primarily from Sokol S: Maturation of visual function studied by visual evoked potentials. In Desmedt JE [ed]: Visual Evoked Potentials. Amsterdam, Elsevier, 1990, p 35.)

electrodes secured with paste are routinely used, although some laboratories use collodion. The head can be wrapped with gauze or a diaper to secure the electrodes. In our experience the ear reference has not been satisfactory since it is often noisy and difficult to maintain. We prefer using the midfrontal electrode and vertex as references. In infants (from premature through about 3 months of age) the electrode position is quite difficult to standardize. The use of four channels with four occipital positions are recommended: (1) low midline—1 cm above the inion; (2) high midline—5 cm above the inion; (3) left lateral—2 cm above the inion and over 3 cm to the left; and (4) right lateral—up 2 cm above the inion and over 3 cm to the right. The montage would be as follows:

- Channel 1—vertex-low midline occipital
- Channel 2—midfrontal-left lateral occipital
- Channel 3—midfrontal-high midline occipital
- Channel 4—midfrontal-right lateral occipital

Impedances of the scalp electrodes should be less than 5 kΩ. Background electroencephalographic (EEG) activity should be monitored visually. It is often best to have the neonate lying in an open crib, whereas the older infant and young child may be more relaxed in the lap of the mother or nurse. It is recommended that the older child with glasses be tested with the glasses in place unless refraction is provided during the evaluation.

Strobe Flash Technique

The most commonly used method for the acquisition of VEPs in infants is the strobe flash. This technique involves the use of a tungsten filament or xenon gas strobe flash, the same type typically used for EEG photic stimulation studies. The light source is placed in front of the infant's head and is flashed sequentially with the computer sweep. In most settings infants are placed on their back and are studied during natural or sedated sleep. The strobe is placed 1 m away from the bridge of the infant's nose. The rate of stimulation is usually about 2/sec, although some authors recommend a rate of 1 to 1.5/sec.[18,19] Others use faster stimulation rates of 5 to 10/sec. The technique is well established and available in nearly every neurophysiology laboratory, and there are a number of sources of normative data.[4,19-22]

However, the strobe flash technique is fraught with several difficulties, as follows:

1. The intensity of the flash bleaches out the receptor protein and can produce an afterimage effect. The intense flash can even produce a photochemical effect on the recording electrodes, particularly those close to the eye, that could produce an artifactual electrical potential.

2. The processing of the flash stimulus at the retinal level consists of a mass response to luminance change, and nearly all of the retinal receptors are stimulated due to the light scatter that occurs. Patterns or colors can be placed in front of the strobe, but this does not provide enough contrast to overcome the scatter effect of the flash stimulus presentation.

3. It is extremely difficult to separately stimulate each eye, and patching of one eye often is disruptive or ineffective.

4. The level of arousal of the infant and the intensity of the flash are difficult to standardize.

5. The infant is usually studied with the eyes closed. The eyelids can attenuate the stimulus as well as act as a red light filter effect.

Light-Emitting Diode Goggle Technique

Another technique for visual stimulation involves the use of light-emitting (LEDs).[23] These LED elements can be placed in goggles and arrayed in a pattern on a grid. The goggles are fitted over the infant's eyes and are taped gently in place for the duration of the examination. LEDs can come in various colors, but the most commonly used is red.[24] The stimulus parameters can be precisely defined as a square wave onset-offset curve that provides an effective nervous system stimulus.[25] The intensity and pattern of the LED array can be standardized easily, and the red color obviates the variability produced by the red filter effect of the eyelid. The use of the goggles allows for stimulation of each eye separately. An alternating grid pattern of LEDs can provide a pattern-shift method of stimulation, rather than an onset-offset method, so that luminance can remain the same. The LED array can be linked to a computer so that various parameters can be changed systematically throughout a recording sequence. The intensity of the LED stimulus is not great enough to bleach the visual pigment,

and there is no photochemical effect at the recording electrodes. This method is gaining more popularity, particularly in the nursery, where it is not disruptive to the other infants and can be performed with the infant lying comfortably in the incubator or warmer.[23] An example of VEPs elicited by goggles is provided in Figure 10-6.

Pattern Reversal Technique

The pattern reversal method for VEP stimulation was developed and popularized in the early 1960s.[1] The pattern is produced on a computer monitor screen. The most effective method for studying central vision is to keep luminance constant and to stimulate only those aspects of the retina that respond to edge detection and orientation of receptor fields. This can be accomplished by the pattern reversal technique. In the most popular method, a checkerboard pattern is presented to the central vision with an equal number of dark and light squares, With reversal, the black squares turn white, and the white turn black. There is no resultant luminance change, but the retinal receptor units experience linear orientation effects as well as edge detection.[26] This produces specific ganglion cell stimulation in a highly efficient manner. Experience has shown that this method produces the most consistent, reproducible, and clinically useful VEP waveforms.[27,28]

The pattern reversal VEP method may be difficult in some children. Although some workers have been able to use it quite successfully with infants,[14,15,29] the most success has been with young children.[2,30-32] The most effective technique involves having the child sit on the parent's lap and attend to a cartoon superimposed on the television screen.[33,34] The screen is placed approximately 1 m away from the bridge of the child's nose. This distance must be determined precisely to keep constant the minutes of arc subtended by the edge of each square—which should be about 50 minutes for infants up to about 12 months of age, and about 20 minutes for young children. It is also wise to carefully measure the degrees of arc subtended by the screen itself. Central vision covers about 5 degrees of arc, and most screens cover from 10 to 15 degrees. The child must attend to the pattern long enough to obtain a reproducible VEP. This requires very close observation of the child so that the VEP data are collected only when the child is looking directly at the screen. Usually the technologist stands behind the screen and observes the reflection off the child's cornea. By the use of a toggle switch the technologist can stop and start the averaging so it occurs only during the interval when the child is adequately focused on the screen. A large screen covering 20 to 30 degrees of arc is generally more effective than the smaller one, since the probability is higher that the child will be looking at the pattern. Each eye can be tested

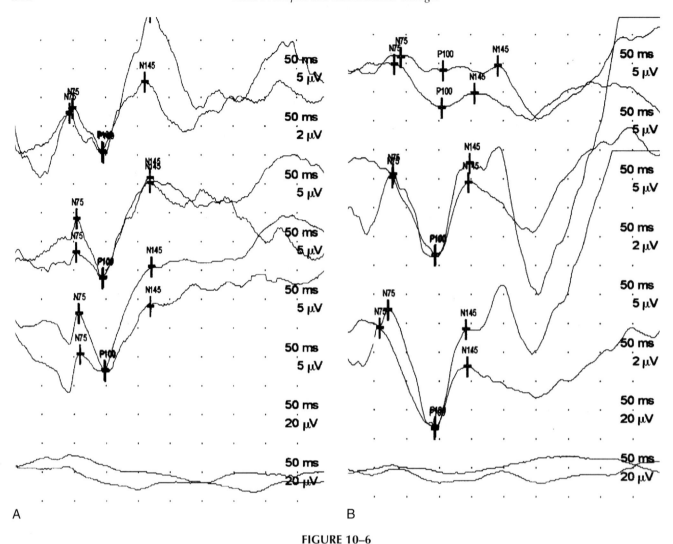

FIGURE 10–6

Example of visual evoked potentials using light-emitting diode goggles. The child was 1 year old and had infantile spasms. There was a question of whether the child could see. A, Right eye stimulated. B, Left eye stimulated. Top channel, Fz-O1; second channel, Fz-Oz; third channel, Fz-O2.

independently by patching the other eye during the study. An example of a VEP evoked by pattern reversal is provided in Figure 10-7.

Sinusoidal Gratings Pattern Technique

Sine wave gratings are alternating light and dark stripes with midlines of maximum and minimum luminance and a gradual transition between the maxima. The change in luminance forms a sine wave.[26] This method is physiologically more simple and stimulates the cells of the retina in a specific manner.[27] The fast Fourier transform of the stimulus is a simple spacial frequency, unlike the checkerboard, which produces a highly complex spatial frequency.[35] Certain ganglion cells of the retina respond to gradual changes of contrast in a manner that enhances the impression of an edge. The sinusoidal pattern represents a high-order stimulus that produces activation of these specific edge-detecting ganglion cells. The pattern can be oriented in different ways, and motion can be added to make it even more complex. The size of the grating is given in terms of cycles per degree, with a grating of 6 cycles per degree being roughly equivalent to a bar pattern with a bar width of 20 degrees. The phasing of the sinusoidal grating pattern can be varied in a sequential manner with simultaneous computer analysis of the resultant evoked potential to define in exact terms the nature of the physiologic effects it exerts on the retina.

However, the sinusoidal method is difficult to perform in most laboratories. It involves a subject who is cooperative

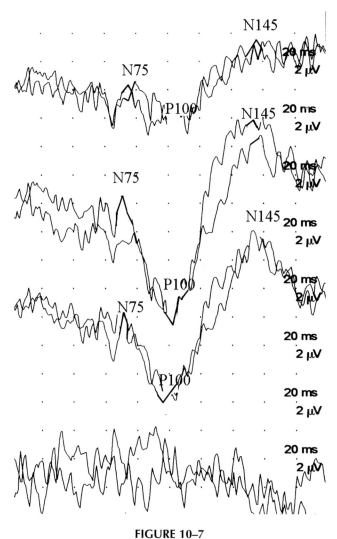

FIGURE 10–7

Pattern reversal evoked potential in a 16-year-old child with suspected multiple sclerosis. Right eye stimulated. Top channel, Fz-O1; second channel, Fz-Oz; third channel, Fz-O2.

and willing to attend to a computer screen for long periods. Although this method could be attempted in the very cooperative older child, it is probably not practical in the young child and infant. Some of the same methods that have been used for testing pattern reversal VEPs in infants and children have also worked with this technique. An excellent review by Sokol and associates[36] has described this method in infants.

Steady-State Visual Evoked Potentials

The typical type of visual stimulation performed during the recording of the EEG involves fast flash rates that produce a driving response. This type of stimulation can be used in an evoked potential setting to record steady-state potentials.[37,38] Flash rates of faster than about 15/sec produce a sinusoidal waveform that is fairly simple and can be analyzed by fast Fourier transform. These waveforms are usually collected on the evoked potential machine by setting the sweep time to be some defined multiple of the interflash interval. If the flash rate is 40/sec, then the interval would be 25 milliseconds. If the sweep time is 100 milliseconds, then there will be four waveforms captured during the sweep. The fast Fourier transform can then provide phase and power values for the resultant sinelike waveform. The individual waveforms vary considerably from those obtained with the single flash method, and more variability is noted in intertrial and intersubject reproducibility. However, this method has been incorporated into a quick method for assessing acuity in the infant that can be processed by computer. This has been discussed in detail in papers by Norcia and Tyler.[39,40]

The Pattern Electroretinogram

The cellular elements of the retina produce electrical fields as the graded potentials elicited by visual stimuli propagate through the various layers up to the ganglion cells. The measurement of these potentials is referred to as the *electroretinogram* (see Fig. 10-5). This has been studied in great detail in the cat, monkey, and adult human.[25,41,42] Although less well understood in the infant and child, clinical studies have been done.[43] The stimulation parameters have to be carefully controlled to extract photopic versus scotopic components. The best studies have been obtained using a patterned stimulus to stimulate more of the macular elements selectively. This technique involves specialized equipment, including a special contact lens or a fine metal wick placed into the conjunctival sac that is used as the recording electrode.[41] The infant is sedated, the pupils are dilated, and the lids are held open with spring clips. The stimulus is carefully focused on the retina in a standardized manner. Data have been obtained concerning the maturation of the receptors of the retina, and normative latency data are now available.[2] It is not recommended that these studies be performed in a routine neurophysiology laboratory.

Critical Periods

Infant perception involves the activation of inborn neural pathways that must be used to remain functional.[11] If there is a period of no visual stimulation, then the visual system may become irreversibly disrupted so that vision will not develop.[9] This is best illustrated by congenital cataracts.[2] If shapes are not perceived by the involved infant for a sufficient period, then shapes will never be perceived, even if the cataracts are successfully removed. Kittens whose eyes are kept closed or who are kept in cages with only specific line orientations will demonstrate limitation of visual function later on in life.[10,44]

A normal infant must receive appropriate and diverse visual stimulation to preserve the complex visual function that is born into the visual system. If a specific form of visual deprivation persists beyond the critical period, then that aspect of visual perception may be lost. In some cases, the VEP can be used to investigate whether the pathways are still intact.[17,45-47] The methods involved in this type of investigation are complex and are outside the scope of this chapter.

CONCLUSION

The VEP can be readily obtained in the infant. The most prevalent VEP method for studying the visual pathways of infants is the strobe flash technique. This has many disadvantages, is crude, provides variable waveforms and latencies, and may not provide clinically useful information. The LED goggle technique has significantly enhanced our ability to provide useful clinical information about the visual pathways in the infant. The pattern reversal technique has been successful in some children and even infants, but this involves specialized methods that may not be possible in some laboratories.

It is best to develop a simple and easily standardized method for each laboratory. I personally use the LED goggle method in all infants. It has provided excellent information. I defer judgment about acuity or visual perception until more objective methods can be used later in life. We are still a long way away from fully understanding the functional visual pathways; however, the VEP is instrumental in increasing our knowledge. VEPs provide an enhancement of the clinical evaluation that can contribute to the clinical management of the patient. It is hoped that this chapter has helped to broaden the reader's understanding of the VEP and how it can be useful in assessing the visual pathways of an infant. In Chapter 27, we assess the VEP results obtained in specific disease processes.

REFERENCES

1. Sokol S: Visual evoked potentials. *In* Aminoff MJ (ed): Electrodiagnosis in Clinical Neurology. New York, Churchill Livingstone, 1986, p 441.
2. Sokol S: Clinical applications of the ERG and VEP in the pediatric age group. *In* Cracco RQ, Bodis-Wollner I (eds): Evoked Potentials. New York, Alan R. Liss, 1986, p 447.
3. Sokol S: The pattern visual evoked potential in the evaluation of pediatric patients. *In* Desmedt JE (ed): Visual Evoked Potentials. Amsterdam, Elsevier, 1990, p 115.
4. Sokol S: Maturation of visual function studied by visual evoked potentials. *In* Desmedt JE (ed): Visual Evoked Potentials. Amsterdam, Elsevier, 1990, p 35.
5. Kaneko A: Physiology of the retina. Annu Rev Neurosci 1979;2:169-191.
6. Schnapf JL, Baylor DA: How photoreceptor cells respond to light. Sci Am 1987;256:40-47.
7. Hubel DH: Eye, brain, and vision. *In* Scientific American Library Series. New York, W. H. Freeman, 1988, p 22.
8. Magoon EH, Robb RM: Development of myelin in human optic nerve and tract: A light and electron microscopic study. Arch Ophthalmol 1981;99:655.
9. Hickey TL: Postnatal development of the human lateral geniculate nucleus: Relationship to a critical period for the visual system. Science 1977;198:836.
10. Wiesel TN, Hubel DH: Effects of visual deprivation on morphology and physiology of cells in the cat's lateral geniculate body. J Neurophysiol 1963;26:978-993.
11. Wiesel TN: Postnatal development of the visual cortex and the influence of environment. Nature 1982;299:583-591.
12. Rodieck RW: Visual pathways. Annu Rev Neurosci 1979;2:193-225.
13. Hubel DH: Exploration of the primary visual cortex, 1955-1978. Nature 1982;229:515-524.
14. Kurtzberg D, Vaughan HG: Electrophysiological assessment of auditory and visual function in newborn. Clin Perinatal 1985;12:277-299.
15. Sokol S, Jones K: Implicit time of pattern evoked potentials in infants: An index of maturation of spatial vision. Vision Res 1979;19:747-755.
16. Lodge A, Armington JC, Barnet AB, et al: Newborn infants' electroretinograms and evoked electroencephalographic responses to orange and white light. Child Dev 1969;40:267.
17. Lambert SR, Kriss A, Taylor D: Delayed visual maturation: A longitudinal clinical and electrophysiological assessment. Ophthalmology 1989;96:524-529.
18. Ellingson RJ: Variability of visual evoked responses in the human newborn. Electroencephalogr Clin Neurophysiol 1970;29:10-19.
19. Fulton AB, Hansen RM, Manning KA: Measuring visual acuity in infants. Surv Ophthalmol 1981;25:325-332.
20. Brown AM, Dobson V, Maier J: Visual acuity of human infants at scotopic, mesopic, and photopic luminances. Vision Res 1987;27:1845-1858.
21. Kurtzberg D: Event-related potentials in the evaluation of high-risk infants. Ann N Y Acad Sci 1982;388:557-571.
22. Schellbe D, Gasser T, Kohler W: The intra-individual reproducibility of flash evoked potentials in a sample of children. Int J Psychopathol 1987;5:135-143.
23. Mushin J, Hogg CR, Dubowitz LMS, et al: Visual evoked responses to light-emitting diode (LED) photostimulation in newborn infants. Electroencephalogr Clin Neurophysiol 1984;58:317-320.
24. Spydell JD: A low-cost light-emitting diode photic stimulator. Electroencephalogr Clin Neurophysiol 1983;55:485-486.

25. Tan CB, King PJL, Chiappa KH: Pattern ERG: Effects of reference electrode site, stimulus mode, and check size. Electroencephalogr Clin Neurophysiol 1989;74:11-18.

26. Bodis-Woller I, Ghilardi MF, Mylin LH: The importance of stimulus selection in VEP practice: The clinical relevance of visual physiology. *In* Cracco RQ, Bodis-Wollner I (eds): Evoked Potentials. New York, Alan R. Liss, 1986, p 15.

27. Bobak P, Bodis-Wollner I, Guillory S: The effect of blur and contrast on visual evoked potential latency: Comparison between check and sinusoidal grating patterns. Electroencephalogr Clin Neurophysiol 1987;68:247-255.

28. Maier J, Dagnelie G, Spekreijse H, Van Dijk BW: Principal components analysis for source localization of visual evoked potentials in man. Vision Res 1987;27:165-177.

29. Sokol S, Moskowitz A, Paul A: Evoked potential estimates of visual accommodation in infants. Vision Res 1983;23:851-860.

30. Fenwick PBC, Brown D, Hennesey J: The visual evoked response to pattern reversal in "normal" 6- to 11-year-old children. Electroencephalogr Clin Neurophysiol 1981;51:49-62.

31. Moskowitz A, Sokol S: Developmental changes in the human visual system as reflected by the latency of the pattern reversal VEP. Electroencephalogr Clin Neurophysiol 1983;56:1-15.

32. Teller DY, Movshon JA: Visual development. Vision Res 1986;26:1483-1506.

33. Shors TJ, Eriksen KJ, Wright KW: Superimposition of a cartoon program as an aid in recording pattern visual evoked potentials in children. J Pediatr Ophthalmol Strabismus 1987;24:224-227.

34. Wright KW, Eriksen KJ, Shors TJ, Ary JP: Recording pattern visual evoked potentials under chloral hydrate sedation. Arch Ophthalmol 1986;104:718-721.

35. Bodis-Wollner I, Brannan JR, Ghilardi MF: The importance of physiology to visual evoked potentials.

In Desmedt JE (ed): Visual Evoked Potentials. Amsterdam, Elsevier, 1990, p 1.

36. Sokol S, Moskowitz A, McCormack G, Augliere R: Infant grating acuity is temporally tuned. Vision Res 1988;28:1357-1366.

37. Orel-Bixler DA, Norcia AM: Differential growth of acuity for steady-state pattern reversal and transient pattern onset-offset VEPs. Clin Vision Sci 1987;2:1.

38. Pinto F, Boschi C, Mencucci R, et al: Frequency analysis of steady state VEPs in developmental amblyopia. Electroencephalogr Clin Neurophysiol 1987;67:6.

39. Norcia AM, Tyler CW: Spatial frequency sweep VEP: Visual acuity during the first year of life. Vision Res 1985;25:1399-1408.

40. Norcia AM, Tyler CW: Infant VEP acuity measurements: Analysis of individual differences in measurement error. Electroencephalogr Clin Neurophysiol 1985;61:359-369.

41. Armington JC: Electroretinography. *In* Aminoff MJ (ed): Electrodiagnosis in Clinical Neurology. New York, Churchill Livingstone, 1986, p 403.

42. Sokol S, Jones K, Nadler D: Comparison of the spatial response properties of the human retina and cortex as measured by simultaneously recorded pattern ERGs and VEPs. Vision Res 1983;23:723-727.

43. Abramov I, Gordon J, Hendrickson A, et al: The retina of the newborn human infant. Science 1982;217:265-267.

44. Hubel DH: Effects of deprivation on the visual cortex of cat and monkey. Harvey Lect 1978;72:51.

45. Lovasik JV: Normalization of binocular VERs after early onset visual deprivation in man. Electroencephalogr Clin Neurophysiol 1984;59:21-28.

46. Mellor DH, Fielder AR: Dissociated visual development: Electrodiagnostic studies in infants who are "slow to see." Dev Med Child Neurol 1980;22:327-335.

47. Jan JE, Farrel K, Wong PK, McCormich AO: Eye and ear improvements of visually impaired children. Dev Med Child Neurol 1986;28:285-293.

II

Disorders of Cerebral Function

11

Age-Specific Seizure Disorders

PAUL A. L. S. HWANG, HIROSHI OTSUBO, JAMES J. RIVIELLO, JR.,
AND GREGORY L. HOLMES

Epileptic seizures are one of the most common and frightening neurologic conditions occurring in children. With the exception of the elderly, the incidence of seizures in children is significantly higher than adults, with the highest incidence occurring during the first year of life.[1] When appropriately used, the electroencephalogram (EEG) is invaluable in supporting the diagnosis of epilepsy, localizing onset of the seizures, and delineating an epileptic syndrome. Since the routine EEG is noninvasive, totally safe, and relatively inexpensive when compared with other diagnostic studies, all patients with suspected seizures should have a study obtained. However, it must be cautioned that the usefulness of the EEG is in direct relationship to the quality of the study and the competence of the individual interpreting the record.

Epileptiform patterns are distinct from the background activity appropriate for the patient's age and state, have an electrical field and configuration indicative of cerebral origin, illustrate characteristic morphologic features, and demonstrate predictable effects with activation procedures.[2,3] Many of the epileptiform patterns seen in neonates and young children are far different from those seen in adolescents, and the electroencephalographer must be aware of these age-specific patterns. For example, rolandic spikes, neonatal ictal patterns, and hypsarrhythmia are EEG features unique to children. In addition, many spikes and sharp waves seen in children may be normal age-dependent phenomena.

In this chapter, EEG abnormalities in the age-specific seizure disorders are reviewed. Neonatal seizures are discussed in Chapter 13 and are not discussed here.

EPILEPTIC SEIZURES

Classification

The International Classification of Epileptic Seizures is presented in Box 11-1. Seizures are first classified into two broad categories: (a) partial seizures (seizures beginning in a relatively small location in the brain) and (b) generalized seizures (seizures that are bilaterally symmetric and without local onset). Seizures are then further classified by the clinical and EEG manifestations of the seizure. The International Classification of Epilepsies and Epileptic Syndromes is presented in Box 11-2. An epileptic syndrome is a constellation of signs and symptoms that occur together in a number of patients sufficiently large to make a chance combination improbable.[3] The EEG features of the various seizure types are presented in Tables 11-1, 11-2, and 11-3. The classification of seizures and epilepsy is evolving as new seizure types and syndromes are further clarified.[4]

Simple Partial Seizures

The signs or symptoms of simple partial seizures depend on the location of the focus of the seizure. Seizures involving the motor cortex most commonly consist of rhythmic to semirhythmic clonic activity of the face, arm, or leg. There is usually no difficulty in diagnosing this type of seizure. Seizures with somatosensory, autonomic, and psychic symptoms (hallucinations, illusions, déjà vu) may be more difficult to diagnose. Psychic symptoms usually occur as a component

BOX 11-1
PARTIAL SEIZURES

Simple Partial Seizures (consciousness not impaired)

With motor symptoms
　　Focal motor without march
　　Focal motor with march (Jacksonian)
　　Versive
　　Postural
　　Phonatory (vocalization or arrest of speech)

With somatosensory or special-sensory symptoms (simple hallucinations, e.g., tingling, light flashes, buzzing)
　　Somatosensory
　　Visual
　　Auditory
　　Olfactory
　　Gustatory
　　Vertiginous

With autonomic symptoms or signs (including epigastric sensation, pallor, sweating, flushing, piloerection and pupillary dilation)

With psychic symptoms (disturbance of higher cerebral function)
　　Dysphasic
　　Dysmnesic
　　Cognitive
　　Affective
　　Illusions
　　Stuctured hallucination

Complex partial seizures (with impairment of consciousness: may sometimes begin with simple symptomatology)
　　Simple partial onset followed by impairment of consciousness
　　With impairment of consciousness at onset

Partial seizures evolving to secondarily generalized seizures
　　Simple partial seizures evolving to generalized seizures
　　Complex partial seizures evolving to generalized seizures
　　Simple partial seizures evolving to complex partial seizures evolving to generalized seizures

Generalized Seizures

Absence seizures
　　Typical absence
　　　　Impairment of consciousness only
　　　　With mild clonic components
　　　　With atonic components
　　　　With tonic components
　　　　With automatisms
　　　　With autonomic components
Atypical Absence
Myoclonic seizures
Clonic seizures
Tonic seizures
Tonic-clonic seizures
Atonic seizures (astatic)

From Commission on Classification and Terminology of the International League Against Epilepsy. Proposal for revised clinical and electroencephalographic classification of epileptic seizures. Epilepsia 1981; 22:249-260.

of a complex partial seizure. Simple partial seizures can occur at any age.

Complex Partial Seizures

Complex partial seizures (CPSs), formerly termed *temporal lobe* or *psychomotor seizures*, are one of the most common seizure types encountered in both children and adults. CPS may be preceded by a simple partial seizure that may serve as a warning to the patient (i.e., aura) that a more severe seizure is pending. The aura may enable the clinician to determine the cortical area from which the seizure is beginning.

By definition, all patients with CPS have impairment of consciousness, which may be subtle. For example, the patient may either not respond to commands or respond in an abnormally slow manner. Although CPS may be characterized by simple staring and impaired responsiveness, behavior is usually more complex during the seizure. Automatisms, semi-purposeful behaviors of which the patient is unaware and subsequently cannot recall, are common during the period of impaired consciousness. The types of automatic behavior are quite variable and may consist of activities such as facial grimacing, gestures, chewing, lip smacking, snapping fingers, and repeating phrases. The patient does not fully recall this activity following the seizure. Although variable, CPSs usually last from 30 seconds to several minutes.[5] This should be contrasted with absence seizures (described later), which usually last less than 15 seconds. Most patients have some degree of postictal impairment (e.g., tiredness or confusion) following a CPS.

BOX 11-2
INTERNATIONAL CLASSIFICATION OF EPILEPSIES AND EPILEPTIC SYNDROMES

Localization-Related (focal, local, partial) Epilepsies and Syndromes
Idiopathic with age-related onset
  Benign childhood epilepsy with central-temporal spikes
  Childhood epilepsy with occipital paroxysms
  Primary reading epilepsy
Symptomatic
  Chronic, progressive epilepsia partialis continua of childhood (Kojewnikow's syndrome)
  Syndromes characterized by seizures with specific modes of precipitation
Cryptogenic

Generalized Epilepsies and Syndromes
Idiopathic (with age-related onset listed in order of age)
  Benign neonatal familial convulsions
  Benign neonatal convulsions
  Benign myoclonic epilepsy in infancy
  Childhood absence epilepsy (pyknolepsy)
  Juvenile absence epilepsy
  Juvenile myoclonic epilepsy (impulsive petit mal)
  Epilepsy with grand mal seizures on awakening
  Other generalized idiopathic epilepsies not defined above
  Epilepsies with seizures precipitated by specific modes of activation
Cryptogenic or symptomatic (in order of appearance)
  West's syndrome (infantile spasms)
  Lennox-Gastaut syndrome
  Epilepsy with myoclonic-astatic seizures
  Epilepsy with myoclonic absences
Symptomatic
  Nonspecific etiology
    Early myoclonic encephalopathy
    Early infantile epileptic encephalopathy with suppression bursts
    Other symptomatic generalized epilepsies not defined above
  Specific syndromes
    Epileptic seizures may complicate many disease states

Epilepsies and Syndromes Undetermined as to Whether They Are Focal or Generalized
With both generalized and focal seizures
  Neonatal seizures
  Severe myoclonic epilepsy in infancy
  Epilepsy with continuous spike-waves during slow-wave sleep
  Acquired epileptic aphasia (Landau-Kleffner syndrome)
  Other undetermined epilepsies not defined above
  Without unequivocal generalized or focal features

Special Syndromes
Situation-related seizures
  Febrile convulsions
  Isolated seizures or isolated status epilepticus
  Seizures occurring only when there is an acute metabolic or toxic event due to factors such as alcohol, drugs, eclampsia, and nonketotic hyperglycemia

From Proposal for revised classification of epilepsies and epileptic syndromes. Commission on Classification and Terminology of the International League Against Epilepsy. Epilepsia 1989;30:389-399.

EEG. The EEG in partial seizures is characterized by focal spikes, sharp waves, or, less commonly, focal slowing (Figs. 11-1 to 11-4). There is often a relationship between the location of the spikes and the seizure type (i.e., occipital lobe spikes are associated with occipital lobe seizures, whereas frontal lobe spikes are associated with frontal lobe seizures). However, patients with well-documented seizures may have normal interictal EEGs.

Generalized Seizures

Generalized Tonic-Clonic Seizures

Generalized tonic-clonic seizures are characterized by loss of consciousness that occurs simultaneously with the onset of a generalized stiffening of flexor or extensor muscle (termed *tonic phase*). Following the tonic phase, generalized jerking of the muscles (clonic activity) occurs. The seizures are dramatic, and there is rarely any difficulty in making the correct diagnosis. Seizures that begin with bilateral tonic posturing without a focal onset are classified as *primary generalized tonic-clonic*.

Some patients may have a simple partial seizure (aura) preceding the loss of consciousness. As described earlier, this indicates that the seizure was simple partial in onset. As the seizure spreads in the cortex, it develops into a

TABLE 11–1

Electroencephalography in Epileptic Syndromes in Infancy and Early Childhood

Syndrome	Interictal EEG	Ictal EEG
Febrile convulsions	Variable	Rhythmic discharges
West's syndrome	Hypsarrhythmia; modified hypsarrhythmia	Variable; spike-wave, slow waves, decremental response
Benign myoclonic epilepsy	Normal or rare spike-waves while awake; spike-waves during sleep	Generalized spike-waves or multiple spike-waves
Severe myoclonic epilepsy	Fast generalized spike-wave and focal abnormalities	Generalized spike-waves or multiple spike-waves
Myoclonic astatic epilepsy	4-7 Hz rhythmic theta; fast, irregular generalized spike-wave or multiple spikes	Generalized 2-3 Hz spike-waves, multiple spikes
Lennox-Gastaut syndrome	Slow (<2.5 Hz) spike-waves; slow background, multifocal spikes	Generalized 2-3 Hz spike-waves, multiple spikes

TABLE 11–2

Electroencephalography in Epileptic Syndromes in Childhood

Syndrome	Interictal EEG	Ictal EEG
Childhood absence epilepsy	Normal	Generalized 3-Hz spike-waves
Epilepsy with myoclonic absences	Normal background; isolated spike-waves	Generalized 3-Hz spike-waves
Childhood partial benign epilepsy with central-temporal spikes of childhood	Blunt, high-voltage central-temporal spikes; activated by sleep; rare generalized spike-waves	Rhythmic central-temporal spikes with or without generalization
Benign partial epilepsy of childhood with occipital paroxysms	High-amplitude spike-waves or sharp waves, recurring in the occipital and posterotemporal areas; occur only with eye closure	Rhythmic occipital, posterotemporal spikes that may spread to central-anterior-temporal area
Landau-Kleffner syndrome	Bilateral spikes, spike-waves, usually temporal in location; often activated by sleep	Rhythmic temporal discharges that may become generalized
Epilepsy with continuous spike-waves during slow sleep	Generalized spike-waves of various frequencies; continuous spike-waves during sleep	Generalized spike-waves

TABLE 11–3

Electroencephalography in Epileptic Syndromes in Adolescents

Syndrome	Interictal EEG	Ictal EEG
Juvenile absence epilepsy	Normal	Generalized (>3 Hz) spike-waves
Juvenile myoclonic epilepsy	Rapid (3.5-6 Hz) generalized spike-wave; frequent photoparoxysmal response	Generalized spike-waves, multiple spike-waves
Epilepsy with generalized tonic-clonic seizures on awakening	Normal	Generalized spike-waves

generalized tonic-clonic seizure. The seizure would then be classified as a *simple partial seizure with secondary generalization*. Other patients may have a CPS with secondary generalization. Generalized tonic-clonic seizures, whether primary generalized or with a partial onset, are always associated with deep postictal sleep.

EEG. The interictal EEG in patients with generalized tonic-clonic seizures that have a partial onset have similar features to what was described earlier for patients with partial seizures. Patients with primary generalized tonic-clonic seizures may have a variety of findings varying from a normal EEG, generalized spike-wave discharges, or multifocal spikes usually in the frontal lobes. Patients may have photoconvulsive responses during photic stimulation (Fig. 11-5). Persistent focal discharges are suggestive of partial seizures with secondary generalization.

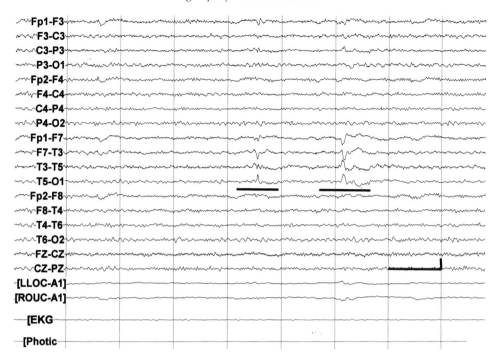

FIGURE 11–1

Left mid-temporal sharp waves (underlined) in a 16-year-old child with complex partial seizures arising from the temporal lobe. Calibration, 1 sec/50 μV.

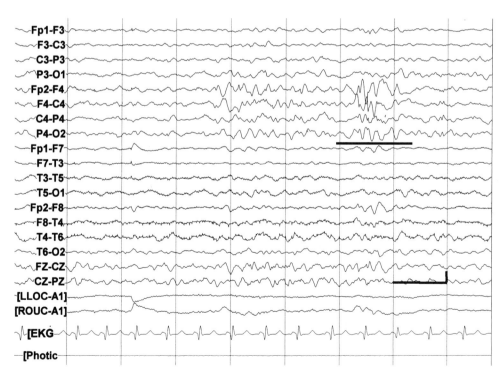

FIGURE 11–2

Right frontal sharp and slow wave complex (underlined) in 9-year-old child with complex partial seizures arising from the frontal lobe. Calibration, 1 sec/50 μV.

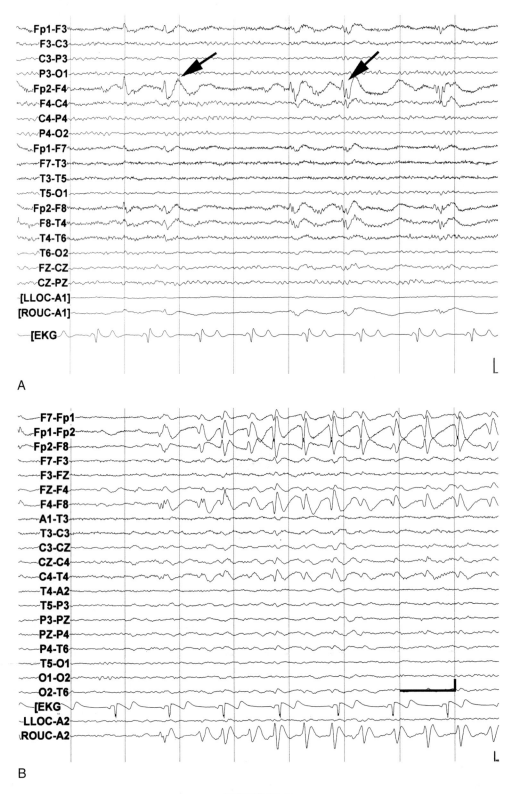

FIGURE 11–3

A, *Right frontal sharp and slow wave complexes (arrows) in an 8-year-old child with complex partial seizures arising from the frontal lobe. B, During drowsiness rhythmic sharp waves arising from the right frontal region (Fp2) occurred. No clinical signs or symptoms accompanied the run of discharges. Calibration, 1 sec/50 μV.*

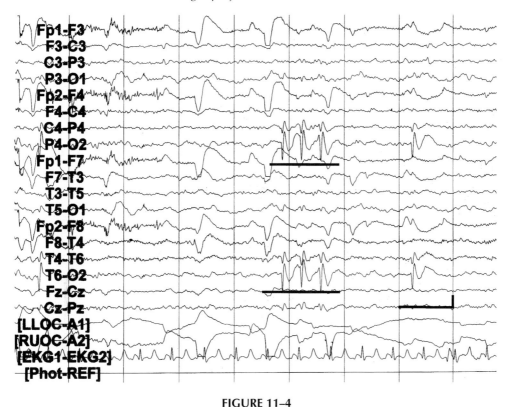

FIGURE 11–4

Right occipital spike and slow wave complexes (underlined) in a 4-year-old child with partial seizures with secondary generalization. Calibration, 1 sec/50 μV.

Absence Seizures

Absence seizures are generalized seizures, indicating bihemispheric initial involvement clinically and electroencephalographically.[6] Absence seizures have an abrupt onset and offset. There is typically a sudden cessation of activities with a "blank" or "distant" look to the face. As the seizure continues, there are often automatisms and mild clonic motor activity such as jerks of the arms and eye blinking.

The terms *typical* and *atypical absence seizures* were used by the International Classification of Epilepsies and Epileptic Syndromes to describe and categorize the various absence types. Many children with absence seizures can be further categorized as having a characteristic epileptic syndrome.

The prototype simple typical absence consists of the sudden onset of impaired consciousness, usually associated with a blank, distant facial appearance without other motor or behavioral phenomena. This subtype is actually relatively rare.[7] The complex typical absence, alternatively, is accompanied by other motor, behavioral, or autonomic phenomena.

Atypical absence seizures are characterized as having more pronounced changes in tone and longer duration than typical absence. However, there is a considerable overlap between typical and atypical absences.[8]

Both typical and atypical absences start abruptly without an aura, lasting from a few seconds to half a minute, and end abruptly.

EEG. The EEG signature of a typical absence seizure is the sudden onset of 3-Hz generalized symmetrical spike- or multiple spike-wave complexes (Fig. 11-6). The voltage of the discharge is often maximal in the frontal-central regions. The frequency tends to be faster, about 4 Hz, at the onset and slows to 2 Hz toward the end of discharges lasting longer than 10 seconds. The spike-and-wave discharge may be precipitated by hyperventilation or photic stimulation. The onset and offset of the spike-waves are usually abrupt although occasionally bifrontal spikes may precede the generalized discharge. EEG abnormalities other than generalized spike-wave are common. Holmes and associates[8] reported that only 44% of 27 patients with typical absences had totally normal EEG backgrounds. Diffuse slowing was seen in 22%, paroxysmal spikes or sharp waves in 37%, and posterior rhythmic delta (<4 Hz) in 15%.

The spike-and-wave discharges are more numerous during all sleep states except rapid eye movement (REM). The spike-wave bursts have a modified appearance in

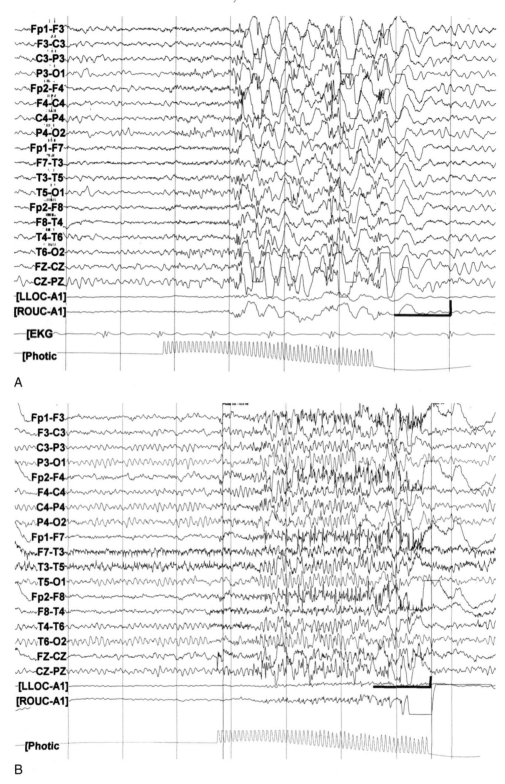

FIGURE 11–5

A, *Photoconvulsive response at 13 Hz in a 12-year-old child with primary generalized tonic-clonic seizures. Note the slow spike-and-wave that continued beyond the end of the photic stimulation. Calibration, 1 sec/50 µV. B, Photoconvulsive response at 13 Hz in a 16-year-old child with primary generalized seizures. The discharges ended before the photic stimulation ended. Calibration, 1 sec/50 µV.*

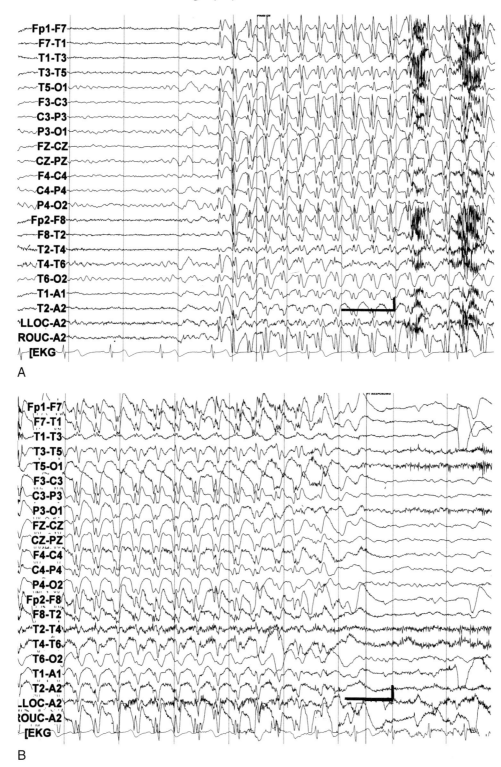

FIGURE 11–6

A *and* B, *Absence seizures demonstrating 3-Hz spike-and-wave activity. The patient is 8 years old. Calibration, 1 sec/50 µV.*

sleep and typically are briefer, irregular, and slow to 1.5 to 2.5 Hz. Hyperventilation, photic stimulation, and hypoglycemia activate typical absence seizures, but hyperventilation is the most effective procedure.

The ictal discharges during an atypical absence seizure are more variable. They typically occur at frequencies between 1.5 and 2.5 Hz and are irregular or asymmetrical in voltage (Fig. 11-7). Only 11% of 27 patients with atypical absences had a normal interictal EEG in the study by Holmes and associates.[8] Diffuse slowing and focal or multifocal spikes or sharp waves were seen in 85%. Sleep often activates the spike-wave discharges.

Clinical effects are generally perceived accompanying discharges lasting longer than 3 seconds. Detailed neuropsychological investigations have demonstrated functional impairment from a spike-and-wave burst of any duration. Auditory reaction times were delayed 56% of the time when a stimulus was presented at the onset of the EEG paroxysm.[9,10] They were abnormal in 80% when the stimulus was delayed 0.5 second. Responsiveness may improve as the paroxysm continues.

Clonic Seizures

Clonic seizures are similar to generalized tonic-clonic seizures, but only have rhythmic or semirhythmic contractions of a group of muscles. These jerks can involve any muscle group although the arms, neck, and facial muscles are most commonly involved. Clonic seizures are much more common in children than adults.

EEG. The interictal EEG pattern seen in patients with clonic seizures is similar to those with generalized tonic-clonic seizures. The ictal pattern usually consists of spike-wave discharges.

Myoclonic Seizures

Myoclonic seizures are characterized by sudden, brief (<350 milliseconds), shocklike contractions that may be generalized or confined to the face and trunk or to one or more extremities, or even to individual muscles or groups of muscles. Myoclonic seizures result in short bursts of synchronized electromyographic activity, which often involves simultaneous activation of agonist and antagonist muscles. The contractions of muscles are quicker than the contractions with clonic seizures. Any group of muscles can be involved in the jerk. Myoclonic seizures may be dramatic, causing the patient to fall to the ground, or be quite subtle, resembling tremors. Because of the brevity of the seizures it is not possible to determine if consciousness is impaired. Myoclonus may occur as a component of an absence seizure or at the beginning of a generalized tonic-clonic seizure. Myoclonic seizures are usually associated with generalized spike-and-wave activity.

EEG. The interictal EEG pattern seen in patients with myoclonic seizures consists of generalized spike-wave or multifocal spikes, or is normal (Figs. 11-8 and 11-9).

Tonic Seizures

Tonic seizures are brief seizures (usually <60 seconds) consisting of the sudden onset of increased tone in the extensor muscles. If standing, the patient typically falls to the ground. The seizures are invariably longer than myoclonic seizures. Electromyographic activity is dramatically increased in tonic seizures. There is impairment of consciousness during the seizure, although in short seizures this may be difficult to assess. Tonic seizures are frequently seen in patients with the Lennox-Gastaut syndrome, a disorder consisting of a mixed seizure disorder, mental retardation, and the EEG findings of a slow spike-and-wave pattern (see later).[11,12]

EEG. The EEG ictal manifestations of tonic seizures usually consist of bilateral synchronous spikes of 10 to 25 Hz of medium to high voltage with a frontal accentuation (Fig. 11-10).[13] Marked suppression—termed *desynchronization*—may also occur (Fig. 11-11). Occasional multiple spike-and-wave or diffuse slow activity may occur during a tonic seizure. The interictal EEG has features similar to those seen in the other generalized seizures (Fig. 11-12).

Atonic Seizures

Atonic (astatic) seizures, or drop attacks, are characterized by a sudden loss of muscle tone. They begin suddenly and without warning and cause the patient, if standing, to fall quickly to the floor. Since there may be total lack of tone, children have no means to protect themselves and injuries often occur. The attack may be fragmentary and lead to dropping of the head with slackening of the jaw or dropping of a limb. In atonic seizures there should be a loss of electromyographic activity. Consciousness is impaired during the fall, although the patient may regain alertness immediately on hitting the floor. Atonic attacks are frequently associated with myoclonic jerks either before, during, or after the atonic seizure.[14,15] This combination has been described as *myoclonic-astatic seizures* (see later). Atonic seizures are rare. Most children with drop attacks have myoclonic or tonic seizures.[16]

EEG. The interictal EEG has features similar to those seen in the other generalized seizures. Atonic seizures are usually associated with rhythmic spike-and-wave complexes varying from slow (1 to 2 Hz) to more rapid, irregular spike- or multiple spike-and-wave activity (Fig. 11-13). Many children with atonic seizures have background slowing as well.

Text continued on p. 233

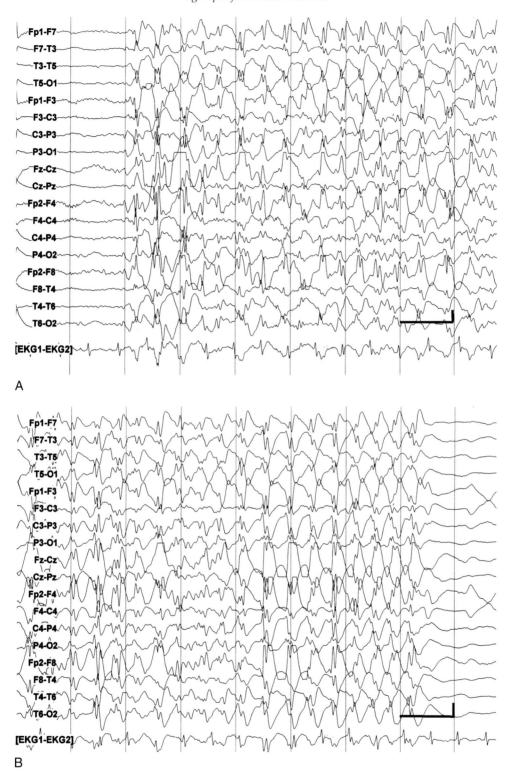

FIGURE 11–7

A and B, *Atypical absence seizure. The spike-and-wave discharges are slower and more irregular than those seen during a typical absence seizure. The patient is 9 years old. Calibration, 1 sec/50 μV.*

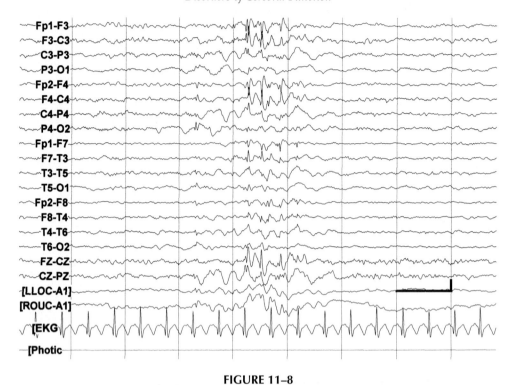

FIGURE 11–8

Irregular spike-and-wave in a 2-year-old child with myoclonic seizures. Calibration, 1 sec/50 μV.

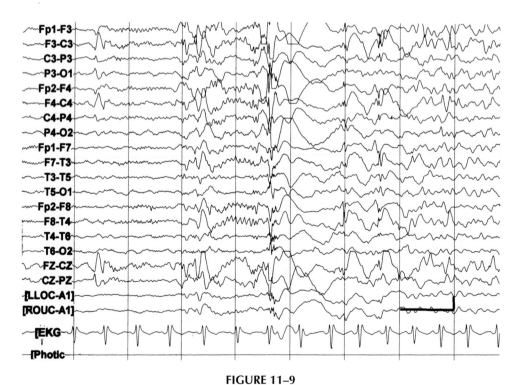

FIGURE 11–9

Irregular spike and multiple spike-and-wave in an 8-month-old infant with myoclonic seizures. Calibration, 1 sec/50 μV.

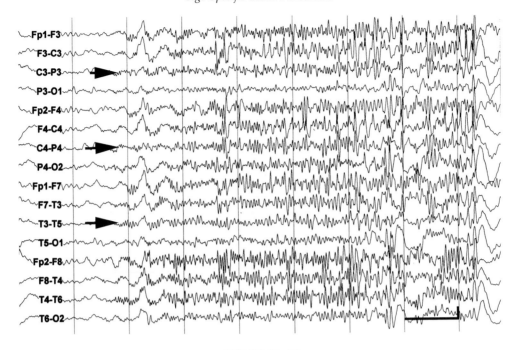

FIGURE 11–10

Rapid spikes in a 9-year-old child with tonic seizures. Arrows mark onset of seizure. Calibration, 1 sec/50 μV.

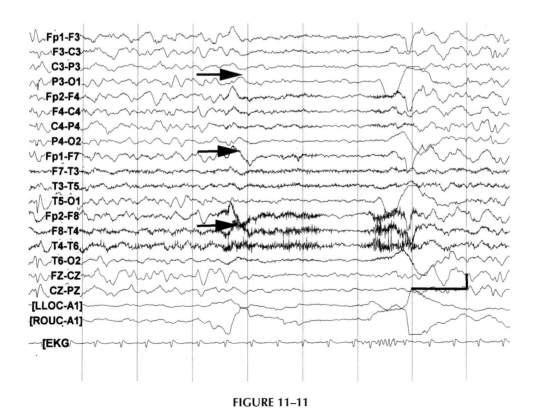

FIGURE 11–11

Brief tonic seizure with an electrodecremental pattern in a 6-year-old girl with tonic seizures. Arrows mark the onset of the seizure. During this seizure the child had subtle trunk flexion and extension of her arms. Calibration, 1 sec/50 μV.

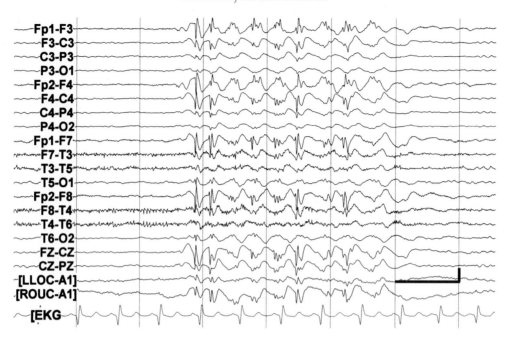

FIGURE 11–12

Interictal irregular spike-and-wave activity in the same 9-year-old child with the tonic seizures depicted in Figure 11-10. Calibration, 1 sec/50 µV.

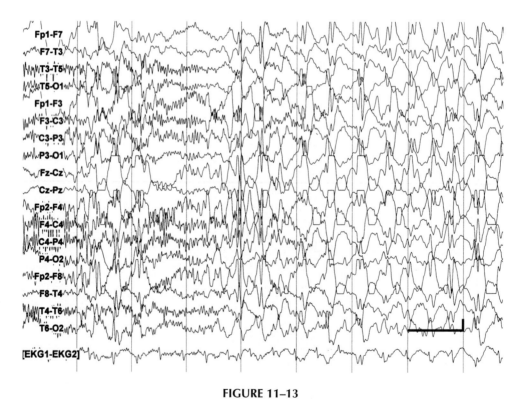

FIGURE 11–13

Irregular spike-and-wave discharges in an 8-year-old child with tonic and atonic seizures. Calibration, 1 sec/100 µV.

EPILEPTIC SYNDROMES

The International Classification of Epilepsies and Epileptic Syndromes (see Box 11-2) divides seizure syndromes into two major categories.[17] The first divides epilepsies with generalized seizures (generalized epilepsies) from epilepsies with partial or focal seizures (localization-related partial or focal epilepsies); the other separates epilepsies of known etiology (symptomatic or secondary epilepsies) from those that are idiopathic (primary) or cryptogenic.

Idiopathic-Related Partial Epilepsies

Although the clinical boundaries of the benign focal epilepsies continue to evolve, the diagnostic criteria include (1) normal neurologic examinations; (2) normal intelligence; (3) normal neuroimaging; (4) a family history of seizures, especially benign types; (5) brief seizures that are stereotyped in clinical manifestation; (6) frequent nocturnal occurrence of the seizures; (7) seizures that are easily controlled with antiepileptic drugs; and (8) frequent remission of the seizures during adolescence.[18] The principal EEG features include (1) normal background activity; (2) spikes with a characteristic morphology and location; (3) activation during sleep; and (4) occasional generalized spike-wave discharges.[19]

Two idiopathic localization-related epileptic syndromes have been delineated: childhood benign epilepsy with central-temporal spikes (BECTS) and childhood epilepsy with occipital paroxysms (CEOP) (benign occipital epilepsy).[17] However, other benign syndromes have been described and likely will be included in further classifications. All of these syndromes are briefly discussed.

Childhood Benign Epilepsy with Central-Temporal Spikes

BECTS is a genetic disorder confined to children that is characterized by nocturnal generalized seizures of probable focal onset and diurnal partial seizures arising from the lower rolandic area and an EEG pattern consisting of a mid-temporal–central spike foci.[20-22] The disorder is also known as *benign rolandic epilepsy*. The disorder always begins during childhood. The age range is from 3 to 13 years, with a peak of age incidence between 7 and 8 years of life. The disorder occurs somewhat more frequently in boys than girls. Most children have normal neurologic examinations and intelligence.

EEG. The characteristic interictal EEG abnormality is a high-amplitude, usually diphasic spike with a prominent following slow wave. The spikes (<70 millisecond) or sharp waves (<200 millisecond) appear singly or in groups at the mid-temporal (T3, T4) and central (rolandic) region (C3, C4) (Figs. 11-14 and 11-15). Using bipolar recording montages, the spikes may be most prominent in the central regions or mid-temporal region and usually occur synchro-

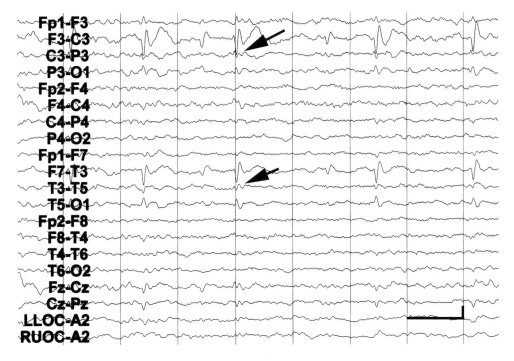

FIGURE 11–14

Central-temporal spikes in a 9-year-old child with benign rolandic epilepsy. Note phase reversals at C3-P3 and T3-T5 (arrows). Calibration, 1 sec/50 μV.

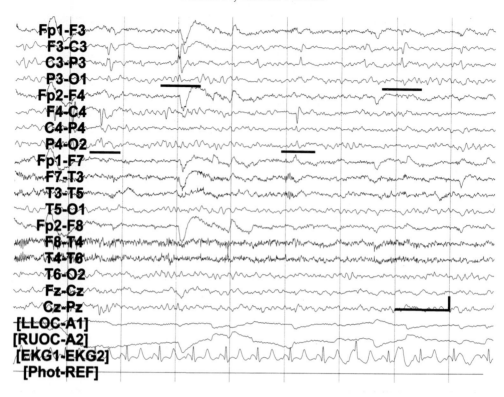

FIGURE 11–15

Bilateral central-temporal spikes (underlined) in an 11-year-old child with benign rolandic epilepsy. Calibration, 1 sec/50 μV.

nously in both the central and mid-temporal region. In a bipolar montage the spike may be very high in amplitude, reflecting a sharp gradient in the dipole. For example, in Figure 11-14, the spike is quite high in amplitude in F3-C3 but of considerable lower amplitude in C3-P3. This suggests that F3 is "seeing" some of the positivity of the dipole while C3 is primarily negative. This results in the high pen deflection. However, in C3-P3 both C3 and P3 are seeing the negative field and pen deflection is less. Although they are typically present in both the central and temporal regions, at times they may shift from one region to the other or only be seen in the mid-temporal or central region.

The spikes may be confined to one hemisphere or occur bilaterally. In approximately 60% of patients the spike focus is unilateral, whereas in 40% there are bilateral spike foci either on the initial EEG or on subsequent recordings.[23] When unilateral, there is an equal representation of spikes in the left and right hemisphere. When bilateral, the spikes can be synchronous or asynchronous, symmetrical or asymmetrical. Magnetoencephalographic analysis of bilaterally synchronous discharges have demonstrated that with bilateral discharges there is a rapid propagation to the contralateral hemisphere, possibly via the corpus callosum.

Rolandic spikes usually occur on a normal background (see Fig. 11-15). However, when the spikes occur frequently, there may be the appearance of focal slowing in the region of the spikes. This "pseudo-slowing" is secondary to the slow waves accompanying the spikes rather than an abnormality of underlying background activity. The spikes are often activated by sleep.[24-27] In approximately 30% of children with BECTS, spikes appear only in sleep.[28] Sleep states are usually normal in BECTS. However, Rose and Duron[29] reported that rolandic spikes were modulated by the type of sleep (REM or non-REM [NREM]), with spikes decreasing during REM sleep.

Rarely, EEGs show generalized spike-wave discharges without any concomitant clinical signs of absence seizures.[30] These diffuse spike-and-wave discharges, which can occasionally occur during the awake state, are strongly activated by sleep. However, children with BECTS with spike-wave discharges rarely have typical absence seizures and have no impairment or alteration of consciousness during the episodes.

Rolandic spikes characteristically have a horizontal dipole (Fig. 11-16).[31-34] Topographic EEG investigations with voltage mapping in children with rolandic spikes have demonstrated maximum negativity of the spikes over the central or mid-temporal electrodes and positivity in the frontal

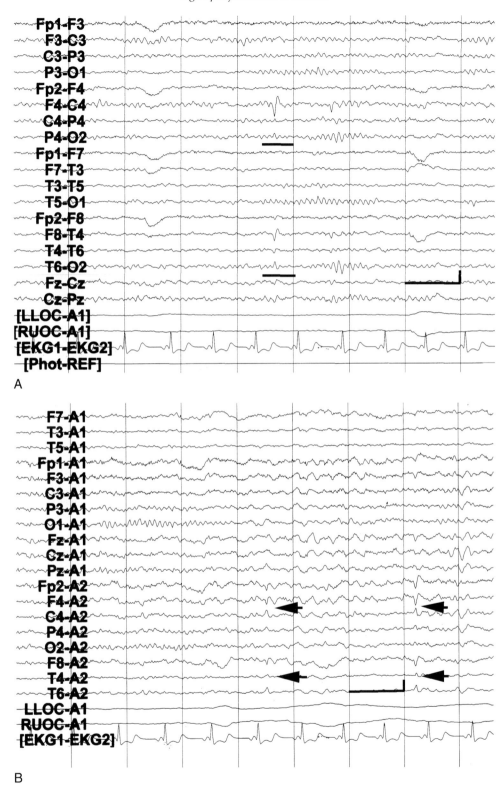

FIGURE 11–16

A, *Right central-temporal spikes (underlined) in a 12-year-old child with benign rolandic epilepsy. Calibration, 1 sec/50 μV.*
B, *Referential montage demonstrating phase reversal at horizontal dipole. F4 and F8 are positive, resulting in downward deflection in F4-A2 and F8-A2. C4 and T6, and to a lesser degree T4, are negative, resulting in upward deflections in C4-A2, T4-A2, and T6-A2. Arrows mark the phase reversals in the average reference montage. Calibration, 1 sec/50 μV.*

regions. Gregory and Wong[35] found a stereotypic dipole field present along the rolandic region in all spikes recorded from children with BECTS. During its most prominent phase, the negative pole of the dipole was maximum at the central-temporal region, with the positive pole in the bifrontal region. A hypothesis was proposed that all discharges arose from a single generator that was oriented tangential to the surface. The generator was most likely situated in the lower rolandic region where the zero potential zone existed, between the frontal positivity and the central-temporal negativity. Gregory and Wong[32] compared the clinical presentation of 99 children with temporal-frontal dipole discharges with 267 children with nondipole rolandic discharges. The clinical profile was substantially different in the two groups: children with a dipole were less likely to have frequent seizures, developmental delay, abnormal neurologic examinations, and school difficulties than the group without a dipole.

Children with BECTS may have spikes in areas other than the central and mid-temporal region. In some patients, occipital spikes are seen, and it is not unusual for EEGs that initially have occipital spikes to evolve into rolandic spikes.[36]

There is not a strong correlation between the frequency and location of the spikes and the frequency, length, and duration of the seizures. Although multiple spikes are unusual, some patients with the typical clinical course of BECTS have multiple-spike discharges. Conversely, some patients with typical rolandic spikes have frequent, medically intractable seizures. Spike frequency varies significantly from patient to patient and may vary, in the same patient, from record to record. Rose and Duron[29] studied the effects of medication on rolandic spikes on the awake EEG before and during treatment. During treatment, the authors found that generalized paroxysmal discharges decreased. However, the presence or absence of either focal or generalized discharges was not related to prognosis.

Physicians rarely have the opportunity to record a seizure from a patient with BECTS since seizure frequency is usually low. Dalla Bernardina and Tassinari[37] recorded a seizure during stage II of sleep. The initial discharge began with low-voltage fast activity in the central-temporal area on one side, then spread to the entire ipsilateral hemisphere and finally to the contralateral side. Gutierrez and colleagues[38] recorded a subclinical seizure from an 8-year-old boy with BECTS. Interictally, the child had typical left central-temporal spikes with a horizontal dipole. The ictal discharges began with left-sided low-amplitude beta, which gradually decreased in frequency and became sharply contoured. This activity was followed by multiple spike-wave discharges.

Not all patients with rolandic spikes or sharp waves have seizures. In a study of focal epileptic EEG discharges in children *without* clinical seizures, Lerman and Kivity-Ephraim[39] reported that 95% had central-temporal spikes. In a large study of 315 patients with rolandic spikes, Beaussart[40] found that 19.3% did not have a history of seizures.

Central spikes also occur commonly in Rett syndrome[41] and fragile X syndrome.[42] In both syndromes the spikes may be similar in location and morphology to BECTS. Focal cortical myoclonus with rolandic cortical dysplasia may be associated with rolandic spikes.[43] Fischer and Clancy[44] reported 21 children with epileptogenic discharges arising from midline electrodes (Fz, Cz, Pz). In five children, midline foci spread preferentially to the adjacent central-parietal region and closely resembled the appearance of benign rolandic foci in the longitudinal EEG montages, a potentially serious cause of EEG misinterpretation. The prognosis for midline spikes is much less favorable than benign rolandic epilepsy.

On rare occasions, typical rolandic spikes may be seen in children with tumors and other structural lesions.[45] Nevertheless, it is highly unlikely that in the presence of a normal neurologic examination and the absence of focal slowing on the EEG that a tumor is the cause of the seizures.

Childhood Epilepsy with Occipital Paroxysms (CEOP)

There are two distinct forms of CEOP. The early-onset type, or Panayiotopoulos syndrome, occurs in young children with a peak of onset of 5 years. The late onset, or Gastaut, type has an age of onset of around 8 to 9 years. Both syndromes are associated with occipital spikes.

The early-onset type (Panayiotopoulos syndrome) is characterized by ictal vomiting and deviation of the eyes, often with impairment of consciousness and progression to generalized tonic-clonic seizures.[46,47] The seizures are infrequent and often solitary, but in about one third of the children the episodes evolve into partial status epilepticus. Two thirds of the seizures occur during sleep. The late-onset (Gastaut) type consists of brief seizures with mainly visual symptoms such as elementary visual hallucinations, illusions, or amaurosis, followed by hemiclonic convulsions. Postictal migraine headaches occur in half of the patients.[48,49]

EEG. The interictal EEG in Panayiotopoulos syndrome is characterized by normal background activity with spikes at a variety of locations. Approximately two thirds of patients have one EEG with occipital spikes.[50] Spikes are similar in morphology and amplitude to those seen in benign rolandic epilepsy and may be eliminated with eye opening.[50,51] The spikes may be activated with drowsiness and sleep. Brief bursts of generalized spike and slow wave activity may occasionally occur. In the Gastaut-type of childhood occipi-

TABLE 11–4
Syndromes Associated with Occipital Spikes

Syndrome	Age, yr	EEG Features
Panayiotopoulos type	4-5	Multifocal spikes, often occipital
Gastaut type	8-10	Occipital spikes with fixation-off sensitivity
Childhood seizures with occipital spikes	<4	Occipital spikes, not altered by fixation
Occipital spikes with calcifications	All ages	Occipital spikes, not altered by fixation

tal epilepsy, the EEG is characterized by high amplitude (200 to 300 μV) spikes demonstrating fixation-off sensitivity. The amplitude is highest over the occipital and posterior temporal regions and can be unilateral or bilateral. When occurring bilaterally, the spikes are frequently asymmetrical. Occipital spikes are activated by darkness as opposed to eye closure per se.[11,51,52] The effect of darkness is due to abolition of central vision and that paroxysms are inhibited by fixation, even when it occurs in darkness.[51] Hyperventilation and photic stimulation rarely activate occipital spikes.[18,51,53] Although spikes on eye closure is a common feature in this syndrome, some patients do not exhibit this characteristic.[50] Generalized bilaterally synchronous spike-wave or multiple spike-wave discharge or central-temporal spikes may occur in the condition.[48,54]

Occipital spikes can also be seen in other seizure disorders in children (Table 11-4). Children younger than 4 years of age often have occipital spikes that occur both during eye opening and eye closure. Only 54.4% of 318 children with occipital spikes studied by Smith and Kellaway[55] had seizures. Unlike in benign CEOP, the seizures typically do not include visual phenomena or postictal headaches.

Gobbi and colleagues[56-58] reported children considered to have benign occipital epilepsy, with occipital spikes, who subsequently showed a mental deterioration and worsening of seizures and who were found to have occipital calcification. Subsequent investigations revealed that these patients had celiac disease and malabsorption of folic acid.

Children with myoclonic, absence, and photosensitive epilepsies may have occipital spikes but would not be classified as having benign occipital epilepsy.[51] Finally, children with visual defects may have occipital spikes and not have seizures.[59,60]

Autosomal Dominant Nocturnal Familial Lobe Epilepsy

Autosomal dominant nocturnal familial lobe epilepsy (ADNFLE) is a disorder in which nocturnal partial sei-

zures begin during the first 2 decades of life.[61-63] Over half of the patients have secondarily generalized seizures. While the motor activity that occurs may be quite severe, usually the seizures are controlled with drug therapy. Normal neurologic examinations and neuroimaging are the rule. Two different mutations have been described in the α_4 subunit of the neuronal nicotinic acetylcholine receptor on chromosome 20q13.2. Phillips and colleagues[64] found linkage of the disorder to 15q24 in one family and exclusion from 15q24 and 20q13.2 in others, demonstrating genetic heterogeneity with at least three different genes for the condition.

EEG. The EEG features in this syndrome are not distinctive. The interictal EEG is often normal or has frontal or temporal spikes.[65]

Benign Epilepsy with Affective Symptoms (Benign Psychomotor Epilepsy)

In benign epilepsy with affective symptoms, children have CPSs in whom affective symptoms, predominately fear, are the major clinical features.[66] Clinically the initial feature of the seizure is sudden fright. This then proceeds to yelling or calling for the mother, clinging to someone nearby, or trying to hide. The terrorized expression on the face is sometimes associated with chewing, swallowing, distressed laughter, pallor, sweating, or abdominal pain. During the seizures some degree of impaired consciousness is apparent. The average duration is 1 to 2 minutes and is frequently followed by sleep. The seizures occur during the wake or sleep states and are often frequent, occurring several times a day. Generalized tonic-clonic seizures are not observed. In most children the course is benign.[66]

EEG. EEG background activity is normal. The most frequent interictal abnormality is a spike with a following slow wave in the frontal-temporal or parietal-temporal area of one or both hemispheres. Other patients have rhythmic sharp waves in the frontal-temporal or the parietal or temporal area of one hemisphere. These abnormalities fluctuate during the course of the disorder and are activated by sleep. In 58% of the cases, brief bursts of generalized spike and wave, alone or in association with focal abnormalities, are seen.

Benign Partial Epilepsy of Adolescence

Benign partial epilepsy of adolescence is a syndrome in which patients between the ages of 10 and 20 years develop one or a cluster of partial seizures, either simple or complex, occurring over a 1 to 2 day period of time.[67,68] The partial seizures become secondarily generalized in some patients. A family history of epilepsy is rare.[67] The outcome is excellent with no recurrences noted.[67]

EEG. EEGs are either normal or show non-specific abnormalities.

Benign Partial Epilepsy with Extreme Somatosensory Evoked Potentials

Benign partial epilepsy with extreme somatosensory evoked potentials is a condition in which tapping the sole of the foot in some children elicits high-voltage evoked potentials, consisting of spikes, up to 400 μV in amplitude, in the contralateral parietal and parasagittal region.[69-72] Tassinari and De Marco[71] described 16 children in which tapping the sole of the feet elicited these spikes, termed *extreme somatosensory evoked potentials*, and seizures. The authors described an evolution from the provocation of these spikes with stimulation, to spontaneous spikes, to partial seizures. The seizures typically are simple partial with versive movements of the head, although other seizure types (tonic, generalized tonic-clonic, and somatosensory) are reported. At times, the seizures are quite frequent, and partial status has been reported. However, in all patients the seizure disorder ends by 9 years of age.

EEG. The EEG is usually normal, except when stimulation of the foot occurs.

Generalized Syndromes

Benign Familial Neonatal Seizures

The diagnosis of benign familial neonatal seizures in a child with seizures[73-75] is based on the following five criteria:

1. Normal neurologic examination
2. Negative evaluation for another etiology of the seizures
3. Normal developmental and intellectual outcome
4. Positive family history of newborn or infantile seizures with benign outcome
5. Onset of seizures during the neonatal or early infantile period

Linkage analysis has demonstrated two loci for the disorder located on chromosomes 20q13.3 and 8q24.[76,77] The genetic markers on chromosomes 20q13.1 and 8q24 has been termed *epilepsy benign neonatal type 1 (EBN1)* and *EBN2*, respectively. The genes, KCNQ2 and KCNQ3, encode subunits of the M-channel, a widely expressed potassium channel that mediates effects of modulatory neurotransmitters and controls repetitive neuronal discharges.[78]

The seizures are usually frequent for a few days and then they stop. The infant is usually alert and vigorous during the interictal period. Clonic seizures, focal or multifocal, are the most frequent type of seizure, although generalized seizures have been reported. The seizures are generally brief, lasting approximately 1 to 2 minutes, but may occur as many as 20 to 30 times a day.

EEG. The EEG is of little assistance in making the diagnosis of benign familial neonatal seizures since it may or may not be abnormal interictally. No diagnostic features have been reported. When abnormal, the findings are frequently transient. Unfortunately, in many of the case reports that were published, infants either had no EEGs performed or the results were not described in sufficient detail. Abnormalities reported include spikes, sharp waves, and slowing.

Hirsch and colleagues[79] recorded 14 seizures from three children with benign neonatal familial convulsions. All the seizures occurred during sleep and were characterized by an initial flattening on the EEG followed by bilateral discharges of spikes and sharp waves. The authors argued that the seizures were a form of generalized tonic-clonic activity whose expression may be asymmetrical.

Neonatal Idiopathic Seizures (Benign Neonatal Convulsions)

Benign neonatal convulsions, also called *benign neonatal idiopathic seizures*, are characterized by seizures occurring in term, otherwise healthy infants. Criteria used to make the diagnosis include the following:

1. Infants born after 39 weeks of gestation
2. Apgar score of 9 or above at 5 minutes of life
3. The presence of a seizure-free interval between birth and the onset of seizures
4. Clonic and/or apneic seizures
5. Negative evaluations for etiology
6. A favorable outcome in regard to neurologic development
7. Lack of seizures outside the neonatal period

Some authors have reported such seizures as "fifth-day fits."[80] It is likely that benign idiopathic neonatal seizures and fifth-day fits are identical syndromes.

Typically, the seizures begin on the fifth day of life, hence the eponym *fifth-day fits*. The seizures are usually partial clonic in type and may be confined to one body part or migrate from one region to another. Apnea may occur with the clonic activity or be the sole manifestation of the seizure. The seizures often occur in a crescendo of activity sometimes culminating in status epilepticus. Initially, the patient is normal between the seizures. The seizures then increase in frequency until status epilepticus. The flurry of seizures usually lasts less than 24 hours, although seizures may continue for a few days.

EEG. Like benign familial neonatal seizures, EEG findings in benign idiopathic neonatal seizures have been variable. In a survey of 101 EEGs from infants with the disorder, the interictal EEG was normal in 10, excessively discontinuous in 6, showed "focal or multifocal" abnormalities in 25, and demonstrated "theta pointu alternant" in 60.[80] The theta pointu alternant pattern consists of dominant theta activity, which is discontinuous, unreactive, and often asynchronous and has intermixed sharp waves. It is present throughout sleep and awaking state and may persist up to the 12th day of life, even after the seizures have ceased. The theta pointu alternant pattern is not specific for benign seizures and can be seen following a variety of neonatal encephalopathies.

Benign Myoclonic Epilepsy in Infancy

Benign myoclonic epilepsy in infants is a rare syndrome in which brief bouts of generalized myoclonus occur during the first or second year of life.[81,82] The EEGs typically show generalized spike-waves occurring in brief bursts during the early stages of sleep. The infants do not have other seizure types although generalized tonic-clonic seizures may occur during adolescence. The seizures are usually easily controlled with antiepileptic drugs and limited to the first few years of life.

Absence Seizures

Absence seizures can be classified into two subtypes: typical and atypical.[6] Typical absence seizures are the primary seizures in two syndromes: childhood absence seizures and juvenile absence seizures. Atypical absence seizures most commonly occur in Lennox-Gastaut syndrome. There are four syndromes in which absence seizures are a major component: childhood absence epilepsy (pyknolepsy), juvenile absence epilepsy, juvenile myoclonic epilepsy (impulsive petit mal), and epilepsy with myoclonic absences. The absence epilepsies appear to have a complex genetic basis; some may be autosomal dominant with an age-dependent, high penetrance.

Childhood Absence Epilepsy (Pyknolepsy)

Pyknolepsy describes typical absence seizures (i.e., both simple and complex) in children between the ages of 3 to 5 years and puberty, who are otherwise normal. There is a strong genetic predisposition, and girls are more frequently affected. The absences are very frequent, occurring at least several times daily, and tend to cluster. The absences typically remit during adolescence, but generalized tonic-clonic seizures may develop.

EEG. The EEG reveals a bilateral, synchronous symmetrical 3-Hz spike-and-wave discharge with normal interictal background activity.

Juvenile Absence Epilepsy

Juvenile absence epilepsy begins around puberty and differs from pyknolepsy in that the seizures are more sporadic and retropulsive movements are less common. This syndrome blurs with juvenile myoclonic epilepsy, as generalized tonic-clonic seizures and myoclonic seizures are often seen on awakening. Sex distribution is equal.

EEG. The EEG findings are similar to childhood absence epilepsy except that the spike-waves are often slightly faster than 3 Hz.

Juvenile Myoclonic Epilepsy (JME)

Juvenile myoclonic epilepsy is a familial disorder that typically begins in the 2nd decade of life and is characterized by mild myoclonic seizures, generalized tonic-clonic or clonic-tonic-clonic seizures (a variation of generalized tonic-clonic seizures in which there is an initial clonic phase), and occasionally, absence seizures. The myoclonic seizures are usually mild to moderate in intensity and involve the neck, shoulders, and arms. They can occur either singularly or repetitively and may cause the patient to drop objects.

Rarely, the jerks may involve the legs and cause the patient to fall to the ground. There have been multiple attempts at determining the gene(s) for the disorder. It now appears clear that there is not a single gene that accounts for all of the cases and that there is considerable genetic and locus heterogeneity in the disorder.

EEG. The interictal EEG in this disorder is distinctive and easily distinguished from other forms of generalized epilepsies. The characteristic feature of the EEG is the fast (3.5- to 6-Hz) spike-and-wave and multiple spike-and-wave complexes (Fig. 11-17). This pattern contrasts with the 3-Hz spike-and-wave complexes seen in classic absence and the slow (1.5- to 2.5-Hz) spike-and-wave complexes of Lennox-Gastaut syndrome. During myoclonic seizures, the ictal EEG consists of 10- to 16-Hz rapid spikes, followed by irregular slow waves. Photosensitivity may activate the epileptiform discharges. If the diagnosis is suspected and the awake EEG is normal, it is imperative that a sleep-deprived EEG be obtained, since this may be the only time the abnormality is present.

Epilepsy with Myoclonic Absences

Epilepsy with myoclonic absences is a syndrome in which patients have rhythmic myoclonic jerks of the shoulders, arms, and legs with a concomitant tonic contraction. Eyelid twitching is usually absent, but perioral myoclonias are frequent. The tonic component mainly affects shoulder and deltoid muscles that may cause elevation of the arms; the duration of the absences varies from 8 to 60 seconds. Myoclonic absences typically occur multiple times daily and last from 8 to 60 seconds.[83]

EEG. The EEG typically shows generalized, rhythmic 3-Hz spike-wave or polyspike-wave.

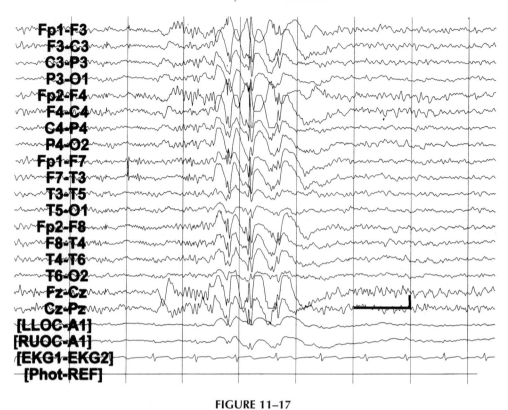

FIGURE 11–17

Rapid spike-and-wave in a patient with juvenile myoclonic epilepsy. Note more rapid spike-and-wave frequency than seen in patients with typical and atypical absence seizures. Calibration, 1 sec/50 μV.

Epilepsy with Grand Mal Seizures on Awakening

Epilepsy with grand mal seizures on awakening is a syndrome in which generalized tonic-clonic seizures occur exclusively or predominantly shortly after awakening.[84,85] The onset is usually in the 2nd decade. If patients have other seizure types, they are usually absence or myoclonic.

EEG. The EEG typically shows generalized spike-wave activity. Photosensitivity is a common feature.

Infantile Spasms

Infantile spasms are a unique and frequently malignant epileptic syndrome confined to infants. The usual characteristic features of this syndrome are tonic or myoclonic seizures, hypsarrhythmic EEGs, and mental retardation.[86] The triad of infantile spasms, hypsarrhythmic EEG, and mental retardation is referred to as *West's syndrome.* Not all infants with infantile spasms conform strictly to this definition. The disorder is also referred to in the literature as *massive spasms*, *salaam seizures*, *flexion* or *flexor spasms*, *jackknife seizures*, and *massive myoclonic jerks.*

Infantile spasms are an age-specific disorder beginning in children only during the first 2 years of life. The peak age of onset is between 4 and 6 months of age. Approximately 90% of infantile spasms begin before 12 months of age.[87] It is rare for infantile spasms to begin during the first 2 weeks of life or after 18 months.

EEG. Infantile spasms are usually associated with markedly abnormal EEGs. The most commonly found EEG pattern is hypsarrhythmia (Fig. 11-18).[88] This pattern consists of high-amplitude slow waves mixed with spikes and sharp waves whose amplitude and topography vary in an asynchronous manner between the two hemispheres. The background activity is completely disorganized and chaotic. During sleep, there are bursts of polyspike and slow waves. Somewhat surprising, in view of the marked background abnormalities, is the presence of sleep spindles in some patients. During REM sleep there may be a marked diminution or complete disappearance of the hypsarrhythmic pattern.[89] Infantile spasms are associated with a decrease of the total sleep time and a decrease in the percentage of REM sleep.[90]

Hrachovy and colleagues[89] reported variations in hypsarrhythmia. These included hypsarrhythmia with interhemispheric synchrony, hypsarrhythmia with a consistent focus of abnormal discharge, hypsarrhythmia with episodes of attenuation, and hypsarrhythmia consisting pri-

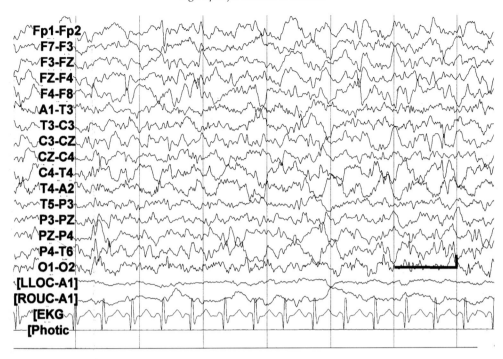

FIGURE 11–18

Hypsarrhythmia in a 5-month-old infant with infantile spasms. Note high-amplitude recording with multifocal spikes and sharp waves. Calibration, 1 sec/100 μV.

marily of high-voltage slow activity with few sharp waves or spikes.

Although a hypsarrhythmic or modified hypsarrhythmic pattern is the most common type of interictal abnormality seen in infantile spasms, this pattern may not be present in some patients with infantile spasms.[91] Some patients with infantile spasms do not have hypsarrhythmia early in the course of the disorder but go on to develop the pattern. Although hypsarrhythmia is primarily associated with infantile spasms, it occurs in other disorders as well.[92,93]

Some patients who eventually develop hypsarrhythmia do not have this pattern at the onset of their clinical spasms. Watanabe and associates[94] described an EEG evolution to hypsarrhythmia with the appearance of focal spikes preceding to multifocal spike or sharp wave discharges prior to hypsarrhythmia. Hypsarrhythmia usually begins during the first year of life, although rarely it can develop after the first year of life.

The ictal EEG changes during infantile spasms are variable.[86,89,95] While Hrachovy and colleagues[89] found 11 different types of ictal EEG patterns that accompanied the clinical seizures, a marked generalized attenuation of electrical activity was a feature of 72% of the seizures. There was not a close correlation between ictal EEG abnormalities and clinical seizure type. The hypsarrhythmic pattern usually disappears between the spasms and reappears at the end of the cluster, or sometimes after it.

In a careful study of the clinical and EEG-polygraphic features of 955 spasms in children with cryptogenic and symptomatic West's syndrome, Fusco and Vigevano[95] found the most characteristic ictal EEG pattern of the spasms consisted of a positive wave over the vertex-central region.

The background EEG activity during a cluster of spasms may vary. In cryptogenic cases hypsarrhythmia usually persists between one spasm and another; disappearance of hypsarrhythmia is observed in symptomatic cases and in infants with cryptogenic spasms who have unfavorable outcomes.[96]

The presence of focality is one of the variations of the basic hypsarrhythmic patterns and may be associated with partial seizures.[89] Partial seizures might precede, accompany, or follow the cluster of spasms.[89,97,98] This observation suggests that cortical "pacemakers" may be important in the development of infantile spasms.[97] Carrazana and colleagues[97,98] reported 16 patients with infantile spasms in whom the onset of the clusters of spasms appeared to be triggered by the close temporal association with partial seizures. Common features included the presence of focal cerebral lesions in 12 infants—3 were classifiable as cryptogenic, and all had partial seizures with EEG localization and clusters of bilateral spasms always preceded by partial seizures.

Although the bilateral spasms were most likely generated at a subcortical level, their close temporal relation with a cortically generated partial seizure strongly suggests that in these 16 patients the infantile spasms were facilitated or possibly induced by the cortical event. The absence of normal interhemispheric connectivity through the corpus callosum in 3 patients mitigated against rapid secondary generalization via this route as a possible explanation for the bilateral spasms.

The EEG is quite useful in differentiating infantile spasms from nonepileptic attacks that clinically resemble infantile spasms. Lombroso and Fejerman[99] described a syndrome that begins in infancy with the flexion spasms. However, the syndrome differed from West's syndrome in the absence of mental retardation or regression and the EEG is normal both during wakefulness and sleep. Dravet and colleagues[100] reported four cases of benign spasms. The infants had short (2- to 4-second) tonic contractions during either the awake or sleep states. The EEGs were normal in all cases. The authors proposed the name *benign nonepileptic infantile spasms* for the syndrome.

Lennox-Gastaut Syndrome

Lennox-Gastaut syndrome is characterized by a mixed seizure disorder of which tonic seizures are a major component along with a slow spike-and-wave EEG pattern.[101-103] The syndrome always begins in childhood. Almost all children with the syndrome are mentally retarded. The child with Lennox-Gastaut syndrome typically has a mixture of seizure types. The most frequently occurring are tonic, tonic-clonic, myoclonic, atypical absences, and "head drops," which represent a form of atonic, tonic, or myoclonic seizures.

Tonic seizures are a major component of this syndrome. They are typically activated by sleep and may occur repetitively throughout the night. They are much more frequent during NREM sleep than during wakefulness and usually do not occur during REM sleep. In Lennox-Gastaut syndrome, tonic seizures are usually brief, lasting from a few seconds to 1 minute, with an average duration of about 10 seconds. The seizures may cause falls and injury. Eyelid retraction, staring, mydriasis, and apnea are commonly associated and may be the most prominent features. During tonic seizures the patient is unconscious, although arousal from light sleep may occur. Since they are often very brief, they often go undetected.

Myoclonic seizures, occurring either in isolation or as a component of an absence seizure, can occur in this disorder. Although atonic seizures are common in this syndrome, they occur less frequently than tonic and myoclonic seizures. Most such seizures are quite brief, lasting 1 to 4 seconds. In the briefest attacks, patients may show only head nodding or sagging at the knees.

Patients with Lennox-Gastaut syndrome typically have very frequent seizures.[103,104] Some children with this syndrome have hundreds of seizures daily.

EEG. The sine qua non of the EEG findings in Lennox-Gastaut syndrome is the slow spike-and-wave discharge superimposed on an abnormal, slow background. The slow spike-and-wave or sharp-and-slow-wave complexes consist of generalized discharges occurring at a frequency of 1.5 to 2.5 Hz (see Figs. 11-7 and 11-13). The morphology, amplitude, and repetition rate may vary both between bursts and during paroxysmal bursts of spike-and-wave activity. Transient and shifting asymmetries of the discharge frequently occur. The area of maximum voltage, while variable, is usually frontal or temporal in location. Although sleep increases the frequency of the discharges, hyperventilation and photic stimulation rarely activate these discharges.

During NREM sleep, slow spike-wave discharges may be replaced by multiple-spike-and-wave discharges, whereas in REM sleep the paroxysmal activity decreases markedly. The typical EEG manifestation of tonic seizures is the occurrence of fast rhythm discharges of 10 to 20 Hz, of progressively increasing amplitude, at times followed by a few slow waves or spike-waves. This has previously been called the *grand mal discharges of Gibbs*. Patients may also have bursts of multiple spike-and-wave during a tonic seizure. In atonic seizures the EEG pattern is most frequently a fast-recruiting discharge, but bursts of slow spike-wave complexes or high-amplitude 10-Hz discharges are sometimes recorded. The EEG correlate of myoclonic seizures consists of bursts of arrhythmic multiple spike-wave or irregular spike-wave activity. Atypical absence seizures are associated with slow (<2.5 Hz), often asymmetrical and irregular spike-and-wave activity.

One unique phenomenon of Lennox-Gastaut during sleep is the frequent occurrence of beta ictal discharges (see Fig. 11-10).[13] This is the key point in differential diagnosis with other epileptic syndromes of the same age. Patients may also have bursts of multiple spike-and-wave during a tonic seizure. In atonic seizures the EEG pattern is most frequently a fast-recruiting discharge, but bursts of slow spike-wave complexes or high-amplitude 10 Hz discharges are sometimes recorded. The EEG correlate of myoclonic seizures consists of bursts of arrhythmic multiple spike-wave or irregular spike-wave activity. Atypical absence seizures have been associated with a variety of patterns: slow (<2.5 Hz), often asymmetrical, irregular spike-and-wave activity, irregular diffuse fast activity occurring at a frequency of 10 to 13 Hz, or a combination of fast spike-and-waves or sharp waves of increasing amplitude followed by synchronous spike-and-wave discharges occurring at 3 Hz.

In atonic or myoclonic-atonic seizures the EEG pattern most frequently demonstrates bursts of slow spike-wave complexes or high-amplitude 10-Hz discharges.[13] The EEG correlate of myoclonic seizures consists of bursts of arrhythmic multiple spike-wave or irregular spike-wave activity. Atypical absence seizures are associated with slow (<2.5 Hz), often asymmetrical and irregular spike-and-wave activity.[8]

Multiple Independent Spike Foci Syndrome

Multiple independent spike foci syndrome is defined as epileptiform discharges (spikes, sharp waves, or both) which, on any single recording, arise from at least three noncontiguous electrode positions with at least one focus in each hemisphere.[105] Excluded are recordings that contained multiple independent spike foci and also have either hypsarrhythmia or sharp-and-slow wave complexes. This syndrome occurs primarily in children with the same clinical features as Lennox-Gastaut syndrome (i.e., mental retardation and multiple seizure types usually refractory to anticonvulsants). The incidence varies minimally with age; in Blume's study,[105] 40% were younger than 6 years, 25% were 6 to 10 years, and 35% were 11 to 15 years of age.

Eighty-four percent of patients with multiple independent spike foci have seizure disorders[105]; generalized tonic-clonic seizures (44%) were the most common form. Other seizures, in decreasing order, are focal or hemiclonic (25%), absence (21%), tonic (19%), bilateral myoclonic (17%), and versive (13%). More than half of the patients had more than one seizure type.

EEG. The background activity in wakefulness is slow and disorganized. Normal sleep patterns are usually absent, and the sleep may lead to greater synchrony of discharges and a slow spike-and-wave appearance, or an increase in the number of foci. Spikes are most frequently seen in the temporal regions and then, in decreasing order of frequency, the occipital, central, frontal, and parietal regions (Fig. 11-19). Hyperventilation and photic stimulation have little or no effect on the EEG.

Epilepsy with Myoclonic-Astatic Seizures

Epilepsy with myoclonic-astatic seizures is characterized by myoclonic and astatic seizures, often in combination with absence, generalized tonic-clonic, and tonic seizures beginning during childhood.[14,83,106] In this syndrome astatic (defined as the inability to stand) seizures occur suddenly, without warning, and children collapse onto the floor as if their legs had been pulled from under them. No apparent loss of consciousness accompanies these seizures. At times the astatic seizures are so short that only a brief nodding of the head and slight flexion of the knees are seen.

With few exceptions, the mental and motor development of the children is normal before the onset of the illness. However, the prognosis is generally unfavorable,

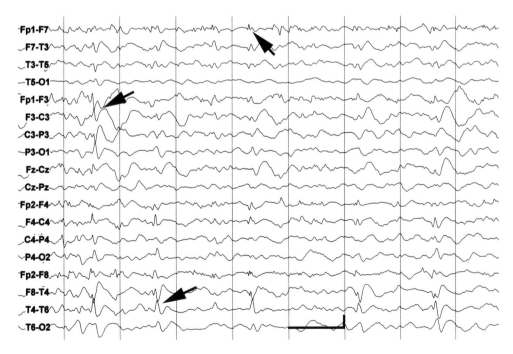

FIGURE 11–19

Multifocal spikes in a 4-year-old child with multiple types of seizures (arrows mark some of the spikes and sharp waves. Calibration, 1 sec/50 μV.

with most patients developing dementia. Absence status is reported to play a role in the pathogenesis of the dementia.

EEG. The characteristic features of the interictal EEG are monomorphic theta rhythms with parietal accentuation as well as occipital 4-Hz rhythm that is blocked by eye opening.[107,108] The EEG is characterized by single or bursts of spike-and-wave activity.[15] The spike-and-wave discharges are irregular in frequency and polymorphic in configuration and usually occur at a frequency of 2 to 3 Hz. Although lateralized discharges occur, typically the discharges shift from hemisphere to hemisphere. Sleep typically activates the spike-and-wave complexes, and photic stimulation results in paroxysmal discharges.

Early Myoclonic Encephalopathy

Early myoclonic encephalopathy is a rare epileptic encephalopathy characterized by erratic, fragmentary myoclonic jerks in association with other types of seizures (especially partial motor seizures and massive myoclonia or infantile spasms, tonic spasm) and suppression-burst pattern on the EEG, occurring within the first 3 months of life.[109,110]

The prognosis is unfavorable. The affected infants are always severely compromised from birth or from the beginning of seizures. There is arrest of psychomotor development and variable neurologic deficits. Death may occur within the first year or two, and most survivors become vegetative if they have not died. Conventional antiepileptic drugs as well as agents such as corticotropin, corticosteroids, and pyridoxine are usually ineffective.

EEG. The EEG features of early myoclonic encephalopathy are quite distinctive. The normal background activity is absent, and the EEG activity in both the waking and sleep states consists of a complex burst of spikes and irregular, arrhythmic spikes, sharp waves, and slow activity lasting for 1 to 5 seconds and alternating with flat periods of 3 to 10 seconds during which there is minimal electrical activity (burst-suppression). The bursts can occur either synchronously or independently over the two hemispheres. Synchronous spike-and-wave activity is never seen. Myoclonic jerks are sometimes, but not always, time linked to the paroxysmal bursts. During partial seizures rhythmic focal spikes or sharp waves are seen. During the seizures the burst-suppression pattern typically continues.

The burst-suppression pattern usually is replaced by atypical hypsarrhythmia or multifocal abnormalities after the first 3 to 5 months of life.[109] The burst-suppression pattern tends to be replaced by atypical hypsarrhythmia after the age of 3 to 5 months. The atypical hypsarrhythmia occurs predominantly during NREM sleep and decreases during REM and the awake states; the suppression-burst

pattern of early myoclonic encephalopathy occurs during both waking and sleep without normal background activity.

Early Infantile Epileptic Encephalopathy

Early infantile epileptic encephalopathy as described by Ohtahara and others[111,112] is characterized by an early onset of tonic spasms and burst-suppression pattern on the EEG. The tonic spasms may or may not occur in flurries. Unlike in early myoclonic encephalopathy, the infants do not have erratic myoclonus. Partial seizures may occur. Neuroimaging frequently demonstrates cerebral dysgenesis.

The prognosis is quite poor with early death or marked psychomotor retardation and seizure intractability with frequent evolution to West's syndrome at 4 to 6 months of age and further to Lennox-Gastaut syndrome in some cases.

EEG. The EEG demonstrates pseudo-periodic burst-suppression with bursts of irregular 150 to 350 μV high-voltage slow waves mixed with spikes, ranging from 1 to 3 seconds in duration followed by an almost flat suppression phase (Fig. 11-20).[111] The burst-burst interval ranges from 5 to 10 seconds. The burst-suppression pattern occurs during the awake and sleep states. Tonic seizures are characterized by diffuse desynchronization of the background.

In infants that survive, the EEG develops into one of several patterns. The records usually evolve from burst-suppression to either focal spikes or generalized polyspike-and-wave activity. Ohtahara and associates[111] noted that in infants that progress to polyspike-and-wave activity a typical sequence is followed: Initially the burst-suppression changes to hypsarrhythmia during the awake state while burst-suppression continues during sleep. As the burst-suppression ends, there is a gradual increase in amplitude of the suppression phase. The next step consists of hypsarrhythmia during both wakefulness and sleep. This is followed by diffuse slow polyspike-and-wave activity during waking state while hypsarrhythmia persists during sleep. Finally, polyspike-and-wave occurs during both wakefulness and sleep.

EPILEPSIES AND SYNDROMES UNDETERMINED AS TO WHETHER THEY ARE FOCAL OR GENERALIZED

Landau-Kleffner Syndrome and Epilepsy with Continuous Spikes and Waves during Slow Sleep

Acquired epileptic aphasia (Landau-Kleffner syndrome) is a rare syndrome characterized by language regression and epileptiform discharges involving the temporal or parietal regions of the brain.[113,114] In this disorder children develop an abrupt or gradual loss of language ability and verbal

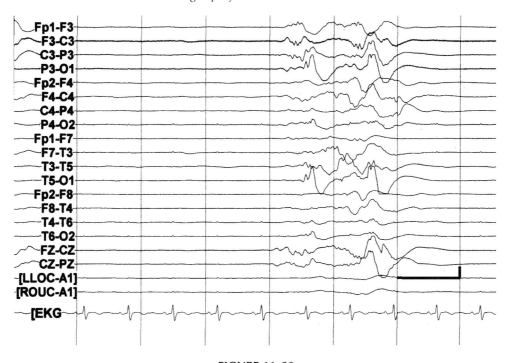

FIGURE 11–20

Burst-suppression pattern in a 4-month-old infant with Ohtahara's syndrome. Calibration, 1 sec/100 μV.

auditory agnosia. This interruption in communication skills is generally closely preceded, accompanied, or followed by the onset of seizures or an abnormal EEG, or both.[115,116] The term *Landau-Kleffner syndrome* variant is used for children with an epileptic aphasia who do not have all the classic features. They include children with pervasive developmental delay with regression and congenital aphasia, with or without regression. Landau-Kleffner syndrome appears to be related to a condition characterized by continuous spikes and waves occurring during sleep, described as *epilepsy with continuous spikes and waves during sleep* (CSWDS) or *electrical status epilepticus of sleep* (ESES). Most children with Landau-Kleffner develop ESES at some point in the course of their disorder.[117]

Although there is a considerable amount of variation in Landau-Kleffner syndrome, the typical history is that a child develops an abrupt or gradual loss of language ability and inattentiveness to sound, with onset during the first decade of life. Some patients have a language disturbance prior to the acquired aphasia.[118] Receptive dysfunction, often referred to as *auditory agnosia*, usually is the dominant feature early in the course of the disorder.[119] In some children the disorder progresses to the point where the child cannot even recognize sounds. The children may become indifferent to auditory stimulation and may not even recognize the sound of a telephone or barking dog, often appearing as though they are deaf or autistic. Reading,

writing, and signing may be relatively spared. In addition to the aphasia, most patients have behavioral and psychomotor disturbances, often appearing autistic. The neurologic examination, other than the mental status assessment, is usually normal.

CSWDS or ESES was first described by Patry and coworkers[120] and later expanded by Tassinari and associates.[121] The original description stressed the importance of defining the syndrome by the amount of spike-wave activity during sleep. In this syndrome spike-wave activity should occupy no less than 85% of the time of slow sleep. Although CSWDS and ESES are often used synonymously, *CSWDS* refers to both the EEG and clinical features of the disorder, whereas *ESES* refers to the spike-wave during sleep. In CSWDS there is a variety of seizure types including partial, generalized tonic-clonic, and myoclonic. As with Landau-Kleffner syndrome, there is often a deterioration in cognitive abilities over time.

EEG. There is not a specific EEG pattern in Landau-Kleffner syndrome. Most commonly there are repetitive spikes, sharp waves, and spike-and-wave activity in the temporal region or parietal-occipital regions bilaterally (Fig. 11-21).[122] Sleep usually activates the record, and at times the abnormality is seen only in sleep recordings. Because of the overlap with CSWDS, Paquier and coworkers[123] suggested that a sleep EEG should be obtained to determine if the patient has spike-wave discharges during slow-wave sleep.

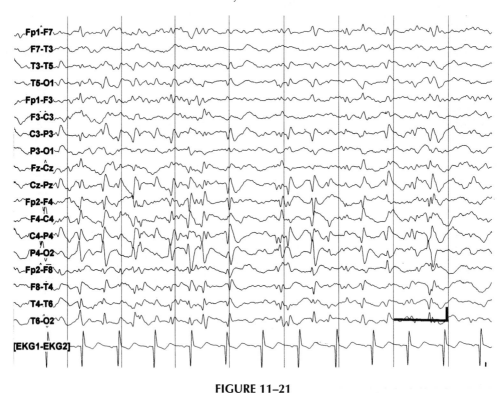

FIGURE 11–21

Frequent right-sided epileptiform discharges in a 9-year-old child with Landau-Kleffner syndrome. Calibration, 1 sec/100 μV.

The distinguishing feature of CSWDS is the continuous bilateral and diffuse slow spike-wave activity persisting through all of the slow sleep stages (see Fig. 11-13). The spike-wave index, calculated by

$$\text{Total minutes of all spike-waves} \times 100 \div \text{total minutes of NREM sleep without spike-wave}$$

ranges from 85% to 100%.[121] EEG abnormalities during the awake state are more variable. Generalized spike-wave, focal, and multifocal spikes can be seen.

Severe Myoclonic Epilepsy in Infancy

Severe myoclonic epilepsy in infancy, also termed *Dravet's syndrome*, is a disorder that typically begins in the first or second year of life with repeat episodes of severe febrile status epilepticus.[124,125] The child then goes on to develop frequent myoclonic seizures. With onset of the afebrile seizures and EEG abnormalities, developmental progression slows and many of the children develop ataxia and corticospinal tract dysfunction. The epilepsy is resistant to all forms of treatment, and the children are mentally retarded.

At the time of the first febrile seizure the EEG is usually normal and without any paroxysmal abnormalities. With onset of the myoclonus, generalized spike-and-wave or polyspike-and-wave activity is seen during the seizures.

The generalized discharges increase during drowsiness. Focal and multifocal spikes and sharp waves are also seen. De novo truncating mutations of the *SCN1A* gene on 2p24 gene coding for the neuronal voltage-gated sodium channel α_1 subunit have been found in severe myoclonic epilepsy in infancy.[126,127]

EEG. At the time of the first febrile seizure the EEG is usually normal and without any paroxysmal abnormalities. Between 1 and 2 years of life the myoclonic seizures begin. The myoclonus can be massive, involving whole muscles, particularly the axial one, or be barely discernible.[125] The jerks can be isolated or occur in flurries. During EEG monitoring generalized spike-and-wave or polyspike-and-wave activity is seen during the seizures. When absence seizures occur they are also associated with generalized spike-and-wave, usually at a frequency of 3 Hz. The generalized discharges increase during drowsiness. Focal and multifocal abnormalities are also seen.

Over time some of the children develop slowing on their EEG with diffuse theta and occasional delta activity. Generalized spike-and-wave activity becomes less frequent during waking. The generalized spike-and-wave is replaced by spikes and spike-and-wave activity usually localized centrally or at the vertex.

Photosensitivity is commonly seen, sometimes early in the course, but is not a uniform feature in all patients.[125,128]

Dravet and colleagues[125] observed photoconvulsive response in 42% of their patients, beginning between 3 months and 5.5 years. Seizures were also precipitated in some of their patients with eye closure, patterns, or television.

Benign Myoclonic Epilepsy in Infancy

Benign myoclonic epilepsy in infancy is characterized by the occurrence of brief myoclonic seizures in otherwise normal infants and toddlers between the age of 4 months to 3 years.[82,100,129] The myoclonic seizures are always brief, involving the arms and head. The legs are rarely involved. The frequency and intensity of the seizures are variable. Often the child has a subtle nod. Unlike infantile spasms, they rarely are precipitated by awakening. However, the seizures are enhanced during drowsiness. Other seizure types do not develop.

Although many children go into remission, some patients develop generalized tonic-clonic seizures. Psychomotor development is typically normal.

EEG. The EEG features are distinctly different from hypsarrhythmia. The interictal EEG is usually normal. Myoclonic jerks are associated with generalized spike-and-wave or polyspike-and-wave activity. The frequency of the discharges is greater than 3 Hz and they usually last 1 to 3 seconds. Some bursts of spike-and-wave activity may rarely occur during the awake state without any accompanying clinical changes. Photosensitivity occurs in some of the patients. Sleep organization appears to be normal. Some patients have generalized spike-and-wave discharges during sleep.

SITUATION-RELATED SEIZURES

Febrile Seizures

Febrile seizures are quite common, affecting approximately 3% of children younger than 6 years of age. Segregation analysis suggests that most cases have complex inheritance, although some families appear to have an autosomal dominant inheritance pattern.[130,131]

Scheffer and Berkovic[132] identified a syndrome termed *generalized epilepsy with febrile seizures plus* (GEFS+). In the families identified, febrile seizure occurred during early childhood, but unlike the typical febrile convulsion syndrome, attacks with fever continued beyond the age of 6 years. Some of the patients also developed afebrile seizures including absences, myoclonic, atonic, or myoclonic-astatic seizures. The seizures typically stop by adolescence.[132,133] In a large family with GEFS+, a linkage has been established to 19q12.1, with a mutation in the regulatory α_1 subunit of the voltage-gated sodium channel.[134] Loss of this allele could lead to hyperexcitability by facilitating an inward depolarizing Na^+ current.[134]

EEG. Somewhat surprisingly, the EEG has not been found to be particularly useful in children with febrile seizures. Although some studies have reported some predictive value of the EEG following febrile seizures,[135,136] other studies have not found the EEG to be a useful prognostic tool.[137] EEGs recorded within a week of a febrile seizure are frequently abnormal with approximately one third of patients, with occipital slowing the most common abnormality.[137] The slowing is common bilaterally, but it is often asymmetrical or even unilateral.

REFERENCES

1. Hauser WA: Epidemiology of epilepsy in children. Neurosurg Clin North Am 1995;6:419-429.
2. Drury I: Epileptiform patterns of children. J Clin Neurophysiol 1989;6:1-39.
3. Holmes GL: Electroencephalographic and neuroradiologic evaluation of children with epilepsy. Pediatr Clin North Am 1989;36:395-420.
4. Engel J Jr: A proposed diagnostic scheme for people with epileptic seizures and with epilepsy: Report of the ILAE Task Force on Classification and Terminology. Epilepsia 2001;42:796-803.
5. Holmes GL: Partial seizures in children. Pediatrics 1986;77:725-731.
6. Pearl PL, Holmes GL: Absence seizures. *In* Pellock JM, Dodson WE, Bourgeois BFD (eds): Pediatric Epilepsy: Diagnosis and Treatment. New York, Demos, 2001, p 219.
7. Penry JK, Porter RJ, Dreifuss FE: Simultaneous recording of absence seizures with videotape and electroencephalography. Brain 1975;98:427-440.
8. Holmes GL, McKeever M, Adamson M: Absence seizures in children: Clinical and electroencephalographic features. Ann Neurol 1987;21:268-273.
9. Porter RJ, Penry JK, Dreifuss FE: Responsiveness at the onset of spike-wave bursts. Electroencephalogr Clin Neurophysiol 1973;34:239-245.
10. Browne TR, Penry JK, Porter RJ, et al: Responsiveness before, during, and after spike-wave paroxysms. Neurology 1974;24:659-665.
11. Lugaresi E, Cirignotta F, Montagna P: Occipital lobe epilepsy with scotosensitive seizures: The role of central vision. Epilepsia 1984;25:115-120.
12. Panayiotopoulos CP: Epileptic Encephalopathies in Early Childhood: A Clinical Guide to Epileptic Syndromes and Their Treatment. Oxfordshire, Bladon, 2002, p 70.
13. Yaqub HA: Electroclinical seizures in Lennox-Gastaut syndrome. Epilepsia 1993;34:120-127.
14. Doose H: Myoclonic-astatic epilepsy. *In* Degen R, Dreifuss FE (eds): Benign Localized and Generalized Epilepsies of Early Childhood. Amsterdam, Elsevier, 1992, p 163.

15. Oguni H, Fukuyama Y, Imaizumi Y, Uehara T: Video-EEG analysis of drop seizures in myoclonic astatic epilepsy of early childhood (Doose syndrome). Epilepsia 1992;33:805-813.

16. Ikeno T, Shigematsu H, Miyakoshi M, et al: An analytic study of epileptic falls. Epilepsia 1985;26:612-621.

17. Proposal for revised classification of epilepsies and epileptic syndromes. Commission on Classification and Terminology of the International League Against Epilepsy. Epilepsia 1989;30:389-399.

18. Lerman P, Kivity S: The benign partial nonrolandic epilepsies. J Clin Neurophysiol 1991;8:275-287.

19. Holmes GL: Benign focal epilepsies of childhood. Epilepsia 1993;34(Suppl 3):S49-S61.

20. Holmes GL: Rolandic epilepsy: Clinical and electroencephalographic features. Epilepsy Res Suppl 1992;6:29-43.

21. Lerman P, Kivity S: Benign focal epilepsy of childhood: A follow-up study of 100 recovered patients. Arch Neurol 1975;32:261-264.

22. Ma CK, Chan KY: Benign childhood epilepsy with centrotemporal spikes: A study of 50 Chinese children. Brain Dev 2003;25:390-395.

23. Lerman P: Benign partial epilepsy with centro-temporal spikes. *In* Roger J, Bureau M, Dravet C, et al (eds): Benign Syndromes in Infancy, Childhood, and Adolescence. London, John Libbey, 1992, p 189.

24. Blom S, Brorson LO: Central spikes or sharp waves (rolandic spikes) in children's EEG and their clinical significance. Acta Paediatr Scand 1966;55:385-393.

25. Clemens B, Majoros E: Sleep studies in benign epilepsy of childhood with rolandic spikes: II. Analysis of discharge frequency and its relation to sleep dynamics. Epilepsia 1987;28:24-27.

26. Clemens B, Majoros E: Sleep studies in benign epilepsy of childhood with rolandic spikes: I. Sleep pathology. Epilepsia 1987;28:20-23.

27. Dieterich E, Doose H, Baier WK, Fichsel H: Long-term follow-up of childhood epilepsy with absences: II. Absence-epilepsy with initial grand mal. Neuropediatrics 1985;16:155-158.

28. Blom S, Heijbel J: Benign epilepsy of children with centro-temporal EEG foci: Discharge rate during sleep. Epilepsia 1975;16:133-140.

29. Rose D, Duron B: Prognostic value of the interictal discharges during nocturnal sleep in children with rolandic spikes. Rev Electroencephalogr Neurophysiol Clin 1984;14:217-226.

30. Dalla Bernardina B, Beghini G: Rolandic spikes in children with and without epilepsy (20 subjects polygraphically studied during sleep). Epilepsia 1976;17:161-167.

31. Graf M, Lischka A, Gremel K: Benign rolandic epilepsy in children: Topographic EEG analysis. Wien Klin Wochenschr 1990;102:206-210.

32. Gregory DL, Wong PKH: Clinical relevance of a dipole field in rolandic spikes. Epilepsia 1992;33:36-44.

33. Yoshinaga H, Amano R, Oka E, Ohtahara S: Dipole tracing in childhood epilepsy with special reference to rolandic epilepsy. Brain Topogr 1992;4:193-199.

34. Jung KY, Kim JM, Kim DW: Patterns of interictal spike propagation across the central sulcus in benign rolandic epilepsy. Clin Electroencephalogr 2003;34:153-157.

35. Gregory DL, Wong PK: Topographical analysis of the centrotemporal discharges in benign rolandic epilepsy of childhood. Epilepsia 1984;25:705-711.

36. Gibbs EL, Gillen HW, Gibbs FA: Disappearance and migration of epileptic foci in childhood. Am J Dis Child 1954;88:596-603.

37. Dalla Bernardina B, Tassinari CA: EEG of a nocturnal seizure in a patient with "benign epilepsy of childhood with rolandic spikes." Epilepsia 1975;16:497-501.

38. Gutierrez AR, Brick JF, Bodensteiner J: Dipole reversal: An ictal feature of benign partial epilepsy with centrotemporal spikes. Epilepsia 1990;31:544-548.

39. Lerman P, Kivity-Ephraim S: Focal epileptic EEG discharges in children not suffering from clinical epilepsy: Etiology, clinical significance, and management. Epilepsia 1981;22:551-558.

40. Beaussart M: Benign epilepsy of children with rolandic (centro-temporal) paroxysmal foci—a clinical entity: Study of 221 cases. Epilepsia 1972;13:795-811.

41. Niedermeyer E, Naidu S: Further EEG observations in children with the Rett syndrome. Brain Dev 1990;12:53-54.

42. Musumecci SA, Colognaola RM, Ferri R, et al: Fragile X syndrome: A particular epileptogenic EEG pattern. Epilepsia 1988;29:41-47.

43. Kuzniecky R, Berkovic S, Andermann F, et al: Focal cortical myoclonus and rolandic cortical dysplasia: Clarification by magnetic resonance imaging. Ann Neurol 1988;23:317-325.

44. Fischer RA, Clancy RR: Midline foci of epileptiform activity in children and neonates. J Child Neurol 1987;2:224-228.

45. Kaschnitz W, Scheer P, Korner K, et al: Rolandic spikes as an electroencephalographic manifestation of an oligodendroglioma. Pediatr Padol 1988;23:313-319.

46. Panayiotopoulos CP: Benign childhood epileptic syndromes with occipital spikes: New classification proposed by the International League Against Epilepsy. J Child Neurol 2000;15:548-552.

47. Caraballo R, Cersosimo R, Medina C, Fejerman N: Panayiotopoulos-type benign childhood occipital epilepsy: A prospective study. Neurology 2000;55:1096-1100.

48. Talwar D, Rask CA, Torres F: Clinical manifestations in children with occipital spike-wave paroxysms. Epilepsia 1992;33:667-674.

49. Gastaut H: A new type of epilepsy: benign partial epilepsy childhood with occipital spike-waves. Clin Electroencephalogr 1982;13:13-22.

50. Panayiotopoulos CP: Benign Childhood Focal Seizures and Related Syndromes: A Clinical Guide to Epileptic Syndromes and Their Treatment. Oxfordshire, Bladon, 2002, p 89.

51. Panayiotopoulos CP: Benign childhood epilepsy with occipital paroxysms: A 15-year prospective study. Ann Neurol 1989;26:51-56.

52. Panayiotopoulos CP: Inhibitory effect of central vision on occipital lobe seizure. Neurology 1981;31:1331-1333.

53. Terasaki T, Yamatgi Y, Otahara S: Electroclinical delineation of occipital lobe epilepsy in childhood. *In* Andermann F, Lugaresi E (eds): Migraine and Epilepsy. London, Butterworth, 1987, p 125.

54. Gastaut H: Benign epilepsy of childhood with occipital paroxysms. *In* Roger J, Bureau M, Dravet C, et al (eds): Epileptic Syndromes in Infancy, Childhood, and Adolescence. London, John Libbey, 1992, p 201.

55. Smith JMB, Kellaway P: The natural history and clinical correlates of occipital foci in children. *In* Kellaway P, Petersen I (eds): Neurological and Electroencephalographic Correlative Studies in Infancy. New York, Grune & Stratton, 1964, p 230.

56. Gobbi G, Sorrenti G, Santucci M, et al: Epilepsy with bilateral occipital calcifications: A benign onset with progressive severity. Neurology 1988;38:913-920.

57. Gobbi G, Ambrosetto P, Zaniboni MG, et al: Celiac disease, posterior cerebral calcifications, and epilepsy. Brain Dev 1992;14:23-29.

58. Gobbi G, Bouquet F, Greco L, et al: Coeliac disease, epilepsy, and cerebral calcifications. Lancet 1992;340:439-443.

59. Levinson JD, Stillerman ML: The correlation between electroencephalographic findings and eye disorders in children. Electroencephalogr Clin Neurophysiol 1950;2:226.

60. Levinson JD, Gibbs EL, Stillerman ML, Perlstein MA: Electroencephalogram and eye disorders: Clinical correlation. Pediatrics 1951;7:422-427.

61. Hayman M, Scheffer IE, Chinvarun Y, et al: Autosomal dominant nocturnal frontal lobe epilepsy: Demonstration of focal frontal onset and intrafamilial variation. Neurology 1997;49:969-975.

62. Scheffer IE, Bhatia KP, Lopes-Cendes I, et al: Autosomal dominant frontal lobe epilepsy: A distinctive clinical disorder. Brain 1995;118:61-73.

63. Scheffer IE: Autosomal dominant nocturnal frontal lobe epilepsy. *In* Berkovic SF, Genton P, Hirsch E, Picard F (eds): Genetics of Focal Epilepsies: Clinical Aspects and Molecular Biology. London, John Libbey, 1999, p 81.

64. Phillips HA, Scheffer IE, Crossland KM, et al: Autosomal dominant nocturnal frontal-lobe epilepsy: Genetic heterogeneity and evidence for a second locus at 15q24. Am J Hum Genet 1998;63:1108-1116.

65. Cho YW, Motamedi GK, Laufenberb I, et al: A Korean kindred with autosomal dominant nocturnal frontal lobe epilepsy and mental retardation. Arch Neurol 2003;60:1625-1632.

66. Dalla Bernardina B, Colamaria V, Chiamenti C, et al: Benign partial epilepsy with affective symptoms ("benign psychomotor epilepsy"). *In* Roger J, Bureau M, Dravet C, et al (eds): Epileptic Syndromes in Infancy, Childhood, and Adolescence. London, John Libbey, 1992, p 219.

67. Loiseau P, Louiset P: Benign partial seizures of adolescence. *In* Roger J, Bureau M, Dravet C, et al (eds): Epileptic Syndromes in Infancy, Childhood, and Adolescence. London, John Libbey, 1992, p 343.

68. Loiseau P, Orgogozo JM: An unrecognized syndrome of benign focal epileptic seizures in teenagers? Lancet 1978;2:1070-1071.

69. De Marco P, Negrin P: Parietal focal spikes evoked by contralateral tactile somatotropic stimulations in four non-epileptic subjects. Electroencephalogr Clin Neurophysiol 1973;34:308-312.

70. Negrin P, De Marco P: Parietal focal spikes evoked by tactile somatotropic stimulation in 60 non-epileptic children: The nocturnal sleep and clinical and EEG evolution. Electroencephalogr Clin Neurophysiol 1977;43:312-316.

71. De Marco P, Tassinari CA: Extreme somatosensory evoked potential (ESEP): An EEG sign forecasting the possible occurrence of seizures in children. Epilepsia 1981;22:569-575.

72. Tassinari CA, De Marco P: Benign partial epilepsy with extreme somatosensory evoked potentials. *In* Roger J, Bureau M, Dravet C, et al (eds): Epileptic Syndromes in Infancy, Childhood, and Adolescence. London, John Libbey, 1992, p 225.

73. Leppert M, Anderson E, Quattlebaum T, et al: Benign familial neonatal convulsions linked to genetic markers on chromosome 20. Nature 1989;337:647-648.

74. Miles DK, Holmes GL: Benign neonatal seizures. J Clin Neurophysiol 1990;7:369-379.

75. Petit RE, Fenichel GM: Benign familial neonatal seizures. Arch Neurol 1991;37:47-48.

76. Charlier C, Singh NA, Ryan SG, et al: A pore mutation in a novel KQT-like potassium channel gene in an idiopathic epilepsy family. Nature Genet 1998;18:53-55.

77. Stoffel M, Jan LY: Epilepsy genes: Excitement traced to potassium channels. Nature Genet 1998;18:6-8.

78. Singh NA, Charlier C, Stauffer D, et al: A novel potassium channel gene, *KCNQ2*, is mutated in an inherited epilepsy of newborns. Nature Genet 1998;18:25-29.

79. Hirsch E, Velez A, Sellal F, et al: Electroclinical signs of benign neonatal familial convulsions. Ann Neurol 1993;34:835-841.

80. Plouin P: Benign idiopathic neonatal convulsions (familial and non-familial). *In* Roger J, Bureau M, Dravet C, et al (eds): Epileptic Syndromes in Infancy, Childhood, and Adolescence. London, John Libbey, 1992, p 3.

81. Dravet C, Bureau M, Roger J: Severe myoclonic epilepsy in infants. *In* Roger J, Dravet C, Bureau M, et al (eds): Epileptic Syndromes in Infancy, Childhood, and Adolescence. London, John Libbey, 1985, p 58.

82. Dravet C, Bureau M, Genton P: Benign myoclonic epilepsy of infancy: Electroclinical symptomatology and differential diagnosis form the other types of generalized epilepsy on infancy. *In* Degen R, Dreifuss FE (eds): Benign Localized and Generalized Epilepsies of Early Childhood. Amsterdam, Elsevier, 1992, p 131.

83. Panayiotopoulos CP: Idiopathic Generalised Epilepsies: A Clinical Guide to Epileptic Syndromes and Their Treatment. Oxfordshire, Bladon, 2002, p 114.

84. Wolf P: Epilepsy with grand mal on awakening. *In* Roger J, Bureau M, Dravet C, et al (eds): Epileptic Syndromes in Infancy, Childhood, and Adolescence. London, John Libbey, 1992, p 329.

85. Janz D, Wolf P: Epilepsy with grand mal on awakening. *In* Engel J Jr, Pedley TA (eds): Epilepsy: A Comprehensive Textbook. Philadelphia, Lippincott-Raven, 1997, p 2347.

86. Holmes GL, Vigevano F: Infantile spasms. *In* Engel J Jr, Pedley TA (eds): Epilepsy: A Comprehensive Textbook. Philadelphia, Lippincott-Raven, 1997, p 627.

87. Kellaway P, Frost JD, Hrachovy RA: Infantile spasms. *In* Morselli PD, Pippenger KF, Penry JK (eds): Antiepileptic Drug Therapy in Pediatrics. New York, Raven Press, 1983, p 115.

88. Gibbs EL, Fleming MM, Gibbs FA: Diagnosis and prognosis of hypsarrhythmia and infantile spasms. Pediatrics 1954;13:66-73.

89. Hrachovy RA, Frost JD Jr, Kellaway P: Hypsarrhythmia: Variations on the theme. Epilepsia 1984;25:317-325.

90. Hrachovy RA, Frost JD, Kellaway P: Sleep characteristics in infantile spasms. Neurology 1981;31:688-694.

91. Bellman M: Infantile spasms. *In* Pedley TA, Meldrum BS (eds): Recent Advances in Epilepsy. Edinburgh, Churchill Livingstone, 1983, p 113.

92. Friedman E, Pampiglione G: Prognostic implications of electroencephalographic findings of hypsarrhythmia in first year of life. BMJ 1971;4:323-325.

93. Baird HW, Borofsky LG: Infantile myoclonic seizures. J Pediatr 1957;50:332-329.

94. Watanabe K, Iwase K, Hara K: The evolution of EEG features in infantile spasms: A prospective study. Dev Med Child Neurol 1973;15:584-596.

95. Fusco L, Vigevano F: Ictal clinical electroencephalographic findings of spasms in West syndrome. Epilepsia 1993;34:671-678.

96. Plouin P, Dulac O, Jalin C, Chiron C: Twenty-four-hour ambulatory EEG monitoring in infantile spasms. Epilepsia 1993;34:686-691.

97. Carrazana EJ, Barlow JK, Holmes GL: Infantile spasms provoked by partial seizures: A case report. J Epilepsy 1990;3:97-100.

98. Carrazana EJ, Lombroso CT, Mikati M, et al: Facilitation of infantile spasms by partial seizures. Epilepsia 1993;34:97-109.

99. Lombroso CT, Fejerman N: Benign myoclonus of early infancy. Ann Neurol 1977;1:138-143.

100. Dravet C, Giraud N, Bureau M, et al: Benign myoclonus of early infancy or benign non-epileptic infantile spasms. Neuropediatrics 1986;17:33-38.

101. Holmes GL: Myoclonic, tonic, and atonic seizures in children. J Epilepsy 1988;1:173-195.

102. Genton P, Dravet C: Lennox-Gastaut and other childhood epileptic encephalopathies. *In* Engel J Jr, Pedley TA (eds): Epilepsy: A Comprehensive Textbook. Philadelphia, Lippincott-Raven, 1997, p 2355.

103. Markand ON: Slow spike-wave activity in EEG and associated clinical features: Often called "Lennox" or "Lennox-Gastaut" syndrome. Neurology 1977;27:746-757.

104. Papini M, Pasquinelli A, Armellini M, Orlandi D: Alertness and incidence of seizures in patients with Lennox-Gastaut syndrome. Epilepsia 1984;25:161-167.

105. Blume WT: Clinical and electroencephalographic correlates of the multiple independent spike foci pattern in children. Ann Neurol 1978;4:541-547.

106. Doose H, Gerken H, Leonhardt R, et al: Centrencephalic myoclonic-astatic petit mal: Clinical and genetic investigations. Neuropaediatrie 1970;2:59-78.

107. Doose H: Myoclonic astatic epilepsy of early childhood. *In* Roger J, Bureau M, Dravet C, et al (eds): Epileptic Syndromes in Infancy, Childhood, and Adolescence. London, John Libbey, 1992, p 103.

108. Doose H, Gundel A: Four to 7 cps rhythms in the childhood EEG. *In* Anderson VE, Hauser WA, Penry JK, Sing CF (eds): Genetic Basis of the Epilepsies. New York, Raven Press, 1982, p 113.

109. Aicardi J: Early myoclonic encephalopathy (neonatal myoclonic encephalopathy). *In* Roger J, Bureau M, Dravet C, et al (eds): Epileptic Syndromes in Infancy, Childhood, and Adolescence. London, John Libbey, 1992, p 13.

110. Lombroso CT: Early myoclonic encephalopathy, early infantile epileptic encephalopathy, and benign and severe infantile myoclonic epilepsies: A critical review and personal contributions. J Clin Neurophysiol 1990;7:380-408.

111. Ohtahara S, Ishida T, Oka E, et al: On the age-dependent epileptic syndromes: The early infantile encephalopathy with suppression-burst. Brain Dev 1976;8:270-288.

112. Murakami N, Ohtsuka Y, Ohtahara S: Early infantile epileptic syndromes with suppression bursts: Early myoclonic encephalopathy versus Ohtahara syndrome. Jpn J Psychiatry Neurol 1993;470:197-200.

113. Landau WM, Kleffner FR: Syndrome of acquired aphasia with convulsive disorder in children. Neurology 1957;7:523-530.

114. Montovani JF, Landau WM: Acquired aphasia with convulsive disorder: Course and prognosis. Neurology 1980;30:524-529.

115. Deonna TW: Acquired epileptiform aphasia in children (Landau-Kleffner syndrome). J Clin Neurophysiol 1991;8:288-298.

116. Sawhney IMS, Suresch N, Dhand UK, Chopra JS: Acquired aphasia with epilepsy—Landau-Kleffner syndrome. Epilepsia 1988;29:283-287.

117. Hirsch E, Marescaux C, Maquet P, et al: Landau-Kleffner syndrome: A clinical and EEG study of five cases. Epilepsia 1990;31:756-767.

118. Soprano AM, Garcia EF, Caraballo R, Fejerman N: Acquired epileptic aphasia: Neuropsychologic follow-up of 12 patients. Pediatr Neurol 1995;11:230-235.

119. Rapin I, Mattis S, Rowan AJ, Golden GS: Verbal auditory agnosia in children. Dev Med Child Neurol 1977;19:192-207.

120. Patry G, Lyagoubi S, Tassinari CA: Subclinical "electrical status epilepticus" induced by sleep in children. Arch Neurol 1971;24:242-252.

121. Tassinari CA, Bureau M, Dravet C, et al: Epilepsy with continuous spikes and waves during slow sleep—otherwise described as ESES (epilepsy with electrical status epilepticus during slow sleep). *In* Roger J, Bureau M, Dravet C, et al (eds): Epileptic Syndromes in Infancy, Childhood, and Adolescence. London, John Libbey, 1992, p 245.

122. Beaumanoir A: The Landau-Kleffner syndrome. *In* Roger J, Dravet C, Bureau M, et al (eds): Epileptic Syndromes in Infancy, Childhood, and Adolescence. London, John Libbey, 1985, p 181.

123. Paquier PF, van Dongen HR, Loonen CB: The Landau-Kleffner syndrome or "acquired aphasia with convulsive disorder": Long-term follow-up of six children and a review of the recent literature. Arch Neurol 1992;49:354-359.

124. Nabbout R, Dulac O: Epileptic encephalopathies: A brief overview. J Clin Neurophysiol 2003;20:393-397.

125. Dravet C, Bureau M, Guerrini R, et al: Severe myoclonic epilepsy in infants. *In* Roger J, Bureau M, Dravet C, et al (eds): Epileptic Syndromes in Infancy, Childhood, and Adolescence. London, John Libbey, 1992, p 75.

126. Claes L, Ceulemans B, Audenaert D, et al: De novo *SCN1A* mutations are a major cause of severe myoclonic epilepsy of infancy. Hum Mutat 2003;21:615-621.

127. Scheffer IE, Wallace R, Mulley JC, Berkovic SF: Clinical and molecular genetics of myoclonic-astatic epilepsy and severe myoclonic epilepsy in infancy (Dravet syndrome). Brain Dev 2001;23:732-735.

128. Renier WO, Renkawek K: Clinical and neuropathological findings in a case of severe myoclonic epilepsy of infancy. Epilepsia 1990;31:287-291.

129. Dravet C, Bureau M, Roger J: Benign myoclonic epilepsy in infants. *In* Roger J, Bureau M, Dravet C, et al (eds): Epileptic Syndromes in Infancy, Childhood, and Adolescence. London, John Libbey, 1992, p 67.

130. Berkovic SF, Scheffer IE: Febrile seizures: Genetics and relationship to other epilepsy syndromes. Curr Opin Neurol 1998;11:129-134.

131. Peiffer A, Thompson J, Charlier C, et al: A locus for febrile seizures (FEB3) maps to chromosome 2q23-24. Ann Neurol 1999;46:671-678.

132. Scheffer IE, Berkovic SF: Generalized epilepsy with febrile seizures plus: A genetic disorder with heterogeneous clinical phenotypes. Brain 1997;120:479-490.

133. Singh R, Scheffer IE, Crossland K, Berkovic SF: Generalized epilepsy with febrile seizures plus: A common childhood-onset genetic epilepsy syndrome. Ann Neurol 1999;45:75-81.

134. Wallace RH, Wang DW, Singh R, et al: Febrile seizures and generalized epilepsy associated with a mutation in the Na$^+$-channel beta$_1$ subunit gene *SCN1B*. Nat Genet 1998;19:366-370.

135. Tsuboi T, Endo S: Febrile convulsions followed by nonfebrile convulsions: A clinical, electroencephalographic, and follow-up study. Neuropadiatrie 1977;8:209-223.

136. Metrakos K, Metrakos JD: Genetics of convulsive disorders: II. Genetic and electroencephalographic studies in centrencephalic epilepsy. Neurology 1961;11:474-483.

137. Frantzen E, Lennox-Buchtal M, Nygaard A: Longitudinal EEG and clinical study of children with febrile convulsions. Electroencephalogr Clin Neurophysiol 1968;24:197-212.

12

Neurophysiology of Language and Behavioral Disorders in Children

Susan K. Klein and Roberto Tuchman

Gibbs and Gibbs[1] were most likely the first investigators who attempted to find robust electrophysiologic correlates for cognitive, language, and psychiatric disorders. Nearly 30 years later, few clear electrophysiologic markers exist for attention deficit disorder (ADD), mental retardation, developmental language disorders, learning disabilities, and autistic spectrum disorders in children.

There are a number of ways in which neurophysiologic techniques can be used to study brain development and higher cortical function.[2] Electroencephalograms (EEGs) of children with deficits can be compared with those of normal children. Transformation of EEG data can be made with the use of advanced statistical techniques to quantify background abnormalities of children with learning disorders in comparison to normal children. Short-latency evoked potentials measuring transmission of information to the primary visual, auditory, or somatosensory cortices can be measured. Finally, event-related potentials (ERPs) that are linked to cognitive processes above the level of the primary sensory cortices can be measured in groups of children with cognitive or learning disorders matched with control children. For example, the P300 (referred to as the *P3*) ERP is widely used as a measure of cognitive functioning and provides a sensitive electrophysiologic index of attentional and working memory demands of a task.

Studies using ERPs are the most challenging technically but provide the most information about cognitive processes because they correlate anatomic localization and behavior. Many studies have measured auditory or visual ERPs in normal infants and children,[3-7] or in babies and children who have been deemed high risk for different reasons (e.g., prematurity, low socioeconomic status).[4,6,7] Identification of positive and negative components of interest is made by comparison of the diverse literature of ERP studies in normal adults.

However, ERPs have been recorded only rarely in groups of children with specific language or learning disorders. There are several reasons for this. Young children with language or cognitive disorders are not as easy to study (partly due to their deficits) using those tasks that often require several hours of focused attention. Second, experimental conditions affect the latency and amplitude of many elicited components.[8] Because no uniform standards have been set for data collection, choice of a different reference electrode may affect the timing or distribution of components.[8]

Age also alters the timing of ERPs. Courschesne[3,9,10] observed that small children generate a negative component to unexpected stimuli, which in older children and adults elicits a P300, or P3. He also observed that the P3 may occur up to 200 milliseconds later in children than adults. Therefore, different laboratories may report different positive and negative components as representative of similar cognitive processes. The methods of choosing components for analysis (often arbitrary), and the different use of statistical techniques offer reasons for varying results from one laboratory to another. For example, Callaway and colleagues[11] showed how different techniques of ERP analyses altered findings in a group of hyperactive children with great individual differences. Thus, individual reports of ERP findings are often limited in significance owing to the lack of adequate control group data or to the different ways in which the data are analyzed.

The greatest methodologic problem in the study of children with disorders of attention, reading, language, and behavior is the failure to define groups of children with behavioral measures. Universal systems of classification for disorders of higher cortical function in children are just being developed. Investigators in this field have difficulty deciding which children meet behavioral criteria for diagnosis, and most define specific disorders in different ways. Thus, it has been nearly impossible to compare ERP findings of "reading-disordered children," for example, because the children are selected on the basis of different criteria. Then their performance on nonstandardized ERP tasks (with varying experimental conditions) is compared to small control groups of differing ages.

This chapter reviews the neurophysiology of higher cortical functions in children. In each section, we have given a brief overview of the major classification issues in the area.

DISORDERS OF ATTENTION

Attention is the gate for higher order formulation of language and memory. It involves the initial selection of a relevant stimulus for further cognitive processing. Attention has been defined as a biphasic quality, incorporating *state* and *channel* operations.[12] State operations are those functions that keep the individual sufficiently aroused to process information. Channel operations are functions that control the selection of specific ideas from the barrage of information presented in the environment. The frontal lobes[13] and the head of the caudate nucleus[14] may be sites of channel operations in humans. Dopamine, norepinephrine, and serotonin play an important role in attention deficit hyperactivity disorder (ADHD) in children.[15-18]

ADHD is the most common neurobehavioral disorder of childhood, with most children maintaining symptoms of ADHD as adolescents and as adults.[19] It is among the most common chronic conditions that primary care pediatricians see. Core behaviors seen in children with ADHD include hyperactivity, impulsivity, and inattention. The *Diagnostic and Statistical Manual of Mental Disorders (DSM)-IV* standard for diagnosis emphasized the importance of documenting that these behaviors occur at school and in the home, the chronicity of symptoms, and the connection between the behaviors and impairments in educational achievement or social development. The complex nature of this disorder is further complicated by the fact that children and adolescents with ADHD have associated conditions, such as learning disorders, anxiety, oppositional behaviors, and depression.

EEG Power Spectral Analysis in Normal Development

There has been a resurgence of interest in examining the emergence of power spectra patterns in normal children. Many studies focus on the relationship of emerging behavior patterns (followed longitudinally) to EEG power spectral patterns observed at a single time point. Temperament studies are a good example. McManis and colleagues[20] studied 56 preadolescent children who had been classified in infancy with respect to temperament. High reactive/fearful children had right frontal activation in the alpha and beta (resting) bands. Henderson and colleagues[21] reported that shy 4-year old children were more likely to show frontal EEG asymmetry.

Others have attempted to characterize normal power spectral patterns across childhood. An interesting report by Yordanova and Kolev[22] related the emergence of stimulus-induced theta bands to the coalescence of endogenous P300 auditory ERP elicited in an oddball paradigm. The latency of mid-central and parietal theta decreased with increasing age and predicted the complementary decrease in latency of late auditory ERP positivity.

EEG Power Spectral Analysis in Children with Attention Deficit Disorders

In the United States, E. Roy John and colleagues have been long-time advocates of the use of quantitative EEG in the evaluation and treatment of children with attention and learning disorders.[23] Russian investigators have long favored quantitative EEG methods, and their experience is becoming more accessible internationally.[24] Chabot and colleagues[23] estimate that up to 25% of children with learning disorders have been reported to show QEEG abnormalities (slowing). Eighty percent of children with ADHD had QEEG abnormalities in frontal/polar regions (primarily an increase in alpha and theta oscillations) in contrast with normal controls.[23,24] Gorbachevskaya and colleagues (reviewed in Kropotov) observed a decrease in low frequency (<20 Hz) beta (right central) and an increase in theta (bitemporal) in children with ADHD.[24]

Some have used EEG biofeedback to change the power spectra of children with ADHD and treat clinical symptoms of the disorder. During EEG biofeedback training, subjects breathe deeply and rhythmically, focus on a picture, and divide their attention between the image and thoughts related to the image. Treatment of ADHD with EEG biofeedback aims to increase low-frequency (<20 Hz) beta and suppress theta and high-frequency (>22 Hz) beta.[25]

Event-Related Negative Components and Selective Attention in Normal Subjects

ERPs have been examined as markers of selective attention (for reviews, see References 26 to 28). Both early negative components and late positive components have been said to define discrete stages of selective attention. Novak and colleagues[29] have reported that in adults early negative waveforms probably reflect sensory processing of stimuli beyond simple detection of the stimulus. Negative components of different topography, called *NA components* when they are derived by subtracting ERP waveforms of unattended stimuli from attended stimuli, occur in response to auditory tasks in a frontal-central distribution (60 to 92 milliseconds) and a posterior-lateral area (132 to 164 milliseconds).[29] Early negative waveforms also mark selective attention in visual tasks (onset = 130 to 150 milliseconds).[30,31] NA may reflect the earliest higher order sensory processing of a stimulus. NA components have been linked to attention because they are insensitive to task complexity and stimulus probability. Novak and colleagues[29] stated that the NA components are different from the processing negativity (PN) components of central and frontal distribution in the same latency ranges described by Naatanen,[32] because the PN components change in latency and amplitude when the subject attends to a stimulus.

However, others have described negative components linked to attention that are affected by stimulus probability and task difficulty. These components are longer in latency and lower in amplitude when elicited by rare stimuli or more difficult tasks. Stages of stimulus selection are marked by N1 (at ≈100 milliseconds),[33-36] and negative difference components (Nd) with onset of 60 to 80 milliseconds and duration of about 150 to 250 milliseconds in auditory[26,37] and visual[34,36,38] modalities. Contingent negative variation (a slow negativity in the central-occipital areas beginning around 350 milliseconds and lasting up to 800 milliseconds) may be related to cortical arousal,[39] and altered in disorders of attention.

Event-Related Negative Components in Children with Attention Deficit Disorders

If early negative waveforms are markers of selective attention, their amplitudes should be decreased in children with ADD. However, conflicting results have been obtained in these children. Loiselle and coworkers[40] studied 12 hyperactive boys selected from a group of children referred to a child development unit and 15 control children. They recorded auditory ERP during three behavioral tasks: (1) a dichotic selective attention task (subject selects signal tone heard in one ear only while stimuli

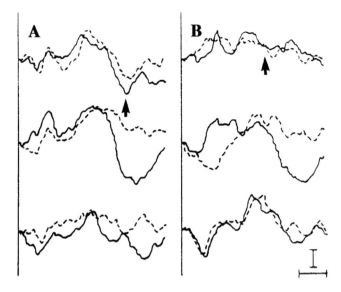

FIGURE 12–1

Auditory event-related potentials to tones for three children with attention deficit disorder (ADD) (B) and three control children (A). Negativity is upward. Target condition is shown by the solid line and the unattended target by the dotted line. Calibration, 2 μV (vertical), 100 milliseconds (horizontal). P300 (arrow) is large in the control children and small in the children with ADD (see text). (A and B, From Loiselle DL, Stamm JS, Maitinsky S, White SC: Evoked potential and behavioral signs of attentive dysfunctions in hyperactive boys. Psychophysiology 1980;17:193-201.)

are presented to either ear); (2) a binaural vigilance task (subject identifies signal tone); and (3) a dichotic listening task (subject reports pair of consonant-vowel syllables). Hyperactive boys scored lower than controls on the selective attention and vigilance tasks and made more errors of commission. These authors found the N100 amplitudes to be larger in controls than in hyperactive boys, with large standard deviations (Fig. 12-1).

Using a stop-signal paradigm with a primary visual task and auditory stop signal, 13 children with ADHD and 13 control children were studied with ERPs.[41] Children with ADHD showed poorer inhibitory performance through a slower inhibitory process. This inhibitory processing of auditory stop signals was marked by a frontal N2 component that was reduced in the ADHD group relative to controls. The authors concluded that the children with ADHD have deficient inhibitory control and that this slower inhibitory processing appears to be due to a specific neural deficiency that manifests in the processing of the stop signal as attenuated negativity in the N2 latency range. In addition, using a cued Go/NoGo task where Go stimuli were presented on 70% of the trials, Smith and associates[42] found that children with ADHD demonstrated atypical early stimulus processing, suggesting problems with sensory registration and identification of stimuli. Compared to the controls, the children with ADHD showed a much larger NoGo>Go effect and an earlier N2 peak, than controls.

Other authors have found enhanced negative waveforms. Klorman and colleagues[43] studied 53 hyperactive children between 6 and 12 years of age identified by clinical rating scales. The children were divided into aggressive (16 children), nonaggressive (20 children), and "not-criterion" (17 children) subgroups, and a 2-week placebo-controlled, double-blind, crossover trial of methylphenidate was carried out. Though the not-criterion children did not meet criteria for ADHD as defined by the investigators, they were viewed by parents and physicians as hyperactive. The children selected either a soft tone or a dim light as targets while both stimuli were presented simultaneously. These authors found larger N100s in all of the subgroups of hyperactive children when the target was a rare tone. The amplitude effect was increased by methylphenidate.

Harter and coworkers[44,45] also did not find a decrease in the amplitudes of early negative waveforms. They studied 24 boys with ADD who were identified by the Diagnostic Interview Schedule for Children. They used visual discrimination tasks requiring selection of letters, nonletter patterns, and colors as targets. Children with ADD did not have an increase in the amplitude of negative waveforms between 200 and 300 milliseconds in different waveforms, as compared with adults who had reduced selective attention when tested similarly by these investigators.[33] However, Harter and colleagues did find a large late negativity (700 milliseconds), which was longer in latency, similar in distribution to the contingent negative variation, and more prominent over the right hemisphere for children with ADD in comparison to reading disabled and control children (Fig. 12-2). The authors concluded that the late negativity signified compensatory cortical arousal in children with ADD. Its distribution, similar to the contingent negative variation which is elicited when a subject waits for future events to occur, suggesting children with ADD may be more dependent on immediate feedback (rewards) than other children.

Treatment with stimulants seems to have mixed effects on negative ERP waveforms in children with ADHD.[28]

Event-Related Potential Positive Components and Attention in Normal Subjects

Late positive ERPs (P3, P300) also have been linked to attention and information processing.[46-48] The P300 is a cognitive evoked potential that evaluates attention and information processing. At least three positive components occur in adults at 300 milliseconds[49]: P3a (peak latency 270 to 350 milliseconds, frontal-central maximum), P3b

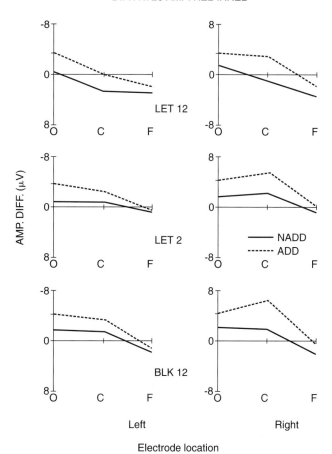

DIFF. N720 AMP: REL-IRREL

FIGURE 12–2

Scalp distribution of PN 720 for children with (dotted line) and without (solid line) attention deficit disorder (ADD). Negativity is upward. Amplitudes are derived from differences in waveforms (relevant minus irrelevant tasks) shown at O (occipital), C (central), and F (frontal) sites for the letter and block tasks. NADD, non-ADD. (From Harter MR, Anllo-Vento L, Wood FB, Schroeder MM: Separate brain potential characteristic in children with reading disability and attention deficit disorder: Color and letter relevance effects. Brain Cogn 1988;7:115-140.)

(peak latency 300 to 600 milliseconds, parietal-central maximum), and positive slow wave (pSW) (peak latency 500 to 1000 milliseconds, parietal-central maximum). In normal adults, the P3b amplitude may be an index of nonspatial attention or selection.[36,38]

Amplitude and Latency of Positive Waveforms in Attention Deficit Disorders

The use of positive ERP waveforms to explain the pathogenesis of disorders of attention in children with ADHD continues to be explored actively. A comprehensive review of this literature is beyond the scope of this chapter, which should provide a framework for additional reading. Investigators seem to agree on the following observations of positive ERP waveforms in children with ADHD in target selection tasks:

1. *Larger amplitude late positivities* (P300 and later) in children with ADHD versus controls—As in other subject groups studied with selective attention tasks, hyperactive children have larger amplitude P300s when they select rare stimuli.[40,44,45] Studies have searched for the significance of this finding in hyperactive children. Even normal children have an increase in P3b amplitude if they are treated with methylphenidate, which presumably increases arousal both in normal and hyperactive children.[50] In target selection, memory, and continuous performance tasks, Peloquin and Klorman[50] observed an increase in P3b amplitude without a corresponding change in latency in 18 normal children who had been treated with methylphenidate.

2. *Variable latency of early positive ERPs* in children with ADHD versus controls—Children with ADHD typically have a prolonged P3b in comparison with age-matched controls; this has been proposed as a sign of impaired stimulus identification.[51] However, children with ADHD can also have normal short latency auditory evoked potentials, absent ERP, or a late positive component with onset longer than 300 milliseconds.[52-54] Klorman[28] has commented that delayed P300 latency may not be a specific marker of attentional dysfunction because it is also seen in children with learning disorders.

   Harter and associates[44,45] concluded that the changes in positive waveform latencies in children with ADHD were more specific than suggested by Klorman's review. They studied 24 boys with ADD as defined by the Diagnostic Interview Schedule for Children (8 boys with ADD alone and 16 boys with ADD and a reading disorder) and compared the performance of these 24 children to that of 11 reading-disabled children and to 17 control children on visual discrimination tasks requiring selection of letters, nonletter patterns, and colors as targets. The children with ADD made more errors than those in other groups on the letter and nonletter selection tasks. There were no other differences among the groups with respect to speed and accuracy of response. They found variable latency of early positive waveforms (240 milliseconds) in children with ADD as compared with controls and children with reading disabilities. They proposed that the P240 may vary more in children with ADD because of variability in negative waveforms that occur at the same time. Harter and colleagues did not find significant

changes in latency or amplitude of intermediate negative waveforms as in adults with reduced selective attention. Because the positive waveforms close in timing to the intermediate negative waveforms were more variable in children with ADD, Harter and coworkers concluded that the change in the P240 may mark reduced selective attention in children with ADHD.

3. *Amplitude by location interactions for positive waveforms* in children with ADHD versus controls—These include observations of larger frontal-central and occipital positivities,[44,45] smaller central-parietal P3 wave-forms,[44] and right hemispheric preponderance[44,45] in children with ADHD versus controls. Harter's group found that the frontal-central positive waveforms elicited by the color relevance task was larger in amplitude for attended stimuli over the right hemisphere for children with ADD in contrast with the reading disabled children, in whom it was larger over the left hemisphere.

4. *Changes in latency for ERP positivities induced by medication*—Not unexpectedly, considering the derivation of ERP from EEG waveforms that are clearly influenced by psychoactive medications, ERP latencies are affected by the use of medications in ADHD.[28] The ratio of the right frontal-central to parietal auditory P300 amplitude has also been demonstrated to predict response to stimulants in children with ADHD, with an FC2-to-P4 auditory P300 amplitude ratio greater than 0.5 seen in children who had a clinical response to medication.[55] Change in the latency of the P300 has also been a predictor of response to imipramine.[46] Whether these latency changes can be used to support or predict a clinical response to medication is still an open question.

DISORDERS OF COGNITION

The American Association of Mental Retardation defines mental retardation as "significantly sub-average general intellectual functioning resulting in or associated with concurrent impairments in adaptive behavior and manifested during the developmental period."[56] Mental retardation implies inability to solve problems of daily living efficiently and is defined in a societal context.[57,58] Cognitive testing, the most commonly used means of classifying children as normal or mentally retarded, was developed to predict school success[59] and may not predict incapability to function in society as an adult, particularly in mildly retarded individuals.[58]

Electrophysiology and Individual Differences in Intelligence

Many investigators have tried to correlate electrophysiologic findings with individual differences in intelligence, but no clear marker of intellectual giftedness or deficit has been identified. Although the routine EEG is abnormal in a wide variety of disorders associated with mental retardation, it has not been possible to use EEG as a surrogate marker of intelligence. Within individual disorders associated with mental retardation there may be some EEG features that correlate with the cognitive function. For example, the ratio of the amplitude of alpha rhythm with eye closure to eye opening has been shown to correlate with neuropsychological test scores.[60] Grabner and colleagues[61] found that a decrease in cortical investment (observed in event-related desynchronization) that followed training on a cognitive task correlated negatively with IQ, suggesting that individuals with higher IQ were more mentally efficient. In disorders such as tuberous sclerosis[62] and Rett syndrome,[63] EEG findings may be related to cognitive outcome.

However, when data are combined for groups of patients with varying degrees of intelligence, some differences have been described.[64-67] In an evaluation of EEGs from 115 student-teachers who varied in intelligence from a mean of 82 to 136 and creativity scores from 38 to 84 it was found that there were only weak correlations between measures based on the level of activity in different areas (mean power, mean frequency, and approximated entropy) and intelligence and creativity.[68] However, coherence measures showed a much more robust relationship with both creativity as well as intelligence.

As with the EEG, ERPs may show intelligence-related differences when individuals are grouped according to their IQ.[69] Chalke and Ertl[70] proposed that IQ could correlate with latency of obligatory auditory ERPs (neural efficiency hypothesis). They studied obligatory long-latency auditory evoked potentials to tones in 35 children (22 with above average, 11 with average, and 4 below-average IQ). Long-latency auditory evoked potential latencies were shorter in the children with superior IQ. Ertl and Schafer[71] found shorter latencies of later peaks (which they labeled *E3* and *E4*) in children of higher IQ within a group of 566 children who underwent flash visual evoked potential (VEP) response testing. Perry and coworkers[72] confirmed these findings in a similar study of 98 5-year-old children whose IQ ranged from 94 to 144 on the Wechsler Preschool Primary Scale Intelligence. Ertl and Schafer[71] also proposed that the complexity of the evoked response may be greater in children with high IQ. The authors reported that 10 children with high IQ "were more complex, characterized by high frequency components in the first 100 ms" than children with normal IQ scores (Fig. 12-3).

Blinkhorn and Hendrickson[73] used a to overlay long-latency obligatory auditory evoked potentials and found correlations of this measure of complexity with higher IQs in 33 adults. Ibatullina[74] elicited obligatory auditory EPs to tones in children and found a complex obligatory response

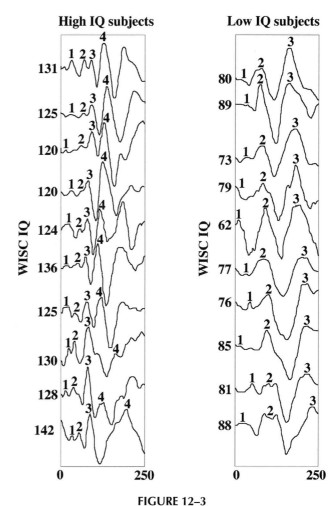

FIGURE 12–3

Averaged obligatory auditory evoked potential to tones for 10 high-IQ and 10 low-IQ subjects. WISC-IQ is listed for each subject. This illustrates the authors' observation that subjects with higher IQs have more complex waveforms. (From Ertl JP, Schafer EWP: Brain response correlates of psychometric intelligence. Nature 1969;223:421-422.)

and a higher amplitude P300 in brighter children compared with retarded children.

Vogel and coworkers[75] tested the complexity-intelligence hypothesis in their study of 236 university students, selected because they had four normal EEG variants (monomorphic alpha, frontal-precentral beta, low-voltage record, beta mixed with alpha). These adults were tested with an intelligence test, with Raven's Standard Progressive Matrices, and also with a test of attention. Passive flash VEP and tone auditory evoked potential testing were carried out, and the waveforms (not shown) were analyzed by a statistical measurement of oscillation as well as the "string measurement" of Blinkhorn and Hendrickson.[73] Vogel and associates[75] found no relationship between intelligence and evoked potential complexity. They explained nonsignificant trends in the data by citing a relationship of the normal EEG variants to the variability (in complexity) of the obligatory auditory and visual evoked responses.

In a study comparing current density measurements in high-intelligence (IQ = 127) and low-intelligence (IQ = 87) individuals using oddball tasks, it was found that in highly intelligent individuals there was a decrease in the volume of activated cortical gray matter between the onset and peak of the P300 and higher current densities were observed compared to individuals with lower intelligence.[65] The same authors[76] evaluated ERP parameters related in 74 individuals (mean IQ =107; range 73 to 135) with average creativity. The subjects passively listened to two tones and performed two auditory and two visual oddball tasks while their EEG was recorded. The approximate entropy parameters, peak latencies, and amplitudes were determined. The correlation coefficients indicated that in the attended conditions, the more intelligent individuals showed more regular ERP waveforms than less intelligent individuals. It was further found that less intelligent individuals showed increased P300 latencies and reduced amplitudes. The authors postulated that the more intelligent individuals used more specific neural networks than less intelligent individuals.

Rust[77] carried out a twin study to test the sensitivity of evoked potentials to measure individual differences in cognition. He studied 40 adult male twin pairs (half monozygotes) with a passive tone-listening task and found no latency differences between the two groups and a small-amplitude difference in P2-N2, N2-P3, and P3-N3 components.[77] No waveforms were shown in the report. He concluded that the amplitude differences were the result of a genetic effect. Whether electrophysiologic probes can be used as indices of intellectual impairment remains to be seen.

Probe Evoked Potentials and Mental Retardation

Molfese and colleagues[78] used the probe technique of Papanicolaou[79] to study language processing in profoundly retarded mute adolescents. Papanicolaou's[79] technique holds certain continuous and intermittent (or probe) stimuli constant while giving the subject different semantic or perceptual tasks. He then presumes that the alterations in waveforms that occur reflect differential activation of brain centers involved in the cognitive demands of the semantic or perceptual task. In the study by Molfese and associates,[78] six individuals viewed familiar and unknown visual-graphic symbols used as words. A series of three probe tones were presented while the subject studied different symbol sets to elicit the evoked potential components of interest. Responses to familiar symbols were significantly different from those for unknown symbols, suggesting that some form of semantic discrimination can occur in profoundly retarded individuals.

ERPs and Mental Retardation Syndromes

Limited electrophysiologic studies have been carried out in individuals with Down syndrome and fragile X syndrome. St. Clair and colleagues[80] studied 40 adults with fragile X syndrome with a tone selection task and compared their results to 90 adults with Down syndrome and 83 controls. Five of the 33 adults with fragile X syndrome (who may not have understood the task) had low-amplitude responses that were un-interpretable. In the remaining 28, a P3 was elicited to frequent and rare stimuli and was split into two components. Topography was not carried out to see if the two components corresponded to P3a and P3b. Like their Down syndrome counterparts, adults with fragile X syndrome had prolonged N2 and P3 latencies and a smaller amplitude P3 for rare tones as compared with controls. St. Clair and associates[80] concluded that these ERP changes may have resulted from generalized malformations in limbic and medial temporal regions and may help to explain the associated language and behavioral disturbances in these individuals.

Electrophysiology and Other Cognitive Processes

Researchers who study the foundations of intelligence grapple with the fundamental question of whether intelligence is a statistically derived first principal component of a given test (*g*) or whether it comprises discrete cognitive processes.[81] A natural outgrowth of this debate is the trend for psychologists who study individual differences in cognition to use neurophysiologic measures to explore the genetics of cognitive processes. Hansell and coworkers[82] recorded memory and sensory slow wave responses from prefrontal and parietal head regions during a delayed memory task in 391 adolescent twin pairs. They found familial resemblance across the twin pairs for both prefrontal (35% to 37% of shared variance) and parietal (51% to 52% of shared variance) sites, suggesting a genetic influence for this electrophysiologic response, supporting a view that delayed memory search (working memory) is an important process underlying general cognitive ability. This group made a similar observation about the variance in amplitude and latency of P3 in normal adolescent twin pairs who completed a working memory task.[83]

DISORDERS OF LANGUAGE

The most widely researched area of ERPs is most likely the study of normal language processing in adults.[27] Study of normal and abnormal language development in children using ERP is a relatively recent application (for a review of the early work, see Reference 84). This brief review attempts to highlight recent advances and provides an introduction to the voluminous literature in this area.

Normal Language Development in Children

Developmental screening instruments such as the revised Denver Developmental Screening Test and the Early Language Milestone Scale emphasize progressive acquisition of language milestones. However, cross-cultural studies suggest that normal language development is not as orderly as previously thought.[85] Although infants recognize language sounds or phonemes at birth,[86] exposure to different languages varies the order in which common language rules are learned. Bates and Marshman[85] observed that since word order is important in English, native-speaking children learn these rules by age 2 to 2 1/2 years. In contrast, Turkish children learn noun and verb endings before word order rules, because tense endings are relatively more important in their language. Thus, environmental exposure to language alters the course of its development.

Although normal language development varies among individuals, there are certain communication skills that should be established by certain ages (Box 12-1).[57,87] If these milestones have not been achieved, a developmental language disorder may be present.

Electrophysiologic Indices of Normal Language Processing

Most of the ERP studies of normal language processing in children have focused on certain aspects of a basic input-processing-output model and have not been tested against

---

BOX 12-1
SIGNS OF A POSSIBLE DEVELOPMENTAL LANGUAGE DISORDER

Criteria for concern with inadequate language development include the following:
1. No meaningful words by age 18 months
2. No meaningful phrases by age 24 months
3. Speech unintelligible out of context at age 3 years
4. Noncommunicative use of language
5. Inability to express specific wants
6. Impaired comprehension

From Rapin I: Disorders of higher cerebral function in preschool children: I. Am J Dis Child 1988;142:1119-1124.

---

any of the proposed nosologies derived from behavioral data. Aspects of auditory reception (perception, discrimination) can be studied by giving tasks that require identification of speech sounds (*phonemes*), words, or sentences that have been read to the subject. Auditory and visual memory can be studied as the subjects hear or see words, nonwords, or sentences that they must compare to a store of what they already know (*lexicon*). Thus, the study of *phonologic* and *semantic* functions comprises the bulk of research in this area. No tasks have been devised to study other aspects of language processing, i.e., *syntax* (grammar), *pragmatics* (the everyday applicability of language to life situations), *prosody* (the melody of speech), or *formulation* (a more complex process during which a subject generates a linguistic response).

Auditory Perception

Early cortical responses to sound are generated in multiple cortical and subcortical sites,[88] reflected in the middle latency response (15 to 100 milliseconds after the stimulus) and exogenous cortical negative waveforms (for review, see Reference 29; also see Chapter 9). These components have been studied using only tones as stimuli, and their latency and topography in speech sound processing are unknown.

Phonologic Processing

ERPs evoked by words show clear developmental changes in the ERP latency and morphology, especially in regard to early negative waveforms like the N1.[89] N400 amplitudes increased with alliterating word primes and beginning readers with opposite effects when alliterating nonwords were used.

Negative waveforms in the 40- to 210-millisecond range may mark cortical processing of phonologic stimuli as one of the first steps in the discriminative processing of speech sounds. Novick and coworkers[90] studied 14 adolescents with two auditory discrimination tasks. These subjects chose a target from a set of five consonant-vowel-consonant stimuli ("phonetic" task) or from a set of five one-syllable words ("verbal" task). Simple response data (in which the subjects responded to each stimulus as soon as they heard it) were also collected for each task. Subjects were classed as "fast" or "slow" responders by their reaction time latencies, so that variability in component latencies could be minimized. Different waveforms were derived by subtracting the simple grand mean ERP from the discriminative grand mean ERP. This eliminated the variability governed by stimulus probability. For the phonetic condition, subjects showed a negative waveform at 40 to 210 milliseconds, largest at PZ, with a 140-millisecond peak at CZ (Fig. 12-4). The negativity was 30 milliseconds later in onset in the verbal task, yet of the same duration and topography. The authors concluded

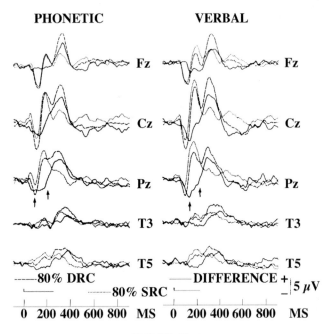

PHONETIC   **VERBAL**

Fz   Fz
Cz   Cz
Pz   Pz
T3   T3
T5   T5

------80% DRC   —— DIFFERENCE +
            ·········80% SRC   _|5 μV
0 200 400 600 800 MS   0 200 400 600 800 MS

FIGURE 12–4

Grand mean event-related potentials of seven fast-responding subjects recorded for phonetic and verbal discrimination (DRC) and simple response conditions (SRC). Differences in waveforms (80% DRC–80% SRC) are depicted by the solid line. Positivity is up. The negative waveforms at 40 to 210 milliseconds, maximal at Pz, are marked with arrows (see text). (From Novick B, Lovrich D, Vaughan HG Jr: Event-related potentials associated with the discrimination of acoustic and semantic aspects of speech. Neuropsychologia 1985;23:87-101.)

that this latency difference corresponded to the difference in stimuli and marked the time when the distinction was first made.

Speech processing probably occurs in multiple areas on the supratemporal plane and the secondary auditory area on the lateral surface of the superior temporal gyrus.[88,91-95] Lovrich and colleagues[91] demonstrated this in adolescents, using nontarget data from the same set of "phonetic" and "verbal" tasks[90] to study the topography of the auditory ERP. The initial negative wave of the auditory ERP (N110) occurred over the superior temporal plane (primary auditory cortex) in both phonetic and verbal conditions (Fig. 12-5). This observation demonstrates that there is concurrent activation of primary and secondary auditory areas in linguistic processing.

Electrophysiologic Studies of Semantic Function

ERP studies using word recognition and classification tasks are easy to devise. Consequently, a large number of studies using ERP probes of semantic functions have been carried out, some of which have been in children.

Auditory Tasks

Novick and coworkers[90] used a "semantic" classification task in their study of 14 adolescents described previously. The subject had to select animal names as targets from a list of 15 words. The authors derived different waveforms by subtracting the nontarget responses for differentiation of words from nonwords ("verbal" task) from those for classification ("semantic" task) and found a large negativity beginning at 185 milliseconds and maximal at 255 milliseconds in the frontal-central region (Fig. 12-6). They proposed that this negativity corresponded to the negative potentials derived from visually presented classification tasks in adults.[30] Some later negative peaks at 310 and 380 milliseconds also occurred in the frontal-central region.[91]

Although increases in cerebral blood flow have been found by others during auditory discrimination tasks,[96] Lovrich and associates[91] concluded that the cortical areas involved in semantic classification tasks presented orally could not yet be mapped definitively.

Visual Tasks

Late parietal negative waveforms in the 400-millisecond range can be elicited by word discrimination and classification tasks presented visually to adults.[97,98] Kutas and Hillyard[97] studied 14 subjects with a sentence reading task in which terminal words of high and low probability were varied. Sentences were written with a high to low probability of use and concluded with a high- to low-probability word at the end of the sentence. An example of a high/high-probability sentence would be "He mailed the letter without a stamp." An example of a low-probability sentence with a low-probability word is "He was soothed by the gentle wind." When a low-probability word ended the sentence (e.g., "The bill was due at the end of the *hour*"), the subjects produced a large negativity at 400 milliseconds (Fig. 12-7).

These observations have been used by Kutas[97,98] and others to study semantic priming, the process by which context enhances speed of response.

Language Processing in Children with Developmental Language Disorders

Courchesne and colleagues[99] studied nine children who had a receptive-developmental language disorder as defined by DSM III with target selection and missing stimulus auditory and visual tasks. They found an increase in the amplitude of the auditory P3b in these children as compared with 16 control children. The authors concluded that the amplitude increase indicated an alteration in language

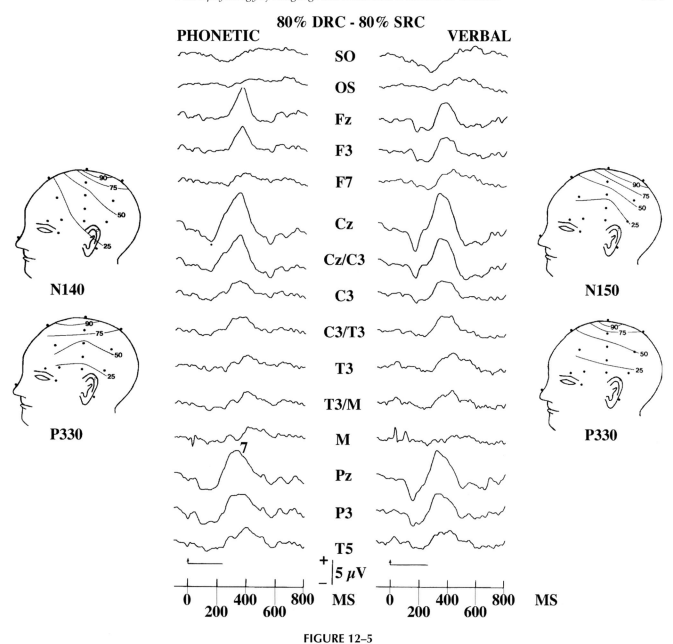

FIGURE 12–5

Grand mean difference event-related potentials were derived by subtracting discriminative responses (DRC) from simple responses (SRC) for the two tasks. Positivity is up. The fields of the components are mapped onto the head, and maxima are marked by a dot. N140 occurs over the supratemporal plane and superior temporal gyrus. (From Lovrich D, Novick B, Vaughan HG Jr: Topographic analysis of auditory event-related potentials associated with acoustic and semantic processing. Electroencephalogr Clin Neurophysiol 1988;71:40-54.)

processing in these children (Fig. 12-8). However, because their interstimulus interval was relatively long (1 second for targets and 2.05 seconds for nontargets), they commented that these findings were inconsistent with the hypothesis that children with receptive language disorders make language errors because they need more time to process stimuli.[100]

Acquired Aphasia in Children

Landau-Kleffner syndrome[101-104] is an acquired aphasia syndrome in children that has been linked to electrophysiologic abnormalities. In 1930, Worster-Drought and Allen[105] observed that some children with normal hearing

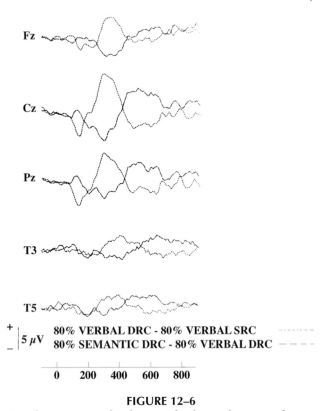

FIGURE 12–6

Grand mean event-related potentials of seven fast-responding subjects recorded for word classification (semantic) and word/nonword discrimination (verbal) tasks. Differences in waveforms were derived by subtracting semantic DRC from verbal DRC, because the acoustic analyses were judged to be similar. Positivity is up. Negative waveforms occurred at 185 to 255 milliseconds and 310 to 830 milliseconds (see text). (From Novick B, Lovrich D, Vaughan HG Jr: Event-related potentials associated with the discrimination of acoustic and semantic aspects of speech. Neuropsychologia 1985;23:87-101.)

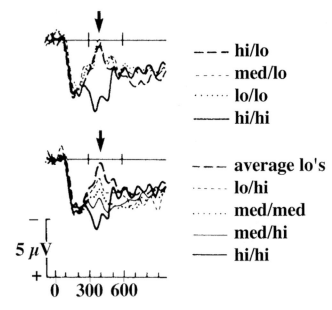

FIGURE 12–7

Sentences of high or low probability in English that end in a noun of high or low probability were presented to the patients (see text). The tracings demonstrated the grand average of event-related potentials of 124 subjects recorded at Pz, showing N400 (marked by arrows). Negativity is up. (From Kutas M, Hillyard SA: Brain potentials during reading reflect word expectancy and semantic association. Nature 1984;307:161-163.)

had selective inability to understand spoken language. Landau and Kleffner[101] made the association of language disturbance with seizures. They described six preschool children with normal language development who lost language milestones after the onset of clinical seizures. The EEGs of these children showed bitemporal spike discharges, though other electrographic patterns (focal temporal spikes, multifocal slow spikes, slow spike bursts, slow spike-wave complexes maximal posteriorly, electrical status epilepticus in sleep) have since been reported in association with the characteristic language disorder (Fig. 12-9; see also Chapter 11).[106-110]

Children with Landau-Kleffner syndrome have a severe receptive and expressive aphasia, with a more severe disturbance of language reception. Children with only an expressive language disorder have been described.[111-113] Some children have an abnormal EEG in association with the receptive and expressive aphasia but have never had a clinical seizure.[114] The etiology of the Landau-Kleffner syndrome is also unknown.

Evoked potential studies of children with Landau-Kleffner syndrome show normal auditory brainstem responses[115-117] and middle latency responses.[116,117] Obligatory cortical auditory event-related potentials (CAEPs) were absent in two individuals with damage to the primary auditory cortex who were tested with pure tone stimuli.[115,118] Klein and colleagues[117] found prolonged P2 latency for pure tone stimuli in two of six subjects tested. These two individuals were the only subjects who had persisting clinical seizures, and neither had damage to the primary auditory cortex on magnetic resonance imaging.

Rapin and associates[87] compared children with verbal auditory agnosia to adults with word deafness and proposed that these children had a specific deficit in decoding phonemes, the smallest distinguishable units of speech. Klein and colleagues[117] compared the performance of 6 recovered young adults and 11 age-range controls on visual and auditory discrimination tasks using an oddball paradigm. Subjects with persisting phonologic discrimination deficits as measured by the Goldman-Fristoe-Woodcock Test of Auditory Discrimination had P2 components larger

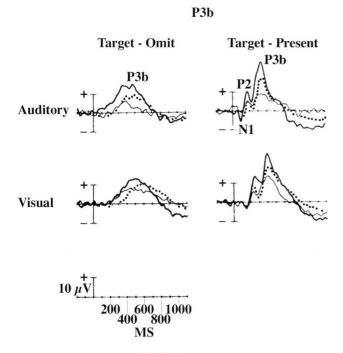

FIGURE 12–8

P3b elicited by auditory and visual tasks in 11 autistic (thin line), *9 receptive-developmental language disordered* (heavy line), *and 16 normal* (dotted line) *subjects, shown at Pz. Positivity is up. P3b is abnormally large in the children with developmental language disorder and abnormally small in autistic children. (From Courchesne E, Lincoln AJ, Yeung-Courchesne R, Elmasian R, Grillon C. Pathophysiologic findings in nonretarded autism and receptive developmental language disorder. J Autism Dev Disord 1989;19:1-17.)*

in amplitude and longer latency P3 components than controls for discrimination of some phonemes, but not in visual or tone tasks. These data support the hypothesis that the underlying pathology in Landau-Kleffner syndrome may be a deficit of phonemic decoding.

Speech deficits in the syndrome may be explained by either disruption of normal connections or an excessive inhibitory reaction to epileptiform discharges. Speech usually does not improve in the syndrome unless the EEG improves. However, the severity of the aphasia does not always have a close correlation with degree of EEG abnormality[107,119] or the severity of clinical seizures.[101] It is possible that the epileptiform activity is an epiphenomenon and simply is reflective of an underlying cortical abnormality.[107,120,121] Even if the EEG parallels speech recovery, this does not prove that epileptiform activity causes aphasia. It is possible that the decreased epileptiform activity during speech recovery simply reflects resolving injury to the speech areas.

Treatment of Landau-Kleffner syndrome and epilepsy with continuous spikes and waves during sleep (CSWDS) can be frustrating. Unless objective evidence of changes in

speech is found by an impartial, blinded observer, separating a placebo effect from drug-related improvement is difficult. Standard antiepileptic drugs such as valproic acid, levetiracetam, and lamotrigine can sometimes both reduce seizure frequency and improve language and cognitive function. Recently there has been success with high-dose diazepam treatment in CSWDS. Administration of corticosteroids resulted in improved speech, suppression of seizures, and normalization of the EEG in several small series of children. Subpial cortical transections have been reported to be useful in patients with Landau-Kleffner syndrome.[122]

The outcome in both Landau-Kleffner syndrome and CSWDS is variable. Recovery of language in LKS is highly dependent on age of onset of the syndrome, with the best recovery seen in children with early onset. Likewise, in CSWDS, outcome varies from full recovery to continued speech and cognitive impairment. Most patients with CSWDS have some amelioration in their cognition and behavioral disorders over time.

Epilepsy and Cognition

A discussion of the effects of epilepsy on cognition (defined as intelligence, academic achievement, or as individual components of cognitive function such as memory, or executive function) is beyond the scope of this chapter. This is an area of active research. Challenges in this area include identifying representative individuals in each epilepsy syndrome; developing a standardized way to quantitate clinical severity; accounting for the effects of age at onset and presence of structural brain lesions; and controlling for the exposure to antiepileptic agents, which may in themselves contribute to cognitive blunting.

DISORDERS OF LEARNING

Kirk[123] proposed the term *learning disabilities* at a conference in 1963 to describe a group of children with normal neurologic examinations who had difficulties in learning to read, spell, and compute. Learning disabilities include reading, spelling, mathematical, nonverbal, and right hemisphere deficits. Several limited studies have attempted to identify electrophysiologic substrates of learning disorders.

Dyslexia and Reading Disorders

Five percent to 10% of school-age children fail to learn to read in spite of normal intelligence, adequate environment, and educational opportunities.[124] See Shaywitz and Shaywitz[125] for a review of the clinical and neuropathologic features of dyslexia.

A   **B**   **C**

D   **E**   **F**

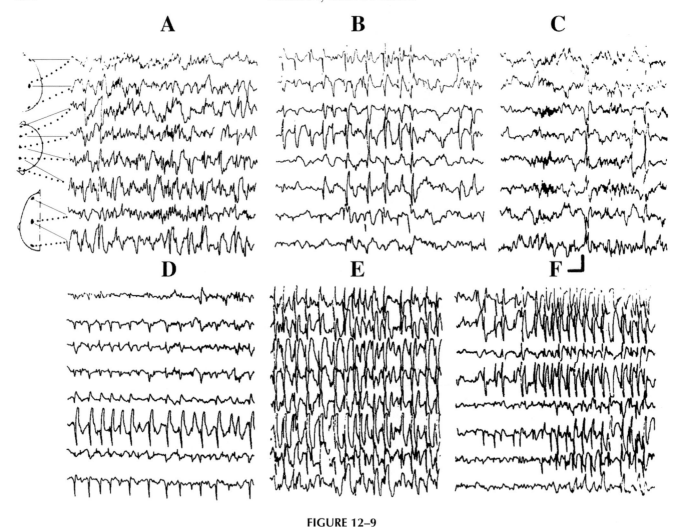

FIGURE 12–9

Serial sleep EEGs in a 5-year, 7-month-old child with Landau-Kleffner syndrome, beginning 7 months after language regression started (A), two 5-month intervals after the initial EEG (B and C), and 3-month intervals subsequently (D-F). (A-F, From Hirsch E, Marescaux C, Maquet P, et al: Landau-Kleffner Syndrome: A clinical and EEG study of five cases. Epilepsia 1990;31:756-767.)

EEG

Results of frequency spectra analysis of EEG in dyslexic children provide some evidence for left hemispheric dysfunction (for a review, see Reference 126). Although Leisman and Ashkenazi[127] found decreased low-frequency EEG activity at rest in the left parietal-occipital region in dyslexic subjects, others have not been able to replicate their results.[128,129] Duffy and coworkers[130] found differences in EEG spectra in the left temporal, temporal-parietal, and medial frontal regions in eight dyslexic boys. However, subtypes of reading disabled boys cannot be distinguished on the basis of spectral EEG analysis alone.

Event-Related Potentials

ERPs have been extensively used in the evaluation of developmental language disorders and dyslexia.[131] Differences in sensory ERPs at the latency range of P1 and N1-P2 components have been reported between children with language disorders and dyslexia and controls.[132] Latency differences between the groups may be related to a common timing deficit suggested as one of the possible underlying mechanisms in both conditions. As noted earlier, N1 amplitude group differences may be partly related to arousal/attentional factors and partly to the "tuning" of the auditory sensory system. In addition, in both children with developmental language disorders and dyslexia the P3 amplitudes are, in general, lower and the latencies longer compared with those in controls. The differences in ERPs may not reflect only maturational lag but also more fundamental processing deficiencies.

Studies using ERP suggest that left hemispheric processing is different in children with dyslexia.[45,133,134]

Children with dyslexia do not have the expected increase in P3 amplitude over left hemispheric central and occipital areas that occurs normally in letter recognition tasks. In addition, children with dyslexia have prolonged P3 latency when compared with controls.[45] Unlike children with ADD with and without reading disorders, children with reading disorders alone do not have a compensatory (possibly right) frontal positive waveforms.[45]

Taylor and Keenan[135] found no evidence of interhemispheric differences in processing of visual and language stimuli in children with dyslexia. In a study of 21 children of normal intelligence with dyslexia with a 2-year discrepancy between achievement scores in reading and chronologic age, the authors reported that the P3 elicited by word/nonword, letter/nonletter, and different symbol discrimination tasks was prolonged and had broader bilateral distribution compared with controls (Fig. 12-10).

A defect in magnocellular function in dyslexia has been postulated.[136-139] Children with dyslexia have been shown

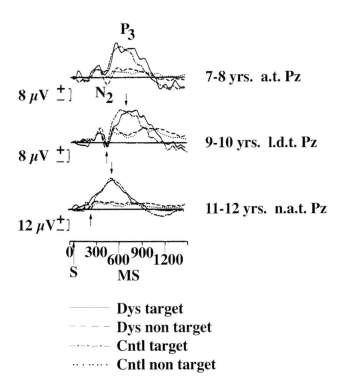

FIGURE 12–10
Grand average event-related potentials of 21 dyslexic and 32 control subjects in word/nonword (lexical decision [ldt]), letter (alphabetic [at] and symbol discrimination (nonalphabetic [nat]) tasks. Positivity is up. P3 is broad in dyslexic children (solid line) in the alphabetic and lexical decision tasks. Waveforms are shown at Pz. Upward arrows mark N2, downward arrows mark P3. (From Taylor MJ, Keenan NK: Event-related potentials to visual and language stimuli in normal and dyslexic children. Psychophysiology 1990;27:318-327.)

to have attenuated amplitudes of motion-onset VEPs but not of the stationary VEPs. The magnocellular deficit theory is one of the prominent hypotheses in dyslexia research. However, recent studies have produced conflicting results. Ten dyslexic children and 12 controls were examined with VEPs elicited by random dot kinematogram. The experiment comprises two sequences: one with randomly moving dots (control condition) and a second sequence where a fraction of the dots were moved coherently at the left or right side (depending on the level of coherence, 10%, 20%, and 40% of the dots). Randomly moving dots elicited two components, a P100 and P200, which were not different between the groups. Coherently moving dots elicited a late positivity between 300 and 800 milliseconds, which was significantly attenuated in dyslexic children. The area of this component becomes larger at a higher level of coherence. This study supports the hypothesis of an impairment of a specific magnocellular function in dyslexia.[138]

Alterations in auditory ERPs may occur early in life in children at risk for dyslexia. Auditory ERPs were studied in newborns and 6-month-old infants, about half of whom had a familial risk for dyslexia.[7] Syllables varying in vowel duration were presented in an oddball paradigm, in which ERPs to deviating stimuli are assumed to reflect automatic change detection in the brain. The ERPs of newborns had slow positive deflections typical of their age, but significant stimulus and group effects were found only by the age of 6 months. However, when the authors made the stimulus presentation rate slower, the ERPs to the short deviant /ka/ were different from those to the long standard/kaa/stimulus in newborns.[6] In addition, clear group differences in the ERPs were found. The results demonstrated that infants born with a high familial risk for dyslexia process speech and auditory stimulus durations differently from control infants at birth.

In summary, there is some ERP evidence for processing dysfunction in dyslexia, but further localization of this dysfunction is still being debated.

DISORDERS OF BEHAVIOR

Autistic and dysphasic children share the common core symptom of impairment of language. They differ because autistic children show impairment in social interaction and a markedly restricted repertoire of activities. The relationship between language dysfunction and the impairment in social interaction and abnormal behaviors present in autistic children remains unclear. DSM III-R[140] suggests that the pervasive disturbance in interpersonal communication accounts for the disordered language present in autism. Allen and coworkers[141,142] have proposed that autistic children have developmental language disorders. They suggested that with the exception of two purely expressive subtypes, the language disorders of nonautistic dysphasic children also occur in the autistic population. Thus, although autism is not simply a disorder of language, autistic children are also dysphasic.

Electrophysiologic studies comparing autistic and nonautistic dysphasic children may provide critical information regarding the different pathways that form the neural bases of these disorders. Both clinical EEG and evoked potential studies have been carried out.

Clinical EEG Studies in Autism

Investigators[143-153] have reported EEG abnormalities in 13% to 83% of autistic children. The heterogeneity of autism itself, the diagnostic criteria used for autism, and the methods of recording and interpreting clinical EEGs are likely to account for these differences. Furthermore, although cognition is not a defining feature of autism, mental deficiency occurs in a large proportion of these children. The abnormalities found in these studies may represent underlying brain dysfunction that is not specific to autism itself.

EEG studies have suggested that abnormal patterns of cerebral lateralization and maturational delay are commonly found in autistic children.[144,146,154,155] Whether the language dysfunction in autism is secondary to diffuse cortical impairment with global attention deficits or whether it is secondary to an atypical pattern of hemispheric specialization is still unclear.

There have been few clinical electrophysiologic studies in autistic children that have attempted to link specific EEG findings to language dysfunction in individual language subtypes. Dorenbaum and coworkers[156] studied 17 children with autism and tried to determine if there was a correlation between the presence and characteristics of EEG changes and the nature of speech and language disturbances. There was no statistically significant correlation between EEG changes and each of the communication variables studied. This study is somewhat limited by the number of children included and the lack of non-autistic dysphasic children as controls. However, it does attempt to address the relationship of EEG findings to language dysfunction.

Tuchman and colleagues[157] compared rates of epilepsy in autistic and nonautistic dysphasic children and found a very high incidence of epileptiform abnormalities in patients with epilepsy (71% of autistic vs. 58% of dysphasic children with EEG data). Furthermore, a high incidence of epilepsy occurred in children with epileptiform EEG abnormalities (73% of autistic and 65% of dysphasic children). This latter finding was biased by the fact that children with seizures were more likely to have been tested with EEG. The great variability in the number of autistic children with epilepsy may be due to differences in associated disabilities among the populations studied. In the Tuchman study, no risk factor

other than language type was associated with an increased risk of epilepsy in autistic children when cognitive and motor deficits were taken into account. Unless children with autism had associated cognitive and motor disabilities, they had no greater risk of developing epilepsy than did nonautistic dysphasic children. Children with the most severe deficit in comprehension of oral language, those with verbal auditory agnosia, were most likely to have epilepsy (48% of all autistic and dysphasic children). However, only 34% of the children with verbal auditory agnosia (5 of 17 autistic children and 5 of 12 dysphasic children) had an epileptiform EEG. Further studies incorporating uniform clinical criteria to identify autistic and nonautistic dysphasic children, appropriate control groups, classification of language subtype, and awake and asleep EEG recordings are needed to determine the relationship of the electrophysiologic abnormalities found in some children with autism and language dysfunction.

Short-Latency Evoked Potential Studies in Autism

Evoked potential studies may be of value in understanding the pathophysiology of language disorders in autistic and nonautistic individuals. Age, gender, body temperature, and mental status all affect the characteristics of the brainstem auditory evoked potential (BAEP). Recent studies that take these factors into account have found no abnormality in either the BAEPs or the middle latency responses (MLRs) of non-mentally retarded autistic individuals.[158] This suggests that the abnormalities of late ERPs reported by several investigators are not due to abnormal sensory processing at the level of the brainstem and auditory cortical structures that generate the BAEP and MLR.[99,158-160]

Event-Related Potential Studies in Autism

Several studies have found smaller P3 amplitudes in autistic compared with nonautistic subjects.[90,99,155,160,161] Although speech-related ERPs are greater in amplitude over the right hemisphere than over the left hemisphere in both autistic and dysphasic subjects, the relationship of these findings to language function is not the same for these two groups of children.[162] Dawson and coworkers[162] found that autistic subjects with increased right hemisphere N1 potential amplitude and shorter right hemisphere N1 latency had the poorest language abilities, suggesting to them that overactivation of the right hemisphere may interfere with normal left hemisphere functions in this population. On the other hand, they found that in dysphasic nonautistic subjects, superior language ability was associated with shorter left hemisphere N1 latency. The short N1 latency over the left hemisphere in dysphasic children suggested inherent left hemisphere dysfunction, accounting for their poor language skills.

Courchesne and associates[99] have also found that nonmentally retarded autistic and receptive developmental language disorder (R-DLD) subjects differ from each other in their endogenous responses (Nc and P3b) to auditory stimuli. Specifically, they found that in the autistic group, the auditory P3b was smaller than normal and in the R-DLD group it was larger than normal. Nc responses were normal in the R-DLD group, whereas in the autistic group Nc was absent or reduced, even when no auditory language or sensory processing was required. In fact, in the autistic group, there was actually a positive potential over frontal scalp regions (of similar distribution and timing to the negative Nc potential) (Fig. 12-11).[99,161]

These results suggest that autism and receptive developmental language disorders are neurally separate syndromes.

SUMMARY

Neurophysiologic study of attention, language, cognitive, and behavioral disorders is an active and rapidly evolving field, with a vast, and not easily condensed, literature. Despite this intensive, often multidisciplinary, and international effort, investigators have identified few electrophysiologic markers for identification of and treatment response for specific disorders. Except for children with Landau-Kleffner syndrome, conventional electroencephalography does not identify children with these disorders or predict their prognosis. The work of Duffy and colleagues[130] in children who have dyslexia raised hopes in the early 1980s that computer-analyzed EEG might be an effective tool to study children with disorders of higher cognitive function. More normative data are needed to clarify whether quantitative EEG methods will be useful in diagnosis and management of behavioral disorders. Evoked potentials and ERPs have best added to our understanding of how children learn. However, evoked potentials and ERPs have many limitations. It is difficult to get children to remain still and to concentrate on the tasks, which are necessarily repetitious. Interpreting results can be challenging, since technical artifacts must be excluded. Normal subjects must be studied with each new task as well, because experimental conditions affect the size and timing of positive and negative components. Magnetoencephalography (see Chapter 39) is a newer and relatively cost-effective alternative that is emerging as another important neurophysiologic method to study behavior. At this time, electrophysiologic tests remain research techniques *only* when used to study children with language, learning, and behavioral problems. However, these tests will continue to complement imaging studies and neuropsychological testing, because they can give us real-time information about the process of learning.

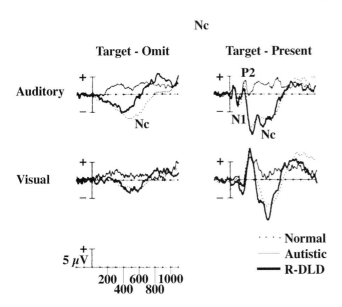

Nc

FIGURE 12–11

Grand average event-related potentials from electrode site midway between Fp2 and F8 for auditory and visual tasks in 8 autistic children, 9 children with receptive-developmental language disorder, and 16 normal subjects. Positivity is up. Autistic individuals (thin line) show no Nc in the target condition. (From Courchesne E, Lincoln AJ, Yeung-Courchesne R, et al: Pathophysiologic findings in nonretarded autism and receptive developmental language disorder. J Autism Dev Disord 1989;19:1-17.)

REFERENCES

1. Gibbs FA, Gibbs EL: Atlas of Electroencephalography, Vol 3: Neurological and Psychiatric Disorders. Reading, MA, Addison-Wesley, 1964.
2. Thomas KM: Assessing brain development using neurophysiologic and behavioral measures. J Pediatr 2003;143(Suppl):S46-S53.
3. Courchesne E: Event-related brain potentials: Comparison between children and adults. Science 1977;197:589-592.
4. Kurtzberg D, Hilpert PL, Kreuzer J, Vaughan HG Jr: Differential maturation of cortical auditory evoked potentials to speech sounds in normal fullterm and very low-birthweight infants. Dev Med Child Neurol 1984;26:466-475.
5. Molfese DL, Molfese VJ: Cortical responses of preterm infants to phonetic and nonphonetic speech stimuli. Dev Psychol 1980;16:574-581.
6. Leppanen PH, Pihko E, Eklund KM, Lyytinen H: Cortical responses of infants with and without a genetic

risk for dyslexia: II. Group effects. Neuroreport 1999;10:969-973.

7. Pihko E, Leppanen PH, Eklund KM, et al: Cortical responses of infants with and without a genetic risk for dyslexia: I. Age effects. Neuroreport 1999;10:901-905.

8. Brandeis D, Lehmann D: Event-related potentials of the brain and cognitive processes: Approaches and applications. Neuropsychologia 1986;24:151-168.

9. Courchesne E: Neurophysiological correlates of cognitive development changes in long-latency event-related potentials from childhood to adulthood. Electroencephalogr Clin Neurophysiol 1978;45:468-482.

10. Courchesne E: Cognitive components of the event-related brain potential: Changes associated with development. *In* Gaillard AWK, Ritter W (eds): Tutorials in ERP Research: Endogenous Components. Amsterdam, North Holland, 1983, pp 329-344.

11. Callaway E, Halliday R, Herning R: A comparison of methods for measuring event-related potentials. Electroencephalogr Clin Neurophysiol 1983;55:227-232.

12. Mesulam MM: Attention, confusional states, and neglect. *In* Mesulam MM (ed): Principles of Behavioral Neurology. Philadelphia, FA Davis, 1985, pp 125-168.

13. Zametkin AJ, Nordahl TE, Gross M, et al: Cerebral glucose metabolism in adults with hyperactivity of childhood onset. N Engl J Med 1990;323:1361-1366.

14. Lou HC, Henriksen L, Borner H, Nielsen JB: Striatal dysfunction in attention deficit and hyperkinetic disorder. Arch Neurol 1989;46:48-52.

15. Volkow ND, Wang GJ, Fowler JS, et al: Evidence that methylphenidate enhances the saliency of a mathematical task by increasing dopamine in the human brain. Am J Psychiatry 2004;161:1173-1180.

16. Tzavara ET, Bymaster FP, Davis RJ, et al: M_4 muscarinic receptors regulate the dynamics of cholinergic and dopaminergic neurotransmission: Relevance to the pathophysiology and treatment of related central nervous system pathologies. FASEB J 2004;18:1410-1412.

17. Eiland LS, Guest AL: Atomoxetine treatment of attention-deficit/hyperactivity disorder. Ann Pharmacother 2004;38:86-90.

18. Cook EH, Stein MA, Krasowski MD, et al: Association of Attention Deficit Disorder and Dopamine Transporter Gene. Am J Hum Genet 1995;56:993.

19. Reiff MI, Stein MT: Attention-deficit/hyperactivity disorder evaluation and diagnosis: A practical approach in office practice. Pediatr Clin North Am 2003;50:1019-1048.

20. McManis MH, Kagan J, Snidman NC, Woodward SA: EEG asymmetry, power, and temperament in children. Dev Psychobiol 2002;41:169-177.

21. Henderson HA, Marshall PJ, Fox NA, Rubin KH: Psychophysiological and behavioral evidence for varying forms and functions of nonsocial behavior in preschoolers. Child Dev 2004;75:236-250.

22. Yordanova J, Kolev V: Brain theta response predicts P300 latency in children. Neuroreport 1996;8:277-280.

23. Chabot RJ, diMichele F, Prichep L, John ER: The clinical role of computerized EEG in the evaluation and treatment of learning and attention disorders in children and adolescents. J Neuropsychiatry Clin Neurosci 2001;13:171-186.

24. Kropotov YD, Ponomarev VA, Grin-Yatsenko VA: EEG-biocontrol method in treating the attention deficit hyperactivity disorder in children. Hum Physiol 2001;27:496-504; translated from Fiziologiya Cheloveka 2001;27:126-135.

25. Othmer SF, Othmer S: Efficacy and remediation of attention deficits. *www.eegspectrum.com/tova92/tova92.htm* (electronic publication), 1992.

26. Knight RT: Electrophysiology in behavioral neurology. *In* Mesulam MM (ed): Principles of Behavioral Neurology. Philadelphia, FA Davis, 1985, pp 327-346.

27. Picton TW, Hillyard SA: Endogenous event-related potentials. *In* Picton TW (ed): Human Event-Related Potentials: EEG Handbook, Vol 3 (revised series). New York, Elsevier, 1988, pp 361-426.

28. Klorman R: Psychophysiological research on childhood psychopathology. *In* Hersen M, Ammerman RT (eds): Advanced Abnormal Child Psychology, 2nd ed. Mahwah, NJ, Lawrence Erlbaum Associates, 2000, pp 57-80.

29. Novak GP, Ritter W, Vaughan HG Jr, Wiznitzer M: Differentiation of negative event-related potentials in an auditory discrimination task. Electroencephalogr Clin Neurophysiol 1990;75:255-275.

30. Ritter W, Simson R, Vaughan HG Jr: Event-related potential correlates of two stages of information processing in physical and semantic discrimination tasks. Psychophysiology 1983;20:168-179.

31. Ritter W, Simson R, Vaughan HG Jr, Macht M: Manipulation of event-related potential manifestations of information processing stages. Science 1992;218:909-911.

32. Naatanen R: Processing negativity: An evoked potential reflection of selective attention. Psychol Bull 1982;92:605-640.

33. Harter MR, Guido W: Attention to pattern orientation: Negative cortical potentials (Oz, Cz, Fz), reaction time, and the selection process. Electroencephalogr Clin Neurophysiol 1980;49:461-465.

34. Hillyard SA, Hink RF, Swchent VL, Picton TW: Electrical signs of selective attention in the human brain. Science 1973;182:177-190.

35. Hillyard SA, Munte T: Selective attention to color and location: An analysis with event-related brain potentials. Percept Psychophys 1984;36:185-198.

36. Neville HJ, Lawson D: Attention to central and peripheral visual space in a movement detection task: I. Normal hearing adults. Brain Res 1987;405:253-294.

37. Hansen JC, Hillyard SA: Endogenous brain potentials associated with selective auditory attention. Electroencephalogr Clin Neurophysiol 1980;49:277-290.

38. Harter MR, Aine C, Schroeder C: Hemispheric differences in the neural processing of stimulus location

and type: Effects of selective attention on visual evoked potentials. Neuropsychologia 1982;20:421-438.

39. Donchin E, Ritter W, McCallum C: Cognitive psychophysiology: The endogenous components of the ERP. *In* Callaway E, Tueting P, Koslow SH (eds): Brain Event-Related Potentials in Man. New York, Academic Press, 1978, pp 349-441.

40. Loiselle DL, Stamm JS, Maitinsky S, White SC: Evoked potential and behavioral signs of attentive dysfunctions in hyperactive boys. Psychophysiology 1980;17:193-201.

41. Dimoska A, Johnstone SJ, Barry RJ, Clarke AR: Inhibitory motor control in children with attention-deficit/hyperactivity disorder: Event-related potentials in the stop-signal paradigm. Biol Psychiatry 2003;54:1345-1354.

42. Smith JL, Johnstone SJ, Barry RJ: Inhibitory processing during the Go/NoGo task: An ERP analysis of children with attention-deficit/hyperactivity disorder. Clin Neurophysiol 2004;115:1320-1331.

43. Klorman R, Brumaghim JT, Salzman LF, et al: Effects of methylphenidate on processing negativities in patients with attention-deficit hyperactivity disorder. Psychophysiology 1990;27:328-337.

44. Harter MR, Diering S, Wood FB: Separate brain potential characteristic in children with reading disability and attention deficit disorder: Relevance-independent effects. Brain Cogn 1988;7:54-86.

45. Harter MR, Anllo-Vento L, Wood FB, Schroeder MM: Separate brain potential characteristic in children with reading disability and attention deficit disorder: Color and letter relevance effects. Brain Cogn 1988;7:115-140.

46. Sangal JM, Sangal RB, Persky B: Prolonged P300 latency in attention deficit hyperactivity disorder predicts poor response to imipramine. Clin Electroencephalogr 1996;27:191-201.

47. Sangal RB, Sangal JM: Topography of auditory and visual P300 in normal children. Clin Electroencephalogr 1996;27:46-51.

48. Overtoom CC, Kenemans JL, Verbaten MN, et al: Inhibition in children with attention-deficit/hyperactivity disorder: A psychophysiological study of the stop task. Biol Psychiatry 2002;51:668-676.

49. Rosler F, Sutton S, Johnson R Jr, et al: Endogenous ERP components and cognitive constructs: A review. *In* McCallum WC, Sappoli R, Denoth F (eds): Cerebral Psychophysiology: Studies in Event-Related Potentials. New York, Elsevier, 1986, pp 51-92.

50. Peloquin LJ, Klorman R: Effects of methylphenidate on normal children's mood, event-related potentials, and performance in memory scanning and vigilance. J Abnorm Psychol 1986;95:88-98.

51. Klorman R, Brumaghim JT, Fitzpatrick PA, Borgstedt AD: Methylphenidate reduces abnormalities of stimulus classification in adolescents with attention deficit disorder. J Abnorm Psychol 1992;101:130-138.

52. Schochat E, Scheuer CI, Andrade ER: ABR and auditory P300 findings in children with ADHD. Arq Neuropsiquiatr 2002;60:742-747.

53. Strandburg RJ, Marsh JT, Brown WS, et al: Continuous-processing-related event-related potentials in children with attention deficit hyperactivity disorder. Biol Psychiatry 1996;40:964-980.

54. Sunohara GA, Voros JG, Malone MA, Taylor MJ: Effects of methylphenidate in children with attention deficit hyperactivity disorder: A comparison of event-related potentials between medication responders and non-responders. Int J Psychophysiol 1997;27:9-14.

55. Sangal RB, Sangal JM: Attention-deficit/hyperactivity disorder: Cognitive evoked potential (P300) topography predicts treatment response to methylphenidate. Clin Neurophysiol 2004;115:188-193.

56. Grossman HJ: Classification in Mental Retardation. Washington, DC, American Association of Mental Deficiency, 1983.

57. Rapin I: Children with Brain Dysfunction: Neurology, Cognition, Language, and Behavior. New York, Raven Press, 1982.

58. Richardson SA, Koller H: Epidemiology. *In* Clarke AM, Clarke ADB, Berg M (eds): Mental Deficiency: The Changing Outlook. London, Methuen, 1985, pp 356-402.

59. Binet A, Simon Th: L'Annee Psychologique, Vol. 2. Cited in: Madge N, Tizard J: Intelligence. *In* Rutter M (ed): Scientific Foundations of Developmental Psychiatry. Baltimore, University Park Press, 1981, pp 245-266.

60. Partanen J, Soininen H, Kononen M, et al: EEG reactivity correlates with neuropsychological test scores in Down's syndrome. Acta Neurol Scand 1996;94:242-246.

61. Grabner RH, Fink A, Stipacek A, et al: Intelligence and working memory systems: Evidence of neural efficiency in alpha band ERD. Cogn Brain Res 2004;20:212-225.

62. Bolton PF, Park RJ, Higgins JN, et al: Neuro-epileptic determinants of autism spectrum disorders in tuberous sclerosis complex. Brain 2002;125:1247-1255.

63. Bashina VM, Simashkova NV, Grachev VV, Gorbachevskaya NL: Speech and motor disturbances in Rett syndrome. Neurosci Behav Physiol 2002;32:323-327.

64. Jausovec N, Jausovec K, Gerlic I: Differences in event-related and induced EEG patterns in the theta and alpha frequency bands related to human emotional intelligence. Neurosci Lett 2001;311:93-96.

65. Jausovec N, Jausovec K: Differences in EEG current density related to intelligence. Brain Res Cogn Brain Res 2001;12:55-60.

66. Jausovec N, Jausovec K: Differences in event-related and induced brain oscillations in the theta and alpha frequency bands related to human intelligence. Neurosci Lett 2000;293:191-194.

67. Martin-Loeches M, Munoz-Ruata J, Martinez-Lebrusant L, Gomez-Jarabo G: Electrophysiology and intelligence: The electrophysiology of intellectual functions in intellectual disability. J Intellect Disabil Res 2001;45:63-75.

68. Jausovec N, Jausovec K: Differences in resting EEG related to ability. Brain Topogr 2000;12:229-240.

69. Brumback CR, Low KA, Gratton G, Fabiani M: Sensory ERPs predict differences in working memory span and fluid intelligence. Neuroreport 2004;15:373-376.

70. Chalke FCR, Ertl J: Evoked potentials and intelligence. Life Sci 1965;4:1319-1322.

71. Ertl JP, Schafer EWP: Brain response correlates of psychometric intelligence. Nature 1969;223:421-422.

72. Perry NW Jr, McCoy JG, Cunningham WR, et al: Multivariate visual evoked response correlates of intelligence. Psychophysiology 1976;13:323-329.

73. Blinkhorn SF, Hendrickson DE: Averaged evoked responses and psychometric intelligence. Nature 1982;295:596-597.

74. Ibatullina AA: Auditory evoked potentials to indifferent and meaningful stimuli in young children. Zh Vyssh Nerv Deiat Im I P Pavlova 1983;33:632-638.

75. Vogel F, Kruger J, Schalt E, et al: No consistent relationships between oscillations and latencies of visually and auditory evoked EEG potentials and measures of mental performance. Hum Neurobiol 1987;6:173-182.

76. Jausovec N, Jausovec K: Correlations between ERP parameters and intelligence: A reconsideration. Biol Psychol 2000;55:137-154.

77. Rust J: Genetic effects in the cortical auditory evoked potential: A twin study. Electroencephalogr Clin Neurophysiol 1975;39:321-327.

78. Molfese DL, Morris RD, Romski MA: Semantic discrimination in nonspeaking youngsters with moderate or severe retardation: Electrophysiological correlates. Brain Lang 1990;38:61-74.

79. Papanicolaou AC: Cerebral excitation profiles in language processing: The photic probe paradigm. Brain Lang 1980;9:269-280.

80. St. Clair DM, Blackwood DHR, Oliver CJ, Dickens P: P3 abnormality in fragile X syndrome. Biol Psychiatry 1987;22:303-312.

81. Deary I: g and cognitive elements of information processing: An agnostic view. In Sternberg RJ, Grigorenko EL (eds): The General Factor of Intelligence: How General Is It? Mahwah, NJ, Lawrence Erlbaum Associates, 2002, pp 151-181.

82. Hansell NK, Wright MJ, Geffen GM, et al: Genetic influences of ERP slow wave measures of working memory. Behav Genet 2001;31:603-614.

83. Wright MJ, Hansell NK, Geffen LB, et al: Genetic influence on the variance in P3 amplitude and latency. Behav Genet 2001;31:555-565.

84. Picton TW, Stuss DT: Event-related potentials in the study of speech and language: A critical review. In Caplan D, Roch Lecours A, Smith A (eds): Biological Perspectives on Language. Cambridge, MA, MIT Press, 1984, pp 303-360.

85. Bates E, Marchman VA: What is and is not universal in language acquisition. In Plum F (ed): Language, Communication, and the Brain. Research Publications,

Vol. 66. Association for Research in Nervous and Mental Disease. New York, Raven Press, 1988, pp 19-38.

86. Elimas PD, Tartter VC: On the development of speech perception: Mechanisms and analogies. Adv Child Dev Behav 1979;13:155-193.

87. Rapin I, Mattis S, Rowan AJ, Golden GS: Verbal auditory agnosia in children. Dev Med Child Neurol 1977;19:192-207.

88. Scherg M, Von Cramon D: Two bilateral sources of the late AEP as identified by a spatiotemporal dipole model. Electroencephalogr Clin Neurophysiol 1985;62:32-44.

89. Bonte M, Blomert L: Developmental changes in ERP correlates of spoken word recognition during early school years: A phonological priming study. Clin Neurophysiol 2004;115:409-423.

90. Novick B, Lovrich D, Vaughan HG Jr: Event-related potentials associated with the discrimination of acoustic and semantic aspects of speech. Neuropsychologia 1985;23:87-101.

91. Lovrich D, Novick B, Vaughan HG Jr: Topographic analysis of auditory event-related potentials associated with acoustic and semantic processing. Electroencephalogr Clin Neurophysiol 1988;71:40-54.

92. Scherg M, Von Cramon D: Evoked dipole source potentials of the human auditory cortex. Electroencephalogr Clin Neurophysiol 1986;65:344-360.

93. Vaughan HG Jr, Ritter W, Simson R: Topographic analysis of auditory event-related potentials. In Kornhuber HH, Deecke L (eds): Motivation, Motor, and Sensory Processes of the Brain. Vol 54. Amsterdam, Elsevier, 1980, pp 278-285.

94. Wolpaw JR, Penry JK: A temporal component of the auditory evoked response. Electroencephalogr Clin Neurophysiol 1975;39:609-620.

95. Wood CC, Wolpaw JR: Scalp distribution of human auditory evoked potentials: II. Evidence for multiple sources and involvement of auditory cortex. Electroencephalogr Clin Neurophysiol 1982;54:25-38.

96. Roland PE, Skinjoj E, Lassen NA: Focal activations of human cerebral cortex during auditory discrimination. J Neurophysiol 1981;45:1139-1151.

97. Kutas M, Hillyard SA: Brain potentials during reading reflect word expectancy and semantic association. Nature 1984;307:161-163.

98. Kutas M, Van Petten C, Besson M: Event-related potential asymmetries during the reading of sentences. Electroencephalogr Clin Neurophysiol 1988;69:218-233.

99. Courchesne E, Lincoln AJ, Yeung-Courchesne R, et al: Pathophysiologic findings in nonretarded autism and receptive developmental language disorder. J Autism Dev Disord 1989;19:1-17.

100. Tallal P: Neurophysiological foundations of specific developmental disorders of speech and language: Implications for theories of hemispheric specialization. In Cavenas JO (ed): Psychiatry: Psychobiological Foundations of Clinical Psychiatry, Vol 3. Philadelphia, JB Lippincott, 1985, pp 1-15.

101. Landau WM, Kleffner FR: Syndrome of acquired aphasia with convulsive disorder in children. Neurology 1957;7:523-530.

102. Nabbout R, Dulac O: Epileptic encephalopathies: A brief overview. J Clin Neurophysiol 2003;20:393-397.

103. Paquier PF, van Dongen HR, Loonen CB: TheLandau-Kleffner syndrome or "acquired aphasia with convulsive disorder": Long-term follow-up of six children and a review of the recent literature. Arch Neurol 1992;49:354-359.

104. Robinson RO, Baird G, Robinson G, Simonoff E: Landau-Kleffner syndrome: Course and correlates with outcome. Dev Med Child Neurol 2001;43:243-247.

105. Worster-Drought C, Allen IM: congenital auditory imperception (congenital word-deafness) and its relations to idioglossia and other speech deficits. J Neurol Psychopathol 1930;10:193-236.

106. Deonna T, Fletcher P, Voumard C: Temporary regression during language acquisition: A linguistic analysis of a 2 1/2-year-old child with epileptic aphasia. Dev Med Child Neurol 1982;24:156-163.

107. Holmes GL, McKeever M, Saunders Z: Epileptiform activity in aphasia of childhood: An epiphenomenon? Epilepsia 1981;22:631-639.

108. Praline J, Hommet C, Barthez MA, et al: Outcome at adulthood of the continuous spike-waves during slow sleep and Landau-Kleffner syndromes. Epilepsia 2003;44:1434-1440.

109. Smith MC, Hoeppner TJ: Epileptic encephalopathy of late childhood: Landau-Kleffner syndrome and the syndrome of continuous spikes and waves during slow-wave sleep. J Clin Neurophysiol 2003;20:462-472.

110. Tuchman R, Rapin I: Epilepsy in autism. Lancet Neurol 2002;1:352-358.

111. Deonna T, Peter C, Ziegler AL: Adult follow-up of the acquired aphasia-epilepsy syndrome in childhood: Report of seven cases. Neuropediatrics 1989;20:132-138.

112. Sato S, Dreifuss FE: Electroencephalographic findings in a patient with developmental expressive aphasia. Neurology 1973;23:181-185.

113. van de Sandt-Koenderman WME, Smit IAC, van Dongen HR, van Hest JBC: A case of acquired aphasia and convulsive disorder: Some linguistic aspects of recovery and breakdown. Brain Lang 1984;21:174-183.

114. Hirsch E, Marescaux C, Maquet P, et al: Landau-Kleffner syndrome: A clinical and EEG study of five cases. Epilepsia 1990;31:756-767.

115. Cole AJ, Andermann F, Taylor L, et al: The Landau-Kleffner syndrome of acquired epileptic aphasia: Unusual clinical outcome, surgical experience, and absence of encephalitis. Neurology 1988;38:31-38.

116. Denes G, Balliello S, Volterra V, Pellegrini A: Oral and written language in a case of childhood phonemic deafness. Brain Lang 1986;29:252-267.

117. Bratlson A, Krevzen JA, et al: Electrophysiologic manifestations of impaired temporal lobe auditory processing in verbal auditory agnosia. Brain Lang 1995;51:383-405.

118. Fejerman N, Medina CS: Afasia epiléptica adquirida en el niño. Arch Arg Ped 1980;78:510-520.

119. Foerster C: Aphasia and seizure disorders in childhood. *In* Penry JK (ed): Epilepsy: The Eighth International Symposium. New York, Raven Press, 1977, pp 305-306.

120. Kellermann K: Recurrent aphasia with subclinical bioelectric status epilepticus during sleep. Eur J Pediatr 1978;128:207-212.

121. Lou HC, Brandt S, Bruhn P: Aphasia and epilepsy in childhood. Acta Neurol Scand 1977;56:46-54.

122. Morrell F, Whisler WW, Smith MC, et al: Landau-Kleffner syndrome: Treatment with subpial intracortical transection. Brain 1995;118:1529-1546.

123. Kirk SA: Behavioral diagnosis and remediation of learning disabilities. Conference on Exploration into the Problems of the Perpetually Handicapped Child. Evanston, IL, Fund for the Perpetually Handicapped Child, 1963, pp 1-7.

124. Habib M: The neurological basis of developmental dyslexia: An overview and working hypothesis. Brain 2000;123:2373-2399.

125. Shaywitz SE, Shaywitz BA: Neurobiological indices of dyslexia. *In* Swanson HL, Harris KR, Graham S (eds): Handbook of Learning Disabilities. New York, Guilford Press, 2003, pp 514-531.

126. Landwehrmeyer B, Gerling J, Wallesch C-W: Patterns of task-related slow potentials in dyslexia. Arch Neurol 1990;47:791-797.

127. Leisman G, Ashkenazi M: Aetiological factors in dyslexia: IV. Cerebral hemispheres are functionally equivalent. Neuroscience 1980;11:157-164.

128. Fein G, Galin D, Yingling CD, et al: EEG spectra in dyslexic and control boys during resting conditions. Electroencephalogr Clin Neurophysiol 1986;63:87-97.

129. Yingling CD, Galin D, Fein G, et al: Neurometrics does not detect "pure" dyslexics. Electroencephalogr Clin Neurophysiol 1986;63:426-430.

130. Duffy FH, Denckla MB, Sandini G: Dyslexia: Regional differences in brain electrical activity by topographic mapping. Ann Neurol 1980;7:412-420.

131. Schulte-Korne G, Deimel W, Bartling J, Remschmidt H: Neurophysiological correlates of word recognition in dyslexia. J Neural Transm 2004;111:971-984.

132. Leppanen PH, Lyytinen H: Auditory event-related potentials in the study of developmental language-related disorders. Audiol Neuro-otol 1997;2:308-340.

133. Lovrich D, Stamm JS: Event-related potential and behavioral correlates of attention in reading retardation. J Clin Neurophysiol 1983;5:13-37.

134. Ollo C, Squires N: Event-related potentials in learning disabilities. *In* Cracco R, Bodis-Wollner I (eds): Frontiers of Clinical Neurosciences: Evoked Potentials. New York, AR Liss, 1986, pp 497-512.

135. Taylor MJ, Keenan NK: Event-related potentials to visual and language stimuli in normal and dyslexic children. Psychophysiology 1990;27:318-327.

136. Farrag AF, Khedr EM, bel-Naser W: Impaired parvocellular pathway in dyslexic children. Eur J Neurol 2002;9:359-363.

137. Schulte-Korne G, Bartling J, Deimel W, Remschmidt H: Motion-onset VEPs in dyslexia: Evidence for visual perceptual deficit. Neuroreport 2004;15:1075-1078.

138. Schulte-Korne G, Bartling J, Deimel W, Remschmidt H: Visual evoked potential elicited by coherently moving dots in dyslexic children. Neurosci Lett 2004;357:207-210.

139. Scheuerpflug P, Plume E, Vetter V, et al: Visual information processing in dyslexic children. Clin Neurophysiol 2004;115:90-96.

140. American Psychiatric Association: Diagnostic and Statistical Manual of Mental Disorders, 3rd ed. Washington, DC, American Psychiatric Association, 1987.

141. Allen DA: Autistic spectrum disorders: Clinical presentation in preschool children. J Child Neurol 1988;3(Suppl):S48-S56.

142. Allen DA, Rapin I, Wiznitzer M: Communication disorders of preschool children: The physician's responsibility. Dev Behav Pediatr 1988;9:164-170.

143. Golden GS: Neurologic functioning. *In* Cohen D, Donnellan AM (eds): Handbook of Autism and Related Developmental Disorders. New York, John Wiley, 1987, pp 133-147.

144. James AL, Barry RJ: A review of psychophysiology in early-onset psychosis. Schizophren Bull 1980;6:506-525.

145. Kolvin I, Ounsted C, Roth M: Cerebral dysfunction and childhood psychoses. Br J Psychiatry 1971;118:407-414.

146. Ornitz EM: Neurophysiology of infantile autism. J Am Acad Child Adolesc Psychiatry 1985;24:251-262.

147. Ornitz EM: Neurophysiologic studies of infantile autism. *In* Cohen D, Donnellan AM (eds): Handbook of Autism and Related Developmental Disorders. New York, John Wiley, 1987, pp 148-165.

148. Rutter M: Autistic children: Infancy to adulthood. Semin Psychiatry 1970;2:435-450.

149. Small JG: EEG and neurophysiological studies of early infantile autism. Biol Psychiatry 1975;10:385-397.

150. Tanguay PE, Edwards RM: Electrophysiological studies of autism: The whisper of the bang. J Autism Dev Disord 1982;12:177-184.

151. Tsai LY, Stewart M: Handedness and EEG correlation in autistic children. Biol Psychiatry 1982;17:595-598.

152. Tsai LY, Tsai MC, August GJ: Brief report: Implications of EEG diagnoses in the subclassification of infantile autism. J Autism Dev Disord 1985;15:339-344.

153. White PT, DeMyer W, DeMyer M: EEG abnormalities in early childhood schizophrenia: A double-blind study of psychiatrically disturbed and normal children during promazine sedation. Am J Psychiatry 1964;120:950-958.

154. Cantor DS, Thatcher RW, Hrybyk M, Kaye H: Computerized EEG analyses of autistic children. J Autism Dev Disord 1986;16:169-187.

155. Dawson G, Warrenburg S, Fuller P: Cerebral lateralization in individuals diagnosed as autistic in early childhood. Brain Lang 1982;15:353-368.

156. Dorenbaum D, Mencel E, Blume WT, Fishman S: EEG findings and language patterns in autistic children: Clinical correlations. Can J Psychiatry 1987;32:31-34.

157. Tuchman R, Rapin I, Shinnar I: Autistic and dysphasic children: II. Epilepsy. Pediatrics 1991;88:1219-1225.

158. Grillon C, Courchesne E, Askhoomoff N: Brainstem and middle latency auditory evoked potentials in autism and developmental language disorder. J Autism Dev Disord 1989;19:255-269.

159. Ciesielski K, Courchesne E, Elmasian R: Effects of focused selective attention tasks on event-related potentials in autistic and normal individuals. Electroencephalogr Clin Neurophysiol 1990;75:207-220.

160. Courchesne E, Courchesne R, Hicks G, Lincoln A: Functioning of the brain-stem auditory pathway in non-retarded autistic individuals. Electroencephalogr Clin Neurophysiol 1985;61:491-501.

161. Novick B, Kurtzberg D, Vaughan HG Jr: An electrophysiologic indication of defective information storage in childhood autism. Psychiatr Res 1979;1:101-108.

162. Dawson G, Finley C, Philips S, et al: Reduced P3 amplitude of the event-related brain potential: Its relationship to language ability in autism. J Autism Dev Disord 1988;18:493-504.

13

Neonatal Electroencephalography: Abnormal Features

MARK S. SCHER

The clinical neurophysiologist's interpretive abilities concerning abnormal neonatal electroencephalographic (EEG) patterns can assist in the neurologic care of the sick neonate. As discussed in the chapter for normal neonatal EEG (see Chapter 2), several guidelines help frame the overall advantages and limitations of such a laboratory tool for diagnostic and prognostic purposes (Box 13–1).

Single EEG recordings obtained randomly during the acute or convalescent neonatal periods may be helpful but are far less advantageous than serial recordings.[1–7] Multiple recordings at appropriate intervals during the acute and convalescent neonatal period offer a wealth of information concerning neurophysiologic maturation and integrity. The resolution or persistence of abnormal encephalopathic patterns has important prognostic implications.

Even though one can follow the progression of an encephalopathy with serial recordings, the onset of an encephalopathic process may have occurred prior to birth. EEG abnormalities, seen shortly after birth, may therefore reflect antepartum as well as intrapartum insults to the central nervous system. Current methods of fetal surveillance (i.e., abnormal fetal heart rate tracings, placental abnormalities, antepartum fetal ultrasound findings) also suggest either intrapartum and/or antepartum difficulties and must be integrated into the clinical correlation of an EEG interpretation.

Abnormal EEG patterns in the neonate are rarely pathognomonic, and a specific diagnosis is infrequently associated with a particular EEG pattern. Diverse etiologies can contribute to the encephalopathic state. Every attempt should be made to incorporate pertinent clinical correlations into the interpretive section of the EEG report, uniting all known clinical and laboratory facts together with the electrographic interpretation. However, it is not necessarily the goal of the clinical neurophysiologist to offer specific diagnoses based on only electrographic interpretations. Rather, EEG studies complement clinical and imaging evaluations to broaden one's diagnostic and prognostic profile of the high-risk infant.

It has been widely observed that even severe EEG pattern abnormalities rapidly disappear over time. This normalization of EEG disturbances occurs even in infants who suffer severe neurologic sequelae.[2,5] It is advisable, therefore, to obtain serial studies beginning early during the acute phase of an illness and systematically repeat studies daily or weekly depending on clinical priorities with respect to the management of the infant. It is not recommended that EEG studies be initially obtained late in the convalescent period prior to discharge. By that time, severe abnormalities may have completely or partially resolved.

ASSESSMENT OF ENCEPHALOPATHY: DIAGNOSTIC AND PROGNOSTIC GOALS

Determination of the sick neonate's level of consciousness is an enormously difficult task. The clinical repertoire

---

BOX 13-1
GUIDELINES FOR THE USE OF EEG TO ASSESS FOR AN ENCEPHALOPATHY IN THE SICK NEONATE

1. Information concerning gestational age, state of arousal, and medical conditions, including medications, needs to be considered before offering an electrographic interpretation.
2. Serial recordings are far more advantageous than single recordings to document the progression or resolution of an encephalopathic process.
3. The EEG abnormality may reflect an encephalopathy due to antepartum, intrapartum, and/or neonatal difficulties.
4. Abnormal EEG patterns are rarely pathognomonic for specific diagnoses and complement clinical and imaging evaluations.
5. Partial or complete normalization of EEG disturbances commonly occurs over time.
6. Both diffuse and focal disturbances can coincidentally affect background EEG activity.
7. Significant EEG abnormalities may be seen in the absence of clinical expression of neurologic disturbances in the neonate.
8. Mild to moderately severe EEG abnormalities are difficult to use for prognostic purposes and should be closely matched with the evolving clinical condition.

---

of the neonate is largely limited to the infant's level of arousal, muscle tone, and postural reflexes. There are also the practical limitations to performing the neonatal examination because of the neonatal intensive care unit (NICU) setting. The neonate, particularly the preterm infant, may be confined to an incubator environment. The newborn infant may be intubated with multiple catheters and require paralytic agents for ventilatory control.

All of these factors seriously disrupt the efficient assessment of the neonate's level and content of arousal. Because of the dearth of clinical findings and the hostile NICU environment, the clinician's ability to assess the level and stability of neurologic state in the sick neonate is significantly limited. Such restrictions, therefore, emphasize the important role of neurophysiologic studies for the assessment of an encephalopathic process.

Many varied medical situations can contribute to the encephalopathic state of the sick neonate either on a diffuse hemispheric, multifocal, or regional basis. It is not uncommon to have multiple events contribute to the expression of

an encephalopathic state. For example, metabolic derangements give more diffuse EEG disturbances, whereas cerebrovascular accidents express more focal abnormalities. These conditions can, in fact, be present concurrently. Comparisons of serial recordings, therefore, may represent a variety of different abnormalities depending on both the time of the recording and the predominate encephalopathic process that is electrographically expressed.

EEG disturbances are generally graded as mild, moderate, or marked. Unfortunately, results may vary from laboratory to laboratory, particularly with respect to the grading of mild or moderate abnormalities.[5] Quantitative measurements of regional and hemispheric activities by computer techniques allow a more reliable threshold for these degrees of abnormality. Nonetheless, certain general categories of abnormalities are listed in the following sections that assist in the assessment of preterm (PT) and fullterm (FT) neonates. Table 13–1 lists the major EEG abnormalities that are used as reference points for the neurophysiologist with respect to the severity of an encephalopathy.

CLASSIFICATION OF BACKGROUND EEG ABNORMALITIES IN FULLTERM INFANTS

There are a number of sources that have highlighted the variety of background disturbances that can be seen in FT infants.[1,2,8] Attempts at grading these abnormalities are also included. Although PT infants may have similar abnormalities, they are discussed separately. A critical discussion of neonatal seizures concludes this chapter.

TABLE 13–1
Major EEG Abnormalities

	Near-Term and Fullterm (36–41+ wk)	Preterm (30–36 wk)
Inactive	X	X
Burst-suppression	X	X
Slow	X	X
Low voltage	X	—
Monorhythmic	X	—
No spatial/temporal organization	X	—
Asymmetry	X	X (>50%)
Interhemispheric asynchrony	X	X
Abnormal superimposed patterns	X	X
Focal spikes	X	X
Seizures	X	X

MARKEDLY ABNORMAL ABNORMALITIES IN FT INFANTS

Electrocerebral Inactivity (Isoelectric Recording)

Cerebral activity below 5 μV despite high sensitivity settings and long interelectrode distances may be noted on neonatal recordings. The lack of reactivity to sensory stimulation usually accompanies this severe degree of abnormality. Minimal amplitude criteria (i.e., < 5 μV) have been used by several authors,[2,9–11] whereas others have required the total absence of all cerebral electrical activity.[12] Once the possibilities of a postictal situation, hypothermia, or a reversible metabolic-toxic disorder are eliminated, this abnormal pattern carries grave prognostic implications.[2,3] Most infants either die or have severe neurologic sequelae.[9–14] These studies indicate that an isoelectric record noted during the early neonatal course is associated with high mortality in a high percentage of patients. Seventeen (90%) of 19 died in one study,[15] with only 1 survivor being developmentally normal at 6 years of age, whereas two others had seizures with developmental delay. Another study involving both PT and FT infants with isoelectric records showed a survival rate of less than 20% (17 of 20) with only 1 normal survivor of 7 years of age.[13]

A neuropathologic study from the same laboratory[12] found that infants with isoelectric records who died had widespread encephalomalacia and ischemic neuronal necrosis. In this study, 10 different anatomic sites were systematically studied in six neonates who had an isoelectric EEG. The cerebral cortex, corpus callosum, thalamus, midbrain, and pons showed moderate to marked injury in all these cases. Other locations such as the white matter, cerebellum, hypothalamus, and medulla were also damaged. These sites, however, were spared in at least one infant, who initially had an isoelectric record with qualitative improvement on a subsequent recording.

A variety of clinical situations ranging from massive intracranial hemorrhage to fulminant meningitis all may be expressed as an inactive or isoelectric EEG. Even major central nervous system malformations such as hydranencephaly as well as severe inborn errors of metabolism disorders such as nonketotic hyperglycinemia may result in such an abnormal recording. These conditions resemble records seen in severe hypoxic-ischemic encephalopathy. This is followed by the re-emergence of seizures and other abnormal background activity.[16]

In one study,[13] 15 of 20 infants had at least one isoelectric record during the first several days of life, with clinical evidence of partially preserved brain function (Figs. 13–1 to 13–3). They, therefore, could not satisfy the criteria of brain death. In addition, 12 of 20 infants had

evidence of antepartum injury. Timing of the insult was based on obstetric (i.e., loss of fetal movements), placental/cord pathology (meconium-laden macrophages, small placental weight), and/or clinical findings (i.e., intrauterine growth retardation, joint contractures). Most infants in this group had demonstrable brain insults that could also be dated to events prior to labor and delivery. All but three infants died in the immediate neonatal period, with only one of the survivors being developmentally normal. Clearly, an antepartum insult that predated the intrapartum obstetric management of the mother and child may also result in an isoelectric EEG pattern rather than an emergent insult during labor and delivery. Furthermore, the presence of brain function on examination puts in question the legitimacy of using an isoelectric EEG to help define brain death in the immediate neonatal period. As with older children, such an electrographic finding can only be confirmatory of the clinical examination of absent brain function in the neonate.

Paroxysmal or Suppression Burst Pattern

The gestational age of the infant must be known before definitely identifying this abnormality, since the PT infant commonly has a discontinuous tracing that superficially may resemble this severely abnormal pattern (sometimes termed *paroxysmal pattern*) (Figs. 13–4 and 13–5). Earlier descriptions of the suppression-burst pattern consisted of a nonreactive discontinuous tracing, with a long period of quiescence greater than 20 seconds in duration[10,17] interrupted by synchronous or asynchronous bursts of poorly organized background activity. More recently, modified forms of this pattern have also been described that comprise better organized bursts of background activity with shorter quiescent periods. Modified forms may in part be due to more aggressively managed clinical situations but could also reflect specific metabolic-toxic encephalopathies that are potentially reversible (i.e., drug intoxication).

The paroxysmal or suppression burst pattern has been traditionally associated with a poor prognosis.[9–12,15] Pezzani and associates[15] found that four of six FT infants with this pattern died, while the survivors had severe neurologic sequelae. Aso and colleagues[12] found that seven infants with suppression-burst patterns had neuronal necrosis in five of the seven cases, periventricular leukomalacia in three, cerebral infarctions in three, and two with pontosubicular necrosis. This neuropathologic study emphasizes the diverse types of severe deficits that can be seen with suppression-burst activity.

Modified forms of the suppression burst pattern have been described.[9] These patients have a pattern that may electrographically demonstrate reactivity with stimulation.

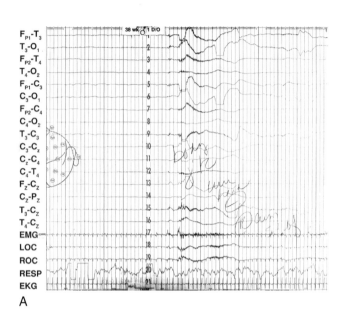

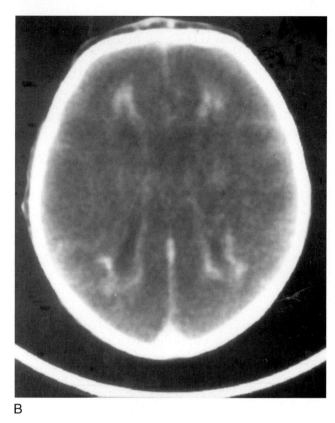

FIGURE 13–1

A, EEG recording of a 38-week, 1-day-old boy with nonimmune hydrops fetalis. The patient demonstrated an isoelectric EEG tracing in the context of a partially preserved neurologic examination. Prominent whole-body jerks with head turning and arm stiffening were noted suggestive of seizures. Preserved neurologic function was documented by clinical examination. However, no electrographic seizure correlate was noted on coincident EEG recordings as depicted in this example. B, CT scan for patient in A documenting significant cortical hypodensities and prominent periventricular enhancement. Postmortem examination revealed widespread cavitation and calcification.

Five infants had discontinuous tracings consistent with suppression-burst that became a continuous pattern with tactile stimulation. Although none of the infants were normal at follow-up, only one of the children had severe deficits.

Hypsarrhythmia

The hypsarrhythmic pattern associated with infantile spasms usually appears by 3 to 4 months of age (see Chapter 11).[18] It is rarely noted during the neonatal period, observed in children less than 44 weeks conceptional age (CA). Asynchronous bursts of high-amplitude slow activity mixed with multifocal spikes and sharp waves have been described. Periods of suppression may vary in duration, may be generalized, but occasionally may be lateralized. Generalized myoclonic movements may appear during periods of attenuation. One group has recently differentiated neonatal hypsarrhythmia from suppression burst by the high amplitude of activity exceeding 1000 μV.[19] Ohtahara[19] suggested a syndrome of infantile spasms and suppression-burst activity in the EEG of the neonate that differs from those in older patients, termed *early infantile epileptic encephalopathy*. Other authors have described a similar syndrome called *neonatal myoclonic encephalopathy*, which begins during the first weeks of life. Such patients have fragmentary myoclonus associated with a variety of seizures other than infantile spasms with a suppression-burst pattern on the EEG.[64] The suppression-burst pattern can be seen with either brain malformations or inborn errors of metabolism.

Spikes and Sharp Waves

In most situations, the electroencephalographer has difficulty assigning clinical significance to sporadic epilep-

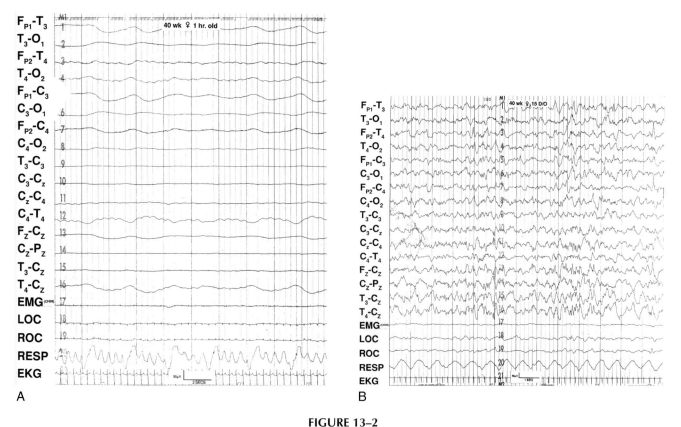

FIGURE 13-2

A, EEG recording of a 40-week, 1-hour-old girl with a history of a severe abruption placenta and velamentous insertion of the umbilical cord. Sudden exsanguinations and cardiac arrest after delivery necessitated cardiopulmonary resuscitation. An EEG was obtained within 30 minutes of life indicating an isoelectric background in the context of agitation, tremulousness, and increased muscle tone on examination. B, Follow-up record for the same patient at 15 days of age showing a well-developed quiet sleep segment. Subsequently, the patient developed spasticity of the lower extremities that resolved by 2 years of age. She is functionally normal at 6 years of age.

tiform features on recordings of either PT or FT neonates. These features (see Chapter 2) can be seen in asymptomatic, apparently healthy infants. However, several features can help distinguish normal from abnormal spike and sharp wave discharges. Principally, epileptiform discharges that are frequent and multifocal, or persistently occur in any state, may have pathologic significance. Several authors[17,20] have suggested that more than five spike or sharp wave discharges per hour may suggest an abnormality (see Fig. 13–5A). Other features such as positive sharp waves, periodic discharges, and midline discharges commonly reflect central nervous system insults. These are discussed later in the section "Background Abnormalities in Preterm Infants."

Spike and sharp wave discharges have been described in several neonatal populations who are at risk because of serious medical disorders, principally seizures. Hughes and associates[21] described spike and sharp wave discharges

in 236 neonates whose CA ranged from 24 to 48 weeks. Fifty-five percent had recordings because of the clinical suspicion of neonatal seizures. Sporadic sharp waves, more frequent in the right hemisphere, were principally located in the centrotemporal region in 85% of the total population. An additional 15% had either positive sharp waves or repetitive discharges. Unfortunately, coincident EEG seizures were not documented, nor was follow-up reported for this population. Figure 13–5B demonstrates vertex and frontal sharp waves.

Rowe and colleagues[20] documented sharp wave discharges in 51% of 74 neonates (30 to 40 weeks CA) with clinical seizures. Follow-up data were available to 33 months of age. The presence of sharp waves was predictive of neurodevelopmental outcome when considered independently. However, the authors stressed that EEG background abnormalities were more helpful in predicting neurologic sequelae than were epileptiform features.

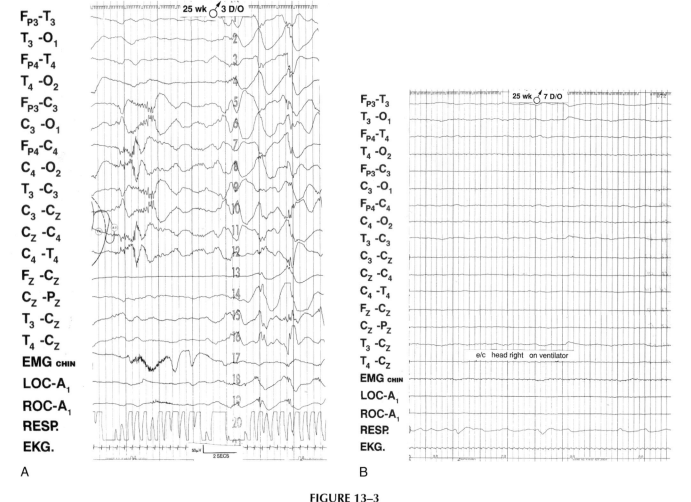

FIGURE 13–3

A, *Portion of an EEG tracing for a 25-week, 3-day-old boy demonstrating an age-appropriate tracé discontinu background..*
B, *Following a severe hypotensive episode secondary to disseminated intravascular coagulation, a repeat record demonstrated an isoelectric background. The patient later died, and postmortem examination was denied.*

Low-Amplitude Recording

Low-amplitude electrographic pattern is characterized by background frequencies that are of 5 to 15 μV in amplitude during the wakeful state and 10 to 25 μV during the sleep states.[2,10] Although differences in amplitude between sleep states may be seen, most records have a persistently low-amplitude background with no state differentiation. This, of course, should take into account the cyclic nature of the ultradian sleep rhythm during which the low-voltage irregular active sleep background comprises approximately 10% to 15% of the record.

This background abnormality has grave prognostic significance,[9–11] particularly if it persists beyond the 1st week of life.[2,3] At times, this low-amplitude recording may have intermixed monotonous, nonreactive theta activity.[10,22]

One should be alert to a variety of situations that can result in low-amplitude records. Postictal records following seizures or barbiturates administration, for example, can result in an inactive record. Ample recording times (i.e., of at least an hour) should help distinguish clinically significant records from nonpathologic situations.

Excessive Discontinuity

Although discontinuity does not imply isoelectric, inactive, or suppression-burst criteria, this background abnormality may also represent a significant encephalopathy. Permanently discontinuous activity has been described[15] consisting of bursts that are less than 3 seconds in duration. This is contrasted by Aso and coworkers[12] who defined an interburst interval to be 60 seconds or greater. Pezzani

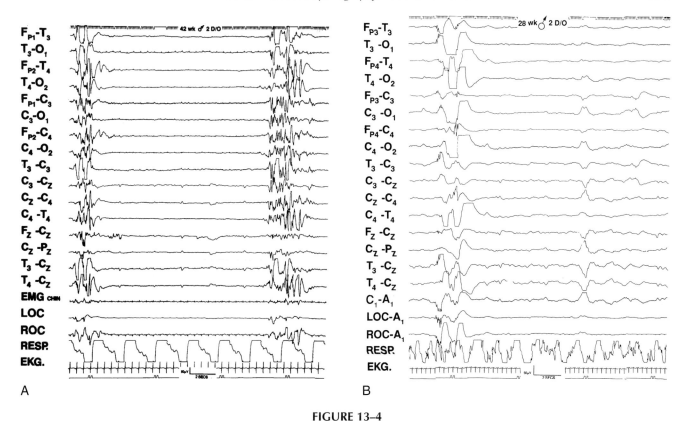

FIGURE 13–4

A, A 42-week, 2-day-old boy with suppression-burst pattern on an EEG recording that did not react to sensory stimulation. Note the low-amplitude sharp wave morphology from respiratory excursion at the midline electrode.
B, An age-appropriate tracé discontinu pattern for a 28-week, 2-day-old boy. Compare with the invariant suppression-burst pattern noted in **A.**

and associates[15] found no children with this background pattern survived without sequelae, and five of eight of these children expired. These authors claimed that the longer the interburst interval, the more compromised the neurologic outcome. No children escaped major sequelae when their interburst intervals were longer than 40 seconds. Fourteen of 15 children (93%) with permanently discontinuous background and absent normal physiologic patterns either died or had severe sequelae.

Diffusely Slow Background

A diffusely slow pattern comprising delta activity either during wakefulness or sleep with little activity in the theta range have been described by several authors.[2,9,11,23] Invariant and diffusely distributed delta rhythms are noted acutely during the 1st week of life but can be seen during the convalescent period several weeks after birth. These patterns initially were described in studies that predated the establishment of the modern NICU;[10] more recently, authors[3] have claimed that this pattern is uncommon.

Hemispheric Amplitude Asymmetry

Hemispheric amplitude asymmetry, defined as greater than 50% difference in amplitude in each hemisphere, has been described with neuropathologic correlates.[12] This pattern is seen with lateralized pathology. Four infants had cerebral lesions that were either hemorrhagic or ischemic in nature, with attenuated voltage over the more pathologically involved hemisphere (Fig. 13–6). Congenital lesions such as porencephaly may also contribute to hemispheric attenuation of background amplitudes. As previously emphasized in Chapter 2, notation of cephalohematomas, scalp edema, or technical conditions such as head positioning, electrode paste smearing, sweat, or asymmetric electrode placement must be documented. With any questions concerning these EEG asymmetries, follow-up records are strongly recommended.

Asymmetries may accompany seizures phenomena with transient suppression of activity in areas where an ictal pattern was recently documented. An asymmetry usually

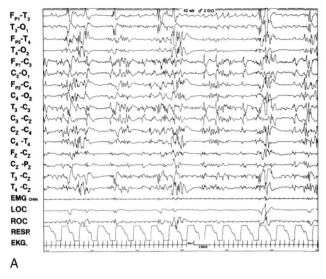

A

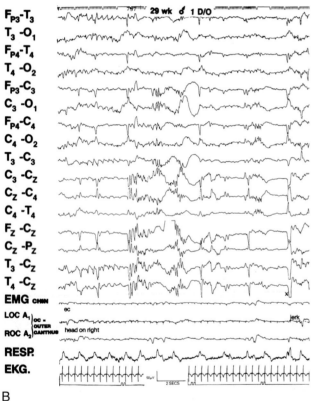

B

FIGURE 13–5

A, *Portion of an EEG tracing for a 42-week, 2-day-old boy*
following a hypoxic-ischemic insult. Multifocal sharp waves and
a disorganized background are noted during tracé alternant.
B, *A portion of an EEG tracing for a 29-week, 1-day-old boy*
twin following twin-to-twin transfusion. The patient was
clinically hypotonic and less responsive. Prominent vertex and
frontal sharp waves were noted. The patient had a CT scan
showing white matter hypodensities. Follow-up examination
was within normal limits at three years of age.

implies that the pathology exists on the more attenuated
regions.

Finally, transient asymmetries have been described in
asymptomatic previously healthy neonates[14,24] and may be
noted during the first several minutes of quiet sleep in the
absence of structural lesions.

Focal Attenuation

There are records that are persistently attenuated over
only one scalp region without involvement of the entire
hemisphere (Fig. 13–7). These have been classified as focal
attenuation and are commonly associated with focal or
lateralized neuropathologic lesions. Aso and coworkers[12]
found that five infants with at least one EEG with a focal
attenuation were noted to have neuropathologic lesions.
Three of these patients had extensive lesions that were
unilateral to the attenuation, and one infant showed more
severe white matter infarction in the opposite hemisphere.
An additional infant showed no pathologic changes that
could be correlated with the attenuation of the EEG.
Conversely, these authors described unilateral lesions on
postmortem examination involving either necrosis or
hemorrhage in the cortex or white matter with the absence
of a demonstrable EEG attenuation. The accuracy of
detecting a morphologic lesion was estimated to be 74%,
with a specificity of 85%.

Intrahemispheric Asynchrony

As described in Chapter 2, the definition of asynchrony
has been arbitrarily assigned. Morphologically similar bursts
that are separated by more than 1.5 seconds have been
defined as *asynchronous.* Although some authors claim that
the infant's CA help predict the degree of asynchrony, this
has been recently challenged.[25] Asynchrony of any degree in
the FT infant, however, is considered abnormal (Fig. 13–8).
The neuropathologic findings associated with patients with
marked asynchrony have also recently been described.[12]
Nine patients with excessive asynchrony included two
patients with lesions within the corpus callosum. In general,
white matter lesions, periventricular hemorrhage, and intraventricular hemorrhage (IVH) were noted in infants with
asynchrony compared with infants who did not manifest this
abnormality.

Normative values for interhemispheric asynchrony need
to be more firmly established for each gestational age range
before assigning specific risks of pathologic significance.

Although it has been emphasized that a rudimentary
sleep cycle in the PT neonate is difficult to ascertain, such
state differentiation can be seen as early as 31 to 32 weeks'
gestation. Certainly by corrected term ages, cycles between active and quiet sleep segments are expected. The

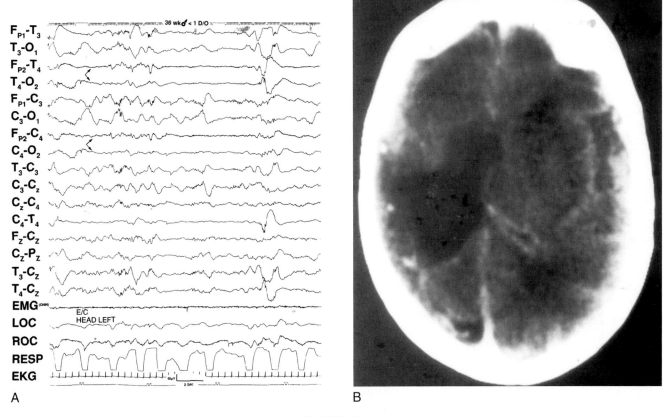

FIGURE 13–6

A, *Portion of an EEG recording of a 36-week, 1-day-old boy infant with congenital porencephaly. Note the attenuation in the right hemisphere both above and below the sylvian fissure* (twin arrow marks). B, *CT scan obtained on the patient in A showing porencephaly in the right hemisphere in the distribution of the right middle cerebral artery.*

absence or disruption of these cycles can be diagnostic of an encephalopathy as well as prognostic for neurologic sequelae (Fig. 13–9).

Pezzani and associates[15] found that EEGs obtained during the first 24 hours of life in 80 FT infants included 24 infants with the absence of sleep state organization. These infants either died or survived with major sequelae. Three additional infants with no sleep state organization only during the first 24 hours of life did develop normally. Clearly, serial studies rather than single studies are preferable to predict outcome based on this type of abnormality. Metabolic toxic states, hypothermia, and other environmental factors can also disrupt the sleep cycling. Certain medications, such as phenobarbital, may alter or abolish state transitions, particularly when in the toxic range. Lombroso[2,3] noted that excessive indeterminate or transitional sleep can be seen with a variety of conditions, but this pattern has variable clinical significance.

Excessively labile EEG sleep states have also been described, with rapid transitions between sleep stages over seconds to minutes. This usually reflects mild to moderate degrees of acute encephalopathy but may also be associated with infants with more chronic brain dysfunction such as with hypoplastic left heart syndrome,[26] maternal substance use,[27] or maternal preeclampsia.[28] Normative values for sleep state segments estimate that active sleep is 50% and quiet sleep 30% to 35% of the cycle. This does not control for antepartum, intrapartum, or neonatal conditions that may influence sleep architecture and continuity measures. Normative values for sleep architecture consisting of percentages of active, quiet, and transitional sleep are needed using appropriate healthy controls to better assess children who are at risk for neurodevelopmental difficulties.

Abnormalities of Maturational Development

As described previously, an experienced electroencephalographer should be able to determine CA within

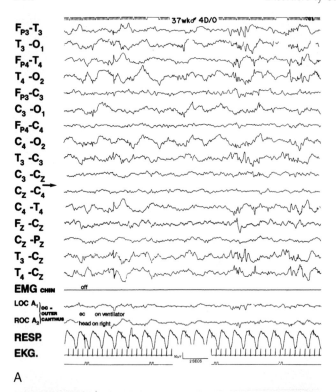

A

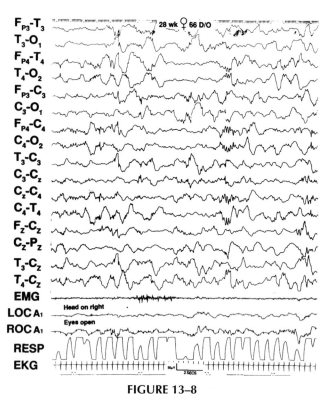

FIGURE 13–8

EEG from a 28-week, 66-day-old girl who suffered a grade IV intraventricular hemorrhage. The patient had a normal neurologic examination. This EEG tracing indicated a significant asynchrony with alternating attenuation in homologous temporal and central regions. At 3 years of age the patient had a significant hemiparesis.

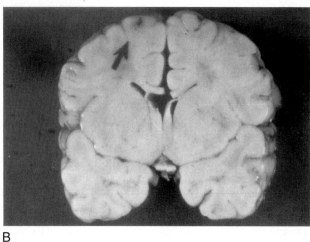

B

FIGURE 13–7

A, *Portion of an EEG for a 37-week, 4-day-old boy with vertex attenuation* (see arrow). *The patient had persistent pulmonary hypertension of the newborn and subsequently died. B, Brain section of the patient described in A showing multifocal infarctions. An arrow indicated one such infarction in the parasagittal region of the right hemisphere, corresponding with the attenuation noted on the EEG described in A.*

2 weeks in the premature infant and within 1 week for the FT infant. Disorders of electrographic maturation suggest cerebral insults during intrauterine life or the immediate neonatal period. Dysmaturity of more than 2 weeks of the stated CA of the infant defines an abnormality (Fig. 13–10). Dysmature patterns may be transient in infants who suffer severe but reversible hyaline membrane disease and have little prognostic significance.[29] However, persistently dysmature patterns based on either electrographic or sleep state criteria are worrisome with respect to neurodevelopmental sequelae. For instance, dysmature patterns on the EEG (i.e., excessive brushes or asynchrony) have been noted in neonates with chronic lung disease who later demonstrate compromised neurodevelopmental milestones at 3 years of age.[30] Dysmature sleep architecture and continuity measures have also been noted in neonates with chronic lung disease.[4]

Strict guidelines for assessing EEG maturation still need to be developed. Although normative values for certain patterns such as delta brush have been suggested, systematic investigations of other discrete wave forms such as occipital and temporal theta bursts are still needed. Computer analyses provide better quantification of regional and hemispheric power spectra at specific EEG frequencies and provide more strict maturational criteria for frequency and amplitude. Normative data based on both analog and

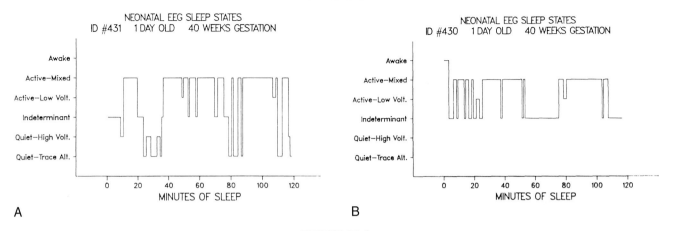

FIGURE 13–9

A, *Histogram of a normal neonatal sleep cycle indicating the alternation between active and quiet sleep segments with intermixed transitional or indeterminate sleep periods. B, Histogram of an abnormal EEG cycle indicating no quiet sleep segments and excessively long transitional sleep periods.*

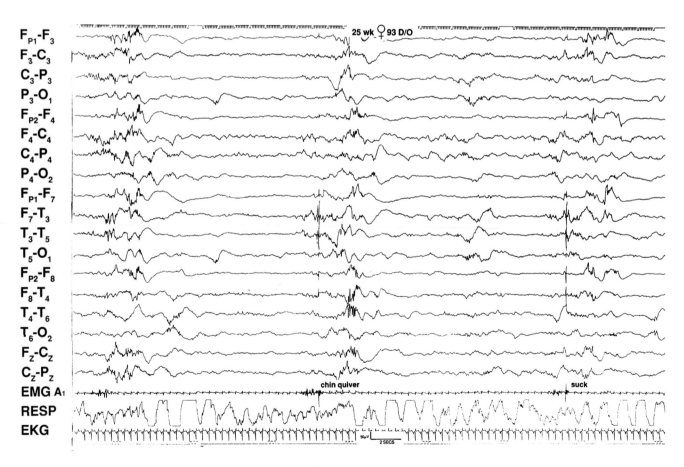

FIGURE 13–10

Portion of an EEG tracing of a 25-week, 93-day-old boy with a dysmature EEG tracing consisting of a lack of background, excessive delta brush patterns, and asynchrony for a corrected term age. The patient was abnormal at 3 years of age with delayed cognitive and motor development.

digital analyses then can be more confidently assessed for dysmaturity.

BACKGROUND ABNORMALITIES IN PT INFANTS

As suggested in Table 13–1, abnormalities in the EEG of the PT infant have not been as widely studied as in FT infants. Yet, several abnormalities overlap with FT infants. Other findings, however, require knowledge of the expected electrographic and polygraphic features for a particular gestational age.

The most comprehensive study of background abnormalities reviewed 181 serial EEGs performed during the neonatal period on 81 infants with an estimated gestational age of less than 36 weeks.[6] These authors found that infants whose serial EEGs were normal in the neonatal period were usually normal or had minor sequelae at follow-up. On the other hand, children with at least one markedly abnormal record either died or had significant dysfunction on follow-up. In this particular study, moderately abnormal records were not noted to be significant. The authors classified severely abnormal records as having at least one of the following patterns: isoelectric backgrounds, positive rolandic sharp (PRS) waves, EEG seizures, paroxysmal discharges on isoelectric background, excessive intrahemispheric asynchrony (i.e., > 50% of the record) persistent hemispheric voltage amplitude asymmetries, and excessively slow background of variable amplitudes that is unreactive to stimulation. The authors classified moderately abnormal records as the following abnormal patterns: generalized low-amplitude activity with normal background; low-amplitude background with permanent asymmetry that is less than 50% of the record; and excessive asynchrony for the age, dysmaturity, and low-amplitude records with preservation of patterns appropriate for the infant's CA.

Isoelectric Pattern

Based on criteria described in the section on FT infants, few PT infants with isoelectric records have been described. Tharp and associates[6] described two infants, both of who expressed this pattern. Barabas and colleagues[13] described seven PT infants with isoelectric records, all of whom died or had major neurologic sequelae (see Fig. 13–3).

Suppression-Burst or Paroxysmal Pattern

Suppression-burst patterns consist of bursts of high-amplitude chaotic delta activity with intermixed spike or faster rhythms on an isoelectric background with interburst intervals greater than 20 seconds. Such a pattern would be difficult to classify in the PT infant because of tracé discontinu, which commonly occurs at more immature gestational ages. If such activity was invariant and unresponsive to stimulation and contained prolonged interburst intervals, such a pattern may be equivalent to the suppression-burst patterns seen at term. Such a pattern was described by Tharp and associates[6] in six infants and resulted in death or severe neurologic sequelae in all patients.

Low-Amplitude Recording

Electrographic studies with background activity below 20 μV, with occasional bursts of rhythmic activity or sharp wave features, have been classified as low amplitude. They can be considered as severely or moderately abnormal, depending on the persistence of patterns that would be expected for that particular CA. Tharp and associates[6] found five infants with unreactive low-amplitude records consisting of delta activity. One child survived with only minor sequelae.

Slow-Frequency Background

Background activity consisting of diffuse delta between 20 to 100 μV in amplitude with superimposed theta activity non-reactive to sensory stimuli would fit this classification. Age-appropriate discrete patterns such as delta brush and theta burst patterns would be diminished or absent during such recordings. As with FT infants, this pattern is unusual in the PT infant. Tharp and associates[6] described two infants with this pattern, both of whom survived with major neurologic sequelae.

Asymmetric Records

EEG studies were considered markedly abnormal with interhemispheric amplitude asymmetries exceeding 50% throughout the entire recording in all demonstrable EEG sleep states. More regional or focal asymmetries were considered only moderately abnormal, with less than 50% difference in amplitude. Asymmetric patterns have been associated with a compromised neurologic outcome.[22] Tharp and associates found that all nine infants with at least one record with a significant amplitude asymmetry either died or had severe sequelae. Aso and coworkers[12] also found that hemispheric asymmetry was associated with significant brain pathology in all four PT patients with this EEG abnormality.

POSITIVE SHARP WAVES IN THE MIDLINE AND CENTRAL REGIONS

Waveforms between 50 and 250 μV that are surface positive lasting 100 to 250 milliseconds are important abnormal features of the PT neonate record. Such discharges occur unilaterally or bilaterally in either the central or midline regions (Fig. 13–11). Waveform morphology can be complex, with surface negative components following the positive phase. Such patterns are seen singly or in brief runs. Historically, authors associated central sharp waves with IVH.[31–35] However, more recently, this finding has also been seen with white matter necrosis associated with meningitis, hydrocephalus, aminoacidopathies, and hypoxic-ischemic insults.[36,37]

Cukier and associates[34] first described PRS waves and the association with IVH. Blume and Dreyfus-Brisac[31] described two types of PRS. The first type occurred singly, clearly differentiated from the background, whereas the second type was admixed with fast and slow background activity. Clancy and colleagues[32,33] found central positive sharp waves in 13 of 22 infants with IVH on 30 EEG studies. Only one other infant had PRS waves without IVH. They therefore suggested that PRS has a high specificity but low sensitivity. These same authors later described 30 premature infants with multifocal white matter necrosis with and without IVH on ultrasound or autopsy with central positive sharp waves.[36] Infants with grade III to IV IVH had a higher prevalence (69.2%) of central positive sharp waves than the entire group of patients (31.8%), with the greatest prevalence occurring between the 5th and 8th postnatal day.

Scher[37] reported that positive sharp waves with a midline field of distribution were associated with a variety of pathologic lesions, including white matter necrosis (Fig. 13–12). Reviewing 25 records on 16 premature infants with a mean gestational age of 27 weeks resulted in the following profile of patients: 14 patients (88%) had cerebral lesions, 8 infants had IVH, 5 infants had periventricular leukomalacia, and 1 infant had cerebral infarction. The amplitude of these discharges ranged from 20 to 180 µV with an anteroposterior electrical field maximal at CZ extending from FZ to PZ. Myoclonic movements were sometimes associated with these discharges. Predominantly biphasic but also triphasic and polyphasic waveforms were noted. In patients with IVH, PRS waves had a mean repetitive rate of 1.3/min, with vertex positive sharp waves displaying a mean repetitive rate of 1.9/min in patients. However, those patients with periventricular leukomalacia displayed midline discharges with a mean repetitive rate of 2.5/min. Seventy-six percent of records with positive vertex sharp waves were obtained on infants who were older than 1 week. This feature was one of several midline electrographic abnormalities that frequently occurred in association with parasagittal cerebral lesions in the newborn. Midline electrographic abnormalities also have been noted in older patients.[38–41] In addition, midline discharges of positive or negative polarity can also occur coincident with myoclonus, suggesting the phenomenon of neonatal cortical myoclonus.[42] This may carry the same clinical significance as myoclonic phenomena noted in older patients.[43–45]

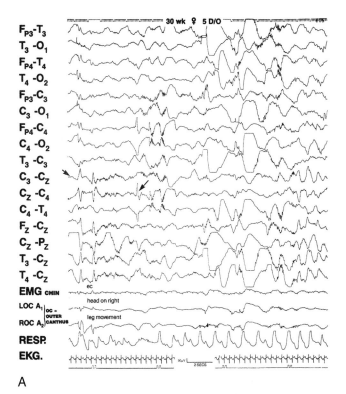

A

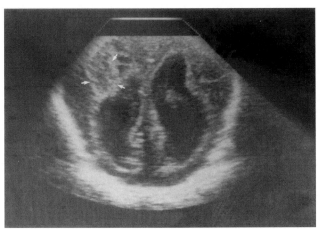

B

FIGURE 13–11

A, EEG recording of a 30-week, 5-day-old girl showing midline and rolandic positive sharp waves in the context of relatively preserved background rhythms. B, Coronal view on cranial ultrasound demonstrating a grade IV intraventricular hemorrhage of the patient noted in A (note arrowheads).

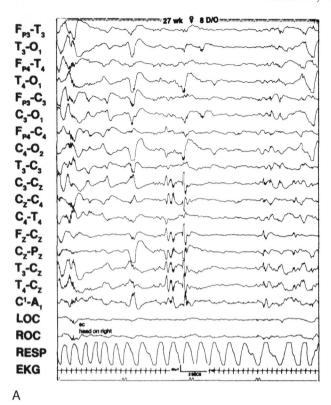

A

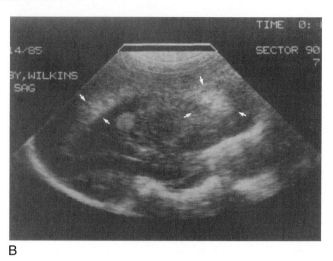

B

FIGURE 13–12

A, Portion of an EEG tracing of a 27-week, 8-day-old girl with a prominent parasagittal positive sharp wave that is also recorded using an adjacent electrode close to the midline. B, Sagittal view on cranial ultrasound of the patient described in A documenting extensive periventricular echodensities in both the anterior and posterior regions. The patient had significant spastic quadriplegia on follow-up examination at 4 years of age.

PROLONGED QUIESCENT PERIODS DURING DISCONTINUOUS SLEEP IN THE PRETERM INFANT

Prolonged quiescent periods during discontinuous sleep in the preterm infant is an abnormality, sometimes seen with monorhythmic theta activity in the PT infant, that was recently described.[46] Three subdivisions of interburst intervals of increasing duration in activity suggest a more unfavorable outcome. These authors reviewed EEGs of infants 25 to 35 weeks CA and divided interburst intervals into 20 seconds, 20 to 29 seconds, and those greater than 30 seconds. Favorable outcome was seen with intervals that were less than 20 seconds with a more unfavorable outcome in intervals greater than 30 seconds. These findings support other reports that also describe interburst intervals for PT infants. All investigators describe an expected interburst interval of less than 20 seconds in duration for the healthy asymptomatic neonate (see Chapter 2 and Table 2–1 in the chapter).

PERIODIC DISCHARGES IN PRETERM AND FULLTERM INFANTS

Periodic EEG patterns are regularly recurrent generalized or focal/lateralized transient complexes, associated with various neurologic disorders.[7,38,40,47–55] Generalized periodic EEG patterns have clinical significance primarily for degenerative disorders in older patients.[47,49,51] Generalized periodic patterns can also be seen with a variety of metabolic encephalopathies.[48,55]

Periodic lateralized epileptiform discharges (PLEDs) are usually associated with acute vascular, infectious, or traumatic lesions of the brain.[40,50,55] Although associated with acute structural brain lesions, PLEDS can also occur following seizures with or without structural lesions[40,56] and in patients with chronic encephalopathies.[7,54]

Children with focal or lateralized periodic patterns have been reported, but descriptions are limited to chronic diffuse lesions of the brain in older children,[54] FT neonates with hypoxic ischemic encephalopathy,[57] or PT and FT neonates with herpes encephalitis.[58–60]

These discharges are stereotypic paroxysmal complexes separated by nearly identical intervals between individual recurrent complexes. PLEDs of at least 10 minutes in duration or 20% of the recording time are defined as PLEDs.[49,50] One report[61] reviewed 1114 recordings from 592 neonates and found focal periodic discharges in 57 (5%) of the recordings for 34 neonates, 26 PT neonates, and 8 FT infants. PLEDs were noted in only 4 of these infants. Sixteen patients (47%) with focal periodic discharges also had electrographic seizures on the same or subsequent record. Stroke was the most common brain lesion (53%) in this

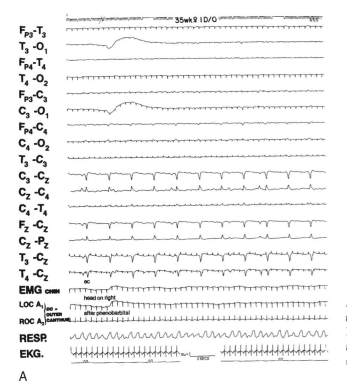

A

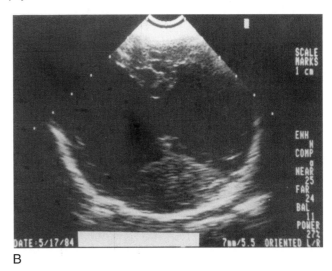

B

FIGURE 13–13

A, *Portion of an EEG tracing for a 35-week, 1-day-old girl with trisomy 13/15 demonstrating a periodic discharge in the midline.* B, *Coronal view of the cranial ultrasound for the patient described in A showing labor holoprosencephaly. The patient died, with verification of this malformation on postmortem examination.*

neonatal population. Figure 13–13 demonstrates periodic discharges in a child with holoprosencephaly. PT neonates had discharges that were less than 60 seconds in duration and located in the parasagittal regions, whereas discharges in FT neonates were longer than a minute and located in the temporal regions. Of the 34 neonates, 15 (44%) died and 58% of the surviving infants were abnormal with respect to neurologic development. The authors argue that focal periodic discharges in the neonate including PLEDs have the same clinical significance as PLEDs recorded on older children and adults. PLEDs are less common in the neonatal population with an incidence rate of 0.3%, which is below the reported range of 0.6% to 8.5% in older patients.[50]

Although these discharges usually indicate a lesion in the neonatal brain, the neurologic examination findings may or may not be helpful depending on the gestational maturity of the infant. FT infants with periodic discharges appear to have decreased levels of arousal or hypotonia in all cases. Only 50% of PT neonates demonstrated a neurologic abnormality at the time the discharges were noted.

Other differences include a higher percentage of seizures in FT infants (80%) than in PT infants (35%). Shewmon[62] recently argued, however, that periodic discharges may represent electrographic seizures with a prolonged duration but a markedly slow evolution that is not easily discernible on the standard EEG recording.

Acute hypoxic ischemic encephalopathy was the predominant etiology associated with periodic discharges in FT infants. More varied etiologies were present in the PT infants. Although some authors[57–60] have described periodic discharges in neonates with either neonatal herpes simplex encephalitis or asphyxia, these authors argue that periodic discharges are not pathognomonic of any specific condition.

Bilateral periodic high-amplitude slow and sharp waves as well as spike and slow wave complexes can also be seen in neonates with severe metabolic encephalopathies due to inborn errors of metabolism.[63] Such complexes are maximally expressed in the frontal regions with intervals between 5 and 20 seconds. Some authors have described these generalized periodic discharges as a *suppression-burst variant of hypsarrhythmia*.[19,64]

Generalized Monorhythmic Background Frequencies

Generalized or focal monorhythmic activities in the theta or alpha range are unusual patterns that are associated with severe neonatal brain disease. These rhythms occur synchronously as well as independently in each hemisphere, sometimes prominently in the central and temporal regions. Although alpha range activity has been seen in chromosomal abnormalities and multiple congenital

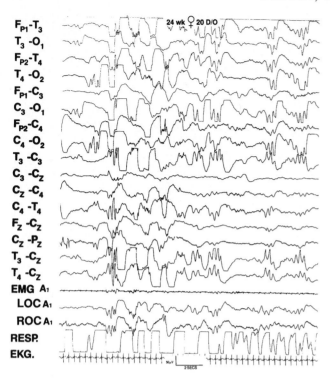

FIGURE 13–14

EEG tracing of a 24-week, 20-day-old girl with a diffuse theta background lacking in other rhythms. The patient had suffered septic shock and disseminated intravascular coagulation and later died. No autopsy was available.

anomalies,[1] more diffuse theta activity can be seen in PT infants following significant hypoxic-ischemic encephalopathies (Fig. 13–14).

ASSESSMENT OF PROGNOSIS IN PRETERM AND FULLTERM INFANTS

As emphasized several times during this discussion, serial EEGs offer more information than an isolated recording. Some reports nonetheless emphasize the prognostic significance of even single recordings that demonstrate severely abnormal features.[28,65,66] Other reports, however, suggest that serial studies provide the clinician with a more sensitive prognostic indication of neurodevelopmental outcome.[6,10] As previously summarized in Table 13–1, the major abnormalities in these two significant studies indicate that a normal neonatal EEG is highly correlated with favorable outcome as well. Major abnormalities were predictive of poor outcomes in both FT and PT infants. Other authors have also relied on the interictal EEG patterns to predict developmental outcome. Rose and Lombroso[11] stated that

the neonates with seizures and a normal EEG had an 86% chance of normal development at 4 years of age regardless of the clinical history at the time of their illness. Rowe and coworkers[20] evaluated the prognostic value of EEG in both FT and PT infants with seizures and also found that in 74 infants between 30 and 43 weeks of age, the background activity was highly correlated with outcome. Watanabe and associates[66] reviewed EEGs of 422 FT infants with neonatal asphyxia, also claiming that background EEG was an excellent predictor of outcome.

Certain authors have stressed the superiority of the EEG over neurologic examination to assess outcome. Holmes and colleagues[9] found that in 38 FT infants with neonatal asphyxia who had EEGs during the first 2 weeks, the EEG was a more sensitive predictor of sequelae than the examination. Tharp and coworkers[30] also emphasized the superiority of EEG over examination findings in PT infants. Scher and Beggarly[61] found that although all PT infants with periodic discharges either expired or had major sequelae, only 50% of PT infants were clinically symptomatic at the time of these discharges. Although early studies stress the clinical criteria to help predict outcome in term infants with asphyxia,[67] such examinations may be difficult to elicit or standardize in a busy NICU. Constant manipulation of the infant, aggressive use of medications that affect muscle tone or strength, and multiple indwelling catheters severely hamper one's ability to examine an ill neonate, masking or altering neurologic findings. EEG examinations can therefore assist when such examinations are difficult or impossible to perform.

Medications can clearly alter EEG activities (see Chapter 14). Few drugs, however, used in neonatal care have been studied. Prolonged inactivity usually occurs following a loading dose of phenobarbital, which may last longer than 1 hour following administration. Staudt and associates[68] argued that in infants phenobarbital plasma levels higher than 6 mg/dL cause significant background suppression. Other authors also reported the appearance of an isoelectric record or invariant discontinuous record with high doses of antiepileptic medications.[15] Benda and colleagues,[46] on the other hand, in studying 46 PT infants found that a mean therapeutic phenobarbital level did not prolong interburst intervals during tracé discontinu in PT infants.

No studies have systematically investigated the effects of other nonepileptic medications that may also affect the EEG tracing. In a case report, nafcillin-induced seizures were reported after intraventricular administration.[69] Yet other commonly used drugs in the neonatal patient, such as morphine, fentanyl, and theophylline, have not been studied. Quantitative analyses using computer techniques will be better able to monitor EEG changes relative to loading and maintenance doses as well as establish dose-response effects on EEG frequencies and amplitudes.

NEONATAL SEIZURES: CONTROVERSIES AND OPPORTUNITIES FOR THE NEUROPHYSIOLOGIST

A seizure in a newborn is one of the few neurologic emergencies in the neonatal age group. There is an urgency to establish a rapid diagnostic and therapeutic plan, and this emphasizes the crucial role played by the clinical neurophysiologist. A neurophysiologic strategy for the recognition and management of neonatal seizures demands heightened diagnostic acumen. The neurophysiologist can be aided by two current technologic advances. Synchronized video-EEG polygraphic monitoring and computer analysis will both occupy a central role in neonatal neurologic intensive care strategies over the next decade. However, as discussed later, controversial aspects concerning this condition must be resolved before a consensus is achieved with respect to the diagnosis and prognosis of neonates with seizures.[70,71]

Despite the need to establish the diagnosis of neonatal seizures, several unique aspects of this condition impede proper recognition. Multiple etiologic possibilities may present themselves with the clinical expression of seizures. Efficacy of antiepileptic drugs and the prediction of outcome are also controversial. These problems impede the establishment of accepted diagnostic and treatment criteria of this neonatal medical emergency.

Previous studies have fallen short of resolving these issues because of limited PT populations, technologic resources, patients pretreated with antiepileptic medications, or limited follow-up capabilities. Certain pioneering investigations predated the development of portable EEG or synchronized video polygraphic monitoring or did not use such systems available at the time of the studies. Traditionally, many centers chose only clinical criteria to diagnose neonatal seizures and therefore could not address the problems of overestimation and underestimation of seizure incidence based on coincident paper EEG or synchronized video-EEG polygraphic recordings.[72–75] Few studies recruited PT infants,[71,74,76] particularly those who were less than 30 weeks' gestation. No center has attempted to study efficacy of treatment by controlling the type of antiepileptic medications used to treat seizures. In fact, studies included patients who were already treated with such medications prior to neurophysiologic assessments.[72,77] Finally, most studies have not included statistical analyses of antepartum, intrapartum, and neonatal conditions that may better predict efficacy of response to medication, survival, or neurologic morbidity in patients with seizures.

All of these mentioned concerns must be kept in mind by the clinical neurophysiologist when approaching detection and managment of the clinical and electrical aspects of neonatal seizures.

CLINICAL VERSUS EEG CRITERIA

The international classification of epileptic seizures does not apply to newborn seizures.[28] Neonates are unable to sustain organized generalized discharges as in older patients and therefore do not manifest tonic-clonic seizures. As a result, clinical seizure phenomena are difficult to detect. Until recently, neonatal seizure criteria have been commonly grouped into five clinical types based on behavioral observation.[16] More recently, studies using EEG and behavioral monitoring by synchronized video-EEG polygraphic technique monitoring have improved these classifications, but more comprehensive diagnostic criteria using both clinical and electrical categories are needed that represent a more balanced approach to neonatal seizure diagnosis.

It is appropriate to first describe the clinical category. Seizures of this clinical type are commonly characterized by repetitive facial activity, unusual cycling or pedaling movements, momentary fixation of gaze, or apnea (Fig. 13–15).[16] Particular subtle behaviors such as apnea (which is also a common respiratory finding) rarely occur as the only clinical expression of a seizure.[78] Convulsive apnea is usually associated with other clinical seizure categories.

In general, subtle seizures are quite unimpressive in their clinical appearance and may be overlooked, but they may reflect significant brain injury. The inconsistent relationship of subtle behaviors with scalp-recorded electrographic seizures[72] emphasizes the need to study more closely the temporal and spatial characteristics of both criteria.

CLONIC SEIZURES

The clonic seizure classification consists of rhythmic movements of muscles that are either focal or multifocal in distribution, involving one or multiple extremities. Tonic components are usually quite subtle and may be absent. Generalized clonic movements may be seen in the absence of any tonic activity. Although multifocal clonic activity has been described to have no predictable anatomic pattern, focal clonic activity may suggest a specific regional or hemispheric brain lesion. Figure 13–16A is an EEG tracing of a 41-week, 1-day-old boy with clonic movements of the left foot seen coincidentally with bihemispheric electrographic seizures, whereas Figure 13–16B demonstrates bilateral discharges without coincident clinical seizure activity.

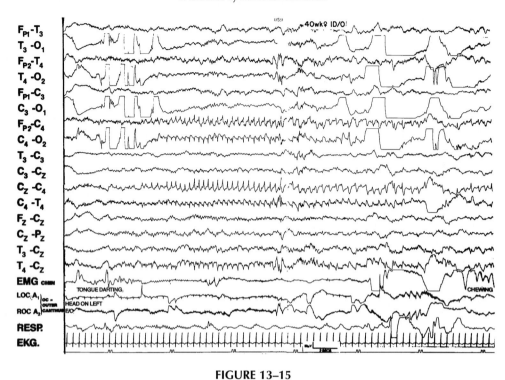

FIGURE 13–15

EEG tracing of a 40-week, 1-day-old girl described in Figure13–2A documenting lingual and lateral eye movements (note eye channels) coincidental with an electrographic seizure in the right central region.

MYOCLONIC SEIZURES

Myoclonic seizure movements are rapid isolated jerks, most frequently noted in PT infants but also seen in severely ill term infants (Fig. 13–17). Consequently, myoclonic seizures are associated with major central nervous system insults. Simultaneous EEG recordings are necessary since nonepileptic pathologic myoclonus of the newborn may also exist in the sick infant. What is more, both healthy PT as well as FT infants may manifest either age-appropriate myoclonus of prematurity or clinically benign sleep myoclonus.[79,80]

TONIC SEIZURES

Tonic seizures involve extension of axial or appendicular muscles. As with myoclonic seizures, EEG confirmation is necessary since tonic activity occurs in the absence of cortical seizures in a high percentage of patients. One study by Kellaway and Hrachovy[81] noted only a 30% correlation between tonic seizures and coincident electrographic correlates. Tonic seizures also respond poorly to antiepileptic drugs and, if associated with electrographic seizures, signify poor prognostic significance.

VIDEO-EEG CORRELATION OF SEIZURES AND OTHER NEONATAL BEHAVIOR

Synchronized video-EEG monitoring is now widely used in pediatric populations at risk for different neurologic diseases.[72] Given the issues that are discussed in the following sections concerning the clinical versus EEG correlation of seizures, such a technique has become extremely useful. Mizrahi and Kellaway[72] proposed a new classification of seizure and nonseizure activity based on the temporal relationships between clinical and electrical criteria documented by synchronized video-EEG correlations. Their investigations using a bedside video-EEG polygraphic monitoring technique provide insights into the interpretation of abnormal clinical findings in relation to electrographic activity. In one study, 415 clinical seizures in 71 infants were monitored, showing that clonic seizure activity had the best correlation with coincident electrographic seizures whereas subtle seizures had an inconsistent relationship with coincident EEG seizure activity.[72] Whether such clinical phenomena should then be interpreted as nonepileptic brainstem release behavior or represent subcortical seizure onset with inconsistent propagation to the surface has yet to be resolved.

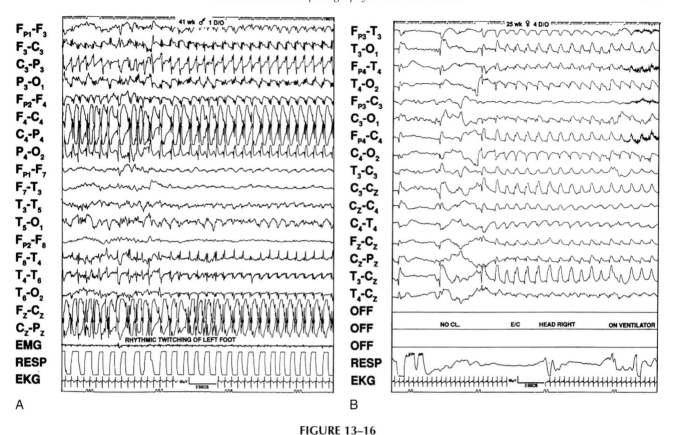

FIGURE 13–16

A, *EEG tracing of a 41-week, 1-day-old boy with clonic movements of the left foot seen coincidentally with bihemispheric electrographic seizures, with higher amplitude in the right central regions.* B, *EEG tracing of a 25-week, 4-day-old girl with an electrographic seizure noted without coincident behavioral changes.*

New technologies that can combine video, audio, and electrographic information will more effectively integrate complicated sets of diagnostic criteria and more accurately define the spatial and temporal components of cortical and subcortical seizures. This is particularly important before prospective, randomized trials of antiepileptic drugs can study the effects of different drug classes on the clinical and electrographic expression of seizures.

INCIDENCE OF NEONATAL SEIZURES

Problems with the recognition of neonatal seizures result from both overestimation and underestimation of the incidence of this disorder. Previous investigations have reported a wide range of incidence, from 0.5% in FT infants to 10.2% in PT infants.[82,83] Such wide discrepancies may in part be due to the varying CAs of newborns included in such studies as well as criteria for selection. Furthermore, hospital-based studies that specialize in evaluating the high-risk infant may report a higher rate than population studies that are based on newborns admitted to general nurseries and who are less medically ill. Most importantly, previous incidence figures have been based on clinical criteria that may not adequately distinguish seizures from normal or pathologic nonepileptic neonatal behavior. A report of the inborn incidence of neonatal seizures in a hospital-based population of high-risk infants[84] estimated that 2% of the neonatal population admitted to a NICU had electrographic seizures. This is 0.2% of all births at this obstetric center. Future studies must compare the incidence of seizures for both inborn and outborn populations, using both electrographic and clinical criteria.

STUDIES OF OVERESTIMATION OF SEIZURES

Studies emphasize the difficulty in identifying suspicious movements without coincident EEG monitoring.

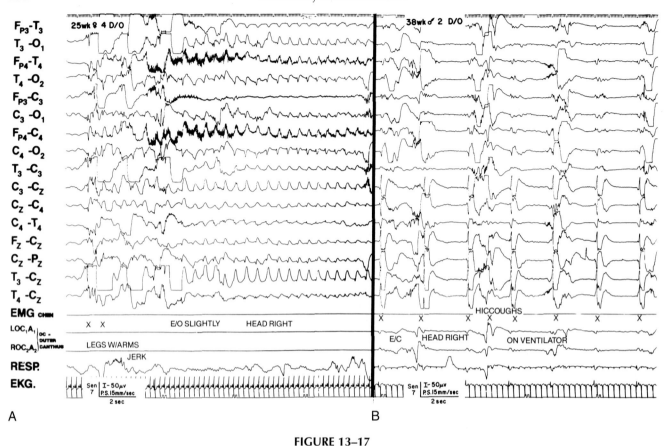

FIGURE 13–17

A, *EEG tracing of a 25-week, 4-day-old girl with brief myoclonic movements prior to an electrographic seizure seen diffusely over both hemispheres.* B, *EEG tracing of a 38-week, 2-day-old boy with prominent midline electrographic seizures, which are temporally related to myoclonic movements of the diaphragm.*

Careful evaluation of suspicious behaviors such as tremors or myoclonus may be abnormal but nonepileptic. Only 30% of infants with tonic behavior have coincident EEG seizure activity,[81] prompting investigators to emphasize the experimental animal evidence for brainstem release phenomena as an explanation for these neonatal behaviors.

In another study from the same center, only 17% with subtle movements had a consistent relationship with EEG seizures in 71 FT and near-FT infants,[72] emphasizing again a nonepileptic pathophysiologic mechanism. Another study also stressed the limitations of scalp recorded EEGs, by reporting that only 10% of the EEGs obtained on 80 neonates with suspicious movements had coincident electrographic seizures.[71] All these studies emphasize the risk of overestimating seizures when suspicious movements are identified without coincident EEG monitoring. In fact, it has been suggested[85] that synchronized video polygraphic monitoring should be required to fully characterize the electrographic and clinical phenomena associated with questionable seizure activity.

UNDERESTIMATION OF SEIZURES

Newborns may have electrographic seizures that would go undetected unless the EEG is used.[71,86] Although some of these patients may be pharmacologically paralyzed for ventilatory support,[86,87] other electrographic seizures have no observable clinical activity.[62,71,76,86] A report has indicated that 50% of electrographic seizures in neonates are unaccompanied by clinical phenomena.[84] Clinical and electrographic criteria were noted in 20 (45%) of 62 PT and 16 (53%) of 30 FT infants. This population was defined over a 4-year period in which 92 neonates with seizures using EEG criteria were identified in the NICU. Seventeen infants in this group had seizures documented while paralyzed.

In part, underestimation of seizures may result because of inadequate monitoring of autonomic changes coincident with electrographic seizures. Autonomic changes may consist of alterations in respiration, blood pressure, or heart rate as well as changes in pupillary size or salivation (Fig. 13–18). Paroxysmal autonomic events that are

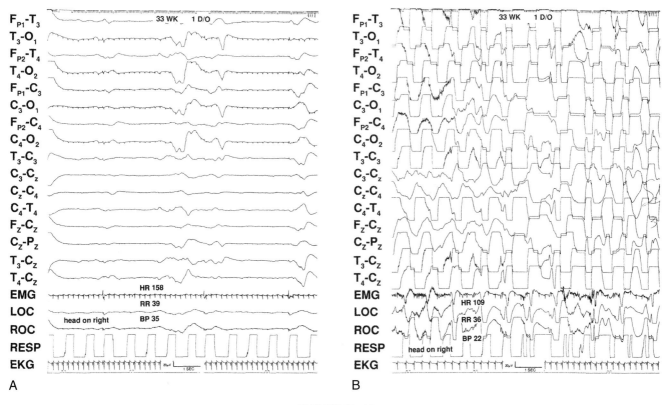

FIGURE 13–18

A, *EEG tracing of a 33-week, 1-day-old girl indicating a lack of normal background. Note the vital sign values for blood pressure, heart, and respiratory rates.* B, *Same patient as described in Figure 13–20A showing a precipitous drop in heart rate and blood pressure coincident with a generalized electrographic seizure. An evolution in this generalized seizure was noted over 3 minutes.*

periodic or recurring should always be treated as possible seizure phenomena when a seizure recording is obtained.

ELECTROCLINICAL DISASSOCIATION OF NEONATAL SEIZURES

The brain is dependent on deep gray matter structures for seizure propagation as well as surface cortical tissue. Although depth recordings in adults and adolescents have documented subcortical seizures, direct or indirect evidence in the neonate has not yet been available. Electroclinical disassociation (ECD)[88] attempts to address this controversial topic. One hundred ten infants with electrographically confirmed seizures were investigated with respect to ECD. A seizure was defined as an electrographic event characterized by the sudden appearance of repetitive waveforms that had a demonstrable evolution in frequency, morphology, amplitude, and field, with a minimum duration of 10 seconds. ECD was defined as a clinical seizure that occurred at times with, and other times without, electrographic signature. Since the study focused on the relationship of clinical move-

ments to their electrographic expression, 34 infants with only electrical seizures and 25 pharmacologically paralyzed infants were excluded.

Of the remaining 51 infants, 33 satisfied the criteria for electroclinical (EC) seizures, having movements consistently coupled to an electrographic discharge. This group was compared to 18 infants who had ECD. The ECD group comprised 16% of infants with electrographically confirmed seizures and 19% of 243 with EC seizures. Extremity movements occurred at a significantly higher rate with EC seizures, whereas clinical features that preceded electrical seizures were associated with the ECD group to a statistically significant degree.

The phenomena of ECD may contribute to a more balanced seizure taxonomy[89] that includes both EEG and clinical seizure criteria. Rather than strictly interpreting clinical behaviors as nonepileptic because of the inconsistent association of these movements with coincident EEG seizure activity, one might alternately suggest that certain clinical activity lacks a consistent EEG correlate because of ECD. The inconsistent electrographic capture on scalp recordings may represent seizures emanating from foci deep within the brain, only inconsistently discharging through final anatomic pathways.[88] Multimedia monitoring equipment using video, audio, and electrographic data may provide the necessary temporal resolution necessary to characterize such behavioral and electrographic events.

SEIZURE DURATION AND TOPOGRAPHY

Little attention has been directed toward quantifying the ictal and interictal periods on an EEG recording. A study[77] measured the exact duration of these periods in primarily FT and near-FT infants. The majority of the population (87%) received one or more antiepileptic medications prior to obtaining the EEG tracings. Seizures were recurrent but relatively brief, lasting 137 seconds, separated by interictal recovery periods of variable duration, but 8 minutes on the average. The minimum duration of seizures was defined as 10 seconds.

In another study,[108] seizure durations were reviewed in 68 neonates consisting of 34 FT neonates and 34 PT neonates. This study considered the effect of gestational age, serial seizures, and antiepileptic medication on seizure durations. Serial seizures were defined as either continuous seizure activity for at least 30 minutes or recurrent seizures for 50% or more of the recording time. Eleven (36%) of 34 FT infants had serial seizures, and this subgroup contributed to a mean duration of series of 14.2 minutes prior to antiepileptic drug use. By contrast, only 3 (9%) of 33 PT had serial seizures, with a mean seizure duration of 3.1 minutes. Excluding patients with serial seizures, mean seizure durations were similar: 2.9 and 4.6 minutes for PT and FT infants, respectively. Interictal durations were shorter in FT than PT infants (10 vs. 24 minutes). However, this longer interval between seizures was noted only in PT infants older than 32 weeks' estimated gestational age (EGA). Surprisingly, PT infants who were less than 32 weeks EGA had interburst intervals comparable with FT infants. Possibly, subcortical neuronal pathways in very PT infants function to suppress the initiation of seizures in a similar manner to neocortical pathways in FT infants. "Older" PT infants may have more dominant inhibitory neuronal circuitry during a particular stage of brain development.

Studies of ictal and interictal durations are needed before automated seizure detection programs can be established. Ultimately, computer techniques may more accurately measure ictal and interictal durations but must first be based on visually analyzed records. Such computer strategies then better assess the efficacy of antiepileptic drugs as measured by their effects on seizure duration, electrographic field, as well as clinical expression.

ICTAL PATTERNS

Ictal patterns in the newborn are rhythmic discharges consisting of waveforms of similar morphology that change an evolution with respect to frequency, amplitude, and electrical field (Fig. 13–19).[90] Four basic categories of ictal patterns have been traditionally described: focal ictal patterns with normal background, focal ictal patterns with abnormal background, focal monorhythmic patterns of various frequencies, and multifocal ictal patterns.

Shewmon[62] stressed the problems defining an electrographic seizure, even among experienced clinical neurophysiologists. The author emphasized the ictal-interictal dichotomy involving both brief and intermittent rhythmic discharges that are less than 10 seconds as well as prolonged periodic discharges that have a slow evolution that cannot be easily discerned as seizures. Although such concerns have not presently been resolved, most electroencephalographers identify ictal patterns as having at least 10 seconds in duration with an evolution in the earlier-mentioned electrographic features (Fig. 13–20).

FOCAL ICTAL PATTERNS

Discharges originating in one region may spread to homologous regions in both PT and FT infants. In general, discharges seen with normal EEG background and the absence of a structural lesion have a more favorable prognosis.[83] Conversely, focal ictal patterns with low amplitude and disorganized backgrounds are associated with structural lesions and a higher risk for sequelae (Fig. 13–21).

FOCAL MONORHYTHMIC CHARGES OF VARYING FREQUENCIES

Such discharges may be in any frequency range. There appears to be no specific association with gestational age, but on rare occasions, specific frequencies have been associated with particular types of clinical phenomena (i.e., alpha frequency seizures associated with apnea). In general, focal seizures at any frequency arise most often in the central and temporal areas.[1] A second most common site would be the occipital region.

MULTIFOCAL ICTAL DISCHARGES

Electrical seizure activity may originate from anatomically unrelated brain regions. Such a pattern is usually associated with a high instance of neurologic sequelae.[1,71]

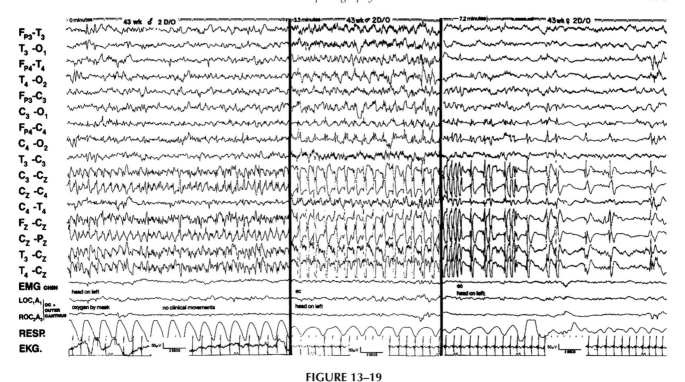

FIGURE 13–19

EEG tracing of a 43-week, 2-day-old boy demonstrating the evolution of electrographic discharge with an onset in the midline spreading to the central and temporal regions. Note the evolution in morphology frequency and field.

ETIOLOGIES OF NEONATAL SEIZURES

Issues exist with respect to the causes of neonatal seizures. As with background EEG abnormalities, seizures are also not disease specific. A neonate who is ill may have a variety of medical difficulties that predispose to seizures.[16] Despite the large number of possibilities that can be associated with neonatal seizures, a small subset of etiologies most commonly are noted. Medical conditions that occur with hypoxic ischemic insults contribute significantly to the seizure diathesis. The presence of hypoglycemia, hypocalcemia, intracranial hemorrhage, or cerebral infarct all can occur in the patient with asphyxia.[67,75] Rarely, a genetic form of neonatal seizures can occur.[91,92] Most asphyxia occurs before or during labor and delivery with only 10% of neonates suffering asphyxia during the neonatal period.[16] Therefore, intrauterine factors that lead to asphyxia may contribute to seizures, including placental or maternal disease. With the advent of more sophisticated fetal ultrasonography, antenatal intracranial brain lesions associated with asphyxia can also be detected.

Cerebral infarction has an important association with neonates with seizures (see Fig. 13–21).[75,93–95] Ischemic brain lesions in one particular study were noted in 77% of FT and 39% of PT infants.[96] Grade III to IV subependymal

hemorrhage was also seen in 45% of PT infants with neonatal seizures. Documentation of these structural lesions are important, together with other clinical and demographic data in relation to immediate and long FT outcome.

PROGNOSIS OF NEONATES WITH SEIZURES

Although it has recently been suggested that the mortality rate for clinical seizures has dropped from 40% to 15%,[16] this trend is not based on the electrographic diagnoses of seizures. In fact, in one report, the EEG criteria for seizures found 50% mortality in PT and 40% in FT infants.[71] Furthermore, the incidence of adverse neurologic sequelae was noted in 65% of survivors.

A change in the etiologies of seizures over the last several decades must be considered before assessing the prognosis of infants with seizures. Although there are substantial reductions in seizures caused by late-onset hypocalcemia or birth trauma, proportionally higher numbers of neonates with hemorrhagic or ischemic cerebrovascular lesions are now associated with neonatal seizures.[52,75,93–95]

Specific clinical criteria of neonatal seizures have prognostic implications. Tonic, myoclonic, and subtle seizures imply a more diffuse or multifocal brain insult

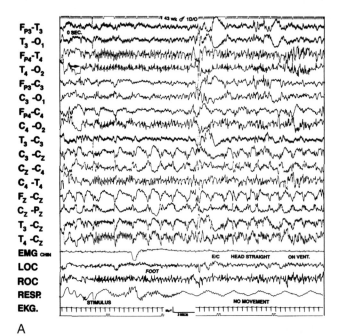

A

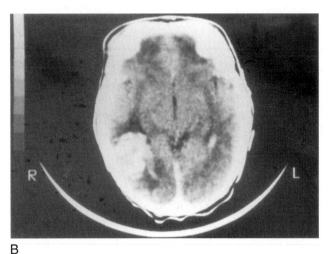

B

FIGURE 13–20

A, *EEG tracing of a 43-week, 1-day-old boy with an onset of a focal seizure in the right posterior quadrant (note arrow). This patient had severe pulmonary hypertension of the newborn.*
B, *CT scan of the patient in A showing a hemorrhagic infarction in the right posterior quadrant. This patient has severe spastic quadriparesis at 7 years of age.*

suggesting a poorer prognosis.[2,71,97] Such seizure types have also been noted in association with inborn errors of metabolism, malformations, and severe asphyxia.

Interictal EEG findings are particularly useful in predicting neurologic outcome in neonates with seizures. Background EEG activity is an excellent indicator of outcome, as emphasized in earlier sections. Certain major

disturbances such as suppression burst are highly predictive of poor outcome. Ictal patterns alone or interictal spikes and sharp waves may not fully predict the risk for sequelae. In a study of 137 FT infants with neonatal seizures, Rose and Lombroso[11] found that neonates with seizures who had a normal EEG had an 86% chance of normal development at age 4 years. Conversely, in neonates with low-amplitude, periodic or multifocal spikes in the interictal EEG background had only a 7% chance for normal development. In a more recent study, Rowe and associates[20] supported these findings in their discussion of prognosis in 74 FT and PT neonates with seizures. They emphasized that EEG background actually was more predictive of outcome than interictal sharp waves.

As previously mentioned, Monod,[10] Tharp,[6] and their groups emphasized for FT and PT infants, respectively, the importance of serial records in assessing neurologic outcome. These authors found that normal neonatal EEGs were highly correlated with favorable outcomes whereas markedly abnormal records are associated with poorer outcomes for both FT and PT infants.

The clinician treating patients with neonatal seizures is appropriately concerned about the risk of epilepsy. Few studies have attempted to predict subsequent epilepsy in neonates with seizures as confirmed by electrographic studies. Using clinical criteria only, some reports estimate that as many as 10% to 30% of neonates with seizures will develop epilepsy.[70,97,98] More recently, excluding seizures with fever, the incidence of epilepsy at 4 years of age appears to be 15% to 20% of neonates with electrographically confirmed seizures.[99]

Brain imaging techniques developed over the last two decades have revolutionized the diagnosis of major structural diseases of the brain, thereby improving the accuracy of predicting outcome. Newer techniques applying both structural-functional studies such as nuclear magnetic resonance (NMR) and positron emission tomography (PET) extend our abilities to detect structural and metabolic disturbances of the brain due to seizures. Comparisons of these techniques will augment our ability to describe the metabolic and neurophysiologic consequences of structural lesions of the brains of neonates with seizures.

EFFICACY OF TREATMENT

A number of issues still remain with respect to the treatment of neonatal seizures.[70,71] Although some argue that neonates should be treated only if seizures are clinically expressed and prolonged in duration, others suggest that all seizures should be treated because of the possibility of their detrimental effects on the immature brain.[100–102] These topics have been recently reviewed.[103–105]

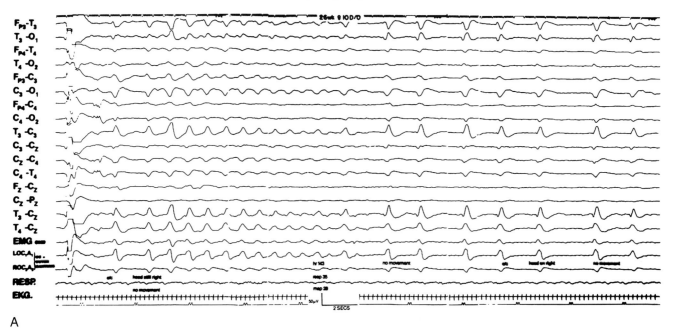

A

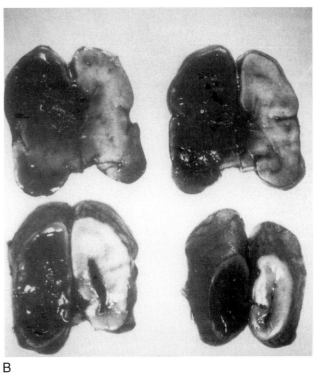

FIGURE 13–21

A, *EEG tracing of a 26-week, 10-day-old girl with necrotizing enterocolitis and disseminated intravascular coagulation. An electrographic seizure was seen predominantly in the left hemisphere both above and below the sylvian fissure with spread to involve the homologous right hemispheric regions. The patient subsequently died, but no autopsy was obtained. B, Coronal section of the brain of the patient described in A, indicating a significant hemorrhagic infarction of the left hemisphere.*

B

Different medications are available that are used to treat neonatal seizures. Phenobarbital and phenytoin remain the most widely used, but the benzodiazepines are also efficacious for treating neonatal seizures. Published studies in which the efficacy of phenobarbital was reported are conflicting. Using clinical seizure criteria, only 36% of neonates at one institution responded to phenobarbital alone.[106,107] Similarly, Lockman and associates[108] found cessation of seizures with phenobarbital in 32%. By contrast, Gal and colleagues[109] reported that seizure control was achieved with phenobarbital monotherapy in 85% of patients with loading doses that were twice that reported in infants. More recently, free drug fractions that determine efficacy and toxicity have been studied in pediatric populations.[71] Binding of drugs in neonates with seizures have only recently been reported. Binding can be significantly altered in a sick neonatal patient. Such alterations may cause toxic side effects by affecting cardiovascular or respiratory functions. Efficacy of treatment must use not only appropriate total, free, and bound fractions to verify the cortical representation of seizures but guard against toxicity if free fractions are dangerously high. Serial drug level determinations combined with analog and digital EEG analyses will better assess efficacy and toxicity of antiepileptic drugs in future studies.

SUMMARY

As already emphasized at the conclusion of Chapter 2, electrophysiologic monitoring is the only technique that can assess cerebral function continuously over time. This advantage must also be stressed in the context of the neurophysiologic assessment of the sick neonate. To identify objectively pathophysiologic concomitants of episodic or periodic diseases, the noninvasive methods of electrophysiologic recordings adapt most readily to the complicated environment of the NICU. Pathophysiologic events may occur intermittently at unpredictable times, (i.e., neonatal seizures). Furthermore, maladaptive physiologic interrelationships among cortical and subcortical neuronal tract systems may subtly herald disturbances of biologic rhythm (i.e., neonatal EEG-sleep) that can be detected only by quantitative EEG recordings over extended periods. Other methods of measuring brain structure and function (i.e., PET and spectral NMR) provide detailed but brief "snapshots" of information that can be better interpreted in the context of continuous electrophysiologic recordings. As with other physiologic monitoring techniques in cardiology, neuroanesthesia, and epilepsy, which rely on long-term monitoring in the intensive care, operating, and epilepsy suites, long-term neurophysiologic monitoring deserves an important place in the NICU.

REFERENCES

1. Hrachovy RA, Mizrahi EM, Kellaway P: Electroencephalography of the newborn. *In* Daly DD, Pedley TA (eds): Current Practice of Clinical Electroencephalography. New York, Raven Press, 1990, p 201.

2. Lombroso CT: Neonatal electroencephalography. *In* Niedermeyer E, Lopes da Silva F (eds): Electroencephalography: Basic Principles, Clinical Applications, and Related Fields. Baltimore, Urban & Schwarzenberg, 1982, p 599.

3. Lombroso CT: Neonatal polygraphy in full-term and premature infants: A review of normal and abnormal findings. J Clin Neurophysiol 1985;2:105-153.

4. Scher MS, Painter MJ, Guthrie RD: Cerebral neurophysiologic assessment of the high-risk neonate. *In* Guthrie RD (ed): Recent Advances in Neonatal Care. New York, Churchill Livingstone, 1987, p 41-69.

5. Tharp BR: Electroencephalography in the assessment of the premature and full-term infant. *In* Stevenson DK, Sunshine P (eds): Fetal and Neonatal Brain Injury: Mechanisms, Management and the Risks of Practice. New York, Cambridge University Press, 1989.

6. Tharp BR, Cukier F, Monod N: The prognostic value of the electroencephalogram in premature infants. Electroencephalogr Clin Neurophysiol 1981;51:219-236.

7. Westmoreland BF, Klass DW, Sharbrough FW: Chronic periodic lateralized epileptiform discharges. Arch Neurol 1986;43:494-496.

8. Holmes GL, Lombroso CT: Prognostic value of background patterns in the neonatal EEG. J Clin Neurophysiol 1993;10:323-352.

9. Holmes GL, Rowe J, Hafford J, et al: Prognostic value of the electroencephalogram in neonatal asphyxia. Electroencephalogr Clin Neurophysiol 1982;53:60-72.

10. Monod N, Pajot N, Guidasci S: The neonatal EEG: Statistical studies and prognostic value in full-term and pre-term babies. Electroencephalogr Clin Neurophysiol 1972;32:529-544.

11. Rose AL, Lombroso CT: Neonatal seizure states: A study of clinical, pathological, and electroencephalographic features in 137 full-term babies with a long-term follow-up. Pediatrics 1970;45:404-425.

12. Aso K, Scher MS, Barmada MA: Neonatal electroencephalography and neuropathology. J Clin Neurophysiol 1989;6:103-123.

13. Barabas RE, Barmada MA, Scher MS: Timing of brain insults in severe neonatal encephalopathies with isoelectric EEG. Pediatr Neurol 1993;9:39-44.

14. O'Brien MJ, Lems YL, Prechtl HF: Transient flattenings in the EEG of newborns—a benign variation. Electroencephalogr Clin Neurophysiol 1987;67:16-26.

15. Pezzani C, Radvanyi Bouvet MF, Relier JP, Monod N: Neonatal electroencephalography during the first twenty-four hours of life in full-term newborn infants. Neuropediatrics 1986;17:11-18.

16. Volpe JJ: Neurology of the Newborn, 3rd ed. Philadelphia, WB Saunders, 1995.

17. Stockard-Pope JE, Werner SS, Bickford RG: Atlas of Neonatal Electroencephalography, 2nd ed. New York, Raven Press, 1992.

18. Watanabe K, Kuroyanagi M, Hara K, Miyazaki S: Neonatal seizures and subsequent epilepsy. Brain Dev 1982;4:341-346.

19. Ohtahara S: Clinico-electrical delineation of epileptic encephalopathies in childhood. Asian Med J 1978;21:7-17.

20. Rowe JC, Holmes GL, Hafford J, et al: Prognostic value of the electroencephalogram in term and preterm infants following neonatal seizures. Electroencephalogr Clin Neurophysiol 1985;60:183-196.

21. Hughes JR, Fino J, Gagnon L: The use of the electroencephalogram in the confirmation of seizures in premature and neonatal infants. Neuropediatrics 1983;14:213-219.

22. Tharp B, Cukier F, Monod M: [The prognostic value of the EEG in premature infants (authors' transl)]. Rev Electroencephalogr Neurophysiol Clin 1977;7:386-391.

23. Monod N, Pajot N: Le sommeil du nouveau-né et du prematuré: I. Analyse des etudés polygraphiques (mouvements oculaires, respiration et EEG chez le nouveau-né á terme). Biol Neonate 1965;8:281-307.

24. Challamel MJ, Isnard H, Brunon AM, Revol M: Asymetrie EEG transitoire a l'entree dans le sommeil calme chez le nouveau-ne: Etude sur 75 observations. Rev Electroencephalogr Neurophysiol Clin 1984;14:17-23.

25. Anderson CM, Torres F, Faoro A: The EEG of the early premature. Electroencephalogr Clin Neurophysiol 1985;60:95-105.

26. Olson DM, Shewmon DA: Electroencephalographic abnormalities in infants with hypoplastic left heart syndrome. Pediatr Neurol 1989;5:93-98.

27. Scher MS, Richardson GA, Coble PA, et al: The effects of prenatal alcohol and marijuana exposure: Disturbances in neonatal sleep cycling and arousal. Pediatr Res 1988;24:101-105.

28. Schulte FJ, Heinze G, Schrempf G: Maternal toxemia, fetal malnutrition, and bioelectric brain activity of the newborn. Neuropadiatrie 1971;2:439-460.

29. Holmes GL, Logan WJ, Kirkpatrick BV, Meyer EC: Central nervous system maturation in the stressed premature. Ann Neurol 1979;6:518-522.

30. Tharp BR, Scher MS, Clancy RR: Serial EEGs in normal and abnormal infants with birth weights less than 1200 grams—a prospective study with long-term follow-up. Neuropediatrics 1989;20:64-72.

31. Blume WT, Dreyfus-Brisac C: Positive rolandic sharp waves in neonatal EEG: Types and significance. Electroencephalogr Clin Neurophysiol 1982;53:277-282.

32. Clancy RR, Tharp BR: Positive rolandic sharp waves in the electroencephalograms of premature neonates with intraventricular hemorrhage. Electroencephalogr Clin Neurophysiol 1984;57:395-404.

33. Clancy RR, Tharp BR, Enzman D: EEG in premature infants with intraventricular hemorrhage. Neurology 1984;34:583-590.

34. Cukier F, André M, Monod N, Dreyfus-Brisac C: Apport de l'EEG au diagnostic des hémorragies intra-

35. Marret S, Parain D, Samson-Dollfus D, et al: Positive rolandic sharp waves and periventricular leukomalacia in the newborn. Neuropediatrics 1986;17:199-202.

36. Novotny EJ Jr, Tharp BR, Coen RW, et al: Positive rolandic sharp waves in the EEG of the premature infant. Neurology 1987;37:1481-1486.

37. Scher MS: Midline electrographic abnormalities and cerebral lesions in the newborn brain. J Child Neurol 1988;3:135-146.

38. de la Paz D, Brenner RD: Bilateral independent periodic lateralized epileptiform discharges: Clinical significance. Arch Neurol 1981;38:713-715.

39. Ehle A, Co S, Jones MG: Clinical correlates of midline spikes: An analysis of 21 patients. Arch Neurol 1981;38:355-357.

40. Kennedy WA: Clinical and electroencephalographic aspects of epileptogenic lesions of the medial surface and superior border of the cerebral hemisphere. Brain 1959;82:147-161.

41. Tukel K, Jasper H: The electroencephalogram in parasagittal lesions. Electroencephalogr Clin Neurophysiol Suppl 1952;4:481-494.

42. Scher MS: Pathologic myoclonus of the newborn: electrographic and clinical correlations. Pediatr Neurol 1985;1:342-348.

43. Halliday AM: The electrophysiological study of myoclonus in man. Brain 1967;90:241-284.

44. Monod N, Dreyfus-Brisac C, Ducas P, Mayer M: L'EEG du nouveau-ne à terme: Étude comparative chez le nouvau-né en présentation céphalique et en présentation de siege. Rev Neurol 1960;102:375-379.

45. Shibasaki H, Neshige R, Hashiba Y: Cortical excitability after myoclonus: Jerk-locked somatosensory evoked potentials. Neurology 1985;35:36-41.

46. Benda GI, Engel RC, Zhang YP: Prolonged inactive phases during the discontinuous pattern of prematurity in the electroencephalogram of very-low-birthweight infants. Electroencephalogr Clin Neurophysiol 1989;72:189-197.

47. Au WJ, Gabor AJ, Vijayan N, Markand ON: Periodic lateralized epileptiform discharges (PLEDs) in Creutzfeldt-Jakob disease. Neurology 1980;30:611-617.

48. Bickford RG, Butt HR: Hepatic coma: The electroencephalographic pattern. J Clin Invest 1955;34:790-799.

49. Celesia GG: Pathophysiology of periodic EEG complexes in subacute sclerosing panencephalitis (SSPE). Electroencephalogr Clin Neurophysiol 1973;35:293-300.

50. Chatrian GE, Shaw C-M, Leffman H: The significance of periodic lateralized epileptiform discharges in EEG: An electrographic, clinical, and pathological study. Electroencephalogr Clin Neurophysiol 1964;17:177-193.

51. Cobb WA: Evidence on the periodic mechanism in herpes simplex encephalitis. Electroencephalogr Clin Neurophysiol 1979;46:345-350.

52. Lesse S, Hoefer PF, Austin JH: The electroencephalogram in diffuse encephalopathies: Significance of periodic

synchronous discharges. Arch Neurol Psychiatry 1958;79:359-375.

53. Markand ON, Daly DD: Pseudoperiodic lateralized paroxysmal discharges in electroencephalogram. Neurology 1971;21:975-981.

54. PeBenito R, Cracco JB: Periodic lateralized epileptiform discharges in infants and children. Ann Neurol 1979; 6:47-50.

55. Schwartz MS, Prior PF, Scott DF: The occurrence and evolution in the EEG of a lateralized periodic phenomenon. Brain 1973;96:613-622.

56. Kuroiwa Y, Celesia GG: Clinical significance of periodic EEG patterns. Arch Neurol 1980;37:15-20.

57. McCutchen CB, Coen R, Iragui VJ: Periodic lateralized epileptiform discharges in asphyxiated neonates. Electroencephalogr Clin Neurophysiol 1985;61:210-217.

58. Estivill E, Monod N, Amiel-Tison C: Etude électroencéphalographique d'un cas d'éncephalite herpetique-neo-natal. Rév EEG Neurophysiol Clin 1977;7:380-385.

59. Mizrahi EM, Tharp BR: A characteristic EEG pattern in neonatal herpes simplex encephalitis. Neurology 1982;32:1215-1220.

60. Sainio K, Granström M-L, Pettay O, Donner M: EEG in neonatal herpes simplex encephalitis. Electroencephalogr Clin Neurophysiol 1983;56:556-561.

61. Scher MS, Beggarly M: Clinical significance of focal periodic discharges in neonates. J Child Neurol 1989;4:175-185.

62. Shewmon DA: What is a neonatal seizure? Problems in definition and quantification for investigative and clinical purposes. J Clin Neurophysiol 1990;7:315-368.

63. Scher MS, Bergman I, Ahdab-Barmada M, Fria T: Neurophysiological and anatomical correlations in neonatal nonketotic hyperglycinemia. Neuropediatrics 1986;17:137-143.

64. Aicardi J: Early myoclonic encephalopathy. In Roger J, Dravet C, Bureau M, Dreifuss FE, Wolf P (eds): Epileptic Syndromes in Infancy, Childhood, and Adolescence. London, John Libbey Eurotext, 1985, p 12.

65. Harris R, Tizard JPM: The electroencephalogram in neonatal convulsions. J Pediatr 1960;57:501-520.

66. Watanabe K, Miyazaki S, Hara K, Hakamada S: Behavioral state cycles, background EEGs, and prognosis of newborns with perinatal hypoxia. Electroencephalogr Clin Neurophysiol 1980;49:618-625.

67. Brown JK, Cockburn F, Forfar JO: Clinical and chemical correlates in convulsions of the newborn. Lancet 1972;1:135-139.

68. Staudt F, Roth JG, Engel RC: The usefulness of electroencephalography in curarized newborns. Electroencephalogr Clin Neurophysiol 1981;51:205-208.

69. Brozanski BS, Scher MS, Albright AL: Intraventricular nafcillin-induced seizures in a neonate. Pediatr Neurol 1988;4:188-190.

70. Camfield PR, Camfield CS: Neonatal seizures: A commentary on selected aspects. J Child Neurol 1987;2:244-251.

71. Scher MS, Painter MJ: Controversies concerning neonatal seizures. Pediatr Clin North Am 1989;36:281-310.

72. Mizrahi EM, Kellaway P: Characterization and classification of neonatal seizures. Neurology 1987;37:1837-1844.

73. Mizrahi EM, Plouin P, Kellaway P: Neonatal seizures. In Engel J Jr, Pedley TA (eds): Epilepsy: A Comprehensive Textbook. Philadelphia, Lippincott-Raven, 1997, p 647.

74. Radvanyi-Bouvet MF, Vallecalle MH, Morel-Kahn F, et al: Seizures and electrical discharges in premature infants. Neuropediatrics 1985;16:143-148.

75. Scher MS, Klesh KW, Murphy TF, Guthrie RD: Seizures and infarction in neonates with persistent pulmonary hypertension. Pediatr Neurol 1986;2:332-339.

76. Hellström Westas L, Rosen I, Svenningsen NW: Cerebral complications detected by EEG-monitoring during neonatal intensive care. Acta Paediatr Scand 1989;360(Suppl):83-86.

77. Clancy RR, Legido A: The exact ictal and interictal duration of electroencephalographic neonatal seizures. Epilepsia 1987;28:537-541.

78. Fenichel GM, Olson BJ, Fitzpatrick JE: Heart rate changes in convulsive and nonconvulsive neonatal apnea. Ann Neurol 1980;7:577-582.

79. Coulter DL, Allen RJ: Benign neonatal sleep myoclonus. Arch Neurol 1982;39:191-192.

80. Miles DK, Holmes GL: Benign neonatal seizures. J Clin Neurophysiol 1990;7:369-379.

81. Kellaway P, Hrachovy RA: Status epilepticus in newborns: A perspective on neonatal seizures. In Advances in Neurology, Vol 34: Status Epilepticus. New York, Raven Press, 1983, p 93.

82. Bergman I, Painter MI, Hirsch RP, et al: Outcome of neonates with convulsions treated in an intensive care unit. Ann Neurol 1983;14:642-647.

83. Hill A, Volpe JJ: Seizures, hypoxic-ischemic brain injury, and intraventricular hemorrhage in the newborn. Ann Neurol 1981;10:109-121.

84. Scher MS, Painter MJ, Bergman I, et al: EEG diagnoses of neonatal seizures: Clinical correlations and outcome. Pediatr Neurol 1989;5:17-24.

85. Volpe JJ: Neonatal seizures: Current concepts and revised classification. Pediatrics 1989;84:422-428.

86. Coen RW, McCutchen CB, Wermer D, et al: Continuous monitoring of the electroencephalogram following perinatal asphyxia. J Pediatr 1982;100:628-630.

87. Goldberg RN, Goldman SL, Ramsay RE, Feller R: Detection of seizure activity in the paralyzed neonate using continuous monitoring. Pediatrics 1982; 69:583-586.

88. Weiner SP, Painter MJ, Geva D, et al: Neonatal seizures: Electroclinical dissociation. Pediatr Neurol 1991;7:363-368.

89. Volpe JJ: Neonatal seizures. In Volpe JJ (ed): Neurology of the Newborn, 3rd ed. Philadelphia, WB Saunders, 1995, p 172.

90. Lombroso CT, Holmes GL: Value of the EEG in neonatal seizures. J Epilepsy 1993;6:39-70.

91. Biervert C, Steinlein OK: Structural and mutational analysis of *KCNQ2*, the major gene locus for benign familial neonatal convulsions. Hum Genet 1999;104:234-240.

92. Leppert M, Anderson E, Quattlebaum T, et al: Benign familial neonatal convulsions linked to genetic markers on chromosome 20. Nature 1989;337:647-648.

93. Clancy R, Malin S, Laraque D, et al: Focal motor seizures heralding stroke in full-term neonates. Am J Dis Child 1985;139:601-606.

94. Levy S, Abroms I: Seizures and cerebral infarctions in the full-term newborn. Ann Neurol 1985;17:366-372.

95. Ment LR, Duncan CC, Ehrenkranz RA: Perinatal cerebral infarction. Ann Neurol 1984;16:559-568.

96. Scher MS: A developmental marker of central nervous system maturation: I. Pediatr Neurol 1988;4:265-273.

97. Brunquell PJ, Glennon CM, DiMario FJ Jr, et al: Prediction of outcome based on clinical seizure type in newborn infants. J Pediatr 2002;140:707-712.

98. Holden KR, Mellits ED, Freeman JM: Neonatal seizures: I. Correlation of prenatal and perinatal events with outcomes. Pediatrics 1982;60:165-176.

99. Scher MS, Painter MJ: Electroencephalographic diagnosis of neonatal seizures: Issues of diagnostic accuracy, clinical correlation, and survival. *In* Wasterlain CG, Vert P (eds): Neonatal Seizures. New York, Raven Press, 1990, p 15.

100. Wasterlain CG, Plum F: Vulnerability of developing rat brain to electroconvulsive seizures. Arch Neurol 1973;29:38-45.

101. Wasterlain CG: Effects of neonatal status epilepticus on rat brain development. Neurology 1976;26:975-986.

102. Wasterlain CG: Neonatal seizures and brain growth. Neuropaediatrie 1978;9:213-228.

103. Holmes GL, Khazipov R, Ben-Ari Y: New concepts in neonatal seizures. Neuroreport 2002;13:A3-A8.

104. Holmes GL, Ben-Ari Y: The neurobiology and consequences of epilepsy in the developing brain. Pediatr Res 2001;49:320-325.

105. Sanchez RM, Jensen FE: Maturational aspects of epilepsy mechanisms and consequences for the immature brain. Epilepsia 2001;42:577-585.

106. Painter MJ, Pippenger C, Wasterlain C, et al: Phenobarbital and phenytoin in neonatal seizures: Metabolism and tissue distribution. Neurology 1981;31:1107-1112.

107. Painter MJ, Scher MS, Stein AD, et al: Phenobarbital compared with phenytoin for the treatment of neonatal seizures. N Engl J Med 1999;341:485-489.

108. Lockman LA, Kriel R, Zaske D, et al: Phenobarbital dosage for control of neonatal seizures. Neurology 1979;29:1445-1449.

109. Gal P, Toback J, Boer HJ, et al: Efficacy of phenobarbital monotherapy in treatment of neonatal seizures: Relationship to blood levels. Neurology 1982;32:101-140.

14

Drug Effects on the Human Electroencephalogram

EDWARD H. KOVNAR, GREGORY L. HOLMES, FAYE MC NALL,
AND JAMES J. RIVIELLO, JR.

Hans Berger (1873–1941), the father of electroencephalography, was the first to describe the effects of drugs on the electroencephalogram (EEG).[1,2] In a paper in 1931, Berger found that the amplitude of the alpha waves increased after the administration of cocaine, at a time when the pupils were dilated, pulse rate increased, and psychic processes enhanced.[2] Following an intramuscular injection of phenobarbital, he noted that "the alpha wave(s) showed an increased length, . . . became strikingly low in voltage . . . and tended to fuse with each other."[3] Berger also found that scopolamine increased the frequency of EEG beta activity during agitation or excitation, slowing of the alpha when the patient was drowsy, and desynchronization of the EEG following caffeine.[2]

Unfortunately, although Berger's theories regarding the relationship between EEG changes and behavior have been generally confirmed, EEG changes following drug administration vary considerably from patient to patient and have not been specific enough to allow prediction of drug effect in individual patients. Nevertheless, the effect of drugs on the EEG is an important concern in the day-to-day interpretation of records. A large percentage of children sent to the clinical neurophysiology laboratory will be taking medications, and it is important that the technician and physician performing and interpreting these studies be aware of the changes in the record that may be responsible for these changes.

EFFECT OF DRUGS ON THE EEG

Drug ingestion or overdosage must be considered in the evaluation of any child with unexplained coma or altered mental status. Equally important is the recognition that changes in the EEG may be induced by a variety of medications even when given at therapeutic and presumably nontoxic dosages.[4,5] Although changes in the EEG may represent incidental findings of no clinical significance, they may also herald idiosyncratic or unanticipated adverse effects of treatment. As with metabolic encephalopathies, no EEG finding or constellation of findings is pathognomonic for a specific class of drug. Furthermore, the type and degree of EEG abnormality in a particular patient may be profoundly influenced by chronicity of exposure, underlying neurologic disorder, effects of other medications, and coexisting metabolic abnormalities. Although drug-induced changes in the EEG are typically diffuse, patients with structural pathology may show either enhanced or suppressed drug-related changes on the side of the lesion.[6,7]

Several drugs have been associated with an increase in the frequency of epileptiform discharges (spikes, sharp waves, and spike-and-wave complexes). Such medications include phenothiazines, butyrophenones, tricyclic antidepressants, lithium, and carbamazepine. These drugs may not only produce activation of epileptiform discharges but also lower the seizure threshold in susceptible individuals.[8,9] Drug withdrawal, especially when abrupt, may result in epileptiform discharges as well as generalized tonic-clonic seizures. This is particularly prevalent following withdrawal of short-acting barbiturates after prolonged use even in individuals with no prior history of seizures.[10]

Antiepileptic Drugs

Intoxication with barbiturates and benzodiazepines provides a model for understanding the clinical and EEG manifestations of the more common sedative-hypnotic drugs. Effects of other centrally acting drugs are reviewed later.

Barbiturates such as phenobarbital and deoxybarbiturates such as primidone produce increased fast activity even at blood concentrations within the therapeutic range.[11,12] The magnitude of EEG abnormalities associated with acute sedative-hypnotic intoxication closely parallels the severity of impaired consciousness.[13,14] With low doses, the most characteristic change is that of increased fast activity within the beta frequency range of 13 Hz or greater (Fig. 14–1).

Brazier and Finesinger[15] administered amobarbital sodium, thiopental sodium, or pentobarbital sodium to adult patients. The initial effect was the appearance of high-voltage fast activity, occurring at a frequency of 21 to 32 Hz, with voltages between 25 and 100 μV. In patients that received larger doses, delta activity (3 to 4 Hz) developed. In all patients the high-voltage fast activity first appeared in the frontal leads, followed by the parietal, temporal, and finally occipital leads, and disappeared in the reverse order. The authors made the interesting observation that the beta activity occurred first in the areas that were of most recent ontogenetic and phylogenetic development.

Since beta activity is so common with barbiturates, the lack of beta may have prognostic significance. Niedermeyer and associates[16] reported that the absence of barbiturate-induced beta activity in patients with seizures on barbiturates was associated with severe cerebral impairment. Focal reduction of benzodiazepine-induced fast activity may occur in the presence of an underlying cerebral lesion such as tumor, infarction, or porencephalic cyst.

There may be an increase in epileptiform activity during the withdrawal of barbiturates.[17] Seizures may also occur with rapid withdrawal of the barbiturates, even in patients without a history of seizures.[18]

Benzodiazepines, like the barbiturates, markedly increase beta activity.[19] With high blood levels, slowing of background activity can also occur. More severe intoxication is associated with runs of high-amplitude, intermittent rhythmic delta activity superimposed on a background of nearly continuous slow activity of less than 4 Hz. Intermittent fast activity may persist over the frontocentral regions. Little reactivity is elicited by stimulation. When present, such reactivity may consist of a paradoxical increase in high-amplitude rhythmic delta. Triphasic waves similar to those seen in hepatic or renal encephalopathies may be observed. Profound sedative-hypnotic intoxication results in either a suppression-burst pattern or electrocerebral silence. Underlying focal pathology may result in a localized burst-suppression pattern.[7] Drug-induced coma with periods of electrocerebral silence lasting as long as 28 hours has been associated with complete neurologic recovery.[13]

Sudden withdrawal of benzodiazepines can lead to an increase in epileptiform activity and seizures.[10,20]

Other Antiepileptic Drugs

As a general rule, the antiepileptic drugs (AEDs) reduce epileptiform activity,[21,22] although on occasion they can exacerbate EEG abnormalities and seizures.[23,24] In patients with generalized spike-and-wave activity on the EEG, there is an inverse relation between AED levels of valproic acid,[25] ethosuximide,[26] and clonazepam[27] and the number of generalized spike-and-wave discharges. However, the relationship between quantity of focal epileptiform discharges and AEDs is less clear.[21,28–30] Despite adequately controlled seizures, epileptiform discharges frequently persist. This is particularly true in benign rolandic epilepsy (benign childhood epilepsy with centrotemporal spikes) and occipital lobe epilepsy.[11,31]

AEDs such as valproate, ethosuximide, clobazam levetiracetam, felbamate, and vigabatrin have been used to reduce epileptiform discharges in conditions such as Landau-Kleffner syndrome and electrical status epilepticus of sleep.[32–37]

Phenytoin and other hydantoin medications at usual therapeutic blood concentrations produce little or no change in the EEG. As phenytoin levels exceed the usual therapeutic range, the EEG may show slowing of the occipital alpha rhythm and decreased abundance of alpha activity.[38] In cases of clinically apparent phenytoin intoxication the EEG may show diffuse slow activity within the delta frequency range.[38]

Riehl and McIntyre[39] found that although intravenous administration of phenytoin to normal patients resulted in no change in the EEG, when the drug was administered to patients with epilepsy, a moderate degree of slowing and increase in amplitude of the EEG was seen 10 to 15 minutes after the injection. The authors postulated that the effect of diphenylhydantoin might be secondary to existing alterations in the blood-brain barrier or due to a preferential effect of the drug on abnormal neurons. There

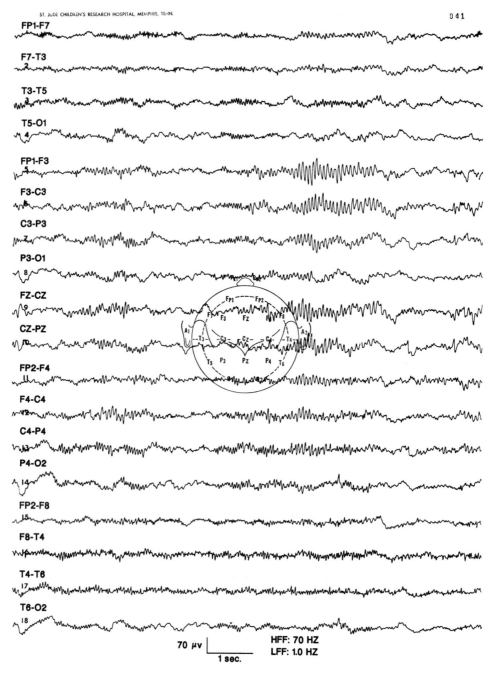

FIGURE 14–1

Frontal dominant 14-Hz fast activity in an 8-year-old boy treated 30 minutes prior to the present EEG recording with intravenous lorazepam GLH.

have been several reports of increased seizures with toxic levels of phenytoin.[40,41]

Carbamazepine, an anticonvulsant structurally related to the tricyclic antidepressants, may produce mild diffuse slowing at therapeutic levels. In susceptible individuals, carbamazepine administration may result in an increase in the number of spikes, sharp waves, and generalized spike-and-wave bursts.[42] Clinically, an increase in one or more seizure types has been observed in children with mixed seizure disorders treated with carbamazepine.[23] Bilaterally synchronous 2.5 to 3/sec spike-and-wave discharges were found to correlate with an increased frequency of atypical absence seizures; generalized bursts of 1 to 2/sec spikes and slow waves suggested an increased risk of generalized convulsive seizures.

Ethosuximide and other succinamides produce little if any changes in the EEG background except at toxic levels where mild slowing may be seen.

Valproic acid has not typically been associated with significant EEG changes when used within the therapeutic range. Bruni and colleagues[25] did not observe consistent changes in the EEG following valproate; nor have changes in the EEG frequency spectra been reported in children treated with valproic acid.[43] As with other AEDs, toxic levels of valproic acid may lead to slowing and decreased voltage of background activity. Pedersen and Juul-Jensen[44] described a series of EEGs from a patient who ingested 75 gm of valproate sodium. The first EEG at the time of a valproate sodium level of 1500 µg/mL (usual therapeutic range, 50 to 150 µg/mL) showed diffuse slowing. Eight hours later when the serum level was 1800 µg/mL, the record consisted of low-voltage delta activity. The following day the EEG was "almost without activity." Six days later, when the patient's clinical condition was normal, the EEG had returned to normal.

Although sedation may occur with the initiation of valproic acid, this effect usually subsides with continuation of therapy. Rare cases of stupor and coma have been reported with valproic acid levels within the accepted therapeutic range. Although hyperammonemia and comedication with other AEDs have been considered as possible causes of this unusual reaction, the mechanism of valproate-induced coma remains poorly understood.[45,46] Carnitine depletion or an inborn error of organic acid metabolism unmasked by valproic acid therapy may be responsible.[47,48] EEG findings observed in cases of valproate-induced coma include high-amplitude frontal delta and theta slowing. In contrast with cases of idiosyncratic fatal hepatic necrosis, the reversible form of valproate-induced coma is typically associated with hyperammonemia but otherwise normal measures of hepatic function.[49]

Felbamate, at therapeutic levels, does not typically alter EEG background activity. Sackellares and colleagues[50] performed automated analyses of generalized spike-wave discharges on patients before and during treatment. A spike-wave index was computed by summing the durations of all spike-wave complexes and dividing by the duration of the recording. Reduction of generalized spike-wave in the felbamate, but not placebo group, provided independent evidence of a statistically significant antiepileptic effect of felbamate in patients with Lennox-Gastaut syndrome.

Lamotrigine is one of the newer generation AEDs which has broad-spectrum efficacy against a variety of seizure types and epileptic syndromes. At therapeutic levels lamotrigine does not alter background rhythms. The drug has been shown to reduce epileptiform activity on the EEG of children.[51]

With *gabapentin*, in most patients there are no discernible changes in EEG background activity; however, quantitative analysis has demonstrated EEG slowing with chronic gabapentin use.[52]

Topiramate typically does not cause dramatic changes in the EEG. Quantitative analysis has shown increases in power in the beta and theta bands in both patients and normal volunteers.[53,54]

Tiagabine has little effect on EEG background activity.[55] There have been a number of reports associating tiagabine with the development of subclinical status epilepticus; however, this is still controversial.[56–59]

Zonisamide and *levetiracetam* have not been associated with any significant EEG changes.

Table 14–1 provides a summary of the major effects of AEDs on the EEG.

Psychotropic Medications

The phenothiazines, butyrophenones, tricyclic antidepressants, and lithium all may induce epileptiform dis-

TABLE 14–1
Effect of Antiepileptic Drugs on the EEG

Antiepileptic Drugs	Low Serum Levels	High Serum Levels
Benzodiazepines	Increased beta	Increased beta, reduction in alpha frequency, increased theta
Phenytoin	No changes	Reduction in alpha frequency, increased theta, increased delta
Carbamazepine	Usually no changes; may reduce alpha frequency and increase theta and delta activity	Reduction in alpha frequency, increased theta, increased delta
Barbiturates	Increased beta	Increased beta, reduction in alpha frequency, increased theta, increased delta
Valproate	Usually no changes; may be associated with increased theta activity	Reduction in alpha frequency, increased theta, increased delta
Ethosuximide	No changes	Reduction in alpha frequency, increased theta, increased delta

charges on the EEG, and in some patients seizures can be precipitated by these drugs. According to Itil and Soldatos[8] chlorpromazine and lithium markedly potentiate epileptiform discharges; thioxanthenes, butyrophenones, and amitriptyline are moderately potentiating; and imipramine, monoamine oxidase inhibitors, thioridazine, meprobamate, chlordiazepoxide, and methylphenidate have slight or no potentiating tendencies. In patients with a history of seizures, increased numbers of epileptiform discharges have been found following intravenous administration of imipramine and amitryptyline.[60] However, these drugs rarely cause seizures in patients without a history of seizures.

Epileptiform activity is more likely to be precipitated during the first weeks of treatment and during withdrawal[8,17] than thereafter and is more commonly observed in children than adults.[9] Logar and colleagues[17] evaluated the EEGs in 31 patients undergoing withdrawal from tranquilizers and found that 35% of the patients had generalized spike activity. In patients who combined tranquilizers with alcohol or barbiturates, a higher rate of abnormal EEGs during withdrawal was found.

Tricyclic Antidepressants

The EEG changes associated with nontoxic levels of heterocyclic antidepressants are minor.[14] Those antidepressants with minimal sedative effect (e.g., desipramine) are associated with increased alpha activity when administered at the usual therapeutic dosage. In contrast, tricyclics with significant sedative effect (e.g., amitriptyline and imipramine) are associated with decreased abundance of alpha rhythm and increased fast and slow activities.[9]

Patients with a history of seizures may show increased numbers of epileptiform discharges following administration of intravenous imipramine[60] and amitriptyline.[61] Due to the lower risk of precipitating seizure activity, desipramine is preferred in patients with known seizure disorders.[62] These drugs rarely cause seizures in children without a history of epilepsy.

Toxic levels of tricyclic antidepressants produce diffuse slowing with superimposed beta or irregular 9- to 10-Hz activity.[63] The alpha coma EEG pattern has also been observed with intoxication due to imipramine.[64]

Major Tranquilizers (Antipsychotic Agents)

Phenothiazines, butyrophenones, and related centrally active dopamine antagonists produce little or no change in the EEG when given at less than toxic doses. Low doses rarely may be associated with an increase in the amplitude and abundance of theta activity and a decrease in the frequency of the dominant alpha rhythm.[65] Other changes may include an increase in beta activity. Toxic levels produce increasing amounts of slow activity in the theta and delta range and a decrease in the amount of alpha rhythm.[14]

Phenothiazines and butyrophenones may induce epileptiform discharges and, in susceptible individuals, lower the threshold for seizures. Intoxication with chlorpromazine is associated with slowing of the background, bursts of bilaterally synchronous high-amplitude slowing, as well as spike and spike-wave complexes.[8,9] Although similar changes may be observed with haloperidol, the potential for producing epileptiform discharges is reported to be greater for phenothiazines such as chlorpromazine in contrast with butyrophenones such as haloperidol.

Central Nervous System Stimulants (Sympathomimetics)

Dextroamphetamine, methylphenidate, cocaine, and other centrally acting adrenergic agents increase the abundance of beta activity and alpha rhythm.[66] They may be associated with attenuation or suppression of delta activity. Xanthine derivatives, theophylline and aminophylline, are associated with a dose-related increase in multifocal spikes and the occurrence of repetitive and focal seizures at toxic levels (>20 μg/mL). Caffeine, although structurally and pharmacologically related to aminophylline, does not appear to cause either epileptiform discharges or seizure activity but may increase beta activity and decrease the voltage of the alpha rhythm.[9]

Lithium, when used in the management of manic-depressive affective disorder, produces significant EEG changes even at therapeutic serum concentrations.[67,68] These changes can include epileptiform discharges and alteration of the background rhythms.[68–70] The slow activity occurs either diffusely, focally, or in generalized bursts.[68,71,72] Small[70] observed that although EEG abnormalities tended to increase with higher plasma levels, no correlation was noted between EEG changes and plasma levels within the therapeutic range.

Struve[67] compared patients treated with lithium carbonate (either alone or in combination with other agents) with patients taking either no medication or other psychotropic medications. The author found EEG abnormalities consisting of generalized or paroxysmal delta activity in 30% to 39% of lithium-treated patients in contrast with only 2% to 5% of medication-free controls. The prevalence of abnormal EEGs was also significantly higher for lithium-treated patients than for patients treated with other psychotropic agents.

Intoxication with lithium may produce a reversible dementia with EEG changes including the presence of periodic complexes similar to those seen in Jakob-Creutzfeldt disease.[70,73,74]

EEG changes associated with lithium therapy occur in both children and adults. Bennett and colleagues[75] compared baseline EEGs with those repeated after treatment with haloperidol, lithium, or placebo in 48 children with aggressive behavior between the ages of 5 and 12 years. During the baseline placebo period 58% of the children had abnormal EEGs. Children receiving haloperidol or lithium at optimal doses were more likely to show paroxysmal or focal abnormalities than those children treated with placebo.

The combination of haloperidol and lithium has been associated with an increased neurotoxic interaction. This combination of treatment may result in photomyoclonic and photoparoxysmal responses.[76]

Table 14–2 lists the major effects of psychotropic medications on the EEG.

Street Drugs

Cannabis Derivatives

Tetrahydrocannabinol (THC) is the antiemetic and psychotomimetic agent in marijuana and hashish. Derived from the plants *Cannabis sativa* and *Cannabis indica*, it varies in potency from hashish (strongest) to marijuana (weakest). There are conflicting findings regarding EEG changes with marijuana.[73,77,78] Volavka and associates[79] reported that delta-9 tetrahydrocannabinol, the active component of marijuana, produced an increase in the amount of alpha activity and decrease in beta and theta activity, whereas other authors report minimal or no changes with inhalation of the street drug.[2,80–82]

Cocaine

Cocaine is one of 14 alkaloids found in the leaves of the *Erythroxylon coca* plant.[83] The most devastating form of the drug is *crack*, a mixture of cocaine, water, and baking soda that is heated to eliminate adulterants. Because of the widespread abuse of cocaine, the effect of the drug on central nervous system (CNS) physiology has been extensively evaluated.[84–91] Herning and coworkers[87] studied the effects of cocaine on the adult awake EEG. Fifty subjects were given one of three intravenous cocaine doses (0.2, 0.4, and 0.6 mg/kg) while 33 volunteers received one of three oral doses of cocaine (2, 3, and 4 mg/kg). The EEG was analyzed as with fast Fourier transformation for delta, theta, alpha, and beta power. At each dose, and for each route, cocaine increased the power of beta. The authors postulated that the increase in beta power was a consequence of a direct stimulation of the central noradrenergic arousal system. The amount of alpha activity has been reported to be increased over the occipital and parietal areas during the euphoric phase that occurs with cocaine.[84,89]

Herning and coworkers[86] also found that cocaine altered long latency evoked potentials. Administration of cocaine by either intravenous or oral routes reduced the amplitude of the P200 and P300 components of the auditory evoked potential during a task requiring attention to an oddball auditory stimulus. The P200 latency decreased and the N100 amplitude was reduced only after intravenous administration of cocaine.

Cocaine is also known to increase brain excitability and epileptiform activity on the EEG and can lead to seizures in both children and adults.[83,92–95] Bateman and Heagarty[96] described four pediatric patients who had passively inhaled the smoke of crack used by their "caretakers." Two of the children had seizures. Chronic administration of cocaine has been used to produce kindling.[88,97,98]

Phencyclidine

Phencyclidine (PCP) and its derivative, the anesthetic agent *ketamine*, produce EEG changes that include a periodic pattern consisting of bursts of generalized slow wave activity at intervals of approximately 4 seconds alternating

---

TABLE 14–2

Effects of Psychotropic Medications on the EEG

Drug	Nontoxic Levels	Toxic Levels
Tricyclic antidepressants: amitriptyline, desipramine, imipramine, nortriptyline, protriptyline	Increased theta and beta; sometimes decreased alpha frequency	Slowing with increased beta
Major tranquilizers: phenothiazines, butyrophenones, thioxanthenes, indoles	Few changes; increased theta, decreased alpha frequency, decreased beta; rarely paroxysmal patterns	Decreased alpha, increased theta and delta
CNS stimulants: methylphenidate, caffeine, nicotine	Mild increase in alpha frequency and increased amounts of beta	Slowing with theta and delta
Lithium	Mild reduction in alpha frequency and amount	Decreased alpha with increased delta and theta; sharp waves; rarely periodic complexes
Alcohol	Little or no change	Slowing with theta and delta

CNS, central nervous system.

TABLE 14–3
Effect of Street Drugs on the EEG

Drug	Nontoxic Levels	Toxic Levels
Lysergic acid diethylamide (LSD)	Little or no change; occasionally increased beta	Continuous rhythmic theta activity with periodic slow-wave complexes
Cocaine	Mild increase in alpha frequency and increased amounts of beta	Slowing with theta and delta
Marijuana	Little or no change	Slowing with theta and delta
Phencyclidine	Rhythmic theta and delta activity and increased voltage of beta activity	Slowing with theta and delta
Psilocybin	Increased voltage of beta activity	Slowing with theta and delta

with a background of sinusoidal 6-Hz theta similar to that seen in subacute sclerosing panencephalitis.[99]

Table 14–3 lists the major effects of street drugs on the EEG.

Chloral Hydrate

Chloral hydrate is often used to sedate children unable to cooperate during investigations such as EEG requiring the patient to be still. Thoresen and associates[100] performed recordings of the EEG before, during, and after rectal administration of chloral hydrate in 13 children aged 1.5 to 13.5 years with severe epilepsy and additional neurologic impairments. All children had frequent spike-wave activity before chloral hydrate. In 9 children chloral hydrate had no effect on the EEG. In 3 children there was a significant reduction in epileptic activity after 20 to 50 minutes and in 1 a significant increase. This study demonstrated that chloral hydrate can generally be used before an EEG recording without loss of information, but in some children there were changes that could alter interpretation.

Narcotics

Morphine, meperidine, codeine, and other opiate derivatives typically produce an initial slowing of the alpha rhythm. Return to near-normal frequencies appears to parallel clinical evidence of tolerance to analgesic effects. Intravenous administration of heroin is associated acutely with an increase in the alpha voltage and decrease in the frequency of the dominant alpha rhythm. Subsequent changes include decreased amounts of alpha activity and increased amounts of theta and delta that are reversed by intravenous naloxone.[79] Meperidine is associated with more prolonged alpha slowing that persists in spite of tolerance to analgesic effects for as long as meperidine or its metabolites remain detectable. Patients with impaired renal function may experience agitation, confusion, and seizures following large or repeated doses of meperidine owing to accumulation of normeperidine, a toxic metabolite of the parent drug.[101]

TABLE 14–4
Effect of Narcotics and Other Drugs on the EEG

Drug	Nontoxic Levels	Toxic Levels
Narcotics: morphine, heroin, methadone, codeine	Minimal changes; may cause slowing of the background	Slowing with theta and delta
Antihistamines: diphenhydramine	Minimal changes; may increase beta	Slowing with theta and delta
Chloral hydrate	Increased beta activity	Slowing with theta and delta

Antihistamines

Antihistamines such as diphenhydramine may increase beta activity at low doses and induce slowing in the theta and delta bandwidths at high doses.

Table 14–4 lists the effects of narcotics, antihistamines, and chloral hydrate on the EEG.

Alcohol

With low levels of ethanol, there is an increase in amount of alpha.[89] With higher levels of alcohol there is a mild shift to slower frequencies in the EEG.[102,103] Krauss and Niedermeyer[104] reported that 56% of 136 patients with chronic alcoholism and normal EEGs had voltages below 25 μVs compared with 13.9% of 1167 patients without a history of alcoholism ($P < 0.001$). However, as noted by the authors, a low-voltage EEG is not specific for alcoholism.

There is some controversy regarding the effects of alcohol withdrawal on the EEG.[10,17,105–107] Some authors have observed that during alcohol withdrawal in unmedicated patients, photic stimulation may produce a photomyogenic response, representing a nonspecific state of neuromuscular irritability.[107] Victor and Brausch[107] reported abnormal EEGs during photic stimulation, including photoparoxysmal responses, during the acute withdrawal phase. These responses developed within 24 hours after the last alcohol intake, peaked during the 2nd day, and disappeared after the 5th day following withdrawal. Hauser and associates[108] studied 117 patients with presumed alcohol withdrawal seizures. In contrast with Victor and Brausch,[107] Hauser and associates[108] demonstrated a photoparoxysmal pattern in only one patient. Vossler and Browne[109] recorded EEGs of 40 patients who had stopped drinking within the preceding 96 hours. They found no photomyoclonic or photoparoxysmal responses. However, since the patients were on benzodiazepines, the paroxysmal responses may have been suppressed. Fisch and colleagues[105] analyzed EEG findings in 49 patients with clinical withdrawal symptoms not treated with benzodiazepines. Two patients had a photomyoclonic response, but none showed photoparoxysmal responses. Spontaneous epileptiform discharges are usually absent in alcohol withdrawal.

General Anesthesia

Anesthetic agents, including ether, nitrous oxide, cyclopropane, pentothal, and enflurane, produce predictable EEG changes that depend on the depth of anesthesia.[110] During the initial stage of anesthesia, the alpha rhythm disappears while beta activity increases in voltage and becomes more widespread. With deepening anesthesia, beta is intermixed with slow activity within the theta and delta frequency range. This slowing increases in amplitude, shifting toward the lower frequency range until a burst-suppression pattern appears. At the deepest level of anesthesia, EEG activity becomes undetectable.

Following enflurane anesthesia, normal subjects will show persistent slowing of the alpha rhythm by 1 to 4 Hz for up to 6 days; intermittent rhythmic delta may persist for 6 to 30 days.[111] Enflurane may also induce epileptiform discharges including spikes and spike-and-slow wave complexes not only in patients with a known history of seizures but also in normal subjects undergoing elective surgery.[111–113]

Ito and colleagues[114] compared the effect of isoflurane and enflurane on the electrocorticogram of patients with intractable epilepsy undergoing temporal lobectomy. The mean frequency of epileptiform spikes decreased during use of isoflurane but not enflurane. When compared with nitrous oxide anesthesia, isoflurane decreased the mean number of electrodes exhibiting spike activity while enflurane increased the mean number of electrodes demonstrating epileptiform activity.

Both phenobarbital and pentobarbital[115] have been used to induce burst-suppression in patients with status epilepticus. As with the general anesthetics noted earlier, there is a progression in the EEG from slowing to complete electrical inactivity as the dosage of the barbiturates is increased.

Antineoplastic Agents

Effective chemotherapy requires a delicate balance between cytoxicity toward neoplastic cells and clinical toxicity. It is not surprising therefore that chemotherapeutic compounds can lead to alteration in cerebral electrical activity. CNS toxicity is limited for many systemically administered agents by restricted access across the blood-brain barrier. Toxic encephalopathies may occur, however, due to administration of chemotherapy in very high doses, by selective intra-arterial injection, or by modification of the blood-brain barrier with osmotic agents such as mannitol or prior cranial irradiation. Intrathecal injection of antineoplastic agents provides a means of delivering drug to sanctuary sites where leukemia cells may escape systemic chemotherapy. Fortunately, adverse effects of intrathecal therapy are not common. CNS toxicity may occur after repeated intrathecal doses or in individuals with abnormal cerebrospinal fluid resorption. Injection of antineoplastic agents through an Ommaya reservoir may, in rare instances, be complicated by extravasation into the surrounding brain parenchyma.

Methotrexate

High-dose intravenous methotrexate may result in an acute, reversible encephalopathy manifested by somnolence, confusion, headache, seizures, and transient focal neurologic deficits.[117–119] Proposed mechanisms include inhibition of cerebral glucose metabolism,[120] or altered concentrations of monoamine neurotransmitters through inhibition of tetrahydrobiopterin biosynthesis.[121,122] EEG changes observed with acute methotrexate-induced encephalopathy include generalized slow activity in the theta-to-delta frequency range as well as focal polymorphic delta activity (Fig. 14–2). Reversal of the encephalopathy by high-dose leucovorin is supported experimentally although not proved clinically.[123]

L-Asparaginase

L-Asparaginase is a hydrolytic enzyme that catalyzes the conversion of L-asparagine to aspartic acid and ammonia. The antineoplastic activity of this enzyme is mediated through depletion of the amount of L-asparagine available to certain tumors cells containing low concentrations of L-asparagine synthetase.[124] L-Asparaginase has been especially useful for the treatment of children with acute lymphoblastic leukemia.[125] A wide range of adverse effects related to inhibition of protein synthesis may occur as a result of treatment with this agent. These effects include coagulation disorders, liver dysfunction, hyperglycemia, and disturbance in level of consciousness. Mental status changes usually occur within 24 hours after administration of L-asparaginase.[126] Serial EEGs before and after

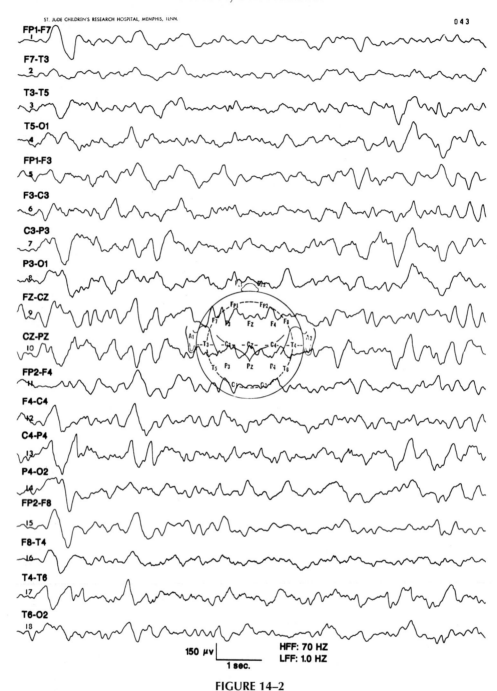

FIGURE 14–2

Diffuse polymorphic slow activity in an 8-year-old boy who received intrathecal methotrexate for treatment of occult central nervous system leukemia 1 week prior to this recording.

administration of L-asparaginase have shown nonspecific abnormalities including decreases in the frequency of the alpha rhythm and increases in the amount of theta and delta activity.[127] Liver dysfunction may result in EEG changes that are similar to those seen in early hepatic coma. These changes do not correlate well with ammonia levels.[128] Alterations of mental status are usually transient and not associated with focal or lateralized clinical or EEG abnormalities. An important exception is the occurrence of either intraparenchymal hemorrhage or cerebral venous thrombosis due to depletion of procoagulation or anti-coagulation factors.[129]

Ifosfamide

Ifosfamide is a structural analog of the alkylating agent cyclophosphamide that has found increasing use in the treatment of a variety of solid tumors of childhood, including osteosarcoma. Neurologic toxicity including transient cerebellar dysfunction, altered mental status, hallucinations, and seizures can occur with a frequency as high as 20% to 50%.[130] Accumulation of chloracetaldehyde, an oxidative metabolite of ifosfamide, may underlie these CNS effects. Serial EEGs in patients receiving ifosfamide show slowing of the alpha rhythm, followed by increase in slow activity within the delta frequency range as well as high-voltage rhythmic delta activity; epileptiform discharges occur rarely.

Immunomodulating Agents

Immunomodulators are a group of agents that include immunosuppressive drugs such as cyclosporine and a growing list of biologic response modifiers such as interferon. Evaluation of CNS toxicity associated with these agents is frequently confounded by the effects of underlying disease, prior therapy, infectious diseases, and intercurrent metabolic disturbances.

Cyclosporine

The introduction of cyclosporine, an antilymphocytic polypeptide, has substantially improved the success of bone marrow and organ transplantation in children as well as adults. Although renal toxicity is the most frequent and important adverse effect of cyclosporine, neurologic toxicity including complex visual hallucinations and seizures may occur.[131,132] The mechanism of such neurologic effects remains a subject of controversy. Concurrent hypomagnesemia and decreased serum cholesterol levels have been suggested as contributing factors.[133,134] EEG findings typically include diffuse slowing, although focal slowing and epileptiform discharges have also been described (Fig. 14–3).[135]

Interferons

The interferons comprise a family of glycoproteins known to possess a broad range of biologic activities that includes modulation of immune responses as well as inhibition of DNA synthesis and cellular replication. Interferons have found use in the treatment of certain viral illness, graft-versus-host disease, and specific neoplastic diseases. Alpha interferon has been shown to have clinical efficacy in the treatment of hairy cell leukemia, chronic myelogenous leukemia, and Kaposi's sarcoma. Adverse effects of this agent commonly include fever, headache, and myalgias. CNS effects include altered mental status, impaired memory, confusion, somnolence, and ataxia that may occur within 2 weeks of initiation of therapy.[136] EEG changes associated with interferon encephalopathy include slowing of the dominant alpha rhythm; diffuse arrhythmic delta activity; and frontally dominant, intermittent rhythmic delta activity.[137]

USE OF MEDICATIONS TO LOCALIZE ABNORMALITIES

Classes of Agents

Barbiturates

Asymmetries of beta activity may have lateralizing or localizing value.[138] Pampiglione[6] administered either secobarbital sodium (Seconal Sodium) orally or amobarbital sodium intravenously to 40 patients with a variety of cerebral lesions. Beta activity, between 18 and 26 Hz, appeared first in the frontal regions, then in the parietal, temporal, and eventually in the occipital regions, and disappeared in the inverse order. The author found decreased beta on the side of the lesion in patients with cerebral lesions.[6]

Methohexital (Brevital Sodium) has been used as an activator of focal and generalized seizures.[139] Wyler and associates[140] used methohexital as an activating agent in 62 patients undergoing focal cortical resections of epileptogenic foci and in 6 patients undergoing chronic EEG and video monitoring with intracranial strip electrodes. In 87% of the patients, methohexital caused selective activation of the epileptogenic focus during acute electrocorticography. The authors did not find activation of epileptiform activity outside the epileptogenic zone. In a study of 50 patients, Musella and colleagues[139] found that intravenous methohexital resulted in activation of temporal lobe spikes in 18 (72%) of 25 patients with complex partial seizures, whereas in control patients methohexital did not produce any epileptiform activity.

Some epilepsy centers have used intracarotid *amobarbital* to localize EEG abnormalities. Amobarbital typically has been used in patients with generalized spike-and-wave activity in which the investigator wishes to determine if there is a focal onset. In theory, if amobarbital is perfused through the hemisphere in which the spike-and-wave originates, it would be expected that the discharges will cease. Conversely, if amobarbital is injected into the internal carotid that perfuses the side opposite of the primary focus, the spike-and-wave activity will continue contralateral to the side of the injection and be reduced or eliminated on the side of injection. If injections of amobarbital into the left and right carotids result in similar findings, bilateral synchrony is suggested.[138]

Benzodiazepines

Brazier and colleagues[15] administered diazepam to 13 patients with intractable seizures in whom unequivocal

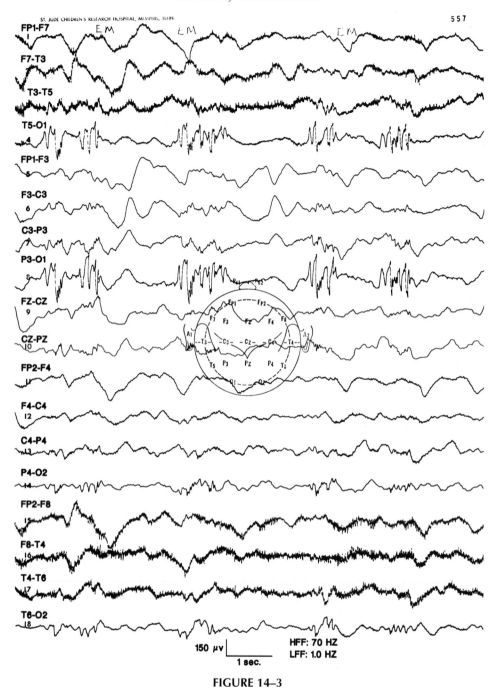

FIGURE 14–3

Diffuse, irregular slowing and bursts of repetitive polyspike activity arising focally from the left occipital derivations in an 8-year-old boy being treated with cyclosporine for graft-versus-host disease following an unrelated donor bone marrow transplantation.

lateralizing signs were not demonstrable. The authors found that in areas of abnormal cortex, diazepam did not result in as much beta activity as normal cortex. Niedermeyer[141] demonstrated that diazepam is more effective in eliminating generalized discharges than focal discharges.

Pentylenetetrazol (PTZ), an activator of epileptiform activity, has been used to localize a seizure focus.[142] Injections of a series of small doses of PTZ through the internal carotid artery on the side of the focus would be expected to elicit epileptiform activity and seizures at lower doses than on the contralateral side. Unfortunately, because of cross-flow across carotid circulations, both hemispheres may be affected by the injections. Since many patients have equivocal or nonreproducible responses, such tests are now infrequently used. Long-term monitoring using either conventional electroencephalography or invasive monitoring (subdural or depth electrodes) has generally replaced this test for localization purposes.

Phenothiazines

The phenothiazines have been used to activate epileptiform activity in some patients with suspected epilepsy.[9] Unfortunately, phenothiazines may activate abnormalities in patients without a previous history of seizures as well. Because of this, the drug is rarely used to activate seizures in patients.

EEG Changes in Acute Drug Poisoning

A number of drugs, when in the toxic range, can produce severe EEG suppression, even to the point of electrocerebral inactivity.[13,143] Haider and coworkers[13] performed continuous EEG monitoring in 127 cases of acute drug poisoning. The drugs included the barbiturates, benzodiazepines, and tricyclic antidepressants as well as an assortment of others. The EEGs were classified as in Table 14–5. As can be seen, the authors found a significant correlation between the EEG grade of coma and the clinical assessment.

Alpha coma, which consists of the presence of a predominate alpha frequency rhythm on the EEG of a clinically comatose patient, can be seen following drug ingestion.[144] Guterman and colleagues[144] reported a patient who had alpha coma following ingestion of a large amount of lorazepam. Despite the presence of an EEG demonstrating nonreactive 9- to 10-Hz alpha frequency over the entire head, the patient fully recovered. The authors emphasize that drug-induced alpha coma has a far better prognosis than alpha coma following anoxic insults or brainstem infarction.

Effect of Drugs on the Neonatal EEG

Although studies on the effects of drugs on the neonatal EEG are few, most authors agree that certain drugs, especially if in the toxic range, can alter background activity.[145,146] The acute administration of AEDs has also been noted to depress cerebral electrical activity. Unfortunately, AEDs, particularly barbiturates, are often administered to infants with seizures prior to their first EEG, raising the question of the prognostic value of the recording. To study this problem, Staudt and coworkers[147] reviewed EEG records from a total of 26 neonates who had an EEG while on phenobarbital treatment. In 5 infants an EEG was available prior to treatment with barbiturates. In 1 infant mild background suppression improved to normal in spite of a high barbiturate level. In the second infant viral encephalitis was thought to be responsible for changing the EEG from excessive slowing and frequent central sharp waves to moderate suppression with multifocal spike activity. In 2 infants no change in background activity occurred, even though barbiturates reduced the number of interictal discharges. In the final infant the EEG improved from a mild suppression with focal seizures to normal. The authors also compared EEG background activity with phenobarbital blood levels. The phenobarbital plasma levels in the group with severe or moderate suppression, mild suppression, and normal background activity were not statistically different. The authors concluded that with

TABLE 14–5
Alteration of EEG Background and Level of Consciousness with Toxic Levels of Drugs

Grade	Description	No. of Patients	Clinical Condition
I	Alpha rhythm or predominant alpha rhythm with beta or some rare theta waves	20	Conscious or drowsy
II	Predominantly theta rhythm with some alpha, beta, or low-voltage delta activity	17	Conscious or drowsy
III	Predominantly low- or high-voltage delta rhythm mixed with some theta waves	24	Unconscious, responded to painful stimulation
IV	Delta waves with or without brief isoelectrical intervals	19	Unconscious, responded to painful stimulation
V	Suppression-burst activity	19	Deep coma
VI	Near silence but with isolated and low-voltage, 3–7 Hz occurring singly or in bursts of 0.5-second duration	12	Deep coma
VII	An isoelectrical record, totally unresponsive to all stimuli	10	Deep coma

From Haider I, Matthew H, Oswald I: Electroencephalographic changes in acute drug poisoning. Electroencephalogr Clin Neurophysiol 1971;30:23–31.

phenobarbital plasma levels of 1.3 to 5.9 mg/dL, background suppression does not occur. Supporting this observation, Benda and colleagues,[148] in a study of 46 premature infants, reported that mean phenobarbital levels at the time of the EEG failed to show a significant relationship with the duration of the inactive phase of discontinuous sleep.

However, Ashwal and Schneider[149] reported that phenobarbital levels greater than 25 μg/mL may suppress EEG activity in sick or young neonates. These authors found a discordance between EEG activity and radionucleotide uptake in infants with levels between 25–35 μg/mL. The lack of EEG activity with the presence of cerebral blood flow suggested that the phenobarbital suppressed EEG activity. One infant who met the clinical criteria for brain death had absent cerebral activity with a level of 30 μg/mL but had some cerebral electrical activity when the level fell to zero. Pezzani and coworkers[150] reported two patients with high AED levels that likely resulted in severely abnormal EEGs. In the first child an isoelectrical record was obtained from a 1-day-old infant whose mother was taking 35 mg/day of diazepam. Four hours after the first recording, the record was only moderately abnormal. In the other infant with a permanently discontinuous record, a high level of phenobarbital (serum level 68 μg/mL) was found. A repeat study, on day 2 of life, demonstrated a moderately abnormal EEG despite the same blood level. The outcome in this child was favorable.

The question of how much AEDs alters the neonatal EEG remains open to question and needs further study. It is wise therefore to be cautious in making prognostic statements about infants with high levels of AEDs or infants that have been acutely loaded with AEDs.

Medications other than AEDs may also alter the neonatal EEG. We have made unpublished observations that opiates may depress background activity, increase the amount of discontinuity, and alter sleep cycles. In addition, drugs consumed during pregnancy may alter the neonatal EEG. An excess of spikes and sharp waves were seen in 17 (45%) of 38 neonates born to mothers abusing cocaine during pregnancy.[151] The abnormalities were multifocal in 14 of 17 of the tracings. On follow-up, 9 of 17 abnormal EEGs remained abnormal during the 2nd week of life; however, by 3 to 12 months of age, 9 of 10 previously abnormal tracings were normal. None of the infants had clinical seizures.

Alcohol consumption during the first trimester of pregnancy has been associated with disturbances in sleep and arousal, whereas marijuana affected sleep and motility regardless of trimester used.[152] Ioffe and Chernick[153] reported that newborn infants of mothers who abused alcohol during pregnancy had hypersynchronous EEGs with total power of spectral analysis higher in quiet,

indeterminate, and rapid eye movement sleep than in control infants. The authors found that the power of the EEG, using linear regression analysis, was significantly higher among infants of mothers who were binge drinkers than in those of mothers who were alcoholics. It was concluded that acute exposure to high quantities of alcohol were even more harmful to the fetal brain than continuous chronic exposure.[153]

Infants born to drug-dependent mothers are at risk for behavioral and developmental abnormalities.[154,155] Van Baar and colleagues[154,155] compared neurobehavioral development and EEGs in 35 infants of drug-dependent mothers with 37 control infants. The drug-dependent mothers had abused a variety of drugs including methadone, heroin, cocaine, tranquilizers, and amphetamines, typically in combination. EEGs and behavioral rating skills were abnormal more frequently in the first month of life in the infants of the drug-abusing mothers. However, by one year of age there were no differences between the two groups.

REFERENCES

1. Gibbs GA: Hans Berger (1873-1941). *In* Haymaker W, Schiller F (eds): The Founders of Neurology. Springfield, IL, Charles C Thomas, 1970, p 171.
2. Fink M: Pharmacoelectroencephalography: A note on its history. Neuropsychobiology 1984;12:173-178.
3. Gloor P: Hans Berger on the electroencephalogram of man: The fourteen original reports on the human electroencephalogram. Electroencephalogr Clin Neurophysiol 1969;28(Suppl):1-350.
4. Holmes GL, Korteling F: Drug effects on the human EEG. Am J EEG Technol 1993;33:1-26.
5. Bear MF, Kirkwood A: Neocortical long-term potentiation. Curr Opin Neurobiol 1993;3:197-202.
6. Pampiglione G: Induced fast activity in the EEG as an aid in the location of cerebral lesions. Electroencephalogr Clin Neurophysiol 1952;4:79-82.
7. Sperling MR, Brown WJ, Crandal PH: Focal burst suppression induced by thiopental. Electroencephalogr Clin Neurophysiol 1986;63:203-208.
8. Itil TM, Soldatos C: Epileptogenic side effects of psychotropic drugs: Practical recommendations. JAMA 1980;244:1460-1463.
9. Itil TM: Psychotropic drugs and the human EEG. *In* Niedermeyer E, Lopes da Silva F (eds): Electroencephalography: Basic Principles, Clinical Applications, and Related Fields. Baltimore, Urban & Schwarzenberg, 1982, p 499.
10. Wickler A, Pescor FT, Fraser HF, Isbell H: Electroencephalographic changes associated with intoxication and withdrawal in alcoholism. Am J Psychiatry 1956;113:106-114.

11. Ambrosetto G, Giovanardi Rossi P, Tassinari CA: Predictive factors of seizure frequency and duration of antiepileptic treatment in rolandic epilepsy: A retrospective study. Brain Dev 1987;9:300-304.

12. Brillman J, Gallagher BB, Mattson RH: Acute primidone intoxication. Arch Neurol 1974;30:255-258.

13. Haider I, Matthew H, Oswald I: Electroencephalographic changes in acute drug poisoning. Electroencephalogr Clin Neurophysiol 1971;30:23-31.

14. Kurtz D: The EEG in acute and chronic drug intoxications. *In* Glaser GH, Rémond A (eds): Handbook of Electroencephalography and Clinical Neurophysiology, Vol 15-C. Amsterdam, Elsevier, 1976, p 88.

15. Brazier MAB, Finesinger JE: Action of barbiturates on the cerebral cortex: Electroencephalographic studies. Arch Neurol Psychiatry 1945;53:51-58.

16. Niedermeyer E, Yarworth S, Zobniw AM: Absence of drug-induced beta activity in the electroencephalogram. Eur Neurol 1977;15:77-84.

17. Logar C, Grabmair W, Reinbacher N, Ladurner G: EEG changes in the withdrawal phase of tranquilizer or drug abuse. EEG-EMG Z Elektroenzephalogr Elektromyogr Verwandte Geb 1986;16:37-40.

18. Wikler A, Essig CF: Withdrawal seizures following chronic intoxication with barbiturates and other sedative drugs. Mod Probl Pharmacopsychiatry 1970;4:170-184.

19. Brazier MAB, Crandall PH, Walsh GO: Enhancement of EEG lateralizing signs in temporal lobe epilepsy: A trial of diazepam. Exp Neurol 1976;51:241-258.

20. Specht U, Boenigk HE, Wolf P: Discontinuation of clonazepam after long-term treatment. Epilepsia 1989;30:458-463.

21. Libenson MH, Caravale B: Do antiepileptic drugs differ in suppressing interictal epileptiform activity in children? Pediatr Neurol 2001;24:214-218.

22. Milligan N, Richens A: Methods of assessment of antiepileptic drugs. Br J Clin Pharmacol 1981;11:443-456.

23. Snead OC, Hosey LC: Exacerbation of seizures in children by carbamazepine. N Engl J Med 1985;313:916-921.

24. Shields WD, Saslow E: Myoclonic, atonic, and absence seizures following institution of carbamazepine therapy in children. Neurology 1983;33:1487-1489.

25. Bruni J, Wilder BJ, Bauman AW, Willmore LJ: Clinical efficacy and long-term effects of valproic acid therapy on spike-and-wave discharges. Neurology 1980;30:42-46.

26. Panayiotopoulos CP: Treatment of typical absence seizures and related epileptic syndromes. Paediatr Drugs 2001;3:379-403.

27. Browne TR: Clonazepam—a review of a new anticonvulsant drug. Arch Neurol 1976;33:326-332.

28. Bielmann P, Levac T, Gagnon MA: Clonazepam: Its efficacy in association with phenytoin and phenobarbital in mental patients with generalized major motor seizures. Int J Clin Pharmacol 1978;16:268-273.

29. Cereghino JJ, Brock JT, Van Meter JC, et al: Carbamazepine for epilepsy: A controlled prospective evaluation. Neurology 1974;24:401-410.

30. Duncan JS: Antiepileptic drugs and the electroencephalogram. Epilepsia 1987;28:259-266.

31. Loiseau P, Strube E, Brousset D, et al: Learning impairment in epileptic patients. Epilepsia 1983;24:183-192.

32. Marescaux C, Hirsch E, Finck S, et al: Landau-Kleffner syndrome: A pharmacologic study of five cases. Epilepsia 1990;318:768-777.

33. Appleton R, Hughes A, Beirae M, Acomb B: Vigabatrin in the Landau-Kleffner syndrome. Dev Med Child Neurol 1993;35:457-458.

34. Glauser TA, Olberding LS, Titanic MK, Piccirillo DM: Felbamate in the treatment of acquired epileptic aphasia. Epilepsy Res 1995;20:85-89.

35. Rintahaka PJ, Chugani HT, Sankar R: Landau-Kleffner syndrome with continuous spikes and waves during slow-wave sleep. J Child Neurol 1995;10:127-133.

36. Deuel RK, Lenn NJ: Treatment of acquired epileptic aphasia. J Pediatr 1977;90:959-961.

37. Holmes GL, Riviello JJ: Treatment of childhood idiopathic language deterioration with valproate. Epilepsy Behav 2001;2:272-276.

38. Roseman E: Dilantin toxicity: A clinical and electroencephalographic study. Neurology 1961;11:912-921.

39. Riehl J-L, McIntyre HB: A quantitative study of the acute effects of diphenylhydantoin on the electroencephalogram of epileptic patients. Neurology 1968;18:1107-1112.

40. Levy LL, Fenichel GM: Diphenylhydantoin-activated seizures. Neurology 1965;15:716-722.

41. Troupin AS, Ojemann LM: Paradoxical intoxication—a complication of anticonvulsant administration. Epilepsia 1975;16:753-758.

42. Sachdeo R, Chokroverty S: Increasing epileptiform activities in the EEG in presence of decreasing clinical seizures after carbamazepine. Epilepsia 1985;26:522.

43. Benninger C, Matthis P, Scheffner D: Spectral analysis of the EEG in children during the introduction of antiepileptic therapy with valproic acid. Neuropsychobiology 1985;13:93-96.

44. Pedersen B, Juul-Jensen P: Electroencephalographic alterations during intoxication with sodium valproate: A case report. Epilepsia 1984;25:121-124.

45. Sackellares JC, Lee SI, Dreifuss FE: Stupor following administration of valproic acid to patients receiving other antiepileptic drugs. Epilepsia 1979;20:697-703.

46. Batshaw ML, Brusilow SW: Valproate-induced hyperammonemia. Ann Neurol 1982;11:319-321.

47. Ohtani Y, Endo F, Matsuda J: Carnitine deficiency and hyperammonemia associated with valproic acid therapy. J Pediatr 1982;101:782-785.

48. Triggs WJ, Bohan TP, Lin S-N, Willmore LJ: Valproate-induced coma with ketosis and carnitine deficiency. Arch Neurol 1990;47:1131-1133.

49. Coulter DL, Allen RJ: Hyperammonemia with valproic acid therapy. J Pediatr 1981;99:317-319.

50. Sackellares JC, Burdette DE, Cunsheng Z, Olson LD: Electroencephalographic measures of antiepileptic drug

effects in the Lennox-Gastaut syndrome. Epilepsia (in press).

51. Akman CI, Holmes GL: The effect of lamotrigine on the EEGs of children and adolescents with epilepsy. Epilepsy Behav 2003;4:420-423.

52. Salinsky MC, Binder LM, Oken BS, et al: Effects of gabapentin and carbamazepine on the EEG and cognition in healthy volunteers. Epilepsia 2002;43:482-490.

53. Wang WW, Li JC, Wu X: Quantitative EEG effects of topiramate. Clin Electroencephalogr 2003;34:87-92.

54. Neufeld MY, Kogan E, Chistik V, Korczyn AD: Comparison of the effects of vigabatrin, lamotrigine, and topiramate on quantitative EEGs in patients with epilepsy. Clin Neuropharmacol 1999;22:80-86.

55. Kalviainen R, Aikia M, Mervaala E, et al: Long-term cognitive and EEG effects of tiagabine in drug-resistant partial epilepsy. Epilepsy Res 1996;25:291-297.

56. de Borchgrave V, Lienard F, Willemart T, van Rijckevorsel K: Clinical and EEG findings in six patients with altered mental status receiving tiagabine therapy. Epilepsy Behav 2003;4:326-337.

57. Imperiale D, Pignatta P, Cerrato P, et al: Nonconvulsive status epilepticus due to a de novo contralateral focus during tiagabine adjunctive therapy. Seizure 2003;12:319-322.

58. Shinnar S, Berg AT, Treiman DM, et al: Status epilepticus and tiagabine therapy: Review of safety data and epidemiologic comparisons. Epilepsia 2001;42:372-379.

59. Fitzek S, Hegemann S, Sauner D, et al: Drug-induced nonconvulsive status epilepticus with low dose of tiagabine. Epilept Disord 2001;3:147-150.

60. Kiloh LG, Davison K, Osselton JW: An electroencephalographic study of the analeptic effects of imipramine. Electroencephalogr Clin Neurophysiol 1961;13:216-223.

61. Davison K: EEG activation after intravenous amitriptyline. Electroencephalogr Clin Neurophysiol 1965;19:298-300.

62. Richardson JW, Richelson E: Antidepressants: Clinical update for medical practitioners. Mayo Clin Proc 1984;59:330-337.

63. Conners CK: The acute effects of caffeine on evoked response, vigilance, and activity level in hyperkinetic children. J Abnorm Child Psychol 1979;7:145-151.

64. Pulst S-M, Lombroso CT: External ophthalmoplegia, alpha, and spindle coma in imipramine overdose: Case report and review of the literature. Ann Neurol 1983;14:587-590.

65. Florio V, Longo VG, Verdeaux G: EEG effects of antipsychotics, tranquilizers, and antidepressants. *In* Longo VG (ed): Handbook of Electroencephalography and Clinical Neurophysiology, Vol 7-C. Amsterdam, Elsevier, 1977, p 40.

66. Fink M: EEG classification of psychoactive compounds in man: A review and theory of behavioral association. *In* Effran DH (ed): Psychopharmacology: A Review of Progress (Publication No. 1836). Washington, DC, U.S. Public Health Service, 1968, p 497.

67. Struve FA: Lithium-specific pathological electroencephalographic changes: A successful replication of earlier investigative results. Clin Electroencephalogr 1987;18:46-53.

68. Helmchen H, Kanowski S: EEG changes under lithium (Li) treatment. Electroencephalogr Clin Neurophysiol 1971;30:269.

69. Schou M, Amdisen A, Trap-Jense J: Lithium poisoning. Am J Psychiatry 1968;125:520-527.

70. Small JG: EEG and lithium CNS toxicity. Am J EEG Technol 1986;26:225-239.

71. Johnson G: Lithium and the EEG: An analysis of behavioral, biochemical, and electrographic changes. Electroencephalogr Clin Neurophysiol 1969;27:656-657.

72. Platman SR, Fieve RR: The effect of lithium carbonate on the electroencephalogram of patients with affective disorders. Br J Psychiatry 1969;115:1185.

73. Glaze DG: Drug effects. *In* Daly DD, Pedley TA (eds): Current Practice of Clinical Electroencephalography, 2nd ed. New York, Raven Press, 1990, p 489.

74. Smith SJM, Kocen RS: A Creutzfeldt-Jakob-like syndrome due to lithium toxicity. J Neurol Neurosurg Psychiatry 1988;51:120-123.

75. Bennett WG, Korein J, Kalmijn M, et al: Electroencephalogram and treatment of hospitalized aggressive children with haloperidol or lithium. Biol Psychiatry 1983;18:1427-1440.

76. Addy RO, Foliart RH, Saran AS, Schubert DS: EEG observations during combined haloperidol-lithium treatment. Biol Psychiatry 1986;21:170-176.

77. Verdeaux G, Longo VG: EEG effects of hallucinogenic drugs. *In* Longo VG (ed): Handbook of Electroencephalography and Clinical Neurophysiology, Vol 7-C. Amsterdam, Elsevier, 1977, p 57.

78. Volavka J, Dornbusch R, Feldstein S, Fink M: Effects of delta-9 tetrahydrocannabinol on EEG, heart rate, and mood. Electroencephalogr Clin Neurophysiol 1972;33:453.

79. Volavka J, Zaks A, Roubicek J, Fink M: Acute EEG effects of heroin and naloxone. Electroencephalogr Clin Neurophysiol 1971;30:165.

80. Deliyannaki SE, Panagopoulos C, Huott AD: The influence of hashish on human EEG. Clin Electroencephalogr 1970;1:128-140.

81. Fink M: EEG profiles and bioavailability measures of psychoactive drugs. Mod Probl Pharmacopsychiatry 1974;8:76-98.

82. Rodin EA, Domino EF: Effects of acute marijuana smoking on the EEG. Electroencephalogr Clin Neurophysiol 1970;29:321.

83. Conway EE Jr, Mezey AP, Powers K: Status epilepticus following the oral ingestion of cocaine in an infant. Pediatr Emerg Care 1990;6:189-190.

84. Alper KR, Chabot RJ, Kim AH, et al: Quantitative EEG correlates of crack cocaine dependence. Psychiatr Res 1990;35:95-105.

85. Castellani S, Ellinwood EH Jr, Kilbey NM, Petrie WM: Cholinergic effects on arousal and cocaine-induced

olfactory-amygdala spindling and seizures in cats. Physiol Behav 1983;31:461-466.

86. Herning RI, Hooker WD, Jones RT: Cocaine effects on electroencephalographic cognitive event-related potentials and performance. Electroencephalogr Clin Neurophysiol 1987;66:34-42.

87. Herning RI, Jones RT, Hooker WD, et al: Cocaine increases EEG beta: A replication and extension of Hans Berger's historic experiments. Electroencephalogr Clin Neurophysiol 1985;60:470-477.

88. Livezey GT, Sparber SB: Hyperthermia sensitizes rats to cocaine's proconvulsive effects and unmasks EEG evidence of kindling after chronic cocaine. Pharmacol Biochem Behav 1990;47:761-767.

89. Lukas SE, Mendelson JH, Amass L, Benedikt R: Behavioral and EEG studies of acute cocaine administration: Comparisons with morphine, amphetamine, pentobarbital, nicotine, ethanol, and marijuana. NIDA Res Monogr 1989;95:146-151.

90. O'Connor S, Kuwada S, DePalma N, et al: Amplitude-modulated frequency response during acute cocaine intoxication in rabbits. NIDA Res Monogr 1989;95:331-332.

91. Pickworth WB, Brown BS, Hickey JE, Muntaner C: Effects of self-reported drug use and antisocial behavior on evoked potentials in adolescents. Drug Alcohol Depend 1990;25:105-110.

92. Kramer LD, Locke GE, Ogunyemi A, Nelson L: Cocaine-related seizures in adults. Am J Drug Alcohol Abuse 1990;16:304-317.

93. Kramer LD, Locke GE, Ogunyemi A, Nelson L: Neonatal cocaine-related seizures. J Child Neurol 1990;5:60-64.

94. Merriam AE, Medalia A, Levine B: Partial complex status epilepticus associated with cocaine abuse. Biol Psychiatry 1988;23:515-518.

95. Pascual-Leone A, Dhuna A, Altafullah I, Anderson DC: Cocaine-induced seizures. Neurology 1990;40:404-407.

96. Bateman DA, Heagarty MC: Passive freebase cocaine (crack) inhalation by infants and toddlers. Am J Dis Child 1989;143:25-27.

97. Kilbey MM, Ellinwood EH, Easler ME: The effects of chronic cocaine pretreatment on kindled seizures and behavioral stereotypes. Exp Neurol 1979;64:306-314.

98. Post RM: Progressive changes in behavior and seizures following chronic cocaine administration: Relationship to kindling and psychosis. Adv Behav Biol 1977;21:353-373.

99. Stockard JJ, Werner SS, Aalbers JA, Chiappa KH: Electroencephalographic findings in phencyclidine intoxication. Arch Neurol 1976;33:200-203.

100. Thoresen M, Henriksen O, Wannag E, Laegreid L: Does a sedative dose of chloral hydrate modify the EEG of children with epilepsy? Electroencephalogr Clin Neurophysiol 1997;102:152-157.

101. Szeto HH, Inturrisi CE, Houde R, et al: Accumulation of normeperidine, an active metabolite of meperidine, in patients with renal failure or cancer. Ann Intern Med 1977;86:738-741.

102. Bergleiter H, Platz A: The effects of alcohol on the central nervous system in humans. *In* Kissin B, Begleiter H (eds): The Biology of Alcoholism, Vol 2. New York, Plenum Press, 1972, p 293.

103. Ehlers CL, Wall TL, Schuckit MA: EEG spectral characteristics following ethanol administration in young men. Electroencephalogr Clin Neurophysiol 1989;73:179-187.

104. Krauss GL, Niedermeyer E: Electroencephalogram and seizures in chronic alcoholism. Electroencephalogr Clin Neurophysiol 1991;78:97-104.

105. Fisch BJ, Hauser WA, Brust JCM, et al: The EEG response to diffuse and pattered photic stimulation during acute untreated alcohol withdrawal. Neurology 1989;39:434-436.

106. Reilly EL, Glass G, Faillace LA: EEGs in an alcohol detoxification and treatment center. Clin Electroencephalogr 1979;10:69-71.

107. Victor M, Brausch C: The role of abstinence in the genesis of alcoholic epilepsy. Epilepsia 1967;8:1-20.

108. Hauser WA, Rich S, Nicolosi A, Anderson VE: Electroencephalographic findings in patients with ethanol withdrawal seizures. Electroencephalogr Clin Neurophysiol 1982;52:64.

109. Vossler DG, Browne TR: Absence of EEG photoparoxysmal responses in alcohol withdrawal seizure patients treated with benzodiazepines. Neurology 1988;38(Suppl 1):404.

110. Clark DL, Rosner BS: Neurophysiologic effects of general anesthetics: I. The electroencephalogram and somatosensory evoked responses in man. Anesthesiology 1973;38:564-582.

111. Burchiel KJ, Stockard JJ, Calverley RK, Smith NT: Relationship of pre- and post-anesthetic abnormalities of enflurane-induced seizure activity. Anesth Analg 1977;56:509-514.

112. Flemming DC, Fitzpatrick J, Fariello RG, et al: Diagnostic activation of epileptogenic foci by enflurane. Anesthesiology 1980;52:431-433.

113. Neigh JL, Garman JK, Harp JR: The electroencephalographic pattern during anesthesia with ethrane. Anesthesiology 1971;35:482-487.

114. Ito BM, Sato S, Kufta CV, Tran D: Effect of isoflurane and enflurane on the electrocorticogram of epileptic patients. Neurology 1988;38:924-928.

115. Osorio I, Reed RC: Treatment of refractory generalized tonic-clonic status epilepticus with pentobarbital anesthesia after high-dose phenytoin. Epilepsia 1989;30:464-471.

116. Bleyer WA: Neurologic sequelae of methotrexate and ionizing radiation: A new classification. Cancer Treat Rep 1981;65(Suppl 1):89-98.

117. Jaffe N, Takaue Y, Anzai T, Robertson R: Transient neurologic disturbances induced by high-dose methotrexate treatment. Cancer 1985;56:1356-1360.

118. Packer RJ, Grossman RI, Belasco JB: High-dose systemic methotrexate-associated acute neurologic dysfunction. Med Pediatr Oncol 1983;11:159-161.

119. Phillips PC, Dhawan V, Strother SC, et al: Reduced cerebral glucose metabolism and increased brain capillary permeability following high-dose methotrexate chemotherapy: A positron emission tomographic study. Ann Neurol 1987;21:59-63.

120. Abelson HT: Methotrexate and central nervous system toxicity. Cancer Treat Rep 1978;62:1999-2001.

121. Silverstein FS, Johnston MV: A model of methotrexate encephalopathy: Neurotransmitter and pathologic abnormalities. J Child Neurol 1986;1:351-357.

122. Phillips PC, Thaler HT, Allen JC, Rottenberg DA: High-dose leucovorin reverses acute high-dose methotrexate neurotoxicity in the rat. Ann Neurol 1989;25:365-372.

123. Ohnuma T, Holland JF, Sinks LF: Biochemical and pharmacological studies with asparaginase in man. Cancer Res 1970;30:2297-2305.

124. Land VL, Sutow WW, Fernbach DJ, et al: Toxicity of L-asparaginase in children with advanced leukemia. Cancer 1972;30:339-347.

125. Pratt CB, Roberts D, Shanks E, et al: Asparaginase in combination chemotherapy for remission induction in childhood acute lymphocytic leukemia. Cancer Res 1973;33:2020-2025.

126. Moure JMB, Whitecar JP, Bodey GP: Electroencephalogram changes secondary to asparaginase. Arch Neurol 1970;23:365-368.

127. Kuroiwa Y, Furukawa T: EEG prognostication in drug-related alpha coma. Arch Neurol 1981;38:200.

128. Priest JR, Ramsay NK, Steinherz PG, et al: A syndrome of thrombosis and hemorrhage complicating L-asparaginase therapy for childhood leukemia. J Pediatr 1982;100:984-989.

129. Pratt CB, Green AA, Horowitz ME, et al: Central nervous system toxicity following the treatment of pediatric patients with ifosfamide/mesna. J Clin Oncol 1986;4:1253-1261.

130. Noll RB, Kulkarni R: Complex visual hallucinations and cyclosporine. Arch Neurol 1984;41:329-330.

131. Joss DV, Barrett AJ, Kendra JR, et al: Hypertension and convulsions in children receiving cyclosporine A. Lancet 1982;1:906.

132. Thompson CB, June CH, Sullivan KM, Thomas ED: Association between cyclosporin neurotoxicity and hypomagnesaemia. Lancet 1984;2:1116-1120.

133. de Groen PC, Aksamit AJ, Rakela J, et al: Central nervous system toxicity after liver transplantation: The role of cyclosporine and cholesterol. N Engl J Med 1987;317:861-866.

134. Rubin AM, Kang H: Cerebral blindness and encephalopathy with cyclosporin A toxicity. Neurology 1987;37:1072-1076.

135. Smedley H, Katrak M, Sikora K, Wheeler T:Neurologic effects of recombinant interferon. BMJ 1983;2860:262-264.

136. Suter CC, Westmoreland BF, Sharbrough FW, Hermann RC: Electroencephalographic abnormalities in interferon encephalopathy: A preliminary report. Mayo Clin Proc 1984;58:847-850.

137. Grabow JD: Optimal recording techniques and activation procedures: Children and adults. In Wada JA, Ellingson RJ (eds): Handbook of Electroencephalography and Clinical Neurophysiology (Revised Series), Vol 4. Amsterdam, Elsevier, 1990, p 39.

138. Musella L, Wilder BJ, Schmidt RP: Electroencephalographic activation with intravenous methohexital in psychomotor epilepsy. Neurology 1971;21:594-602.

139. Wyler AR, Richey ET, Atkinson RA, Hermann BP: Methohexital activation of epileptogenic foci during acute electrocorticography. Epilepsia 1987;28:490-494.

140. Niedermeyer E: Electroencephalographic studies on the anticonvulsive action of intravenous diazepam. Eur Neurol 1970;3:88-96.

141. Ambrosetto G, Lugaresi E: EEG effects of convulsants and anticonvulsants in man. In Longo VG (ed): Handbook of Electroencephalography and Clinical Neurophysiology, Vol 7-C. Amsterdam, Elsevier, 1977, p 78.

142. Kubicki ST, Rieger H, Busse G: EEG in fatal and near-fatal poisoning with soporific drugs: I. Typical EEG patterns. Clin Electroencephalogr 1970;1:5-13.

143. Guterman B, Sebastian P, Sodha N: Recovery from alpha coma after lorazepam overdose. Clin Electroencephalogr 1981;12:205-208.

144. Lombroso CT: Neonatal polygraphy in full-term and premature infants: A review of normal and abnormal findings. J Clin Neurophysiol 1985;2:105-153.

145. Rung GW, Wickey GS, Myers JL, et al: Thiopental as an adjunct to hypothermia for EEG suppression in infants prior to circulatory arrest. J Cardiothorac Vasc Anesth 1991;5:337-342.

146. Staudt F, Scholl ML, Coen RW, Bickford RB: Phenobarbital therapy in neonatal seizures and the prognostic value of the EEG. Neuropediatrics 1982;13:24-33.

147. Benda GI, Engel RC, Zhang YP: Prolonged inactive phases during the discontinuous pattern of prematurity in the electroencephalogram of very-low-birthweight infants. Electroencephalogr Clin Neurophysiol 1989;72:189-197.

148. Ashwal S, Schneider S: Brain death in the newborn. Pediatrics 1989;84:429-437.

149. Pezzani C, Radvanyi Bouvet MF, et al: Neonatal electroencephalography during the first twenty-four hours of life in full-term newborn infants. Neuropediatrics 1986;17:11-18.

150. Doberczak TM, Shanzer S, Senie RT, Kandall SR: Neonatal neurologic and electroencephalographic effects of intrauterine cocaine exposure. J Pediatr 1988;113:354-358.

151. Scher MS, Richardson GA, Coble PA, et al: The effects of prenatal alcohol and marijuana exposure: Disturbances in neonatal sleep cycling and arousal. Pediatr Res 1988;24:101-105.

152. Ioffe S, Chernick V: Development of the EEG between 30 and 40 weeks' gestation in normal and alcohol-exposed infants. Dev Med Child Neurol 1988;30:797-807.

153. van Baar AL, Fleury P, Soepatmi S, et al: Neonatal behaviour after drug-dependent pregnancy. Arch Dis Child 1989;64:235-240.

154. van Baar AL, Fleury P, Ultee CA: Behaviour in first year after drug-dependent pregnancy. Arch Dis Child 1989;64:241-245.

15

Electroencephalography and Structural Disease of the Brain

WILLIAM N. MAY

It was determined relatively early in the clinical use of the electroencephalogram (EEG) that structural disease in the central nervous system, specifically hemispheric brain tumors, produced recognizable and predictable changes in the EEG signal. Following the introduction of this concept, the EEG developed rapidly as an important clinical tool in the diagnosis of structural brain disease.

With development of neuroimaging techniques, including computed tomography (CT) and magnetic resonance imaging (MRI) technology, the EEG is no longer as useful in the evaluation of patients with structural brain disease. However, EEG does remain important as a measure of brain function in monitoring patients with various types of structural disease, including structural injury as a result of head trauma, stroke, and brain neoplasm. The analog EEG signal as well as digitally processed and averaged EEG signals are employed in patients with structural brain disease as an indication of response to treatment for prognostication and for monitoring side effects of treatment. This chapter reviews the types of EEG abnormalities seen in structural brain disease and the correlation of EEG abnormalities with underlying neuropathologic changes.

NEUROPHYSIOLOGY OF STRUCTURAL LESIONS

The maintenance of the normal cortical rhythm is dependent on the interaction between cortical and subcortical structures via white matter pathways. Structural disruption of the brain may arise as a result of failure of developmental processes in utero or as a result of acquired brain insult such as stroke, abscess, trauma, or neoplasm. The EEG may show a change as a result of these disruptions and generally reflect varying degrees of involvement of cortical gray matter, white matter, or subcortical gray matter. Processes that change the relationships of this system because of neuronal destruction pathway disruption may produce EEG dysrhythmia or changes in the voltage of the scalp EEG. EEG abnormalities associated with structural brain disease include changes in background amplitude or frequency or epileptiform discharges, either ictal or interictal. Typically, a combination of abnormalities is present. The voltage fluctuations of the scalp EEG are due to the activities of cortical neurons.

The power of the scalp EEG depends on the summed voltages generated by the ionic current flow around large numbers of cortical neurons. The power of the scalp EEG also depends on characteristics of the volume through which the currents pass and the voltages are measured (i.e., the cerebral spinal fluid, skull and scalp) and also by the number of generators in the view of the exploring electrode at the scalp. It follows that reduction in the number of generators (neuronal loss) or changes in the conducting medium such as scalp edema and subgaleal or extra-axial intracranial fluid collections would be causes for the reduction in voltage reductions in the scalp EEG.

Common conditions leading to reduction of neuronal generators include diffuse insults such as global hypoxic or

320

ischemic injury, or more focal insults such as cerebral infarcts, cerebritis or abscess, trauma, or neoplasm. Focal and diffuse voltage reductions may be seen with cerebral dysgenesis of the brain as in the case of migrational disorders including lissencephaly and schizencephaly, and encephalomalacia. Structural damage to the brain may result in loss of cortical neuronal loss and voltage reductions may result. In addition, changes in the frequency spectrum with shifts to the slower frequencies may occur. Slowing of the EEG is the most frequent marker of structural brain insults.

RHYTHM DISTURBANCES IN STRUCTURAL BRAIN DISEASE

One of the earliest discoveries in EEG relates to rhythm disturbances associated with tumors of the cerebral hemispheres.[1,2] Two rhythm disturbances have been proposed as indicators of underlying structural brain disease. They are focal polymorphic delta slowing (PDS), which usually arises from one hemisphere, and rhythmic intermittent slowing, usually arising from both hemispheres with either a frontal or occipital emphasis. Although focal slowing is often a reliable indicator of underlying structural brain disease, intermittent rhythmic slowing appears to be a poor prediction of structural disease.

Polymorphic Delta Slowing

PDS is helpful in the localization of focal structural brain disease (Figs. 15–1 and 15–2).[3–8] Polymorphic delta activity (PDA) is generated as a result of injury to subcortical white matter and/or subcortical nuclear structures.[9–11]

In animal studies, PDA can be elicited by subcortical brain lesions.[12,13] Experimental focal lesions of subcortical white matter produced by thermocoagulation produces delta slowing overlying the area of injury. These waves are polymorphic, with maximum amplitudes of 500 µV and a dominant frequency of 1 to 2 Hz mixed with 3- to 4-Hz activity. The fast activities in the area of the lesion are depressed, and the slow components are four or five times higher in amplitude than the surrounding desynchronized background arising from cortex overlying normal white matter. The delta activity appears immediately after producing lesions in these animals. Thalamic lesions also produce slowing, although the slowing is more variable than in animals with white matter lesions.

Focal slowing may occur in the absence of structural brain disease. Commonly, focal slowing is seen in patients with paroxysmal conditions such as seizures and migraine.[5,14–16] It has been shown that PDA may be seen in children without evidence of focal structural disease on MRI or CT scan.[8]

After an acute condition such as a migraine or seizure, the slow wave focus dissipates.[14]

The EEG detects abnormalities quickly after acute insults.[14,17] Although the MRI is the most valuable test used in the detection of structural abnormalities, the EEG can be a useful complementary test. In addition to slowing, the EEG may demonstrate epileptiform activity.

Size of the area encompassing slow activity, amplitude of the slow activity, and frequency of the focal slow activity does not correlate well with the size of the lesion using neuroimaging.[18] The amplitude or degree of slowing or the size of the area of slowing was not as consistently indicative of the significance of the lesion as was the lack of reactivity or persistence of the slow wave activity. A low-voltage theta focus with a small field of distribution that is consistently present and does not vary with changes in patient state would be more likely associated with a significant destructive lesion with mass effect than a higher voltage widespread delta focus, which is intermittently present in a tracing, or shows reactivity to changes in patient alertness.[18,19] Focal slowing that is continuous and nonreactive is most indicative of the presence of significant focal destructive brain disease.

Generalized Continuous Slow Activity

The presence of generalized diffuse slowing has been reported in patients with disease involving primarily the white matter of both hemispheres or a combination of gray and white matter disease. For the most part, these types of changes would be expected with hypoxic-ischemic injury, toxic-metabolic disturbances, or progressive degenerative disease. Generalized polymorphic delta has been reported clinically with diffuse white matter encephalopathies, thalamic tumors, and lesions of the upper brainstem. Continuous generalized slow activity is seen in patients with lesions limited to the upper brainstem and diencephalon.[9]

Intermittent Rhythmic Slow Activity

"Distant rhythms" consist of rhythmic slow waves in the delta range manifested in the scalp EEG in brain areas distant to the primary pathology. These rhythms are intermittent in nature occurring in brief bursts with sinusoidal morphology (Fig. 15–3). The intermittent periods of slowing may be of significant voltage and may even be within the delta range in frequency. These monorhythmic bursts have come to be known as the *intermittent rhythmic delta activity* (IRDA) in contradistinction to the polymorphic slowing. The nonspecificity and nonlocalizing characteristic of these rhythmic patterns have been subsequently confirmed.[20] When such slowing is seen in the absence of structural brain disease, the slowing tends to be intermittent and

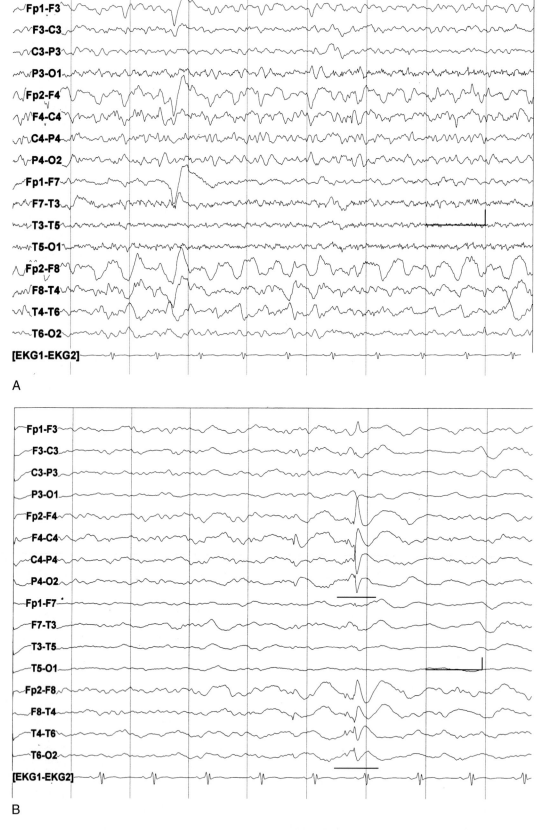

FIGURE 15–1

A, *Right-sided polymorphic slowing in a 14-year-old child with focal cortical dysplasia involving the right hemisphere.* B, *Patient had partial seizures with intermittent central and midtemporal spikes (underlined). Calibration, 1 sec/50 μV.*

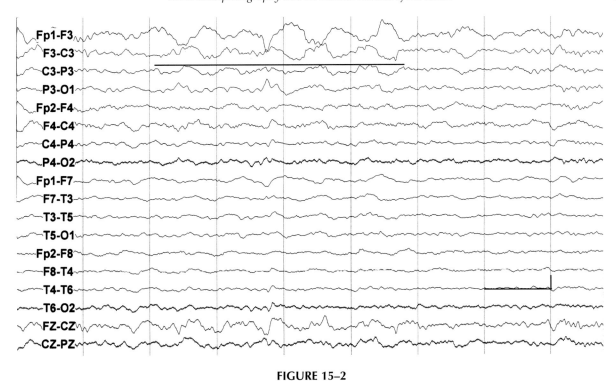

FIGURE 15–2

Polymorphic slowing (underlined) in a 16-year-old patient with a low-grade left frontal lobe glioma. Calibration, 1 sec/50 μV.

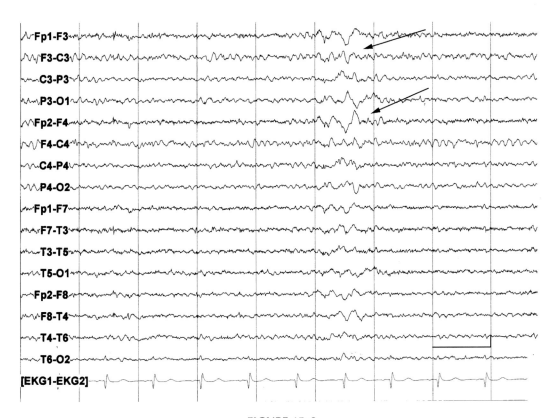

FIGURE 15–3

Brief bursts of delta activity (arrows) in an 8-year-old child with a hypothalamic hamartoma. Calibration, 1 sec/50 μV.

may shift from side to side, showing considerable reactivity to stimulation with varying levels of alertness in the patient. Distant or projected rhythms are best thought of as very nonspecific manifestations of brain dysfunction resulting from a wide range of pathologic processes, either diffuse or focal in nature. Intermittent rhythmic slowing may appear as either rhythmic high-voltage theta or delta activity and may be seen arising from the occipital, frontal, or vertex head regions.

In the adult patient, IRDA tends to be seen in the frontal leads of the EEG and is known as *frontal IRDA* (FIRDA), whereas, in children, the slowing tends to occur in the posterior head regions and is known as *occipital IRDA* (OIRDA).[21,22] Although IRDA is most often a non-localizing finding, FIRDA, which appears to be accentuated over one hemisphere, may point to an ipsilateral hemispheric lesion. When FIRDA is associated with a deep frontal lobe tumor, the frequency tends to be in the range between 1.5 and 2.0 Hz and may be accentuated on the side of the tumor.[23]

BRAIN TUMORS IN CHILDREN

Brain tumors represent the most common type of solid malignancy of childhood, with 1200 to 1500 new cases per year in children younger than 15 years of age. In children between the age of 2 years and adolescence, the most common tumors are those arising from the posterior fossa. Tumors of glial origin are the most common; tumors of primitive neuroectodermal origin are the second most common type of tumor seen.

The EEG has been obsolete as a tool for evaluating patients who were thought to have brain tumors, at least from the standpoint of diagnostic importance. The EEG, however, may give the clinician additional knowledge as to the stability of the nervous system in a patient with a tumor.[24] The child with a tumor that is producing hydrocephalus, shifting brain structures, secondary vascular compromise, or impending herniation may show signs of a disturbed EEG rhythm that might indicate change in the patient's status. Serial EEG studies in patients undergoing radiation treatment may give clinical insight into the status of the brain's response to treatment.

Tumors of the Posterior Fossa

The most significant childhood tumors of the posterior fossa include cerebellar medulloblastoma, cerebellar astrocytoma, ependymoma, and brainstem glioma. As early as 1944, Walter and Dovey[25] described 4- to 7-Hz activity associated with deep-seated midline tumors in the infratentorial regions. The concept of projected EEG rhythms associated

with posterior fossa tumors was introduced by Faure and associates in 1951.[26] In a series of EEG from 154 children with posterior fossa neoplasms, 76% of the records were considered abnormal, with abnormalities divided into four categories: (1) posterior rhythmic delta activity (27%); (2) generalized, bilateral bursts of rhythmic slow waves (32%); (3) posterior arrhythmic slow waves (51%); and (4) rhythmic theta or delta waves on vertex or anterior quadrants (11%).[27] Patients often had more than one type of abnormality. The first two categories were represented in 59% of the abnormal EEGs and were thought to represent projected or distant rhythms. These IRDA may be dominant frontally (FIRDA) or occipitally (OIRDA).

IRDA, when present in the EEG of young children, tends to appear more frequently as OIRDA more than FIRDA and has been attributed to earlier maturation of occipital cortex and its subcortical connections.[28] OIRDA is characterized by its large amplitude, simple wave form, and reactivity to arousing stimuli.

The third rhythm listed earlier, posterior arrhythmic slow waves, is less reactive and more continuous than the intermixed rhythmic delta activity just described.[27] The transmitted monorhythmic activity is attributed to the presence of third ventricle enlargement due to hydrocephalus. The arrhythmic posterior slow activity is a result of a more regional disturbance of occipital lobe function, perhaps as a result of upward anatomic distortion or as a result of altered vascular supply to the posterior pole. This hypothesis is supported by the greater incidence of the arrhythmic posterior regional slowing in patients with more rapidly growing medulloblastomas and is thought to be due to the likelihood of the tumor influencing posterior circulation.

EEG abnormalities are common in children with posterior fossa lesions.[29] In a series of EEGs from 120 children with posterior fossa tumors, both diffuse and localized EEG abnormalities with generalized background abnormalities were seen in 100 cases, and these changes were symmetrical in 21 cases. Forty-six cases showed more prominent changes in the posterior head regions, and 7 cases showed more prominent changes in the anterior head region. EEGs were normal in only 14 cases. These authors concluded that tumors located more rostrally in the posterior fossa tended to show more anterior EEG disturbances, and more posterior lesions seemed to produce more posterior changes. In all but one instance of the 15 cases in which the findings were clearly more prominent in one hemisphere, the tumor was ipsilateral to the more involved hemisphere. In one case, the tumor was located in a posterior fossa position contralateral to the involved hemisphere. Normal EEGs were seen in patients less frequently if eye findings suggested increased intracranial pressure. Tumors of the cerebellar hemispheres and vermis are more likely to result in EEG abnormalities than tumors of the brainstem.[27,29]

Supratentorial Tumors

Supratentorial neoplasms are the most frequent type of brain tumor seen in children younger than 18 months and older than 14 years. Among the tumors of glial origin (astrocytomas, oligodendrogliomas, and ependymomas and tumors of the choroid plexus), astrocytomas are the most common. In younger children, tumors of neuroectodermal origin may be seen. Tumors may arise from meninges, neuroendocrine tissue, germ cell rests, vascular tissue, or nerve sheaths, or they may be a result of cystic malformations, such as craniopharyngiomas. EEG abnormalities are common in children with supratentorial tumors.[30]

Focal background slowing is one of the most important EEG signs of focal structural brain disease. The details of slowing are as follows: (1) slowing may be seen in less severe and deeper lesions, (2) slowing may be in the theta range of moderate to low voltage, and (3) slowing may be intermittent. PDA that is seen in association with structural brain disease is characteristically in the 0.5- to 2.5-Hz frequency range and the continuous irregular slow waves are virtually nonreactive to visual stimuli, arousal, or sleep.[23] Hyperventilation may activate slow activity on the EEG.

Although there is not an exact relationship between EEG abnormalities and size of the tumor, as the lesion increases in size, the PDS becomes continuous and higher in voltage.[24] EEG abnormalities associated with supratentorial tumors consist of features such as focal or lateralized epileptiform activity, focal or lateralized slowing, generalized or multifocal epileptiform activity, or diffuse slowing.

Tumors of childhood exerting their effects on the scalp EEG do so by several mechanisms. The first effect might be direct destruction or replacement of neuronal elements. Lesions that affect cortex alone do not cause slowing of the EEG but rather a suppression of voltage.[10] Second, neoplastic tumors may undercut cerebral cortex and produce deafferentation of cortical neurons. Also, the tumor may interpose itself between cortical neurons and the scalp electrode, or produce fluid collections that distance the scalp electrode from the cortical voltage source. With these basic mechanisms understood, it becomes easy to predict the types of effects that supratentorial tumors may have on the scalp EEG. Supratentorial brain tumors are likely to produce more direct and focal changes in the EEG frequency and voltage than tumors located below the tentorium.

Changes in the EEG in supratentorial lesions tend to reflect more accurately the focal location of the tumor with better anatomic correlation than in the case of infratentorial lesions. As previously discussed, posterior fossa lesions produce remote changes while supratentorial tumors often produce well-localized EEG manifestations. In an EEG study of 198 children with tumors, it was found that in 40% of the patients the EEG abnormalities were lateralized to the side of the tumor; in 14% of the patients the EEGs revealed generalized abnormalities; and in only 4% of these patients the EEGs were normal.[31] Likewise, in a series of patients reported by Backus and Millichap,[32] EEGs were of localizing value in 22 (92%) of 24 children with tumors of the cerebral cortex. Shady and colleagues[30] reviewed the records of 98 consecutive patients, 18 years of age or younger, with pathologically confirmed supratentorial astroglial neoplasms. The preoperative EEG accurately lateralized to the tumor side in 88% of the cases and localized to the correct lobe in 56% of the cases.

SUMMARY

Despite advances in neuroimaging techniques over the past three decades that have dramatically improved our ability to identify structural lesions of the brain, the EEG continues to provide valuable information about brain function by demonstrating focal or diffuse background abnormalities as well as epileptiform activity. Structural neuroimaging combined with the EEG measure of functionality provide clinicians with powerful diagnostic tools.

REFERENCES

1. Walter WG, Camb MA: The location of cerebral tumours by electro-encephalography. Lancet 1936;2:305-308.
2. Cobb WA: Rhythmic slow discharges in the electroencephalogram. J Neurol Neurosurg Psychiatry 1945;8:65-78.
3. Arfel G, Fischgold H: EEG signs in tumours of the brain. Electroencephalogr Clin Neurophysiol 1961;19(Suppl):36-50.
4. Drift JHA, van der Magnus O: The value of the EEG in the differential diagnosis of cases with cerebral lesions. Electroencephalogr Clin Neurophysiol 1961;19(Suppl):183-196.
5. Marshall DW, Brey RL, Morse MW: Focal and/or lateralized polymorphic delta activity: Association with either "normal" or "nonfocal" computed tomographic scans. Arch Neurol 1988;45:33-35.
6. Daly DD, Thomas JE: Sequential alterations in the electroencephalograms of patients with brain tumors. Electroencephalogr Clin Neurophysiol 1958;10:395-404.
7. Markand ON: Pearls, perils, and pitfalls in the use of the electroencephalogram. Semin Neurol 2003;23:7-46.
8. Maytal J, Novak GP, Knobler SB, Schaul N: Neuroradiological manifestations of focal polymorphic delta activity in children. Arch Neurol 1993;50:181-184.

9. Jasper H, Van Buren J: Interrelationship between cortex and subcortical structures: Clinical electroencephalographic studies. Electroencephalogr Clin Neurophysiol 1953;(Suppl 4):168-188.

10. Gloor P, Ball G, Schaul N: Brain lesions that produce delta waves in the EEG. Neurology 1977;27:326-333.

11. Lukashevich IP, Shklovskii VM, Kurkova KS, et al: The effects of lesions to subcortical conducting pathways on the electrical activity of the human cerebral cortex. Neurosci Behav Physiol 2004;29:283-287.

12. Humphreys P, Kaufmann WE, Galaburda AM: Developmental dyslexia in women: Neuropathological findings in three patients. Ann Neurol 1990;28:727-738.

13. Ulett G: Electroencephalogram of dogs with experimental space-occupying intracranial lesions. Arch Neurol Psychiatry 1945;54:141-149.

14. Gilmore PC, Brenner RP: Correlation of EEG, computerized tomography, and clinical findings: Study of 100 patients with focal delta activity. Arch Neurol 1981;38:371-372.

15. Ramelli GP, Sturzenegger M, Donati F, Karbowski K: EEG findings during basilar migraine attacks in children. Electroencephalogr Clin Neurophysiol 1998;107:374-378.

16. Jan MM, Sadler M, Rahey SR: Lateralized postictal EEG delta predicts the side of seizure surgery in temporal lobe epilepsy. Epilepsia 2001;42:402-405.

17. Masdeu JC, Azar-Kia B, Rubino F: Evaluation of recent cerebral infarction by computerized tomography. Arch Neurol 1977;34:417-421.

18. Schaul N: Pathogenesis and significance of abnormal nonepileptiform rhythms in the EEG. J Clin Neurophysiol 1990;7:229-248.

19. Schaul N, Green L, Peyster R, et al: Structural determinants of EEG findings in acute hemispheric lesions. Ann Neurol 1986;20:707-711.

20. Watemberg N, Alehan F, Dabby R, et al: Clinical and radiologic correlates of frontal intermittent rhythmic delta activity. J Clin Neurophysiol 2002;19:535-539.

21. Niedermeyer E: Electrophysiology of the frontal lobe. Clin Electroencephalogr 2003;34:5-12.

22. Gullapalli D, Fountain NB: Clinical correlation of occipital intermittent rhythmic delta activity. J Clin Neurophysiol 2003;20:35-41.

23. Goldensohn ES: The use of the EEG for evaluation of focal intracranial lesions. *In* Klass DW, Daly DD (eds): Current Practice of Clinical Electroencephalography. New York, Raven Press, 1979, p 308.

24. Niedermeyer E, Lopes da Silva F: Brain tumors and other space-occupying lesions. *In* Niedermeyer F, Lopes da Silva F (eds): Electroencephalography: Basic Principles, Clinical Applications, and Related Fields. Baltimore, Urban & Schwarzenberg, 1987, p 229.

25. Walter WG, Dovey VJ: Electroencephalography in cases of subcortical tumor. J Neurol Neurosurg Psychiatry 1944;7:57-65.

26. Faure J, Droogleever-Fortuyn J, Gastaut H, et al: De la geneses et de la signification des rythmes recuelillis a distance dans les cas de tumeurs cerebrales. Electroencephalogr Clin Neurophysiol 1951;3:429-434.

27. Martinius J, Matthes A, Lombroso CT: Electroencephalographic features in posterior fossa tumors in children. Electroencephalogr Clin Neurophysiol 1968;25:128-139.

28. Smith JMB, Kellaway P: The natural history and clinical correlates of occipital foci in children. *In* Kellaway P, Petersen I (eds): Neurological and Electroencephalographic Correlative Studies in Infancy. New York, Grune & Stratton, 1964, p 230.

29. Bacia T, Fryze C, Wocjan J: EEG changes in cases of posterior fossa tumors in children. Pol Med J 1969;8:464-470.

30. Shady JA, Black PM, Kupsky WJ, et al: Seizures in children with supratentorial astroglial neoplasms. Pediatr Neurosurg 1994;21:23-30.

31. Chiofalo N, Armengol V, Fuentes A, et al: Electroencephalographical-anatomical correlation of brain tumours in infancy and childhood. Child Brain 1991;8:417-422.

32. Backus RE, Millichap JG: The seizure as manifestation of intracranial tumor in childhood. Pediatrics 1962;29:978-984.

16

Manifestations of Metabolic, Toxic, and Degenerative Diseases

EDWARD H. KOVNAR

This chapter reviews the electroencephalographic (EEG) findings associated with various types of diffuse encephalopathies of childhood.

Markand[1] has skillfully reviewed the EEG changes typically seen in diffuse encephalopathies. The role of EEG in the evaluation of childhood encephalopathies has many facets. In a child with subtle or evanescent changes in mental status, the EEG may provide early clues of an organic brain syndrome as opposed to a functional or psychogenic disorder. The EEG can help narrow the differential diagnosis for a particular set of neurologic signs and symptoms by suggesting focal versus generalized disturbances of function. Although few EEG abnormalities are pathognomonic, some are characteristic enough to change the direction of the diagnostic evaluation. Periodic lateralized epileptiform discharges (PLEDs) in a child with abrupt onset of behavioral changes must prompt consideration of a focal encephalitis. Conversely, laboratory evidence of renal or hepatic failure should be sought in an acutely ill child with unexplained obtundation accompanied by the presence of triphasic waves. The EEG is sufficiently accessible to allow bedside recordings on ventilator-dependent neonates in the intensive care unit and anesthetized patients in the operating room. Serial EEG recordings may provide an objective, albeit nonspecific, indicator of prognosis or response to therapy in patients with previously diagnosed neurologic disorders. Computed frequency analysis and topographic mapping may one day refine the electroencephalographer's ability to provide quantitative measures of neurologic function.

The diseases discussed in this chapter have little in common with respect to pathogenesis, treatment, or prognosis. What they do share is the potential for producing signs and symptoms of diffuse impairment of cerebral function. Although susceptible to the effects of a wide variety of systemic diseases, the brain has a narrow repertoire of reactions to such conditions. Similarly, the abnormalities manifested in the EEG as a result of these disorders comprise a brief list of characteristic findings.

TYPES OF EEG ABNORMALITIES

Alterations in Normal Background. Alpha rhythm, as defined by the International Federation of Societies for Encephalography and Clinical Neurophysiology, is the 8- to 12-Hz rhythmic activity recorded over the posterior region of the head during wakefulness. Alpha rhythm is enhanced by eyelid closure, physical relaxation, and relative mental inactivity and is blocked or attenuated by visual attention and mental effort. Developmental features of the occipital alpha rhythm include its slower frequency at younger ages. As discussed earlier, in Chapter 4, the occipital rhythm has a frequency of 3.5 to 4.5 Hz at 3 to 4 months, 5 to 7 Hz at 1 year, 6 to 8 Hz at 2 years, 7 to 9 Hz at 3 years, and 9 Hz by age 7 to 9 years. A dominant occipital rhythm that falls below the accepted normal range for age suggests the presence of a diffuse encephalopathy due to metabolic abnormalities (hypoglycemia, renal or hepatic insufficiency), endocrine deficiency (hypothyroidism), or drug effects (benzodiazepines, barbiturates, or tricyclic antidepressants).[1] An invariant, frontally dominant rhythm, with little or no reactivity to stimulation, and yet within the alpha frequency range may be seen in comatose patients following hypoxic-ischemic brain injury, brainstem infarction, or drug intoxication.[2]

Theta activity comprising those frequencies from 5 to 7 Hz may occur normally in the awake resting EEG. Such normal theta includes the slow alpha variant, a subharmonic of the occipital alpha rhythm that is reactive to eye opening and eye closure and attenuated during mental activity and drowsiness. In contrast, nonreactive slowing within the theta frequency range provides nonspecific but useful evidence of a diffuse encephalopathy of metabolic or toxic etiology.

Beta activity, which includes all EEG frequencies above 13 Hz, varies in topography and relative abundance depending on age and level of alertness. Barbiturates, benzodi-

azepines, and other sedative-hypnotic drugs are known to produce widespread and bilaterally symmetrical increases in beta activity (Fig. 16-1). Increased beta activity is associated less consistently with psychotropic drugs, including phenothiazines, tricyclic antidepressants, antihistamines, and sympathomimetics.

Episodic Low-Amplitude Events. Defined as brief epochs of relative attenuation of background activity with synchronous hemispheric or bihemispheric onset, episodic low-amplitude events are not uncommonly seen in patients with coma from a variety of etiologies.[3] These episodes are usually brief, lasting less than 5 seconds, and are not associated with high-amplitude bursts of activity, which differentiates this pattern from burst-suppression patterns. In coma due to entities other than status epilepticus, prognosis is poor.[3]

Abnormal Response to Activating Procedures. Reactivity to stimulation is a critical aspect of the EEG evaluation of diffuse encephalopathies.[1] A patient whose

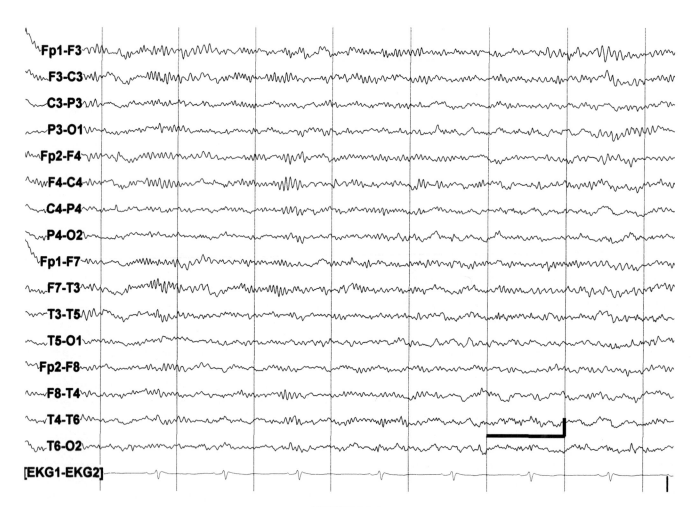

FIGURE 16–1

Excessive beta activity in an 8-year-old child taking clonazepam. Calibration: 50 µV/1 sec.

mentation is only mildly impaired may show a reduction in the amount of slow activity and an increase in the frequency of background activity in response to eye opening or tactile stimulation. Patients with deepening coma may respond to painful stimuli with a prolonged increase in diffuse high-amplitude slowing called a *paradoxical arousal* or *alerting response*. The comatose patient with a severe metabolic, anoxic, or toxic encephalopathy often shows neither clinical nor EEG evidence of reactivity to any form of stimulation.

An exaggerated or prolonged response to hyperventilation is typical of hypoglycemia and hypocalcemia. Photomyoclonic and photoparoxysmal responses may be seen in metabolic encephalopathies such as that seen with renal insufficiency.[4] So-called giant or large-amplitude occipital spikes (visual evoked responses) may be induced by single stroboscopic flashes or repetitive photic stimulation in neuronal ceroid lipofuscinosis.

Continuous Irregular Slow Activity. Diffuse polymorphic slow activity in the delta frequency range, also called *arrhythmic delta activity*, has been correlated in clinical studies with disease processes that produce extensive injury to cerebral white matter or both white and gray matter.[5] Polymorphic delta activity (PDA) is rarely seen in diseases affecting only gray matter. Such observations have led to the concept that deafferentation or disconnection of cortical neurons underlies the mechanism of PDA. Focal PDA is discussed in greater detail in Chapter 15. Typically, PDA is poorly reactive to stimulation.

Intermittent Rhythmic Slow Activity. Intermittent rhythmic delta activity (IRDA) consists of runs of high voltage slow waves which occur serially with a frequency of 2 to 4 Hz. These bursts of rhythmic slow activity may be unilateral or bilateral but, when bilateral, they tend to arise synchronously from both cerebral hemispheres. Frontally dominant bursts of rhythmic delta activity (FIRDA) were once considered to be characteristic of deep, midline structural lesions. FIRDA may, in fact, be seen in a variety of toxic and metabolic encephalopathies as well as conditions associated with widespread structural damage affecting subcortical and cortical gray matter.[6] Posteriorly dominant or occipital IRDA (OIRDA) is more frequently seen in children than in adults. Whether frontal or occipital, IRDA is characteristically suppressed by stimulation and may be present even in clinically subtle encephalopathies.

Periodic Patterns. *Periodic EEG patterns* refer to either slow or sharp activity that recurs at regular intervals with similar morphology within one or more derivations in a given EEG. Periodic patterns may be classified as either diffuse or localized and may be characterized as having either short or long intervals between discharges.[7] Serially recurrent focal discharges with sharply contoured morphology are referred to as PLEDs (Fig. 16-2). PLEDs may

arise in a bilateral but independent manner from both cerebral hemispheres (referred to as *BIPLEDs*). Whether unilateral or bilateral, PLEDs are typically associated with acute, destructive lesions of the cerebral cortex such as focal encephalitis, anoxia, or vascular occlusion.

Serially recurrent waveforms arising synchronously from both cerebral hemispheres are classified as diffuse periodic discharges. Depending on the length of time between discharges, such patterns may be subdivided into periodic short-interval diffuse discharges or periodic long-interval diffuse discharges. Periodic diffuse discharges are nonspecific findings associated with a variety of acute and subacute encephalopathies. Once considered characteristic of slowly progressive encephalitis, periodic diffuse discharges may also be observed in drug intoxication, acquired metabolic disorders, as well as nonconvulsive status epilepticus. The EEG characteristics and clinical correlates of these periodic patterns have been summarized by Brenner and Schaul (Table 16-1).[8]

Restriction in the supply of substrates required for energy-dependent neuronal and glial processes and other alterations in metabolic homeostasis are well known causes of acute and subacute encephalopathies. Although typically reversible, prolonged or irreversible changes accompanied by evidence of structural damage may ensue in certain types of metabolic encephalopathy, such as severe hypoglycemia or hyponatremia. The EEG changes seen in metabolic disorders are typically diffuse and may be roughly correlated with the severity of impaired neurologic function. As discussed previously, the EEG may therefore provide a means of grading the degree of metabolic encephalopathy for prognostic purposes or for assessment of response to therapeutic maneuvers.

Hypoglycemia and Hyperglycemia. Hypoglycemia has been long known to be capable of producing depressed levels of alertness and seizures. Although dramatic EEG changes may accompany hypoglycemia, considerable variation exists between individuals in the degree of such changes. Therefore, the correlation between blood glucose concentrations, level of alertness, and EEG changes is weak.[9] The earliest EEG change consists of an increased sensitivity to hyperventilation. High-amplitude generalized slowing occurs early in hyperventilation in a fasting subject and persists after resumption of normal respiratory rate. The resting EEG often remains normal until the blood glucose level drops to 50 mg/dL. Mild slowing of the occipital alpha rhythm may occur with mild degrees of hypoglycemia. Further decreases in the blood glucose concentration result in generalized slowing in the theta-delta frequency range and bursts of high-amplitude rhythmic 1- to 3-Hz slow waves arising synchronously from both cerebral hemispheres. Severe hypoglycemia with resulting coma may be associated with high-amplitude irregular

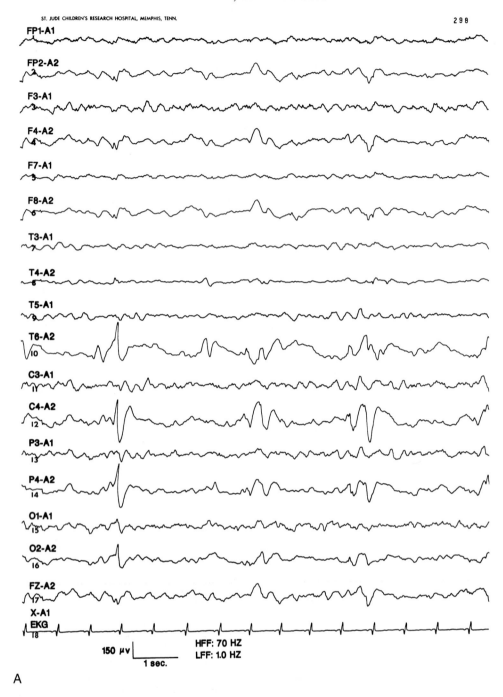

FIGURE 16–2

A and B, Periodic lateralized epileptiform discharges arising from the right temporal, central, and parietal derivations in a 6-year-old girl with an infarction in distribution of the middle cerebral artery following removal of a meningioma of the right middle cranial fossa.

delta or diffuse voltage suppression. Although EEG changes in hypoglycemia are usually symmetrical, focal or lateralized slow waves may appear, often in the setting of a preexisting focal cerebral injury. Administration of intravenous glucose results in rapid reversal of mild to moderate EEG changes. Profound hypoglycemia with coma or repeated hypoglycemic episodes may be followed by prolonged slowing and the emergence of epileptiform activity.

Hyperglycemia produces nonspecific changes in the EEG unless accompanied by other metabolic disturbances such as ketoacidosis, electrolyte disturbances, or hyperosmolarity. Patients with severe or brittle diabetes mellitus

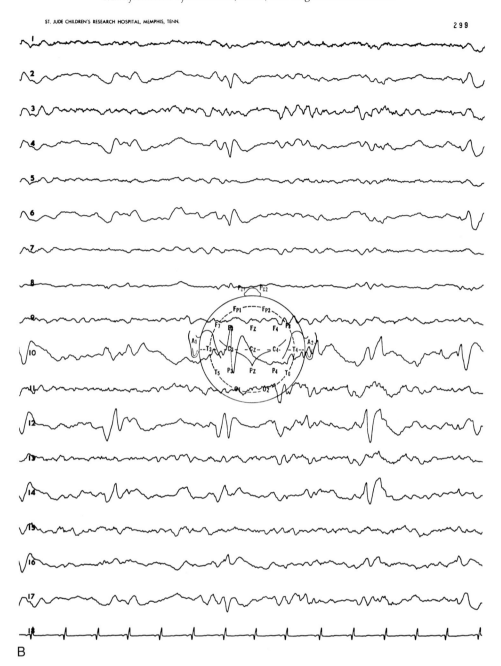

B

FIGURE 16–2 *Cont'd*

may exhibit mild EEG abnormalities, including an increase in theta activity.[10] Hyperosmolarity seen with severe non-ketotic hyperglycemia (blood glucose > 400 mg/dL) may result in coma and seizures and may also unmask focal EEG abnormalities associated with preexisting cerebral lesions.[11]

Hypocalcemia and Hypercalcemia. Unlike in adults, hypocalcemia in children is rarely a manifestation of primary hypoparathyroidism and is more often a consequence of renal or hepatic disease, intestinal malabsorption, excessive phosphorous intake ("cow's milk tetany") or secondary

hypoparathyroidism as seen in perinatal asphyxia or maternal diabetes. Clinical manifestations of hypocalcemia in the newborn period include vomiting, lethargy, apnea, cyanosis, and seizures. Older children complain of paresthesias, muscle stiffness, or cramping and exhibit irritability, tremor, and hyperreflexia. Severe hypocalcemia is associated with agitation, confusion, carpopedal spasms, tetany, and seizures.

In mild degrees of hypocalcemia the resting EEG may be normal or show a modest amount of diffuse slowing in the

TABLE 16–1. PERIODIC COMPLEXES

Characteristic	PLEDs or BIPLEDs	PSIDDs	PLIDDs
Interval duration	0.5-4 sec	0.5-4 sec	4-40 sec
Topography	Focal or lateralized (PLEDs) Bilateral, independent (BIPLEDs)	Diffuse	Diffuse
Morphology	Sharp waves (includes biphasic, triphasic waves); spikes, polyspikes	Sharp waves (includes biphasic, triphasic waves); spikes, polyspikes	Complex, stereotyped, polyphasic
Etiology	Varied, often vascular (PLEDs) CNS infection, anoxia (BIPLEDs)	CJD Metabolic (hepatic or renal) Toxic (baclofen, lithium) Anoxia NGSE	SSPE Toxic (anesthetic) Anoxia
Seizures (focal or generalized tonic-clonic)	Common	Rare	Rare
Myoclonic jerks	Rare	Common (CJD)	Common (SSPE)
Altered mental status	Common	Common	Common

(From Brenner RP, Schaul N: Periodic EEG patterns: Classification, clinical correlation, and pathophysiology. J Clin Neurophysiol 1990;7:249-267.)
PLED, periodic lateralized epileptiform discharge; BIPLED, bilateral independent PLED; PSIDD, periodic short-interval diffuse discharge; PLIDD, periodic long-interval diffuse discharge; CNS, central nervous system; CJD, Creutzfeldt-Jakob disease; SSPE, subacute sclerosing panencephalitis; NGSE, nonconvulsive generalized status epilepticus.

theta frequency range. An exaggerated and prolonged response to hyperventilation is typical of mild hypocalcemia. More severe hypocalcemia is associated clinically with tetany and seizures. EEG correlates include suppression of alpha rhythm and the presence of diffuse slowing in the theta-delta frequency range. Bursts of high-amplitude rhythmic delta activity as well as spikes, sharp waves, and spike-wave complexes appear when the serum calcium level drops below 6.5 mg/dL.[12] Administration of intravenous calcium gluconate results in improvement in tetany and seizures as well as in EEG abnormalities.[13]

Hypercalcemia is an unusual pediatric problem but may occur due to excessive intake of vitamin D or as a result of malignant neoplasms with or without skeletal metastases. Severe hypercalcemia rarely occurs in isolation. Therefore, signs and symptoms provoked by coexistent metabolic and endocrine disturbances may incorrectly be attributed to elevated calcium concentrations. Muscle weakness has been described in adults with hypercalcemia due to hyperparathyroidism. Children may exhibit lethargy and confusion as the only signs of significant hypercalcemia. EEG findings in patients with hypercalcemia are nonspecific and include excessive amounts of slowing in the theta-delta frequency range and bursts of generalized high-amplitude bilaterally synchronous delta activity. Triphasic waves may also be recorded.[12] Although EEG abnormalities usually appear at calcium concentrations higher than 13 mg/dL, the correlation between degree of hypercalcemia and EEG abnormalities is poor.[14]

Hypomagnesemia and Hypermagnesemia. The neurologic manifestations of hypomagnesemia are similar to those of hypocalcemia and include irritability, agitation, confusion, tremor, hyperreflexia, tetany, and convulsions.[15]

Convulsive phenomena in the affected newborn may be focal, both clinically and electrographically.[16] The usual causes of hypomagnesemia include decreased oral intake, intestinal malabsorption, and increased renal loss due to impaired tubular reabsorption as seen in renal tubular acidosis. Signs and symptoms of hypomagnesemia usually occur at a serum concentration less than 0.8 mEq/L.[17]

Hypermagnesemia is an uncommon occurrence and is typically encountered in the setting of excessive intake with impaired renal clearance.[18] The predominant neurologic manifestation of severe hypermagnesemia is muscular paralysis due to blockade of neuromuscular transmission.[19] If untreated, this weakness may produce respiratory insufficiency resulting in hypoxia, CO_2 retention, coma, and death. Experimentally, elevation of serum magnesium in human subjects has been reported to produce slowing of the EEG but *no* central nervous system (CNS) depression at concentrations as high as 15 mEq/L.[20] Although lethargy and confusion typically occur at serum concentrations of 8 to 10 mEq/L, this may reflect concomitant hypoxia and hypercarbia due to respiratory compromise.[21]

Hyponatremia and Hypernatremia. Hyponatremia may occur as a result of inadvertent water intoxication (improper mixing of infant formula or administration of large volumes of hypotonic intravenous solution), impaired water elimination (renal or cardiac insufficiency), inadequate mineralocorticoid secretion (adrenal insufficiency), certain drugs (narcotics, carbamazepine, oxycarbazepine, general anesthetics, or antineoplastic agents) or inappropriate antidiuretic hormone secretion. Clinical manifestations include headache, lethargy, seizures, and coma. Severity of symptoms and signs is related not only to the degree of hyponatremia but also to the rate at which the lowering of serum sodium occurs.[22] EEG abnormalities correlate closely with reduction in level of alertness. Initial findings include suppression of the alpha rhythm and increase in theta activity (Fig. 16-3). More severe depression in consciousness is associated with runs of diffuse high-amplitude delta activity.[23]

Hypernatremia per se produces minimal EEG abnormalities. Rapid correction of hypernatremia, however, may be associated with clinical signs and EEG findings similar to those associated with acute water intoxication.

Hypokalemia and Hyperkalemia. Disturbances of potassium concentration may have profound effects on the

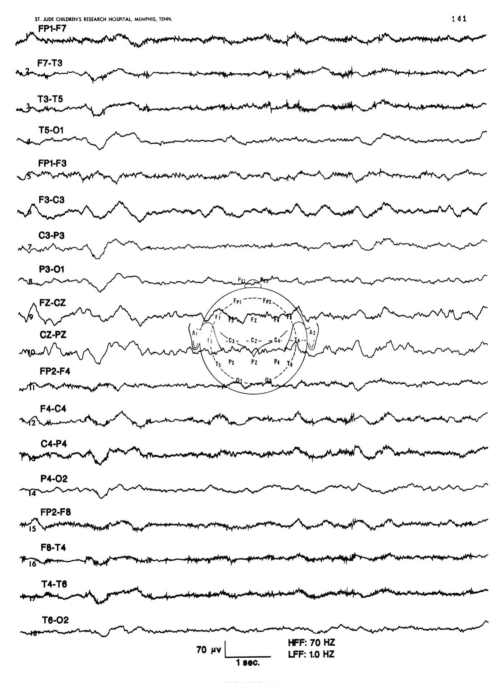

FIGURE 16–3

Diffuse irregular slow activity and suppression of the occipital alpha rhythm in a 12-year-old girl with stupor due to hyponatremia (serum sodium = 120 mEq/L).

excitability of striated and smooth muscle fibers. Clinical manifestations of hypokalemia include weakness of trunk and proximal limb muscles and decreased intestinal peristalsis. In the absence of superimposed respiratory insufficiency, hypokalemia produces little or no change in CNS function. Changes in the EEG associated with either hyperkalemia or hypokalemia are minimal unless accompanied by other metabolic disturbances.[18]

Hypoxic-Ischemic Encephalopathy. Cerebral hypoxia can occur as a result of reduced blood oxygen content (hypoxemia), decreased cerebral blood flow (ischemia), or impaired oxygen extraction. Hypoxemia rarely occurs in isolation but frequently is accompanied by ischemia due to decreased cerebral perfusion as a result of compromised cardiovascular function. Asphyxia, which occurs more often in infants and children than in adults, implies the interruption of pulmonary exchange of oxygen and carbon dioxide. Normal compensatory mechanisms include increased systemic blood pressure and cerebral vasodilation in response to decreased arterial oxygen or increased carbon dioxide. Cerebral blood flow is also maintained within a narrow range despite fluctuation in systemic blood pressure through compensatory changes in cerebrovascular tone (autoregulation). Autoregulation may be ineffective in premature infants due to developmental factors and may be compromised at any age due to lactic acidosis or vascular endothelial injury. When compensatory mechanisms fail to provide sufficient cerebral perfusion and oxygen, delivery, a series of metabolic events ensue including an increase in anaerobic glycolysis and accumulation of lactic and pyruvic acid. Depletion of high-energy phosphate molecules leads to a failure to maintain Na^+-K^+ concentration gradients and transmembrane potentials. With prolonged hypoxia, function and structural integrity of cerebral neurons are imperiled.

The EEG provides a sensitive means of following the neurophysiologic events that accompany cerebral hypoxia. Total interruption of both blood flow and oxygen delivery during cardiac arrest in adults is accompanied by sequential changes in the EEG.[24] During the first 6 seconds of the arrest, neither clinical nor EEG changes are detected. Within 7 to 13 seconds, however, slow waves of increasing amplitude appear. With cessation of circulation lasting longer than 13 seconds, high-amplitude rhythmic delta appears diffusely. Further interruption in cerebral perfusion results in attenuation and ultimately flattening of all EEG activity. Restoration of cerebral perfusion after a brief arrest is followed by reversal of the previously described EEG changes in a reverse order to which they occurred.

Although hypothermia may provide some protective effects, normothermic patients who sustain profound hypoxic-ischemic insults lasting longer than 4 to 8 minutes suffer irreversible brain damage. The EEGs in such patients show a variety of patterns, some of which have significance in predicting neurologic outcome. A variety of schemata have been proposed for prediction of outcome in adults.[25,26] Typically, patients with normal or near-normal EEG tracings have an excellent prognosis for survival and neurologic recovery. Patients with bursts of polymorphic delta alternating with periods of voltage attenuation (suppression-burst pattern) or unremitting voltage suppression have a poor prognosis for survival and meaningful neurologic recovery. Patients with mild or moderate EEG abnormalities show variable outcomes that may be clarified with serial recordings. Rapidly improving EEGs correlate with better neurologic outcomes. Serial EEGs have prognostic value in children suffering uncomplicated cardiac arrest.[26]

Caution must be exercised in interpretation of EEGs obtained soon after cardiac arrest. EEG activity may return after electrocerebral silence lasting as long as 1 hour.[27] EEGs obtained to provide prognostic information should, therefore, be delayed 5 to 6 hours after a hypoxic-ischemic insult. The potential for drug intoxication and hypothermia to produce profound but reversible EEG abnormalities must also be considered in the interpretation of the EEG obtained after a hypoxic-ischemic insult.

Less common EEG abnormalities associated with anoxic encephalopathy include tracings with frontally dominant triphasic waves similar to those seen with hepatic encephalopathy or short-interval periodic sharp waves similar to those of Creutzfeldt-Jakob disease.[28] Patients with periodic complexes often exhibit myoclonic jerks in conjunction with the sharp waves.[29] The prognosis of patients with this pattern is extremely grave. Other patterns that may follow hypoxic-ischemic brain injury include long-interval periodic complexes resembling those in subacute sclerosing panencephalitis. PLEDs similar to those in herpes simplex encephalitis may also occur.[30]

Patients rendered comatose after cardiopulmonary arrest may exhibit diffuse invariant fast activity within the alpha frequency range with little or no reactivity to stimulation. Originally described in adults, this pattern has also been observed in infants and young children.[31,32] Although cardiopulmonary arrest is the most common cause of alpha coma, other etiologies include brainstem infarction and drug intoxication.[33] Patients with alpha coma due to drug intoxication may recover uneventfully;[34] those having suffered a cardiopulmonary arrest almost always do poorly.[2,34,35]

Hypothermia and Hyperthermia. Significant reduction in core body temperature, below 90°F (32.2°C) may occur accidentally, such as a result of drug intoxication or cold water immersion, or iatrogenically during cardiac surgery. Patients undergoing iatrogenic hypothermia during open heart surgery have been studied with serial EEGs.[36-38] At core body temperatures less than 30°C, the EEG initially shows high-amplitude slowing followed by voltage attenuation.[27] Suppression-burst patterns become evident at 20°C to 22°C. Complete electrocerebral silence usually appears below 17°C. It is possible that a combination of illness, treatment (anesthetics, anticonvulsants), and hypothermia might produce a reversibly isoelectric EEG above 17°C. Such temperatures, however, would be well below those seen in most clinical situations.[39]

Elevated body temperature, without complicating systemic illness, produces mild EEG changes. Hyperthermia (as high as 42°C) may result in reversible slowing and voltage suppression.[39]

ENCEPHALOPATHIES RELATED TO SPECIFIC ORGAN FAILURE

Liver Disease. Hepatic encephalopathy is characterized clinically by a continuum of changes in mental status from apathy, euphoria, and irritability to impaired cognitive function, lethargy, stupor, and coma. Asterixis is a characteristic sign consisting of recurrent abrupt loss of muscle tone of the outstretched and dorsiflexed hands that appears early in the course of disease. The biochemical mechanisms of hepatic encephalopathy remain controversial. Severity of signs and symptoms usually parallels concentrations of blood ammonia. Altered metabolism of free fatty acids, amino acids, as well as accumulation of false neurotransmitters have been implicated in the pathogenesis of hepatic encephalopathy.[40-44]

The EEG abnormalities associated with hepatic encephalopathy usually correlate well with changes in mental status. Patients with mild encephalopathy (lethargy and confusion) have EEG findings that include slowing of the alpha rhythm and progressive replacement of the background by slower frequencies. Bursts of medium- to high-amplitude delta activity may be superimposed on well-preserved alpha rhythm. With the onset of moderate encephalopathy, the patient is stuporous but briefly arousable to stimulation. It is during this precomatose state that triphasic waves are commonly seen.

Originally described as *blunt spike-waves,* triphasic waves are recurrent high-amplitude transients with an initial low-voltage surface-negative component followed by a surface-positive sharp wave and a long-duration slow wave that recur with a frequency of 2 to 4 Hz (Fig. 16-4).[45] Although characteristic of hepatic encephalopathy, triphasic waves may also be seen in renal insufficiency, postanoxic encephalopathy, hyponatremia, hypercalcemia, hyperthyroidism, and drug intoxication.[12,22,28,46,47] The following features have been described as typical triphasic waves in

hepatic encephalopathy: anteriorly predominant, bilaterally symmetrical, and synchronous, occurring in groups or runs with a progressive time lag in the surface-positive component from anterior to posterior head regions.[48,49]

With progressive obtundation, the EEG is characterized by frontally dominant, high-amplitude rhythmic delta activity. Profound coma is heralded by progressive voltage attenuation, occasional periods of generalized flattening, and, ultimately, electrocerebral silence.

Reye's syndrome is an acute systemic illness of childhood associated not only with hepatic dysfunction but also with cerebral edema due to incompletely understood toxic or metabolic factors. Its incidence has seen a sharp decline in parallel with the decline in the use of aspirin and antiemetics in the pediatric age group.[50] Biochemical abnormalities include hyperammonemia, hypoglycemia, and increased levels of short-chain fatty acids. Clinical features vary from vomiting and headache in mild cases to coma with increased intracranial pressure in severe cases. Death may occur due to transtentorial herniation and brainstem compression. EEG abnormalities associated with this illness have been studied in detail by Aoki and Lombroso.[51] Various degrees of EEG slowing on tracings obtained shortly after hospital admission were found to correlate not only with mental status but also with eventual outcome. Mild EEG changes (grade 1 or 2), manifested by slowing of the background activity to the theta-delta range, were associated with a 100% survival rate. Patients showing severe EEG abnormalities (grade 4 or 5) including an invariant background of low-amplitude delta activity or a suppression-burst pattern either died or survived with profound neurologic sequelae. An intermediate degree of EEG changes (grade 3) was associated with a 50% chance of recovery. Although EEGs obtained before institution of therapy were helpful as prognostic indicators, serial EEG studies were even more useful in predicting outcome.

Triphasic waves are rarely observed in this disorder despite the presence of significant hepatic dysfunction. Interictal epileptiform features are also uncommon even in those children who experience clinically apparent seizures during their acute illness. An interesting EEG phenomenon of uncertain clinical significance is the occurrence of bursts of 14/ and 6/sec positive spikes in as many as 50% of children with Reye's syndrome.[52] Fourteen/ and 6/sec positive spikes are not unique to Reye's syndrome and may be seen in other diffuse encephalopathies as well as in normal subjects.[53]

Renal Insufficiency. Although a variety of metabolic abnormalities can be seen in renal insufficiency, no single metabolic disturbance is directly correlated with the degree of encephalopathy or the type of EEG changes. Nonetheless, elevation of the blood urea nitrogen concentration is a strong biochemical predictor for the degree of EEG

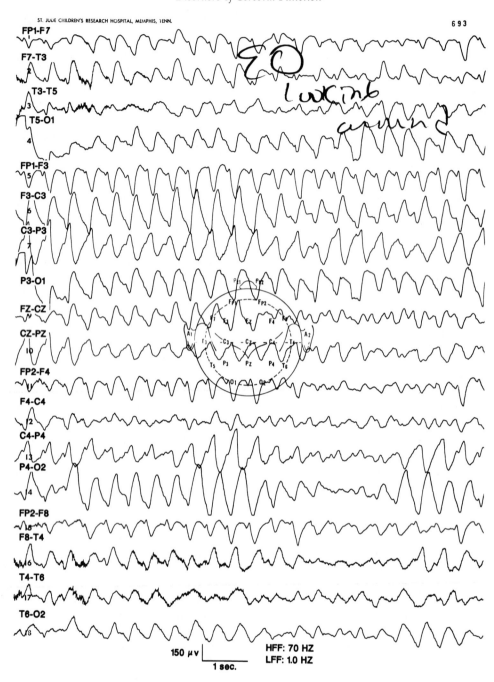

FIGURE 16–4

Triphasic waves in a 10-year-old boy with lethargy and hepatic dysfunction following treatment with L-asparaginase for acute lymphoblastic leukemia.

abnormality.[6] The EEG typically remains normal despite biochemical evidence of mild uremia. By the time the patient exhibits clinically evident changes in mental status (agitation, confusion, and tremor), the EEG shows slowing of the alpha rhythm and scattered runs of generalized theta activity. With progression to moderate encephalopathy (lethargy, fasciculations, and myoclonus), the background is replaced by generalized theta with superimposed bursts of anteriorly dominant, bilaterally synchronous delta activity. There may be a paradoxical response to alerting maneuvers such as accentuation of the occipital background rhythm with eye opening.[54] Triphasic waves can also be observed in renal encephalopathy.[46] Photomyoclonic or photoparoxysmal responses may be elicited with photic stimulation. There also may be an exaggerated response to hyperventilation manifested by prolonged high-amplitude generalized delta activity.[4] Bilaterally synchronous bursts of spikes and spike-wave activity are reported in some children with progressive renal encephalopathy.[55] Multifocal myoclonic jerks may occur with or without apparent association to recorded EEG discharges.[56]

Dialysis disequilibrium syndrome is a term applied to a clinical condition in which patients with renal failure develop headache, fatigue, nausea, vomiting, and, in some cases, convulsive seizures during or shortly after hemodialysis. This syndrome may be related to abrupt changes in osmotic gradients between the intracellular fluid compartment of the brain and the extracellular fluid compartment of blood and cerebrospinal fluid (CSF). A lag in the removal of urea or other osmotically active molecules presumably results in an osmotic gradient across the blood-brain barrier that favors movement of water into the brain. EEG changes include the presence of high-amplitude rhythmic delta activity superimposed on either a normal background or a background of irregular slowing.[57] These changes may occur during dialysis even without clinical signs or symptoms. Improvements in dialysis technique have resulted in reduction in the incidence of dialysis disequilibrium syndrome.[4]

Subacute progressive dialysis encephalopathy (dialysis dementia) is a slowly progressive, potentially fatal condition manifested clinically in patients with chronic renal failure by dementia, speech impairment, behavioral disturbances, and myoclonic jerks. Although histologic changes in the brain are nonspecific, elevated concentrations of aluminum in the gray matter of affected patients have been reported.[58] Aluminum accumulation in the brain is presumably related to elevated concentrations of aluminum in dialysis fluid or ingestion of excessive amounts of antacid preparations containing aluminum hydroxide. Patients with dialysis dementia have abnormal EEG findings, including diffuse slowing of the background with superimposed bursts of bilaterally synchronous FIRDA and generalized bursts of repetitive frontally dominant sharp and slow wave complexes. These EEG abnormalities may be present several months before the onset of clinical signs or symptoms.[59]

Thyroid Function. Infants with congenital hypothyroidism have EEG changes including slowing of the background activity and voltage attenuation.[60,61] Delay in the ontogeny of sleep spindles has also been reported.[62] In adults, hypothyroidism is associated with slowing of the alpha rhythm and generalized decrease in amplitude of the background activity.[63] Discontinuation of thyroid replacement therapy has been reported to produce a decrease in the frequency of the alpha rhythm and a decrease in the amplitude of photic driving.[64] Coma is a rare but serious complication of profound hypothyroidism. The EEG in this condition shows low-amplitude generalized slowing in the theta-delta frequency range.

Hyperthyroidism is associated with an increase in the frequency of alpha rhythm and accentuation of beta activity in the 15- to 30-Hz range.[65,66] EEG changes often persist after initiation of appropriate therapy despite establishing a euthyroid state. Thyroid crisis precipitated by surgery or infection may result in the appearance of slowing in the theta-delta range and bursts of either irregular or rhythmic delta activity.[9] Triphasic waves have also been reported in patients with hyperthyroidism and altered mental status.[47]

Cranial Irradiation. Radiation therapy constitutes the backbone of treatment for primary and metastatic tumors of the CNS. Lower doses of so-called prophylactic irradiation are also used in childhood leukemia for the elimination of occult residual disease within sanctuary sites shielded from systemic chemotherapy by the blood-brain barrier. Somnolence syndrome is a transient disorder following cranial irradiation at doses as low as 1800 cGy. Symptoms range from mild drowsiness to marked lethargy, anorexia, nausea, vomiting, headache, ataxia, and low-grade fever.[67,68] Acute lymphoblastic leukemia (ALL) may be associated with EEG slowing at the time of diagnosis even in the absence of detectable CNS involvement.[69] Although an increase in the mean alpha frequency has been noted following induction therapy and prophylactic cranial irradiation, an abrupt drop in mean alpha frequency typically occurs at the onset of somnolence syndrome.[67] Slowing of the background EEG becomes less marked as clinical symptoms of somnolence syndrome resolve; however, the mean alpha frequency remains significantly lower than normal controls up to 4 years after diagnosis.

In contrast with the mild, transient symptoms of the somnolence syndrome, late effects of therapeutic irradiation are potentially more severe and often irreversible. The most common late effects of irradiation associated with childhood cancer therapy are a consequence of injury to glial cells, especially oligodendroglia, and damage to cerebral vasculature. Neurons are comparatively insensitive to doses of ionizing irradiation within the usual therapeutic range. The clinicopathologic correlates of delayed radiation effects include subacute leukoencephalopathy and mineralizing microangiopathy.[70,71]

Subacute leukoencephalopathy is an uncommon form of delayed neurotoxicity that occurs primarily in children treated with cranial irradiation together with intrathecal or systemic methotrexate.[70,72,73] Children with ALL treated with all three modalities appear to be at greatest risk for developing this complication.[73] Leukoencephalopathy may, however, also occur in children treated with either intrathecal or intravenous methotrexate or cranial irradiation alone, especially when given at high doses. Cumulative methotrexate dose and prior cranial irradiation (>2000 cGy) are major risk factors for leukoencephalopathy. Other potential contributing factors include the presence of CNS leukemia, meningitis, hydrocephalus, or other causes of delayed CSF resorption.[74] Demyelination, focal areas of white matter necrosis, and reactive gliosis are the characteristic histopathologic features of leukoencephalopathy.[70] Axonal swelling and fragmentation may also occur, although gray matter is largely spared. In fulminant cases, focal areas of necrosis become confluent, leading to extensive areas of white matter degeneration and cavitation.

Clinically, leukoencephalopathy becomes evident within 4 to 12 months after completion of cranial irradiation. Early symptoms include decline in school performance, personality changes, and gait disturbance. Mild confusion, lethargy, dysarthria, aphasia, and ataxia may be followed in severe cases by progressive dementia, spasticity, and seizures. Although decerebration, coma, and death may ensue, neurologic signs and symptoms more often become stabilized. Although some improvement occurs over time, most affected individuals are left with static neurologic deficits.

The EEG is almost always abnormal in patients with clinically evident leukoencephalopathy. EEG changes comprise diffuse and generalized slowing, with or without focal findings. Epileptiform features are often seen in late survivors of severe leukoencephalopathy (Fig. 16-5).

Mineralizing microangiopathy is a specific histopathologic lesion attributable to radiation-induced injury to the cerebral vasculature. Histologic findings include the accumulation of calcium and mucopolysaccharides within and around smaller arteries, arterioles, capillaries, and venules within the brain.[71] Occlusion of affected vascular structures is associated with necrosis of adjacent brain parenchyma and deposition of calcified debris. In contrast with subacute leukoencephalopathy, mineralizing microangiopathy involves primarily the gray matter. The basal ganglia, especially the putamen, are most commonly affected, followed in frequency by the cerebral and cerebellar cortex along the junction between gray and white matter.

In contrast with subacute leukoencephalopathy, mineralizing microangiopathy usually produces mild or transient neurologic symptoms. Affected individuals may show no signs of neurologic dysfunction despite extensive calcifications.[71] In patients with both microangiopathy and leukoencephalopathy, the predominant clinical features are those of leukoencephalopathy. In general, the EEG has not proved to be useful in predicting which patients are at higher risk for developing microangiopathy, leukoencephalopathy, or other late treatment effects.[75,76]

INBORN ERRORS OF METABOLISM

This section reviews representative examples of heritable metabolic disorders caused by disturbances of intermediary metabolism. Those inborn errors related to peroxisomal, mitochondrial, or lysosomal enzyme defects are discussed under the section on neurodegenerative diseases.

Phenylketonuria (PKU). Phenylalanine is an essential amino acid which is a constituent of the normal diet. Once absorbed, this amino acid is used either directly for protein synthesis or converted to tyrosine via phenylalanine hydroxylase. Tyrosine in turn serves as a substrate for the synthesis of thyroxine, melanin, and the neurotransmitters dopamine, epinephrine, and norepinephrine. Deficiency of phenylalanine hydroxylase results in an accumulation of phenylalanine, which, at sufficiently high concentrations, is converted into phenylpyruvic acid via phenylalanine transaminase. Elevated plasma levels of phenylalanine in the presence of normal dietary intake plus urinary excretion of phenylpyruvic acid, phenylacetic acid, and other metabolites constitute the biochemical hallmarks of the relatively common and potentially devastating illness, PKU. Brain injury in patients with PKU appears to be mediated by the inhibitory effects of phenylalanine on the transport of large neutral amino acids such as tyrosine and tryptophan. Postmortem examination of inadequately treated older patients reveals demyelination involving the white matter of the cerebral hemisphere, optic tracts, and cerebellum. Decreased numbers of cortical neurons and disordered synaptic organization may also play an important role in the pathogenesis of clinically evident mental retardation, seizures, and behavioral disturbance.

Untreated patients with PKU frequently appear normal at birth. Delay in acquisition of developmental milestones, both social and motor, is usually evident by 6 months of age. Physical signs include skin color that is lighter than other family members, eczema, and a musty odor caused by phenylacetic acid excretion. Mandatory screening of newborn blood permits early detection of elevated phenylalanine levels and referral of patients with suspected PKU to appropriate centers for confirmation and initiation of dietary restriction.

Patients with PKU diagnosed and treated early have normal or minimally abnormal EEGs.[77] Most patients in whom diagnosis is delayed beyond 6 months or dietary restriction is inadequate have abnormal EEGs.[77] EEG findings often include slowing of the background activity and epileptiform features such as multifocal sharp waves and spike-and-wave discharges. Analysis of EEG activity by fast Fourier transformation in patients given a diet containing higher amounts of phenylalanine has shown reversible decreases in mean power frequency.[78]

Branched-Chain Amino Aciduria (Maple Syrup Urine Disease [MSUD]). Catabolism of the amino acids

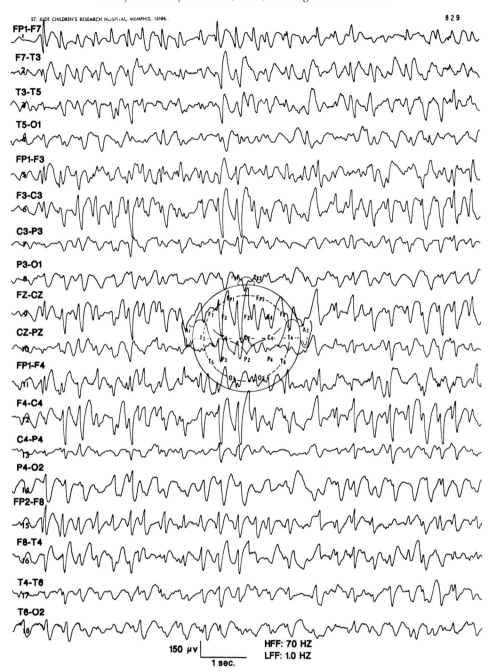

FIGURE 16–5

Generalized irregular slow activity and repetitive sharp and slow wave complexes arising synchronously from the right and left frontal derivations in an 18-year-old male with dementia and seizures due to subacute leukoencephalopathy following cranial irradiation and both systemic and intrathecal methotrexate.

leucine, valine, and isoleucine is mediated by the enzyme complex, branched-chain ketoacid decarboxylase (BCKD). Deficiency of BCKD activity results in the accumulation of the branched-chain amino acids and their ketoacid analogs. Hypoglycemia and profound ketoacidosis in affected infants

ensue, producing lethargy, poor feeding, seizures, increased intracranial pressure, opisthotonos, and coma within the first few weeks of life. The name *MSUD* is derived from the sweet odor of ketoacids in the sweat and urine. Now that MSUD is included in newborn blood screening in many states, its early diagnosis permits appropriate referral for evaluation and initiation of dietary restriction of branched-chain amino acids to an amount that maintains growth with the least ketoacidosis. Intermittent and intermediate forms of branched-chain amino aciduria occur, presenting with ataxia, unusual odor, and ketoacidosis, usually precipitated by infection or other stress.

In the past, untreated patients with classic MSUD usually succumbed to their disease within a year. Pathologic findings in such patients include cystic degeneration of the white matter and arrest of normal myelination. Laminar architecture of the cerebral cortex is disordered, implying a prenatal disturbance of neuronal migration despite the observation that affected infants appear normal at birth.

EEG recordings in patients with MSUD have typically shown high-voltage slowing. Patients with symptomatic disease have been noted to have epileptiform activity including independent multifocal spikes, polyspikes, and sharp wave discharges.[79]

Nonketotic Hyperglycinemia. Glycine, the simplest of all amino acids, plays a central role in a variety of synthetic pathways. This amino acid constitutes an important component in structural proteins such as collagen and also an important inhibitory neurotransmitter in the spinal cord and brainstem. Glycine catabolism provides a source of single carbon units for the synthesis of purines and porphyrins. A block in the enzymatic system for glycine cleavage is the presumed defect leading to nonketotic hyperglycinemia. This life-threatening condition results in the accumulation of large amounts of glycine in the blood, urine, and, in particular, CSF. In contrast with disorders of organic acid metabolism such as propionic acidemia, this inborn error is distinguished by the absence of marked ketosis.

The clinical phenotype of nonketotic hyperglycinemia is that of an overwhelming neonatal illness presenting within the first few days of life with lethargy, vomiting, anorexia, and seizures. Rapid deterioration into unresponsiveness, apnea, and coma often follows within 48 hours of the onset of symptoms. Vigorous metabolic and ventilatory support averts early demise. Despite such measures, survivors usually exhibit profound mental retardation and intractable seizures. Neuropathologic findings include cystic degeneration of the white matter, vacuolation, and loss of prenatally acquired myelin and delay in formation of new myelin.

The EEG in newborns with nonketotic hyperglycinemia typically shows a markedly discontinuous background or suppression-burst pattern.[80] Older infants may show diffuse high-voltage irregular slowing or hypsarrhythmia. Recordings in late survivors usually show multifocal spikes and spike-and-wave discharges.

Urea Cycle Defects. To prevent the accumulation of ammonia and other toxic nitrogenous compounds, excess nitrogen is incorporated into urea through a series of five enzymatic steps known as the *urea cycle*. Heritable defects in each of these steps are associated with well-documented clinical phenotypes. The time of onset and severity of symptoms are related to the magnitude of reduction in enzyme activity and the site of the enzyme within the urea cycle.[81] Urea cycle defects include carbamoylphosphate synthetase deficiency (CPSD), ornithine transcarbamylase deficiency (OTCD), argininosuccinate synthetase deficiency (ASD), argininosuccinate lyase deficiency (ALD), and arginase deficiency. Those enzymatic deficiencies closest to the entry of ammonia in the cycle (e.g., CPSD and OTCD) are associated with the highest levels of hyperammonemia and the most intense symptomatology.

Patients with CPSD, OTCD, ASD, and ALD may present in one of two ways: either acutely in the newborn period or as an episodic illness in late infancy, childhood, or early adulthood.[82] In the neonatal presentation, the affected infant appears normal at birth but exhibits lethargy and poor feeding between 24 to 72 hours. Additional signs and symptoms include irritability, vomiting, hypothermia, and hyperventilation. A bulging fontanelle and increasing head circumference may lead to the mistaken impression of intracranial hemorrhage. Cranial imaging typically reveals cerebral edema. Blood urea nitrogen is usually low and plasma ammonia is markedly elevated. Symptoms in the late-onset presentation may be precipitated by weaning from breast milk, introduction of cow's milk, or consumption of a high-protein meal. Stress or infection may also produce onset of symptoms that include vomiting, lethargy, agitation, disorientation, or ataxia. Seizures and developmental delay are also common.

EEG findings in the neonatal-onset group have been reported to include multifocal spikes, spike-and-wave complexes, sharp waves, and generalized slowing.[83] Restriction of dietary intake of protein in patients with symptoms due to episodic illness may lead to normalization of the EEG.

Disorders of Purine Metabolism (Lesch-Nyhan Syndrome). Guanine and hypoxanthine are generated by the catabolism of nucleic acids associated with normal cell lysis or turnover. Salvage of these purine bases is catalyzed by the enzyme hypoxanthine phosphoribosyl transferase (HPRT). The phosphorylated purines inosine monophosphate and guanine monophosphate are in turn precursors, not only for the synthesis of DNA and RNA but also for the synthesis of cofactors required for a variety of other enzymatic reactions. Deficiency of HPRT results in the accumulation of hypoxanthine, which is converted into uric acid by the enzyme xanthine oxidase. Partial deficiency of HPRT activity results in hyperuricemia and gouty arthritis. Complete deficiency is associated with the X-linked disorder known as *Lesch-Nyhan syndrome*.

Clinical manifestations of Lesch-Nyhan syndrome are absent at birth. Developmental delay becomes evident, however, by 6 months of age. Neurologic signs including hypotonia and fine athetoid movements of the hands and feet usually appear by 12 months. Later, spasticity, choreo-athetosis, dysarthria, mental retardation, and compulsive self-mutilation ensue. Seizures are not a prominent feature of this disease.

Consistent pathologic findings are absent on routine histologic examination of brain tissue obtained at the time of autopsy. Brown pigmentation of the cerebral cortex, loss of cells in the granular layer of the cerebellar cortex, and cerebellar atrophy have been reported. Depletion of dopamine within nerve terminals in the basal ganglia may play a role in the development of extrapyramidal signs in this disorder.[84]

The EEGs in patients with Lesch-Nyhan syndrome are either normal or mildly abnormal due to excessive slowing for age. In polysomnographic studies of the amount of slow wave and rapid eye movement (REM) sleep, the REM density and the frequency of REM bursts are decreased.[84a]

Disorders of Copper Transport. Copper is an integral component of several essential enzymes.[85] Examples include cytochrome oxidase, dopamine β-hydroxylase, and lysyl oxidase. Dietary copper is absorbed through the intestine at a site that is as yet unknown. On entering the plasma, copper is temporarily bound to albumin. After transport to the liver, copper is incorporated into ceruloplasmin, in which form more than 90% of serum copper is found. Two distinct diseases are associated with disorders of copper transport: Wilson's and Menkes'.

Wilson's Disease (Hepatolenticular Degeneration). In this disease biliary excretion and incorporation of copper into ceruloplasmin are both impaired.[86] Defective biliary excretion of copper leads to toxic accumulation in the liver and subsequently overflow of non-ceruloplasmin copper into the plasma and brain. Clinical manifestations begin in childhood or early adolescence with either liver disease or neurologic symptoms. Liver disease may present at any age beyond 6 years.[87] Neurologic symptoms are more frequent in young adults and are usually referable to basal ganglia involvement. These include slow, dysarthric speech, rigidity, masklike facies, and tremor. Deposition of copper in Descemet's membrane results in a yellow-brown stain at the limbus of the cornea referred to as a *Kayser-Fleisher ring*. This sign may be absent in children presenting with acute hepatic disease.

A diagnosis of Wilson's disease is supported by the laboratory findings of decreased serum ceruloplasmin, increased non-ceruloplasmin copper, and reduced total serum copper levels. Urinary excretion of copper is increased and is augmented by penicillamine. Analysis of tissue obtained by liver biopsy also shows increased levels of the metal.[87] Effective treatment consists of chelation of excessive free copper with penicillamine.[88] Postmortem examination of the

brain of patients with Wilson's disease is usually normal, although the basal ganglia may have a reddish discoloration. Neuropathologic changes in advanced cases include atrophy and cavitation of the basal ganglia.

The EEG in Wilson's disease has been described as either normal or nonspecifically abnormal. EEG changes, when present, parallel the severity of the underlying disease.[89] Markedly abnormal recordings are usually seen as a result of severe hepatic insufficiency.[90] Asymptomatic but affected siblings may have abnormal EEGs that improve with chelation therapy.

Menkes' Disease (Trichopoliodystrophy). This disorder is associated with a pervasive abnormality of intracellular copper transport that blocks incorporation of this metal into several critical enzymes.[91] Intracellular copper accumulates in the form of metallothionein. Defective intestinal absorption leads to systemic copper deficiency. Despite parenteral supplementation, however, copper enzyme activity remains deficient. Reduction of lysyl oxidase activity results in failure to form cross-linkages between collagen and elastin molecules. This produces extensive connective tissue changes involving the skin, joints, and large arteries. Defective formation of disulfide bonds in keratin leads to structural changes of the hair. Lack of tyrosinase activity causes depigmentation of the skin as well as hair. Deficient dopamine β-hydroxylase activity, required for the synthesis of dopaminergic neurotransmitters, may underlie the profound neurologic impairment associated with this disease.

Signs and symptoms of Menkes' disease often begin at birth with premature delivery, hypothermia, and hyperbilirubinemia. Other than fine hair texture, affected infants may otherwise appear normal until 3 months of age when seizures and developmental regression become evident. Characteristically the hair becomes twisted, brittle, and colorless. Skeletal radiographs show osteoporosis, flared metaphyses, and fractures, particularly of the ribs. Cerebrovascular complications including subdural hematoma may occur during the first year of life. Computed tomographic imaging shows cerebral atrophy and focal areas of decreased attenuation.[91,92] Arteriography demonstrates lengthening, tortuosity, and variable caliber of major arteries of the brain, viscera, and limbs.

The diagnosis of Menkes' disease is usually suspected on the basis of clinical findings alone. Supportive biochemical data include low levels of serum copper and ceruloplasmin and reduced copper content within liver tissue. Pathologic changes in the brain include neuronal loss in the cerebral cortex and cerebellum. Myelin is deficient presumably due to neuronal loss. Infarction and hemorrhage may be evident due to arterial changes. Findings within arteries of the brain and systemic vascular tree include aneurysmal dilation, rupture, stenosis, and thrombosis.

The EEG in Menkes' disease shows diffuse as well as focal abnormalities, including irregular slowing, spike-and-wave complexes, and hypsarrhythmia.[93]

Neurodegenerative Diseases

In the early stages of disease, neurodegenerative disorders usually express themselves by affecting primarily white matter or gray matter.[94] Disorders producing diffuse cerebral white matter damage result in abnormalities of the background EEG including continuous high-amplitude PDA with little epileptiform or paroxysmal activity. Those diseases that cause primarily gray matter damage produce bursts of intermittent rhythmic slow activity as well as epileptiform activity such as multifocal spikes and spike-and-wave discharges. With end-stage disease, diffuse cerebral injury results in EEG abnormalities consistent with both white and gray matter involvement.

The type of EEG abnormalities observed in a particular child with neurodegenerative disease reflects the pattern of neuroanatomic involvement, extent of disease progression, and level of brain maturation. In the neonatal period, diffuse gray matter injury is typically associated with a markedly discontinuous EEG or burst-suppression pattern. Later in infancy, a similar disease process may result in a background consisting of high-voltage irregular delta activity with superimposed multifocal spike and spike-wave discharges consistent with hypsarrhythmia. Diffuse gray matter disease in older children is frequently associated with a diffusely slow background with bursts of IRDA and frequent epileptiform discharges. Thus, the EEG findings depend not only on the type of neurodegenerative process but also on the age of the affected child and duration of disease at the time the recording is obtained.

Modern electrophysiologic techniques permit assessment of function of both the central and peripheral sensory pathways as well as that of sensory organs including the retina and cochlea. The electroretinogram (ERG) and visual evoked response (VER) help define whether visual loss is due to degeneration of the photoreceptive rods or cones versus disease affecting retinal ganglion cells or the central visual pathways. The ERG is attenuated in those diseases that are associated with retinal pigmentary degeneration. In contrast, the ERG is preserved in diseases in which there is lipid storage within the retinal ganglion cells and sparing of the rods and cones. VERs become abnormal as a result of retinal ganglion cell degeneration due to lipid accumulation. Abnormal VERs are also observed in diseases associated with either abnormal myelin formation or diffuse central white matter destruction. Brainstem auditory evoked responses (BAERs), somatosensory evoked potentials (SSEPs), and nerve conduction velocity (NCV) provide additional data regarding involvement of central and peripheral myelin.

Evoked potentials are considered in greater detail in the chapters devoted to each modality. Where appropriate, these neurophysiologic techniques are discussed in the context of particular neurodegenerative disorders.

Peroxisomal Diseases

Peroxisomes are important ultrastructural components of all mammalian cells except mature erythrocytes. Although especially abundant in the liver and kidney, they are also numerous in the cytoplasm of steroid-secreting cells of the adrenal cortex and myelin-forming cells of the central and peripheral nervous system. Anabolic functions of peroxisomes include synthesis of plasmalogens, ether phospholipids found in high concentration in myelin. Catabolic functions include beta oxidation of very long-chain fatty acids (VLCFAs) and peroxidative clearance of polyamines, pipecolic acid, and oxalate. Hydrogen peroxide generated by the latter reactions is converted to oxygen and water by the peroxisomal enzyme, catalase.

Peroxisomal dysfunction is associated with three groups of genetically determined diseases.[95] Group 1 includes those disorders with absent or decreased numbers of peroxisomes and deficiency of multiple peroxisomal enzymes. Group 2 comprises disorders with normal numbers of peroxisomes and a single enzyme deficiency. Those disorders with multiple peroxisomal enzyme defects despite normal numbers of peroxisomes are included in group 3. The clinical, pathologic, and EEG findings in diseases typical of the first two groups are reviewed in this section.

Zellweger's Syndrome and Variants (Group 1). Zellweger's syndrome is the prototype of disorders with defective peroxisomal biogenesis. Originally designated as cerebrohepatorenal syndrome, affected infants present in the newborn period with dysmorphic facial features, severe weakness, hypotonia, seizures, cataracts, glaucoma, and retinal pigmentary degeneration. The presumed defect in this disorder is a failure to import peroxisomal enzymes from the cytosol into their target organelles. As a result, peroxisomes are present but exist as nearly empty membranes or ghosts.

Biochemically, patients with Zellweger's syndrome have increased levels of VLCFAs in plasma and tissues, increased excretion of medium- and long-chain dicarboxylic acids, increased tissue accumulation of phytanic acid, and increased plasma levels of pipecolic acid.

In addition to the absence of normal peroxisomes, pathologic findings in Zellweger's syndrome include migrational abnormalities involving neurons destined to populate the cerebral cortex.[96] These migrational abnormalities cause the cerebral convolutions to be abnormally small (microgyria) or thick (pachygyria). Prominent white matter involvement is manifested by severe myelin deficiency and accumulation of sudanophilic lipids. Inclusions composed of cholesterol esters of VLCFAs are found in both white and gray matter.

Defective plasmalogen synthesis is thought to contribute to the severe myelin deficiency.

EEG recordings from infants with Zellweger's syndrome show repetitive spike and sharp wave activity during both wakefulness and sleep.[97] The ERG is abnormal or absent as a result of retinal pigmentary degeneration. Absent or delayed BAER waveforms and prolonged SSEP latencies are consistent with defective central and peripheral myelin formation.

Other examples of defective peroxisomal biogenesis include neonatal adrenoleukodystrophy (NALD), infantile Refsum's disease, and hyperpipecolic acidemia. NALD appears to be a variant of Zellweger's syndrome with less pronounced facial dysmorphism and longer survival. In addition to hypotonia and seizures, affected children also exhibit retinal pigmentary degeneration and sensorineural hearing loss. Biochemical and pathologic changes are similar to Zellweger's syndrome, only milder.

EEG findings in infants with NALD include high-amplitude slow activity as well as multifocal and generalized spike-and-wave discharges consistent with hypsarrhythmia.[98] The ERG in NALD is abnormal due to retinal pigmentary degeneration.[99] NCV is also prolonged, reflecting peripheral myelin involvement.[100]

X-Linked Adrenoleukodystrophy (ALD) (Group 2). This category of diseases is characterized by a defect involving a single peroxisomal enzyme. The most common example of this disease group is X-linked ALD. An impaired capacity to degrade saturated, unbranched fatty acids of 24- to 30-carbon chain length results in abnormally high levels of saturated VLCFAs in plasma as well as accumulation of cholesterol esters of VLCFAs in the adrenal gland, central white matter, and Schwann cells.[101] Several clinical phenotypes of this disorder have been described, including childhood ALD, adolescent ALD, adult-onset ALD, adrenomyeloneuropathy (AMN), and Addison's disease (adrenal insufficiency) without neurologic involvement.

The most common type of X-linked ALD is the childhood form, which typically presents between 3 and 8 years of age with behavioral changes, emotional lability, impaired attention, and school failure. These symptoms are rapidly followed by dementia, visual loss, focal or generalized seizures, and, ultimately, a vegetative state. Adrenal insufficiency is manifested by diminished secretion of cortisol and by skin hyperpigmentation due to the effects of increased production of adrenocorticotropic hormone and melanocyte-stimulating hormone.

Postmortem studies of the brain from patients with ALD show confluent and bilaterally symmetrical demyelination. Demyelination is most prominent within the parietooccipital region and centrum semiovale. White matter structures that are characteristically involved include the corpus callosum, posterior limb of the internal capsule, and optic tracts. In contrast, the cerebral cortex remains intact to gross inspection. Ultrastructural findings include the presence of electron-dense inclusions within macrophages of the central white matter, Schwann cells, and cells within the adrenal cortex. Gray matter is largely spared.

The EEG in childhood ALD often shows high-voltage irregular slowing that is most prominent over the posterior head regions. The ERG is normal, whereas the VER is abnormal in approximately a third of cases.[102] BAER findings include either increased latency to wave V or absence of waves III-V.[103] Abnormal BAER findings have also been reported in women who are heterozygous for ALD.[104] SSEP latencies are characteristically prolonged in patients with ALD and AMN and may also be prolonged in female ALD heterozygotes.[105]

Mitochondrial Encephalopathies

Although mitochondrial diseases involve multiple organ systems, the dependence of the brain and muscle on oxidative metabolism results in predominance of neurologic symptoms in the clinical presentation of these disorders.[106,107] The underlying biochemical defects associated with this group of diseases involve pyruvic acid metabolism, the citric acid cycle, and the respiratory chain. Lactic acidosis is the biochemical hallmark of many of these disorders. The characteristic histologic finding is the accumulation of abnormal mitochondria that can be seen in appropriately stained muscle biopsy specimens as "ragged red fibers." Although the list of neuromuscular diseases attributable to mitochondrial dysfunction is growing, three deserve specific mention.

Myoclonus Epilepsy and Ragged Red Fibers (MERRF). This disorder is characterized clinically by normal early development and the onset of myoclonus and ataxia beginning between 5 and 40 years of age.[107-109] Less consistent clinical features include dementia, hearing loss, and seizures (other than myoclonic). In addition to the presence of ragged red fibers on muscle biopsy, postmortem examination of the brain may show cystic cavitation of the periventricular white matter, demyelination, and neuronal loss described as spongiform degeneration.[110] EEG recordings in patients with MERRF have been reported to show slowing of the background activity and multifocal epileptiform discharges.[111,112] Enhanced photic driving and progressive deterioration of the background are not typical of this disorder.

Mitochondrial Encephalomyopathy, Lactic Acidosis, and Strokelike Episodes (MELAS). The occurrence of alternating hemiparesis, hemianopsia, or aphasia distinguishes this disorder from other mitochondrial encephalopathies.[107,113] Postmortem examination of brain tissue from affected individuals has reportedly shown multiple cerebral infarctions that were not in the distribution of specific cerebral arteries. Microcytic liquefaction, focal softening, and basal ganglia calcification are also prominent. EEG findings in MELAS have included diffuse as well as focal slowing and multifocal epileptiform discharges.

Kearns-Sayre Syndrome. This disorder is characterized by the occurrence of progressive external ophthalmoplegia and pigmentary retinopathy, typically before 20 years of age.[114] Common, but not invariant, findings include cardiac conduction defects, ataxia, and elevated CSF protein. Notably *absent* are myoclonus, seizures and strokelike episodes, although dementia and spongy degeneration of the brain may occur. EEG recordings have shown nonspecific slowing of the background activity.

Lysosomal Disease

Lysosomal disease is a group of disorders that includes those heritable diseases in which a normal lipid component of biologic membranes accumulates due to a defect in the sequential degradation of the stored lipid. Although usually classified on the basis of the type of stored material, the clinical presentation of various subtypes also depends on the extent of CNS versus visceral involvement and the specific enzymatic defect.

GM$_2$ Gangliosidosis (Tay-Sachs Disease). The ganglioside GM$_2$ is a complex glycolipid from which *N*-acetyl galactosamine is cleaved in normal individuals by the enzyme hexosaminidase A.[115] Deficient activity of this enzyme results in accumulation of GM$_2$ in neurons and astrocytes. The earliest clinical signs appear between 3 and 5 months of age and include mild weakness and irritability. Exquisite sensitivity to auditory stimuli results in a massive startle reflex in response to even subtle noises. Progressive weakness, hypotonia, and poor head control are usually evident between 6 and 10 months of age. Attention to visual cues and visual tracking may either begin to decline by 6 months or fail to develop. Progressive loss of vision becomes apparent by 12 months of age. Degeneration of affected retinal ganglion cells results in a gray appearance of the retina surrounding the normally pink fovea. Referred to as a "cherry red spot," this finding on funduscopic examination usually appears in the first few months of life. Seizure activity typically becomes manifest between 12 and 18 months of age. Progressive deterioration during the second year of life leads to decerebrate posturing, swallowing dysfunction, and unresponsiveness.

The EEG in infants with Tay-Sachs disease is often normal during the first year of life.[116] EEG findings during the second year include slowing of the background activity and the appearance of bursts of high-amplitude intermittent rhythmic delta (Fig. 16-6). With disease progression, there is gradual attenuation of the background voltage. Multifocal sharp waves and spike discharges as well as prolonged bursts of spikes or sharp waves may be observed with or without clinically evident seizure activity.

The ERG is characteristically normal in Tay-Sachs disease, reflecting the absence of retinal pigmentary degeneration.[117] The VER elicited by stroboscopic flash is preserved early in disease. Progressive visual loss due to lipid storage within retinal ganglion cells leads to attenuation and delay of VER waveforms. Giant VERs in response to photic stimulation are notably absent.

Generalized GM$_1$ Gangliosidosis. Absence of GM$_1$ β-galactosidase results in the accumulation of GM$_1$ ganglioside in neuronal and glial cells as well as liver and spleen. In the infantile form of this disease (type 1), mucopolysaccharide is also accumulated in the liver, bones, and soft tissues, resulting in an appearance similar to Hurler's syndrome. Neurologic manifestations in type I disease include severe retardation of intellectual and motor development with diffuse weakness despite brisk reflexes. Hyperacusis and macular cherry-red spots similar to Tay-Sachs disease are often present. Seizures occur after 6 months of age and gradually become a dominant feature of the disease. The juvenile form of this disease (type II) is characterized by a later onset of symptoms, slower course, and milder soft tissue and bony abnormalities. EEG usually demonstrates generalized slowing with occasional spike-and-wave discharges.[118]

Sphingomyelin Lipidosis (Niemann-Pick Disease). This disorder comprises several different subtypes that differ in age of onset of symptoms, extent of CNS involvement, and biochemical defect. The underlying biochemical defect in the acute or infantile form (type IA), subacute or juvenile form (type IS), and chronic or adult form (type IC) is a deficiency in the activity of sphingomyelinase. This enzyme catalyzes the hydrolysis of sphingomyelin to sphingosine and phosphoric acid. Accumulation of sphingomyelin occurs within the reticuloendothelial cells of the liver, spleen, lymph nodes, and bone marrow in all three forms of type I disease. Lack of sphingomyelinase activity in the CNS in children with type IA disease results in accumulation of lipid within neurons and glial cells of the brain, spinal cord, and retina.

Neurologic involvement in types IS and IC disease is either absent or minimal compared with the acute infantile form. Clinical manifestations of infantile Niemann-Pick disease include progressive intellectual and motor deterioration as well as hepatosplenomegaly. Macular degeneration results in the cherry-red spot in approximately 50% of cases. Seizures occur but not as commonly as in GM$_1$ or GM$_2$ lipidoses.

EEG findings in Niemann-Pick disease include background slowing, diffuse slow wave, and spike-wave discharges.[118] As in Tay-Sachs, the ERG is normal; progressive loss of VER amplitude occurs late in disease.

Galactoceramide Lipidosis (Krabbe's Disease). Galactocerebroside β-galactosidase normally catalyses the

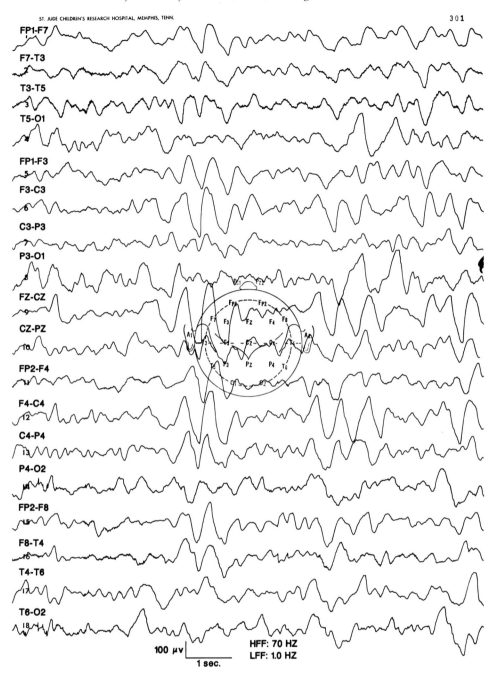

FIGURE 16–6

Intermittent high-voltage (100 to 200 μV) rhythmic slow activity in an 18-month-old boy with GM$_2$ gangliosidosis (Tay-Sachs disease).

cleavage of galactose from galactocerebroside. Deficiency of this enzyme activity results in a histologically distinctive pattern of white matter destruction described as globoid cell leukodystrophy. The characteristic finding in brain tissue from children with Krabbe's disease is the presence of perivascular clumps of reactive cells presumed to represent macrophages. The stimulus for invasion of macro-

phages (globoid cells) appears to be the presence of free galactocerebroside. Reactive macrophages in turn destroy myelin-producing oligodendroglia, resulting in extensive demyelination. It is this demyelination that is responsible for the clinical expression of this disorder.

Symptoms usually begin between 3 and 6 months of age with intermittent fevers of unknown origin, irritability, and hypertonicity of the lower extremities. Hepatosplenomegaly is notably absent. Episodes of tonic hyperextension of the extremities may be difficult to distinguish from generalized seizure activity. Although optic atrophy is usually present due to demyelination, lack of substantial lipid accumulation in retinal ganglion cells explains the absence of the cherry-red spot. With disease progression, the child usually becomes blind, deaf, and opisthotonic. Late in the disease, demyelination of the peripheral nerves may result in loss of muscle stretch reflexes.

The EEG in Krabbe's disease may be normal in the early stages of disease but later demonstrates moderate to large amounts of high-voltage polymorphic slowing consistent with diffuse white matter involvement.[119] Episodes of screaming with hyperextension of the trunk and either flexion or extension of the extremities may occur in the absence of EEG changes.

The ERG is reportedly normal in Krabbe's disease.[118] The VER shows a progressive decrease in waveform amplitude consistent with demyelination involving the optic nerve or pathway. Abnormal central auditory conduction is demonstrable with BAER.[120] Although central white matter involvement is the predominant feature of this disease, peripheral nerve conduction has also been documented electrophysiologically to be abnormal with NCV.[121]

Sulfatide Lipidosis (Metachromatic Leukodystrophy [MLD]). Deficient activity of aryl sulfatase A results in the accumulation of cerebroside sulfate due to a block in cleavage of the sulfate moiety from the parent lipid. When biopsy material or urinary sediment is stained with toluidine blue, this lipid exhibits a brown or gold color. This tinctorial property constitutes the basis of the name MLD.

MLD is a systemic disease affecting both central and peripheral myelin as well as kidney, pancreas, adrenal gland, liver, and gallbladder. Several variants of this disease are described, differing primarily in age of onset of symptoms. The late infantile form presents between 1 and 2 years of age with developmental delay, ataxia, and hypotonia. Progressive quadriparesis, bulbar signs, and intellectual decline proceed over the next 1 to 2 years. Muscle stretch reflexes are lost. Decerebrate posturing, optic atrophy, and seizures are occasionally seen late in the disease. The juvenile form of MLD results in symptoms beginning between 5 and 10 years of age with spasticity, ataxia, and dementia. Decerebrate posturing and generalized seizures occur late.[122] Patients with the adult form of MLD usually present with dementia and, occasionally, psychosis.

As with other progressive white matter diseases, the EEG in MLD may be normal early in the disease. Generalized polymorphic slow activity is seen with onset of clinical symptomatology. Spikes and sharp wave discharges are uncommon in MLD, although they may occur late in the

disease.[123] The BAER in late infantile MLD shows prolongation of interpeak latencies and loss of wave components consistent with delay or block in conduction in the eighth cranial nerve and brainstem.[124] Abnormalities in the VER and SSEP have also been reported.[125] NCV is slow in most cases and may provide evidence of MLD before the onset of clinical symptoms.[126]

Neuronal Ceroid-Lipofuscinoses (Batten's Disease). The neuronal ceroid-lipofuscinoses (NCLs) represent a group of disorders with similar histopathologic findings and clinical features.[127] Despite the lack of a clearly defined biochemical defect, the NCLs are linked by the characteristic finding of autofluorescent lipopigments in neurons in the CNS as well as in non-neural tissues outside the CNS. Four major varieties of NCL have been delineated on the basis of age of onset, initial symptomatology, and course of illness. Two forms present acutely with myoclonus, both epileptic and nonepileptic, visual loss, and dementia. The infantile form (Santavuori-Haltia disease, Finnish type) becomes symptomatic between 1 and 2 years of age with myoclonus, blindness, and retinal degeneration. The late infantile form (Bielschowsky-Jansky disease) typically presents between 2 and 3 years with intractable myoclonic seizures, ataxia, and dementia; visual loss is apparent later.

Although death by 10 to 12 years of age is common with the acute forms of NCL, slow progression and prolonged survival are associated with the chronic forms of this disease. Visual loss due to retinal degeneration beginning between 5 and 10 years of age is characteristic of the juvenile form of NCL (Spielmeyer-Vogt-Sjögren syndrome); dementia and seizures occur later. Adult NCL (Kufs' disease) usually presents in the 2nd or 3rd decade of life but may present in adolescence. Clinical features of adult NCL include extrapyramidal signs, ataxia, and myoclonus; visual loss and dementia are less prominent than in juvenile or infantile NCL.

Pathologic changes vary depending on the duration and severity of disease. Postmortem examination of the brain after advanced disease shows marked cerebral atrophy involving both gray and white matter. Neuronal loss is prominent in areas of severe atrophy. Ultrastructural findings include fusiform enlargement of the proximal segments of pyramidal neurons within the cerebral cortex. Cytosomal bodies containing either globular or lamellated deposits of lipopigment can be identified within cells of the nervous system as well as within non-neural tissues.

Electrophysiologic studies provide important supportive data in the evaluation of suspected NCL. In contrast to Tay-Sachs disease, the EEG is abnormal early in the course of NCL.[128] Normal occipital background activity is replaced by irregular slow activity over the posterior derivations. Bursts of diffuse, bilaterally synchronous slow activity are often observed. Spike-and-wave discharges are present during the early stages of disease and become increasingly prominent with disease progression. Slow spike-and-wave discharges may also be seen.

A characteristic feature of NCL is the presence of large-amplitude spikes in response to slow photic stimulation (≤ 3 flashes/sec) that is maximal over the posterior head regions and may reach 50 to 500 μV.[128-130] These giant flash VERs are sometimes accompanied by jerks of the limbs and face and occasionally by convulsive seizure activity. Late in the disease, the VER becomes attenuated and ultimately extinguished as blindness becomes clinically evident. The ERG is of low amplitude or absent altogether, reflecting the extent of retinal degeneration. In Tay-Sachs disease, the ERG is characteristically normal. Thus, the presence of exaggerated flash VERs and an attenuated ERG help distinguish early NCL from Tay-Sachs disease.

Rett Syndrome. The second most common cause of mental retardation in females, has been associated with mutations in MeCP2, the archetypical member of the methyl-CpG binding domain family of proteins.[130a] Although elevated blood ammonia levels were initially reported, no specific biochemical or histologic abnormalities in this disease have been confirmed.[131] Reduced levels of certain biogenic amines including 3-methoxy-4-hydroxyphenylethylene glycol (MHPG) and homovanillic acid (HVA) have been found in the CSF of girls affected with Rett syndrome.[132] MHPG is a metabolite of norepinephrine, and HVA, a metabolite of dopamine. Postmortem neuropathologic changes in Rett syndrome are nonspecific; they include mild cerebral atrophy, neuronal cell loss, and the presence of Alzheimer type II astrocytes.[133]

Clinical manifestations of Rett syndrome are usually noted between 6 and 18 months of age and include developmental delay and decreased head growth. Between 1 and 4 years of age, affected girls exhibit progressive dementia, autistic behavior, and stereotyped handwringing movements. Other symptoms include ataxia, intermittent hyperventilation, and seizures. After a period of apparent stabilization, progressive intellectual and motor impairment are evident between 5 and 15 years of age.

The EEG in Rett syndrome is abnormal in virtually all patients older than 3 years of age.[131] Findings consist of slowing of the background and progressive decrease in background voltage. Bursts of spike-and-wave complexes are noted occasionally during wakefulness and become especially prevalent during sleep.

Leukodystrophies of Unknown Etiology. This is a heterogenous group of disorders that have as their common feature a predilection for white matter destruction. Their infrequent occurrence and uncertain classification may explain the paucity of published data regarding the electrophysiologic findings associated with these disorders.

Spongy Degeneration of the Brain (Canavan's Disease). This progressive disease occurs with an autosomal dominant pattern of inheritance and produces extensive myelin destruction by an uncertain pathogenetic mechanism. Elevated levels of N-acetylaspartic acid have been reported in the urine of affected individuals.[134] Activity of the enzyme aspartoacylase also may be decreased in cultured fibroblasts. The significance of these biochemical changes has not been established. The definitive diagnosis of this disease has been made on the basis of characteristic neuropathologic findings. These include severe myelin loss, multiple vacuoles in the subcortical white matter and deeper layers of the cerebral cortex, and the presence of enlarged, often bizarre astrocytes (Alzheimer type II cells) within all layers of the cerebral cortex. Peripheral nerves appear normal. Loss of neurons within the cerebral cortex and cerebellum occurs as a late finding after longstanding disease.

Clinical manifestations vary depending on the age of presentation. The neonatal form presents acutely with impaired sucking and swallowing, frequent crying, and reduction of spontaneous movement. Respiratory compromise and death ensue within weeks. The infantile form constitutes the most common presentation with subacute onset within the first year of life. In retrospect, symptoms such as lethargy and hypotonia may be recognized as early as 3 months of age. Poor head control and macrocephaly are typical findings on physical examination. As the disease progresses, flaccidity gives way to spasticity and extensor posturing. The juvenile form of Canavan's disease presents after 5 years of age with progressive ataxia, spasticity, dementia, visual loss, and optic nerve atrophy.

The EEG may be paradoxically normal despite extensive demyelination.[135,136] Although evoked potential studies have not been examined extensively, abnormalities of the BAER and VER would be anticipated.

Alexander's Disease. This is a rare disorder with unproved genetic origin, unknown pathogenesis, and no consistent biochemical abnormalities. Clinical features include macrocephaly, spasticity, developmental arrest, and regression. The diagnosis of this disease rests on the neuropathologic findings of myelin destruction, arrest of myelin formation, and increased numbers of Rosenthal fibers. Rosenthal fibers are not specific for Alexander's disease and may be seen in a variety of diseases including low-grade astrocytomas, diffuse cerebral gliomatosis, neurofibromatosis, and multiple sclerosis.[137]

The EEG in Alexander's disease has not been reported to show significant or specific changes.

Pelizaeus-Merzbacher Disease. This X-linked disorder represents, in all likelihood, several different diseases with shared clinical and pathologic features. The neuropathologic findings include patchy demyelination with preservation of islands of intact myelin. Within demyelinated areas, neurons and axons are usually well preserved. Lipid products of myelin breakdown (triglycerides and cholesterol esters) stain positively with Sudan black. This has led to the term *sudanophilic leukodystrophy*. The absence of myelin breakdown products in certain cases suggests lack of myelin formation rather than myelin destruction.

This loosely defined group of disorders has been subdivided on the basis of age of onset and rate of disease progression.[138] Classic Pelizaeus-Merzbacher disease (type I) usually presents within the first few months of life. Early clinical features include nystagmus and head tremor. Disease progression is accompanied by developmental delay, ataxia, dysarthria, spasticity, and choreoathetosis. Optic atrophy and seizures may also occur. The connatal form (type II) presents at birth with involuntary (extrapyramidal) movements, nystagmus, and spasticity. Other forms include transitional (type III), adult (type IV) and variant (type V) presentations.

The EEG in Pelizaeus-Merzbacher disease shows nonspecific generalized slowing of the background with no focal or epileptiform features.[139] The ERG is reported to be normal, whereas the flash VER and BAER show conduction abnormalities consistent with demyelination within the visual and central auditory pathways.[120,125]

SUMMARY

One of the fascinations that the study of pediatric neurology brings to its practitioners is the constant demand to consider a variety of etiologies when faced with a child with an explained neurologic complaint. The experienced clinician regards each symptom and abnormal sign in the context of the child as a whole. Similarly, the EEG must be interpreted in the setting of the patient's age, symptomatology, onset of illness, tempo of progression, and concurrent therapy. Interpretation of the EEG without ancillary data and an awareness of developments in other areas of neurobiology are an invitation to error. A broad perspective allows the electroencephalographer to maintain clinical neurophysiology as an evolving science and prevent it from becoming an arcane art.

REFERENCES

1. Markand ON: Electroencephalography in diffuse encephalopathies. J Clin Neurophysiol 1984;1:357-407.
2. Austin EJ, Wilkus RJ, Longstreth WT: Etiology and prognosis of alpha coma. Neurology 1988;38:773-777.
3. Rae-Grant AD, Strapple C, Barbour PJ: Episodic low-amplitude events: An under-recognized phenomenon in clinical electroencephalography. J Clin Neurophysiol 1991;8:203-211.
4. Cadilhac J: The EEG in renal insufficiency. *In* Remond A (ed): Handbook of Electroencephalography and Clinical Neurophysiology. Amsterdam, Elsevier, 1976, p 51.
5. Gloor P, Kalaby O, Giard N: The electroencephalogram in diffuse encephalopathies: Electroencephalographic correlates of grey and white matter lesions. Brain 1968;91:779-802.
6. Hughes JR: Correlations between EEG and chemical changes in uremia. Electroencephalogr Clin Neurophysiol 1980;48:583-594.
7. Prensky AL, Coben LA: Electroencephalography. *In* Baker AB, Baker LH (eds): Clinical Neurology. Philadelphia, Harper & Row, 1983, p 143.
8. Brenner RP, Schaul N: Periodic EEG patterns: Classification, clinical correlation, and pathophysiology. J Clin Neurophysiol 1990;7:249-267.
9. Cadilhac J, Ribstein M: The EEG in metabolic disorders. World Neurol 1961;2:296-308.
10. Wilson DR: Electroencephalographic studies in diabetes mellitus. Can Med Assoc J 1951;65:462-465.
11. Maccario M, Messis CP, Vastola EF: Focal seizures as a manifestation of hyperglycemia without ketoacidosis: A report of seven cases with review of the literature. Neurology 1965;15:195-206.
12. Swash M, Rowan AJ: Electroencephalographic criteria of hypocalcemia and hypercalcemia. Arch Neurol 1972;26:218-228.
13. Glaser GH, Levy LL: Seizures and idiopathic hypoparathyroidism: A clinical-electroencephalographic study. Epilepsia 1960;1:454-465.
14. Cohn R, Sode J: The EEG in hypercalcemia. Neurology 1971;21:154-161.
15. Fishman RA: Neurological aspects of magnesium metabolism. Arch Neurol 1965;12:562-569.
16. Volpe JJ: Neurology of the Newborn, 3rd ed. Philadelphia, WB Saunders, 1995.
17. Shils ME: Experimental human magnesium depletion. Medicine 1969;48:61-85.
18. Riggs JE: Neurologic manifestations of fluid and electrolyte imbalances. Neurol Clin 1989;7:509-523.
19. Layzer RB: Mineral and electrolyte disorders. *In* Layzer RB (ed): Neuromuscular Manifestations of Systemic Disease. Philadelphia, FA Davis, 1985, p 47.
20. Somjen G, Hilmy M, Stephen CR: Failure to anesthetize human subjects by intravenous administration of magnesium sulphate. J Pharmacol Exp Ther 1966;154:652-659.
21. Alfrey AC, Terman DS, Brettschneider L: Hypermagnesemia after renal homotransplantation. Ann Intern Med 1970;73:367-371.
22. Crawford JD, Dodge PR: Complications of fluid therapy in neurologic disease: Water intoxication and hypertonic dehydration. Pediatr Clin North Am 1964;11:1029-1052.
23. Zwang HJ, Cohn D: Electroencephalographic changes in acute water intoxication. Clin Electroencephalogr 1981;12:35-40.

24. Meyer JS, Sakamoto K, Akiyama M, et al: Monitoring cerebral blood flow, metabolism, and EEG. Electroencephalogr Clin Neurophysiol 1967;23:497-508.

25. Hockaday JM, Potts F, Epstein E, et al: Electroencephalographic changes in acute cerebral anoxia from cardiac or respiratory arrest. Electroencephalogr Clin Neurophysiol 1965;18:575-586.

26. Pampiglione G, Harden A: Resuscitation after cardiovascular arrest: Prognostic evaluation and early electroencephalographic features. Lancet 1968;1:1261-1264.

27. Prior PF: The EEG in Acute Cerebral Anoxia. Amsterdam, Excerpta Medica, 1973.

28. Kuroiwa Y, Celesia GG, Chung HD: Periodic EEG discharges and status spongiosus of the cerebral cortex in anoxic encephalopathy: A necropsy case report. J Neurol Neurosurg Psychiatry 1982;45:740-742.

29. Nilsson BY, Olsson Y, Sourander P: Electroencephalographic and histopathologic changes resembling Jacob-Creutzfeld disease after transient cerebral ischemia due to cardiac arrest. Acta Neurol Scand 1972;48:416-426.

30. de la Paz D, Brenner RD: Bilateral independent periodic lateralized epileptiform discharges: Clinical significance. Arch Neurol 1981;38:713-715.

31. Homan RW, Jones MG: Alpha-pattern coma in a 2-month-old child. Ann Neurol 1981;9:611-613.

32. Yamada T, Stevland N, Kimura J: Alpha-pattern coma in a 2-year-old child. Arch Neurol 1979;36:225-227.

33. Kuroiwa Y, Furukowa T: EEG prognostication in drug-related alpha coma. Arch Neurol 1981;38:200.

34. Kaplan PW, Genoud D, Ho TW, Jallon P: Etiology, neurologic correlations, and prognosis in alpha coma. Clin Neurophysiol 1999;110:205-213.

35. Iragui VJ, McCutchen C: Physiologic and prognostic significance of "alpha coma." J Neurol Neurosurg Psychiatry 1983;46:632-638.

36. Fischer-Williams M, Cooper RA: Some aspects of the electroencephalographic changes during open heart surgery. Neurology 1964;14:472-482.

37. Harden A, Pampiglione G: EEG studies in children with circulatory arrest during hypothermia. Electroencephalogr Clin Neurophysiol 1966;21:202.

38. Reilly EL, Brunberg JA, Doty DB: The effect of deep hypothermia and total circulatory arrest on the electroencephalogram in children. Electroencephalogr Clin Neurophysiol 1974;36:661-667.

39. Reilly EL: Electroencephalographic inactivity as a temperature effect: unlikely as an isolated etiology. Clin Electroencephalogr 1981;12:69-71.

40. Gabuzda GJ: Ammonium metabolism and hepatic coma. Gastroenterology 1967;53:806-810.

41. Zieve L: The mechanism of hepatic coma. Hepatology 1981;1:360-365.

42. Jones EA, Schafer DF, Ferenci P, Pappas SC: The neurobiology of hepatic encephalopathy. Hepatology 1984;4:1235-1242.

43. Fraser CL, Arieff AL: Hepatic encephalopathy. N Engl J Med 1985;313:865-873.

44. Fischer JE: False neurotransmitters and hepatic coma. In Plum F (ed): Brain Dysfunction in Metabolic Disorders. New York, Raven Press, 1974, p 53.

45. Foley JM, Watson CW, Adams RD: Significance of the electroencephalographic changes in hepatic coma. Trans Am Neurol Assoc 1950;75:161-164.

46. Simsarian JP, Harner RN: Diagnosis of metabolic encephalopathy: Significance of triphasic waves in the electroencephalogram. Neurology 1972;22:456.

47. Hirano M, Endo M, Kubo T: Triphasic waves in a case of hyperthyroidism with psychotic symptoms. Clin Electroencephalogr 1982;13:97-102.

48. Reiher J: The electroencephalogram in the investigation of metabolic coma. Electroencephalogr Clin Neurophysiol 1970;28:104.

49. Karnaze DS, Bickford RG: Triphasic waves: A reassessment of their significance. Electroencephalogr Clin Neurophysiol 1984;57:193-198.

50. Casteels-van Daele M, Van Geet C, Wouters C, Eggermont E: Reye syndrome revisited: A descriptive term covering a group of heterogeneous disorders. Eur J Pediatr 2000;159:641-648.

51. Aoki Y, Lombroso C: Prognostic value of electroencephalography in Reye's syndrome. Neurology 1973;23:333-343.

52. Yamada T, Young S, Kimura J: Significance of positive spike bursts in Reye syndrome. Arch Neurol 1977;34:376-380.

53. Drury I: 14 and 6 positive bursts in childhood encephalopathies. Electroencephalogr Clin Neurophysiol 1989;72:479-485.

54. Jacob JC, Gloor P, Elwan OH, et al: EEG changes in chronic renal failure. Neurology 1965;15:419-429.

55. Stockard JJ, Trauner DA: Distinctive EEG abnormalities in progressive renal encephalopathy of childhood: Similarity to those in progressive dialysis dementia (PDA). Electroencephalogr Clin Neurophysiol 1984;57:60P.

56. Tyler HR: Neurologic disorders in renal failure. Am J Med 1968;44:734-748.

57. Kennedy AC, Linton AL, Luke RG, Renfrew S: EEG changes during hemodialysis. Lancet 1963;1:408-411.

58. Alfrey AC, LeGendre GR, Kaehny WD: The dialysis encephalopathy syndrome: Possible aluminum intoxication. N Engl J Med 1976;294:184-188.

59. Hughes JR, Schreeder MT: EEG in dialysis dementia. Neurology 1980;30:1148-1159.

60. Nieman EA: The electroencephalogram in congenital hypothyroidism: A study of 10 cases. J Neurol Neurosurg Psychiatry 1961;24:50-57.

61. Harris R, Della-Rovere MD, Prior P: Electroencephalographic studies in children with hypothyroidism. Arch Dis Child 1965;40:612-617.

62. Schultz MA, Schulte FJ, Akiyama Y, Parmelee AH: Development of sleep phenomenon in hypothyroid infants. Electroencephalogr Clin Neurophysiol 1968;25:351-358.

63. Browning TB, Atkins R, Weiner M: Cerebral metabolic disturbances in hypothyroidism: Clinical and EEG studies of the psychosis of myxedema and hypothyroidism. Arch Intern Med 1954;93:939-950.

64. Lansing RW, Trunnell JB: Electroencephalographic changes accompanying thyroid deficiency in man. J Clin Endocrinol Metab 1963;23:470-480.

65. Condon JV, Becka DR, Gibbs FA: Electroencephalographic abnormalities in endocrine disease. N Engl J Med 1954;251:638-641.

66. Wilson WP, Johnson JE: Thyroid hormone and brain function: I. The EEG in hyperthyroidism with observations on the effect of age, sex, and reserpine in the production of abnormalities. Electroencephalogr Clin Neurophysiol 1964;16:321-328.

67. Freeman JE, Johnson PGB, Voke JM: Somnolence after prophylactic cranial irradiation in children with acute lymphoblastic irradiation. BMJ 1973;4:523-525.

68. Ch'ien LT, Aur RA, Stagner S, et al: Long-term neurologic implications of somnolence syndrome in children with acute lymphoblastic leukemia. Ann Neurol 1980;8:273-277.

69. Epstein CM, Humphries LL, Alvarado CS, et al: Sequential quantitative EEG analysis in acute lymphocytic leukemia of children. Clin Electroencephalogr 1985;16:208-212.

70. Price RA, Jamieson PA: The central nervous system in childhood leukemia: II. Subacute leukoencephalopathy. Cancer 1975;35:306-318.

71. Price RA, Birdwell DA: The central nervous system in childhood cancer: III. Mineralizing microangiopathy and dystrophic calcification. Cancer 1978;42:717-728.

72. Rubinstein LJ, Herman MM, Long TF, Wilbur JR: Disseminated necrotizing leukoencephalopathy: A complication of treated central nervous system leukemia and lymphoma. Cancer 1975;35:291-305.

73. Bleyer WA: Neurologic sequelae of methotrexate and ionizing radiation: A new classification. Cancer Treat Rep 1981;65(Suppl 1):89-98.

74. Duffner PK, Cohen ME, Brecher ML, et al: CT abnormalities and delayed methotrexate clearance in children with CNS leukemia. Neurology 1984;34:229-233.

75. Ochs J, Mulhern R, Fairclough D, et al: Comparison of neuropsychologic functioning and clinical indicators of neurotoxicity in long-term survivors of childhood leukemia given cranial radiation or parenteral methotrexate: A prospective study. J Clin Oncol 1991;9:145-151.

76. Carli M, Perilongo G, Laverda AM, et al: Risk factors in long-term sequelae of central nervous system prophylaxis in successfully treated children with acute lymphocytic leukemia. Med Pediatr Oncol 1985;13:334-340.

77. Rolle-Daya H, Pueschel SM, Lombroso CT: Electroencephalographic findings in children with phenylketonuria. Am J Dis Child 1975;129:896-900.

78. Krause W, Epstein C, Averbook A, et al: Phenylalanine alters the mean power frequency of electroencephalograms and plasma L-dopa in treated patients with phenylketonuria. Pediatr Res 1986;20:1112-1116.

79. Schwartz JF, Kolendrianos ET: Maple syrup urine disease: A review with a report of an additional case. Dev Med Child Neurol 1969;11:460-470.

80. Markand ON, Garg BP, Brandt IK: Nonketotic hyperglycinemia: Electroencephalographic and evoked potential abnormalities. Neurology 1982;32:151-156.

81. Breningstall GN: Diseases of ammonia metabolism. *In* Swaiman KF (ed): Pediatric Neurology: Principles and Practice. St. Louis, Mosby, 1989, p 959.

82. Brusilow SW, Horwich AL: Urea cycle enzymes. *In* Scriver CR, Beaudet AL, Sly WS, Valle D (eds): The Metabolic Basis of Inherited Disease. New York, McGraw-Hill, 1989, p 629.

83. Zhang L, Spigelman I, Carlen PL: Development of GABA-mediated, chloride-dependent inhibition in CA_1 pyramidal neurones of immature rat hippocampal slices. J Physiol 1991;444:25-49.

84. Lloyd KG, Hornykiewicz O, Davidson L, et al: Biochemical evidence of dysfunction of brain neurotransmitters in the Lesch-Nyhan syndrome. N Engl J Med 1981;305:1106-1111.

84a. Saito Y, Hanaoka S, Fukumizu M, et al: Polysomnographic studies of Lesch-Nyhan syndrome. Brain Dev 20:579-585.

85. Danks DM: Disorders of copper transport. *In* Scriver CR, Beaudet AL, Sly WS, Valle D (eds): The Metabolic Basis of Inherited Disease. New York, McGraw-Hill, 1989, p 1411.

86. Gibbs K, Walshe JM: Biliary excretion of copper in Wilson's disease. Lancet 1980;2:538-539.

87. Danks DM, Stevens BJ: Diagnosis of Wilson's disease in children with liver disease: A report of two families. Lancet 1969;1:22-25.

88. Walshe JM: Copper chelation in patients with Wilson's disease. Q J Med 1973;42:441-452.

89. Westmoreland BF, Goldstein NP, Klass DW: Wilson's disease: Electroencephalographic and evoked potential studies. Mayo Clin Proc 1974;49:401-404.

90. Hansotia P, Harris R, Kennedy J: EEG changes in Wilson's disease. Electroencephalogr Clin Neurophysiol 1969;27:523-528.

91. Danks DM: Copper transport and utilization in Menkes' syndrome and in mottled mice. Inorg Perspect Biol Med 1986;1:73.

92. Farrelly C, Stringer DA, Daneman A, et al: CT manifestations of Menkes' kinky hair syndrome (trichopoliodystrophy). J Can Assoc Radiol 1985;35:406-408.

93. Friedman E, Harden A, Koivikko M, Pampiglione G: Menkes' disease: Neurophysiological aspects. J Neurol Neurosurg Psychiatry 1978;41:505-510.

94. Freeman JM, McKhann GM: Degenerative diseases of the central nervous system. Adv Pediatr 1969;16:121-175.

95. Lazarow PB, Moser HW: Disorders of peroxisome biogenesis. *In* Scriver CR, Beaudet AL, Sly WS, Valle D (eds): The Metabolic Basis of Inherited Disease. New York, McGraw-Hill, 1990, p 1479.

96. Volpe JJ, Adams RD: Cerebro-hepato-renal syndrome of Zellweger: An inherited disorder of neuronal migration. Acta Neuropathol 1972;20:175-198.

97. Govaerts L, Colon E, Rotteveel J, Monnens L: A neurophysiologic study of children with the cerebro-hepato-renal syndrome of Zellweger. Neuropediatrics 1985;16:185-190.

98. Verma NP, Hart ZH, Nigro M: Electrophysiologic studies in neonatal adrenoleukodystrophy. Electroencephalogr Clin Neurophysiol 1985;60:7-15.

99. Aubourg P, Scotto J, Rocchiccioli F, et al: Neonatal adrenoleukodystrophy. J Neurol Neurosurg Psychiatry 1986;49:77-86.

100. Kelley RI, Datta NS, Dobyns WB, et al: Neonatal adrenoleukodystrophy: New cases, biochemical studies, and differentiation from the Zellweger and related peroxisomal polydystrophy syndromes. Am J Med Genet 1986;23:869-901.

101. Moser HW, Moser AB: Adrenoleukodystrophy (X-linked). *In* Scriver CR, Beaudet AL, Sly WS, Valle D (eds): The Metabolic Basis of Inherited Disease. New York, McGraw-Hill, 1990, p 1511.

102. Battaglia A, Harden A, Pampiglione G, Walsh PJ: Adrenoleukodystrophy: Neurophysiological aspects. J Neurol Neurosurg Psychiatry 1981;44:781-785.

103. Ochs R, Markand ON, DeMyer WE: Brainstem auditory evoked responses in leukodystrophies. Neurology 1979;29:1089-1093.

104. Moloney JBM, Masterson JC: Detection of adrenoleukodystrophy by means of evoked potential. Lancet 1982;2:852.

105. Garg BP, Markand ON, DeMyer WE, Warren C: Evoked response studies in patients with adrenoleukodystrophy and heterozygous relatives. Arch Neurol 1983;40:356-359.

106. DeVivo DC, DiMauro S: Mitochondrial encephalomyopathies. Int Pediatr 1990;5:112-120.

107. Garaschuk O, Linn J, Eilers J, Konnerth A: Large-scale oscillatory calcium waves in the immature cortex. Nature Neurosci 2000;3:452-459.

108. Fukuhara N, Tokiguchi S, Shirakawa S, Tsubaki T: Myoclonus epilepsy associated with ragged red fibers (mitochondrial abnormalities): Disease entity or syndrome? Light and electron microscopic studies of two cases and review of the literature. J Neurol Sci 1980;47:117-133.

109. Berkovic SF, Carpenter S, Evans A, et al: Myoclonus epilepsy and ragged-red fibers (MERRF): I. A clinical, pathological, biochemical, magnetic resonance spectrographic, and positron emission tomographic study. Brain 1989;112:1231-1260.

110. Fukuhara N: Myoclonus epilepsy and mitochondrial myopathy. *In* Scarlato G, Cerri C (eds): Mitochondrial Pathology in Muscle Diseases. Padova, Piccin, 1983.

111. Serra G, Piccinnu R, Tondi M, et al: Clinical and EEG findings in eleven patients affected by mitochondrial encephalomyopathy with MERRF-MELAS overlap. Brain Dev 1996;18:185-191.

112. Canafoglia L, Franceschetti S, Antozzi C, et al: Epileptic phenotypes associated with mitochondrial disorders. Neurology 2001;22:1340-1346.

113. Pavlakis SG, Phillips PC, DiMauro S, et al: Mitochondrial myopathy, encephalopathy, lactic acidosis, and strokelike episodes: A distinctive clinical syndrome. Ann Neurol 1984;16:481-488.

114. Rowland LP, Blake D, Hirano M, et al: Clinical syndromes associated with ragged red fibers. Rev Neurol 1991;147:473.

115. Kolodny EH: The GM$_2$ gangliosidoses. *In* Rosenberg RN, Prusiner SB, DiMauro S, et al (eds): The Molecular and Genetic Basis of Neurological Disease. Boston, Butterworth-Heinemann, 1993, p 531.

116. Pampiglione G, Privett G, Harden A: Tay-Sachs disease: Neurophysiological studies in 20 children. Dev Med Child Neurol 1974;16:201-208.

117. Pampiglione G, Harden A: Neurophysiological investigations in GM$_1$ and GM$_2$ gangliosidoses. Neuropediatrics 1984;15(Suppl):74-84.

118. Percy AK: The inherited neurodegenerative disorders of childhood: Clinical assessment. J Child Neurol 1987;2:82-97.

119. Kliemann FAD, Harden A, Pampiglione G: Some EEG observations in patients with Krabbe's disease. Dev Med Child Neurol 1969;11:475-484.

120. De Meirleir LJ, Taylor MJ, Logan WJ: Multimodal evoked potential studies in leukodystrophies of children. Can J Neurol Sci 1988;15:26-31.

121. Hogan GR, Gutmann L, Chou SM: The peripheral neuropathy of Krabbe's (globoid) leukodystrophy. Neurology 1969;19:1094-1100.

122. Haltia T, Palo J, Haltia M, Icen A: Juvenile metachromatic leukodystrophy: Clinical, biochemical, and neuropathologic studies in nine new cases. Arch Neurol 1980;37:42-46.

123. Mastropaolo C, Pampiglione G, Stephens R: EEG studies in 22 children with sulphatide lipidosis (metachromatic leucodystrophy). Dev Med Child Neurol 1971;13:20-31.

124. Doose H, Spranger J, Warner M: EEG in mucolipidosis I. Neuropädiatrie 1975;6:98-101.

125. Markand ON, Garg BP, DeMyer WE, et al: Brain stem auditory, visual, and somatosensory evoked potentials in leukodystrophies. Electroencephalogr Clin Neurophysiol 1982;54:39-48.

126. Clark JR, Miller RG, Vidgoff JM: Juvenile-onset metachromatic leukodystrophy: Biochemical and electrophysiologic studies. Neurology 1979;29:346-353.

127. Dyken PR: Neuronal ceroid lipofuscinoses. *In* Swaiman KF, Wright FS (eds): The Practice of Pediatric Neurology. St. Louis, CV Mosby, 1982, p 902.

128. Pampiglione E, Harden A: So-called neuronal ceroid lipofuscinosis: Neurophysiological studies in 60 children. J Neurol Neurosurg Psychiatry 1977;40:323-330.

129. Vas GA, Cracco JB: Diffuse encephalopathies. *In* Daly DD, Pedley TA (eds): Current Practice of Clinical

Electroencephalography, 2nd ed. New York, Raven Press, 1990, p 371.

130. Rapin I: Myoclonus in neuronal storage and Lafora diseases. *In* Fahn S, Marsden CD, Van Woert MH (eds): Myoclonus. New York, Raven Press, 1986, p 65.

130a. Amir RE, Van dV I, Wan M, et al: Rett syndrome is caused by mutations in X-linked MECP2, encoding methyl-CpG-binding protein 2. Nat Genet 1999;23:185–188.

131. Hagberg B, Aicardi J, Dias K, Ramos O: A progressive syndrome of autism, dementia, ataxia, and loss of purposeful hand use in girls—Rett's syndrome: Report of 35 cases. Ann Neurol 1983;14:471-479.

132. Zoghbi H, Percy AK, Glaze DG, et al: Reduction of biogenic amine levels in the Rett syndrome. N Engl J Med 1985;313:921-924.

133. Rett A: Cerebral atrophy associated with hyperammonemia. *In* Vinken PJ, Bruyn GW, Klawans HL (eds): Metabolic and Deficiency Diseases of the Nervous System, Part III. Handbook of Clinical Neurology, Vol. 29. Amsterdam, North Holland, 1977, p 305.

134. Matalon R, Michals K, Sebasta D, et al: Aspartoacylase deficiency and *N*-acetylaspartic aciduria in patients with Canavan disease. Am J Med Genet 1988;29:463-471.

135. Kamoshita S, Rapin I, Suzuki K, Suzuki K: Spongy degeneration of the brain: A chemical study of two cases including isolation and characterization of myelin. Neurology 1968;18:975-985.

136. Buchanan DS, Davis RL: Spongy degeneration of the nervous system. Neurology 1965;15:207-222.

137. Trommer BL, Naidich TP, Dal Canto MC, et al: Noninvasive CT diagnosis of infantile Alexander disease: Pathologic correlation. J Comput Assist Tomogr 1983;7:509-516.

138. Stark G: Pelizaeus-Merzbacher disease. Dev Med Child Neurol 1972;14:806-809.

139. Wilkus RJ, Farrell DF: Electrophysiologic observations in the classical form of Pelizaeus-Merzbacher disease. Neurology 1976;26:1042-1045.

17

Infectious Diseases

JAMES J. RIVIELLO, JR., AND EDWARD H. KOVNAR

Although the electroencephalogram (EEG) is not commonly thought of as an important diagnostic test in infectious diseases, the study can provide insight into the etiologic agent responsible for the central nervous system (CNS) infection. In addition, the EEG can provide information regarding risk of seizures and prognosis.

INFECTIOUS CENTRAL NERVOUS SYSTEM DISORDERS WITH EEG ABNORMALITIES

Meningitis

Acute purulent meningitis is the most common bacterial infection of the CNS in childhood.[1] In the newborn period, group B beta-hemolytic streptococcus and gram-negative enteric bacilli are the most prevalent causative organisms. In older children, *Haemophilus influenzae*, *Streptococcus pneumoniae*, and *Neisseria meningitides* predominate. Early neurologic complications of bacterial meningitis may include seizures, increased intracranial pressure, and hyponatremia due to inappropriate secretion of antidiuretic hormone. Subdural effusions are common but usually insignificant clinically. Serious but infrequent neurologic sequelae include cerebral infarction, subdural empyema, and brain abscess. Brief, generalized convulsions or prolonged focal motor episodes (epilepsia partialis continua) may occur early in the disease.

EEG. The EEG in acute childhood meningitis typically shows diffuse slow wave abnormalities (Fig. 17-1).[2] High-

voltage rhythmic slowing may be prominent over the frontal or occipital derivations; occipital intermittent rhythmic delta is especially common in childhood.[3] The EEG usually returns to normal over several weeks; rapid improvement is characteristic of meningococcal meningitis.[4] Subdural effusions rarely produce specific EEG changes, although voltage suppression may occur. Focal features, especially when persistent, suggest the possibility of either a cerebral abscess or infarction. Persistence of a focally abnormal EEG carries an increased risk for the occurrence of late seizures in children with bacterial meningitis.[5]

Aseptic Meningitis

Aseptic meningitis is typically a self-limited illness in which meningeal inflammation is caused by a viral infection. Symptoms consist of headache, fever, stiff neck, as well as drowsiness, nausea, vomiting, and photophobia.

EEG. The EEG in uncomplicated cases may be normal or show mild slowing that usually resolves within 1 to 2 weeks.[6] Younger children are more likely to exhibit slowing than are older children. The presence of focal or persistent abnormalities implies involvement of not only the meninges but also the underlying cerebral cortex, in which case a diagnosis of meningoencephalitis may be inferred.[7]

Brain Abscess

Localized purulent infection of the brain parenchyma usually occurs by direct extension from a parameningeal source, such as sinusitis and mastoiditis, or by hematogenous

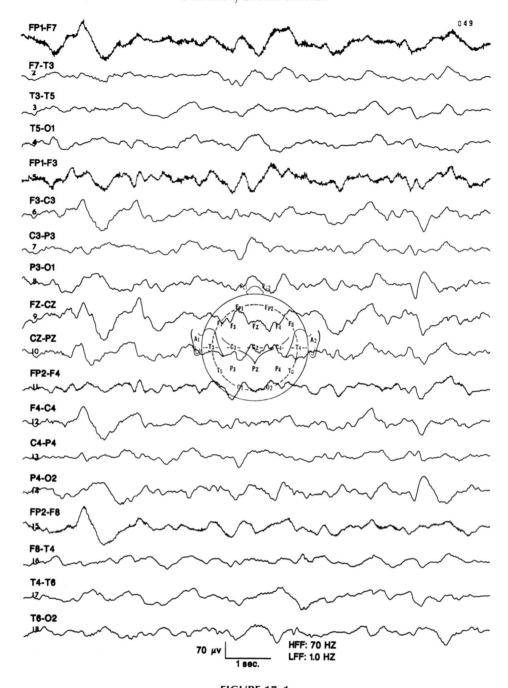

0 4 9

70 μv

1 sec.

HFF: 70 HZ
LFF: 1.0 HZ

FIGURE 17–1

Diffuse, irregular slow activity in a 17-year-old girl with meningitis due to Candida tropicalis.

spread, such as bacterial endocarditis and pneumonia. In the era of effective antibiotic therapy, brain abscess is a rare complication of adequately treated meningitis.

EEG. EEG changes associated with brain abscess depend in part on the location of the infection. An infratentorial abscess is likely to produce only diffuse slowing of

moderate degree or intermittent rhythmic delta without localizing features.[2] A supratentorial abscess may also produce diffuse slowing but often shows focal slowing as the inflammatory process becomes localized (Fig. 17-2). Focal or lateralized epileptiform discharges over the involved area of brain may also occur.[8] Epileptiform features

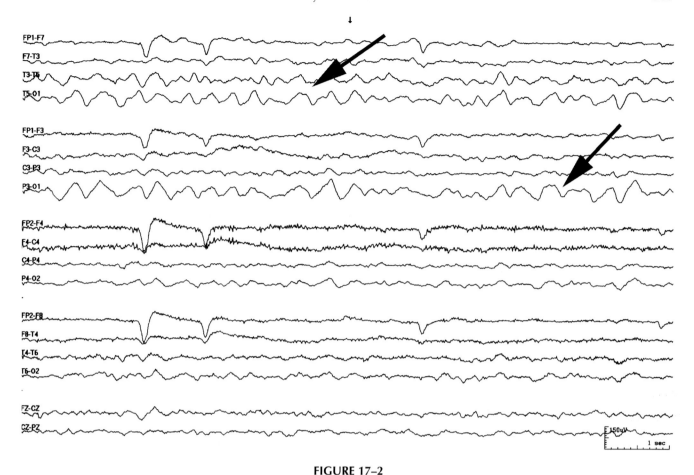

FIGURE 17–2

EEG from a 5-year-old patient with an abscess in the left temporal lobe. Note focal slowing in left temporal and parietal region (arrows).

are associated with an increased risk of seizures as a late complication of brain abscess.[9] Focal voltage suppression or attenuation may also occur.[10] Chronic abscesses are likely to behave as a slowly growing tumor, producing focal slow wave abnormalities or asymmetry of the background activity.[11]

Encephalitis

Most of the viruses known to cause infections of the CNS in humans are common pathogens for which involvement of the brain represents an unusual complication.[12] Although such viruses may be acquired through insect bites (arboviruses) or animal contact (lymphocytic choriomeningitis), most cases of encephalitis are associated with organisms transmitted through person-to-person contact. Access to the brain by these viruses is most often accomplished through hematogenous spread or, less commonly, by transneuronal migration. The route of CNS penetration

is usually dictated by the type of virus. Some viruses exhibit a tropism for specific cell types within the CNS; for example, rabies virus preferentially infects neurons within the limbic system. Localization of other viruses reflects spread from adjacent anatomic structures. It is postulated that in some cases of herpes simplex, type 1, virus activated within the trigeminal ganglion may migrate through nerves within the dura of the middle and anterior cranial fossa into the overlying temporal and orbital-frontal cortex.[13]

The clinical hallmark of encephalitis is the occurrence of altered mental status, ranging from mild lethargy to confusion, stupor, and coma. Seizures, focal neurologic deficits, and increased intracranial pressure are also commonly seen. Signs and symptoms vary from patient to patient and are related, in part, to the specific viral pathogen.

EEG. During the acute phase of viral encephalitis, the EEG is almost always abnormal.[2] Typical findings include diffuse, high-voltage slowing that may be either irregular or rhythmic (Fig. 17-3). Epileptiform features are commonly

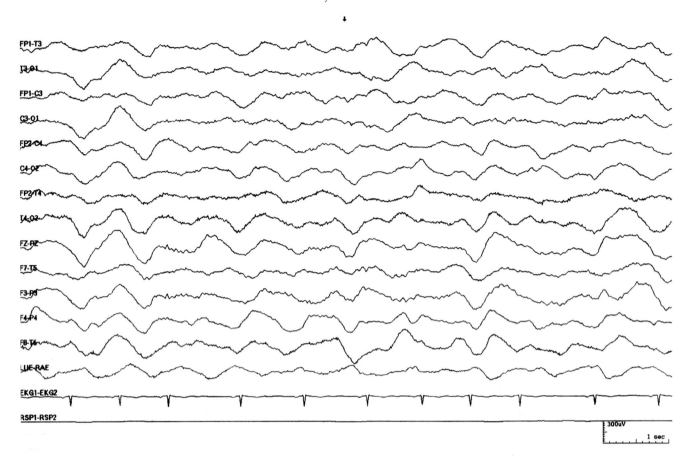

FIGURE 17–3

EEG from a patient with viral encephalitis of unknown etiology. Note the severe slowing in the delta range. The record was nonreactive without change to toe pinching or auditory stimulation.

associated with cortical involvement (Fig. 17-4). Diffuse involvement of the cortical gray matter is associated with bursts of intermittent rhythmic slow activity (Fig. 17-5).[14] The degree of slowing reflects the severity of infection, the level of consciousness, and the presence or absence of associated systemic complications, including hypoxia and disturbances in fluid and electrolyte balance.[3,15] Slow wave abnormalities may also accompany otherwise uncomplicated childhood viral infections such as measles (rubeola), rubella, and chicken pox (varicella) without overt signs or symptoms of CNS infection.[16]

Herpes Simplex Encephalitis

The EEG can be quite helpful in the diagnosis of herpes simplex encephalitis. This type of encephalitis produces acute necrosis with a predilection for the inferior temporal and orbital-frontal lobes. Fever and headache are early clinical features followed within several days by altered behavior,

hallucinations, seizures, aphasia, focal motor deficits, stupor and, in severe cases, coma.[17,18]

EEG. Early in the course of the infection the EEG typically demonstrates focal or lateralized irregular slow wave activity.[19-21] With disease progression, irregular slowing becomes diffuse, although there is often a focal emphasis over the temporal or frontal-temporal derivations. Periodic lateralized epileptiform discharges (PLEDs), consisting of sharp or sharp-and-slow wave complexes, appear over the area of maximal involvement within 2 to 5 days of the onset of illness.[22,23] The appearance of PLEDs may, however, occur as late as day 24 to 30 of the illness.[21] The sharp wave component of the periodic complexes typically recurs every 1 to 5 seconds. Involvement of both cerebral hemispheres may produce bilateral periodic complexes occurring in either a synchronous or independent pattern.[20,24] Serial EEGs show PLEDs in more than two thirds of pathologically proven cases.[25] In nonfatal herpes simplex encephalitis, the periodic complexes are gradually replaced by focal

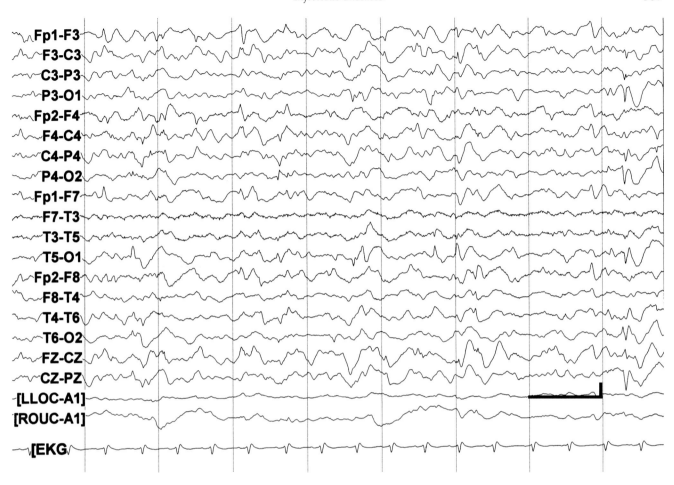

FIGURE 17–4

Polymorphic slow activity with intermixed spikes and sharp waves in a 12-year-old child with viral encephalitis. Calibration 50 μV/1 sec.

or lateralized slow wave abnormalities or voltage suppression over the area of maximal involvement.[3,15] EEG abnormalities often persist despite clinical improvement.[26]

Periodic complexes also occur in a high percentage of cases of neonatal herpes simplex encephalitis. Focal or multifocal periodic complexes, often shifting from side to side, are a prominent feature in affected infants (Fig. 17-6).[27] In infants who succumb to their disease, serial EEGs often show progressive voltage suppression and ultimately isoelectric tracings.[27]

Subacute Sclerosing Panencephalitis

Subacute sclerosing panencephalitis (SSPE) represents a chronic, slowly progressive disease caused by measles virus. This form of postinfectious encephalitis is associated with persistence of virus within the brain after primary infection in early childhood due to an abnormal host immune response.[28] The incidence of this disease has decreased dramatically in recent years due to effective immunization programs.[29] The usual age of onset is between 5 and 15 years. Symptoms begin insidiously with behavioral problems and decline in school performance. This initial phase (stage I) may last for weeks to months and occasionally longer. The next phase (stage II) is characterized by the appearance of myoclonic jerks and progressive dementia. Other features noted during this phase may include seizures, chorioretinitis, optic atrophy, ataxia, and dystonia. Relentless neurologic deterioration accompanies the third phase (stage III); stupor, spasticity, extrapyramidal signs, and temperature instability are frequent signs. After a period of 3 to 12 months, the patient lapses into a vegetative state (stage IV).[30]

EEG. As with herpes simplex encephalitis, the EEG in SSPE may provide an early clue of the nature of the disease process.[31] Serial EEGs in patients with SSPE demonstrate

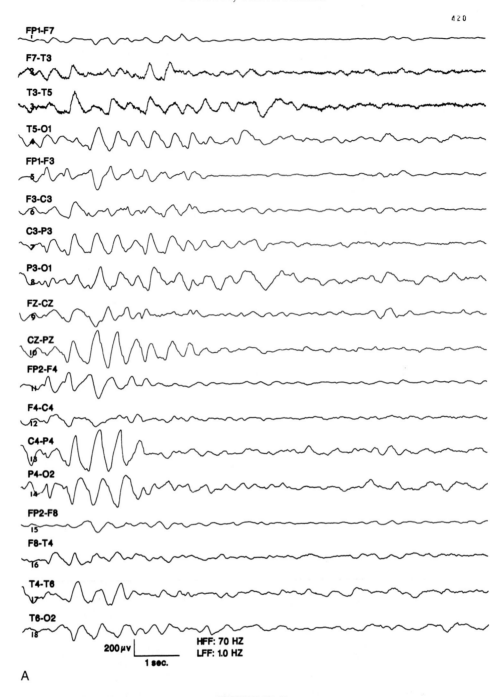

FIGURE 17–5

A and B, Diffuse high-voltage (200 to 300 μV) intermittent rhythmic slow activity in a 16-month-old male infant with chronic enteroviral encephalitis due to subacute combined immunodeficiency.

highly characteristic, although nondiagnostic, changes. During stage I, nonspecific slowing is usually present. Periodic complexes with long interburst intervals are typically observed during stage II. These discharges consist of high-voltage (300 to 1500 μV) polyphasic, sharp-and-slow wave complexes ranging from 0.5 to 2 seconds, recurring every 4 to 15 seconds (Fig. 17-7).[32] The complexes are usually generalized and bilaterally synchronous, although they may be focal or lateralized early in the disease.[2,33,34] Stereotyped motor spasms (slow myoclonic jerks) may precede, accompany, or follow the periodic complexes.[35] Increasing amounts of irregular slow activity are observed in stages III and IV of

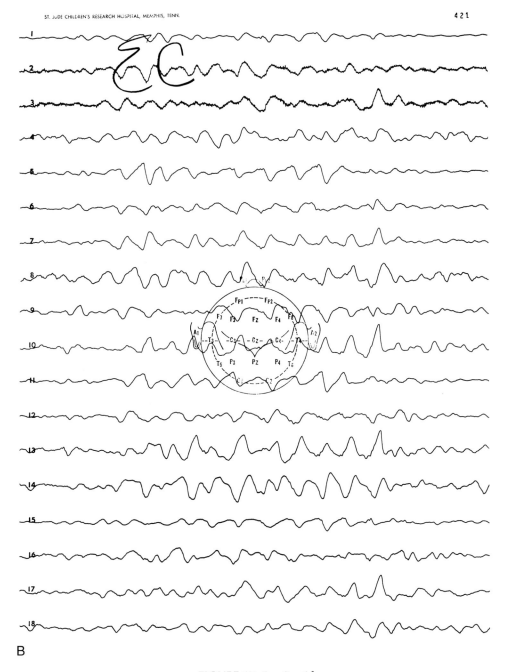

B

FIGURE 17–5   *Cont'd*

disease, during which periodic complexes may persist.[36] The EEG during the terminal stage of disease consists of low-voltage irregular slow activity, approaching an isoelectric recording in some cases.[36]

HUMAN IMMUNODEFICIENCY VIRUS

Human immunodeficiency virus (HIV) is associated with a wide variety of neurologic disorders related either to primary infection of the brain and spinal cord or secondary infectious or neoplastic complications.

EEG. EEG recordings in patients with acquired immunodeficiency syndrome (AIDS) dementia typically show diffuse slowing of the background.[37] Focal slowing suggests the presence of a superimposed opportunistic infection such as toxoplasmosis or neoplasm such as lymphoma. Electrophysiologic testing, including EEG and evoked potentials, may detect changes in asymptomatically infected individuals. Visual inspection and computed

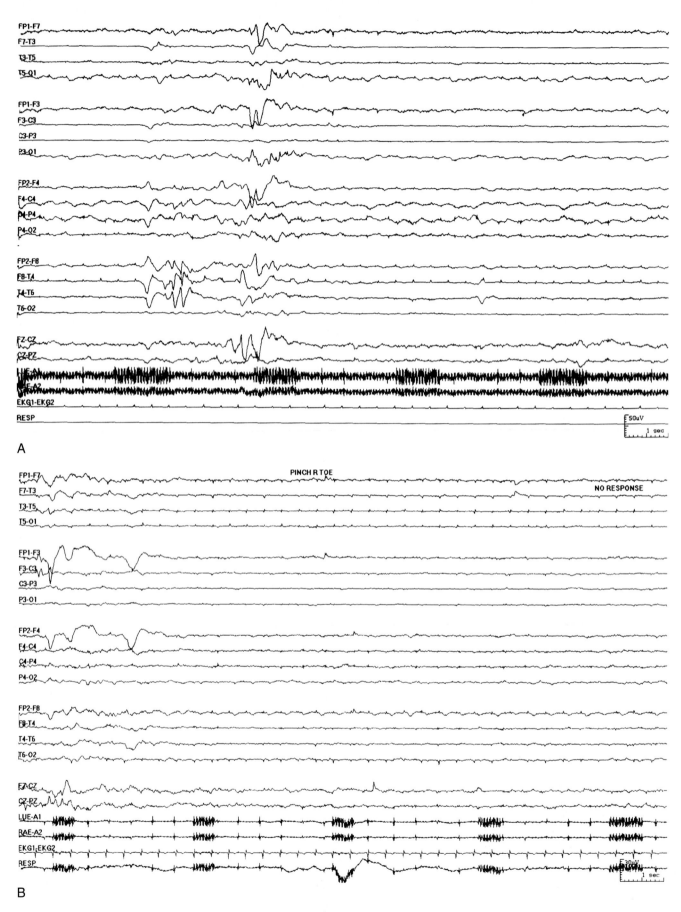

FIGURE 17–6

EEG from a newborn with herpes simplex encephalitis. A, Interictal EEG showing burst-suppression pattern. B, Low-voltage pattern. Note the lack of EEG response to pinching of the right toe.

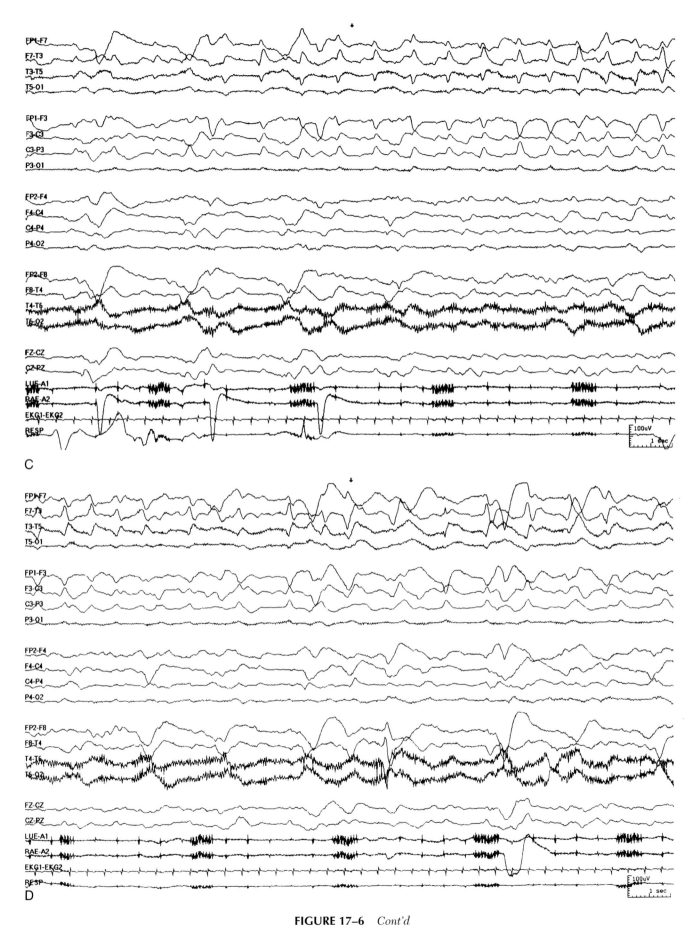

FIGURE 17–6 *Cont'd*

C, Onset of left temporal/central seizure. Note sharply contoured rhythmic delta activity in the left temporal and central region.

D, Electrographic seizure continues.

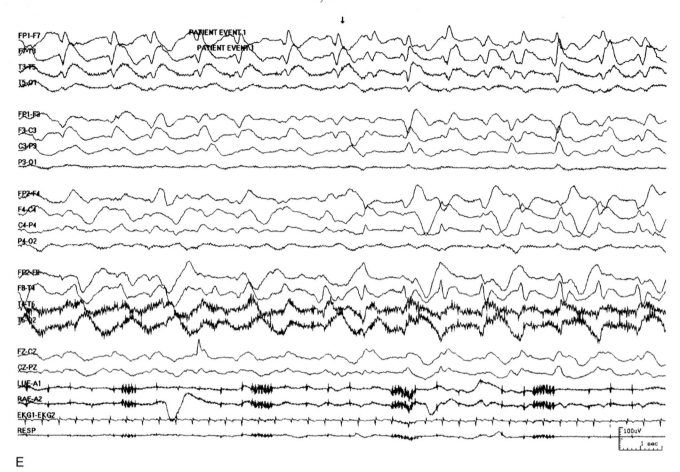

FIGURE 17–6 *Cont'd*

E, *Electrographic seizure continues. Note the spread of seizure to the right central and temporal regions.*

analysis of serial EEGs have shown background slowing in 30% to 40% of asymptomatic carriers of HIV despite the absence of demonstrable changes on either magnetic resonance imaging or neuropsychological testing.[38] Serial EEGs may also help assess the effects of antiviral drugs on the nervous system.[39]

The EEG usually becomes abnormal in patients with progressive encephalopathy,[40-42] consisting of background slowing, spikes, or attenuation of the background activity. In 18 patients reported by Belman and colleagues,[43] 6 of 18 developed encephalopathy when followed for 14 months. The EEG was normal in 1 patient with a static encephalopathy, whereas mild to moderate background slowing occurred in all patients with a progressive encephalopathy.

In a comprehensive neurophysiologic evaluation, Schmitt and associates[42] evaluated 47 HIV-seropositive children with EEG and brainstem and somatosensory evoked potentials.

Twenty-three children were symptomatic, 8 were seropositive without symptoms, and 16 children were younger than 15 months of age. Some of them were investigated at different stages of HIV infection. During the neonatal period, 7 newborns of drug-addicted mothers had seizures and frequent spikes and sharp waves in their EEGs. Among symptomatic children, 6 of 23 showed background slowing and 1 had rhythmic theta activity. In the brainstem evoked potential, bilateral prolonged interpeak latencies were found in 1 child with severe AIDS encephalopathy. Side differences greater than or equal to 0.4 milliseconds in interpeak latencies were seen in 2 children. Median somatosensory evoked potentials were normal in 24 of 26 patients; the N20/N13 amplitude ratio was reduced in only 2 patients. For monitoring the effectiveness of zidovudine treatment in HIV encephalopathy, the authors recommended the use of EEG.

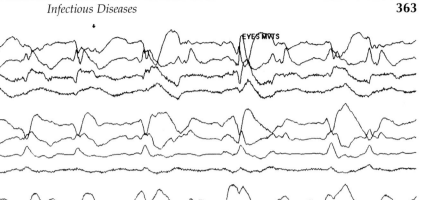

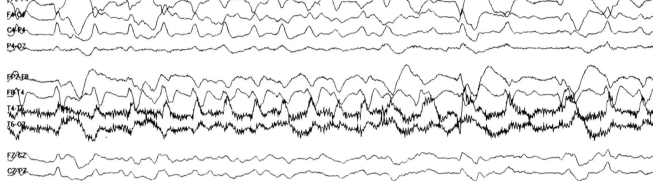

F

FIGURE 17–6   *Cont'd*

F, *Electrographic seizure continues. Note the involvement of the right hemisphere.*

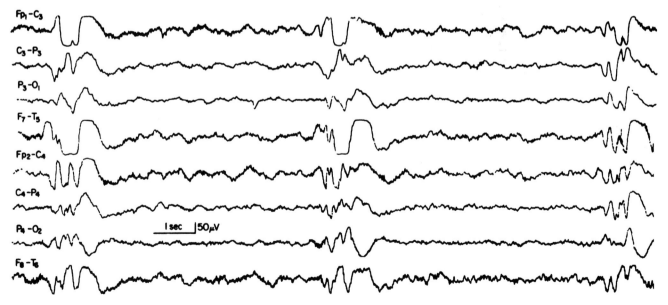

FIGURE 17–7

Periodic discharges in subacute sclerosing panencephalitis in an 8-year-old child. (From Niedermeyer E: Abnormal EEG patterns: Epileptic and paroxysmal. In Niedermeyer E, Lopes-Cendas I [eds]: Electroencephalography: Basic Principles, Clinical Applications, and Related Fields. Philadelphia, Williams & Wilkins, 1999, p 235.)

REFERENCES

1. Kovnar EH, Golden GS: Central nervous system infections. *In* Summit RL (ed): Comprehensive Pediatrics. St. Louis, Mosby, 1990, p 926.

2. Kooi KA, Tucker RP, Marshall RE: Infectious disorders. *In* Fundamentals of Electroencephalography. Hagerstown, MD, Harper & Row, 1978, p 163.

3. Kiloh LG, McComas AJ, Osselton JW: Infective and non-infective encephalopathies. *In* Kiloh LG, McComas AJ, Osselton JW (eds): Clinical Electroencephalography. Boston, Butterworths, 1972, p 141.

4. Turrell RC, Roseman E: Electroencephalographic studies of the encephalopathies: IV. Serial studies in meningococcal meningitis. Arch Neurol Psychiatry 1955;73:141-148.

5. Pomeroy SL, Holmes SJ, Dodge PR, Feigin RD: Seizures and other neurologic sequelae of bacterial meningitis in children. N Engl J Med 1990;323:1651-1657.

6. Gibbs FA, Carpenter PR, Spies HW: Electroencephalographic study of patients with acute aseptic meningitis. Pediatrics 1962;29:181-186.

7. Gibbs FA, Gibbs EL, Spies HW, Carpenter PR: Common types of childhood encephalitis—electroencephalographic and clinical relationships. Arch Neurol 1964;10:1-11.

8. Le Beau J, Dondey M: Importance diagnostique de la certaines activites électroencéphalographiques latéralisées, périodiques, ou à tendance périodique au cours des abcés du cerveau. Electroencephalogr Clin Neurophysiol 1959;11:43-58.

9. Legg NJ, Gupta PC, Scott DF: Epilepsy following cerebral abscess: A clinical and EEG study of 70 patients. Brain 1973;96:259-268.

10. Pine I, Atoynatan TH, Margolis G: The EEG findings in eighteen patients with brain abscess: Case reports and a review of the literature. Electroencephalogr Clin Neurophysiol 1952;4:165-179.

11. Westmoreland BF: The EEG in cerebral inflammatory processes. *In* Neidermeyer E, Lopes da Silva F (eds): Electroencephalography: Basic Principles, Clinical Applications, and Related Fields. Baltimore, Urban & Schwarzenberg, 1987, p 259.

12. Johnson RT: Meningitis, encephalitis, and poliomyelitis. *In* Viral Infections of the Nervous System. New York, Raven Press, 1982, p 87.

13. Johnson RT: Herpesvirus infections. *In* Viral Infections of the Nervous System. New York, Raven Press, 1982, p 129.

14. Hughes JR: Correlations between EEG and chemical changes in uremia. Electroencephalogr Clin Neurophysiol 1980;48:583-594.

15. Cobb WA: Electroencephalographic changes in viral encephalitis. *In* Illis LS (ed): Viral Diseases of the Central Nervous System. Baltimore, Williams & Wilkins, 1975, p 76.

16. Gibbs FA, Gibbs EL, Carpenter PR, Spies HW: Electroencephalographic abnormality in "uncomplicated" childhood diseases. JAMA 1959;171:1050-1055.

17. Drachman DA, Adams RD: Herpes simplex and acute inclusion body encephalitis. Arch Neurol 1962;7:61-79.

18. Olson LC, Buescher EL, Artenstein MS, Parkman PD: Herpesvirus infection of the human central nervous system. N Engl J Med 1967;277:1271-1277.

19. Misra UK, Kalita J: Neurophysiological studies in herpes simplex encephalitis. Electromyogr Clin Neurophysiol 1998;38:177-182.

20. Gupta PC, Seth P: Periodic complex in herpes simplex encephalitis: A clinical and experimental study. Electroencephalogr Clin Neurophysiol 1973;35:67-74.

21. Illis LS, Taylor FM: The electroencephalogram in herpes simplex encephalitis. Lancet 1972;1:718-721.

22. Upton A, Grumpert J: Electroencephalography in diagnosis of herpes simplex encephalitis. Lancet 1970;1:650-652.

23. Ch'ien LT, Boehm RM, Robinson H, et al: Characteristic early EEG changes in herpes simplex encephalitis: Clinical and virologic studies. Arch Neurol 1977;34:361-364.

24. Smith JB, Westmoreland BF, Reagan TJ, Sandok BA: A distinctive clinical EEG profile in herpes simplex encephalitis. Mayo Clin Proc 1975;50:469-474.

25. Whitley RJ, Soong S-J, Linneman C Jr, et al: Herpes simplex encephalitis: Clinical assessment. JAMA 1982;247:317-320.

26. Whitley RJ: Viral encephalitis. N Engl J Med 1990;323:242-250.

27. Fujikawa DG, Dwyer BE, Lake RR, Wasterlain CG: Local cerebral glucose utilization during status epilepticus in newborn primates. Am J Physiol 1989;256:C1160-C1167.

28. Johnson RT: The pathogenesis of acute viral encephalitis and postinfectious encephalomyelitis. J Infect Dis 1987;155:359-364.

29. Centers for Disease Control: Subacute sclerosing panencephalitis and measles. MMWR Morb Mortal Wkly Rep 1977;26:309-310.

30. Dyken PR: Subacute sclerosing panencephalitis. Neurol Clin 1985;3:179-196.

31. Kubota T, Okumura A, Takenaka J, et al: A case of subacute sclerosing panencephalitis preceded by epileptic seizures: Evolutional EEG changes. Brain Dev 2003;25:279-282.

32. Cobb W: The periodic events of subacute sclerosing leucoencephalitis. Electroencephalogr Clin Neurophysiol 1966;21:278-294.

33. Yemisci M, Gurer G, Saygi S, Ciger A: Generalised periodic epileptiform discharges: Clinical features, neuroradiological evaluation, and prognosis in 37 adult patients. Seizure 2003;12:465-472.

34. Shivji ZM, Al-Zahrani IS, Al-Said YA, Jan MM: Subacute sclerosing panencephalitis presenting with unilateral periodic myoclonic jerks. Can J Neurol Sci 2003;30:384-387.

35. Metz H, Gregoriou M, Sandifer P: Subacute sclerosing pan-encephalitis: A review of 17 cases with special reference to clinical diagnostic criteria. Arch Dis Child 1964;39:554-557.

36. Rabending G, Radermecker FJ: Encephalitis due to slow virus infections. *In* Remond A (ed): Handbook of Electroencephalography and Clinical Neurophysiology, Vol 15-A. Amsterdam, Elsevier, 1977, p 28.

37. Gabuzda DH, Levy SR, Chiappa KH: Electroencephalography in AIDS and AIDS-related complex. Clin Electroencephalogr 1988;19:1-6.

38. Sinha S, Satischchandra P: Nervous system involvement in asymptomatic HIV seropositive individuals: A cognitive and electrophysiological study. Neurol India 2003;51:466-469.

39. Parisi A, Perri G, Strosseli M, et al: Instrumental evidence of zidovudine effectiveness in the treatment of HIV-associated subacute encephalitis. AIDS 1988;2:482-483.

40. Epstein LG, Sharer LR, Joshi VV, et al: Progressive encephalopathy in children with acquired immune deficiency syndrome. Ann Neurol 1985;17:488-496.

41. Schmitt B, Seeger J, Kreuz W, et al: Central nervous system involvement of children with HIV infection. Dev Med Child Neurol 1991;33:535-540.

42. Schmitt B, Seeger J, Jacobi G: EEG and evoked potentials in HIV-infected children. Clin Electroencephalogr 1992;23:111-117.

43. Belman AL, Ultmann MH, Horoupian D, et al: Neurological complications in infants and children with acquired immune deficiency syndrome. Ann Neurol 1985;18:560-566.

18

Head Trauma

PHILIP J. BRUNQUELL

Using electroencephalography (EEG) to study patients with head trauma dates from the inception of the technique. Hans Berger's original apparatus, an optical recording system without electrical amplification, was barely adequate to detect the alpha rhythm.[1] Cognizant of the technical limitations of his equipment, Berger initially selected patients with defects of the calvarium to permit a closer proximity of the recording electrodes to the brain.[2] Since this pioneering work, large numbers of head injured patients have been investigated with more sophisticated methodologies, including computerized methods of data acquisition and analysis. Although the corresponding medical literature is vast, the proportion of studies devoted exclusively to pediatric patients is relatively small, and the percentage of pediatric studies designed with a strict sense of academic rigor is smaller still. These latter studies serve as the focus of this discussion.

The paucity of pediatric studies belies the magnitude of the clinical problem. Head trauma is the most common form of accidental injury among children.[3,4] Approximately 1 in 10 children experience traumatic loss of consciousness prior to adulthood.[5] A population-based study found that the average annual incidence of head trauma is 220 per 100,000 children.[6] The incidence of inflicted traumatic brain injury in the first 2 years of life is 17.0 per 100,000 person-years.[7] There is an impressive sex predilection: Boys sustain closed head injury three times as often as girls,[8] and boys with a prior history of head trauma have a twofold risk of incurring subsequent head trauma.[9] Maltreatment of children constitutes an important subset of the disease spectrum. During the first year of life, more than 95% of serious intracranial injuries are due to child abuse.[10] Each year 10 of every 100,000 children in this country die from head trauma.[9] Even minor head injury in children can be associated with serious sequelae,[11] including long-term neuropsychological deficits.[12,13]

Despite the extent of the problem and the realization that head trauma can give rise to significant alterations of electrocortical function, many authors believe that the EEG is of limited or no diagnostic use in the acute assessment of the head-injured child.[12,14] This position may be based at least partly on the higher specificity and sensitivity of imaging studies such as computed tomography (CT) and magnetic resonance imaging (MRI) in excluding structural pathology.[15] Since the likelihood of mortality increases directly with the length of time between impact and the removal of progressive space-occupying lesions such as an expanding subdural hematoma, EEGs are not usually obtained prior to surgery. However, once surgically amenable lesions have been excluded or addressed, the EEG can provide valuable information while the child is still acutely ill.

As an indicator of the functional integrity of the nervous system, the EEG offers a quantifiable measure of the severity of the insult as well as a means to follow the natural course of the condition and monitor the rate of recovery. These data may be of particular benefit when there are discrepancies among the history, the findings on the neurologic examination, and/or the results of imaging studies. The insidious onset of complications such as vasospasm, abscess, hematoma, or hydrocephalus may be heralded by alterations on sequential EEG tracings. The advent of continuous EEG monitoring in the intensive care unit may be especially helpful in detecting these changes.[16,17] In children whose findings on the neurologic examination are obliterated by pharmacologically induced neuromuscular blockade, the EEG may reveal signs of improvement or decline that are otherwise unobtainable. The effectiveness of medical and surgical interventions can be evaluated by EEG, and in some cases, such as the use of pharmacologic agents to control intracranial hypertension, dosages and dosing intervals may in large part be determined by EEG findings.[18,19] Although the EEG is not helpful in predicting post-traumatic seizures in both mild[20] and severe[21] head injury, it can provide important information in establishing an overall prognosis.

Obtaining this information may demand considerable effort, for the technical difficulties of recording EEGs in children are commonly magnified in the head-injured child.[22,23] Excessive muscle and movement artifact may result from the child's being restless from pain or uncooperative from delirium or confusion. Scalp lacerations, bandages, and cranial deformities may dictate unconventional electrode placements that may result in spurious asymmetries. Asymmetries may also be produced by subgaleal hematoma or scalp edema, including that produced by extravasations from scalp intravenous lines. Cranial injury may be followed by increased pulsatility of scalp arteries that may introduce slow wave artifact in the delta frequency range. Life support systems and other monitoring devices may introduce a baffling variety of other artifacts. In such circumstances, the electroencephalographer is aided by a technician who not only is well versed in dealing with critically ill children but who also thoroughly understands the recording environment and is willing and able to provide the interpreter with meticulous notations regarding the clinical status of the child during the progress of the recording.

This chapter begins with a short discussion of the biomechanical factors that lead to the electrophysiologic abnormalities seen in childhood head trauma. Attention is then given to the cardinal EEG abnormalities: slow wave activity, epileptiform features, asymmetries, and certain stereotypic patterns. The postconcussion syndrome and also the role of quantitative EEG are reviewed. Finally, the prognostic value of EEG and the electrophysiologic effects of various forms of injury due to interventions are considered. Table 18-1 is a summary of the relationship between various forms of head injury and the primary EEG findings.

BIOMECHANICAL ANTECEDENTS

There are many types of head injury.[24] *Impact* injury refers to the direct application of mechanical force to the cranium, whereas *impulse* injury occurs when the force is transmitted indirectly to the cranium from its application

TABLE 18–1. RELATIONSHIP BETWEEN LESION AND EEG CHANGES

Lesion	Expected EEG Changes
Scalp edema	Local attenuation of amplitude
Subgaleal hematoma	Local attenuation of amplitude
Skull defect	Local increase in amplitude
Epidural hematoma	Same as for subdural hematoma
Subdural hematoma	Focal slow; focal slow with diminished amplitude; bilateral changes may also occur; PLEDs
Subarachnoid hemorrhage	Generalized slow, especially with fluctuating level of consciousness; amplitude asymmetry and focal slow if local cortical damage/vasospasm
Cortical contusions, lacerations, intracerebral hematoma	Continuous focal polymorphic delta activity; focal absence or depression of fast activity; epileptiform discharges

PLED, periodic lateralized epileptiform discharge.

elsewhere on the body (e.g., whiplash). *Dynamic* head injury results when forces are applied quickly (usually < 200 milliseconds) as in acceleration/deceleration types of insult. With *static* head injury the force is applied much more slowly (e.g., crushing injuries to the cranium). The dural covering remains intact in *closed* head trauma but is penetrated in *open* trauma. Most childhood head trauma studied electrophysiologically has been of the closed, dynamic impact type, and so this form of injury serves as the major focus of this discussion.

The pathophysiology of head trauma differs in children and adults.[25-27] Children are anatomically predisposed to brain injury from dynamic inertial loading.[28] Compared with adults, the head mass in children is relatively larger in proportion to body and extremity size.[26] This results in a higher center of gravity; hence, children tend to "lead with the head" when dynamic forces are applied.[29] A differential in the movement between the skull and the intracranial contents ensues. This was first demonstrated by the elegant studies of Pudenz and Shelden.[30] Brain movement following impact was observed in animals fitted with Lucite calvaria. Following dynamic loading, rotatory movements of the brain within the cranial cavity were observed. In contrast, static impact (in which the calvarium was fixed and not permitted to move following impact) did not produce such movements, and a much greater force was required to render clinical signs of unconsciousness.

The rotational movements of the brain following dynamic loading produce strains within the brain parenchyma and also promote contact between the cortical surface and the bony prominences of the inner table of the skull.[31,32] Strains may cause a change in brain shape without alteration in volume (shear injury), a change in volume without alteration in shape (compression-rarefaction injury), or both. The pathologic consequences depend on the severity of the impact. In mild injuries, there may be no demonstrable lesions or only subtle ballooning of axis cylinders in the white matter immediately subjacent to the cortex and possibly in the corpus callosum.[33] In more severe cases, contusion, laceration, and hematoma may result. Overall, neuropathologic changes tend to evolve in a centripetal direction. In experimentally concussed primates, for example, mild impact results in lesions confined to the cortical regions; with increasing severity of impact, the diencephalon and ultimately the mesencephalon become affected.[34] Such animal models predict that brainstem lesions do not occur in isolation but are associated with diffuse injury elsewhere in the brain, a finding that has been closely corroborated in human autopsy material.[35]

Although the EEG changes that ensue from such events may be simplistically construed as the result of the mechanical disruption of neural generators, the precise cellular and subcellular mechanisms are far from clear. Traumatic impact of nervous tissue initiates multiple primary and secondary biochemical and ultrastructural changes that singly or in combination could contribute to alterations in EEG frequency, amplitude, and waveform. Concussive injury, for example, produces a dramatic increase in the rate of energy consumption, as signaled by a depletion of adenosine triphosphate and a rise in lactate.[36] Swollen mitochondria with leaky outer membranes, as demonstrated by electron microscopic examination of traumatized tissue, are probably the morphologic substrates of this process.[37] In the face of increased metabolic need, there is a sharp decline in substrate delivery due to cytotoxic edema and a loss of autoregulation of cerebral blood flow.[38] The former is promoted by calcium entry into cells with resulting membrane failure. The latter process, especially pronounced in young children, can lead to a state of diffuse cerebral hyperemia with vascular stasis ("malignant brain edema").[39] The consequent drop in cerebral profusion pressure further potentiates brain swelling and tissue hypoxia.[40] Neuronal responses include the release of increased amounts of excitatory neurotransmitters[41] that could possibly facilitate the appearance of post-traumatic seizures. In addition, the release of arachidonic acid leads to the release of free radicals that covalently bind to lipoproteins, macromolecules, and nucleic acids and promote neuronal destruction.[42]

SLOW WAVE ACTIVITY

The most common EEG abnormality following head injury in children is slowing of background rhythms

(Fig. 18-1). Compared with adults who sustain a similar degree of injury, the slow wave activity in children is more pronounced and persists for a longer period.[43] Consequently, significant slow wave activity in the head-injured child does not necessarily stipulate the presence of irreversible brain damage.

Regardless of the site of cranial impact, there is a striking proclivity for the slow wave activity to be maximally expressed over the posterior head regions. Strauss,[44] for example, in an analysis of slow wave foci after head trauma, noted a posterior distribution in 80% of children in contrast with 29% of adults. Silverman[45] studied 100 consecutive children younger than 16 years of age within 4 weeks of head injury. Sixty percent of the 66 patients who had abnormal EEGs showed parieto-occipital slowing, the most frequently observed abnormality. Most of the 294 children between 1 and 18 years of age in the series of Gibbs and coworkers were studied within 6 days of injury.[46] Single-area slow wave foci (left, right, or bilateral) were the most common abnormalities occurring in 46% of the patients. Furthermore, 84% of this group manifested slowing in an occipital distribution. Enomoto and associates[47] restricted their series to 280 children younger than 15 years of age who had mild head injury. This was defined as the absence of a depressed skull fracture or a subdural hematoma necessitating surgical intervention. All children were examined within 1 week of injury. Nonparoxysmal abnormalities were the most common EEG disturbance, occurring in 78% of patients with abnormal EEGs. Sixty-one percent of the nonparoxysmal group showed slowing confined to the occipital head regions or more widespread slowing with an occipital emphasis.

In children, the tendency of slow wave activity to achieve an occipital maximum is not confined to instances of head trauma. A similar distribution is seen in children with hypoxia, encephalitis, and leukemia, as well as during the physiologic response to hyperventilation.[48] It is imperative, however, to distinguish pathologic slowing from the expected age-dependent changes in the frequency of the posterior head rhythm and from the physiologic posterior slow waves of youth (see Chapter 4). The latter waveforms are intermixed with the ongoing dominant posterior head rhythm, do not exceed 120% of the voltage of this rhythm, do not show an interhemispheric asymmetry greater than 50%, and block with eye opening.[48] In examining the tracing of a head-injured child, the greater the tendency of occipital slow wave activity to deviate from these parameters, the more likely this activity represents a pathologic finding.

Once abnormal slow wave activity is identified, a much more difficult task is to determine when such findings evolved. The typical lack of a preinjury baseline recording makes this distinction exceedingly difficult, particularly if

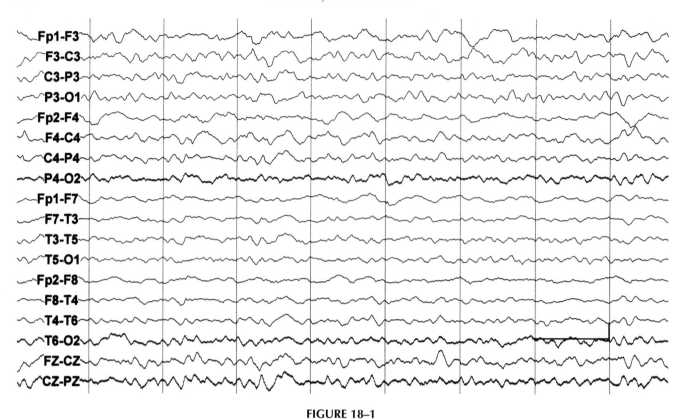

FIGURE 18–1

Diffuse, continuous EEGs in an 8-year-old boy who sustained severe bifrontal contusions following a fall from a skateboard. Calibration: 1 second, 50 μV.

the child has had a history of recurrent trauma or other preexisting neurologic deficit. Obtaining an EEG as early as is reasonable in the post-traumatic period, comparing the results of this study with serial recordings during convalescence, and placing these findings in the context of the clinical history are necessary to begin to approach this vexatious problem, but even then, serious question may remain regarding the genesis of the EEG abnormality.

Despite these problems, recognition of abnormal slow wave activity is of fundamental importance in the evaluation of the EEG of the head-injured child because it can serve as an important marker to trace the natural course of the disease. This was demonstrated by Mizrahi and Kellaway[20] in their elegant study of 371 children who had sustained concussion, defined as "transient loss of consciousness with or without subjective sequelae and without neurologic abnormalities after recovery of consciousness." There was close correlation between the degree and distribution of slowing and the clinical state of the patients. In the more mildly affected patients, records were either normal or showed some occipital slow wave activity. With increasing evidence of clinical insult (determined by the length of altered consciousness and the severity and duration of ensuing symptoms such as amnesia, dizziness, headache, and vomiting),

slow wave activity became more pronounced and widely distributed, extending from the posterior to the anterior head regions. The most severely affected patients showed generalized very slow wave activity. The interval of time between the traumatic insult and the recording was critical in the detection of these abnormalities; for each degree of severity of concussion, the length of this interval was inversely related to the degree of EEG abnormality. The earlier the record was obtained in relationship to the traumatic insult, the greater was the degree of EEG abnormality.

The resolution of slow wave activity occurred in a predictable fashion. First, slow wave activity became more rhythmic and organized and of higher frequency. Following this, the slowing diminished anteriorly, the posterior alpha rhythm reappeared, and some posterior slow wave activity typically remained. The sequence of changes during resolution was independent of the degree of concussion, although the rate of appearance of these EEG changes was closely coupled with the clinical state. Specifically, children with more severe degrees of concussion proceeded through the stages of resolution more slowly.

This study[20] underscored the value of systematic observation versus random EEG sampling in head-injured children. Since prominent slow wave activity can occur following minor trauma in a child who appears relatively neurologically intact, there may be a tendency to reject the slow wave activity as carrying any significance. However, when serial tracings are obtained using consistent grading of both clinical and electrophysiologic abnormalities, the relevance of slow wave activity becomes readily apparent.

EPILEPTIFORM ACTIVITY AND POST-TRAUMATIC SEIZURES

Following head injury, the prevalence of epileptiform activity (Fig. 18-2) is higher in children compared with adults, and the youngest children show the greatest amount of this abnormality.[49] Nonetheless, the overall prevalence of spikes and sharp waves in children is low, particularly in comparison with the previously described slow wave activity. When epileptiform activity is encountered, it must be recalled that up to 2% of normal children have spike foci in their EEGs.[47,50] Hence, Mizrahi and Kellaway[20] concluded that the occurrence of spikes in the initial EEGs of 2.2% of their series of 371 children with concussion was most likely

unrelated to the trauma. None of this subgroup went on to experience clinical seizures, emphasizing the benign nature of the finding.

Other authors have reported a similar low incidence of epileptiform abnormalities. Only 9.3% of the series of Enomoto and colleagues[47] of 280 children with minor head injury showed "paroxysmal" changes on initial tracings. Most of these changes represented epileptiform activity. The authors did not view this figure as elevated compared to a reference population.[51] However, serial tracings revealed prognostically useful information. The prevalence of paroxysmal discharges increased directly with the persistence of clinical neurologic abnormalities. Discharges occurred in 19% of the children who recovered within 3 months, in 42.8% of those who normalized between 3 and 12 months, and in 90% of those with persistent deficits.

None of the 100 consecutive children studied by Silverman[45] had focal or generalized spike-wave patterns, although follow-up was less than 1 year for most of the subjects. None of the 294 children studied by Gibbs and associates[46] was reported to show generalized spike-wave discharges. The prevalence of focal spikes on both initial

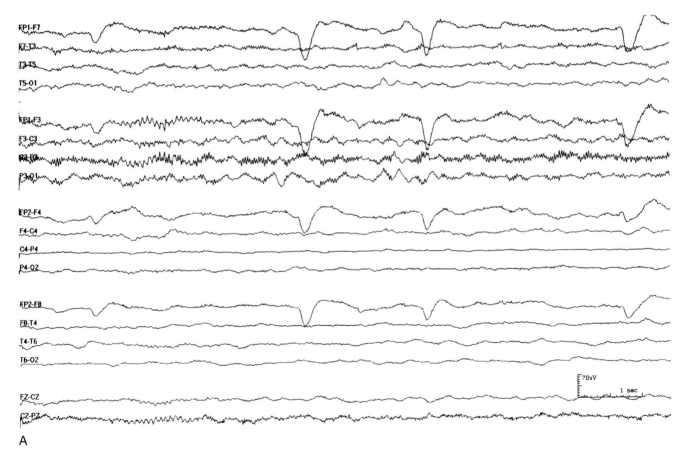

A

FIGURE 18–2

A 6-year-old girl with right subdural hematoma. A, Marked voltage suppression is noted over the right hemisphere.

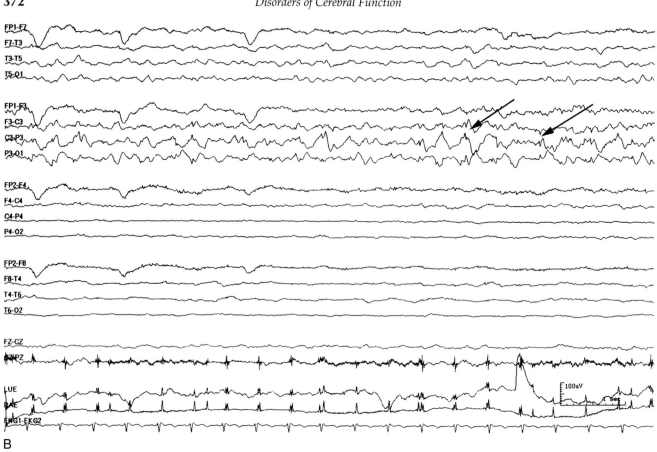

FIGURE 18–2   *Cont'd*

B, *Spikes can be seen arising from the left central region* (arrows).

and follow-up studies for children with all grades of severity of injury was less than 10%.

Because epileptiform activity and clinical seizures each occur in only a few head-injured children, it is logical to ask whether the two are linked. To place this question in context, the unique childhood features of posttraumatic seizures is reviewed, followed by a comparison of the role of EEG versus clinical findings in seizure prediction.

The epidemiology of seizures following head injury is much different in children than adults. In a large population-based study,[52] the incidence of early post-traumatic seizure (i.e., those occurring within 1 week of injury) was more common in children (2.6%) than in adults (1.8%), whereas late post-traumatic seizures (i.e., those occurring more than 1 week following injury) were slightly more common in adults (1.9%) than in children (1.6%). Seizures as a response to head injury occur more immediately in children than in adults. Up to 70% of children with early seizures sustain them within the first 24 hours following injury, whereas approximately 50% of the adults do the same.[53] In adults, the appearance of early seizures is closely correlated with the severity of the injury, but children may experience early

seizures after only trivial head injury.[11] Late-onset seizures, however, are closely correlated with the severity of injury in both groups. The incidence of late seizures rose from 0.2% to 7.4% in children with mild and severe injuries, respectively, whereas for adults the increase was from 0.8% to 13.3%.[52]

As with early post-traumatic seizures, post-traumatic status epilepticus is more common in children than in adults. In one series[53] it was seen in 16.4% of 177 children compared with 7.5% of 288 adults; the highest incidence occurred in the youngest patients, that is, 22.1% in children younger than 5 years of age. Status epilepticus can occur even after minor impact in children and does not necessarily indicate the presence of a space-occupying lesion.[54] In contrast, post-traumatic status epilepticus in adults constitutes a grave prognostic sign.[55] Most episodes of status epilepticus in children occur shortly after the injury and require prompt treatment. Thus, it is not surprising that studies on the ictal signatures of such events are lacking.

The morbidity that accompanies late post-traumatic epilepsy has prompted a search for factors that predict its development. EEG findings are not particularly helpful in

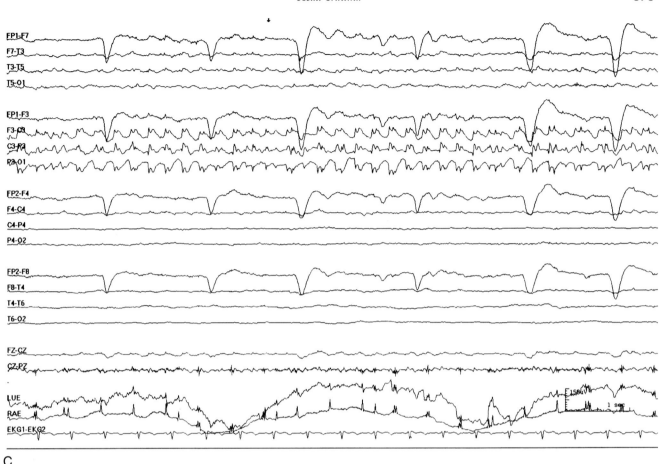

FP1-F7
F7-T3
T3-T5
T5-O1

FP1-F3
F3-C3
C3-P3
P3-O1

FP2-F4
F4-C4
C4-P4
P4-O2

FP2-F8
F8-T4
T4-T6
T6-O2

FZ-CZ
CZ-PZ
LUE
RAE
EKG1-EKG2

C

FIGURE 18–2 *Cont'd*
C *and* D, *Electrographic seizure arising in the left central region. No behavioral changes were noted during the ictal event.*

predicting outcome in post-traumatic epilepsy.[56,57] Although the EEG is abnormal in 60% of children following head injury,[58] it is normal in one third of those who ultimately develop epilepsy.[59] Although focal abnormalities are more common in those who go on to develop epilepsy, they are also seen when this complication does not develop.[60] However, Angeleri and colleagues[61] found that an EEG focus 1 month after head injury substantially increased the risk for seizures compared with individuals without a focus.

Clinical rather than EEG criteria remain the mainstays of prediction.[62] Jennett defined the following independent risk factors for late post-traumatic epilepsy: intracranial hematoma, early post-traumatic seizures, and depressed skull fracture.[63] Feeney and Walker,[64] using a constant probability model, identified the following major risk factors: intracranial hemorrhage; hemiplegia, hemiparesis, or aphasia; injury in the central-parietal area; and penetration of the dura by either a bone fragment or missile. For both individual patients as well as groups of subjects, their mathematical model offered a prediction accuracy of 95%.

The appearance of epilepsy following head injury may be related more to the child's premorbid genetic susceptibility to seizures than to the injury itself.[65] The EEG may sometimes be helpful in making this distinction. For example, the appearance of generalized bisynchronous 3-Hz spike-and-wave discharges would make it highly unlikely that a child's seizures are due to trauma. Obtaining tracings on the proband's first-degree relatives may provide further support for a genetic diathesis. In other cases, the distinction may not be so clear, and the child's clinical condition may result from a combination of factors. For example, traumatic insult might further depress a child's seizure threshold that is already genetically lowered, thus permitting seizures to be clinically expressed.

ASYMMETRIES

Regional and lateralized asymmetries of voltage and/or frequency may arise from technical problems (see earlier)

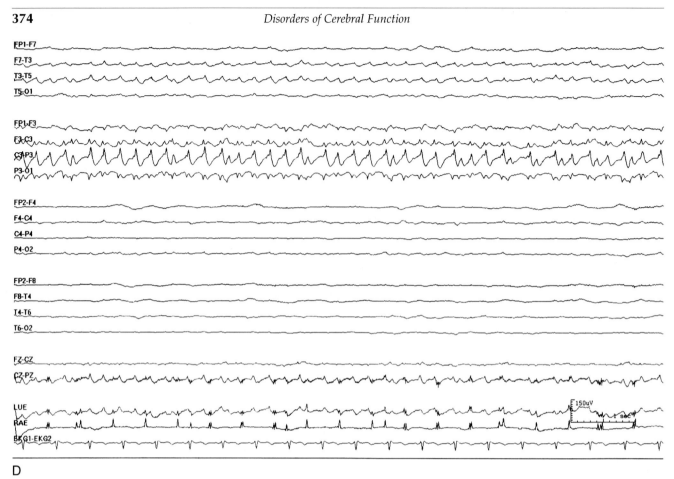

FIGURE 18–2 *Cont'd*

or from structural lesions (Fig. 18-3; see also Fig. 18-2). These lesions vary from those with no lasting significance (e.g., scalp edema) to those with profound prognostic implications (e.g., extra-axial and intracerebral hematomas).

Scalp Edema and Subgaleal Hematoma

Scalp edema can arise directly from the traumatic impact or from infiltration of scalp intravenous lines. The latter may be particularly common in neonates, in whom extravasations of small volumes of fluid can lead to fluid collections that are large relative to cranial size.[66] The expected change is a localized voltage attenuation of background rhythms. Similar EEG findings are seen with subgaleal hematoma. Chatrian and coworkers[67] have suggested that the amplitude changes may be due to the fluid collection's increasing the distance between the cortex and the recording electrodes and/or to its forming a salt bridge between electrodes. In examining the scalp prior to the recording, it should be noted that although both scalp edema and subgaleal hematoma cross suture lines, the former is soft and pitting and the latter is firm and fluctuant.[68]

Skull Defects

Because the axes of neural generators in the cerebral cortex are aligned at right angles to the overlying skull, skull defects, whether occasioned by trauma or neurosurgical interventions, produce a regional increase in amplitude.[69] There is no accompanying change in frequency; the contention that the skull acts as a high-pass filter and that circumscribed removal of bone would therefore introduce a frequency asymmetry was never proved.

The amplitude increase may be seen not only from electrodes overlapping the defect but also from electrodes adjacent to it. The asymmetry is seen with circumscribed burr holes as well as with larger cranial defects. When the burr hole fills in with fibrous tissue or when the bone flap is replaced, the asymmetry commonly persists, suggesting that the impedance characteristics of the tissue remain altered.

The morphology of the enhanced activity may appear spikelike. This is especially true of the mu-shaped 6- to 11-Hz activity noted over the rolandic or mid-temporal regions that Cobb and associates[69] referred to as "breach rhythm." This pattern is not related to epilepsy. The central breech

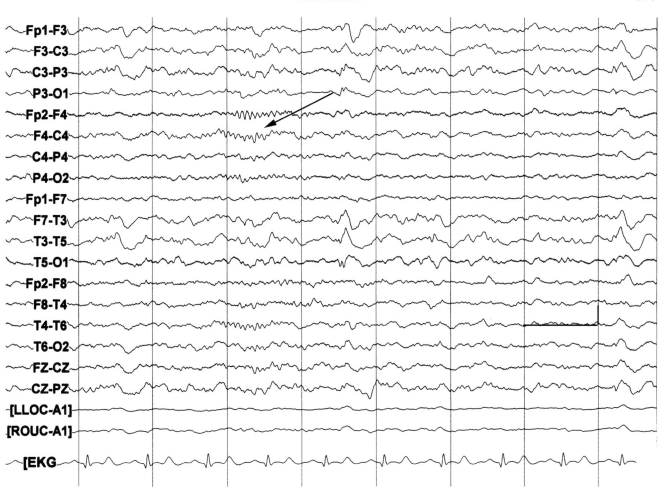

FIGURE 18–3

A 12-year-old boy with left subdural hematoma. Note slowing over the left hemisphere. Spindles could be seen over the right hemisphere (arrow) *but not the left. Calibration: 1 second, 50 μV.*

rhythm blocks to fist clenching whereas the mid-temporal form does not.

In deciding whether an asymmetry over a bone defect is associated with subjacent cerebral pathology, Spehlman[70] has offered the following guidelines:

- A cerebral process is more likely if the asymmetry involves frequency and waveform as well as amplitude
- Abnormalities are seen when recording from electrodes placed distant from the margin of the bone defect
- The amplitude differences develop gradually after the removal of bone

Subdural Hematoma

Subdural hematomas can occur as a consequence of impulse as well as impact injury (see "Biomechanical Antecedents"). The former is exemplified by babies who are violently shaken and thus incur tearing of their bridg-

ing cerebral veins with formation of subdural collections.[71] Retinal hemorrhages are commonly associated and there may be "grab mark" bruises on the trunk or extremities.

Acute unilateral subdural hematomas are correctly lateralized 60% to 75% of the time by EEG findings.[33] Local slow wave activity with or without amplitude reduction comprises the classic findings[72] but these may not always be present.[73,74] The amplitude reduction may be explained by shunting of electrocortical activity between regions subjacent to the hematoma, increased impedance between cortex and the recording electrodes due to the interposed hematoma, and depressed activity of the underlying cortical neurons. CT, MRI, and, if necessary, angiography are the diagnostic procedures of choice. With expansion of the hematoma and secondary compression of brainstem structures, diffuse slow wave activity supervenes and serves as an ominous sign. Local spikes, periodic lateralized epileptiform discharges (PLEDs), and triphasic waves have also been reported with subdural hematoma (see "Stereotypical Patterns").

The EEG findings of epidural hematoma are considered to be the same as those of subdural hematoma.[75]

Subarachnoid Hemorrhage

Much of our knowledge of the EEG changes in subarachnoid hemorrhage comes from studies on patients with ruptured intracranial aneurysms.[76] Trauma-induced subarachnoid hemorrhage is thought to produce the same effects.[77] Diffuse arrhythmic slow wave activity, the amplitude and frequency of which parallel the degree of impaired consciousness, is the cardinal manifestation. Superimposed focal or lateralized slowing with amplitude suppression usually indicates subjacent cerebral injury or vasospasm.[78]

Cortical Contusions and Intracerebral Hematoma

Cortical contusions and intracerebral hematoma are lesions that have as their hallmark continuous focal polymorphic delta activity that exhibits little or no reactivity to the application of external stimuli. Such activity is indicative of subcortical white matter injury[79] and as such is seen with a variety of conditions other than traumatic lesions, including abscesses, infarcts, and neoplasms. The severity and acuteness of the traumatic lesion are related directly to the persistence and degree of polymorphism of the waveforms and indirectly to the "equivalent frequency" of the pattern.[80] Intermittent rather than continuous polymorphic delta activity may sometimes be seen in the early stages of evolution of the hematoma or conversely, during its resolution.

Another, more subtle, index of a traumatic cerebral lesion may be lateralized depression of spontaneous and drug-induced fast activity.[48] Abnormality on the side of lower voltage is probable when the asymmetry exceeds 30%. Interictal and ictal epileptiform activity is also possible.[23,81]

Early in their evolution, intracerebellar hematomas may produce no EEG change. Later, when surrounding mass effect leads to compression of the brainstem and tonsillar herniation, there is impairment of consciousness with diffuse EEG slowing.

From this brief survey of asymmetrical EEG changes in children with head injuries, some generalizations can be abstracted as follows:

1. Careful demarcation of scalp lesions at the time of electrode placement is essential. If it is unclear to what extent a superficial lesion, such as scalp edema or subgaleal hematoma, is contributing to an area of regional attenuation, the EEG should be repeated when the superficial lesion has resorbed.

2. The EEG changes for each lesion are not etiologically specific; that is, an intracerebral hematoma can produce a focus of continuous polymorphic delta activity, but so can an abscess complicating a penetrating head wound.

3. Lesions may coexist and interact in complex ways. For example, the regional enhancement caused by a skull defect may be offset by the amplitude attenuation caused by subjacent cortical damage, with the net EEG pattern representing a balance of these two processes.[82]

4. Given the varied mixture of waveforms that can develop following childhood head trauma, assessing the presence of a frequency asymmetry in the setting of a prominent amplitude asymmetry may be difficult. Adjusting the sensitivity in those channels recording over the involved area so that the displayed amplitude equals that from surrounding regions assists in making this distinction.

5. The results of EEG investigations should be correlated with neuroimaging findings. Controversies regarding the appropriateness of EEG versus neuroimaging are now antiquated and largely irrelevant. The two types of investigations offer complementary information; both are available in most referral centers and their combination can be exploited for the best interests of the patient. Most often it is not a matter of "either/or," but of "when." In excluding neurosurgically amenable lesions, imaging procedures should be performed first.

STEREOTYPICAL PATTERNS

In interpreting the EEGs of head-injured children, certain patterns may occasionally be distinguished from, or are conjoined with, the previously described abnormalities of slowing, epileptiform discharge, and asymmetry. Although the patterns exhibit relatively stereotypical waveform morphology and distribution, their occurrence is not unique to the setting of head trauma. Nonetheless, their appearance in a head-injured child may at times herald significant clinical change and also be of prognostic value.

Periodic Lateralized Epileptiform Discharges

PLEDs may occur in children as a result of injuries including acute subdural hematoma, cortical contusion, and laceration.[83] The morphologic characteristics are similar to those of adults.[84] The discharges are biphasic, triphasic, or polyphasic with the major component being a surface-negative spike or sharp wave that is frequently followed by a slow wave. The repetition rate averages 1/sec (range once every 0.5 to 5 seconds) and is fairly consistent for a given patient. Although a lateralized distribution is characteristic, bilateral independent discharges (BIPLEDs) have been reported.[85]

The temporal profile of PLEDs in children is also similar to adults. The discharges are usually transitory and are ultimately replaced by focal spikes or slowing. Despite their evanescent nature, they are indicative of severe underlying brain dysfunction.

Like adults, PLEDs occur in clinical contexts other than trauma. They have been reported with acute infarction due to sickle cell disease, metabolic imbalance, perinatal brain injury, cerebral cysticercosis, encephalitis, tumor, and brain abscess.[83,86,87] The latter would be of particular concern if PLEDs developed during the convalescent phase of a child with a penetrating head wound.

Animal models suggest that in response to an acute traumatic insult, children may not develop PLEDs as readily as adults.[88] Periodic bursts do not develop in acute preparations of the isolated cortex of immature animals, although they do occur in chronically isolated cortex, suggesting that brain maturational factors may be necessary for their expression.

Triphasic Waves

Triphasic waves are generalized, bilaterally synchronous, bifrontally predominant complexes recurring at a rate of approximately 2/sec and having distinctive morphology.[89] An initial, small-amplitude, sharp negative component is followed by a large-amplitude sharp wave and ends with a slow negative wave. The pattern is commonly associated with metabolic disturbances, including hepatic coma,[90] but can also be seen with structural lesions, including subdural hematoma.[91] In children, the incidence of triphasic waves of any cause is extremely low.[90] Their close association with metabolic derangements means that if triphasic waves are noted in the record of a head-injured child, the prospect of concurrent disturbances such as anoxia or water and electrolyte imbalance should be considered.

Spindle Coma

The spindle coma pattern consists of spindles that bear the same morphology as those of state II sleep, except that they tend to be more widespread and are not confined to a specific portion of the sleep cycle (Fig. 18-4).[92] It has been reported in traumatized children as well as adults.[93-95] If the pattern can be interrupted by the application of external stimuli, the prognosis is considered better than if the pattern is unreactive. Horton and colleagues[95] found that the frequency of the invariant, nonreactive, diffuse cortical

activity seen in children with coma was not confined to a single frequency and proposed the term *rhythmic coma* as a unified concept for alpha, beta, spindle, and theta coma in children.

As with the other previously described stereotypical patterns, spindle coma is not relegated to cases of head trauma. Furthermore, it is imperative to distinguish spindle coma from the increased beta activity induced by sedative-hypnotic drugs; the physiologic fast activity of early sleep that commences at age 5 to 6 months, peaks at 12 to 18 months, and declines thereafter; and the pattern of extreme spindles. The latter pattern is characterized by 8- to 15-Hz spindles that are more continuous than normal sleep spindles and may be present in wakefulness as well as in sleep.[96] It may be seen in as many as 18% of children with mental retardation or cerebral palsy who are between the ages of 1 and 12 years, with maximum expression occurring at age 3 years.

Alpha Coma

Series of children exhibiting the alpha coma pattern due to head injury have not been reported. It is mentioned here because of its established occurrence in adults with head trauma[92,97] and the propensity of the immature brain to produce this pattern in other, sometimes coexisting circumstances, including anoxia and drug overdose.[31,98-101] Unlike the physiologic posterior head rhythm, the alpha frequency activity tends to be more diffusely distributed, with a centrofrontal emphasis, is most often unreactive to external stimulation, and is manifest in comatose and stuporous states.[77] There is consensus that it is an abnormally generated pattern, not merely a modification of the posterior alpha rhythm.[102] At least in postanoxic states, it may originate in the amygdaloid nuclei and be propagated by relatively intact thalamocortical pathways.[103] Although some attempt has been made to distinguish features of the alpha coma pattern that would indicate either diffuse cortical versus primary brainstem pathology,[97] such distinctions are not uniformly tenable.[54] The alpha coma pattern must be distinguished from the ictal alpha discharge (pseudoalpha) seen in neonates who are having seizures.[104]

Burst-Suppression

Burst-suppression activity consists of brief bursts of spike, sharp and slow-wave activity alternating with longer periods of relative electrocortical flattening that may last from seconds to many minutes. The pattern is usually bilateral but may be asymmetrical and is unreactive to external stimuli.[77] Both human and experimental data have shown that the pattern occurs when cortex has been isolated from its connections with other cortical regions and from subcortical

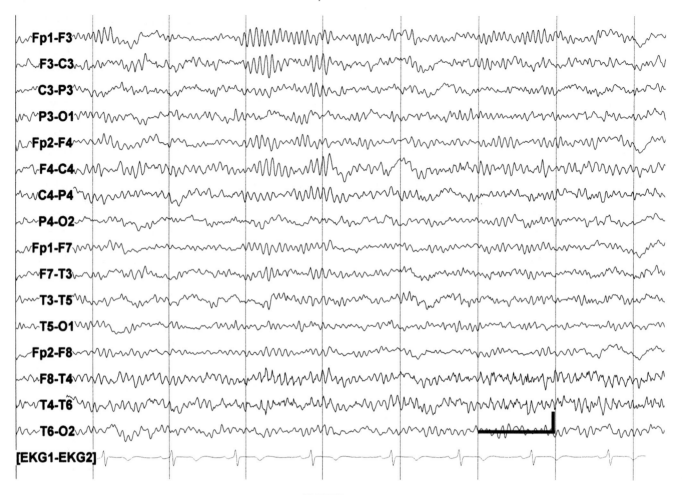

FIGURE 18–4

Spindle coma in an 18-year-old girl following a closed head injury. Calibration: 1 second, 50 µV.

nuclei.[47,105] Hence, burst-suppression may arise from pathologic processes that produce cortical deafferentation. This could account for its occurrence in a variety of conditions including anoxia, encephalitis, hypothermia, Reye's syndrome, deep anesthesia, and depressant drug overdoses as well as head trauma.[70] In neonates, it must be distinguished from the physiologic tracé alternant pattern of quiet sleep. In patients with infantile spasms, it may be seen as a component of the hypsarrhythmic EEG. Some authors have indicated that burst-suppression occurs only when cerebral anoxia complicates head trauma,[23,106] thus portending a poor prognosis. In dealing with children, it is perhaps best to take a more cautious approach. Serial tracings may be particularly beneficial in this instance. If the bursts become briefer, lower in amplitude, and simpler in morphology as the periods of suppressed activity lengthen, the prognosis is poor and the pattern may likely give way to one of electro-

cerebral inactivity. Conversely, if the bursts become longer with corresponding diminishment of the suppressed periods and physiologic background rhythms begin to make their reappearance, the outlook is improved.

ELECTROCEREBRAL INACTIVITY AND THE LOW-VOLTAGE OUTPUT RECORD

Electrocerebral inactivity is defined as "no EEG activity over 2 µV when recording from scalp electrode pairs 10 cm or more apart with interelectrode impedances under 10,000 Ω but over 100 Ω."[107] The particular difficulties of applying electrocerebral inactivity criteria to the pediatric age group are discussed in Chapter 20. The precursor of electrocerebral inactivity, the low-voltage record, consists of remnants of

EEG activity less than 20 μV.[108] In the absence of reversible causes of electrocortical depression, such as hypothermia, central nervous system depressants, hypotension, and various metabolic and endocrine disorders,[109] these patterns are grave prognostic signs and represent the ultimate effects of progressive increased intracranial pressure. Although studies of patients with pseudotumor cerebri have indicated that increased intracranial pressure per se does not alter the EEG,[71,110] in the setting of post-traumatic coma, pressure changes are associated clinically with secondary midbrain and bulbar syndromes that reflect the rostrocaudal deterioration of neurologic function[111] and express themselves electrophysiologically in a defined sequence.[112] The variety of EEG patterns (slow wave abnormalities, sleep or sleeplike activity, and alternating patterns) and the reactivity of these patterns to external stimulation decrease with progression of the rostrocaudal deterioration, with the low-voltage and electrocerebral inactivity signatures representing the latter phases of this process.

POSTCONCUSSION (POST-TRAUMATIC) SYNDROME

In adults, the postconcussion syndrome consists of a spectrum of symptoms including headache, vertigo, inability to concentrate, irritability, impaired memory, nervousness, fatigue, and insomnia.[113,114] A similar syndrome has been reported in children, but there are some important differences.[115] Children tend to complain less of headache, but sleep disturbances, enuresis, personality changes, and psychiatric symptoms are more common. Whether the postconcussion syndrome results from traumatic disruption of nervous tissue or from a conscious exercise on the part of the patient to win litigation has been long debated. That the syndrome occurs in children who cannot fathom the prospect of legal reward has been taken by some as proof of the former and refutation of the latter.[116] Regardless of the mechanism, there is a typical lack of objective physical findings on the neurologic examination, and this has led investigators to seek laboratory confirmation of the diagnosis. The EEG, however, can neither prove nor disprove the presence of the syndrome.[117] A normal EEG may be seen in children with significant brain injury, whereas severe EEG abnormalities may occur in children who do not manifest any of the aforementioned symptoms.[81] Several researchers have claimed that other electrophysiologic parameters, such as visual[118] and auditory[119] evoked potentials and long latency auditory event-related potentials[120] provide objective markers of the syndrome, but for the most part, these studies have involved small numbers of patients and the results await verification by other laboratories.

QUANTITATIVE EEG

The term *quantitative EEG* refers to a variety of computer-assisted methods of EEG analysis and display including spectral analysis, compressed spectral array (CSA), significance probability mapping, and topographic brain mapping.[121] Potential advantages of these techniques are that they may reveal abnormalities that are missed by visual inspection of the routine EEG, they may assist in determining whether particular EEG features are present to an abnormal degree, and they may permit the reformatting of conventional EEG data in a way that is more understandable to those who are unfamiliar with methods of routine EEG interpretation.[122] These features suggest that quantitative EEG holds great promise for the assessment of head-injured children. Some preliminary studies, conducted with mainly adult patients, are encouraging in this regard. In a series of comatose patients, Karnaze and associates[123] found that the presence of alternating patterns on CSA was significantly associated with survival. The prognostic value of CSA was equal to the Glasgow Coma Scale and the neurologic examination, and occasionally it added prognostic information. Bricolo and colleagues[124] noted that an unfavorable outcome occurred in 95% of patients with a slow and monotonous CSA but in only 30% of patients with changeable CSA patterns. Sironi and coworkers[82] also correlated CSA patterns with outcome. Mortality was 88% with a slow unchanging CSA, 59% with diphasic CSA patterns that alternated between the alpha and delta frequency ranges, and 13% with a changeable sleeplike CSA.

Thatcher and associates[125] evaluated the ability of power spectral analysis of EEG to discriminate between mild head-injured patients and a group of age-matched controls. The former showed diminished alpha power in the posterior head regions, decreased power differences between anterior and posterior head regions, and increased coherence and decreased phase in frontal and frontotemporal regions. Cant and Shaw[126] monitored CSA in a combined series of comatose adults and children. The etiology of coma in most of these patients was head trauma. Persistence or return of peak activity within the alpha or theta frequency ranges in the first 10 days of coma occurred in all patients who made a good recovery. Continued absence of this peak for 10 days or its return and loss was associated with residual disability or death. Similarly, Tebano and colleagues[127] found a shift of mean alpha frequency toward lower values and a reduction of fast beta in patients with mild head injuries compared with age- and sex-matched controls.

The primary difficulty in translating the results of these studies into guidelines for clinical practice is that differences noted between groups of subjects (e.g., those with changing vs. unchanging CSA patterns) do not necessarily predict the prognosis of the individual patient.[128] Furthermore, the currently available computer-assisted techniques have limited specificity and sensitivity.[122] Normal variants may be read as abnormal; transient slowing may be obscured; epileptogenic spikes may be ignored or identified as artifact; and true artifact rejection is more problematic than with routine EEG.[129] Techniques vary widely among laboratories, and there is a pressing need to establish normative databases. This is especially true for the pediatric population in whom the usual variables such as the state of alertness and the effects of medication are compounded by the influences of age.

These limitations indicate that the same recommendations that apply to the use of quantitative EEG in other clinical areas be followed in the assessment of children with head trauma.[130] Quantitative EEG studies should always be accompanied by the unprocessed data, that is, standard EEGs performed according to established pediatric guidelines.[107] The interpreter of such studies must have experience not only in routine EEG interpretation but also in the technical and statistical aspects of computer data processing. A normative data base spanning the age ranges of the children being studied must be available to the interpreter. Finally, quantitative EEG studies should be considered an adjunct and not a substitute for conventional EEG recording. As further refinements in the specificity and sensitivity of quantitative EEG are made, the technique can be expected to assume a more visible role in the assessment of the head-injured child.

PROGNOSIS

Whether EEG findings provide prognostic information for head-injured children is controversial. That these findings fail to predict the development of posttraumatic epilepsy should not necessarily imply that other prognostically useful data cannot be obtained. On the other hand, patients frequently demonstrate a lack of spatial and temporal concordance between their anatomic lesions and EEG abnormalities,[131] and such discrepancies may be magnified in children.[23,132,133] As indicated earlier, children have a higher proportion of abnormal EEGs compared with adults with similar injury. These abnormalities persist for a longer period and are frequently noted even after trivial impact. Given these observations, it is possible that EEG findings may not only fail to prognosticate for children but also provide information that is misleading. Such conclusions, however, become less tenable when careful attention is given to principles of study design. A single sample of EEG activity obtained at a random interval after injury without consideration of the patient's coexisting medical conditions can hardly be expected to delineate clinical events that occur weeks or months later. To truly determine the usefulness of EEG, serial studies on nonselected patients must be obtained

with a consistent system of grading both the clinical severity of trauma and the EEG abnormalities. Allowances must be made for concurrent conditions such as hypoxia, hypotension, and metabolic imbalance that might contribute to the EEG findings. The timing of the recordings in relationship to the injury needs to be specified, and an effort must be made to assess the potential influences of interreader variability.

A number of studies have sought to address these important issues. The meticulous study of Mizrahi and Kellaway[20] discussed earlier showed that children with severe degrees of concussion demonstrated a delayed resolution of slow wave activity coupled with a more protracted course of clinical recovery compared with children with milder insults. Dusser and colleagues[21] studied 24 children with severe closed head injury, defined as impact resulting in immediate or secondary loss of consciousness lasting for at least 6 hours. If EEGs were obtained during the first 3 days following injury, they showed variable findings that were not clearly linked to outcome. In contrast, EEGs obtained after the 3rd day were more stable and provided more prognostically useful information. A prewaking pattern, consisting of monomorphic synchronous 2- to 3-Hz activity in the posterior derivations with lower voltage faster activity anteriorly, was never seen in nonsurvivors. This pattern uniformly predicted complete clinical awakening with reestablishment of organized waking EEG rhythms. On the other hand, a monotonous pattern of continuous, diffusely distributed high-voltage 0.5- to 3.0-Hz activity was associated with a longer period of coma and awakening compared with other EEG patterns and predicted intellectual and motor deficits in half of the survivors.

Rather than correlating overall EEG patterns with outcome, some workers have adopted a different approach, that is, examining the relevance of specific aspects of EEG activity. The association of epileptiform discharges with the persistence of neurologic defects, delineated by Enomoto and coworkers,[47] has already been mentioned. Another salient example is the work of Rumpl and associates.[112] These researchers examined the incidence and prognostic value of sleep spindles in a mixed group of head-injured children and adults who were comatose with signs of brainstem dysfunction. Recordings were obtained in the acute phase (1 to 2 days after injury) and during prolonged coma (3 to 12 days after injury). Spindles were detected more frequently in acute coma (91% of EEGs) than in prolonged coma (30% of EEGs). During the acute phase, typical symmetrical spindles (defined as well-organized, easily recognizable 12- to 14-Hz activity) portended a good prognosis regardless of whether coma was due to supratentorial lesions with early signs of secondary brainstem impairment or to primary lesions of the brainstem. In the latter group, spindles heralded a good outcome even in the presence of decerebrate posturing. With worsening of outcome, not only did the percentage of spindles decrease, but the spindles that were identified became increasingly asymmetrical and distorted. Although small contusions detected on CT scan did not influence spindle activity, more severe intracerebral lesions produced decomposition and ultimately disappearance of the spindles. During prolonged coma, spindles were reduced independent of outcome. However, when they were present, asymmetrical and distorted forms were significantly increased in patients with an unfavorable outcome.

Thus far we have examined how general EEG characteristics (frequency and distribution of background rhythms) and specific EEG patterns (epileptiform discharges, sleep spindles) can aid in providing prognostic information for the head-injured child. Recently, there has been an effort to combine both general and specific EEG findings into prognostic models using standardized rating scales. The system of Rae-Grant and colleagues,[134] for example, is based on dichotomous variables. Various features of the post-traumatic EEG, including background activity, symmetry, reactivity, variability, and specific abnormal patterns, are scored as present or absent (the dichotomy). Each of the features marked as present is then weighted according to its prognostic value based on the available literature on a scale from +10 (good) to –10 (poor). For each EEG, the weightings of the individual features are summed for an overall dichotomous score. The authors retrospectively scored the initial EEGs of 57 adults with head trauma. There was high intrareader and interreader reliability as well as a high correlation between the Glasgow Outcome Score at discharge and the dichotomous EEG score.

Synek[135] graded EEG abnormalities among adults with diffuse anoxic and traumatic encephalopathies. The EEG findings stratified into three outcome categories. Favorable outcome occurred in patients whose EEGs showed any of the following patterns: predominant alpha with some theta, predominant theta that attenuated by external stimulation, and frontal monorhythmic delta. Prognostically uncertain were patients with EEGs that showed diffuse theta that did not attenuate to stimulation, diffuse delta that reacted to stimulation, and the reactive type of alpha coma pattern. Prognostically malignant patterns were small-amplitude diffusely distributed irregular delta, burst-suppression (particularly when associated with epileptiform discharges and a "low-output" EEG), theta pattern coma, the nonreactive type of alpha pattern coma, and electrocerebral silence.

The Rae-Grant[134] and Synek[135] scales have been directed exclusively toward adult patients. There is a pressing need to devise a pediatric counterpart to these scales and to apply it prospectively to large numbers of nonselected head-injured children. Such efforts may hopefully assist in the accurate prognostication that is a necessary basis for the delivery of rational health care to this group of patients.

IATROGENIC INTERVENTIONS

Although most childhood head trauma that comes under electrophysiologic scrutiny results from unpredicted events such as motor vehicle accidents and falls, significant alterations of electrocortical activity can also arise from the planned iatrogenic disruption of nervous tissue. Two areas of particular concern are shunt placement and ablative surgery.

Shunt Placement

The most common procedure for the surgical treatment of hydrocephalus is placement of a ventriculoperitoneal shunt. The proximal end of the shunt is usually inserted through the right posterior parietal region to enter the ipsilateral lateral ventricle. A number of studies have investigated the possibility that shunt placement irritates surrounding cortex and produces an epileptogenic focus.[136] In an uncontrolled study, 40 children who had shunts for hydrocephalus underwent EEG testing following the onset of clinical seizures.[137] Specific abnormalities (spikes, sharp waves, and spike wave discharges) and nonspecific abnormalities (monomorphic and polymorphic slow wave activity) both occurred more frequently over the shunted hemisphere.

Laws and Niedermeyer[138] compared 18 shunted with 25 unshunted hydrocephalic patients. Although abnormal EEGs occurred in both groups, lateralization of abnormalities to the "correct" side occurred in most of the shunted group; in none of the unshunted patients was significant lateralization seen. Ines and Markand[139] compared the EEGs of 81 shunted hydrocephalic children with those of 11 children with nonshunted hydrocephalus. Shunted patients had a significantly higher prevalence of abnormal EEGs and seizures. All types of focal abnormalities and especially slow wave foci were more frequently lateralized over the shunted hemisphere. In more than one half of patients with focal abnormalities, localization to the region of the shunt itself was evident. Seizures in shunted patients uniformly occurred following shunt placement, and left-sided motor seizures were the most common type of focal seizure in patients with right-sided shunts.

Graebner and Celesia[140] compared 21 nonshunted children with hydrocephalus with 26 of their shunted counterparts. Adults and children were included in this study. Again, the shunted group showed a higher prevalence of abnormal EEGs, focal paroxysmal discharges, and clinical seizures. In the shunted group, focal discharges were seen most frequently over the shunted hemisphere.

The pattern of EEG abnormalities was studied in 68 patients (41 male, 27 female, age range 1 month to 17 years) with hydrocephalus by Al-Sulaimann and Ismail.[141] They all had standardized EEG recordings that were read by the same electroencephalographer. In 48 children the EEG was performed after ventriculoperitoneal shunting. The EEG abnormalities in the shunted group included slow waves in 26 patients (focal, 2 [4.2%]; generalized asynchronous, 22 [45.8%]; generalized synchronous, 2 [4.2%]); amplitude abnormalities in 2 (focal, 1; generalized, 1); epileptiform activity in 26 (partial, 11 [22.9%]; generalized, 15 [31.3%]) and hypsarrhythmia in 4 (8.3%). Only four (8.3%) traces were normal, giving an overall percentage abnormality of 92%. In the unshunted group, generalized asynchronous slow waves were found in 12 patients (60%), generalized amplitude abnormality in 1, focal epileptiform activity in 3 (15%), and generalized epileptiform activity in 6 (30%); two tracings in this group were normal, giving an overall percentage abnormality of 90%. The conclusion of the study was that hydrocephalus in children, regardless of the cause, may be associated with generalized or focal EEG abnormalities.

These studies have several obvious limitations. They were not prospective, and presurgical EEGs were not routinely available. Attempts to exclude patients with gross structural lesions such as tumors, cysts, and hematomas did not eliminate the possibility of cortical microdysgenesis, microscopic hypoxic-ischemic cell damage, or the hydrocephalus itself from contributing to the observed EEG abnormalities. Nonetheless, the studies do provide evidence that shunt placement can cause focal cortical irritability with seizures and that not all children who sustain seizures following shunt placement may do so because of their underlying disease.

Ablative Surgery

The effects of ablative surgery on the EEG have been most extensively studied in patients undergoing operative procedures for control of intractable epilepsy. Four procedures will be briefly considered: corpus callosotomy, amygdalohippocampectomy, traditional hemispherectomy, and functional hemispherectomy.

Corpus callosotomy tends to produce some asymmetry of the background rhythms but does not significantly alter the frequency of the posterior dominant head rhythm.[142] In the majority of patients, the abundance of the generalized discharges is reduced[142,143] and epileptiform activity becomes asymmetrical and/or asynchronous[142] often in a multifocal or bifrontal distribution. Neither the number of discharges nor the number of epileptiform foci on the postoperative EEG appears to be related to outcome.

Following selective amygdalohippocampectomy, the postoperative EEG tends to show improvement in background abnormalities, ipsilateral and contralateral focal slowing, and ipsilateral and contralateral epileptogenic activity.[144] Postoperative normalization of the EEG is more pronounced in patients with tumors and dysplasias including arteriovenous malformations, compared with patients with mesiotemporal lobe sclerosis. In contrast to patients undergoing corpus callosotomy, patients undergoing selective amygdalohippocampectomy show a strong correlation between improvement in the EEG and clinical seizure outcome.

Hemispherectomy produces attenuation of electrocortical activity on the operated side but does not eliminate all activity.[145] The attenuation of activity is presumably due to the short circulating effect of the CSF which accumulates in the evaluated space, since the conductivity of CSF is approximately five times that of brain. In a series of elegant experiments, Cobb and Sears[146] concluded that the presence of residual activity on the side of the removed hemisphere was due to potential field changes arising from surgical alteration of the shape of the conducting medium. The activity is most likely generated from the remaining deep structures of the operated hemisphere or from the non-operated side and transmitted to the recording electrodes by volume conduction.

In functional hemispherectomy, the central strip and the parietal and temporal lobes are removed. The frontal or occipital lobes, or both, are left in situ with initial blood supply, although commissural and brainstorm connections are divided.[147] The majority of patients undergoing this procedure show complete resolution of epileptogenic activity. In a minority, discharges are noted from the isolated cortical slabs, but these waveforms are different from those evident in the preoperative EEG, being isolated rather than rhythmic, and they do not stipulate the presence of clinical seizure behavior. In general, there is a good correlation between EEG findings and outcome. Patients whose preoperative EEGs showed epileptogenic abnormalities arising independently from the better hemisphere continued to experience recurrent seizures postoperatively. In contrast, bilaterally synchronous spike-and-wave discharges that were unaccompanied by independent discharges from the "good" hemisphere resolved after functional hemispherectomy and presumably represented cases of secondary bilateral synchrony. Those patients all experienced good outcomes.

The use of EEG in the evaluation of epilepsy surgery patients is discussed in more detail in Chapters 22 and 23.

CONCLUSION

Head trauma is the most common form of serious accidental injury in childhood, and children are anatomically predisposed to head trauma. Most of the head injury that has come under EEG investigation has been of the closed, dynamic impact type. The ensuing EEG changes cannot be construed as simply the mechanical disruption of cerebral neural generators; head injury incites a variety of primary and secondary biochemical and ultrastructural changes that can potentially contribute to the observed alterations in EEG frequency, amplitude, and waveforms.

Slowing of background rhythms is the most common abnormality. Compared with adults who sustain a similar degree of injury, the slow wave activity is more pronounced and persists for a longer period. Epileptiform activity is less common, although the prevalence of epileptiform activity is higher in children compared with adults, and the youngest children show the greatest amount of this abnormality. Certain asymmetries and stereotypical patterns may occur and enhance our understanding of the child's functional state. On the other hand, EEG findings can neither prove nor disprove the presence of postconcussion syndrome, nor do they predict the development of post-traumatic epilepsy. Quantitative EEG holds promise in the investigation of the head-injured child. Currently, however, it should be considered an adjunct and not a replacement for conventional EEG recording.

Although it has been debated whether EEG findings can assist in prognostication for head-injured children, a number of studies have shown that general as well as specific EEG features may be helpful in this regard. EEG rating scales using dichotomous variables hold promise for combining both general and specific findings in a prognostically meaningful way. Finally, EEG findings can enhance our understanding of clinical phenomena following iatrogenic disruption of nervous tissue such as shunt placement and ablative surgery.

REFERENCES

1. Gloor P: Hans Berger on the electroencephalogram of man: The fourteen original reports on the human electroencephalogram. Electroencephalogr Clin Neurophysiol 1969;(Suppl 28):1-350.
2. Berger H: Über das Electroenkephalogram des Menchen. J Psychol Neurol 1930;40:160-179.
3. Casey R, Ludwig S, McCormick MC: Morbidity following minor head trauma in children. Pediatrics 1986;78:497-502.
4. Lam WH, MacKersie A: Paediatric head injury: Incidence, aetiology, and management. Paediatr Anaesth 1999;9:377-385.
5. Epstein FJ: Head trauma: Issues and answers. Issues Pediatr Neurosurg 1992;1:1-4.
6. Annegers JF, Grabow JD, Kurland LT, Laws ER: The incidence, causes, and secular trends of head trauma in Olmstead County, Minnesota, 1935-1974. Neurology 1980;30:912-919.
7. Keenan HT, Runyan DK, Marshall SW, et al: A population-based study of inflicted traumatic brain injury in young children. JAMA 2003;290:621-626.
8. Menkes JH, Batzdorf U: Postnatal trauma and injuries by physical agents. *In* Menkes JH (ed): Textbook of Child Neurology. Philadelphia, Lea & Febiger, 1990, p 462.
9. Annegers JF: The epidemiology of head trauma in children. *In* Shapiro K (ed): Pediatric Head Trauma. Mt. Kisco, NY, Futura, 1983, p 1.
10. Schmitt BD, Krugman RD: Abuse and neglect of children. *In* Behrman RE, Vaughan VC (eds): Nelson Textbook of Pediatrics. Philadelphia, WB Saunders, 1987, p 81.
11. Snoek JW, Minderhoud JM, Wilmink JT: Delayed deterioration following mild head injury in children. Brain 1984;107:15-36.
12. Singer HS, Freeman JM: Head trauma for the pediatrician. Pediatrics 1978;62:819-825.
13. Klonoff H, Low MD, Clark C: Head injuries in children: A prospective five-year follow-up. J Neurol Neurosurg Psychiatry 1977;40:1211-1219.
14. Menkes JH, Batzdorf U: Postnatal trauma and injuries by physical agents. *In* Menkes JH (ed): Textbook of Child Neurology. Philadelphia, Lea & Febiger, 1980, p 411.
15. Alfonso I, Curless RG, Holzman BH, et al: Computerized tomography and electroencephalography in childhood coma: Which test should be performed first? J Fla Med Assoc 1985;72:843-845.
16. Jordan KG: Continuous EEG monitoring in the neuroscience intensive care unit and emergency department. J Clin Neurophysiol 1999;16:14-39.
17. Jordan KG: Continuous EEG and evoked potential monitoring in the neuroscience intensive care unit. J Clin Neurophysiol 1993;10:445-475.
18. Pichlmayr I, Lips U, Künkel H: The Electroencephalogram in Anesthesia: Fundamentals, Practical Applications, Examples. Berlin, Springer-Verlag, 1984.
19. Raphaely RC, Swedlow DB, Downes JJ, Bruce DA: Management of severe pediatric head trauma. Pediatr Clin North Am 1980;27:715-727.
20. Mizrahi EM, Kellaway P: Cerebral concussion in children: Assessment of injury by electroencephalography. Pediatrics 1984;73:419-425.
21. Dusser A, Navelet Y, Devictor D, Landrieu P: Short- and long-term prognostic value of the electroencephalogram in children with severe head injury. Electroencephalogr Clin Neurophysiol 1989;73:85-93.
22. Bickford RG, Klass DW: Acute and chronic EEG findings after head injury. *In* Caveness WV, Walker AE (eds): Head Injury: Conference Proceedings. Philadelphia, JB Lippincott, 1966, p 63.
23. Stockard JJ, Bickford RG, Aung MH: The electroencephalogram in traumatic brain injury. *In* Vinken PJ, Bruyn GW (eds): Handbook of Clinical Neurology, Vol. 23. Amsterdam, North Holland, 1975, p 317.
24. Ommaya AK: Experimental head injury. *In* Vinken PJ, Bruyn GW (eds): Handbook of Clinical Neurology, Vol. 23. Amsterdam, North Holland, 1975, p 67.

25. Greenwald BD, Burnett DM, Miller MA: Congenital and acquired brain injury: I. Brain injury: Epidemiology and pathophysiology. Arch Phys Med Rehabil 2003;84(Suppl 1):S3-S7.

26. James HE: Pediatric head injury: what is unique and different. Acta Neurochir 1999;73(Suppl):85-88.

27. Ommaya AK, Goldsmith W, Thibault L: Biomechanics and neuropathology of adult and paediatric head injury. Br J Neurosurg 2002;16:220-242.

28. Charles S: Stepchild of American pediatrics: Child transportation safety. Pediatr Annu 1977;6:77-101.

29. Siegel AW: Injuries to children in automobile collisions. *In* Proceedings, 12th Stapp Car Crash. New York, Society of Automotive Engineers, 1968, p 1.

30. Pudenz RHA, Shelden CH: The lucite calvarium—a method for direct observation of the brain: II: Cranial trauma and brain movement. J Neurosurg 1946;3:487-505.

31. Holbourn AHS: Mechanics of head injuries. Lancet 1943;2:438-441.

32. Prange MT, Coats B, Duhaime AC, Margulies SS: Anthropomorphic simulations of falls, shakes, and inflicted impacts in infants. J Neurosurg 2003;99:143-150.

33. Sullivan JF, Abbott JA, Schwab RS: The electro-encephalogram in cases of subdural hematoma and hydroma. Electroencephalogr Clin Neurophysiol 1951;3:131-139.

34. Ommaya AK, Gennarelli TA: Cerebral concussion and traumatic unconsciousness: Correlation of experimental and clinical observations of blunt head injuries. Brain 1974;97:633-654.

35. Adams JH, Mitchell DE, Graham DI, Doyle D: Diffuse brain damage of immediate impact type: Its relationship to primary brainstem damage in head injury. Brain 1977;100:489-502.

36. Yang MS, DeWitt DS, Becker DP, Hayes RL: Regional brain metabolite levels following mild experimental head injury in the cat. J Neurosurg 1985;63:617-621.

37. Bakay L, Lee JC, Lee GC, Peng J-R: Experimental cerebral concussion: I. An electron microscopic study. J Neurosurg 1977;47:525-531.

38. Lewelt W, Jenkins LW, Miller JD: Autoregulation of cerebral blood flow after experimental fluid percussion injury to the brain. J Neurosurg 1980;53:500-511.

39. Bruce DA, Alavi A, Bilaniuk LT, et al: Diffuse cerebral swelling following head injuries in children: The syndrome of "malignant brain edema." J Neurosurg 1981;54:170-178.

40. Overgaard J, Tweed WA: Cerebral circulation after head injury: I. Cerebral blood flow and its regulation after closed head injury with emphasis on clinical correlatives. J Neurosurg 1974;41:531-541.

41. Becker DP, Verity MA, Povlischock J, Cheung M: Brain cellular injury and recovery: Horizons for improving medical therapies in stroke and trauma. West J Med 1988;148:670-684.

42. Ellis EF, Wright KF, Wei EP, Kontos HA: Cyclooxygenase products of arachidonic acid metabolism in cat cerebral cortex after experimental concussive brain injury. J Neurochem 1981;37:892-896.

43. Blume WT: Atlas of Pediatric Electroencephalography. New York, Raven Press, 1982.

44. Strauss H: The electroencephalogram in the evaluation of head injuries without gross neurologic deficit. J Hillside Hosp 1956;5:268-281.

45. Silverman D: Electroencephalographic study of acute head injury in children. Neurology 1962;12:273-281.

46. Gibbs EL, Gibbs EL, Gibbs FA: Electroencephalographic findings among children with head injuries. Clin Electroencephalogr 1982;13:162-177.

47. Enomoto T, Ono Y, Nose T, et al: Electroencephalography in minor head injury in children. Child Nerv Syst 1986;2:72-79.

48. Kellaway P: An orderly approach to visual analysis: Characteristics of the normal EEG of adults and children. *In* Daly DD, Pedley TA (eds): Current Practice of Clinical Electroencephalography. New York, Raven Press, 1990, p 139.

49. Frantzen E, Harvald B, Haugsted H: Fresh head injuries. Acta Psychiatr Neurol Scand 1958;33:417-428.

50. Eeg-Olofsson O, Petersén I, Selldén U: The development of the electroencephalogram in normal children from the age of 1 through 15 years: Paroxysmal activity. Neuropädiatrie 1971;2:375-404.

51. Fukushima Y, Kawaguchi S, Ohsawa T, Onuma T: A study of EEG abnormality in normal children. Folia Psychiatr Neurol Jpn 1973;27:106-115.

52. Annegers JF, Grabow JD, Groover RV, et al: Seizures after head trauma: A population study. Neurology 1980;30:683-689.

53. Jennett B: Trauma as a cause of epilepsy in childhood. Dev Med Child Neurol 1973;15:56-62.

54. Grindal AB, Suter C, Martinez AJ: Alpha-pattern coma: Twenty-four cases with nine survivors. Ann Neurol 1977;1:371-377.

55. Oxbury JM, Whitty CW: Causes and consequences of status epilepticus in adults: A study of eighty-six cases. Brain 1971;94:733-744.

56. Jennett B, van de Sande J: EEG prediction of post-traumatic epilepsy. Epilepsia 1975;16:251-256.

57. Scherzer E, Wessely P: EEG in posttraumatic epilepsy. Eur Neurol 1978;17:38-42.

58. Courjon J, Mauguiere F: L'EEG dans le epilepsies post-traumatiques. Boll Lega It Epil 1982;39:19-22.

59. Kennedy CR: Posttraumatic seizures in childhood. Pediatr Epilepsy 1988;1:3-9.

60. Hendrick EB, Harris L: Post-traumatic epilepsy in children. J Trauma 1968;8:547-555.

61. Angeleri F, Majkowski J, Cacchio G, et al: Posttraumatic epilepsy risk factors: One-year prospective study after head injury. Epilepsia 1999;40:1222-1230.

62. Chiaretti A, De Benedictis R, Polidori G, et al: Early post-traumatic seizures in children with head injury. Child Nerv Syst 2000;16:862-866.

63. Jennett B: Posttraumatic epilepsy. *In* Vinken PJ, Bruyn GW (eds): Handbook of Clinical Neurology, Vol. 24. Amsterdam, North Holland, 1976, p 445.

64. Feeney DM, Walker AE: The prediction of posttraumatic epilepsy: A mathematical approach. Arch Neurol 1979;36:8-12.

65. Caveness WF, Meirowsky AM, Rish BL, et al: The nature of posttraumatic epilepsy. J Neurosurg 1979;50:545-553.

66. Stockard-Pope JE, Werner SS, Bickford RG: Atlas of Neonatal Electroencephalography, 2nd ed. New York, Raven Press, 1992.

67. Chatrian GW, Somasundaram M, Foltz EL: EEG changes in subgaleal hematomas. Electroencephalogr Clin Neurophysiol 1969;26:524-527.

68. Volpe JJ: Neurology of the Newborn, 3rd ed. Philadelphia, WB Saunders, 1995.

69. Cobb WA, Guiloff RJ, Cast J: Breach rhythm: The EEG related to skull defects. Electroencephalogr Clin Neurophysiol 1979;47:251-271.

70. Spehlmann R: EEG Primer. Amsterdam, Elsevier, 1981.

71. Caffey J: The whiplash shaken-infant syndrome: Manual shaking by the extremities with whiplash-induced intracranial and intraocular bleedings, linked with residual permanent brain damage and mental retardation. Pediatrics 1974;54:396-403.

72. Chusid JG, de Gutierrez-Mahoney CG: The electroencephalogram in head injuries with subdural hematoma. Neurology 1956;6:11-21.

73. Pampiglione G: Some criteria of maturation in the EEG of children up to the age of 3 years. Electroencephalogr Clin Neurophysiol 1972;32:463.

74. Rodin EA: Contribution of the EEG to prognosis after head injury. Dis Nerv Sys 1967;28:595-601.

75. Kooi KA, Tucker RP, Marshall RE: Fundamentals of Electroencephalography. Hagerstown, MD, Harper & Row, 1978.

76. Roseman E, Bloor BM, Schmidt RP: The electroencephalogram in intracranial aneurysms. Neurology 1951;1:25-38.

77. Tyner FS, Knott JR, Mayer WB Jr: Fundamentals of EEG Technology, Vol. 2: Clinical Correlates. New York, Raven Press, 1989.

78. Rumpl E, Bauer G, Stampfel G: Der Angiospasmus bei der Subarachnoidalblutung als wichtige Ursache für fokale Veränderungen im EEG. Z EEG-EMG 1977;8:200-204.

79. Gloor P, Ball G, Schaul N: Brain lesions that produce delta waves in the EEG. Neurology 1977;27:326-333.

80. Daly DD, Markand ON: Focal brain lesions. *In* Daly DD, Pedley TA (eds): Current Practice of Clinical Electroencephalography. New York, Raven Press, 1990, p 335.

81. Courjon J, Scherzer E: Traumatic disorders. *In* Remond A, Magnus O, Courjon J (eds): Handbook of Electroencephalography and Clinical Neurophysiology, Vol. 14. Amsterdam, Elsevier, 1972, p 8.

82. Sironi VA, Ravagnati L, Signoroni G, et al: Diagnostic and prognostic value of EEG compressed spectral analysis in post-traumatic coma. *In* Villani R, Papo I, Giovanelli M, et al (eds): Advances in Neurotraumatology. Amsterdam, Excerpta Medica, 1983, p 328.

83. PeBenito R, Cracco JB: Periodic lateralized epileptiform discharges in infants and children. Ann Neurol 1979;6:47-50.

84. Chatrian GE, Shaw C-M, Leffman H: The significance of periodic lateralized epileptiform discharges in EEG: An electrographic, clinical, and pathological study. Electroencephalogr Clin Neurophysiol 1964;17:177-193.

85. de la Paz D, Brenner RD: Bilateral independent periodic lateralized epileptiform discharges: Clinical significance. Arch Neurol 1981;38:713-715.

86. Illis LS, Taylor FM: The electroencephalogram in herpes simplex encephalitis. Lancet 1972;1:718-721.

87. Virmani V, Roy S, Kamala G: Periodic lateralised epileptiform discharges in a case of diffuse cerebral cysticercosis. Neuropaediatrie 1977;8:196-203.

88. Purpura DP, Housepian EM: Morphological and physiological properties of chronically isolated immature cortex. Exp Neurol 1961;4:377-401.

89. Bahamon-Dussan JE, Celesia GC, Gigg-Damberger MM: Prognostic significance of EEG triphasic waves in patients with altered state of consciousness. J Clin Neurophysiol 1989;6:313-319.

90. MacGillivay BB: The EEG in liver disease. *In* Rémond A (ed): Handbook of Electroencephalography and Clinical Neurophysiology, Vol. 15-C. Amsterdam, Elsevier, 1976, p 26.

91. Watson CW, Flynn RE, Sullivan JF: A distinctive electroencephalographic change associated with subdural hematoma resembling changes which occur with hepatic encephalopathy. Electroencephalogr Clin Neurophysiol 1958;10:780.

92. Chatrian GE, White LE, Shaw C-M: EEG pattern resembling wakefulness in unresponsive decerebrate state following traumatic brain stem infarct. Electroencephalogr Clin Neurophysiol 1964;16:285-289.

93. Kaplan PW, Genoud D, Ho TW, Jallon P: Clinical correlates and prognosis in early spindle coma. Clin Neurophysiol 2000;111:584-590.

94. Kaplan PW, Genoud D, Ho TW, Jallon P: Etiology, neurologic correlations, and prognosis in alpha coma. Clin Neurophysiol 1999;110:205-213.

95. Horton EJ, Goldie WD, Baram TZ: Rhythmic coma in children. J Child Neurol 1990;5:242-247.

96. Gibbs EL, Gibbs FA: Extreme spindles: Correlation of electroencephalographic sleep pattern with mental retardation. Science 1962;138:1106-1107.

97. Westmoreland BF, Klass DW, Sharbrough FW, Reagan TJ: Alpha coma: Electroencephalographic, clinical, pathologic, and etiologic correlations. Arch Neurol 1975;32:713-718.

98. Carroll WM, Mastaglia FL: Alpha and beta coma in drug intoxication uncomplicated by cerebral hypoxia. Electroencephalogr Clin Neurophysiol 1979;46:95-105.

99. Frischer S, Herishanu Y: Mu and alpha rhythm in comatose children. Child Nerv Syst 1985;1:208-210.

100. Lersch DR, Kaplan AM: Alpha-pattern coma in childhood and adolescence. Arch Neurol 1984;41:68-70.

101. Pulst S-M, Lombroso CT: External ophthalmoplegia, alpha, and spindle coma in imipramine overdose: Case report and review of the literature. Ann Neurol 1983;14:587-590.

102. Collins AT, Chatrian GE: EEG rhythm of alpha frequency in a 22-month-old child after strangulation. Neurology 1980;30:1316-1319.

103. Gurvitch AM, Zarzhetsky Yu V, Trush VD, Zonov VM: Experimental data on the nature of post-resuscitation alpha frequency activity. Electroencephalogr Clin Neurophysiol 1984;58:426-437.

104. Lombroso CT: Neonatal polygraphy in full-term and premature infants: A review of normal and abnormal findings. J Clin Neurophysiol 1985;2:105-153.

105. Echlin FA, Arnett V, Zoll J: Paroxysmal high-voltage discharges from isolated and partially isolated human and animal cerebral cortex. Electroencephalogr Clin Neurophysiol 1952;4:147-164.

106. Rumpl E, Lorenzi E, Hackl JM, et al: The EEG at different stages of acute secondary traumatic midbrain and bulbar brain syndromes. Electroencephalogr Clin Neurophysiol 1979;46:487-497.

107. American Electroencephalographic Society: Guidelines in EEG and Evoked Potentials: Guideline Two. Minimum technical standards for pediatric electroencephalography. J Clin Neurophysiol 1986;3(Suppl 1):7-11.

108. Bauer G: Coma and brain death. *In* Niedermeyer E, Lopes da Silva F (eds): Electroencephalography Basic Principles, Clinical Applications, and Related Fields. Baltimore, Urban & Schwarzenberg, 1987, p 391.

109. Chatrian GE: Coma, other states of altered responsiveness, and brain death. *In* Daly DD, Pedley TA (eds): Current Practice of Clinical Electroencephalography. New York, Raven Press, 1990, p 425.

110. Boddie HG, Banna M, Bradley WG: "Benign" intracranial hypertension. Brain 1974;97:313-326.

111. Gerstenbrand F, Lücking CH: Die akuten traumatischen Hirnstammschäden. Arch Psychiatr Nervenkrankh 1970;213:264-281.

112. Rumpl E, Prugger M, Bauer G, et al: Incidence and prognostic value of spindles in post-traumatic coma. Electroencephalogr Clin Neurophysiol 1983;56:420-429.

113. Caveness WF: Posttraumatic sequelae. *In* Caveness WF, Walker AE (eds): Head Injury: Conference Proceedings. Philadelphia, JB Lippincott, 1966, p 209.

114. Savola O, Hillbom M: Early predictors of post-concussion symptoms in patients with mild head injury. Eur J Neurol 2003;10:175-181.

115. Dillon H, Leopold LR: Children and the post-concussion syndrome. JAMA 1961;175:86-92.

116. Symonds C: Concussion and its sequelae. Lancet 1962;1:1-5.

117. Courjon J: La place de l'electroencephalographie en traumatologie cranienne. Cah Méd Lyon 1962;38:315-317.

118. Feinsod M, Hoyt WF, Wilson WB, Spire J-P: Visually evoked response: Use in neurologic evaluation of posttraumatic subjective visual complaints. Arch Ophthalmol 1976;24:237-240.

119. Noseworthy JH, Miller J, Murray TJ, Regan D: Auditory brainstem responses in postconcussion syndrome. Arch Neurol 1981;38:275-278.

120. Drake ME, John K: Long-latency event-related potentials in postconcussion syndrome. Clin Evoked Potentials 1987;5:19-21.

121. Nuwer MR: Quantitative EEG: I. Techniques and problems of frequency analysis and topographic mapping. J Clin Neurophysiol 1988;5:1-43.

122. Therapeutics and Technology Assessment Subcommittee of the American Academy of Neurology: Assessment: EEG brain mapping. Neurology 1989;39:1100-1101.

123. Karnaze DS, Marshall LF, Bickford RG: EEG monitoring of clinical coma: The compressed spectral array. Neurology 1982;32:289-292.

124. Bricolo A, Turazzi S, Faccioli F, et al: Clinical application of compressed spectral array in long-term EEG monitoring of comatose patients. Electroencephalogr Clin Neurophysiol 1978;45:211-225.

125. Thatcher RW, Walker RA, Gerson I, Geisler FH: EEG discriminant analyses of mild head trauma. Electroencephalogr Clin Neurophysiol 1989;73:94-106.

126. Cant BR, Shaw NA: Monitoring by compressed spectral array in prolonged coma. Neurology 1984;34:35-39.

127. Tebano MT, Cameroni M, Gallozzi G, et al: EEG spectral analysis after minor head injury in man. Electroencephalogr Clin Neurophysiol 1988;70:185-189.

128. Duffy FH: Clinical value of topographic mapping and quantified neurophysiology. Arch Neurol 1989;46:1133-1134.

129. Nuwer MR: Uses and abuses of brain mapping. Arch Neurol 1989;46:1134-1136.

130. American Electroencephalography Society: American Electroencephalographic Society statement on the clinical use of quantitative EEG. J Clin Neurophysiol 1987;4:75.

131. Hauser WA: EEG and head trauma. Am J EEG Technol 1979;19:145-151.

132. Dumermuth G: Elecktroencephalographie im Kindesalter. Stuttgart, Thieme, 1965.

133. Lenard HG: EEG: Veränderungen bei frishen Schädeltraumen im Kindesalter. Med Wochenschr 1965;107:1820-1827.

134. Rae-Grant AD, Barbour PJ, Reed J: Development of a novel EEG rating scale for head injury using dichotomous variables. Electroencephalogr Clin Neurophysiol 1991;79:349-357.

135. Synek VM: Prognostically important EEG coma patterns in diffuse anoxic and traumatic encephalopathies in adults. J Clin Neurophysiol 1988;5:161-174.

136. Sato O, Yamguchi T, Kittaka M, Toyama H: Hydrocephalus and epilepsy. Child Nerv Syst 2001;17:76-86.

137. Ligouri G, Abate M, Buono S, Pittore L: EEG findings in shunted hydrocephalic patients with epileptic seizures. Ital J Neurol Sci 1986;7:243-247.

138. Laws ER, Niedermeyer E: EEG findings in hydrocephalic patients with shunt procedures. Electroencephalogr Clin Neurophysiol 1970;29:325.

139. Ines DF, Markand ON: Epileptic seizures and abnormal electroencephalographic findings in hydrocephalus and their relation to the shunting procedures. Electroencephalogr Clin Neurophysiol 1977;42:761-768.

140. Graebner RW, Celesia GG: EEG findings in hydrocephalus and their relation to shunting procedures. Electroencephalogr Clin Neurophysiol 1973;35:517-521.

141. Al-Sulaimann AA, Ismail HM: Pattern of electrographic abnormalities in children with hydrocephalus: A study of 68 patients. Child Nerv Syst 1998;14:124-126.

142. Goldberg WE, Holmes GL, Gould J: Effects of anterior corpus callosotomy on the electroencephalogram. *J Epilepsy* 1989;2:73-81.

143. Gates JR, Leppik IE, Yap J, Gumnit RJ: Corpus callosotomy: Clinical and electroencephalographic effects. *Epilepsia* 1984;25:308-316.

144. Siegel AM, Wieser HG: Comparative pre- and postoperative interictal scalp electroencephalographic examinations in patients with selective amygdalohippocampectomy. *J Epilepsy* 1989;2:65-72.

145. Marshall C, Walker AE: The electroencephalographic changes after hemispherectomy in man. *Electroencephalogr Clin Neurophysiol* 1950;2:147-156.

146. Cobb W, Sears TA: A study of the transmission of potentials after hemispherectomy. *Electroencephalogr Clin Neurophysiol* 1960;12:371-383.

147. Rasmussen T: Hemispherectomy for seizures revisited. *Can J Neurol Sci* 1983;10:71-78.

19

Childhood Sleep-Wake Disorders

Suresh Kotagal

Sleep-wake disorders are common, affecting 17% to 21% of all children.[1] They are of diverse etiology. Some such as narcolepsy and parasomnias are related to intrinsic central nervous system dysfunction, whereas others such as limit-setting disorder are due to extrinsic factors. Childhood sleep disorders may adversely impact the sleep and quality of life of not only the patient but also other family members. Many sleep disorders are treatable. This chapter addresses techniques commonly used in the clinical neurophysiologic assessment of common childhood sleep disorders. A glossary of commonly used terms is provided before embarking on a discussion of technical issues. Sleep ontogeny is not reviewed because it has been covered elsewhere in this book.

POLYSOMNOGRAPHY NOMENCLATURE

Periodic breathing   This a normal variant that is defined as three or more central apnea episodes of ≥ 3 seconds with an intervening period of ≤ 20 seconds. It is most prevalent in premature infants during active sleep.

Central apnea   Cessation of oronasal airflow/nasal pressure signal along with simultaneous loss of the thoracic and abdominal respiratory effort lasting ≥ 20 seconds (Fig. 19-1)

Mixed apnea   Simultaneous cessation of oronasal airflow/nasal pressure signal, and thoracic and abdominal respiratory effort, but with recovery of the respiratory effort prior to that of the nasal airflow/nasal pressure recording (Fig. 19-2)

Obstructive sleep apnea   Cessation of oronasal airflow/nasal pressure signal but with preservation of the thoracic and abdominal respiratory effort

Arousals   These are electroencephalographic (EEG) events of ≥ 3 seconds that are characterized by an abrupt shift in the EEG background from a slower frequency to a faster frequency (e.g., from delta to theta). They are an index of sleep fragmentation. There may be simultaneous augmentation of electromyographic (EMG) activity and an increase in heart rate. Arousals generally need to be separated from each other by a minimum of 10 seconds (Fig. 19-3).

Hypopneas   Children frequently manifest partial upper airway obstructions or hypopneas rather than true obstructive apneas. Hypopneas are defined as respiratory events of ≥ 5 seconds during which there is an approximately 50% reduction in amplitude of the oronasal airflow/nasal pressure signal, along with 3% to 4% oxygen desaturation (Fig. 19-4).

Sleep-related hypoventilation   The end-tidal carbon dioxide ($ETCO_2$) level is measured at the level of the anterior nares and correlates well with the alveolar CO_2 levels. Patients with shallow chest wall motion such as those with Down syndrome, neuromuscular disorders, and obesity frequently show elevated $ETCO_2$ levels. The physiologic $ETCO_2$ is generally between 35 and 45 mm Hg. Hypoventilation is defined as $ETCO_2$ of > 50 mm Hg for ≥ 10% of the total recording time.

Nocturnal oxygen desaturation   The physiologic oxygen saturation is ≈ 96%, whereas saturation values < 92% are considered abnormal in children. Low

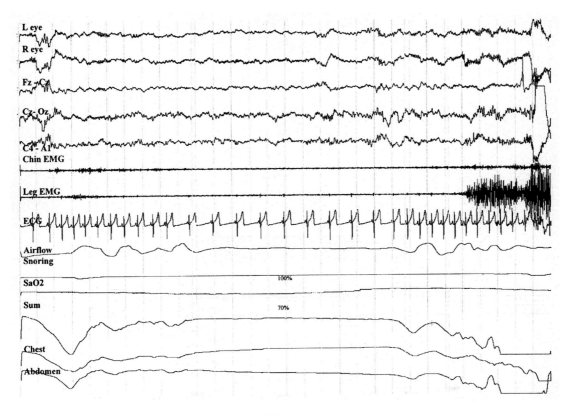

FIGURE 19–1

Central apnea in a child with a pilocytic astrocytoma of the brainstem. Note the simultaneous loss of signal in the airflow as well as thoracic and abdominal respiratory effort channels. The EKG channel shows bradycardia. In the final third of the graph, the EEG channels Fz-Cz, Cz-Oz, and C4-A1 show an arousal response on the termination of the apnea, with appearance of an alpha rhythm. Paper speed: 10 mm/sec.

levels are common in patients with sleep-related upper airway obstruction.

Periodic limb movements (PLMs) A series of three or more events of activation of leg or arm EMG activity, each of 0.5- to 5-second duration, separated by 4- to 90-second interval that is generally seen during non-rapid eye movement (NREM) sleep. PLMs may provoke arousals. The normal PLM index (events per hour of sleep) is generally < 5 (Fig. 19-5).

Sleep latency time Time between lights out and sleep onset during polysomnography

Rapid eye movement (REM) latency Time between the onset of sleep and the onset of the first epoch of REM sleep

Cyclic alternating patterns Periodic EEG activity during NREM sleep that is characterized by sequences of transient electrocortical events distinct from the EEG background that recur at (1-minute) intervals. They constitute another marker for sleep fragmentation.

Vertex sharp transients EEG transients of 50- to 200-millisecond duration and of variable amplitude

($\leq$ 250 μV); generally seen in stages I and II of NREM sleep

K-complexes Biphasic or triphasic high-amplitude transients of 0.5- to 2-second duration; most often observed during stage II of NREM sleep and also infrequently during stages III and IV

NOCTURNAL POLYSOMNOGRAPHY

Methodology

Nocturnal polysomnography is the technique of simultaneous recording of multiple physiologic parameters during sleep. It is indicated in the assessment of intrinsic sleep disorders such as suspected upper airway resistance syndrome, obstructive sleep apnea, parasomnias, idiopathic hypersomnia, and narcolepsy.

Typically, the EEG, eye movements, chin and leg EMG, oronasal airflow/nasal pressure, thoracic and abdominal respiratory effort, electrocardiogram (ECG), oxygen saturation,

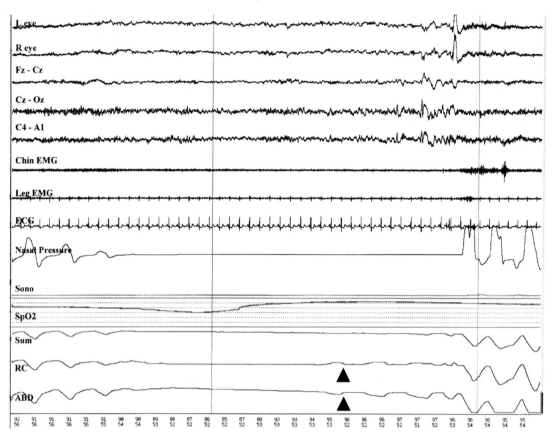

FIGURE 19–2

Mixed apnea. There is loss of signal in the nasal pressure, rib cage (RC), and abdominal respiratory effort channels, quite like that seen in central apneas. However, there is recovery of signal in the rib cage and abdominal effort channels (arrowheads) well prior to the recovery of signal in the nasal pressure channel. An arousal response is also seen at the termination of the mixed apnea, with a burst of eye movement and tonic activation of the chin EMG. Paper speed: 10 mm/sec.

esophageal pH, and end-tidal CO_2 are sampled. The addition of an esophageal balloon, though somewhat intrusive, is helpful in excluding upper airway resistance syndrome. Two or three channels of EEG generally suffice for routine polysomnography (C3-A2/C4-A1, O1-A2/O2-A1, Fz-Cz and Cz-Oz). The central leads are useful for detecting sleep spindles and K-complexes that are generally seen during stages I and II of NREM sleep. The occipital leads help in detecting the transition from the alpha rhythm of quiet wakefulness into the theta-delta mixture of sleep. An expanded, 16-channel EEG montage combined with digital synchronized videotaping is recommended when parasomnias are suspected. The scalp EEG electrodes are applied according to the standard International 10-20 System.[2] Whenever possible, electrodes are secured using collodion to ensure firm electrode contact with the skin and to maintain electrode impedance below 10 kΩ. Pen sensitivity is kept at 50 µV/cm but may be reduced if EEG activity is of very high amplitude and is leading to pen blocking. Respiratory inductive plethys-

mography is the preferred method for recording thoracic and abdominal respiratory effort, although mercury-filled strain gauges have also been used. A pressure transducer is used for measuring nasal pressure. Reductions in the nasal pressure correlate with increases in the negative intra-esophageal pressure that is seen during obstructive sleep apnea and upper airway resistance syndrome events recorded using esophageal balloons. The nasal pressure transducer is therefore a useful device for detecting upper airway resistance events. Oronasal thermocouples or thermistors can be used if the nasal pressure transducer is not tolerated, as happens sometimes with toddlers. Oxygen saturation is sampled using a probe that is clipped onto a finger. Both oxygen saturation and end-tidal CO_2 should be sampled in patients with suspected hypoventilation secondary to obesity, Down syndrome, Prader-Willi syndrome, or neuromuscular disorders. Slow biopotentials such as respiratory effort, oxygen saturation, esophageal pH, and end-tidal CO_2 are generally recorded on direct-current preamplifiers, whereas EEG,

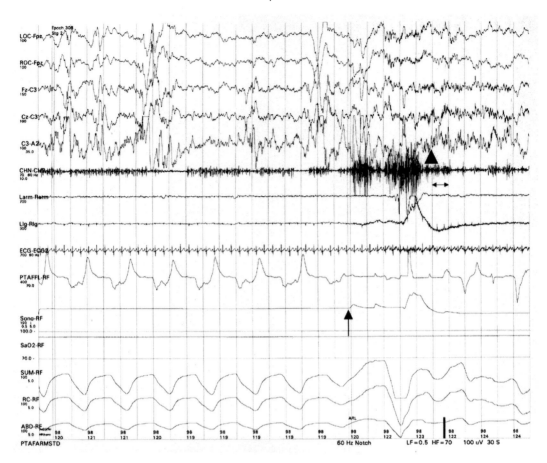

FIGURE 19–3

Arousal provoked by crescendo snoring (arrow) *during stage II of non-rapid eye movement sleep. There is a shift in the EEG frequency (FZ-C3, Cz-C3, C3-A2 channels) from 2- to 3-Hz delta to 7 to 8 Hz* (arrowhead), *along with augmentation of the chin EMG.*

eye movements, EMG, and ECG are recorded on alternate-current preamplifiers.[3,4,5] Recommended settings for various polygraphic channels are shown in Table 19-1.

The data are recorded on moving graph paper or using a computed storing and analysis system. In contrast with standard EEG recordings where the recording paper speed is 30 mm/sec, the general "paper" speed for polysomnography is 10 mm/sec. Frequent notations made throughout the recording about body position, awakenings, involuntary movement, snoring, application of continuous positive airway pressure, and so forth by the sleep technologist help accurate scoring. The attending sleep technologist has to be mindful of artifacts throughout the recording and is required to make an effort to minimize them. The artifacts may be biologic (e.g., sweating), related to the equipment (e.g., a loose electrode), or due to environmental factors (e.g., 60-cycle interference from a fluorescent lamp).[6]

Except in newborns, nap studies are of limited value because they do not adequately sample REM and NREM sleep; thus, all-night polysomnography is the procedure of choice. The validity of unattended polysomnography for the assessment of sleep-related breathing problems has been established only in children older than 5 years of age. At this point, therefore, attended polysomnography within the sleep laboratory remains the gold standard.

Scoring of Polygraphic Data

Computerized systems permit flexibility in varying the epoch length during analysis. The Anders manual[7] is used as a guide for scoring sleep in newborns—sleep is categorized simply into active, quiet, or indeterminate states. From 6 weeks to 6 months, the criteria of Guilleminault and Souquet[8] are used—sleep is categorized into REM and NREM stages I + II and NREM stages III + IV. Beyond 6 months, the standard criteria of Rechtschaffen and Kales[9] are applied, with classification into REM and NREM sleep stages I, II, III, and IV (Table 19-2, Figs. 19-6 and 19-7). Sleep latency may be prolonged in sleep-onset insomnias,

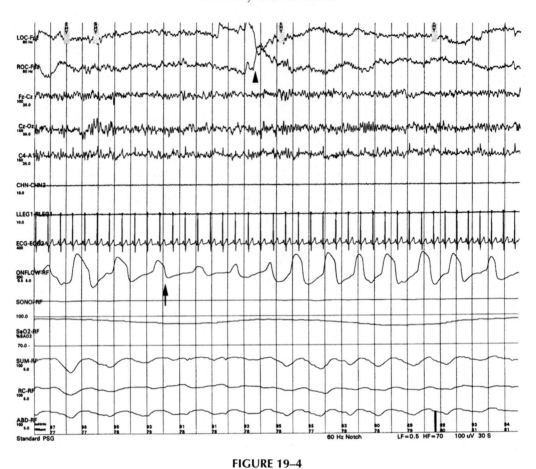

FIGURE 19–4

Hypopnea during non-rapid eye movement sleep. There is an approximately 50% reduction in the amplitude of the oronasal airflow channel and oxygen desaturation, but with preservation of thoracic and abdominal respiratory effort (arrow). There is an isolated eye movement toward the termination point of the hypopnea (arrowhead). Paper speed: 10 mm/sec.

including restless leg syndrome. A short initial nocturnal REM latency (< 70 minutes; normal 120 to 140 minutes) in a teenager is suspicious for depression or narcolepsy.[3] Arousals are scored using the criteria established by the American Sleep Disorders Association.[10] There is unfortunately no clear consensus on scoring respiratory events such as hypopneas, but the reader will find the guidelines established by the American Thoracic Society helpful.[11] The arousal index (events per hour of sleep) is generally less than 12. An increased number of arousals, especially those triggered by snoring, is characteristic of upper airway resistance syndrome. The scoring of hypopneas in children remains arbitrary and somewhat problematic. Specifically, there has been no agreement whether to use 3% or 4% oxygen desaturation to score hypopneas and whether the decrease in the amplitude of the nasal airflow/nasal pressure signal needs to be 30% of the baseline or 50% of the baseline. With regard to obstructive apneas, in contrast with adults who frequently show obstructive apnea events of 10 or more seconds,

the duration of these events in childhood is generally 5 to 10 seconds.[12,13] Reference values for some key polysomnographic findings are given in Table 19-3.

MULTIPLE SLEEP LATENCY TEST

The multiple sleep latency test (MSLT) is a standard, validated (in adults) tool for assessing suspected daytime sleepiness.[14] It measures the speed with which the patient falls asleep in a darkened, quiet environment during the daytime and also whether the transition is from wakefulness into NREM sleep (physiologic; Fig. 19-8) or from wakefulness into REM sleep (pathologic; Fig. 19-9). The MSLT is indicated in the assessment of suspected narcolepsy, idiopathic hypersomnia, and Klein-Levin syndrome.[3,15] As a prerequisite, the individual should be withdrawn from all psychostimulants and REM sleep-suppressing drugs such as antidepressants for at least 2 to 3 weeks. A polysomnogram

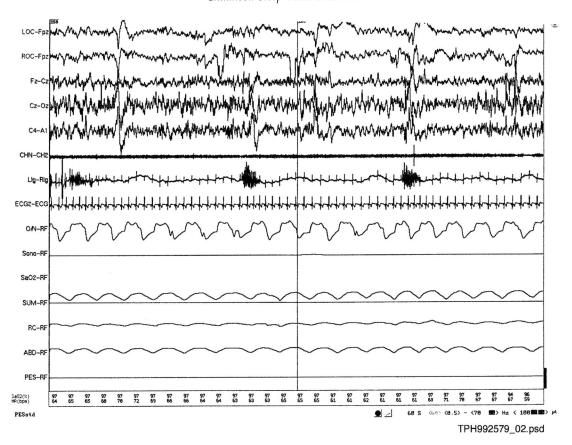

TPH992579_02.psd

FIGURE 19–5

Periodic limb movements. The left leg–right leg channel shows three shorts bursts of EMG activation occurring about 10 seconds apart, with burst lasting approximately 2 seconds; the patient is in non-rapid eye movement sleep. Paper speed: 10 mm/sec.

TABLE 19–1. RECOMMENDED AMPLIFIER SETTINGS

Parameter	Low-Filter Setting, Hz	High-Filter Setting, Hz	Time Constant, sec	Sensitivity, µV/mm
EEG: C3-A2/C4-A1; O1-A2/O2-A1	0.3	90	0.25	7
Eye movements: ROC-A1/A2; LOC-A1/A2	0.3	90	0.25	7
Chin EMG: Right chin-left chin	10	90	0.01	2
EKG: lead II	0.3-1	90	0.25	500

ROC, right outer canthus; LOC, left outer canthus.
Adapted from Shepard JW (ed): Atlas of Sleep Medicine. Mt. Kisco, NY, Futura, 1991, p 5.

is obtained the night before to exclude nocturnal sleep disorders such as obstructive sleep apnea that could impact daytime sleepiness. The test provides valid results in subjects usually 6 years of age and older.

Methodology

Two or three channels of EEG (Fz-Cz, C4-A1/C3-A2, O2-A1/O1-A2) are used for gathering central and occipital EEG information. Two or three eye movement channels (right outer-left outer canthus, left supraorbital-left infraorbital, and right supraorbital-right infraorbital) are used for capturing both horizontal and vertical eye movements. ECG and submental EMG are also sampled. Nap opportunities are provided at two hourly intervals during the day, for example, at 1000, 1200, 1400, and 1600 hours. The patient is asked to remain in street clothes and to try to fall asleep in a darkened, quiet room with the above montage hook-up. If no sleep occurs, the nap opportunity is terminated 20 minutes after lights out. If the patient falls

TABLE 19–2. POLYGRAPHIC FEATURES OF SLEEP STAGES

Sleep Stage	Polygraphic Features
NREM stage I or drowsiness	Mixed frequency (theta, alpha, and delta) EEG activity, isolated vertex sharp transients, and slow, rolling eye movements; regular respiration; tonic EMG activity
NREM stage II	Sleep spindles and K-complexes are prominent; EEG background shows a mixture of theta and delta frequency activity; regular respiration; tonic EMG activity
NREM stage III	EEG shows an increasing amount of high amplitude (>75 μV) delta, which comprises 20-50% of a 30-second sleep epoch; respiration remains regular; tonic EMG activity
NREM stage IV	EEG shows almost continuous high-amplitude delta activity, which now constitutes > 50% of a 30-second sleep epoch; respiration remains regular; tonic EMG activity
REM sleep	EEG shows low-amplitude and mixed-frequency activity (generally theta-delta) and presence of sawtooth waves; irregular respiration, chin EMG is absent or phasic

REM, rapid eye movement; NREM, non-REM.

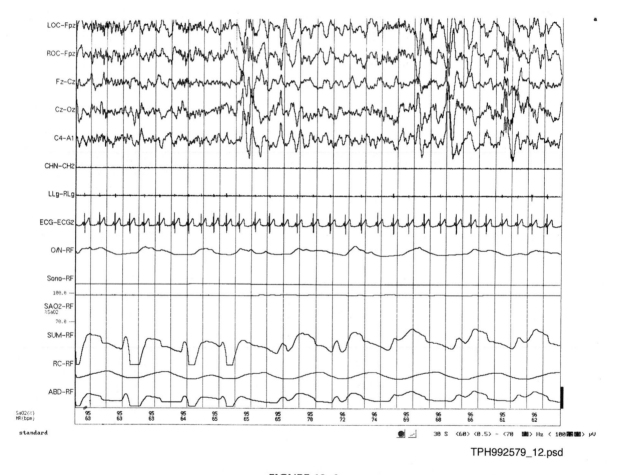

TPH992579_12.psd

FIGURE 19–6

Stage III non-rapid eye movement sleep. Note that the EEG channels Fz-Cz, Cz-Oz, and C4-A1 show high-amplitude delta activity in 20% to 50% of this 30-second epoch; respiration is regular. Paper speed: 10 mm/sec.

asleep, the nap is terminated 15 minutes from sleep onset. The time from lights out to sleep onset is calculated and constitutes the sleep latency. A mean value is derived from the average of sleep latencies of all of the four or five naps.

The help of parents or guardian is needed to keep the patient awake between the nap opportunities; when indicated, a urine drug screen may be obtained during those times.

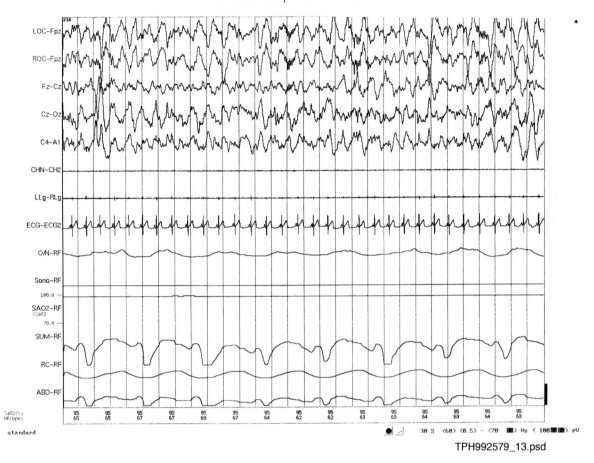

FIGURE 19–7

Stage IV non-rapid eye movement (NREM) sleep. The EEG channels Fz-Cz, Cz-Oz, and C4-A1 show high-amplitude, 2- to 3-Hz continuous delta activity for greater than 50% of this 30-second epoch. Respiration is regular. Stages III and IV NREM sleep are also termed slow wave sleep; nocturnal growth hormone release occurs during slow wave sleep.

TABLE 19–3. NORMAL POLYSOMNOGRAPHIC VALUES IN CHILDREN

Parameter	Value	Comments
TST (hr)	>6	"Acceptable" value during laboratory conditions
Sleep efficiency (%)	>90	"Acceptable" value during laboratory conditions
REM sleep (% of TST)	15-30	Higher values of REM sleep are seen during infancy
Slow wave sleep° (% of TST)	10-40	—
Apnea index†	<1	—
Peak $ETCO_2$ (mm Hg)	<53	—
Duration of hypoventilation‡ (%)	<8	Normal peak CO_2 may be lower during infancy
Oxygen saturation nadir (%)	92	—
Desaturation index§	1.4	—

Adapted from Marcus CR, Loughlin GM: Childhood obstructive sleep apnea. *Semin Pediatr Neurol* 1996;3:23-28.
° Stages III and IV of NREM sleep.
† Events per hour of sleep.
‡ $ETCO_2$ > 50 mm Hg as percent of TST.
§ Oxygen desaturations > 4% per hours of TST.
TST, total sleep time; REM, rapid eye movement; NREM, non-REM; $ETCO_2$, end-tidal carbon dioxide level.

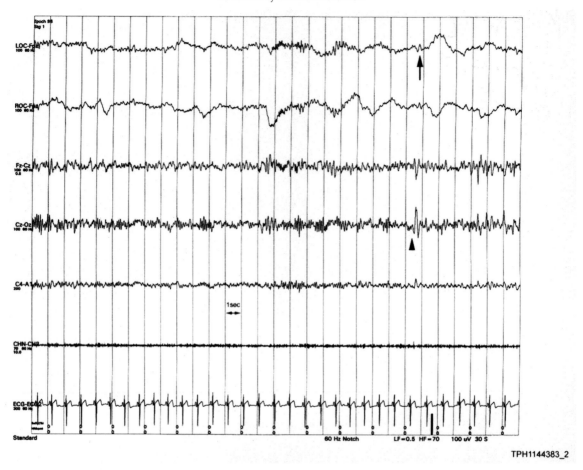

FIGURE 19–8

Multiple sleep latency test showing the normal transition from wakefulness into non-rapid eye movement (NREM) sleep. The Cz-Oz lead shows an alpha rhythm of fluctuating amplitude during the initial two thirds of the graph, which slows to a 4- to 5-Hz theta rhythm in the final third of the graph (arrowhead). *Sleep onset coincides with appearance of slow eye rolling movements characteristic of drowsiness or stage I NREM sleep* (top two channels, arrow).

Clinical Application

The mean sleep latency is closely linked to the Tanner stages of sexual development and varies from 16 to 18 minutes in preadolescents (Tanner stages I, II) to 12 to 14 minutes in older adolescents (Tanner stages IV, V.)[16] In patients with pathologic daytime sleepiness, the mean sleep latency is invariably less than 10 minutes. Patients with narcolepsy generally exhibit mean sleep latencies of less than 5 minutes, along with REM-onset sleep on at least two of four nap opportunities. Making a definitive diagnosis of narcolepsy in childhood at times necessitates obtaining serial MSLTs over a matter of 2 to 3 years to capture a progressive decrease in the mean sleep latency and increase in the number of REM-onset sleep periods.[17] Caution must be exercised in applying the test to teenagers who may frequently show one physiologic sleep-onset REM period during the first MSLT nap. Ambiguous sleep with admixture of features of REM and NREM sleep can also be seen on occasions during the early stages of evolution of narcolepsy (Fig. 19-10). In adults, mean sleep latency below 5 minutes in association with two or more REM-onset sleep periods has 70% sensitivity and 97% specificity for the diagnosis of narcolepsy.[15] Comparable data are not available for children. There is no major difference in the diagnostic sensitivity of the test between patients with narcolepsy with cataplexy and narcolepsy without cataplexy. It is likely that over the next few years, radioimmunoassay of cerebrospinal fluid (CSF) hypocretin will gradually replace the MSLT as a diagnostic tool at least as far as narcolepsy-cataplexy is concerned—CSF hypocretin levels below 110 pg/mL have a 97% specificity and 87% sensitivity for this disorder.[18]

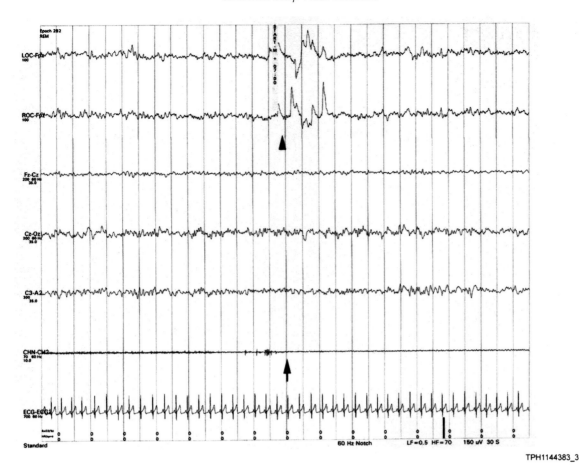

FIGURE 19–9

Multiple sleep latency test showing a sleep-onset rapid eye movement period (SOREMP) and the transition from non-REM (NREM) to REM sleep. The transition may be directly from wakefulness into REM sleep, or from wakefulness into NREM sleep, and then into REM sleep. In this patient, the onset of REM sleep is heralded by drop-off in the amplitude of the chin EMG (arrow) and a burst of REMs (arrowhead). Patients with narcolepsy generally exhibit two or more SOREMPs during the multiple sleep latency test, combined with a mean sleep latency (derived from all the four or five daytime nap opportunities) of less than 5 minutes.

Merits and Limitations of the Multiple Sleep Latency Test

The MSLT has been reliably validated as a measure of daytime sleepiness following sleep loss, sleep disruption, and hypnotic and alcohol effects. It measures the propensity for daytime sleepiness at multiple times of the day and provides mean sleep latency figures that correlate well with the degree of daytime sleepiness. It does not, however, correlate strongly with subjective estimates of daytime sleepiness. Although used extensively even in children, it has not been validated in this age group. It is also somewhat counterintuitive in that it measures the ability to fall asleep in a darkened, quiet environment, whereas most sleepy individuals are trying to stay awake in a bright, and perhaps noisy,

daytime environment. It is also not able to control for the emotional state of the patient that might impact sleep onset (e.g., presence of anxiety). Nevertheless, it remains the most commonly used tool in the assessment of daytime sleepiness in childhood.

MAINTENANCE OF WAKEFULNESS TEST (MWT)

The maintenance of wakefulness test (MWT) is a mirror image opposite of the MSLT. It measures how long a patient can stay awake in a darkened, quiet environment and is used for evaluating the efficacy of stimulant treatment on daytime sleepiness (e.g., to determine if it is safe for a person with a

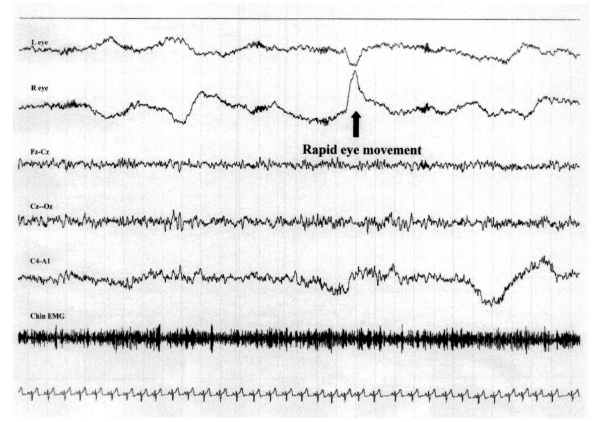

L eye

R eye

Fz-Cz

Cz--Oz

C4-A1

Chin EMG

Rapid eye movement

TPH1142508_10

FIGURE 19–10

Ambiguous sleep in an adolescent with narcolepsy that was in its early stages of evolution. That the patient had demonstrated pathologic daytime sleepiness but did not show two or more sleep-onset rapid eye movement (REM) periods is characteristic of narcolepsy. Notice the intrusion of an REM onto drowsiness (non-REM stage I sleep).

sleep disorder to drive or operate machinery).[19] The hook-up is exactly like that of the MSLT. The patient is provided four or five nap opportunities at two hourly intervals throughout the day, during which the subject is seated upright in a chair and asked to stay awake after lights out. The duration of each opportunity can be either 20 or 40 minutes. The average mean sleep latency for an adult is 35.2 minutes. Normative values have not been established for children and adolescents.

ACTIGRAPHY

The actigraph is a wrist watch–shaped microcomputer that senses linear acceleration and translates it into a numer-ic and graphic representation.[20,21] There is generally good correlation between the level of body movement and sleep-wake states, with increased muscle activity during wake-fulness and relative quiescence during sleep. Information can be gathered reliably in the ambulatory setting about total recording time, total sleep time, and sleep efficiency, continuously 24 hours a day, and longitudinally for 1 to 2 weeks. Wrist actigraphy is useful in the evaluation of ado-lescents with daytime sleepiness, especially those with circa-dian rhythm sleep disorders such as delayed sleep-phase syndrome (Fig. 19-11). Actigraphy has also been used in the evaluation of children with suspected attention deficit hyperactivity disorder to monitor response to therapy in terms of a reduction in motor activity.[22]

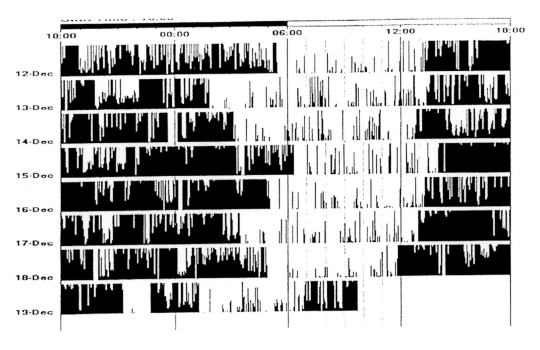

FIGURE 19–11

Wrist actigraph on an adolescent with a circadian rhythm disorder (delayed sleep-phase syndrome). Time on the 24-hour clock is displayed over the top on the horizontal axis. Days of the month are shown on the vertical axis. For each day, the shaded area denotes presence of muscle activity that coincides with wakefulness, whereas the clear areas indicate lack of muscle activity that coincides with sleep. The graph suggests that sleep onset is occurring between 1:30 AM and 6:00 AM, whereas the final awakening from sleep is between 12:00 noon and 1:00 PM.

REFERENCES

1. Blader SC, Koplewicz HS, Abikoff H, Foley C: Sleep problems in elementary school children: A community survey. Arch Pediatr Adolesc Med 1997;151:473-480.
2. Harner PF, Sannit T: A review of the International 10-20 System of Electrode Placement. Quincy, MA, Grass Instrument, 1974.
3. Kotagal S, Goulding PM: The laboratory assessment of daytime sleepiness in children. J Clin Neurophysiol 1996;13:208-221.
4. Shepard JW (ed): Atlas of Sleep Medicine. Mt. Kisco, NY, Futura, 1991.
5. McGregor PA: Updates in polysomnographic recording techniques used for the diagnosis of sleep disorders. Am J EEG Technol 1989;29:107-136.
6. Butkov N: Polysomnography. *In* Lee-Chiong TL, Sateia MJ, Carskadon MA (eds): Sleep Medicine. Philadelphia, Hanley & Belfus, 2002, pp 605-637.
7. Anders T, Emde R, Parmelee A (eds): A Manual of Standardized Terminology, Techniques, and Criteria for Scoring of Sleep States and Wakefulness in Newborn Infants. Los Angeles, UCLA Brain Information Service, NINDS Neurological Network, 1971.
8. Guilleminault C, Soquet M: Appendix II. *In* Guilleminault C (ed): Sleeping and Waking Disorders: Indications and Techniques. Menlo Park, CA, Addison-Wesley, 1982, pp 415-426.
9. Rechtschaffen A, Kales A (eds): A Manual of Standardized Terminology, Techniques, and Scoring System for Sleep Stages of Human Subjects. Los Angeles, Brain Information Service/Brain Research Institute, 1968.
10. Polysomnography Task Force, American Sleep Disorders Association Standards of Practice Committee: Practice parameters for the indications for polysomnography and related procedures. Sleep 1997;20:406-422.
11. American Thoracic Society: Cardiorespiratory sleep studies in children: Establishment of normative data and polysomnographic predictors of morbidity. Am J Resp Crit Care Med 1999;160:1381-1387.
12. Marcus CL, Loughlin GM: Obstructive sleep apnea in children. Semin Pediatr Neurol 1996;3:23-28.
13. Rosen CL, D'Andrea L, Haddad GG: Adult criteria for obstructive sleep apnea do not identify children with serious obstruction. Am Rev Respir Dis 1992;146:1231-1244.
14. American Sleep Disorders Association: The clinical use of the multiple sleep latency test. Sleep 1992;15:268-276.

15. Aldrich MS, Chervin RD, Malow BA: Value of the multiple sleep latency test (MSLT) for the diagnosis of narcolepsy. Sleep 1997;20:620-629.

16. Carskadon MA: The second decade. *In* Guilleminault C (ed): Sleeping and Waking Disorders: Indications and techniques. Menlo Park, CA, Addison-Wesley, 1982, pp 99-125.

17. Kotagal S, Swink TD: Excessive daytime sleepiness in a 13-year-old. Semin Pediatr Neurol 1996;3:170-172.

18. Mignot E, Lammers GJ, Ripley B, et al: The role of cerebrospinal fluid hypocretin measurement in the diagnosis of narcolepsy and other hypersomnias. Arch Neurol 2002;59:1553-1562.

19. Doghramji K, Mitler MM, Sangal RB, et al: A normative study of the maintenance of wakefulness test (MWT). Electroencephalogr Clin Neurophysiol 1997;103:554-562.

20. Sadeh A, Hauri PJ, Kripke DF, Lavie P: The role of actigraphy in the evaluation of sleep disorders. Sleep 1995;18:288-302.

21. American Sleep Disorders Association: Practice parameters for the use of actigraphy in the clinical assessment of sleep disorders. Sleep 1995;18:285-287.

22. Corkum P, Tannock R, Moldofsky H, et al: Actigraphy and parental ratings of sleep in children with attention deficit–hyperactivity disorder. Sleep 2001;24:303-312.

20

The Diagnosis of Brain Death

ALEXIS D. BORO AND SOLOMON L. MOSHÉ

There is a moral, legal, and ethical consensus that a person is dead if he or she "has sustained either irreversible cessation of circulatory and respiratory functions or irreversible cessation of all functions of the entire brain, including the brain stem."[1,2] At present there is a generally accepted approach to the diagnosis of death on the basis of brain-based criteria; however, details of the procedures used in arriving at this diagnosis, and the use of ancillary tests, particularly in children, remain subjects of discussion. Among children who have sustained severe cerebral insults, the prognosis varies significantly between age groups and even between individuals in the same age group. Furthermore, the emotional components involved in the care of children make the issue of brain death determination even more sensitive in this patient population.[3-5] The steps in determining brain death commence with identifying the cause of the presenting coma, establishing the irreversibility of the state of coma, and excluding conditions that masquerade as brain death. Brain death is established when motor responses, brainstem reflexes, and respiratory drive are absent in a patient with a known irreversible massive brain lesion in whom hypothermia, hypotension, drug intoxication, and profound metabolic derangement have been excluded.[6]

DETERMINATION OF BRAIN DEATH IN ADULTS

A detailed, practical description of the examination for brain death, including the apnea test, may be found in the American Academy of Neurology practice parameter.[7] These guidelines are summarized in Box 20-1.

The American Academy of Neurology practice parameter does not specify a waiting period after an anoxic insult. There is a consensus that a 24-hour period of observation is required to assess prognosis in this setting.[8] If drug intoxication is suspected but the drug has not been identified, some authorities recommend both a minimum observation period of 48 hours and ancillary testing prior to determination of brain death.[9] There are few data to guide the timing of brain death examinations in the presence of therapeutic or subtherapeutic concentrations of sedating medications in adults.

In practice, institutions formulate specific policies for determination of brain death that conform to state law and guidelines. These policies may differ in detail from those outlined here. For example, according to New York State guidelines, brain death cannot be declared in the setting of a core temperature lower than 32.2°C or a mean arterial blood pressure lower than 55 mm Hg.[10] The required interval between the two clinical evaluations differs from institution to institution. More substantive differences exist regarding the interpretation of an apnea test terminated prior to completion because of hemodynamic instability. At some institutions, early termination of the apnea test precludes the determination of brain death. At others, such an apnea test is regarded as positive, as equivalent to one demonstrating apnea in the presence of the requisite increase in $PaCO_2$.[11] According to the American Academy of Neurology practice parameter, such an apnea test should be regarded as indeterminate, in which case an ancillary test can be used to confirm the diagnosis of brain death.[7]

BOX 20-1
CLINICAL CRITERIA FOR BRAIN DEATH DETERMINATION IN ADULTS

1. Clinical or neuroimaging evidence of an acute central nervous system catastrophe compatible with the clinical diagnosis of brain death
2. Core temperature ≥ 32°C (90°F)
3. Systolic blood pressure ≥ 90 mm Hg
4. Coma
5. Absence of motor responses to noxious stimuli. The presence of responses mediated by the spinal cord is not incompatible with the diagnosis of brain death.
6. Absence of pupillary response to light
7. Absence of corneal reflexes
8. Absence of caloric response
9. Absence of gag reflex and absence of response to tracheal suctioning
10. Absence of spontaneous respirations during prolonged apnea with oxygenation ($PaCO_2$ of 60 mm Hg or 20 mm Hg above baseline values)*
11. Repeat clinical evaluation after an interval of 6 hours

From the Quality Standards Subcommittee of the American Academy of Neurology. Practice Parameters for determining brain death in adults (summary statement). Neurology 1995;45:1012-1014.
* The American Academy of Neurology Practice Parameters require a core temperature of ≥ 36.5°C (97°F) for the performance of the apnea test.

ANCILLARY TESTS

In most settings, brain death can be established by clinical criteria, and ancillary tests are not necessary. At times, however, the clinical examination does not provide the requisite degree of certainty and ancillary testing is indicated. In some patients, there may be concern that cortical function remains despite an absence of brainstem function—a pontine lesion may raise the question of a deafferented (locked-in) state. There may be doubt regarding the interpretation of the clinical examination. The classification of complex movements in response to noxious stimulation may be uncertain. In some patients, specific components of the clinical examination cannot be performed; extensive facial injury occasionally precludes caloric testing. In some states, ancillary testing can shorten the required period between brain death examinations and facilitate more rapid organ transplantation.

Cerebral Angiography

A cerebral angiogram confirms brain death by demonstrating a lack of effective blood flow to the brain. Iodinated contrast material is injected into the anterior and posterior circulation. A patent external carotid circulation should be demonstrated. The absence of filling of the carotid and vertebral arteries beyond the level of entry into the skull is pathognomonic of brain death. False-negative results have occurred in patients who have undergone craniotomy, previous intraventricular shunting procedures, and decompressing skull fractures.[12-14] This is a time-consuming, invasive procedure that must be performed in the radiology suite. The injection of contrast is associated with a risk of nephrotoxicity and may compromise organ donation.

Electroencephalography

The scalp electroencephalogram (EEG) is a readily available, safe, noninvasive ancillary test. The EEG should be recorded according to the criteria in Box 20-2. These criteria were developed in 1976 by the Committee on Cerebral Death at the American Clinical Neurophysiology Society (ACNS), known then as the American Electroencephalographic Society.[15] The Committee chose the term *electrocerebral silence* (ECS) to characterize tracings in which electrocerebral activity cannot be detected. The technical standards recommended by the ACNS have become generally accepted as the norm for the determination of brain death, having proven to be highly effective in minimizing the likelihood of false-positive and false-negative results.

The two most innovative recommendations set forth by the Committee were the sensitivity criteria, which require that tracings be performed at 2.0 μV/mm, and the recommended interelectrode distance, which must be at least 10 cm. The theory underlying the low sensitivity setting is that since current EEG machines produce noise levels of 2 μV, cerebral activity has to exceed this voltage to be distinguished from the background noise. Thus, ECS does not necessarily imply that the brain is "silent" or inactive but rather that the cortical activity generated is so attenuated that it cannot be distinguished from the noise of the recording instrument. Although the technical standards of the ACNS are precise, a specific montage is not defined and laboratories can devise their own montages to suit their own requirements. With the current availability of computed EEG, the theory that the electrodes should be placed at least 10 cm apart has become a testable hypothesis. Figure 20-1 compares a conventional EEG recording and a reformatted recording using an interelectrode distance of 10 cm. Both show ECS.

The interpretation of an isoelectric EEG is relatively easy when appropriate guidelines are used. The main difficulty is

BOX 2-2
MINIMUM TECHNICAL STANDARDS FOR EEG RECORDING IN SUSPECTED CEREBRAL DEATH

1. A minimum of eight scalp electrodes and earlobe references covering the major brain areas should be used. A ground electrode should not be used if the patient is in the intensive care unit or if electrical monitoring equipment is in place.

2. Disk electrodes should be applied. Interelectrode impedances should be kept between 100 and 10,000 Ω, and the distance between electrodes should be at least 10 cm.

3. Each electrode should be touched separately to create an artifact potential on the record.

4. Sensitivity should be increased from 7 to 2 μV/mm during most of the recording, with inclusion of appropriate calibration.

5. High frequency filters should not be set below 30 Hz and low-frequency filters should not be set above 1 Hz.

6. The EEG should be tested for reactivity with a loud noise and a pinch.

7. Recording should be done for at least 30 minutes.

8. A pair of electrodes should be applied on the dorsum of the right hand separated by a distance of 6 to 7 cm; an electrocardiographic monitor should be applied.

9. Electromyographic artifacts can sometimes be seen in a patient with electrocerebral silence; if these obscure the recording, a neuromuscular blocking agent such as pancuronium or succinylcholine should be used.

10. The recording should be performed only by a qualified technologist; a repeat EEG should be obtained if there is doubt about the presence of electrocerebral silence.

From American Electroencephalographic Society Guidelines in EEG and Evoked Potentials. Guideline Three: Minimum technical standards for EEG recording in suspected cerebral death. J Clin Neurophysiol 1986;3(Suppl 1):12-17.

in eliminating artifacts or recognizing them as such. The main sources of artifact are muscle, heart, respirator activity, and exogenous electrical activity from surrounding equipment in the patient's room, usually an intensive care unit.

The artifacts produced by the heart, usually in the electrocardiogram (ECG) and pulse, are readily identifiable because of their stereotypic configuration and frequency (Figs. 20-2 and 20-3). High-amplitude electromyographic (EMG) potentials generated from the scalp can easily obscure a significant portion of the background EEG activity (Fig. 20-4). Like ECG activity, EMG activity can be readily recognized and differentiated from cortical activity. Both the ECG artifact and EMG activity can obscure background activity to the point of preventing accurate interpretation of the recording. If muscle artifact cannot be eliminated, the usual recommendation is to administer a paralytic agent. Succinylcholine (20 to 40 mg) is used most frequently. Complications associated with succinylcholine include hypertension, tachycardia, bradycardia, and cardiac arrest.[16]

The ventilator can produce a variety of movement artifacts. These are usually present in the more anterior electrodes and are often periodic (Fig. 20-5). They can be removed momentarily by briefly disconnecting the ventilator. This should be done cautiously since some patients, particularly those with unstable cardiovascular status, may not tolerate prolonged interruption of ventilation. If the artifacts are diffuse, it may be impossible to obtain 30 minutes of interpretable EEG.

Other easily identifiable artifacts, such as the intravenous drip artifact, can be readily detected and removed, whereas others, such as the 60-Hz electrical artifact (see Fig. 20-1B), may or may not be removed by notch filters and can prevent accurate interpretation of the record. Some artifacts can resemble activity of cerebral origin. Identifying the source of these artifacts and differentiating them from true cortical activity can present a challenge to the electroencephalographer (Fig. 20-6).

Isoelectric EEG tracings obtained using the technical standards of the ACNS can serve to support a diagnosis of brain death, but only after the clinical criteria have been met. ECS is not pathognomonic of brain death. ECS can occur in patients with residual brainstem function after anoxic injury.[17] Many of the conditions that can cause reversible global loss of brain function can also cause transient ECS. These include drug intoxication, hypothermia, profound hypotension, and severe metabolic or endocrine disarray.[18] The EEG therefore adds little to the clinical examination when these conditions are present or when the mechanism of coma is uncertain. Conversely, because the EEG is a test of cortical function that does not depend on an intact brainstem, the EEG can be a valuable adjunct to the clinical examination when the mechanism of coma suggests the possibility of preserved cortical function in the presence of significant brainstem dysfunction.[19] There are several reports, for example, of patients with Guillain-Barré syndrome in whom clinical findings were consistent with brain death criteria.[20]

In previous years, when standard EEG montages were being used for the determination of brain death, the return of EEG activity after an initial "flat" EEG tracing was

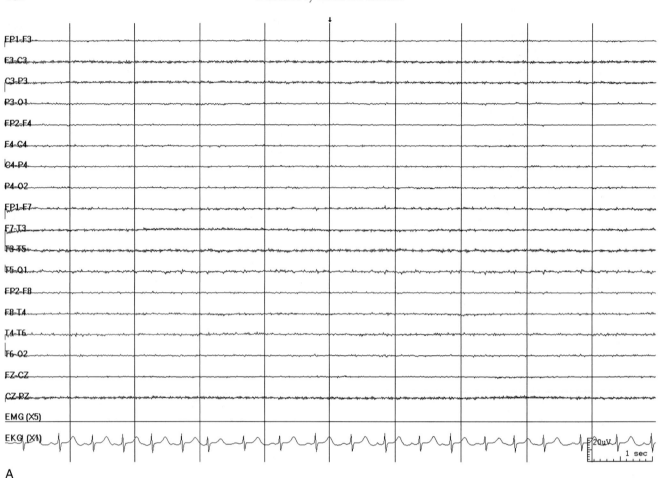

A

FIGURE 20–1

An EEG viewed in a longitudinal bipolar montage (A) and after the data were reformatted using a 10-cm interelectrode distance.

often reported. However, the recordings suggestive of brain death that were followed by subsequent recordings in which cerebral activity was clearly demonstrated did not meet the clinical criteria later suggested by the ACNS. We could not find a single report of a patient outside of the neonatal age group with a return of EEG activity after an initial isoelectric EEG recording when the appropriate clinical criteria and technical standards were met. Thus, the EEG remains an excellent noninvasive diagnostic tool for the confirmation of brain death in the clinical setting. In one series, however, at least 20% of clinically brain-dead patients had evidence of residual EEG activity.[21]

Cerebral Scintigraphy

Technetium-99m hexamethylpropyleneamineoxime (Tc-99 HMPAO) is a lipid-soluble compound that diffuses across the blood-brain barrier where it is taken up by living neurons in cortical and brainstem structures and enzymati-

cally converted to a nondiffusible species.[20] The absence of uptake of intravenously injected Tc-99m HMPAO into the brain parenchyma supports the diagnosis of brain death. Successful injection of the isotope may be confirmed by obtaining additional images of the liver.[9] The images can be acquired at the bedside with a portable gamma camera. The isotope must be injected within 30 minutes of its reconstitution. Single-photon emission computed tomography has been advocated as an alternative;[22] this requires transfer of the patient from the intensive care unit to the radiology suite.

Evoked Potentials

In contrast with the EEG, somatosensory evoked potentials can be used to assess both brainstem and cortical function. Bilateral absence of the P14-N20 responses to median nerve stimulation supports the diagnosis of brain death.[7, 23-25] Peripheral and spinal cord lesions can abolish the N9 and

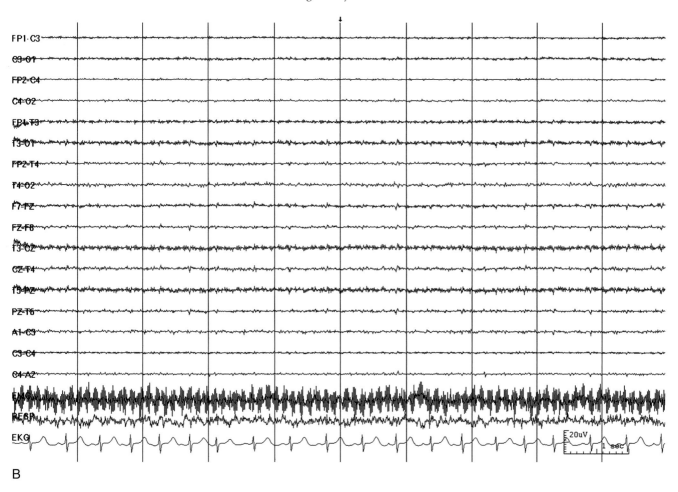

FP1-C3
C3-O1
FP2-C4
C4-O2
FP1-T3
T3-O1
FP2-T4
T4-O2
F7-FZ
FZ-F8
T3-CZ
CZ-T4
T5-PZ
PZ-T6
A1-C3
C3-C4
C4-A2
EMG
RESP
EKG

FIGURE 20–1 *Cont'd*

(B) *Both show electrocerebral silence. A technician who suspects the possibility of brain death should place respiratory and EMG leads and perform a 30-minute recording in accordance with the American Clinical Neurophysiology Society standards. If the technician's suspicions are not borne out, the EEG can be reviewed in conventional montages. B also demonstrates a prominent 60-Hz electrical artifact, best seen in derivations containing the T3 and T5 electrodes.*

N13 responses. Somatosensory evoked potentials cannot be used to confirm the diagnosis of brain death in patients without these responses. This occurs in fewer than 5% of cases.[25]

Brainstem auditory evoked potentials have been used as well. In most brain-dead patients, wave I is absent in addition to the medullary components.[23,25] This is a liability because it is important to establish that the input signal has reached the central nervous system (CNS).

Visual evoked potentials in response to flash stimulation are abolished in brain death. However, these potentials are sensitive to the effects of hypothermia and CNS depressant medications.[26] Because the retina is more resistant than the cortex to hypoxic damage, a retinal response may be obtained in the absence of a cortical contribution to the visual evoked potential.[18]

Transcranial Doppler Ultrasonography

The increased intracranial pressure associated with brain death and the consequent increased vascular resistance result in small, early systolic peaks and reverberating or absent diastolic flow. Since 10% of patients do not have adequate insonation windows, the complete absence of flow on an initial study does not confirm the diagnosis of brain death.[7,9,27]

DETERMINATION OF BRAIN DEATH IN CHILDREN

The clinical evaluation of children is similar to that of adults, although the absence of sucking and rooting reflexes

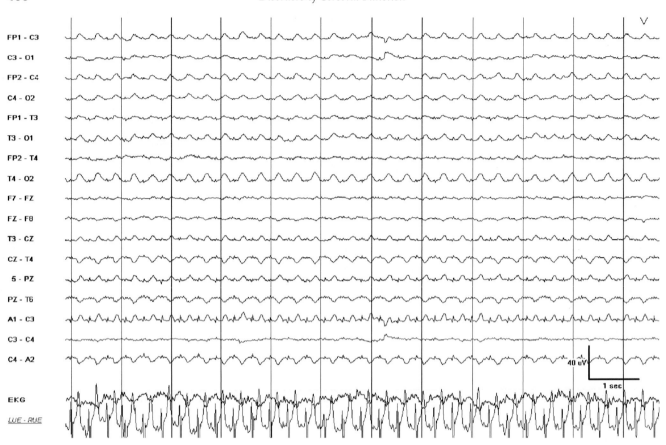

FIGURE 20–2

Prominent ECG artifact. This is readily identifiable because of its stereotypical configuration.

should be specifically demonstrated. The examination of preterm and fullterm neonates can be limited by the fact that the cranial nerve responses are not fully developed in this age group, and observations of an infant in an incubator may be less certain.[9] Because the brains of infants and young children have increased resistance to damage and may recover substantial function even after prolonged comatose states, the criteria for declaring brain death in young children are more stringent. Longer durations of observation are recommended for children, and ancillary testing has a greater role (Table 20-1).

As in adults, hypothermia, hypotension, intoxication, and profound metabolic derangement must be excluded. The possibility that an unrecognized metabolic disorder is present must be excluded. The effects of paralytic agents must not be overlooked. Often, therapeutic and subtherapeutic concentrations of sedating medications are present. In a study of clinically brain-dead children with therapeutic levels of barbiturates and isoelectric EEGs, ECS persisted when follow-up EEGs were done with lower barbiturate levels.[28]

The guidelines issued by the Task Force for the Determination of Brain Death in Children, adopted by the American Academy of Neurology, the American Academy of Pediatrics, the American Neurologic Association, and the Child Neurology Society, recommend a minimum observation period of 12 hours in children older than 1 year of age.[29] A minimum of 24 hours of observation is appropriate if the coma is due to a hypoxic or ischemic event or another cause in which the extent and reversibility of brain damage can be difficult to assess. Although ancillary testing is not required in this age group, it is often done because of its role in determining the irreversibility of the coma.

In children aged 2 months to 1 year, the Task Force recommends two clinical examinations with two EEGs performed 24 hours apart. Repeat examination and EEG are not necessary if a concomitant cerebral radionuclide angiographic study demonstrates absence of visualization of the cerebral arteries. In patients between 7 days and 2 months of age, the Task Force recommends two examinations and two EEGs at least 48 hours apart.

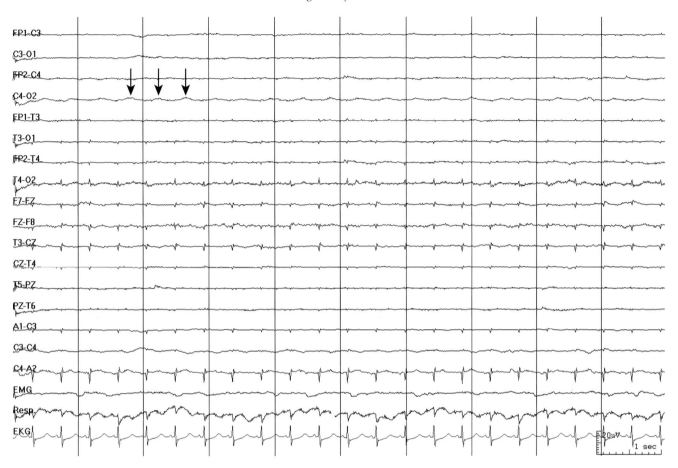

FIGURE 20–3

Ballistocardiographic artifact seen in C4-O2 (arrows). This is readily identified by its occipital location and frequency. It was eliminated by repositioning the head.

The Task Force did not make recommendations for children younger than 7 days of age. It is difficult to establish a state of irreversibility in this age group, particularly if the infant is premature, and clinical determination of brainstem death is likewise difficult. In some institutions, determination of brain death may not be made before 7 to 8 days of life.[11]

ANCILLARY TESTS IN CHILDREN

Angiography

In most situations, as in adults, the cerebral angiogram is the definitive ancillary test. Residual cortical blood flow occasionally occurs in brain-dead children as a result of skull defects[12] or, in the newborn, the presence of open sutures and fontanelles.[30] Radionucleotide angiograms have demonstrated preserved cortical blood flow in clinically brain-dead patients with severe atrophy.[31]

EEG

Electrical artifacts are often problematic in neonates receiving intensive care. Artifacts associated with mechanical ventilation are often most prominent in the smallest patients. Head and chest movements associated with respiration can produce rhythmic and sometimes complex transient effects that may suggest paroxysmal discharges or a burst-suppression pattern. The ventilator can produce vibratory artifacts that may not be periodic and are sometimes difficult to differentiate from the background. The small head size of the infant limits the electrode locations and combinations that meet the requirement for a 10-cm electrode separation. The Task Force guidelines recommend decreasing the interelectrode distance in proportion to head size.[29]

In addition to technical challenges, a variety of interpretive problems limit the value of the EEG as an ancillary test for neocortical death in children younger than 2 to 3 months of age. The EEG in children younger than 3 months is highly sensitive to insults.[19] The electrocerebral activity in

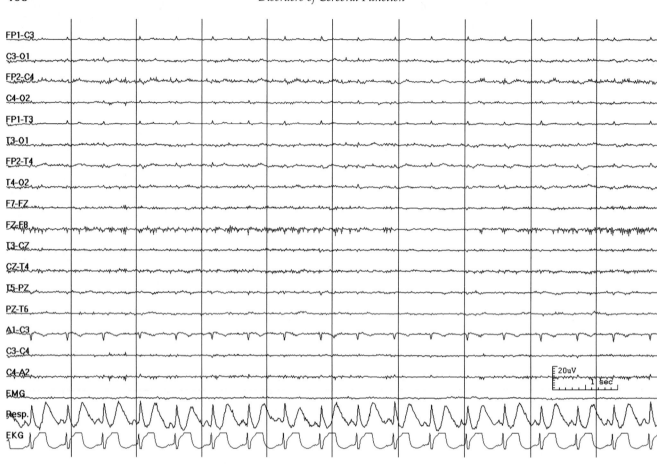

FIGURE 20–4

High-amplitude EMG potentials best seen in Fp2-C4, Fz-F8, and Cz-T4. These are generated from the scalp and could easily obscure a significant portion of the background EEG activity.

this age group can be suppressed, albeit transiently, by extrinsic and intrinsic factors. The normal neonatal EEG is discontinuous. Transient ECS has been observed in very young children during the administration of diazepam and in hypotension, hypoxia, hypothermia, and metabolic disorders, as well as postictal states.[18,32] In patients between 2 and 3 months of age, the EEG shares the characteristic features of both infants and neonates. It does not usually present all of the characteristic background features of infants and children until after the age of 3 months. A thorough knowledge of the ontogenesis of the neonatal EEG is required to interpret these studies. An electroencephalographer who primarily interprets adult EEGs may not possess these skills.[18]

Infants between the ages of 3 months and 1 year represent a more homogeneous group than that of infants between 2 months and 1 year. For this reason Alvarez and associates argued that the brain death criteria recommended for patients between 7 days and 2 months of age should be extended to include infants up to 3 months of age.[19] They also suggested, on the basis of a retrospective study of 52 brain-dead patients younger than 5 years of age, 28 of whom had repeat EEGs, that a single EEG with ECS at the end of the observation period was sufficient to corroborate the diagnosis of brain death in children older than 3 months of age.[19]

Evoked Potentials

Some limited data support the use of brainstem auditory evoked potentials and somatosensory evoked potentials as ancillary tests for the determination of brain death in the pediatric population.[33] There are few data validating their use in very young children. Transient loss of brainstem auditory evoked potentials has been documented in newborns, infants, and small children who did not meet the clinical criteria for brain death following anoxic episodes.[18,34]

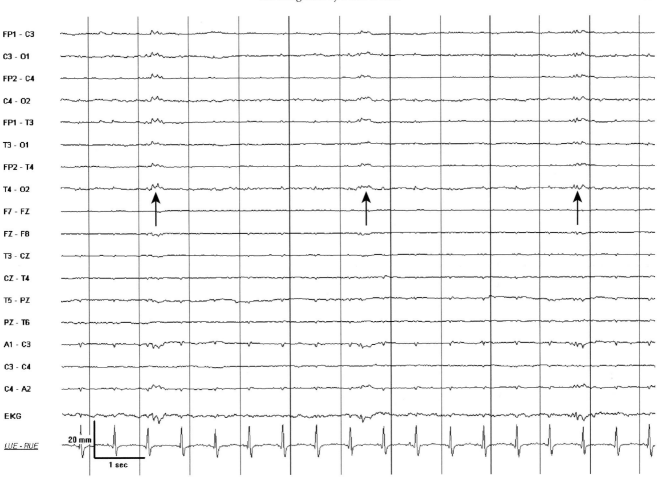

FIGURE 20–5

A periodic artifact that could be mistaken for a burst-suppression pattern (arrows). *The suspicion that it represented an artifact produced by the ventilator was confirmed by briefly switching the ventilator off.*

Transcranial Doppler Ultrasonography

False-negative examinations (studies failing to demonstrate absent cerebral blood flow in a brain-dead patient) can occur in the setting of skull defects.[35] Doppler alterations consistent with brain death, such as absent or retrograde flow during diastole, can be seen in patients with congenital heart disease.[36]

CONCLUSION

The determination of brain death must satisfy both medical criteria and institutional and legal requirements. Its diagnostic criteria, particularly with regard to the role of ancillary testing, are still evolving. Although it is never obligatory in adults to perform an EEG to confirm the diagnosis of brain death, there are data that indicate that 20% of clinically brain-dead patients demonstrate residual EEG activity.[21] Similarly, although the preservation of pupillary light reflexes is inconsistent with the diagnosis of brain death, the preservation of neurologic regulation of water homeostasis is not.[37] The issue here is not one of prognosis. There is no doubt that the remaining cortical neurons supporting residual EEG activity and the hypothalamic neurons supporting the regulation of water homeostasis eventually die in patients who meet current criteria for brain death. The question is rather how should we define the point at which the individual is dead? Uncertainty at the margins should not be used to justify continued support of brain-dead patients or prevent expeditious organ donation. As a society we acknowledge the concept of brain death, although the criteria by which it is diagnosed may continue to be refined. Indeed, not only are new diagnostic methods becoming available but the medical community continues to

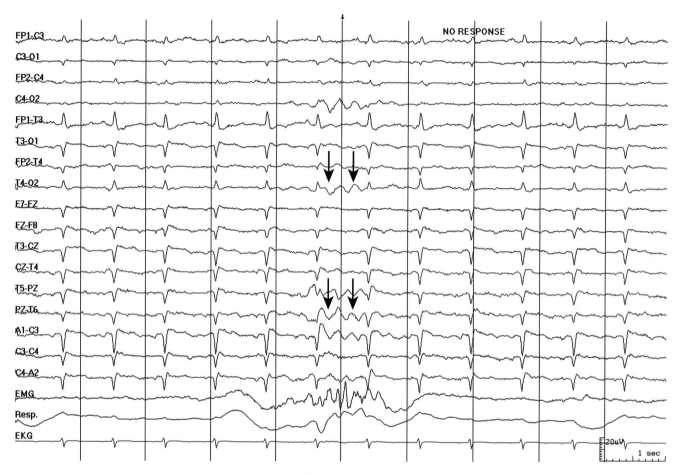

FIGURE 20–6

The transients in the 5th and 6th seconds were produced by a brief sternal rub (arrows). The distribution of their field, as well as the technician's comment, suggests that these transients represent artifacts. The fact that the artifact was produced by a sternal rub suggests that the transients in the respiratory channel most likely represent movement artifact rather than a change in respiratory pattern in response to noxious stimulation. This EEG does not support the diagnosis of brain death because it exhibits activity on the order of 4 μV.

TABLE 20–1. STUDIES AND OBSERVATION PERIODS RECOMMENDED FOR DETERMINATION OF BRAIN DEATH IN CHILDREN

Patient's Age	*Types of Studies and Observation Periods*
7 days to 2 months	Two physical examinations and two EEGs demonstrating electrocerebral inactivity at least 48 hours apart
2 months to 1 year	Two physical examinations and two EEGs showing electrocerebral inactivity at least 24 hours apart, or a physical examination and an EEG demonstrating electrocerebral inactivity, and a cerebral radionucleotide angiogram demonstrating absent cerebral circulation
>1 year	Two physical examinations fulfilling criteria of brain death 12 hours apart. The period of observation should be prolonged to at least 24 hours if extent and irreversibility of brain damage are uncertain.

gain experience with more familiar techniques. The data of Alvarez and associates,[19] which suggest that a single EEG demonstrating ECS is sufficient to corroborate the diagnosis of brain death in children older than 3 months of age, were not available when the Task Force recommended that two confirmatory EEGs be performed in children between the ages of 2 months and 1 year.

REFERENCES

1. Uniform Determination of Death Act, 12 Uniform Laws Annotated (U.L.A) 589 (West 1993 and West Supp. 1997).
2. Guidelines for the determination of death: Report of the medical consultants on the diagnosis of death to the President's Commission for the Study of Ethical Problems in Medicine and Biomedical and Behavioral Research. JAMA 1981;246:2184-2186.

3. Chang MY, McBride LA, Ferguson MA: Variability in brain death declaration practices in pediatric head trauma. Pediatr Neurosurg 2003;39:7-9.

4. Banasiak KJ, Lister G: Brain death in children. Curr Probl Pediatr 2003;15:288-293.

5. Mejia RE, Pollack MM: Variability in brain death determination practices in children. JAMA 1995;274:1761-1762.

6. Wijdicks EF: Brain death worldwide: Accepted fact but no global consensus in diagnostic criteria. Neurology 2002;58:20-25.

7. Quality Standards Subcommittee of the American Academy of Neurology: Practice Parameters for Determining Brain Death in Adults (summary statement). Neurology 1995;45:1012-1014.

8. President's Commission for the Study of Ethical Problems in Medicine and Biomedical and Behavioral Research: Defining death: A report on the medical, legal, and ethical issues in the determination of death. Washington, DC, U.S. Government Printing Office, 1981.

9. Wijdicks EF: The diagnosis of brain death. N Engl J Med 2001;344:1215-1221.

10. New York State Department of Health's Recommended Voluntary Consensus Guidelines for Determination of Death. New York, State Department of Health, 1997.

11. Montefiore Medical Center, Bronx NY, Administrative Policy and Procedure JD01.1, 2001. Los Angeles County and University of Southern California Medical Center, Brain Death Declaration Policy ASA 106, 2003.

12. Alvarez LA, Lipton RB, Hirschfeld A, et al: Brain death determination by angiography in the setting of a skull defect. Arch Neurol 1988;45:225-227.

13. Braum M, Ducrocq X, Hout JC, et al: Intravenous angiography in brain death: Report of 140 patients. Neuroradiology 1997;39:400-405.

14. Flowers WM Jr, Patel BR: Persistence of cerebral blood flow after brain death. South Med J 2000;93:364-370.

15. American Electroencephalographic Society Guidelines in EEG and Evoked Potentials: Guideline Three: Minimum technical standards for EEG recording in suspected cerebral death. J Clin Neurophysiol 1986;3(Suppl 1):12-17.

16. Verma A, Bedlack RS, Radtke RA, et al: Succinylcholine-induced hyperkalemia and cardiac arrest death related to an EEG study. J Clin Neurophysiol 1999;16:46-50.

17. Heckmann JG, Lang CJ, Pfau M, Neudorfer B: Electrocerebral silence with preserved but reduced cortical brain perfusion. Eur J Emerg Med 2003;10:241-243.

18. Chatrain GE, Giorgio ST: Electrophysiological evaluation of coma, other states of diminished responsiveness, and brain death. *In* Ebersole JS, Pedly TA (eds): Current Practice of Clinical Electrophysiology, 3rd ed. New York, Raven Press, 2003, pp 405-462.

19. Alvarez LA, Moshé SL, Belman AL, et al: EEG and brain death determination in children. Neurology 1988;38:227-230.

20. Harding JW, Chatterton BE: Outcomes of patients referred for confirmation of brain death by 99m Tc-exametazime scintigraphy. Intensive Care Med 2003;29:539-543.

21. Grigg MM, Kelly MA, Celesia GG, et al: Electroencephalographic activity after brain death. Arch Neurol 1987;44:948-954.

22. Facco E, Zucchetta P, Munari M, et al: 99m Tc-HMPAO SPECT in the diagnosis of brain death. Intensive Care Med 1998;24:911-917.

23. Goldie WD, Chiappa KH, Young RR, Brooks EB: Brainstem auditory and short-latency somatosensory evoked responses in brain death. Neurology 1981;31:248-256.

24. Facco E, Casartelli Liviero M, Munari M, et al: Short latency evoked potentials: New criteria for brain death? J Neurol Neurosurg Psychiatry 1990;53:351-353.

25. Facco E, Munari M, Gallo F, et al: Role of short latency evoked potentials in the diagnosis of brain death. Clin Neurophysiol 2002;113:1855-1866.

26. Russ W, King D: Effect of hypothermia on visual evoked potentials (VEP) in humans. Anesthesiology 1984;61:207-210.

27. Ducrocq X, Braun M, Debouverie M, et al: Brain death and transcranial Doppler: Experience in 130 cases of brain dead patients. J Neurol Sci 1998;160:41-46.

28. LaMancusa J, Cooper R, Vieth R, Wright F: The effects of falling therapeutic and subtherapeutic barbiturate blood levels on electrocerebral silence in clinically brain-dead children. Clin Electroencephalogr 1991;22:112-117.

29. Task Force for the Determination of Brain Death in Children: Guidelines for the determination of brain death in children. Ann Neurol 1987;22:616-617.

30. Altman DI, Perlman JM, Powers WJ, et al: Exuberant brainstem blood flow and intact cerebral blood flow despite clinical and pathological evidence for brainstem and cerebral necrosis in an asphyxiated newborn infant. Ann Neurol 1986;20:409.

31. Alvarez LA, Lipton RB, Moshé SL: Normal cerebral radionucleotide angiogram and electrocerebral silence in the presence of severe cerebral atrophy. Neuropediatrics 1987;18:112.

32. Moshé SL, Alvarez LA, Davidoff BA: Role of EEG in brain death determination in small children. *In* Kaufman HH (ed): Pediatric Brain Death and Organ/Tissue Retrieval: Medical, Ethical, and Legal Aspects. New York, Plenum, 1989, pp 165-175.

33. Ruiz-Lopez MJ, Martinez de Azagra A, Serrano A, Casado-Flores J: Brain death and evoked potentials in pediatric patients. Crit Care Med 1999;27:412-416.

34. Taylor MJ, Houston BD, Lowry NJ: Recovery of auditory brainstem responses after a severe hypoxic insult. N Engl J Med 1983;309:1169-1170.

35. Cabrer C, Dominguez-Roldman JM, Manyalich M, et al: Persistence of intracranial diastolic flow in transcranial Doppler sonography exploration of patients in brain death. Transplant Proc 2003;35:1642-1643.

36. Rodriguez RA, Cornel G, Alghofaili F, et al: Transcranial Doppler during suspected brain death in children: Potential limitation in patients with cardiac "shunt." Pediatr Crit Care Med 2002;3:153-157.

37. Traug RD, Robinson WM: The diagnosis of brain death [Letter]. N Engl J Med 2001;345:617.

21

Ambulatory Electroencephalography

SAMUEL L. BRIDGERS

Ambulatory electroencephalography is now widely used in the evaluation of children with seizures and other neurologic conditions. Over the past decade, the technical capabilities of ambulatory recording have expanded considerably and the test is now widely applied in the evaluation of both children and adults with neurologic disorders.

Some of the characteristics of ambulatory electroencephalography have made it an especially promising method for the clinical neurophysiologic evaluation of infants and children. The small size of the ambulatory recorder has made it particularly suitable for electroencephalographic (EEG) monitoring in the setting of crowded neonatal intensive care units, where unimpeded access to the patients at all times makes traditional EEG difficult. The capacity for EEG recording in the home is important in the evaluation of children for whom a hospital admission and separation from the security of familiar surroundings may be undesirable. Ambulatory EEG provides a useful means of monitoring and quantifying seizure activity and medication effects in absence epilepsy, a type often occurring in childhood. Ambulatory EEG monitoring can almost always be performed during extended sleep without the need for sedation, and it has an enhanced opportunity for detecting epileptiform abnormalities, even in the absence of seizures.

On the other hand, ambulatory EEG clearly has its drawbacks for the general population as well as pediatrics. Unless ambulatory video recordings are incorporated, there is no monitoring by trained personnel to provide sophisticated behavioral observation or to ensure continuing technical integrity. The data being collected cannot be practically analyzed "on-line." Patient cooperation is necessary to maintain the array of meticulously applied electrodes, which is essential for a recording of high quality. For older children, the ambulatory recorder itself is sometimes an object of intense curiosity that can result in loss of the recording and damage to the recorder. Even when recording is successful, ambulatory EEG interpretation requires specialized expertise and is fraught with opportunities for error.

Despite these qualifications, ambulatory EEG is a useful diagnostic technique in children as well as in adolescents and adults, and it is a valuable addition to the diagnostic armamentarium. Most importantly, the initial limitation of ambulatory EEG that hampered its general acceptance is no longer an issue. That is, the requirement for recording with a fixed montage of relatively few channels has been met with the development of devices that permit the recording of 16 channels.

In this chapter, the technical development of ambulatory EEG; its clinical validation, recording, and interpretive methods; its general clinical utility; and specific considerations for its application in seizure assessment in the pediatric population are reviewed. A comprehensive work on ambulatory EEG has been published that provides more detailed information.[1]

TECHNICAL DEVELOPMENT OF AMBULATORY EEG

The original ambulatory EEG devices recorded analog signals on audio tape. Using a slow turnstile speed (≈2 mm/sec), 24 hours of data could be acquired on a

$\frac{1}{8}$-inch audio tape cassette. Initially, analysis required printing out the entire 24 hours of recorded data on EEG paper for conventional review. Commercial systems were then developed that used an alternative and novel "page mode display" playback unit. With this device, the data could be examined as rapidly advancing "pages" on a video screen. With playback speeds up to 60 times that of actual time, EEG activity entered the audible frequency range, and the EEG could be heard as well as seen.[2]

The original 4-channel system was quickly succeeded by the development of 8 and 16 channels for physiologic data. These ambulatory recorders weighed approximately 0.7 kg and were easily worn with a belt or strap by most patients, including small children. Replay units provided a video display of data at chosen page lengths and speeds of review, plus simultaneous audio on one channel. At the fastest replay speed, typically 60 times that of actual time, 24 hours of EEG could be reviewed in 24 minutes. By connecting the playback unit to a standard EEG machine, a paper record could be obtained.

Ives and colleagues developed a solid-state 16-channel EEG event recorder that stored EEG events in solid-state memory.[3] The use of solid-state technology eliminated mechanical problems associated with audio cassettes as well as signal deterioration or dropout when recording on a magnetic media. The digitized EEG events could be stored or written on standard EEG paper or on a printer. In addition, the EEG could interconnect with an automatic seizure detection unit. Over the past decade technology has enabled portable recordings with sampling rates of more than 200 Hz. Although analog systems remain available, most commercial companies are now marketing digital recorders.

TECHNIQUES

As noted by Ebersole,[4] one of the advantages of ambulatory EEG monitoring is that the procedure can be performed as an outpatient without medical supervision. However, any electrode difficulty or mechanical failure during the recording will not be detected. As with routine EEG, it is critical that the electrodes be placed correctly and securely. Guidelines for the practice of ambulatory EEG have been published by the American EEG Society.[5] A detailed guide of techniques has been provided by Clenney.[6]

Electrodes

Only disk electrodes applied with collodion should be used for outpatient monitoring. For emergency recordings and neonatal and nonambulatory studies, self-adhering "stick-on" electrodes can be useful. In addition to securing the electrodes, the wires should also be secured to the scalp using collodion.[6] An impedance of less than 5000 Ω for all electrodes should be obtained.

The patient's scalp can be wrapped in gauze or elastic material with the lead wires gathered and tacked to reduce traction on the electrodes.

Calibration

At the beginning of each tape, a calibration signal of 50 to 100 µV square wave should be introduced in all channels. The initial calibration signal should be reviewed from tape on video playback or monitored on-line by EEG printout to assess the functioning of the system prior to beginning the EEG recording. A similar period of calibration at the end of the recording is also recommended because this serves as a test for problems that may have developed during the recording.

Before beginning the recording, the integrity of the recording system from electrode to storage medium should be checked. This can be accomplished by observing the ongoing EEG, tapping electrodes or connectors, and having the patient generate physiologic artifacts such as eye blinking, swallowing, and chewing. Recording amplifier sensitivity may have to be decreased in those patients with high-amplitude baseline rhythms or previously recognized paroxysmal abnormalities to prevent amplifier blocking.

When the patient returns to the laboratory for removal of the device, the end of the recording should be reviewed to ensure that signal recording was maintained.

Patient Diaries

The importance of keeping an accurate diary cannot be overstated. Since there are no technician's notes to benefit the reader, the patient log becomes important. In addition to making notes regarding possible seizures, the patient should also record other activities, such as eating, exercising, relaxing, and sleeping. Encouraging the patient or parents to begin notations while still in the laboratory enhances compliance on leaving the laboratory.

Activation Procedures

As with routine EEGs, it is useful to have the patient hyperventilate for 3 minutes and perform photic stimulation before leaving the laboratory.

Montages

During the past, when using 4- and 8-channel EEG, montage design was critically important for detecting interictal and ictal events and rejecting artifacts. With the newer digital systems, standard EEG montages are adequate, since digital reformatting is always an option.

AMBULATORY EEG MONITORING

Depending on the recording and data display system employed, ambulatory EEG interpretation may be either virtually identical to or radically different from the traditional EEG interpretation. When the EEG is printed on paper with a recording montage consisting of standard longitudinal chains, the analysis is quite similar to routine EEGs. However, today that technique is rarely used. Rather, the ambulatory EEG is reviewed using digital or analog analysis. When one's effort is directed toward use of the rapid analysis of EEG data on a video or computer screen, a strategy of recording and interpretation is necessary to ensure that pertinent abnormalities can be rapidly and reliably identified and that artifact that dominates ambulatory recording can be quickly and confidently dismissed.

Because ambulatory EEG records a vast amount of data, scanning techniques are necessary to decrease time. Cassette 8-channel systems now allow scanning at 20, 40, and 60 times real time. Although isolated interictal spikes and sharp waves may be missed at these speeds, ictal events are usually detected. In systems in which the analog signal is recorded onto audio tape, listening to the sounds can also be useful. Spikes and sharp waves have typical sounds: Bursts of 3-Hz spike-wave activity have a "Bronx cheer" sound, whereas runs of polyspike-wave activity are more "scratchy" on auditory review.[2] Both generalized convulsive seizures and partial seizures typically feature orderly and gradual evolution of frequencies, usually from high to low, with an accompanying increase in volume. Even when the visual presentation of the seizure is obscured by muscle and movement artifact, these auditory characteristics can still be perceived.

Digital EEG models reduce reviewing time by using ictal and interictal computer dictation software.[7] The software identifies epileptiform discharges on the basis of changes in amplitude, frequency, and rhythm (Fig. 21-1). Further refinements have reduced the incidence of false-positive and false-negative results, although errors continue to occur.

Since seizures may occur during wakefulness, they must be accurately differentiated from a wide variety of rhythmic artifacts. The electroencephalographer reviewing ambulatory records will find a host of artifacts that are not typically seen during routine EEGs. The artifacts encountered during a daytime recording from an active child are quite varied. Activities such as rubbing the face, scratching, tooth brushing, and shivering may present unusual, paroxysmal artifact. Mechanical devices such as an electric toothbrush or shaver can also produce artifact. Most of these artifacts lack the typical frequency evolution, and they often stop and start suddenly, occurring in a discontinuous fashion, which is most unusual for seizure activity. Seizure detection software often falsely identifies such artifacts as epileptiform activity, and the reader must be able to distinguish between artifact and epileptiform activity.

Features that are useful in detecting ictal discharges from artifact include the observation that the spikes are time locked to slow waves and postictal slowing following the discharge. Epileptiform discharges typically occur throughout the record. If the only abnormality occurs when the child is engaged in some activity, it is unlikely that the abnormality is epileptiform.

Partial seizures may produce a lateralized rhythmic discharge that does not contain spikes. The ictal discharge associated with partial seizures almost always has an evolution. For example, the discharge may begin with low-amplitude beta activity that increases in voltage and slows in frequency as the seizure progresses. On other occasions the discharge starts with slow waves that increase with frequency as the seizure progresses. This frequency shift is often more apparent on audio analysis than visually. In addition to a change in frequency and morphology, ictal events often spread to involve more electrodes as the seizure progresses.

During sleep, normal transients must be differentiated from epileptiform discharges. Vertex sharp waves and K-complexes may present a difficulty when only a limited electrode array is available. In young children, vertex sharp waves may be very frequent and have a very sharp configuration. When symmetrical and associated with sleep spindles, there is usually no difficulty in differentiating these from epileptiform discharges. The problem arises when they are asymmetrical and very frequent. Caution is necessary in the interpretation of any sharp transients seen only during sleep.

USE OF AMBULATORY EEG MONITORING IN CHILDREN

Ambulatory EEG is particularly useful in children, since they have many benign behaviors that may resemble seizures.[8] Paroxysmal events such as syncope, breath-holding attacks, shuddering attacks, and episodic rage attack may frequently resemble seizures. The small size of the ambulatory recorders, the resultant mobility, and the outpatient setting all are ideal for the pediatric patient.[4,9,10] Ambulatory EEG has also been found to be helpful in the evaluation of sleep disorders.[11,12]

Although ambulatory EEG was originally touted as an intermediate technology, offering something more than routine EEG because of the expanded temporal sample, yet not truly the equal of the gold standard of intensive inpatient monitoring, it has proven reasonably easy to use

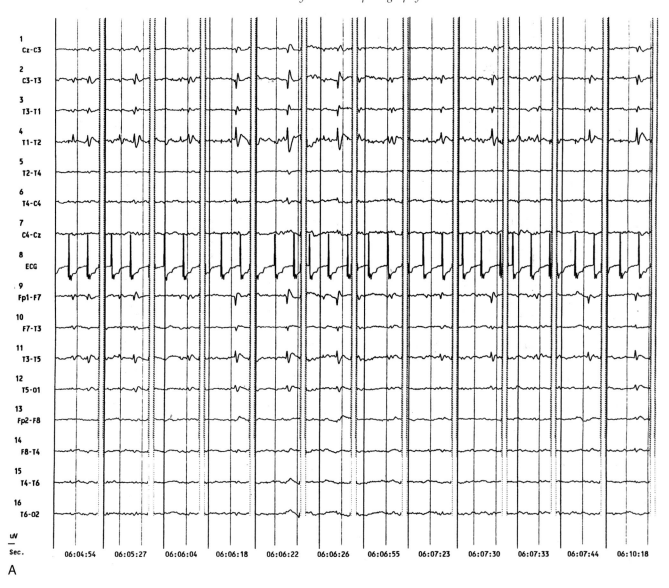

A

FIGURE 21–1

Example of spikes detected with spike detection software. Individual spikes and times recorded are presented. (Courtesy of Sleep Med, Peabody, MA, http://www2.sleepmed.md.)

the system to achieve much of the diagnostic capability of a dedicated inpatient monitoring unit by combining ambulatory EEG with portable video recording equipment to provide simultaneous EEG and behavioral monitoring.[13]

Box 21-1 provides some of the indications where ambulatory EEG may be useful. Figures 21-2 to 21-7 provide some examples of the usefulness of ambulatory EEG monitoring.

AMBULATORY EEG IN NEONATES

Ambulatory EEG seems a natural addition to the high-technology environment of the neonatal intensive care unit.

It offers the opportunity to provide EEG monitoring in circumstances when it would seem certain to be useful, yet without encroaching on critical access to these acutely ill patients. Regrettably, though, it is an area in which ambulatory EEG has received only limited investigation.

Eyre and colleagues[14] reported initially on a series of 25 neonates, all neurologically compromised and most having experienced birth asphyxia. Seizures were documented in 80%, including 5 who had only subclinical seizure activity and 4 with EEG seizure activity while paralyzed to assist in artificial ventilation. Among the 11 patients with clinically evident seizures, ambulatory EEG revealed substantial additional subclinical seizure activity. Three newborns in this

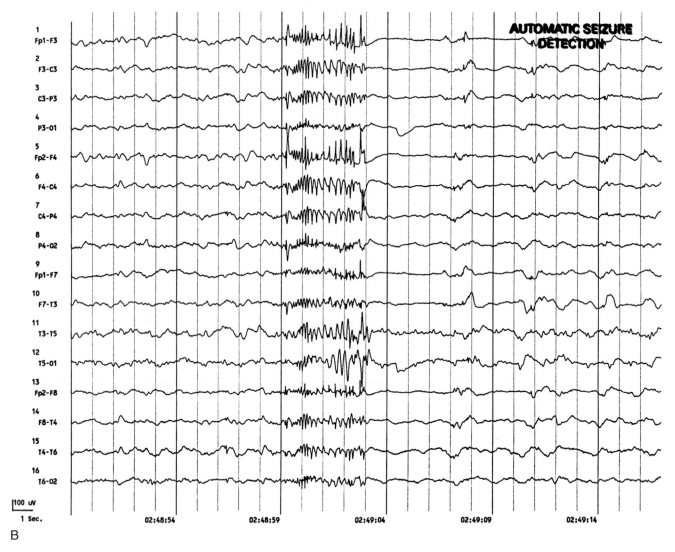

FIGURE 21–1 *Cont'd*

BOX 21-1
SUMMARY OF CLINICAL APPLICATIONS FOR AMBULATORY EEG

Confirm clinical suspicion of seizures
Determine seizure type
Quantify seizure number
Assess response to antiepileptic drug therapy
Identify interictal epileptiform activity
Evaluate nocturnal or sleep-related events
Evaluate rage attacks
Evaluate suspected pseudoseizures
Evaluate etiology of syncope
Evaluate unusual behaviors

series had continuous EEG seizure activity for hours that was clinically not apparent. Ambulatory EEG monitoring of patients in this series was initiated as soon as possible after neurologic compromise was apparent and was continued for as long as 16 hours. In all, 3619 episodes of ambulatory EEG seizure activity were recorded.

Eyre and colleagues[15] monitored a series of 80 newborns requiring mechanical ventilation within hours after birth and thus at high risk for neurologic complications. Ambulatory EEG recording was initiated on the day of birth and continued for 5 days. A control group of 25 low-risk neonates was similarly monitored for the first 5 days following birth. No clinical or ambulatory EEG seizures occurred in the low-risk group, but the yield was high in the high-risk group, with a total of 2825 episodes detected in 34 neonates (46%). Again, all patients with ambulatory EEG seizure activity

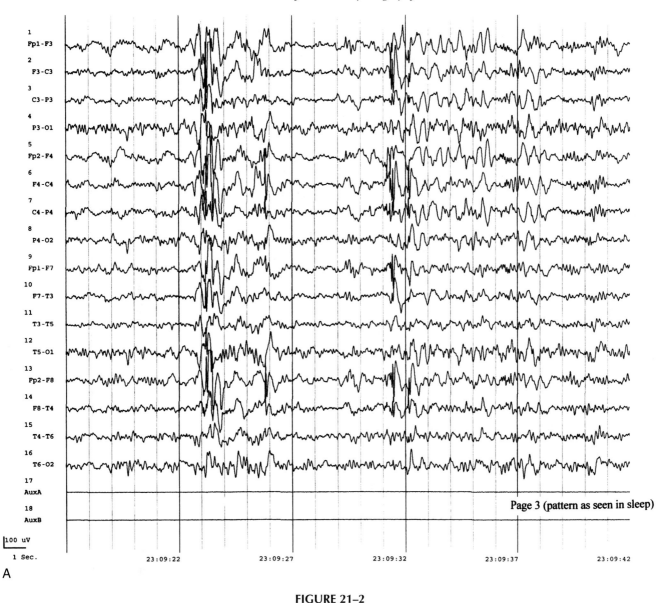

FIGURE 21–2

A 10-year-old girl with episodes of dizziness with visual distortion that she referred to as her "sideways spells" because the world seemed to turn sideways for a few seconds. A, Bursts of generalized, high-voltage >500 μV 3-Hz spike-wave were recorded. Note slow paper speed.

experienced at least some subclinical seizures and a substantial number (10) had only subclinical seizures. These investigators further found that total seizure activity was most abundant on the day of seizure onset and subsequently declined, with half of the patients experiencing seizures for 2 days or less. Seizures began within 24 hours of birth in 68% and within 3 days in 91%. In general, neonates with ambulatory EEG seizure activity were smaller, more premature, and more likely to have experienced birth asphyxia. Further, the findings of ambulatory EEG monitoring were compared to independently assessed outcome at 18 months, with the result that both increased numbers of discrete

ambulatory EEG seizures and increased duration of seizure activity correlated significantly with poorer outcome.

In reviewing her own experience, Eyre concluded that ambulatory EEG monitoring for the first 5 days of extrauterine life would identify most high-risk newborns destined to experience neonatal seizures. Our own experience with ambulatory EEG recording in neonates with seizures underscores the loss of diagnostic information that can be anticipated with reactive rather than expectant monitoring.[16] We performed ambulatory EEG on 37 neonates with a clinical diagnosis of seizures or suspected seizure activity and found seizure activity in only 7 (19%).

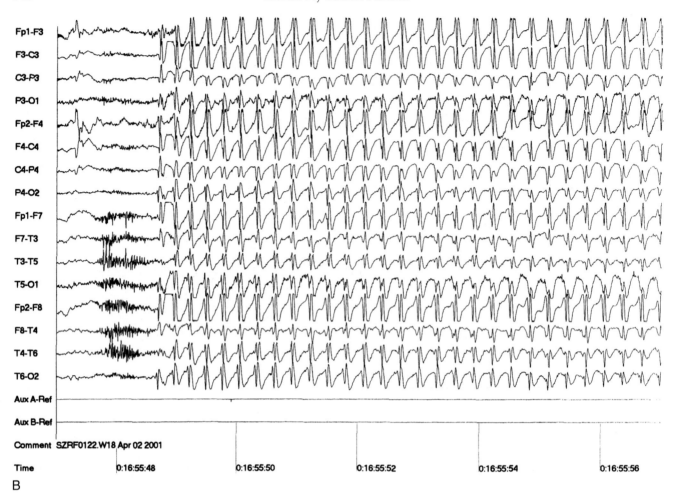

Fp1-F3

F3-C3

C3-P3

P3-O1

Fp2-F4

F4-C4

C4-P4

P4-O2

Fp1-F7

F7-T3

T3-T5

T5-O1

Fp2-F8

F8-T4

T4-T6

T6-O2

Aux A-Ref

Aux B-Ref

Comment SZRF0122.W18 Apr 02 2001

Time   0:16:55:48   0:16:55:50   0:16:55:52   0:16:55:54   0:16:55:56

B

FIGURE 21–2   *Cont'd*

B, Longer burst at faster paper speed. (Courtesy of Sleep Med, Peabody, MA, http://www2.sleepmed.md.)

Ambulatory EEG seizure activity was recorded in 50% of the neonates who had experienced clinical seizures within 24 hours of recording but in only 6% of those who had not. Among 9 patients with ongoing clinical events thought less likely to be seizures, we were able to provide ambulatory EEG support by correlating clinical events with an absence of EEG change in all.

One can draw the following tentative conclusions regarding the use of ambulatory EEG in neonates:

1. Rapidly instituted and extended monitoring in high-risk neonates yields a high incidence of both clinical and subclinical seizures, which may prove useful in guiding therapy and predicting outcome.

2. In neonates who experience apparent clinical seizures, rapidly instituted ambulatory EEG monitoring may accomplish the same ends, whereas delayed institution of monitoring yields little positive information.

3. Monitoring of infants with ongoing events unlikely to be seizures is helpful in confirming the nature of such episodes.

SEIZURE QUANTIFICATION WITH AMBULATORY EEG

Traditionally, measures such as seizure counting and serial standard EEG recording have been used to monitor effectiveness of anticonvulsant medications in absence epilepsy. Neither is truly suitable, since the former is inaccurate and the latter captures only a brief period that may not reflect the true frequency of 3-Hz spike-wave paroxysms, which exhibit considerable diurnal variability.[17-19] Ambulatory EEG, capturing a full day's activity, offers a better opportunity to quantify spike-wave activity objectively. Keilson and coworkers[17] have demonstrated the relative ease with which

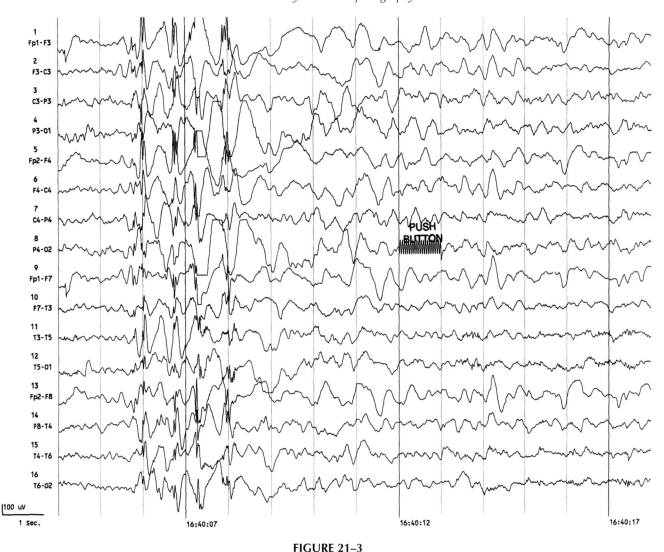

FIGURE 21–3

A 3-year-old boy with a history of generalized seizures consisting of myoclonic jerks and tonic-clonic seizures. Note frontal maximal generalized polyspike and spike-wave discharges. (Courtesy of Sleep Med, Peabody, MA, http://www2.sleepmed.md.)

spike-wave paroxysms can be tabulated using ambulatory EEG. Ambulatory EEG is particularly useful in evaluating drug response in absence seizures and is becoming a standard outcome measure for efficacy.[18,20-22]

Most experience with quantification has relied on direct observation and counting, although the prospect exists that computerized systems may eventually prove reliable enough to perform, or assist with, this task.[7]

CONCLUSIONS

Much can be accomplished with the employment of ambulatory EEG in diagnosing seizures in infants and children and in monitoring the effectiveness of therapy. Ambulatory EEG is by no means an ideal technique in its current state of development, but it is a technique of proven use and accuracy that has yet to receive the attention it deserves, particularly in the area of neonatal neurology. Those of us who have been active in the clinical development of ambulatory EEG have been consistently disappointed by our relatively small numbers, particularly in the United States. One can only hope that as the advantages of electronic storage lead electroencephalographers away from the tradition of paper write-out, and EEG on a video screen comes to seem more the norm than a novelty, ambulatory EEG will generate a new level of interest.

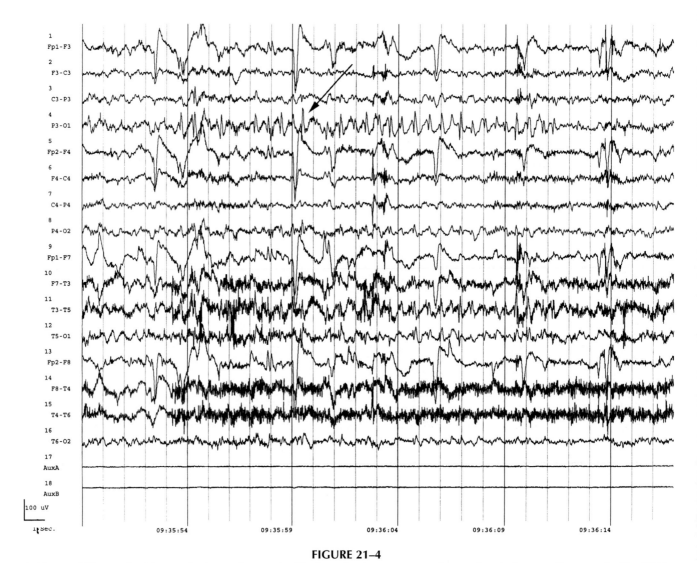

FIGURE 21–4

A 10-year-old boy with a history of seizures characterized by loss of vision, nausea, and stomach pain lasting a few seconds. The EEG demonstrates the presence of focal epileptiform activity in the left occipital region (arrow). (Courtesy of Sleep Med, Peabody, MA, http://www2.sleepmed.md.)

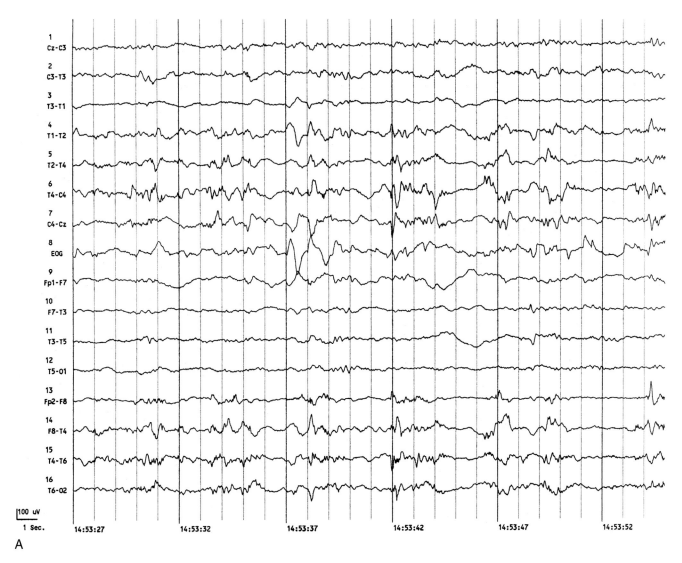

FIGURE 21–5

A 4-month-old girl with Aicardi's syndrome. A, Interictal record with intermittent bursts over the right lateral hemisphere and attenuation over the left hemisphere.

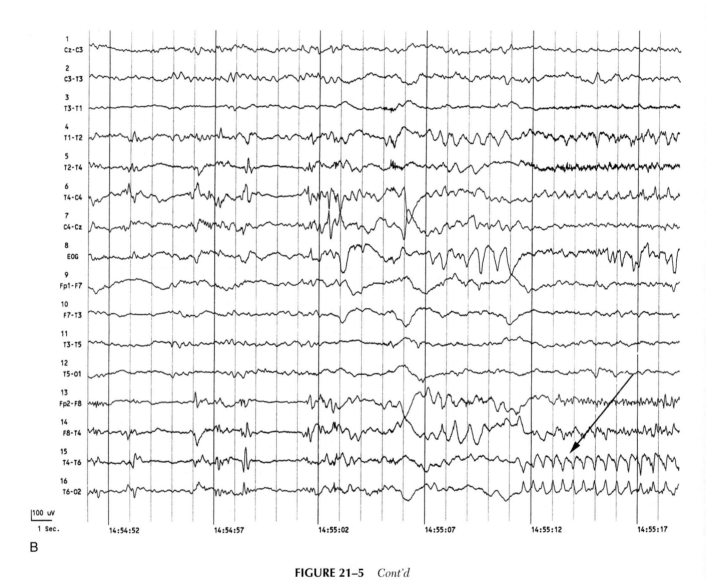

FIGURE 21–5 *Cont'd*
B, *Electrographic seizure starting in the right temporal region* (arrow).*(Courtesy of Sleep Med, Peabody, MA, http://www2.sleepmed.md.)*

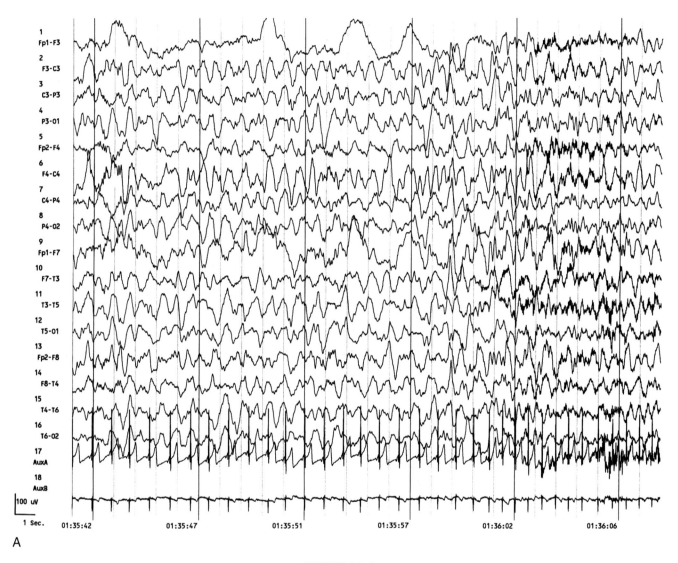

A

FIGURE 21–6

An 11-year-old boy with night terrors. A and B, Note onset in stage III sleep. During the event the child appeared confused. During the episode there is abundant EMG muscle artifact and sinus tachycardia. No epileptiform activity is present. (Courtesy of Sleep Med, Peabody, MA, http://www2.sleepmed.md.)

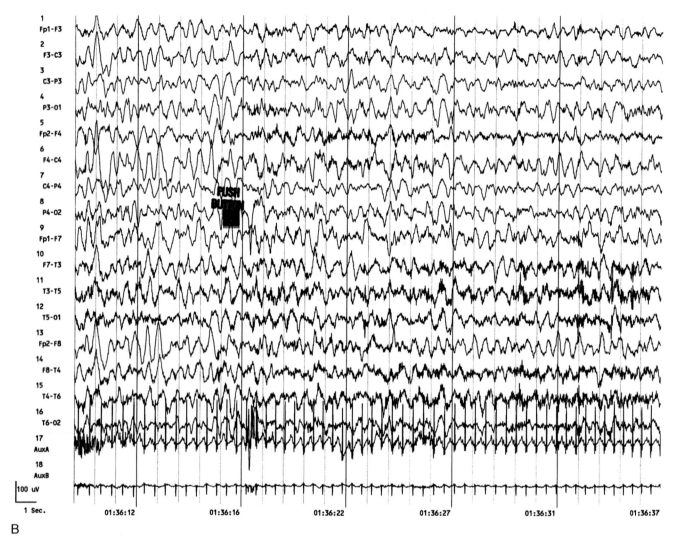

FIGURE 21–6 *Cont'd*

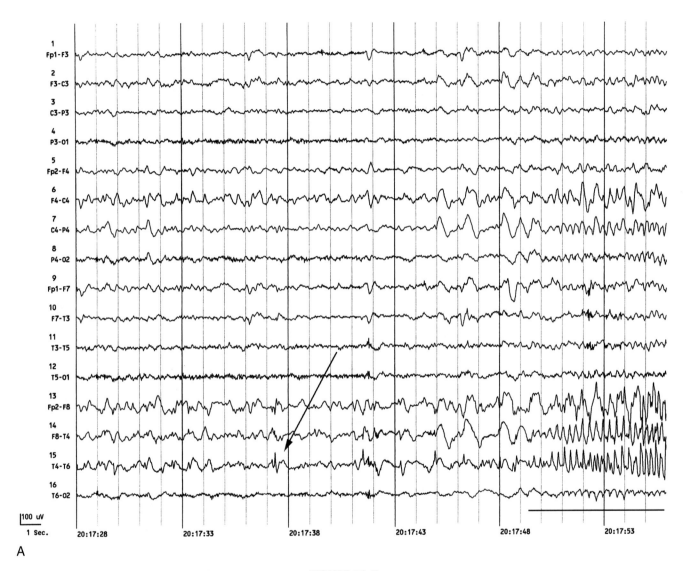

FIGURE 21–7

A 7-year-old girl with right-sided temporal lobe seizures. A, Note interictal spikes in the right temporal lobe (arrow) *and the ictal event* (underline) *beginning in the right temporal region. B, Continuation of right temporal lobe seizure. (Courtesy of Sleep Med, Peabody, MA, http://www2.sleepmed.md.)*

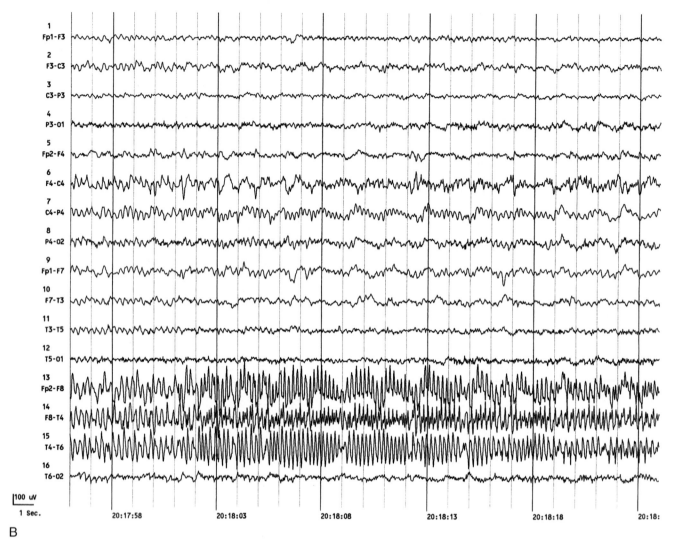

FIGURE 21–7 *Cont'd*

REFERENCES

1. Ebersole JS: Ambulatory EEG Monitoring. New York, Raven Press, 1989.
2. Ebersole JS: Audio-video analysis of cassette EEG. *In* Ebersole JS (ed): Ambulatory EEG Monitoring. New York, Raven Press, 1989, p 69.
3. Ives JR, Mainwaring NR, Schomer DL: SEER: A solid-state EEG event recorder for the ambulatory monitoring of epileptic patients. Epilepsia 1990;31:661.
4. Ebersole JS: Outpatient monitoring: Ambulatory cassette recording. *In* Wada JA, Ellingson RJ (eds): Clinical Neurophysiology of Epilepsy. New York, Elsevier, 1990, p 155.
5. American EEG Society: Guideline twelve: Guidelines for long-term monitoring for epilepsy. J Clin Neurophysiol 1994;11:88-110.
6. Clenney SL: Techniques of cassette EEG recording. *In* Ebersole JS (ed): Ambulatory EEG Monitoring. New York, Raven Press, 1989, p 27.
7. Gotman J: Automated analysis of ambulatory EEG recordings. *In* Ebersole JS (ed): Ambulatory EEG Monitoring. New York, Raven Press, 1989, p 97.
8. Olson DM: Success of ambulatory EEG in children. J Clin Neurophysiol 2001;18:158-161.
9. Aminoff MJ, Goodin DS, Berg BO, Compton MN: Ambulatory EEG recordings in epileptic and nonepileptic children. Neurology 1988;38:558-562.
10. Saravanan K, Acomb B, Beirne M, Appleton R: An audit of ambulatory cassette EEG monitoring in children. Seizure 2001;10:579-582.
11. Oseas-McNamara ME, Rosner B, Regestein QR: Excessive daytime sleepiness associated with idiopathic

alterations of consciousness. Clin Electroencephalogr 1997;28:207-213.

12. Mariotti P, Della Marca G, Iuvone L, et al: Sleep disorders in Sanfilippo syndrome: A polygraphic study. Clin Electroencephalogr 2003;34:18-22.

13. Leroy RF, Rao KK, Voth BJ: Intensive neurodiagnostic monitoring in epilepsy using ambulatory cassette EEG with simultaneous video recording. *In* Ebersole JS (ed): Ambulatory EEG Monitoring. New York, Raven Press, 1989, p 157.

14. Eyre JA, Oozeer RC, Wilkinson AR: Diagnosis of neonatal seizure by continuous recording and rapid analysis of the electroencephalogram. Arch Dis Child 1983;58:785-790.

15. Eyre JA, Oozeer RC, Wilkinson AR: Continuous electroencephalographic recording to detect seizures in paralyzed newborns. BMJ 1983;286:1017-1018.

16. Bridgers SL, Ebersole JS, Ment LR, et al: Cassette electroencephalography in the evaluation of neonatal seizures. Arch Neurol 1986;43:49-51.

17. Keilson MJ, Hauser WA, Magrill JP, Tepperberg J: Ambulatory cassette EEG in absence epilepsy. Pediatr Neurol 1987;3:273-276.

18. Powell TE, Harding GFA: Twenty-four hour ambulatory EEG monitoring: Development and applications. J Med Eng Tech 1986;10:229-238.

19. Horita H, Uchida E, Maekawa K: Circadian rhythm of regular spike-wave discharges in childhood absence epilepsy. Brain Dev 1991;13:200-202.

20. Frank LM, Enlow T, Holmes GL, et al: Lamictal (lamotrigine) monotherapy for typical absence seizures in children. Epilepsia 1999;40:973-979.

21. Coppola G, Licciardi G, Sciscio N, et al: Lamotrigine as first-line drug in childhood absence epilepsy: A clinical and neurophysiological study. Brain Dev 2004;26:26-29.

22. Cross JH: Topiramate monotherapy for childhood absence seizures: An open label pilot study. Seizure 2002;11:406-410.

22

Electroencephalography in the Evaluation for Epilepsy Surgery in Children

ELAINE WYLLIE

Since the pioneering work of Mr. Murray Falconer at the Maudsley Hospital in London, England, in the 1960s and 1970s,[1-5] it has been clear that children as well as adults may benefit from epilepsy surgery. Series from various centers have reported good outcome, with patients seizure free, with auras only, or with only very rare attacks, for 57% to 100% of children and adolescents.[6-9] Within certain subgroups, the frequency of good outcome may be especially high. In one predominantly adult series, the frequency of good outcome among patients with unilateral anterior temporal epileptogenic foci was 91%.[10] In a recent pediatric series,[6] the frequency of seizure-free outcome was higher among patients with low-grade tumor or hippocampal sclerosis than among those with malformation of cortical development.

The success of surgery coupled with the high incidence of pharmacoresistant epilepsy in children has resulted in increasing use of intracranial electroencephalographic (EEG) monitoring to determine the location of the epileptic focus. This review focuses on the approach to pediatric candidates for temporal or extratemporal resection.

TEMPORAL LOBECTOMY

Noninvasive EEG Evaluation

Noninvasive video EEG recording is the cornerstone of the evaluation for epilepsy surgery.[11-13] Its results form the basis for all further steps toward operation. For this reason it is critical to perform a detailed and careful noninvasive EEG evaluation in every case.

Extra electrodes, in addition to those of the standard International 10-20 System,[14] may be useful for detailed analysis of areas with focal epileptiform discharges. Closely spaced scalp electrodes may be placed between and below the standard International 10-20 positions,[11,15] and sphenoidal or nasopharyngeal electrodes may be inserted to record from basal temporal regions.[16-20] With simultaneous bipolar and referential recording using multiple EEG machines, the relative amplitude of focal epileptiform discharges at different electrodes may be compared (Figs. 22-1 and 22-2). These data may be used to generate voltage distribution maps, with relative amplitudes at each electrode expressed by isoelectric lines (Fig. 22-3). Detailed maps of focal interictal sharp waves may be especially helpful in defining the epileptogenic zone, because ictal discharges recorded with noninvasive electrodes often have a more widespread lobar or hemispheric distribution (Fig. 22-4).

Sphenoidal electrodes may be inserted inside a 22-gauge lumbar puncture needle into the muscles of the cheek, through the space between the zygomatic process and the angle of the mandible. In place, the sphenoidal electrodes lie near the region of the foramen ovale and provide increased sensitivity to discharges from mesiobasal temporal regions.

Insertion of sphenoidal electrodes in children may be accomplished more comfortably with conscious sedation.[20] In one series, children were premedicated with intravenous

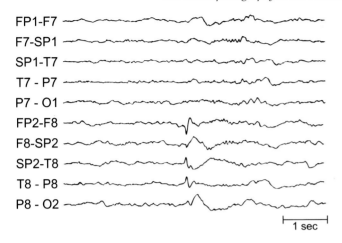

FIGURE 22–1

Bipolar EEG showing a sharp wave from the right anterior temporal lobe in a 17-year-old patient with intractable complex partial seizures since early childhood.

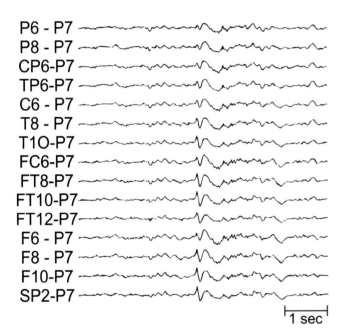

FIGURE 22–2

Referential EEG of the same sharp wave shown in Figure 22-5, with maximum amplitude at the right sphenoidal electrode.

meperidine and midazolam in small aliquots over about 10 minutes. Doses were titrated to a level of conversant relaxation, so that during insertion patients either showed no signs of discomfort or just winced slightly but were not asleep. An added benefit of the midazolam was amnesia, so that afterward none of the children remembered the insertion. This was especially helpful to prevent later anxiety when children returned for repeat EEG evaluations.

Maximum amplitude of epileptiform discharges at sphenoidal or anterior temporal scalp electrodes suggests origin of seizures from the anteromesial temporal area.[15,17] When these results are congruent with clinical, neuroimaging, and positron emission tomography (PET) findings, it may be appropriate to proceed directly to anterior temporal lobectomy.[17] When the noninvasive EEG evaluation does not show that all the epileptiform discharges are localized to the anterior temporal lobe on one side, or when clinical, EEG, and neuroimaging findings are not convergent, then further evaluation with invasive neurophysiologic techniques may be necessary.

Invasive Neurophysiologic Evaluation

With the advent of modern neuroimaging, the need for invasive neurophysiologic techniques has markedly decreased. Surgical strategy may sometimes be decided based on the extent of an epileptogenic lesion seen on magnetic resonance imaging (MRI), even in the presence of less well defined ictal and interictal discharges on scalp EEG. However, in some cases, invasive neurophysiologic techniques may provide important information.

In general, as electrodes become more invasive, they tend to provide more detailed and precisely localized information, at the expense of more limited sampling. Depth electrodes and subdural grids are helpful to answer specific neurophysiologic questions about a highly restricted cortical area, but they are less helpful to explore more widespread localization problems between large cortical areas.[21] Therefore, these techniques should be reserved for cases where basic regional localization problems have already been resolved by scalp and sphenoidal EEG.

Depth Electrodes

Depth electrodes may be helpful when noninvasive EEG suggests more than one epileptogenic area, for example in patients with independent sharp waves from both anteromesial temporal lobes, from the temporal and frontal lobes on one side, or from other temporal or extratemporal areas.[2,22-27] These electrodes are implanted directly into cortical tissue under general anesthesia with stereotactic MRI guidance, to define more precisely the location of seizure onset (Fig. 22-5). Depth electrodes implanted bilaterally into amygdala and hippocampus may be especially helpful for patients with bitemporal independent epileptiform discharges on scalp and sphenoidal EEG. When several seizures are recorded with bilateral depth EEG over days or weeks, it may be possible to determine that one temporal lobe generates a predominance of the clinical attacks. There are data to suggest that when at least 70% of the seizures are from one side, it may be appropriate to proceed to temporal lobectomy, even though the likelihood

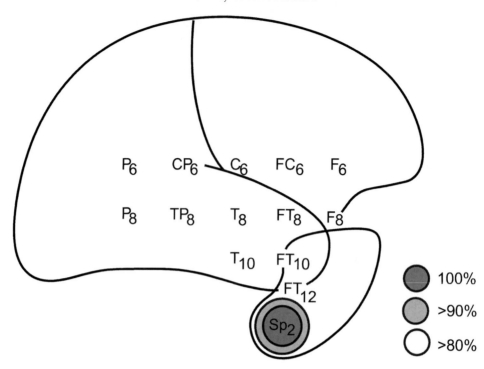

FIGURE 22–3

Distribution map showing the relative amplitude at different electrodes of the sharp wave shown in Figures 22-5 and 22-6. Two years after right anterior temporal lobectomy, the patient remains seizure free.

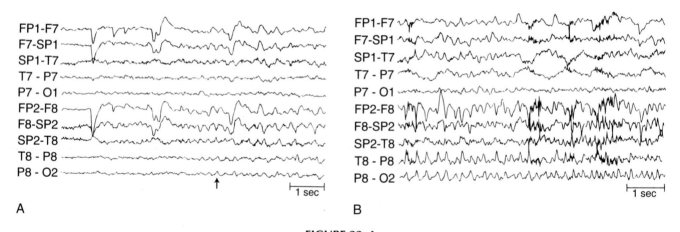

FIGURE 22–4

EEG during a complex partial seizure from the same patient as in Figure 22-3 showing an EEG seizure pattern from the right anterior temporal region. A, EEG at clinical onset (arrow). B, EEG 10 seconds after clinical onset.

of complete seizure control after operation may be lower than in the setting of only unilateral temporal epileptiform discharges.[26]

Disadvantages of depth electrodes include invasion of normal cortex to reach suspected epileptogenic areas and sampling limitations when surveying large areas such as the frontal lobe. In addition, there is a low risk for intracerebral hemorrhage or infection. Although depth electrode series

have occasionally included children, no extensive pediatric series are currently available.

Subdural or Epidural Electrode Grids

Subdural or epidural electrode grids may be helpful in planning safe, effective resection for patients with an epileptogenic region near functional cortex.[10,28-30] For example, in patients with left hemisphere language

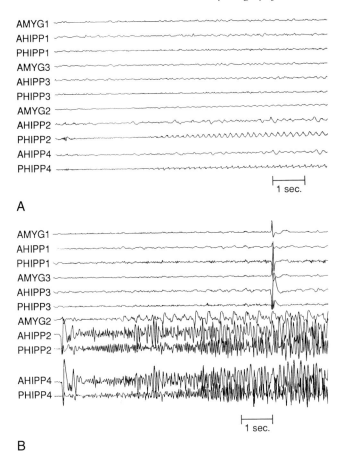

AMYG1
AHIPP1
PHIPP1
AMYG3
AHIPP3
PHIPP3
AMYG2
AHIPP2
PHIPP2
AHIPP4
PHIPP4

1 sec.

A

AMYG1
AHIPP1
PHIPP1
AMYG3
AHIPP3
PHIPP3
AMYG2
AHIPP2
PHIPP2
AHIPP4
PHIPP4

1 sec.

B

FIGURE 22–5

Depth EEG during a complex partial seizure. Previous scalp and sphenoidal EEG showed bitemporal independent interictal sharp waves and poorly lateralized EEG seizures. Depth EEG showed seizure onset in the right hippocampus. A, EEG at clinical onset. B, EEG 20 seconds after clinical onset. AMYG, amygdala; AHIPP, anterior hippocampus; PHIPP, posterior hippocampus; 1, the most mesial contact of a depth electrode in the left hemisphere; 3, the next most mesial contact of a depth electrode in the left hemisphere; 2 and 4, the homologous contacts in the right hemisphere.

tical area to be covered. Subdural electrode grids have the advantage that they may be slipped under the edges of the open craniotomy, including under the temporal or frontal lobe or in the interhemispheric fissure; whereas epidural electrode grids can cover just the exposed area. In addition, unless the dura is excised and then replaced as a graft, cortical stimulation with epidural electrodes may cause pain due to stimulation of meningeal nerve fibers. Stimulation with subdural electrodes is painless unless the plate is near the trigeminal nerve.

Mapping of language areas is accomplished by passing a very small electric current into single subdural or epidural electrodes. Typically the stimulus includes alternating polarity pulses with 0.3-millisecond duration, repetition rate of 50 Hz, and maximum duration less than 20 seconds.[29] Stimulation is usually started at 1 mA and then increased gradually on subsequent trials until signs or symptoms occur or until afterdischarges appear on EEG, to a maximum of 15 mA. Common findings with stimulation of electrodes over language areas include interruption or impairment of speech, anomia, agraphia, or inability to follow spoken commands. Stimulation of extratemporal regions is described later in that section.

Cortical stimulation studies for mapping of language areas are effective in older children, adolescents, and adults but may be less effective in infants and young children. However, developmentally normal children may have successful language mapping as young as 4 or 5 years of age. Children can be encouraged to repeat nursery rhymes or sing songs to provide ongoing verbal output for testing with cortical stimulation.

In one series, the overall risk for infection with subdural electrode grids was 14%.[30] Signs and symptoms range from fever, headache, and cloudy cerebrospinal fluid drainage from the cable site to late failure of incision healing and underlying chronic osteomyelitis. Infections do not generally result in irreversible sequelae, but they do prolong the postoperative hospital course and necessitate intravenous antibiotics or occasionally cranioplasty.[30] Increased intracranial pressure may also occur with placement of subdural or epidural electrode grids. This problem is usually controlled with corticosteroids and fluid restriction, but rarely the evaluation has to be terminated by early removal of the subdural electrode grids. Because of these risks, subdural electrode grids should be reserved for cases when detailed functional localization studies are necessary for a safe and effective resection.

Intraoperative Electrocorticography and Cortical Stimulation

The techniques discussed earlier involve implantation of electrodes for chronic extraoperative invasive EEG. Electrocorticography, evoked potential studies, and cortical

dominance and epileptiform discharges maximum in the mid or posterior temporal region, it may be useful to map the epileptogenic zone in relation to Wernicke's language area (Fig. 22-6). Subdural electrodes also may have utility in the planning of extratemporal resection, as discussed later in that section.

One version of subdural electrode grids consists of stainless steel discs embedded 1 cm apart from center to center in a sheet of Silastic with electrode wires emerging together in a cable from a separate incision (Fig. 22-7). Arrays may be formed in various configurations such as four rows of four electrodes, five rows of eight electrodes, or eight rows of eight electrodes, depending on the size and shape of the cor-

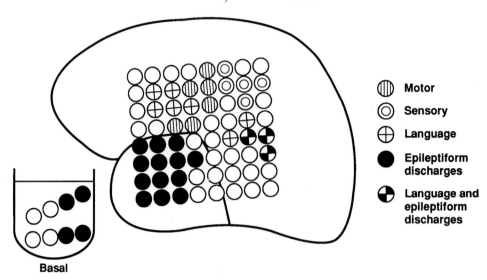

FIGURE 22–6

Subdural EEG and cortical stimulation studies in a 13-year-old boy with intractable complex partial seizures. Invasive studies were performed because surface EEG showed sharp waves from left anterior and posterior temporal regions. The posterior region with interictal epileptiform discharges was not removed in the 7.5-cm resection because it overlapped with Wernicke's language area. During the 6 years since surgery, the patient has had only one complex partial seizure.

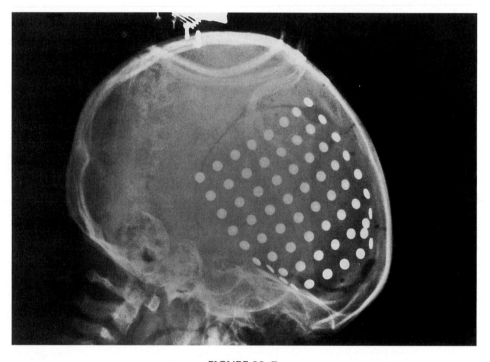

FIGURE 22–7

A subdural electrode grid in place over the right frontal lobe in a 2-year-old boy.

stimulation can also be performed intraoperatively under local anesthesia.[31-33]

Advantages include avoidance of chronic indwelling electrodes, and disadvantages include minimal opportunity for ictal recording and a hectic setting for functional localization studies. Intraoperative localization techniques have been highly successful in adults and mature adolescents but are more difficult to accomplish in children.[34,35]

EXTRATEMPORAL RESECTIONS

Patient Selection and Timing of Operation

Seizures arising from frontal, central, parietal, or occipital areas may have a variety of clinical features, depending on the cortical areas activated by ictal discharges. These features have been described elsewhere.[36-39] Signs and symptoms suggesting involvement of one cortical area, however, may not mean that the seizure began in that region but instead could be a manifestation of spread of the ictal discharge or other process. In the first 2 years of life, for example, focal epileptogenic processes may manifest as infantile spasms with hypsarrhythmia.[9,21,40,41]

Temporal lobectomy is the most frequent type of epilepsy surgery in adults, but extratemporal resections and hemispherectomies are more common among infants and children.[6-9,41] Patients with temporal lobe epilepsy tend not to fulfill all the severity, disability, and intractability criteria for operation until at least 6 or 8 years of age, so operation is unusual before that time. However, infants and children with devastating, intractable, daily focal-onset extratemporal seizures often qualify for operation earlier in life.

Noninvasive EEG Evaluation

The principles for a detailed noninvasive video EEG evaluation for extratemporal epilepsy are similar to those for temporal lobe epilepsy. Closely spaced scalp electrodes over the area of interest are frequently helpful, and sphenoidal electrodes are useful if the suspected epileptogenic area could include the temporal lobe. Plans for resection or invasive EEG may be based on distribution, maps of extratemporal ictal and interictal epileptiform discharges, along with other clinical, neuroimaging, and PET findings.

Invasive Neurophysiologic Evaluation

For extratemporal as well as temporal resections, the need for invasive neurophysiologic studies has decreased with the advent of high-resolution MRI. However, in nonlesional or otherwise difficult cases, invasive studies may be helpful. Intraoperative electrocorticography or extraoperative depth or subdural or epidural grid electrodes may assist in determining the extent of the extratemporal epileptogenic zone in relation to nearby functional areas. However, for frontal resections, experienced surgeons may have good success sparing rolandic motor areas based on anatomic landmarks alone.[26]

Problems with mapping language areas in young children have been described earlier. Mapping of somatosensory areas may also provide challenges in infants and young children because of inadequate verbal skills to describe unusual sensations during cortical stimulation. In these cases, median, tibial, or lip somatosensory evoked potential studies using the subdural electrodes may be helpful at any age.

Findings during cortical stimulation of positive motor areas include involuntary posturing or movement of the affected body part, so this mapping does not require verbal skills. However, mapping of rolandic motor areas may also be unsuccessful in infants and young children, even though verbal skills are not required, for reasons that are not well understood.[28,42]

Jayakar and colleagues[43] described their technique for mapping the cortex in children. The authors stimulated using a biphasic pulse delivered at a frequency in trains lasting up to 5 seconds and used a dual-increment paradigm. Stimulation started at an intensity of 1 mA and pulse duration of 0.3 millisecond. In each subsequent trial, the intensity and pulse duration were adjusted by 1 or 2 mA or 0.1 to 0.2 millisecond, respectively. The highest intensity and duration was an amperage of 15 mA and a duration of 1.0 millisecond. The authors calculated that at this setting the charge per phase was 15 μC/ph; for subdural electrodes, the maximum charge density per phase was 119 μC/cm^2/ph. The authors noted that in adults, the clinical response threshold is usually at or below the afterdischarge threshold, whereas in children, clinical responses may only be obtained at thresholds higher than the afterdischarge threshold.

CONCLUSION

The cornerstones of the evaluation for epilepsy surgery are MRI and noninvasive video EEG. Invasive neurophysiologic techniques may be required in selected cases. However, modern MRI techniques have led to appreciation of a broader spectrum of candidates who can successfully undergo epilepsy surgery without invasive neurophysiology. Encouraging results from recent pediatric series indicate that epilepsy surgery should be considered, even at an early age, for patients with severe intractable epilepsy, a focal epileptogenic zone, and a low risk for new postoperative neurologic deficits.

REFERENCES

1. Davidson S, Falconer MA: Outcome of surgery in 40 children with temporal-lobe epilepsy. Lancet 1975;1:1260-1263.
2. Falconer M: Significance of surgery for temporal epilepsy in childhood and adolescence. J Neurosurg 1970;33:233-252.
3. Falconer M: Temporal lobe epilepsy in children and its surgical treatment. Med J Aust 1972;1:1117-1121.
4. Falconer MA, Hill D, Meyer A, Mitchell W: Treatment of temporal-lobe epilepsy by temporal lobectomy: A survey of findings and results. Lancet 1955;2:827-835.

5. Falconer MA, Serafetinides EA: A follow-up study of surgery in temporal lobe epilepsy. J Neurol Neurosurg Psychiatry 1963;26:154-165.

6. Wyllie E, Comair YG, Kotagal P, et al: Seizure outcome after epilepsy surgery in children and adolescents. Ann Neurol 1998;44:740-748.

7. Duchowny M: Epilepsy surgery in children. Curr Opin Neurol 1995;8:112-116.

8. Duchowny M, Jayakar P, Resnick T, et al: Epilepsy surgery in the first three years of life. Epilepsia 1998;39:737-743.

9. Chugani HT, Shewmon A, Shields WD, et al: Surgery for intractable infantile spasms: Neuroimaging perspectives. Epilepsia 1993;34:764-771.

10. Wyllie E, Lüders H, Morris HH III, et al: Clinical outcome after complete or partial cortical resection for intractable epilepsy. Neurology 1987;37:1634-1641.

11. Lesser RP, Dinner DS, Lüders H, Morris HH: Differential diagnosis and treatment of intractable seizures. Cleve Clin J Med 1984;51:227-240.

12. Lüders H, Dinner DS, Morris HH III, et al: EEG evaluation for epilepsy surgery in children. Clev Clin J Med 1989;56:S53-S61.

13. Wyllie E: Cortical resection for children with epilepsy: Perspectives in pediatrics. Am J Dis Child 1990;145:314-320.

14. Cooper R, Osselton JW, Shaw JC: Electrodes: EEG Technology. Boston, Butterworth, 1980, p 15.

15. Morris HH III, Lüders H: Electrodes. *In* Gotman J, Ives JR, Gloor P (eds): Long-Term Monitoring in Epilepsy. Amsterdam, Elsevier, 1985, p 3.

16. Kristensen O, Sindrup EH: Sphenoidal electrodes: Their use and value in the electroencephalographic investigation of complex partial epilepsy. Acta Neurol Scand 1978;58:157-166.

17. Morris HH III, Kanna A, Lüders H, et al: Can sharp waves localized at the sphenoidal electrode accurately identify a mesio-temporal epileptogenic focus? Epilepsia 1989;30:532-539.

18. Pampiglione G, Kerridge J: EEG abnormalities from the temporal lobe studied with sphenoidal electrodes. J Neurol Neurosurg Psychiatry 1956;19:117-129.

19. Sperling MR, Mendius JR, Engel J Jr: Mesial temporal spikes: A simultaneous comparison of sphenoidal, nasopharyngeal, and ear electrodes. Epilepsia 1986;27:81-86.

20. Wyllie E, Wyllie R, Kotagal P, et al: Comfortable insertion of sphenoidal electrodes in children. Epilepsia 1990;31:521-523.

21. Wyllie E: Intracranial EEG and localization studies. *In* Wyllie E (ed): The Treatment of Epilepsy: Principles, and Practice. Baltimore, Williams & Wilkins, 1996, p 988.

22. Bancaud J: Surgery of epilepsy based on stereotactic investigations—the plan of SEEG investigations. Acta Neurochir 1980;30:S25-S34.

23. King DW, Flanigin HF, Gallagher BB, et al: Temporal lobectomy for partial complex seizures: Evaluation, results, and 1-year follow-up. Neurology 1986;36:334-339.

24. Lieb JP, Engel J Jr, Gevins A, Crandall PH: Surface and deep EEG correlates of surgical outcome in temporal lobe epilepsy. Epilepsia 1981;22:515-538.

25. So N, Gloor P, Quesney LF, et al: Depth electrode investigations in patients with bitemporal epileptiform abnormalities. Ann Neurol 1989;25:423-431.

26. Rasmussen T: Extratemporal cortical excisions and hemispherectomy. *In* Engel J (ed): Surgical Management of the Epilepsies. New York, Raven Press, 1987, p 417.

27. Chugani HT, Shewmon A, Shields WD, et al: Pediatric epilepsy surgery: Preoperative and postoperative evaluation with PET. J Epilepsy 1990;3(Suppl 1):75-82.

28. Goldring S, Gregorie EM: Surgical management using epidural recordings to localize the seizure focus: Review of 100 cases. Neurosurgery 1984;60:457-466.

29. Lüders H, Lesser RP, Dinner DS, et al: Chronic intracranial recording and stimulation with subdural electrodes. *In* Engel J (ed): Surgical Treatment of the Epilepsies. New York, Raven Press, 1987, p 297.

30. Wyllie E, Lüders H, Morris HH, et al: Subdural electrodes in the evaluation for epilepsy surgery in children and adults. Neuropediatrics 1988;19:80-86.

31. Green JR: Surgical treatment of epilepsy during childhood and adolescence. Surg Neurol 1977;8:71-80.

32. Meyer FB, Marsh WR, Laws ER, Sharbrough FW: Temporal lobectomy in children with epilepsy. J Neurosurg 1986;64:371-376.

33. Whittle IR, Ellis HJ, Simpson DA: The surgical treatment of intractable childhood and adolescent epilepsy. Aust N Z J Surg 1981;51:190-196.

34. Meglio M, Cioni B, Cruccu G, Inghilleri M. The "foramen ovale" electrode: A safe tool to study temporal lobe epilepsy. Electroencephalogr Clin Neurophysiol 1987;66:327-330.

35. Rapport RL, Ojemann GA, Wyler AR, Ward AA Jr: Surgical management of epilepsy. West J Med 1977;127:185-189.

36. Meck WH, Smith RA, Williams CL: Prenatal and postnatal choline supplementation produces long-term facilitation of spatial memory. Dev Psychobiol 1988;21:339-353.

37. Lesser RP, Lüders H, Dinner DS, Morris H: Simple partial seizures. *In* Lüders H, Lesser RP (eds): Electroclinical Syndromes. New York, Springer-Verlag, 1987, p 223.

38. Wyllie E, Lüders H: Complex partial seizures in children: Clinical manifestations and identification of surgical candidates. Cleve Clin J Med 1989;56:S43-S52.

39. Kudo Y, Ogura A: Glutamate-induced increase in intracellular Ca^{2+} concentration in isolated hippocampal neurons. Br J Pharmacol 1986;89:191-198.

40. Chugani HT, Shields WD, Shewmon DA, et al: Infantile spasms: I. PET identifies focal cortical dysgenesis in cryptogenic cases for surgical treatment. Ann Neurol 1990;27:406-413.

41. Wyllie E: Epilepsy surgery in infants. *In* Wyllie E (ed): The Treatment of Epilepsy: Principles and Practice. Baltimore, Williams & Wilkins, 1996, p 1087.

42. Nespeca M, Wyllie E, Lüders H, et al: EEG recording and functional localization studies with subdural electrodes in infants and young children. J Epilepsy 1990;3(Suppl):107-124.

43. Jayakar P, Alvarez LA, Duchowny MS, Resnick TJ: A safe and effective paradigm to functionally map the cortex in childhood. J Clin Neurophysiol 1992;9:288-293.

23

Long-Term Electroencephalogram and Video Monitoring

TREVOR J. RESNICK, PRASANNA JAYAKAR, AND MICHAEL DUCHOWNY

Epilepsy is a common problem in pediatric practice, often diagnosed by clinical history alone. However, descriptions of epileptic symptoms by patients and their families are often imprecise, requiring further characterization of clinical features and electrographic correlates to establish the diagnosis and classify the type of epilepsy.

Since epilepsy is by definition episodic in nature, it is only possible to analyze seizures by continuously monitoring the electroencephalogram (EEG) and behavior for extended periods. The inherent limitations of historical information for reaching a diagnosis has spawned technologies that facilitate longer monitoring of EEG and behavior. *Long-term monitoring* (LTM) refers to the continuous assessment of electrophysiologic and behavioral activity over several states with a goal of capturing and characterizing episodic disturbances. Although LTM is time consuming, labor intensive, and expensive, it has proven to be cost-effective by reducing the enormous social and financial burdens of chronic epilepsy.[1-3] It is rapidly becoming standard at most epilepsy centers throughout North America, Europe, and Japan.

In this chapter, we discuss the various methodologies and clinical applications of LTM, with particular emphasis on the evaluation of infants and children.

METHODOLOGY

Pediatric LTM facilities are similar in design to adult units. Pediatric recording rooms should be near monitoring and nursing stations[4,5] and are often located within a general neurology/neurosurgery unit.

Close proximity of the rooms to nursing stations allows prompt intervention during seizures and careful supervision of patients implanted with intracranial electrodes. Unlike adult facilities, in pediatric settings, patient compliance is rarely optimal and parental involvement is usually required. Pediatric monitoring facilities must therefore be designed with the family in mind. Single patient rooms are preferable on pediatric units to accommodate parents, siblings, or guardians.

Child cooperation may need to be enhanced by counseling, especially if invasive monitoring is contemplated. Simple toys and games such as a monitoring doll may help alleviate some of the anxiety and boredom related to these procedures.

Pediatric LTM can also be enhanced by a few simple modifications of the recording environment. Since children need to move around frequently, the nearest playroom area should be equipped to record children, thereby permitting greater freedom of movement. The metallic railings and the sides of the crib that obstruct the view of a patient during a seizure present another pediatric issue and should be replaced by a clear plastic sheet (Fig. 23-1). Neonates and critically ill children in the intensive care unit may be monitored with portable LTM equipment or alternately by transmitting the video/EEG data via a cable to a central monitoring unit.

Admission to the hospital can be frightening for children. Compliance with LTM in a pediatric setting is often improved by preparing the child and family using informational brochures and procedural outlines before hospitalization. Child life specialists or clinical nurse specialists should be

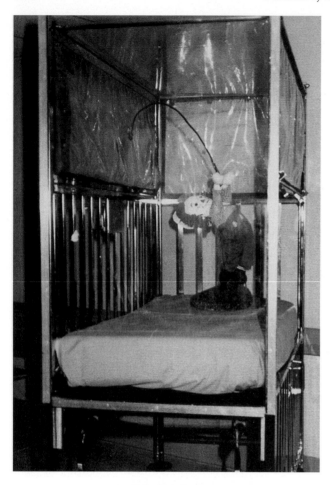

FIGURE 23–1
A sheet of clear plastic replaces the metallic railings and permits an unobstructed view of the child being monitored.

available to discuss monitoring routines. Following admission, hospital-based recreational activities and specially designed play objects such as a monitoring doll or cartoon video monitoring tapes are additional measures to allay anxiety associated with LTM.

Monitoring Equipment

Formal LTM guidelines have been published by the American EEG Society, but there are no specific recommendations for pediatric patients.

Electrodes

Scalp EEG recordings are generally obtained with silver chloride or gold-plated disk electrodes similar to electrodes in conventional recording. Holes in the electrodes allow electrode paste to be introduced to maintain con-

ductivity and impedance levels within acceptable limits. LTM electrodes must be secured with collodion and gauze to prevent dislodgment. Needle electrodes and electrode caps are unsuitable.

Invasive and semi-invasive EEG recordings generally employ stainless-steel electrodes that are flexible and biologically inert. The electrodes are configured to suit specific placements (Fig. 23-2) and their location can be confirmed extraoperatively on plain radiographs or computed tomographic scans. Although platinum and Nichrome electrodes are magnetic resonance imaging compatible, they are considerably more expensive.

Subdural electrodes consist of 4 to 8 contact strips or 20 to 128 contact electrode grids embedded in thin Silastic sheets. These are implanted via burr holes (strips) or under direct observation at craniotomy (grids or strips).[6-9] Depth electrodes, configured as 4 to 8 contacts on thin depthalon wires, are placed stereotaxically using three-dimensional coordinates. Depth electrodes have the advantage of being able to sample deep hemispheric sites.[10,11]

Recording electrodes are connected to amplifiers via specially designed connector cables. Since children are at greater risk to pull out implanted electrodes, it is advisable to employ cable connectors that disengage whenever traction is applied (Fig. 23-3).

Amplifiers, Cameras, and Audio Unit

Amplifiers

The EEG amplifiers of LTM systems comply with performance and safety standards established for routine EEGs. They may be mounted on the head, carried in a pouch, or placed remotely, the latter offering the greatest flexibility of gain, filter, and montage selection.

Video

Video-recorded information is optimally recorded with cameras fitted with automatic irises, remote zoom, and pan and tilt capabilities. Automatic tracking devices, which keep the patient on camera, are of obvious utility for active and mobile children. A battery-powered source infrared generator attached to the patient's collar drives sensors that control the Vpan-tilt mechanism on the camera mounts.

Color cameras require at least 25 foot candles of illumination and provide excellent quality images that allow identification of subtle manifestations during seizures. Monochrome or infrared cameras require only 0.03 foot candles of illumination and generate acceptable images at night even when the room lights are off.

Audio

A microphone suspended from the ceiling records speech or sounds that may help define ictal semiology. The

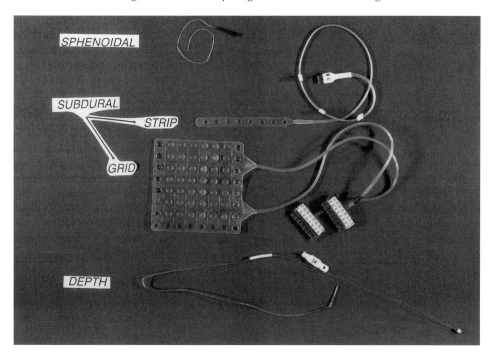

FIGURE 23–2

Sphenoidal, subdural, and depth electrodes.

microphone can also serve as a tool for attending personnel to describe the patient's behavior during an episode.

Data Transmission, Storage, and Review

Cassette EEG Recording Systems

Cassette EEG recording systems record episodic electrographic events in ambulatory patients (see Chapter 21). Twenty-four hours of EEG data can be stored on a single magnetic cassette that is housed in a small recorder carried by the patient. Typically, 8 to 16 channels of EEG are recorded. An event button can be pressed by the patient or an observer at the time of an episode. The EEG data can then be reviewed off-line on a monitor screen. Playback is controlled at 20 to 60 times real time while selected data segments can be printed for further review. Newer systems employ optical storage media.

Cassette EEG recording systems have the advantage of being extremely lightweight and are designed for unrestricted mobility. However, the number of recording channels is often limited, and localization of the seizure focus often proves difficult. Prominent yet unknown artifacts are inevitable in an ambulatory setting and may be easily mistaken for true seizure discharges.[12] Furthermore, data cannot be monitored while being recorded. The major application of cassette EEG recording in childhood has therefore been quantifying seizure frequency in situations where localization data is already known.

Radio Telemetry

Radio telemetry transmission also allows full patient mobility, but within a restricted range. Up to 128 channels of EEG can be recorded.[11] However, radio transmission is both expensive and especially prone to interference and signal dropout beyond range.[13] Radio telemetry is used less commonly than cable telemetry.

Cable Telemetry

Cable telemetry is the most widely used LTM system because of its low level of interference and reliability and is favored at most pediatric LTM centers. Amplified EEG signals are encoded by analog or digital multiplexers, the latter facilitating transmission of the signal without degradation. Up to 256 channels of EEG can be multiplexed and relayed via a shielded cable to a central monitoring facility, a decided advantage when multiple electrodes have been placed during a presurgical evaluation.

At the central monitoring unit, the EEG is demultiplexed to individual channels and time-synchronized to the video image before being displayed on a split-screen cathode ray tube monitor. It is possible to display two video images (one wide angle and one close-up) with the EEG. Time, date, and alphanumeric character generators help identify patients and the time of events. An event marker pressed by the patient or observer tags the recording and an event log is displayed on the screen. This feature, along with the time scale display, allows quick review of events.

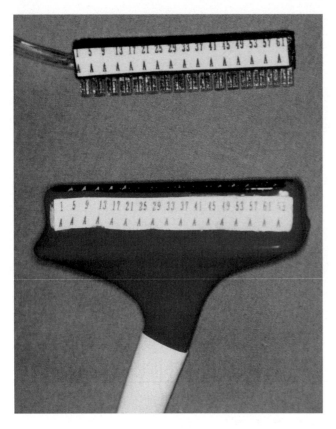

FIGURE 23–3

Illustration of a specially designed connector plug that releases the electrode cable when traction is applied and thus prevents the electrodes from being avulsed.

Newer equipment also allows simultaneous review of past data while current data are being recorded with added features such as frame-by-frame advance and digital zoom–facilitating electroclinical correlations.

Although the video image is generally clear on the monitor screen, the resolution of certain EEG patterns such as low-voltage fast activity may be inadequate and paper printouts are necessary for accurate interpretation. Digital systems allow post-hoc montage reformatting and are immune to problems associated with pen malalignment.

Recording Procedure

Extracranial Electrodes

Although the standard International 10-20 System of electrode placement is adequate for routine EEG, more precise localizing information may be necessary in patients being evaluated for epilepsy surgery. As illustrated by the example in Figure 23-4, additional electrodes help define the field of the epileptic discharge[14,15] and may even identify spikes that are missed on routing electrode montages. The American EEG Society[16] has recommended an elec-

trode placement system based on intermediate electrode designations obtained by combining two neighboring electrodes. For example, FC represents the electrode between frontal and central, and CP, that between central and parietal electrodes.

The anatomic relationship between the scalp recording and underlying cortical region varies according to skull shape.[17] In children, these relationships are further distorted by the late maturation of the frontal lobes.[18] For example, the F7/8 electrodes that overlie the temporal lobes in children appear to "move" over to the inferior frontal convexity in adults.

LTM data can be enhanced by placing additional electrodes in the anterior temporal (T1/T2) region,[19] sphenoidal or supraorbital regions.[20] The T1/T2 electrodes are placed 1 cm above a point lying one third the distance from the external auditory meatus to the outer canthi. Sphenoidal electrodes are inserted immediately below the zygomatic arch between the mandibular rami toward the region of the foramen ovale.[21-23] Sphenoidal electrodes are especially sensitive to epileptiform discharges arising from the anterior-mesial temporal regions and are remarkably well tolerated by children.

Sphenoidal recording is generally artifact free and can record well for several weeks. Occasionally, small pieces of the wire can break and remain in the tissue after the electrode is pulled. This complication has not been harmful. Subdermal electrodes[23] or skin electrodes at the same site[24] can detect spikes comparable to sphenoidal electrodes but are more prone to artifact. By contrast, nasopharyngeal and tympanic electrodes are poorly tolerated in children and subject to significant artifact. Along with nasoethmoidal electrodes, they rarely yield information beyond what can be obtained by scalp or sphenoidal recording and thus have limited clinical utility.[20,25,26]

There is no single ideal reference for scalp EEG studies, and the selection of a reference must be individualized following a baseline EEG. For example, to localize a focus in the temporal lobe, a "distant" scalp reference such as Pz is usually adequate. However, even the contralateral ear, which is more distant from the focus than Pz, may be involved in the temporal spike field and should not be assumed to always be "inactive." The neck-chest reference with a balancing potentiometer or a ring electrode around the neck that can cancel out the electrocardiogram artifact may be useful. However, noncephalic reference options have generally been found to be impractical for LTM. EEG machines with off-line reformatting capabilities that allow the reference to be changed post hoc have decided utility.

Intracranial Electrodes

Intracranial electrodes are often used in surgery candidates who require clearer localization of their seizure foci

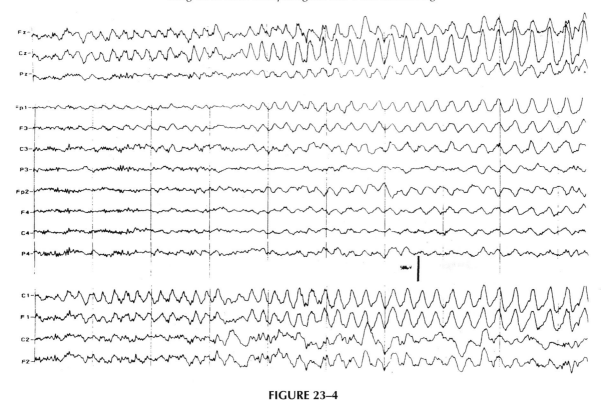

FIGURE 23–4

Scalp EEG demonstrating a focal seizure onset over the vertex (Cz) midline. Lateralization of the seizure focus is difficult on the standard electrode placement but is clearly left hemispheric (C1/F1) on closely spaced derivations.

(see Chapter 22). The recordings are obtained by referencing to a subgaleal electrode located at a distance from the region being monitored. Depth electrode recordings have traditionally been used in adult temporal lobectomy candidates where they are inserted stereotactically. Depth electrodes can be inserted stereotactically without an open craniotomy but provide only limited spatial coverage of epileptogenic regions.

In comparison with adults, children have a higher proportion of medically intractable extratemporal epilepsy. Subdural electrodes that allow widespread spatial sampling and the ability to functionally map eloquent cortex have thus become increasingly popular. Subdural electrodes configured as strips or rectangular grids are placed over the cortical convexity; strips and smaller grids can also be inserted to localize deep basal or interhemispheric seizure foci (Fig. 23-5).

Epidural peg electrodes are easily inserted through burr holes and are therefore semi-invasive. However, they sample a restricted region compared to subdural or depth electrodes and cannot be used for functional mapping. Epidural pegs have been used to guide subsequent subdural or depth electrode placement.

Specially designed multicontact electrodes can also be inserted through the foramen ovale on to the floor of the middle cranial fossa.[27] These foramen ovale electrodes provide good coverage of the mesial temporal region, but there is little experience with this modality in young children.

The choice of invasive electrodes must be based on the clinical data and routine scalp recordings. Unlike adults, epileptogenic zones in children are usually extensive. For example, mesial temporal sclerosis is rarely the exclusive pathologic finding, and epileptogenic zones often extend well beyond the anterior-mesial temporal region to include the posterobasal and lateral temporal neocortex.[4] Thus, sphenoidal electrodes are seldom maximally involved in childhood, and foramen ovale electrodes or temporal depth electrodes alone are often unsuitable. A combination of subdural electrodes and strategically placed depth electrodes is often required for optimal coverage of the neocortex and mesial temporal or deep-seated foci, respectively.

Activation Procedures

Seizures or nonepileptic events tend to be either infrequent or unpredictable and may thus need to be provoked during LTM. Hyperventilation and photic stimulation, as used conventionally, should also be tried during LTM. Interictal discharges are often activated by slow wave sleep, but

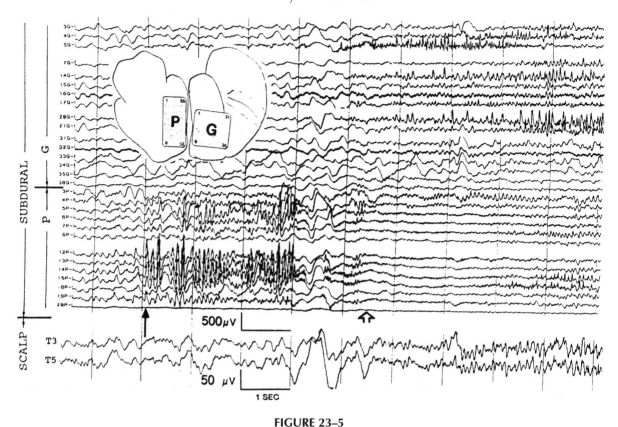

FIGURE 23–5

Subdural EEG recording with ictal onset in the basal temporo-occipital grid (P) characterized by high-amplitude spike/fast activity (solid arrow). The onset is missed at the scalp electrodes T3 and T5, which become active only when the convexity subdural grid (G) becomes involved more than 4 seconds later.

their distribution tends to be extensive and thus misleading. By comparison, the field during rapid eye movement sleep tends to be more reliable and consistent.[28] Sleep deprivation can be a more effective activator than natural sleep and may be achieved in children by either keeping the child awake until midnight or waking the child earlier in the morning. Psychogenic seizures can often be provoked by simple verbal encouragement or by the use of saline injection.

Withdrawal of anticonvulsant medication prior to monitoring may be used to provoke seizures, although seizure foci thus activated may differ from the patient's habitual seizures.[29] Convulsant agents such as pentylenetetrazol are only of historic interest now since these can provoke abnormal activity even in normal subjects. Induction by focal electrical or chemical stimulation may also be falsely localizing.[30]

Computer-Based Techniques

Computers have a multifaceted role in LTM systems. Storage and archiving of large amounts of LTM data and the detection of spikes and seizures can be simplified through use of computers. Computers also achieve considerable data reduction and allow information to be formatted in several different ways. Spikes and seizure frequency counts can be displayed as topographic diagrams. Commercially available interpolation algorithms yield attractive voltage topography but may not be an accurate representation of the raw data.

Automated spike or seizure detection programs are primarily designed for use in adults. The error rate in children where the complexity of waveforms is greater and the background (e.g., spindle activity) is often sharply contoured is therefore high. Artifacts, which are also especially common in children, are a major hurdle for current automated systems. Computer-based spike detection still awaits further technologic development before it can be applied widely in children.

Computers are also useful for reformatting data into various montages such as Laplacian[31] or reference-subtraction montages,[32] which assist in localization. With more sophisticated programming, coherence-phase analysis for studying seizure propagation[33] or an inverse solution for dipolar source localization[34] is possible. Although such mathematical manipulations are attractive, they have several practical limitations that restrict their widespread clinical use.

Cortical Mapping

As the number of young children with intractable partial seizures being considered for excisional surgery increase, it is becoming evident that their epileptogenic regions are often widespread or contiguous with functional cortex. Accurate delineation of eloquent cortex therefore takes on added importance in the presurgical evaluation of the child. Although immature cortex is capable of significant functional recovery, excision of the rolandic motor cortex leads to a lifelong deficit in the contralateral extremities.

The stimulation paradigm that is generally effective for extraoperative mapping in adults[25] rarely elicits clinical responses or afterdischarges in infants and young children.[35,36] One approach to this problem is to employ a paradigm where current intensity and pulse duration are sequentially adjusted so that the energy increment at each step is minimized (Fig. 23-6).[35] This approach also minimizes the energy increments at each step and is thus safe for young children. In some children, clinical responses may only be obtained at thresholds higher than the afterdischarge threshold. The absence of clinical manifestations during an afterdischarge does not therefore conclusively exclude the presence of eloquent cortex in the stimulated region.

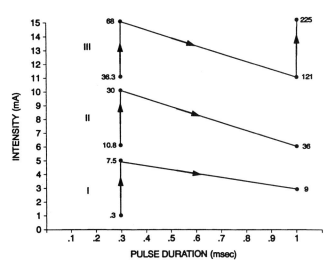

FIGURE 23–6

A graphic illustration of a stimulation paradigm that starts at an intensity of 1 mA and pulse duration of 0.3 milliseconds, corresponding to an energy level of 0.3 nJ (beginning of sequence I). In each subsequent trial, the intensity and pulse duration are adjusted by 1 to 2 mA or 0.1 to 0.2 millisecond, respectively (arrows), to minimize energy increment at each step and ensure convergence to the chronaxie.

Malformations of cortical development are the most common underlying substrate in children with intractable partial epilepsy. The distribution of critical cortex, especially that related to motor function, may be atypical with a homunculus revealing inversion of duplication of body representation. Also, unlike the destructive lesions, cortical dysplasia does not necessarily lead to relocation or transfer of language function to the contralateral side.[37]

CLINICAL APPLICATIONS

Therapeutic intervention based on LTM analysis has been shown to reduce seizure frequency and drug toxicity in most adult patients; many also show improved social skills.[2] LTM is equally cost-effective in children since parental descriptions of clinical events are often imprecise and may occasionally lead to an erroneous diagnosis of epilepsy.[5,38-42] LTM helps to establish a diagnosis of nonepileptic events and obviates the inappropriate use of antiepileptic medications. Parents may also miss brief seizures in disorders such as infantile spasms or absence epilepsy. LTM assists in the characterization and quantification of seizures while also helping to identify special circumstances where they may be activated or missed.

Seizure focus localization with video/EEG monitoring is also vital for children being evaluated for surgical treatment of epilepsy. The overall reduction in morbidity and increase in diagnostic accuracy afforded by LTM reaffirms its place in the management of episodic childhood disorders.[2,42-46]

Differential Diagnosis

The symptomatology of many of the seizures overlaps with nonepileptic events in early childhood. Nonepileptic events present a wide variety of motor manifestations or behaviors that resemble different seizure types (Table 23-1). The diagnosis of epilepsy can usually be established on LTM by demonstrating seizure discharges accompanying the clinical events. The absence of ictal epileptiform activity does not necessarily exclude a seizure disorder. Partial seizures may not have scalp EEG correlates and complex partial seizures and nonconvulsive generalized seizures may show abnormal EEG patterns that are not clearly epileptiform.

Psychogenic Seizures

LTM has been extensively used to evaluate psychogenic seizure manifestations in adolescents and older children.[5,40,41,47] In the adolescent, psychogenic episodes typically mimic tonic-clonic, partial, or atonic seizures[47] and may be associated with incontinence or injury. By contrast, younger patients display behaviors that mimic absences or partial seizures with uncomplicated automatisms;[39,48] pseudo-

TABLE 23–1. SEIZURE TYPES AND NONEPILEPTIC EVENTS THAT MIMIC THEM

Complex Partial	Tonic-Clonic	Myoclonic	Atonic
Pseudoseizures	Pseudoseizures	Benign nocturnal myoclonus	Nonepileptic head drops
Pavor nocturnus	Paroxysmal dystonias	Subcortical myoclonus	Cardiogenic syncope
Episodic dyscontrol	Paroxysmal torticollis	Tics	Cataplexy
Somnambulism	Sandifer's syndrome		
Self-stimulation			

generalized tonic-clonic seizures are extremely rare in young children. Allowing parents to review the video/EEG findings often helps educate them about their child's symptoms. Psychogenic attacks are easily diagnosed on review of the video/EEG data. There is a lack of true synchrony in the motor manifestations, which typically consist of non-physiologic or bizarre sequences. The EEG demonstrates prominent ballistic and muscle artifact superimposed on an otherwise normal background.

Nonepileptic Motor Events

Paroxysmal events such as the sleep dystonias and Sandifer's syndrome can be differentiated from seizures by their lack of EEG correlates. Furthermore, a higher incidence of interictal discharges occurs in patients with true seizures. In patients who have head drops, a careful analysis of the video can also help establish the nature of the events.[49] In epileptic head drops, slow replay analysis reveals rapid descent and slow recovery phase, whereas, in nonepileptic drops, there are equal descent and recovery phases.

Aberrant Repetitive Behaviors

A wide variety of childhood behaviors can appear epileptic in origin. They are often remarkably diverse in their clinical presentation, and their repetitive occurrence and stereotyped appearance are easily mistaken for seizures. Since the historic data and routine EEG are usually noncontributory, LTM constitutes the only means of obtaining an accurate diagnosis.

Stereotyped mannerisms including rocking, shaking, or grimacing are common in young children and often provoke considerable parental anxiety.[5] Shuddering attacks (rapid low-amplitude tremors of the head and arms) are frequent in toddlers.[50] LTM is useful in demonstrating that these events are not seizures. On the other hand, LTM can be helpful in making the diagnosis of epilepsy in patients who appear to have benign disorders such as night terrors.[51]

The cause of most repetitive behaviors is unclear. Self-stimulation is common in retarded patients, and in young girls, masturbation in conjunction with irregular breathing, facial flushing, and diaphoresis may sometimes be diagnosed as seizure activity.[52] Since masturbatory activity can usually be observed daily, LTM diagnosis is usually achieved relatively quickly. Undoubtedly, many of the behaviors are enacted for purposes of seeking attention, and a high level of parental anxiety probably acts as a feedback.

Seizure Classification

The diversity of seizure syndromes in childhood have been clarified and refined through video/EEG analysis techniques. The analysis of the origin and spread of the seizure discharge has permitted more precise formulation of the electroclinical seizure sequence. Unlike adults, in whom the seizure patterns remain stable, seizure manifestations in children often evolve in parallel with brain maturation. In the neonate, for example, focal clonic seizures during the neonatal period may predate infantile spasms that subsequently develop into Lennox-Gastaut syndrome. Evolving seizure patterns may also occur in the genetically determined epilepsies, for example, the appearance of childhood absences before myoclonus in juvenile myoclonic epilepsy (JME).[53]

Absence Seizures

LTM studies of absence seizures have been instrumental in establishing the clinical nosology of absence seizures.[54,55] Uncomplicated ("pure") absences are now recognized to constitute only a small fraction of all absence episodes. In an LTM study of 48 absence seizure patients, only 1 exhibited a classic "blank stare" with accompanying unawareness and amnesia, whereas virtually all episodes were complicated by automatisms, clonic movements, or a reduction in postural tone.[55]

LTM studies have also helped redefine our concept of the "typical" versus "atypical" absence seizure. Although both show considerable clinical and epileptogenic overlap, typical absences are usually observed in neurologically normal children with normal EEG background activity, are shorter in duration, and are more likely to be accompanied by stereotyped automatisms.[54]

Through video/EEG analysis of the absences of JME, it is now clear that automatisms are extremely rare and that myoclonus occurs as an independent seizure pattern.[56] Furthermore, both the spike and multiple spike-and-wave discharges of JME are now recognized to consist of 2- to 7-Hz components rather than stereotyped 3-Hz discharges. Electrographic JME seizures are fragmentary or even discontinuous in contrast with the well-organized rhythmic sequences of the typical absence discharge. These features are particularly helpful when confronted with a child with absences who is thought to have JME but is not yet manifesting myoclonus.

LTM has also been used to study the neuropsychological effects of generalized spike-wave discharges. Bursts greater than 3 seconds in duration are now recognized to consistently interrupt continuous motor performance.[57] When motor reaction time is studied, almost half of all responses obtained during the early phases of the discharge were shown to be abnormal.[58] The rate of abnormality increases further at longer intervals after paroxysmal onset. Auditory responsiveness may also be impaired by generalized discharges, even if they are of very brief duration.[59] These findings suggest that to be effective, therapy for absence seizures must suppress all epileptiform activity.

Atonic Seizures

Routine EEG recording is obviously unsuitable for evaluating epileptic falls lasting a fraction of a second, and LTM studies of clinical and EEG features are of considerable utility.

In a careful video/EEG analysis of falls in 15 children with Lennox-Gastaut syndrome, Ikeno and associates[60] refuted the widely held belief that epileptic falling was predominantly atonic or myoclonic-atonic in origin. Pure lapses of muscle tone accounted for very few falls, whereas falls were more likely to be a consequence of vigorous muscle contraction during tonic seizures or flexor spasms. Many of the children with flexor spasms had West's syndrome in infancy and may thus have been exhibiting a developmental sequence rather than a new-onset seizure pattern.[61]

LTM studies of epileptic falls involving truncal flexion (axial spasms) have revealed a complicated sequence in which the spasm is preceded or followed by alteration of consciousness, athetoid postures, or tonic seizures.[62]

Rarely, partial seizures may manifest as atonic seizures.[63] However, in these cases, the falls tend to be slow, taking 2 to 5 seconds for the child to fall.

Myoclonic Seizures

LTM can help establish the diagnosis of JME in patients believed to have other seizure types.[64] Recording the EEG on awakening was the key to the diagnosis since early morning events had routinely been ignored by the patients ("nervousness on waking up") and their physicians. Since JME responds favorably to antiepileptic drug therapy, prompt diagnosis is of considerable therapeutic importance.

Partial Seizures

Partial seizures tend to be sporadic, unprovoked events. LTM is therefore essential for their accurate electroclinical characterization. In a video/EEG study of children with par-

tial seizures, Holmes[65] showed that simple partial seizures are more common in the very young child or retarded patient and consist of brief motor events, often with forced tonic postures. Their ictal EEG patterns are readily identified and usually overlie regions of structural pathology. By contrast, complex partial seizures last longer, are more complicated, and are followed by postictal unresponsiveness.[65]

Temporal lobe seizures in the infant and younger child reveal a higher incidence of motor involvement.[66-68] Forced deviation of the head and eyes and extensor tonic postures of the upper extremities are common and easily mistaken for generalized seizure patterns. Infants with multifocal EEG discharges may still have localized seizure origin on LTM.[66]

LTM studies of older children and adolescents are similar to those described in adults.[65] Seizures consist of a motionless stare, automatized behaviors, or more rarely, a loss of body tone.

Neonatal Seizures

Prior to the advent of LTM in the newborn nursery, neonatal seizures were classified primarily on the basis of clinical observation and the interictal EEG. "Subtle" but unexplained movements or behaviors were regarded as seizures without correlative ictal EEG documentation.[69]

Using cribside video/EEG polygraphic recording techniques, Mizrahi and Kellaway[70] studied the electroclinical patterns of 349 newborns believed to be experiencing true seizures. The EEG discharge rate correlated with focal tonic-clonic seizure activity and some forms of myoclonic seizures. Electrographic discharges were especially likely to correlate with clonic movements and were shown to be time synchronized to sharp-wave EEG discharges. By contrast, generalized tonic seizures and "subtle" seizure patterns (oral, buccal, facial, ocular movements, and cycling automatisms) showed a much lower electrographic correlation. Conversely, electrographic seizure activity often occurred without clinical manifestations (Fig. 23-7).

Preterm infants also exhibit patterns that may be construed as epileptic in origin.[71] However, in contrast to the term newborn, electrographic and clinical seizure activity was more often dissociated with clonic movements often lacking EEG correlates.

Apnea can accompany tonic or clonic movements or motor automatisms, or it may occur as an isolated symptom.[72] The apnea usually correlates with rhythmic alpha discharges in the temporal regions.

Infantile Spasms

The clinical and EEG characteristics of infantile spasms have been extensively and precisely documented with LTM.[73-76] The patterns of spasms and their relationship to behavioral states, as well as the interictal and ictal EEG patterns, are well known.

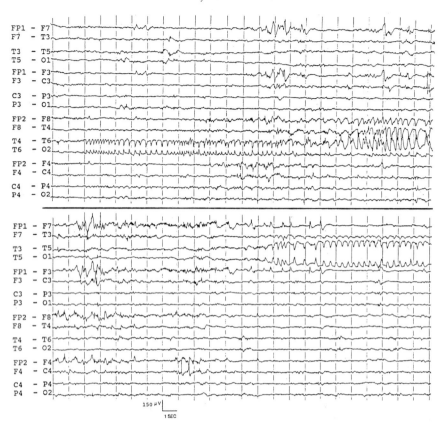

FIGURE 23–7

A routine EEG in a neonate showing independent electrographic seizure discharges initially over the right temporal region and subsequently over the left, without associated clinical accompaniments.

Quantification

Infants and children are unable to report seizure frequency or the nature of their episodes. In some cases, parental anxiety results in over-reporting of behavioral patterns that could be misconstrued as seizures. Alternately, parental observation may be limited and many seizures missed, as, for example, with infantile spasms and/or frequent absence seizures.

Circadian LTM studies reveal considerable variation in the frequency of spike and wave discharging during a 24-hour period.[77] Circadian variation is the result of complex interactions between endogenous, time-modulated processes and exogenous factors such as environmental changes and drug-related effects. Such extremes of discharge variation suggest that the brief sampling provided by a single outpatient EEG could yield unrealistically high or low estimates of mean discharge rates.

Seizure Focus Localization

Video/EEG analysis, in conjunction with neuroimaging, is used to localize seizure foci at most centers.[3,44,45,78-81]

From the standpoint of ictal semiology, manifestations occurring at seizure onset are most reliable for localizing information. For example, the automatisms of anterior lobe seizures often appear more restrained in comparison to the wild "thrashing" observed with orbitofrontal foci. Automatisms are also less common and occur later in the ictal sequence of posterior temporal seizures. Analysis of patterns of head deviation have also been used to lateralize seizure foci.[82]

The scalp EEG is usually adequate for determining the region of the seizure focus in most patients. However, the complexities of scalp data interpretation predispose to several pitfalls. Discharges that involve small cortical areas or those arising from deeper regions are often not evident on the scalp (see Fig. 23-5). Thus, the electrographic onset of partial seizures may go unrecognized, and their clinical manifestation may precede electrographic changes.[32] The scalp EEG may likewise remain silent when seizures arise from severely damaged or deformed cortex.[83] As an example, in the patient with a large left hemispheric schizencephaly illustrated in Figure 23-8, the scalp EEG revealed an apparent seizure onset over the right hemisphere,

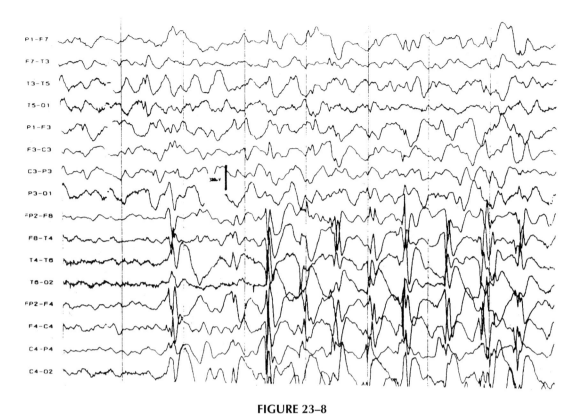

FIGURE 23–8
Scalp EEG showing an apparently right hemispheric partial seizure onset in a patient with a left hemispheric schizencephalic cleft.

whereas intracranial recording conclusively demonstrated seizure onset from the left frontal lobe.

Seizures arising from noneloquent cortex may become manifest clinically only on spread to eloquent regions. Since seizures arising from a silent focus may spread along different pathways, they may give rise to varying ictal semiologies that falsely suggest multiple seizure foci. For example, parietal lobe seizures are usually silent at onset but give rise to sensorimotor manifestations with anterior spread, and behavioral arrest and automatisms with temporal-limbic propagation.[84]

Certain pitfalls of localizing seizure foci are more specific to childhood epilepsy. As emphasized previously, neonatal seizures are more likely to be electroclinically dissociated; that is, seizure patterns may occur without clinical correlation and vice versa, a phenomenon even more frequent if anticonvulsants have been administered.

Infantile spasms often reveal a generalized high-voltage slow wave followed by voltage attenuation with superimposed beta frequencies.

Despite the apparently generalized distribution, focality may still be evident in the interictal background or in the structural and functional imaging studies. These observations suggest that focal brain dysfunction in infants can give rise to "generalized" EEG and clinical seizure patterns.

Finally, the benign partial epileptic syndromes of childhood can have stereotyped spike foci that shift among the central, parietal, and occipital regions. This pattern must be distinguished from the multifocal independent spiking associated with a considerably less favorable outcome.

REFERENCES

1. Gumnit RJ: Intensive neurodiagnostic monitoring: Role in the treatment of seizures. Neurology 1986;36:1340-1346.
2. Porter RJ, Penry JK, Lacy JR: Diagnostic and therapeutic reevaluation of patients with intractable epilepsy. Neurology 1977;27:1006-1011.
3. Thompson JL, Ebersole JS: Long-term inpatient audiovisual scalp EEG monitoring. J Clin Neurophysiol 1999;16:91-99.
4. Duchowny M, Levin B, Jayakar P, et al: Temporal lobectomy in early childhood. Epilepsia 1992;33:298-303.
5. Duchowny M, Resnick TJ, Deray M: Video/EEG diagnosis of repetitive behavior in early childhood and its relationship to seizures. Pediatr Neurol 1988;4:162-164.

6. Lüders H, Lesser RP, Dinner DS, et al: Chronic intracranial recording and stimulation with subdural electrodes. *In* Engel J (ed): Surgical Treatment of the Epilepsies. New York, Raven Press, 1987, p 297.

7. Nespeca M, Wyllie E, Lüders H, et al: EEG recording and functional localization studies with subdural electrodes in infants and young children. J Epilepsy 1990;3(Suppl): 107-124.

8. Wyler AR, Walker G, Richet T, Hermann BP: Chronic subdural strip electrode recordings for difficult epileptic problems. J Epilepsy 1988;1:71-78.

9. Wyllie E, Lüders H, Morris HH, et al: Subdural electrodes in the evaluation for epilepsy surgery in children and adults. Neuropediatrics 1988;19:80-86.

10. Delgado-Escueta AV, Walsh GO: The selection process for surgery of intractable complex partial seizures: Surface EEG and depth electrocorticography. *In* Ward AA Jr, Penry JK, Purpura DP (eds): Epilepsy: Proceedings of the Association for Research in Nervous and Mental Diseases, Vol 61. New York, Raven Press, 1983, p 295.

11. Porter RJ, Theodore WH, Schulman EA: Intensive monitoring of intractable epilepsy: A two-year follow-up. *In* Dam M, Gram L, Penry JK (eds): Advances in Epileptology: XIIth Epilepsy International Symposium. New York, Raven Press, 1981, p 265.

12. Jayakar P, Resnick TJ, Duchowny MS, Alvarez LA: Pitfalls and caveats of localizing seizure foci. J Clin Neurophysiol 1991;8:414-431.

13. Kamp A, Aitnik JW: Improved telemetric EEG monitoring in epileptic patients. Electroencephalogr Clin Neurophysiol 1983;56:254-255.

14. Chatrian GE, Lettich E, Nelson PL: Ten percent electrodes system for topographic studies of spontaneous and evoked EEG activities. Am J EEG Technol 1985;25:83-91.

15. Morris HH III, Lüders H, Lesser RP, et al: The value of closely spaced scalp electrodes in the localization of epileptiform foci: A study of 26 patients with complex partial seizures. Electroencephalogr Clin Neurophysiol 1986;63:107-111.

16. American Electroencephalographic Society: Guidelines for standard electrode position nomenclature. J Clin Neurophysiol 1991;8:200-202.

17. Binnie CD, Dekker E, Smit A, Van der Linden G: Practical considerations in the positioning of EEG electrodes. Electroencephalogr Clin Neurophysiol 1982;53:453-458.

18. Blume WT, Buza RC, Okazaki H: Anatomic correlates of the ten-twenty electrode placement system in infants. Electroencephalogr Clin Neurophysiol 1974;36:303-307.

19. Silverman D: The anterior temporal electrode and the ten-twenty system. Electroencephalogr Clin Neurophysiol 1960;12:735-737.

20. Lesser RP, Lüders H, Morris HH, et al: Extracranial EEG evaluation. *In* Engel J Jr (ed): Surgical Treatment of the Epilepsies. New York, Raven Press, 1987, p 173.

21. Ives JR, Gloor P: New sphenoidal electrode assembly to permit long-term monitoring of the patient's ictal or interictal EEG. Electroencephalogr Clin Neurophysiol 1977;42:575-580.

22. Pampiglione G, Kerridge J: EEG abnormalities from the temporal lobe studied with sphenoidal electrodes. J Neurol Neurosurg Psychiatry 1956;19:117-129.

23. Wilkus RJ, Thompson PM: Sphenoidal electrode positions and basal EEG during long-term monitoring. Epilepsia 1985;26:137-142.

24. Sadler M, Goodwin J: The sensitivity of various electrodes in the detection of epileptiform potentials (EPs) in patients with partial complex (PC) seizures. Epilepsia 1986;27:627.

25. Lesser RP, Lüders H, Klem G, et al: Extraoperative cortical functional localization in patients with epilepsy. J Clin Neurophysiol 1987;4:27-53.

26. Sperling MR, Engel J Jr: Electroencephalographic recording from the temporal lobes: A comparison of ear, anterior temporal, and nasopharyngeal electrodes. Ann Neurol 1985;17:510-513.

27. Wieser HG, Moser S: Montage and recording with bilateral M-FO electrodes. J Epilepsy 1988;1:16-22.

28. Sammaritano M, Gigli GL, Gotman J: Interictal spiking during wakefulness and sleep and the localization of foci in temporal lobe epilepsy. Neurology 1991;41:290-297.

29. Engel J Jr, Crandall PH: Falsely localizing ictal onset with depth EEG telemetry during anticonvulsant withdrawal. Epilepsia 1983;24:344-355.

30. Wieser HG, Bancaud J, Talairach J, et al: Comparative value of spontaneous and chemically and electrically induced seizures in establishing the lateralization of temporal lobe seizures. Epilepsia 1979;20:47-59.

31. Hjorth B: An on-line transformation of EEG scalp potentials into orthogonal source derivations. Electroencephalogr Clin Neurophysiol 1975;39:526-530.

32. Jayakar P, Duchowny M, Resnick TJ, Alvarez LA: Localization of seizure foci: Pitfalls and caveats. J Clin Neurophysiol 1991;8:414-431.

33. Gotman J: Measurement of small time differences between EEG channels: Method and application to epileptic seizure propagation. Electroencephalogr Clin Neurophysiol 1983;56:501-514.

34. Smith DB, Sidman RD, Flanigin H, et al: A reliable method for localizing deep intracranial sources of the EEG. Neurology 1985;35:1702-1707.

35. Alvarez LA, Jayakar PB: Cortical stimulation with subdural electrodes: Special considerations in infancy and childhood. J Epilepsy 1990;3:125-130.

36. Alvarez LA, Moshé SL, Belman AL, et al: EEG and brain death determination in children. Neurology 1988;38:227-230.

37. Duchowny M, Jayakar P, Harvey AS, et al: Language cortex representation: Effects of developmental versus acquired pathology. Ann Neurol 1996;40:31-38.

38. Donat JF, Wright FS: Episodic symptoms mistaken for seizures in the neurologically impaired child. Neurology 1990;40:156-157.

39. Carmant L, Kramer U, Holmes GL, et al: Differential diagnosis of staring spells in children: A video/EEG study. Pediatr Neurol 1996;14:199-202.

40. Carmant L, Kramer U, Mikati MA, et al: Pseudoseizure manifestations in two preschool-age children. Seizure 1995;4:147-149.

41. Kramer U, Carmant L, Riviello JJ, et al: Psychogenic seizures: Video telemetry observations in 27 patients. Pediatr Neurol 1995;12:39-41.

42. Bhatia M, Sinha PK, Jain S, et al: Usefulness of short-term video/EEG recording with saline induction in pseudoseizures. Acta Neurol Scand 1997;95:363-366.

43. Sutula TP, Sackellares JC, Miller JQ, Dreifuss FE: Intensive monitoring in refractory epilepsy. Neurology 1981;31:243-247.

44. Sinclair DB, Aronyk K, Snyder T, et al: Extratemporal resection for childhood epilepsy. Pediatr Neurol 2004;30:177-185.

45. Sinclair DB, Aronyk K, Snyder T, et al: Pediatric temporal lobectomy for epilepsy. Pediatr Neurosurg 2003;38:195-205.

46. Karenfort M, Kruse B, Freitag H, et al: Epilepsy surgery outcome in children with focal epilepsy due to tuberous sclerosis complex. Neuropediatrics 2002;33:255-261.

47. Holmes GL, Sackellares JC, McKiernan J, et al: Evaluation of childhood pseudoseizures using EEG telemetry and video tape monitoring. J Pediatr 1980;97:554-558.

48. Rosenow F, Wyllie E, Kotagal P, et al: Staring spells in children: Descriptive features distinguishing epileptic and nonepileptic events. J Pediatr 1998;133:660-663.

49. Brunquell P, McKeever M, Russman BS: Differentiation of epileptic from nonepileptic head drops in children. Epilepsia 1990;31:401-405.

50. Holmes GL, Russman BS: Shuddering attacks: Evaluation using electroencephalographic frequency modulation radiotelemetry and videotape monitoring. Am J Dis Child 1986;140:72-73.

51. Lombroso CT: Pavor nocturnus of proven epileptic origin. Epilepsia 2000;41:1221-1226.

52. Fleisher DR, Morrison A. Masturbation mimicking abdominal pain or seizures in young girls. J Pediatr 1990;22:810-814.

53. Wirrell EC, Camfield CS, Camfield PR, et al: Long-term prognosis of typical childhood absence epilepsy: Remission or progression to juvenile myoclonic epilepsy. Neurology 1996;47:912-918.

54. Holmes GL, McKeever M, Adamson M: Absence seizures in children: Clinical and electroencephalographic features. Ann Neurol 1987;21:268-273.

55. Penry JK, Porter RJ, Dreifus FE: Simultaneous recording of absence seizures with videotape and electroencephalography. Brain 1975;98:427-440.

56. Panayiotopoulos CP, Obeid T, Waheed G: Absences in juvenile myoclonic epilepsy: A clinic and video-electroencephalographic study. Ann Neurol 1989;25:391-397.

57. Goode DJ, Penry JK, Dreifuss FE: Effects of paroxysmal spike-wave on continuous visual-motor performance. Epilepsia 1970;11:241-254.

58. Porter RJ, Penry JK, Dreifuss FE: Responsiveness at the onset of spike-wave bursts. Electroencephalogr Clin Neurophysiol 1973;34:239-245.

59. Brown TR, Penry JK, Porter RJ, Dreifuss FE: Responsiveness before, during, and after spike-wave paroxysms. Neurology 1974;24:659-665.

60. Ikeno T, Shigematsu H, Miyakoshi M, et al: An analytic study of epileptic falls. Epilepsia 1985;26:612-621.

61. Donat JF, Wright FS: Seizures in series: Similarities between seizures of the West and Lennox-Gastaut syndromes. Epilepsia 1991;32:504-509.

62. Egli M, Mothersill I, O'Kane M, O'Kane F: The axial spasm—the predominant type of drop seizure in patients with secondary generalized epilepsy. Epilepsia 1985;26:401-415.

63. Satow T, Ikeda A, Yamamoto J, et al: Partial epilepsy manifesting atonic seizure: Report of two cases. Epilepsia 2002;43:1425-1431.

64. Delgado-Escueta AV, Enrile-Bascal FE: Juvenile myoclonic epilepsy of Janz. Neurology 1984;34:285-294.

65. Holmes GL: Partial complex seizures in children: An analysis of 69 seizures in 24 patients using EEG FM radiotelemetry and videotape recording. Electroencephalogr Clin Neurophysiol 1984;57:13-20.

66. Duchowny MS: Complex partial seizures of infancy. Arch Neurol 1987;44:911-914.

67. Jayakar P, Duchowny MS: Complex partial seizures of temporal lobe origin in early childhood. J Epilepsy 1990;3:41-45.

68. Yamamoto N, Watanabe K, Negoro T, et al: Complex partial seizures in children: Ictal manifestations and their relation to clinical course. Neurology 1987;37:1379-1382.

69. Volpe J: Neonatal seizures. N Engl J Med 1973;289:413-415.

70. Mizrahi EM, Kellaway P: Characterization and classification of neonatal seizures. Neurology 1987;37:1837-1844.

71. Scher MS, Painter MJ, Bergman I, et al: EEG diagnoses of neonatal seizures: Clinical correlations and outcome. Pediatr Neurol 1989;5:17-24.

72. Watanabe K, Hara K, Miyazaki S, et al: Apneic seizures in the newborn. Am J Dis Child 1982;136:980-984.

73. Dulac O, Plouin P, Jambaque I, Motte J: Spasmes infantiles epileptiques benins. Rev Electroenceph Neurophys Clin 1986;16:371-382.

74. Hrachovy RA, Frost JD Jr, Kellaway P: Hypsarrhythmia: Variations on the theme. Epilepsia 1984;25:317-325.

75. Fusco L, Vigevano F: Ictal clinical electroencephalographic findings of spasms in West syndrome. Epilepsia 1993;34:671-678.

76. Kellaway P, Hrachovy RA, Frost JD Jr, Zion T: Precise characterization and quantification of infantile spasms. Ann Neurol 1979;6:214-218.

77. Kellaway P, Frost JD, Crawley JW: Time modulation of spike-and-wave activity in generalized epilepsy. Ann Neurol 1980;8:491-500.

78. Cascino GD, Trenerry MR, So EL, et al: Routine EEG and temporal lobe epilepsy: Relation to long-term EEG monitoring, quantitative MRI, and operative outcome. Epilepsia 1996;37:651-656.

79. Fogarasi A, Janszky J, Faveret E, et al: A detailed analysis of frontal lobe seizure semiology in children younger than 7 years. Epilepsia 2001;42:80-85.

80. Fogarasi A, Boesebeck F, Tuxhorn I: A detailed analysis of symptomatic posterior cortex seizure semiology in children younger than seven years. Epilepsia 2003;44:89-96.

81. Stuve O, Dodrill CB, Holmes MD, Miller JW: The absence of interictal spikes with documented seizures suggests extratemporal epilepsy. Epilepsia 2001;42:778-781.

82. Jayakar P, Resnick TJ, Duchowny MS, Alvarez LA: Ictal head-deviation: Lateralizing significance of the pattern of head movement. Neurology 1992;42:1989-1992.

83. Samaritano M, de Lobtiniere A, Andermann F, et al: False lateralization by surface EEG of seizure onset in patients with temporal lobe epilepsy and focal cerebral lesions. Epilepsia 1984;25:664.

84. Williamson PD, Boon PA, Thadani VM, et al: Parietal lobe epilepsy: Diagnostic considerations and results of surgery. Ann Neurol 1992;31:193-201.

24

Intraoperative Neurophysiologic Monitoring Using Evoked Potentials

Sandra L. Helmers

Intraoperative monitoring has become widely available in the last 10 to 15 years.[1-5] Monitoring of the spinal cord and central nervous system is useful in assessing functional integrity, allowing early detection of injury, identifying potential mechanisms of injury, and possibly preventing permanent damage during procedures that carry a high risk of morbidity. Over the last several years, as clinical neurophysiologists and surgeons have gained experience with intraoperative neurophysiologic techniques and monitoring, it has been used in the younger patient and has become increasingly useful in the pediatric age group.

This chapter is a review of some of the more common neurophysiologic techniques used in the operating room. Appropriate selection of the type of patient who should be monitored and the techniques most applicable are briefly discussed. In addition, technical and patient-related problems are discussed, with an emphasis on children and young adults younger than 20 years of age.

SPINAL CORD MONITORING

The most common type of spinal cord monitoring is done with somatosensory evoked potentials (SSEPs). When performing SSEPs intraoperatively, posterior tibial nerves or median nerves are most commonly used. The peroneal, ulnar, and radial nerves are less commonly used. Figure 24-1 shows the anatomy of the large-fiber sensory system that is being monitored. When planning to monitor the somato-

sensory system, it is important to know the level at which one is monitoring. Median SSEPs reflect function from the cervical cord to the somatosensory cortex, whereas posterior tibial SSEPs reflect function from the lower lumbar–upper sacral cord to cortex. It is also important to remember that SSEPS measure function in the posterior columns.

The techniques of stimulating and recording intraoperative SSEPs are similar to routine SSEPs except for the ability and sometimes necessity of using invasive electrodes. This can include needle electrodes for stimulating and recording and brain and spinal cord epidural recording electrodes.

SSEPs can be used to monitor the integrity of somatosensory pathways in a wide variety of brain and spinal cord disorders. Intraoperative monitoring is often done during surgery for idiopathic and neuromuscular scoliosis, cervical instability, and repair of Arnold-Chiari malformation.[4-7] In addition, SSEPs have been useful in monitoring patients undergoing resection of brain,[8] spinal cord,[9] and peripheral nerve or plexus tumors.[6]

In most pediatric reports scoliosis surgery is the most common reason for obtaining intraoperative SSEPs.[6] This type of surgery involves instrumentation and distraction of the spine, and one of the most feared complications is paraplegia. The incidence of paraplegia with Harrington rod placement or other instrumentations and distractions is 0.5% to 1.6%.[10] Prior to the availability of intraoperative SSEPs the orthopedic surgeons used the wake-up test.[6,11] The wake-up test involves waking the patients during the procedure and telling them to move their toes and then reanesthetizing them.

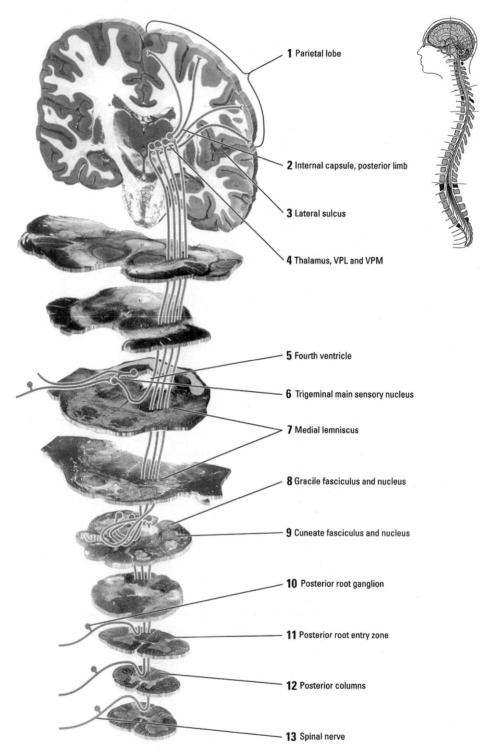

1 Parietal lobe

2 Internal capsule, posterior limb

3 Lateral sulcus

4 Thalamus, VPL and VPM

5 Fourth ventricle

6 Trigeminal main sensory nucleus

7 Medial lemniscus

8 Gracile fasciculus and nucleus

9 Cuneate fasciculus and nucleus

10 Posterior root ganglion

11 Posterior root entry zone

12 Posterior columns

13 Spinal nerve

FIGURE 24–1

Anatomy of the somatosensory pathways measured with somatosensory evoked potentials. Myelinated spinal nerve axons, the first-order neurons, from posterior root ganglion cells enter the medial aspect of the posterior root entry zone of the spinal cord. They climb to the brainstem in the posterior (dorsal) columns with sacral fibers closer to the midline and cervical fibers closer to the dorsal horn. The first synapse is in the posterior column nuclei of the caudal medulla. Lumbosacral fibers synapse in the gracile fasciculus and nucleus and thoracocervical fibers in the cuneate fasciculus and nucleus. Second-order axons from the posterior column nuclei cross in the ventral medulla to form the medial lemniscus, which ascends on the contralateral side. These axons terminate in the ventral posterolateral (VPL) and ventral posteromedial (VPM) nuclei of the thalamus. From the thalamus, third-order axons ascend through the internal capsule to terminate in the somatosensory cortex of the postcentral gyrus and parietal operculum of the parietal lobe. (From Woolsey TA, Hanaway J, Gado MH: The Brain Atlas: A Visual Guide to the Human Central Nervous System, 2nd ed. Hoboken, NJ, John Wiley, 2003.)

The risks involved include movement of or injury from the surgical hardware, extubation, vital sign instability, and psychological trauma to the patient. The wake-up test can be performed only a few times during the procedure, and some patients cannot cooperate with the test. With the introduction of SSEPs into the operating room, the wake-up test can be averted in many of the cases.

One might argue that since only the posterior spinal cord or somatosensory tracts are being monitored, SSEPs would be of little value in predicting damage to the motor pathways.[2,3,7,12-15] With compression or vascular compromise there tends to be involvement in multiple areas of the cord resulting in changes in the SSEPs that correspond to the damage. If discrete areas of the cord are injured, there are unlikely to be changes in the SSEPs unless the somatosensory pathways are involved. Lesions occurring below the level of monitoring will also not be detected. For example, monitoring median nerve SSEPs does not detect thoracic cord compromise. Despite these limitations, intraoperative evoked potential monitoring can be quite useful to the surgeon in preventing complications in many surgical procedures.[2,4,6,14,16-18]

Although much of the early literature dealing with intraoperative SSEP monitoring dealt with the adult population,[19-22] over the past decade SSEPs have become routinely used in monitoring children in the operating room.[3,4,7,23,24]

In a series of 343 children monitored with SSEPs at Children's Hospital in Boston, idiopathic scoliosis comprised the largest group of patients (63.7%) to be monitored during corrective surgery (Tables 24-1 and 24-2). Of interest were the 107 monitored patients with neuromuscular scoliosis. The most commonly associated condition was cerebral palsy. Many other conditions were seen in association with neuromuscular scoliosis such as myelodysplasia and mental retardation. This large group of patients is at higher risk for neurologic sequelae according to MacEwen and colleagues,[10] who reported an incidence of 0.72% for neurologic complications in the surgical treatment of scoliosis, with the true incidence perhaps being higher. With certain conditions there was an increased risk for neurologic injury such as a preexisting neurologic deficit, congenital scoliosis, or scoliosis of a severe degree. Certain procedures also carry an increased risk for neurologic injury such as skeletal traction, Harrington rod instrumentation, or the use of sublaminar wires.[25] Therefore, the most likely patients to benefit from intraoperative SSEP monitoring are the high-risk patients as defined by the underlying or associated neurological disorder or the risk of the procedure.[10,25]

Other types of procedures that benefit from intraoperative SSEP monitoring during surgery include selective rhizotomy, resection of tumors of selected peripheral nerves or plexus, spinal cord tumors, epilepsy, cortical and subcortical masses, carotid endarterectomy, and aortic surgery.

TABLE 24–1. SURGICAL PROCEDURES MONITORED AT CHILDREN'S HOSPITAL —1989 TO 1991[6]

Surgical Procedure	No. of Patients	Type of Evoked Potential Used
Orthopedic Procedures	(95%)	
Instrumentation + distraction	253 (77.6%)	PT SSEP
Fusion	73 (22.4%)	PT SSEP
Neurosurgical Procedures	(5%)	
Tethered cord with lipoma	4	PT SSEP
Cortical mapping	3	MN SSEP
Intramedullary cord tumor	3	PT/MN SSEP
Extramedullary cord tumor	2	PT/MN SSEP
Brainstem glioma	2	PT/MN SSEP, BAEP
Posterior fossa meningioma	1	PT/MN SSEP, BAEP
ACM type 1 decompression	1	PT/MN SSEP, BAEP
Peripheral neurofibroma	1	MN SSEP
Brachial plexus repair	1	MN SSEP

ACM, Arnold-Chiari malformation; SSEP, somatosensory evoked potential; BAEP, brainstem auditory evoked potential; PT, posterior tibial; MN, median nerve.

TABLE 24–2. UNDERLYING DISEASES OF THE PATIENTS MONITORED INTRAOPERATIVELY AT CHILDREN'S HOSPITAL—1989 TO 1991[6]

Procedure	No. of Patients	Instrumentation and Distraction	Fusion Only
Idiopathic scoliosis	219	253	73
Neuromuscular scoliosis	107		
Cerebral palsy			
Myelodysplasia			
Mental retardation			
Spondylolisthesis			
Myopathy/dystrophy			
Neurofibromatosis			
Post-traumatic			
Rett's syndrome			
Tethered cord/lipoma			
Marfan syndrome			
Dwarfism			
Friedreich's ataxia			
Syringomyelia			
Peripheral sensory neuropathy			
Postradiation			
Klippel-Trenaunay-Weber syndrome			
Other procedures	17	—	—
Brainstem/cord neoplasm			
Cervical instability			
Arnold-Chiari malformation			
Brachial plexus injury			

Somatosensory Evoked
Potential Methods

SSEPs should be performed according to the guidelines of the American EEG Society (now named the American Clinical Neurophysiology Society) for intraoperative monitoring.[26,27] After marking electrode sites in accordance with the 10-20 International System (C3′, C4′, Cz′, Fpz, Fz, A1, A2), the recording sites are prepared with a commercially available pumice-based solution. Gold-cup electrodes are affixed using gauze and collodion. Additional gold-cup electrodes are affixed to C2 and C3 cervical spine in the same manner and a ground electrode is placed on the left shoulder. Electrode impedances should be maintained between 2000 and 5000 Ω.

A monophasic stimulus of 0.1- to 0.3-millisecond duration and 10 to 20 mA is delivered to the ankle and/or wrist.[6,28,29] The rate of stimulation is 2 Hz for posterior tibial nerve testing and 5 Hz for the median nerve evoked potential, delivered to each limb separately.[6]

Posterior tibial nerve SSEP recordings are obtained from the popliteal fossa (PF) referenced to an electrode located 4 cm above the popliteal fossa (PFr), upper cervical cord (CS) referenced to Cz′ and ipsilateral ear, and scalp (Cz′) referenced to Fpz. In median nerve SSEPs electrodes are placed over Erb's point (EP) referenced to the contralateral EP, mid-cervical cord (C5) referenced to Cz, and contralateral cortex (C3′, C4′) referenced to contralateral EP and Fpz.

There have been difficulties in obtaining reliable median nerve SSEPs in patients undergoing procedures in the semi-sitting position.[30] However, adding temporal electrodes has been shown to be useful in providing stable recordings and decreasing the rate of false-positive alarms.[31]

Waveforms are recorded approximately every 15 to 30 minutes or more frequently during the critical period of instrumentation or distraction, using filter settings of 30 to 2000 Hz with a gain of 1 K. The analysis time is 120 milliseconds, and responses are identified after 350 to 500 repetitions using a digital averaging system. Up-going potentials are labeled as "negative." Peak latency and amplitude for all waveforms are measured using the digital cursor on the averaging system.

Because cortical responses can be so unreliable in children, it has become imperative to add additional recording sites. In addition to recording from the popliteal fossa and scalp, additional sites include the cervical spine. Unlike the cortical potential, the cervical response is more resistant to the effects of anesthesia, allowing one to monitor spinal cord integrity above the surgery level despite the absence of a scalp response. When the posterior neck recording electrode lies in the operative field, one can record from the anterior neck using a surface electrode, referring to Cz′ or Fpz.[6]

When monitoring children with SSEPs intraoperatively, a number of important differences unique to this group must be recognized. Of particular concern is the small body size of the very young patient making electrode application and stimulation difficult. However, with careful attention to technical detail and measurement, satisfactory recordings can be obtained. To avoid stimulus artifact that can interfere with the recording, careful positioning of the stimulator and extremities is necessary. Use of a smaller stimulating electrode may also be helpful. In a number of other instances we have been unable to record responses owing to the neurologic disorder. In a small number of these cases we have been able to use invasive electrodes to record epidurally.

There have been several patterns of change described in the literature that have been correlated to postoperative outcome. It is generally thought that if the cortical and cervical components of the SSEPs return to baseline within 15 minutes of an acute change, there is unlikely to be postoperative sequelae. If there is a prolonged disappearance of the evoked potentials, the patient has a significant chance of neurologic impairment postoperatively. Nuwer and Dawson[22] reported that if there is a greater than 50% attenuation of the evoked potential, there is perhaps a 25% chance of postoperative impairment. An attenuation of less than 50% is probably not associated with a significant risk of a deficit, although the patient should be watched closely in the postoperative period. Our experience in children has been similar. I consider a consistent increase in the latency by 2.0 milliseconds or greater than the baseline and a decrease in the amplitude of 50% or more from the baseline at the neck and scalp as a warning that the patient is at risk for neurologic injury. Figure 24-2 is an example of a SSEP recording from a patient who had a marked decrease in amplitude following placement of instrumentation for scoliosis. Note that the improvement was when the instrumentation was removed.

In a series of 343 surgical procedures performed at Children's Hospital in Boston, outcome was reviewed.[6] Figures 24-3 and 24-4 show the surgical procedures performed and the age of the patients. Of these 343 patients, 18 had changes in the cervical response that occurred gradually over a 30- to 60-minute period (Table 24-3). The changes occurred prior to instrumentation and consisted of an increase in latency less than 2.0 milliseconds or a decrease in amplitude between 30% and 50% from baseline, both of which are less than the suggested parameters for significant changes.[22] Some of these changes were thought to be due to increasing hypotension, hemodilution, or hypothermia. When these factors were corrected, the latencies and amplitude of the waveforms returned to baseline values.

In another 9 patients, significant changes in the cervical and cortical responses (latency increase > 2 milliseconds, amplitude decrease > 50%) were seen acutely during

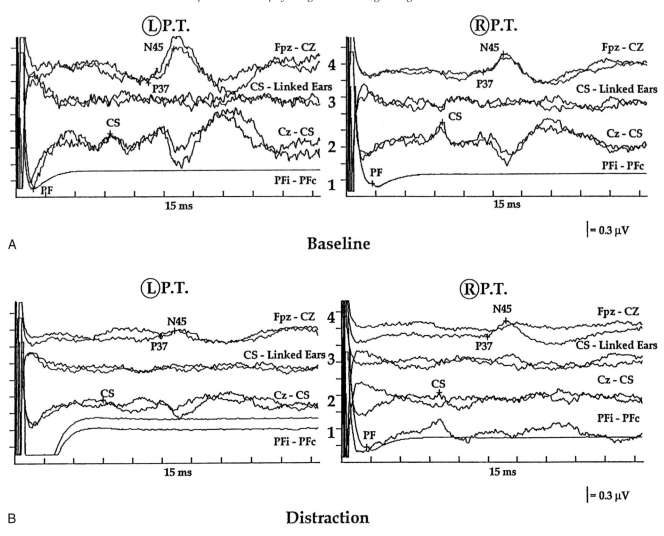

FIGURE 24–2

Somatosensory evoked potential recording from an 18-year-old woman with mental retardation, spastic left hemiparesis, and neuromuscular thoracic scoliosis who underwent Harrington-Luque instrumentation. A, Postinduction baseline recording. Four-channel, bilateral posterior tibial nerve somatosensory evoked potential. Channel 1, PFi-PFc = ipsilateral popliteal fossa to reference electrode. Channels 2 and 3 recorded at the level of the cervical spine, Cz'-CS and CS-A1/A2, C2 = cervical spine; A1/A2 = linked ears reference; channel 4, Fpz-Cz', recorded from the midline scalp. B, Recording during instrumentation. Amplitude has significantly decreased in both cervical and cortical responses, as compared with baseline recordings.

instrumentation. The surgeon was alerted and measures were taken to identify the cause and level affected. Further instrumentation was halted and distraction loosened with a return of the waveforms to baseline within 15 to 20 minutes. There were no changes in blood pressure, temperature, or anesthetic regimen in the time surrounding the SSEP changes in all patients. The patients were carefully monitored throughout the remainder of the operation. A wake-up test was possible in 5 of these patients and was satisfactory. The remaining 4 patients were either mentally retarded or were unable to cooperate with the wake-up test for other reasons. Postoperatively, 8 of these 9 patients had no new neurologic sequelae.

This group of 9 patients illustrates one of the major differences in children with scoliosis: the associated pathologic conditions and neurologic abnormalities that are not commonly seen in adults with scoliosis. All of the monitored patients, with the exception of 1, who had either a significant change during the testing or had postoperative neurologic sequela without SSEP changes were in a high-risk group due to preexisting neurologic abnormalities or surgical procedures. Of the 9 patients who had significant changes,

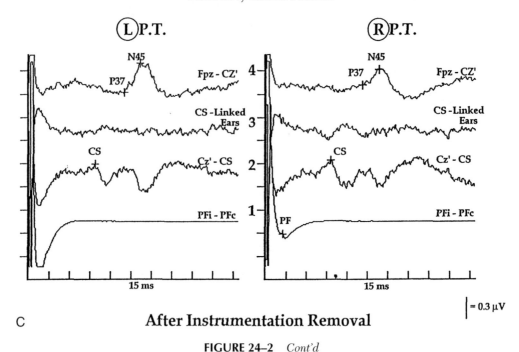

After Instrumentation Removal

C

FIGURE 24–2 *Cont'd*

C, Recording after instrumentation has been removed. Amplitude and latency of cervical and cortical responses have returned to baseline values.

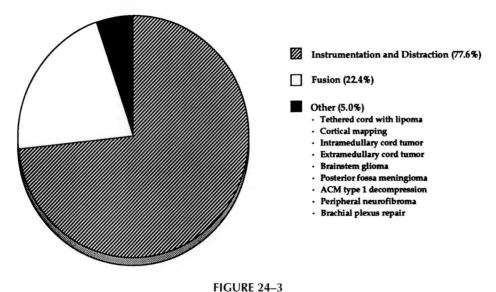

FIGURE 24–3

Survey of surgical procedures monitored at Children's Hospital in Boston over a 3-year period.

6 patients had congenital scoliosis, another had a neuroenteric cyst, and another had a myelomeningocele. Two patients had severe spondylolisthesis requiring osteotomy and correction. One additional patient had a previously resected diastematomyelia. In addition, 2 of these patients were severely retarded, and 1 had a spastic quadriparesis. Only 1 patient had idiopathic scoliosis, and when significant changes were noted during the monitoring, correction was halted, with no neurologic sequelae.

Three patients developed new neurologic deficits within 48 hours of surgery, without a change in the surgical SSEP monitoring, and were considered "false negatives." The first was a patient thought to have an L5 root injury that occurred intraoperatively owing to traction of

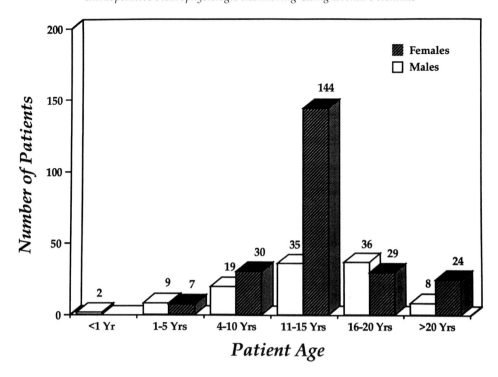

FIGURE 24–4

Survey of ages of patients monitored with somatosensory evoked potentials at Children's Hospital in Boston over a 3-year period.

TABLE 24–3. OUTCOME OF THE PATIENTS MONITORED INTRAOPERATIVELY[6]

Change in SSEP	No. (%) of Patients	Outcome
Gradual	18 (5.5)	18—no neurologic sequelae
Acute	9 (2.8)	9—no neurologic sequelae
		1—Postoperative paraplegia due to cord tumor
No change	296 (90.8)	293—no neurologic sequelae
	3 (0.9)	1—unilateral footdrop due to L5 injury; resolved in 3 mo
		1—urinary retention; resolved in 1 wk
		1—bilateral L4, L5 weakness due to root compression from loose lamina; resolved with correction at reoperation

SSEP, somatosensory evoked potential.

the root. As has been reported by Harper and colleagues,[32] lumbar radiculopathy may be a more common occurrence following scoliosis surgery than has been reported, and SSEPs of the lower extremity are an insensitive method for detection of a radiculopathy. A second patient developed urinary retention that resolved spontaneously in a week. This may have been due to mild intraoperative trauma, narcotics, or overdistention of the bladder postoperatively.

The last patient was found to have suffered direct trauma to several roots due to compression by a displaced lamina. Each of these patients illustrates some of the limitations of the test and the adaptations one can make to better monitor neurophysiologic function.

As can be seen, when interpreting significant changes intraoperatively, many factors need to be considered. Technical problems such as stimulator failure, electrode problems, and computer failures need to be quickly detected and corrected. Because of the operating suite environment, interference from other equipment may distort the waveforms. The patient's underlying pathologic condition may contribute to absent responses. Physiologic changes also need to be considered such as hypotension, hypothermia, and hemodilution. When these factors are ruled out or corrected, and the significant changes persist, the surgeon should be notified. Table 24-4 lists possibilities to be considered when there is a change in waveform morphology, amplitude, or latency during surgery.

There are a number of technical and patient-related problems in addition to the electronic noisy recording environment of the operating room and the effects of hypothermia and hypotension that we have encountered over the last few years that were specific to this age group. In addition to underlying neurologic conditions more commonly seen in children, there are additional unique technical and

TABLE 24–4. SUGGESTED APPROACH TO INTERPRETATION OF SIGNIFICANT CHANGES IN INTRAOPERATIVE SSEPs

Technical Causes	Surgical Manipulation
Hypotension	Instrumentation
Artifact	Ischemia
Hypothermia	Spinal cord trauma
Hemodilution	

SSEP, somatosensory evoked potential.

TABLE 24–5. PATIENTS UNABLE TO BE MONITORED INTRAOPERATIVELY DUE TO THEIR UNDERLYING DISEASE[6]

Pathologic Process	No. of Cases
Myelodysplasia and myelomeningocele	7
Spastic quadriparesis with lower extremity atrophy	4
Cervicothoracic spinal cord trauma	2
Severe scoliosis with myelopathy	2
Friedreich's ataxia	1
Peripheral neuropathy	1
Spinal cord tumor	1
Total	18

patient-related problems when performing intraoperative SSEP monitoring in children. Small body size makes stimulation more difficult, but with smaller stimulating electrodes, this problem can be alleviated.

Another problem that may occur is absence of all responses due to the patient's underlying disease. In the series from Children's Hospital in Boston, we were unable to obtain responses using surface recording electrodes in 18 patients due to their underlying disease (Table 24-5). We had difficulty in recording any potentials, including the popliteal fossa from patients with myelodysplasia and myelomeningocele or severe spastic quadriparesis with atrophy of the lower extremities. In several of these patients we were able to record responses using epidural electrodes placed above and below the operative site by the surgeon. Other pathologies associated with difficulty in obtaining responses were spinal cord trauma, spinal cord tumors, myelopathy, and peripheral neuropathies.

A major difference encountered in children is the sensitivity of the cortical response to volatile anesthetics.[33-36] Gugino and Chabot[33] reviewed the effects of anesthetic agents on the cortical response of the SSEP in adults. Most of the conventional inhalation agents significantly prolong the latency and decrease the amplitude, and narcotics to a lesser extent may also alter the responses. The time when one sees the most variability of the cortical potential is dur-

ing induction of anesthesia or when the patient receives a large bolus of anesthetic.[36,37] Daube[37] evaluated a group of 140 older patients undergoing thoracic-lumbar spine surgery and during induction noted a mean amplitude reduction of one third, and in 5% of their patients the scalp response was lost during induction. Through the course of the surgical procedure there was a gradual reduction (mean reduction 17%) in the amplitude of the scalp responses and an increase in the latency (4% to 6%). An additional 5% of their subjects lost scalp responses with continued anesthesia.

I have found that the combination of nitrous oxide (<60%) or isoflurane (<0.5%) in combination with fentanyl during induction and low-dose nitrous oxide (<50% to 60%) or isoflurane (<0.6%) throughout the rest of the procedure allows for the best SSEP recordings.[6]

These effects may be more profound and more common in children. In our monitored patients, 46% had unreliable cortical responses as defined by a decrease in amplitude greater than 50%, an increase in latency greater than 2 milliseconds, or absence of the response, with a stable cervical potential. This variability was most evident in children younger than 15 years of age and was also dependent on the anesthetic regimen used. Isoflurane in combination with nitrous oxide most consistently abolished or reduced the cortical potentials (Fig. 24-5). With agents such as propofol (Diprivan) or etomidate, the latency of the cortical response remains unchanged or is only slightly prolonged with the amplitude actually increasing. Another agent that has caused some variability in the cortical response when delivered in a bolus is lidocaine, the effect of which is short lived but must be recognized.[38]

In addition to the technical problems, hypothermia, hypotension, hemodilution, smaller body size, and absence of responses due to underlying pathology, the effect of anesthesia on the cortical potential must be realized. With high concentrations or boluses of inhalation agents or narcotics, the cortical response can become markedly attenuated, making it unreliable for monitoring. The clinical perception is that this effect is more prominent in patients younger than 10 years of age. The higher sensitivity and increased variability in young children may be related to maturational changes that take place in the somatosensory system in the 1st decade of life. These changes are thought to be a combination of asynchronous myelination and synaptogenesis.[39] This inherent instability of the cortical response due to immaturity in this age group seems to be greatly increased by anesthetic agents. With the use of a single inhalation agent, with or without a narcotic, the cortical response becomes more stable. Thus, combinations such as nitrous oxide with isoflurane are generally avoided in this age group. In addition, using concentrations of nitrous oxide less than 50% or isoflurane of less than 0.6% allows for the best scalp recordings.

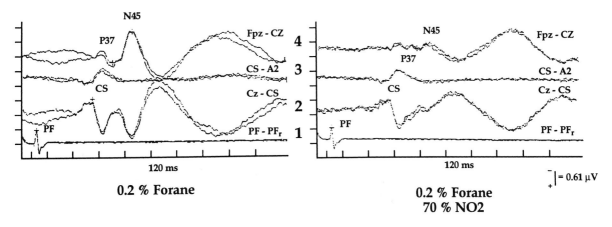

FIGURE 24–5

Change in the cortical potential due to inhalation agents. Four-channel right posterior tibial nerve somatosensory evoked potentials from one patient. The first recording was during the use of a small concentration of a single inhalation agent (isoflurane 0.2%). The second recording was during the use of a combination of agents (isoflurane and nitrous oxide) and the cortical potential in channel 4 has become attenuated, with the cervical and popliteal fossa responses remaining stable. Channel 1, PF- PF$_r$ = ipsilateral popliteal fossa to reference electrode. Channels 2 and 3, Cz'-CS and CS-A2, CS = cervical spine, A2 = right ear, recorded at the level of the cervical spine. Channel 4, Fpz-Cz', is recorded from midline scalp.

With respect to a more specific or sensitive testing modality to detect a root injury, dermatomal SSEPs have been used with variable results in adults.[40] The amplitude of the waveforms is very small as compared to the mixed nerve SSEPs, and reproducibility of dermatomal stimulations is difficult to obtain. This technique has not been studied in children. The summary report of the American Academy of Neurology's Therapeutics and Technology Assessments subcommittee stated that dermatomal SSEPs should still be investigational due to insufficient evidence of reliability and utility cases.

Another technique is EMG monitoring of muscles innervated by particular lumbosacral, cervical, thoracic, and cranial nerves.[41,42] With placement of wire electrodes into the specific muscles of interest, spontaneous muscle activity can be monitored continuously. With injury to the nerve, neurotonic discharges can be heard and seen. Electromyographic (EMG) monitoring is also used in selective dorsal rhizotomy for spasticity. Using 50-Hz stimulation of dorsal rootlets, the neurophysiologist looks for "abnormal" responses such as sustained activity or afterdischarges, lower stimulus thresholds, and spread of responses to distant muscles. Standard EMG recording settings used in the operating room include a gain of 200 to 500 μV, Low frequency filter (LFF) of 30 Hz, High frequency filter (HFF) of 16 KHz, and sweep of 10 msec/cm.

Pedicle screw stimulation is yet another monitoring technique used intraoperatively during spinal instrumentation. The technique is used in the assessment of screw placement and presence of breach of pedicle cortex with associated spinal nerve root injury. By passing electrical current through the pedicle screw head and monitoring for compound muscle action potentials from innervated muscles, one is provided with a real-time window during placement of the screws.

Observing evoked EMG thresholds greater than 15 mA provides evidence of good screw placement.[43] Thresholds less than 10 mA were often associated with breach of pedicle cortex and potential nerve root injury.[44,45]

A relatively new technique, transcranial motor evoked potentials (TcMEP), has evolved over the last decade. TcMEPs are elicited by using high-intensity electrical or magnetic pulsed stimulations that elicit motor responses recorded either from the spinal cord or limb muscles.[46] Used in concert with SSEPs, there is improved capability to assess not only the posterior spinal cord but also the anterior motor tracts directly.

The use of TcMEPs is slowly developing due to inherent difficulties in performance of the test. Such things as reliability in recording from muscles are not as good as recording from the spinal cord. Therefore, accepted criteria for interpretation is still being developed, with complete loss of potentials being the most accepted criteria of significance.[47,48] General anesthesia also greatly affects and degrades the TcMEP.[49,50]

POSTERIOR FOSSA MONITORING

Posterior fossa surgery, although not as common in the pediatric population, can use several techniques to monitor brainstem function and certain cranial nerves.[51]

Intraoperative Brainstem Auditory Evoked Potential Monitoring

Since the brainstem auditory evoked potentials (BAEPs) test the brainstem auditory structures from the peripheral eighth nerve to the midbrain, they are used in monitoring posterior fossa surgeries in patients at risk for loss of hearing. The anatomy is the same as that being tested routinely. As with routine laboratory evoked potentials, the proposed anatomic correlates of the waveform generators are the following:

• Wave I—distal acoustic nerve
• Wave II—proximal acoustic nerve or cochlear nucleus
• Wave III—superior olivary nucleus (lower pons)
• Wave IV—lateral lemniscus
• Wave V—inferior colliculus (upper pons/lower midbrain)
Cortical and subcortical function cannot be assessed using this modality.

The types of procedures intraoperative BAEPs are used in include excision of acoustic neuromas, posterior fossa meningiomas, posterior fossa microvascular decompression, arteriovenous malformations, aneurysms of the posterior circulation, and masses of the fourth ventricle.[8,24,52-55] Surgeons have used BAEPs in the operating room to program cochlear implants in children.[56] BAEPs have also been used to monitor the effects of cooling and rewarming on the core-brain during pediatric cardiopulmonary bypass.[57]

Techniques for stimulating and recording are also similar in regard to the click features and recording parameters. The delivery of the click may be by several types of transducers, earphones, and ear inserts. Additional recording techniques include direct nerve recordings with electrodes placed on the acoustic nerve.[58] As with SSEP monitoring there are several factors that can alter BAEPs. The most important patient factor is age. The normal developmental changes one sees are shorter latency and better formed waves. This is most apparent in patients younger than 3 to 5 years of age. Body temperature also has an effect on BAEPs. With hypothermia (<35°C), the latencies of the waveforms become delayed, wave V being the most sensitive of the waveforms. Wave V disappears at a body temperature below approximately 28°C.

Realizing the changes that can take place due to these factors, there are three types of changes that have been associated with surgical monitoring. The first is a gradual and persistent prolongation of the later waveforms of 1 millisecond or longer. The latencies may or may not return to baseline. Postoperatively, there is no clinical deficit in hearing, but audiologic testing may show abnormalities. The second type of change that may be observed is a sudden loss of all the waveforms without return of responses. This occurs ipsilateral to the side of the surgery. This change is associated with postoperative hearing impairment. Finally, one might see changes contralateral to the side of surgery, intraoperatively. This can be associated with other signs of brainstem disturbances and is associated with a poor outcome.

Somatosensory Evoked Potentials

Monitoring of the posterior fossa can also be supplemented by the use of SSEPs. Either upper or lower extremity SSEPs can be used based on the structures at risk for injury. The procedures, limitations, and interpretations are the same as with spinal cord monitoring.

EMG

Recording from cranial nerve function can also be monitored, in addition to sensory evoked potentials. Wire electrodes can be inserted into muscles innervated by cranial nerves III (inferior rectus), IV (superior oblique), V (masseter), VI (lateral rectus), VII (orbicularis oris), IX (stylopharyngeal), X (cricothyroid, vocalis), XI (trapezius), and XII (tongue). Injury to particular nerves can be detected by neurotonic or injury potentials. Monitoring the EMG also allows one to identify nerves of interest. Standard EMG recording settings are used in the operating room, are a gain of 200 to 500 μV, LFF 30 Hz, HFF 16 KHz, and a sweep of 10 msec/cm.

CORTICAL MONITORING

A number of surgical procedures involve the cortex, sensory and motor, that benefit from intraoperative neurophysiologic applications.

Intraoperative Somatosensory Evoked Potentials

For cortical localization in tumor or epileptic focus resection, SSEP monitoring is used to localize the sensorimotor cortex. The recording is from subdural strips or grid and can be done two ways: either using a bipolar montage looking for a phase reversal or using a referential montage looking for the maximal response compared with the scalp recordings.

Intraoperative Visual Evoked Potential Monitoring

The last sensory evoked potential that has been used intraoperatively is the visual evoked potential (VEP), which monitors the anterior or prechiasmal visual system.[59] Visual testing during operation is technically difficult to do for a number of reasons.

Stimulation is the first problem. Since a patient is not able to fixate on a pattern, a flash or strobe must be used. To deliver the stimulus, light-emitting diode (LED) glasses are easiest to use. They remain out of the operative field and are not disruptive to the operating personnel. The types of procedures VEPs have been used for center mainly around the sellar and suprasellar region. This would include pituitary tumors, suprasellar masses, aneurysms, optic nerve decompression, and craniopharyngiomas.

There is a significant amount of variability of the waveform intraoperatively. This is due to many factors. During hypothermia and hypotension there is a progressive fall in the amplitude and prolongation of the latency. As with the other sensory modalities, the latency is normally longer in very young patients. Another patient factor that affects the recordings is the visual acuity or impairment, both of which can affect the amplitude and latency of the VEP.

Many drugs can alter the waveforms such as barbiturates and halothane, which at low doses may increase the amplitude but at high doses, abolish the response. Nitrous oxide causes a dose-dependent attenuation of the response.

As one can see from the factors discussed and the random variability over time of the waveform itself, VEPs tend to have a high false-positive and false-negative rate. In addition, the full-field strobe is a nonspecific stimulus that can only detect defects anterior to the chiasm. Therefore, VEPs are much more difficult to interpret and generally are not performed intraoperatively.

SUMMARY

In summary, as in adults, intraoperative monitoring has become quite useful in children. It has become an integral part of many of the orthopedic and neurosurgical procedures done in children at my institution owing to the large number of patients at higher risk for surgical morbidity associated with preexisting neurologic impairment or who are undergoing a high-risk procedure. The benefits of intraoperative monitoring to the children identified as being at risk for developing postoperative deficits during surgery are therefore difficult to estimate.

REFERENCES

1. Iwasaki H, Tamaki T, Yoshida M, et al: Efficacy and limitations of current methods of intraoperative spinal cord monitoring. J Orthop Sci 2003;8:635-642.
2. Wiedemayer H, Fauser B, Sandalcioglu IE, et al: The impact of neurophysiological intraoperative monitoring on surgical decisions: A critical analysis of 423 cases. J Neurosurg 2002;96:255-262.
3. Noonan KJ, Walker T, Feinberg JR, et al: Factors related to false- versus true-positive neuromonitoring changes in adolescent idiopathic scoliosis surgery. Spine 2002;27:825-830.
4. Sala F, Krzan MJ, Deletis V: Intraoperative neurophysiological monitoring in pediatric neurosurgery: Why, when, how? Childs Nerv Syst 2002;18:264-287.
5. Strahm C, Min K, Boos N, et al: Reliability of perioperative SSEP recordings in spine surgery. Spinal Cord 2003;41:483-489.
6. Helmers SL, Hall JE: Intraoperative somatosensory evoked potential monitoring in pediatrics. J Pediatr Orthop 1994;14:592-598.
7. Wilson-Holden TJ, Padberg AM, Lenke LG, et al: Efficacy of intraoperative monitoring for pediatric patients with spinal cord pathology undergoing spinal deformity surgery. Spine 1999;24:1685-1692.
8. Grant GA, Farrell D, Silbergeld DL: Continuous somatosensory evoked potential monitoring during brain tumor resection: Report of four cases and review of the literature. J Neurosurg 2002;97:709-713.
9. Quinones-Hinojosa A, Gulati M, Lyon R, et al: Spinal cord mapping as an adjunct for resection of intramedullary tumors: Surgical technique with case illustrations. Neurosurgery 2002;51:1199-1206.
10. MacEwen GD, Bunnell WP, Sriram K: Acute neurological complications in the treatment of scoliosis: A report of the Scoliosis Research Society. J Bone Joint Surg Am 1975;57:404-408.
11. Vauzelle C, Stagnara P, Jouvinroux P: Functional monitoring of spinal cord activity during spinal surgery. Clin Orthop 1973;93:173-178.
12. Chatrian GE, Berger MS, Wirch AL: Discrepancy between intraoperative SSEPs and postoperative function: Case report. J Neurosurg 1988;69:450-454.
13. Lesser RP, Raudzens P, Luders H, et al: Postoperative neurological deficits may occur despite unchanged intraoperative somatosensory evoked potentials. Ann Neurol 1986;19:22-25.
14. Wiedemayer H, Sandalcioglu IE, Armbruster W, et al: False-negative findings in intraoperative SEP monitoring: Analysis of 658 consecutive neurosurgical cases and review of published reports. J Neurol Neurosurg Psychiatry 2004;75:280-286.
15. Papastefanou SL, Henderson LM, Smith NJ, et al: Surface electrode somatosensory-evoked potentials in spinal surgery: Implications for indications and practice. Spine 2000;25:2467-2472.
16. Dawson EG, Sherman JE, Kanim LE, Nuwer MR: Spinal cord monitoring: Results of the Scoliosis Research Society and the European Spinal Deformity Society survey. Spine 1991;16:S361-S364.
17. Nuwer MR, Dawson EG, Carlson LG, et al: Somatosensory evoked potential spinal cord monitoring reduces neurologic deficits after scoliosis surgery: Results of a large multicenter survey. Electroencephalogr Clin Neurophysiol 1995;96:6-11.
18. More RC, Nuwer MR, Dawson EG: Cortical evoked potential monitoring during spinal surgery: Sensitivity,

specificity, reliability, and criteria for alarm. J Spinal Disord 1988;1:75-80.

19. Loder RT, Thomson GJ, LaMont RL: Spinal cord monitoring in patients with nonidiopathic spinal deformities using somatosensory evoked potentials. Spine 1991;16:1359-1364.

20. Lubicky JP, Spadaro JA, Yuan HA, et al: Variability of somatosensory cortical evoked potential monitoring during spinal surgery. Spine 1989;14:790-798.

21. Luders H, Lesser R, Gurd A, Klem G: Recovery functions of spinal cord and subcortical somatosensory evoked potentials to posterior tibial nerve stimulation: Intrasurgical recordings. Brain Res 1984;309:27-34.

22. Nuwer MR, Dawson E: Intraoperative evoked potential monitoring of the spinal cord: Enhanced stability of cortical recordings. Electroencephalogr Clin Neurophysiol 1984;59:318-327.

23. Anderson RC, Emerson RG, Dowling KC, Feldstein NA: Improvement in brainstem auditory evoked potentials after suboccipital decompression in patients with Chiari I malformation. J Neurosurg 2003;98:459-464.

24. Anderson RC, Dowling KC, Feldstein NA, Emerson RG: Chiari I malformation: Potential role for intraoperative electrophysiologic monitoring. J Clin Neurophysiol 2003;20:65-72.

25. Wilber RG, Thompson GH, Shaffer JW, et al: Postoperative neurological deficits in segmental spinal instrumentation: A study using spinal cord monitoring. J Bone Joint Surg Am 1984;66:1178-1187.

26. Guideline eleven: Guidelines for intraoperative monitoring of sensory evoked potentials. American Electroencephalographic Society. J Clin Neurophysiol 1994;11:77-87.

27. American Electroencephalographic Society guidelines for intraoperative monitoring of sensory evoked potentials. J Clin Neurophysiol 1987;4:397-416.

28. Luk KD, Hu Y, Lu WW, Wong YW: Effect of stimulus pulse duration on intraoperative somatosensory evoked potential (SEP) monitoring. J Spinal Disord 2001;14:247-251.

29. Hu Y, Luk KD, Wong YW, et al: Effect of stimulation parameters on intraoperative spinal cord evoked potential monitoring. J Spinal Disord 2001;14:449-452.

30. Wiedemayer H, Schaefer H, Armbruster W, et al: Observations on intraoperative somatosensory evoked potential (SEP) monitoring in the semi-sitting position. Clin Neurophysiol 2002;113:1993-1997.

31. Wiedemayer H, Sandalcioglu IE, Regel J, et al: Enhanced stability of somatosensory evoked potentials attained in the median nerve by using temporal electrodes for intraoperative recording in patients in the semisitting position. J Neurosurg 2003;99:986-990.

32. Harper CM Jr, Daube JR, Litchy WJ, Klassen RA: Lumbar radiculopathy after spinal fusion for scoliosis. Muscle Nerve 1988;11:386-391.

33. Gugino V, Chabot RJ: Somatosensory evoked potentials. Int Anesthesiol Clin 1990;28:154-164.

34. Ku AS, Hu Y, Irwin MG, et al: Effect of sevoflurane/nitrous oxide versus propofol anaesthesia on somatosensory evoked

potential monitoring of the spinal cord during surgery to correct scoliosis. Br J Anaesth 2002;88:502-507.

35. da Costa VV, Saraiva RA, de Almeida AC, et al: The effect of nitrous oxide on the inhibition of somatosensory evoked potentials by sevoflurane in children. Anaesthesia 2001;56:202-207.

36. Laureau E, Marciniak B, Hebrard A, et al: Comparative study of propofol and midazolam effects on somatosensory evoked potentials during surgical treatment of scoliosis. Neurosurgery 1999;45:69-74.

37. Daube JR: Intraoperative monitoring by evoked potentials for spinal cord surgery: The pros. Electroencephalogr Clin Neurophysiol 1989;73:374-377.

38. Chaves-Vischer V, Brustowicz R, Helmers SL: The effect of intravenous lidocaine on intraoperative somatosensory evoked potentials during scoliosis surgery. Anesth Analg 1996;83:1122-1125.

39. Gilmore RL, Bass NH, Wright EA, et al: Development assessment of spinal cord and cortical evoked potentials after tibial nerve stimulation: Effects of age and statue on normative data during childhood. Electroencephalogr Clin Neurophysiol 1985;62:241-251.

40. Tsai RY, Yang RS, Nuwer MR, et al: Intraoperative dermatomal evoked potential monitoring fails to predict outcome from lumbar decompression surgery. Spine 1997;22:1970-1975.

41. Staudt LA, Nuwer MR, Peacock WJ: Intraoperative monitoring during selective posterior rhizotomy: Technique and patient outcome. Electroencephalogr Clin Neurophysiol 1995;97:296-309.

42. Van de Wiele BM, Staudt LA, Rubinstien EH, et al: Perioperative complications in children undergoing selective posterior rhizotomy: A review of 105 cases. Paediatr Anaesth 1996;6:479-486.

43. Shi YB, Binette M, Martin WH, et al: Electrical stimulation for intraoperative evaluation of thoracic pedicle screw placement. Spine 2003;28:595-601.

44. Bose B, Wierzbowski LR, Sestokas AK: Neurophysiologic monitoring of spinal nerve root function during instrumented posterior lumbar spine surgery. Spine 2002;27:1444-1450.

45. Toleikis JR, Skelly JP, Carlvin AO, et al: The usefulness of electrical stimulation for assessing pedicle screw placements. J Spinal Disord 2000;13:283-289.

46. DiCindio S, Theroux M, Shah S, et al: Multimodality monitoring of transcranial electric motor and somatosensory-evoked potentials during surgical correction of spinal deformity in patients with cerebral palsy and other neuromuscular disorders. Spine 2003;28:1851-1855.

47. Calancie B, Harris W, Brindle GF, et al: Threshold-level repetitive transcranial electrical stimulation for intraoperative monitoring of central motor conduction. J Neurosurg 2001;95:161-168.

48. Calancie B, Harris W, Broton JG, et al: "Threshold-level" multipulse transcranial electrical stimulation of motor cortex for intraoperative monitoring of spinal motor tracts:

Description of method and comparison to somatosensory evoked potential monitoring. J Neurosurg 1998;88:457-470.

49. Pechstein U, Nadstawek J, Zentner J, Schramm J: Isoflurane plus nitrous oxide versus propofol for recording of motor evoked potentials after high-frequency repetitive electrical stimulation. Electroencephalogr Clin Neurophysiol 1998;108:175-181.

50. Ubags LH, Kalkman CJ, Been HD: Influence of isoflurane on myogenic motor evoked potentials to single and multiple transcranial stimuli during nitrous oxide/opioid anesthesia. Neurosurgery 1998;43:90-94.

51. Raudzens PA, Shetter AG: Intraoperative monitoring of brain-stem auditory evoked potentials. J Neurosurg 1982;57:341-348.

52. Staecker H, Nadol JB Jr, Ojeman R, et al: Hearing preservation in acoustic neuroma surgery: Middle fossa versus retrosigmoid approach. Am J Otol 2000;21:399-404.

53. Brackmann DE, Owens RM, Friedman RA, et al: Prognostic factors for hearing preservation in vestibular schwannoma surgery. Am J Otol 2000;21:417-424.

54. Tonn JC, Schlake HP, Goldbrunner R, et al: Acoustic neuroma surgery as an interdisciplinary approach: A neurosurgical series of 508 patients. J Neurol Neurosurg Psychiatry 2000;69:161-166.

55. Anderson RC, Dowling KC, Feldstein NA, Emerson RG: Chiari I malformation: Potential role for intraoperative electrophysiologic monitoring. J Clin Neurophysiol 2003;20:65-72.

56. Shallop JK, Peterson A, Facer GW, et al: Cochlear implants in five cases of auditory neuropathy: Postoperative findings and progress. Laryngoscope 2001;111:555-562.

57. Rodriguez RA, Edmonds HL Jr, Auden SM, Austin EH III: Auditory brainstem evoked responses and temperature monitoring during pediatric cardiopulmonary bypass. Can J Anaesth 1999;46:832-839.

58. Moller AR, Jannetta PJ: Monitoring auditory functions during cranial nerve microvascular decompression operations by direct recording from the eighth nerve. J Neurosurg 1983;59:493-499.

59. Wiedemayer H, Fauser B, Sandalcioglu IE, et al: Observations on intraoperative monitoring of visual pathways using steady-state visual evoked potentials. Eur J Anaesthesiol 2004;21:429-433.

60. Woolsey TA, Hanaway J, Gado MH: The Brain Atlas: A Visual Guide to the Human Central Nervous System, 2nd ed. Hoboken, NJ, John Wiley & Sons, 2003.

Abnormal Evoked Potentials

25

Somatosensory Evoked Potentials in Pediatrics—Abnormal

Robin L. Gilmore

Clinical occasions when somatosensory evoked potentials (SSEPs) are useful occur frequently. It is not necessary to have sensory loss to have abnormal SSEPs. There is, however, a good correlation between spinal cord/brainstem lesions involving dorsal column/lemniscal structures and proprioception abnormalities in the adult: If position sense is impaired more than modestly, then the SSEP is likely to be abnormal.[1] Additionally, there may be abnormalities of the SSEP even in the face of a normal sensory examination. This, of course, is what leads to its usefulness in conditions such as multiple sclerosis.

Abnormalities may consist of prolonged latencies (compared with normal control data), absence of obligatory potentials, or prolongation of interpeak intervals or central conduction times (CCT), or slowing of conduction velocities. Decreased amplitude, by itself, is not a criterion for abnormality.

COMA AND ENCEPHALOPATHIES

The value of median nerve SSEPs (MN-SSEPs) for prognosis has been examined in comatose infants and children.[2-4] Early prognosis of outcome in comatose children is difficult based on clinical criteria alone. Physical examination findings may be significantly altered by paralysis and/or sedation. SSEPs, by monitoring neurologic pathways from the peripheral nerve to the cortex, provide an objective and reproducible means to follow the children.

De Meirleir and Taylor[5] classified SSEPs in a large series of 73 comatose children. Coma resulted from a variety of etiologies. SSEPs were graded as normal, increased interpeak latencies, and unilaterally or bilaterally absent cortical responses. The authors found that SSEPs were useful for predicting outcome regardless of coma etiology. Generally, children with totally absent SSEPs died or had severe neurologic sequelae, such as spastic quadriparesis; none were normal. Unilaterally, abnormal cortical SSEPs predicted a residual hemiparesis, although often only of mild degree. Of those with normal SSEPs, most had a normal outcome, and the rest (25%) had only minimal neurologic sequelae. Those patients who had normal outcomes had normal or only mildly abnormal SSEPs that normalized within a few days.

As has been seen with adults, repeated SSEPs also are of value in refining prognosis,[6] especially in children with Reye's syndrome (see later). Investigators have concluded that SSEPs alone are much more useful than brainstem auditory evoked potentials (BAEPs) alone in prognostication.[5] However, SSEPs are especially helpful when combined with BAEPs in providing predictive information. In one group of comatose children with hypoxic insults, BAEPs and MN-SSEPs were better predictors of chronic vegetative state than the electroencephalograms (EEGs) and clinical assessments.[4]

HYPOXIC-ISCHEMIC ENCEPHALOPATHY

SSEPs are useful in evaluating children in coma. In a series of 43 children in coma from head trauma or hypoxic-ischemic encephalopathy in which all children had

MN-SSEP and BAEP, it was found that patients surviving with neurologic sequelae had either unilateral loss or a latency prolongation of the cortical SSEP.[7] Patients who had normal outcomes had initially normal or mildly delayed cortical EPs. Of the patients with bilateral absence of cortical potentials, most died, and one was left with neurologic deficits. Patients with loss of BAEP and SSEP components had a poor prognosis also. Only patients with the most severe condition, who did not survive, showed severe latency prolongations of components. Barbiturates did not influence either the N20 or the CCT. In cases of children with brainstem pathology, the combined recordings of BAEP and MN-SSEP together have provided more information than either test alone.[8,9]

REYE'S SYNDROME

An investigation of electrophysiologic techniques in children with Reye's syndrome indicated that longitudinal SSEPs were more accurate in prognostication than the EEG.[10] In one patient, the cortical components were abnormal in the initial recordings. Patient survival was correlated with early progressive recovery of short-latency (<50 millisecond) scalp-recorded components. Clinical recovery without neurologic sequelae was associated with recovery of later (>100 millisecond) components.

AIDS

Neurologic dysfunction has been described frequently in children with acquired immunodeficiency syndrome (AIDS). SSEPs have been found to be useful in some asymptomatic patients in assessing central somatosensory function[11]; they have not been reported to be helpful in assessing effectiveness of treatment.[12]

DEVELOPMENTAL DELAY

The application of the SSEP in the evaluation of infants and children with developmental delay or static encephalopathies has not been extensively studied. This, in part, relates to the fact that SSEPs are difficult to record in these children. When recordable, they are frequently normal. When abnormal, they may provide clues to the nature of the underlying cerebral dysfunction but rarely provide a diagnosis.[13] It is not clear whether SSEPs, in combination with BAEPs and visual evoked potentials (VEPs), differentiate children with static encephalopathies at early ages from patients with neurodegenerative disease. Experience with EP abnormalities in definite neurodegenerative

diseases suggests that there is a role in the diagnostic evaluation of these children.[14]

NEURODEGENERATIVE DISORDERS

Several investigators have reported abnormalities in SSEPs in a variety of neurodegenerative disorders.[15-20] Abnormalities of spinal and cortical components have been found (Figs. 25-1 and 25-2). Severe abnormalities have been described in children with both gray and white matter diseases. In most of these disorders, the peripheral components are normal, whereas more rostral components are delayed or absent.[15,17] Cracco and associates[15] studied the MN-SSEPs and peroneal SSEPs in 17 children with a variety of neurodegenerative diseases, including Tay-Sachs disease, Canavan's disease, Sandhoff's disease, Hunter's disease, gangliosidosis, and neuronal ceroid lipofuscinosis. In all patients the cauda equina and peripheral nerve conduction

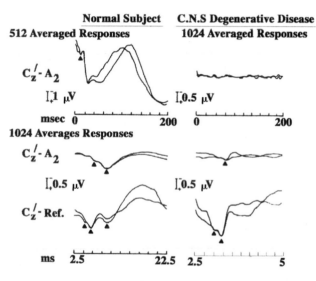

FIGURE 25–1

Comparison of the median nerve evoked short latency (bottom two traces) and longer latency (top traces) potentials in a normal child and a child with degenerative disease. In the bottom two traces the analysis time is 20 milliseconds. In the normal child, three short-latency positive potentials are recorded in the Cz'-hand reference lead (arrowheads). In the Cz'-ear lead only the second two potentials are seen (arrowheads). In the patient, only the first two positive potentials are recorded in the Cz'-hand reference lead (arrowheads). Only the second positive potential is seen in the Cz'-ear lead (arrow). The analysis time in the top traces is 200 milliseconds. In the normal child the Cz'-ear lead yields prominent longer latency potentials. No response is recorded in the patient. (From Cracco JB, Bosch VV, Cracco RQ: Cerebral and spinal somatosensory evoked potentials in children with CNS degenerative disease. Electroencephalogr Clin Neurophysiol 1980;49:437-445.)

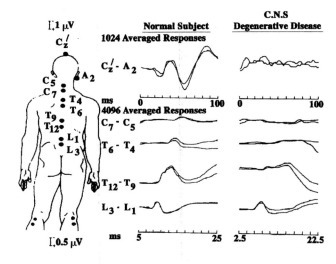

FIGURE 25–2

Comparison of spinal (bottom four traces) and cerebral (top traces) evoked potentials to bilateral peroneal nerve stimulation in a normal subject and a patient with degenerative disease. Electrode placement (L3-C5) refers to spinous process level. Two recordings are superimposed in each trace. In the patient very broad low-voltage responses are recorded over the caudal spinal cord. Potentials over the rostral cord are poorly defined or absent. The cerebral potentials recorded in the normal subject are absent in the patient. (From Cracco JB, Bosch VV, Cracco RQ: Cerebral and spinal somatosensory evoked potentials in children with CNS degenerative disease. Electroencephalogr Clin Neurophysiol 1980;49:437-445.)

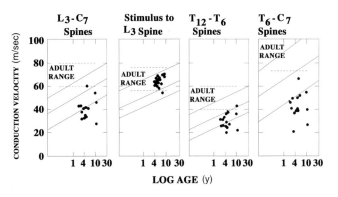

FIGURE 25–3

Distribution of the overall spinal conduction velocities (L3-C7 spines) and the segmental conduction velocities over peroneal nerve and cauda equina (stimulus to L3 spine), caudal spinal cord (T12-T6 spines), and rostral spinal cord (T6-C7 spines) in the patients with degenerative disease. The regression lines with 95% confidence limits for these conduction velocities are presented from 95 normal subjects. The range of conduction velocities in normal adults is indicated by the dashed lines. (From Cracco JB, Bosch VV, Cracco RQ: Cerebral and spinal somatosensory evoked potentials in children with CNS degenerative disease. Electroencephalogr Clin Neurophysiol 1980;49:437-445.)

velocities were normal. The responses over spinal cord segments, brainstem, and cortex were abnormal (Fig. 25-3). Responses were seen over the spinal cord in most instances, but these potentials were considerably greater than normal in duration in many of these patients, suggesting the occurrence of increased temporal dispersion. Many showed slowing over the spinal cord. Slowing of conduction velocity was greater over the rostral segments. This suggested a central "dying back process" within the spinal cord. One patient with myoclonus showed enhancement of cerebral potentials (Fig. 25-4). Additionally this patient showed a high-amplitude positive potential that was larger in amplitude and duration than normal (Fig. 25-5). The authors further speculated that this might reflect activation of polysynaptic spinal cord segmental reflexes.

Leukodystrophies

Patients with Pelizaeus-Merzbacher disease (PMD), adrenoleukodystrophy (ALD), and metachromatic leukodystrophy (MLD) frequently have abnormal SSEPs.[17] In patients with MLD, there may be an absence of Erb's point

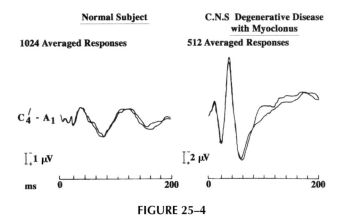

FIGURE 25–4

Comparison of cerebral somatosensory evoked potentials to median nerve stimulation in a normal child and a child with degenerative disease and myoclonus. The response in the patient is about 10 times greater in amplitude than that in the normal subject. CNS, central nervous system. (From Cracco JB, Bosch VV, Cracco RQ: Cerebral and spinal somatosensory evoked potentials in children with CNS degenerative disease. Electroencephalogr Clin Neurophysiol 1980;49:437-445.)

potential, reflecting peripheral nerve involvement. Patients with ALD may have prolongation of the CCT, whereas in patients with MLD, peripheral and more rostral components are abnormal.[16] In a study of 22 children with leukodystrophies including MLD, PMD, Krabbe's disease,

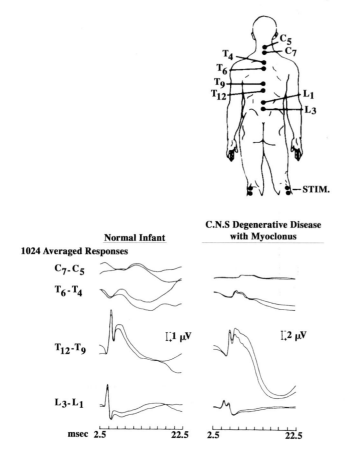

Normal Infant

C.N.S Degenerative Disease with Myoclonus

1024 Averaged Responses

C_7-C_5

T_6-T_4

T_{12}-T_9

L_3-L_1

msec 2.5   22.5   2.5   22.5

FIGURE 25–5

Comparison of spinal evoked potentials in a normal infant and in the same patient illustrated in Figure 25-4. The positive potential that follows the large complex negative potential recorded over the caudal spinal cord (T12-T9 spines) is much greater in amplitude in the patient (note the calibration difference). CNS, central nervous system; STIM, stimulus system. (From Cracco JB, Bosch VV, Cracco RQ: Cerebral and spinal somatosensory evoked potentials in children with CNS degenerative disease. Electroencephalogr Clin Neurophysiol 1980;49:437-445.)

ALD, Canavan's disease, Alexander's disease, and multiple sulfatase deficiency, none of the SSEPs were normal (Fig. 25-6).[21] Cortical components were absent in all except the most mildly affected children. In these children the peripheral or cortical component latencies were prolonged depending on the type of leukodystrophy.[21] Tobimatsu and coworkers[20] have demonstrated that MN-SSEPs are valuable in differentiating adrenomyeloneuropathy (AMN) from ALD.[20] In both of these conditions CCT is prolonged, but in AMN the EP potential is also prolonged. SSEP may be more sensitive than the BAEP in demonstrating abnormalities associated with the ALD gene.[16]

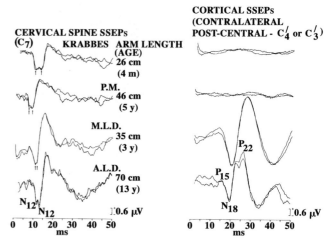

FIGURE 25–6

SSEPs recorded from 4 leukodystrophy patients revealing normal peripheral responses only in the patient with Pelizaeus-Merzbacher disease (PM), and delayed cervical responses in 10 patients with Krabbe's disease, metachromatic leukodystrophy (MLD), and adrenoleukodystrophy (ALD). Cortical SSEPs were absent in the infant-onset leukodystrophies and were delayed in MLD and ALD. (From Fagan ER, Taylor M, Logan WJ: Somatosensory evoked potentials: II. A review of the clinical applications in pediatric neurology. Pediatr Neurol 1987;3:249-255.)

Ataxias

SSEPs have been studied in a variety of neurodegenerative disorders in which ataxia is a major component[18,19] including Friedreich's ataxia, hereditary motor sensory neuropathies (HMSN) I and II, familial spastic paraplegia, olivopontocerebellar atrophy, and ataxia-telangiectasia. Patients with Friedreich's ataxia, olivopontocerebellar atrophy, HMSN-II, and ataxia-telangiectasia frequently have impaired central conduction and normal or slightly prolonged peripheral potential latencies of their MN-SSEPs. In patients with Friedreich's ataxia and HMSN-II, the amplitudes of peripheral nerve potentials were low. Lower extremity SSEPs in patients with Friedreich's ataxia had normal or nearly normal peripheral potential latencies with impairment of transmission within spinal cord afferent pathways. Patients with olivopontocerebellar atrophy usually have normal MN-SSEPs but abnormal lower extremity SSEPs. The patients with HMSN-II and ataxiatelangiectasia usually have normal MN-SSEPs with increased CCT of SSEP with lower extremity testing. Patients with HMSN-I have prolonged latency of EP potential and absence of more rostral potentials consistent with the peripheral disease process. In this study, patients with familial spastic paraplegia had normal SSEPs. Individuals with Friedreich's ataxia had much more severely abnormal SSEPs than those with ataxiatelangiectasia (Fig. 25-7).[19]

FIGURE 25–7

SSEPs from a child with ataxia-telangiectasia (left side) *and a child with Friedreich's ataxia* (right side) *revealing the somewhat poor and noisy recordings typically obtained in these patients. The top traces are from the cervical spine demonstrating the latency of N13 to be within normal limits for both children; however, central conduction was delayed in both, although the abnormality was far more pronounced in the patient with Friedreich's ataxia. Note also the poor morphology and amplitude of the cortical component in Friedreich's ataxia; the SSEPs deteriorate further in this group, such that in the more severely affected patients no SSEP components can be reliably determined. (From Fagan ER, Taylor M, Logan WJ: Somatosensory evoked potentials: II. A review of the clinical applications in pediatric neurology. Pediatr Neurol 1987;3:249-255.)*

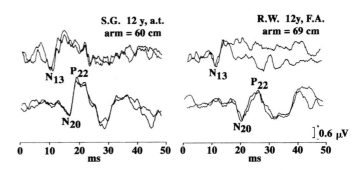

In children with acute cerebellar ataxia the SSEP is usually normal. In children with nonprogressive ataxia, the SSEP is also usually normal.[14] Thus, if a child has an abnormal SSEP in the setting of ataxia, neurodegenerative diseases should be suspected.

Huntington's Chorea

Huntington's disease is a neuropsychiatric disorder caused by the expansion of a CAG trinucleotide repeat. MN-SSEPs and posterior tibial nerve (PTN)-SSEPs are often abnormal in Huntington's chorea.[22-25] An enlarged SSEP has been reported by one group of investigators[25] but not others.[22] A correlation between the decrease in the early component amplitudes (N20 and N30) of the median nerve SEP and the CAG repeat length has been reported, suggesting that these SSEP alterations are related to the genetically determined pathologic process.[24] Children at risk for Huntington's chorea may have amplitude reduction of the cortical EP for the MN-SSEP and PTN-SSEP.[26]

Other Diseases

Metabolic disorders such as aminoacidopathies, neuronal storage diseases, and organic acidemias may demonstrate mild prolongations of CCT. The most profound CCT delays have been seen in Leigh's disease and Krabbe's disease.[27] Abnormalities in spinal cord conduction in patients with juvenile diabetes have been reported.[28]

ASSESSMENT OF HIGH-RISK NEWBORNS

The assessment and prognosis of high-risk newborns can be quite difficult.[29] Assessment via evoked potentials is attractive because it is noninvasive, can be done at the bedside, and can provide quantitative information that can be acquired serially. Numerous studies that evaluate the SSEP in this setting are now provided. Long-latency abnormal cortical components have been reported to occur in 65% of asphyxiated newborns.[30] All patients with persistent abnormalities have clinical evidence of brain injury. In a combined SSEP and BAEP study of 10 infants with hypoxic-ischemic encephalopathy, when studied at 3 months BAEPs were normal or only slightly abnormal while no SSEP cortical components could be detected.[7] Willis and colleagues[31] studied the MN-SSEP in 10 asphyxiated term infants aged 2 to 6 months with subsequent follow-up evaluations to a mean age of 20 months to determine if SSEP findings were predictive of future clinical findings. All children with prolonged latency or unilateral or bilateral absence of the cortical response after MN stimulation experienced subsequent neurologic sequelae. The results of the MN-SSEP correlated with outcome in all patients but were not predictive of the degree of disability.

SSEPs have also been used in the assessment of motor disabilities in children. They reported that the SSEP was more accurate than the EEG in localizing or lateralizing the lesion.[32] Gorke[33] evaluated the prognostic value of the SSEP in infants with cerebral palsy and neurodegenerative and central nervous system (CNS) metabolic diseases. Many infants had prolonged or absent cortical potentials; all of these infants demonstrated fixed disabilities after the 1st year of life. It was concluded that the SSEP was a valuable early indicator of severe motor impairment. However, it was noted that there was a high false-negative rate that was probably related to the exclusive testing of the afferent pathway.

In a study of high-risk neonates, it was found that approximately one third of newborns at risk for neurologic and/or developmental sequelae had abnormal SSEPs consisting of prolongation of absolute cortical latency or CCT, or absence of the scalp-recorded potentials.[34] Patients were subsequently tested at 2 to 3 months of age. Children with prolonged latencies at birth and later normal latencies had mild neurologic deficits; those with absent potentials initially and 3 months later all had spastic quadriparesis.

Bilateral abnormal SSEPs in the neonatal period have also been shown to be associated with developmental delay.[35]

STRUCTURAL AND COMPRESSIVE LESIONS

Structural and compressive lesions may also give rise to abnormal SSEPs depending on the site. Cervical spine lesions such as foramen magnum stenosis are frequently associated with abnormal SSEPs. The extent of abnormality has correlated well with motor delay, hypotonia, and the propensity toward apnea.[27] Patients with extrinsic lesions such as spinal canal stenosis and foramen magnum stenosis secondary to achondroplasia have also been studied. Nelson and coworkers[36] studied the MN-SSEPs and PTN-SSEPs of 23 patients who had achondroplasia with and without symptoms. All symptomatic patients had at least one abnormal SSEP, and 7 (44%) of 16 of asymptomatic patients also had abnormal SSEPs. It was suggested that SSEPs might serve to alert the clinician early in the course about potential problems so that decompressive surgery could be done before serious neurologic compromise occurred.

Intrinsic cervical spine lesions such as those seen in spinal cord gliomas are associated with SSEP abnormalities that have correlated with the severity of clinical involvement. As might be anticipated, structural spinal cord lesions of thoracic and lumbar spine are frequently associated with abnormalities in PTN-SSEPs.[37]

SSEPs continue to play an important role in the evaluation of patients with myelodysplasia and occult spinal dysraphism.[38-40] The large spinal potential normally recorded over the lower thoracic spine is displaced caudally in these children and may be absent altogether (Figs. 25-8 and 25-9). Others have recorded PTN-SSEPs in patients with tethered spinal cord syndrome.[41] To determine the diagnostic usefulness of the SSEP-PTN in tethered cords, Roy and associates[41] studied 22 consecutive children with symptoms of tethered cord syndrome. Results were correlated with clinical, myelographic, and operative findings. In patients with clinical symptoms but no myelographically demonstrable lesions, PTN-SSEPs were within normal limits, suggesting normal function. In patients with myelographically and operatively confirmed tethering dysraphic lesions, PTN-SSEPs were predictive of the level or laterality of the lesion. Similarly, ranking the severity of neurologic

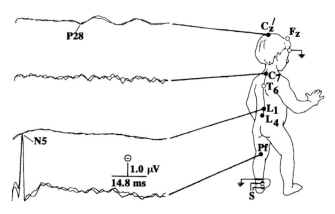

FIGURE 25–8

Abnormal posterior tibial nerve somatosensory evoked potentials of a child with a tethered spinal cord. No potentials from the spinal cord were recorded. Interestingly, the cerebral P28 (equivalent to P37 in the adult) was normal.

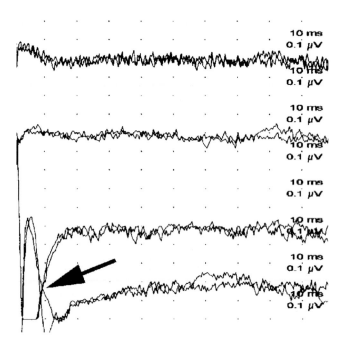

FIGURE 25–9

Absent posterior tibial nerve somatosensory evoked potentials of a child with severe congenital scoliosis with cord compression. No potentials above the popliteal fossa (arrow) were recorded. From top to bottom: CPZ-FPZ, C5s-FPZ, T12-IC, PF-Ref.

impairment and extent of dysraphism at operation, as well as the extent of SSEP abnormality, revealed a significant ($r = 0.81$, $P < 0.001$) correlation between clinical severity and SSEP abnormalities.[41] It has been suggested that tethered cord syndrome produces signs of neurologic impairment by producing subacute hypoxia superimposed on chronic hypoxia of the lumbosacral spinal cord (Fig. 25-10).[42] The

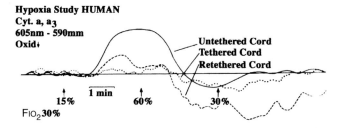

FIGURE 25–10

Redox changes during hypoxia in one group of the human tethered cords (type 1). No redox change is seen before untethering (dotted line), but reduction occurs while the cord is *temporarily retethered (interrupted line).* FIO_2, *fraction of oxygen in the inspired gas mixture.*

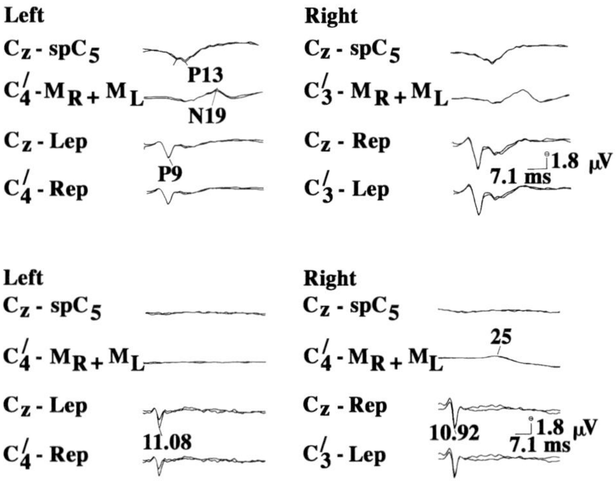

FIGURE 25–11

Top, *Normal median nerve somatosensory evoked potential.* Bottom, *Abnormal median nerve somatosensory evoked potential. On the left in channel 1, note the absence of the obligatory P13, and in channel 2 the absence of the obligatory N19. On the right, note the absence of the obligatory P13 and the prolongation of N19 to 25.0 milliseconds. (From Gilmore RL, Kasarskis EJ, Carr WA, Norvell E: Comparative impact of paraclinical studies in establishing the diagnosis of multiple sclerosis. Electroencephalogr Clin Neurophysiol 1989;73:433-442.)*

effect of hypoxia manifests itself by altered spinal and cortical SSEPs. If the traction is relieved, the SSEP may change in animals[43] as well as in humans.[41]

Structural brainstem lesions such as neoplasms have been frequently associated with abnormalities in both the MN-SSEPs[9] and PTN-SSEPs.[8] They are probably most helpful when used in conjunction with BAEPs. Infants with Möbius' syndrome may have abnormal MN-SSEPs as well.[27] In the evaluation of children suspected of harboring supratentorial brain tumors, SSEPs have been found useful in detecting tumor recurrence.[44]

MULTIPLE SCLEROSIS

Although few patients develop multiple sclerosis during childhood, it is important to be aware of the diagnostic approach. In the last decade the evaluation of patients with suspected multiple sclerosis has been enhanced by the development of multimodality evoked potentials and magnetic resonance imaging (MRI). The diagnosis is based on the clinical demonstration of CNS white matter disease, with multiple lesions occurring at different times in separate anatomic sites. The use of paraclinical studies such as EPs (Fig. 25-11) and MRI permits the clinician to probe the brain and spinal cord in regions which may be clinically "silent" to the examiner. Prior to the introduction of MRI, the role of EPs was well established.[45-50] Of 1000 patients with varying classifications of MS reported in the literature, 58% had abnormal median or digital SSEPs and 76% had abnormal peroneal or tibial SSEPs. In cases classified as definite, probable, or possible multiple sclerosis, the average abnormality rates were 77%, 67%, and 49%, respectively.[51]

Many abnormalities are described in the SSEPs of patients with multiple sclerosis, including absence of centrally generated potentials, preservation of N19 with normal latency and absent N13, and preservation of N13 with absent N19. MRI has been shown to be better than EPs and computed tomography in revealing multiple lesions in the CNS.[43,45] However, VEPs and PTN-SSEPs are methods of choice to evaluate the optic nerve[47,52] and spinal cord[47] in the evaluation of patients suspected of having multiple sclerosis. Hence, the paraclinical evaluation includes MRI, VEPs, and SSEPs.

PERIPHERAL LESIONS

Peripheral nerve plexus and root lesions can also be assessed with SSEPs. Several groups of investigators have reported the findings in patients with Erb's palsy.[14,27,28] If there is a root avulsion, the dorsal root ganglion is intact, an EP potential is recorded, and more rostral components are abnormal (Fig. 25-12).[28] If there is a plexus lesion, the EP potential and more rostral components are absent.

Guillain-Barré Syndrome

Spine-to-scalp "propagation velocities" may be useful for evaluation of proximal peripheral nerves. Schiff and associates[53] reported slowed propagation velocities in Guillain-Barré syndrome. Combinations of prolongation or absence

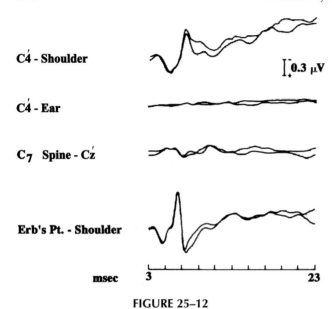

C4 - Shoulder

$\int 0.3 \, \mu V$

C4 - Ear

C7 Spine - Cz

Erb's Pt. - Shoulder

msec   3   23

FIGURE 25–12

Median nerve somatosensory evoked potentials in a 7-year-old girl with severe injury to the brachial plexus at birth. Note that this child has no avulsion, the dorsal root ganglion is intact, and a sensory potential is recorded over Erb's point. Only a P9 is recorded in the C4'-shoulder lead and a barely detectable N9 in the C7 spine-Cz' lead. Potentials are absent in the C4'-ear lead. (From Cracco JB, Bosch VV, Cracco RQ: Cerebral and spinal somatosensory evoked potentials in children with CNS degenerative disease. Electroencephalogr Clin Neurophysiol 1980;49: 437-445.)

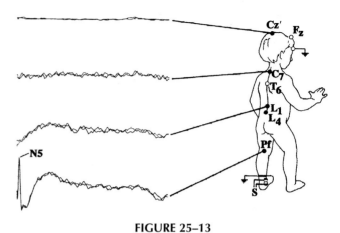

FIGURE 25–13

Posterior tibial nerve somatosensory evoked potentials from a young child with Guillain-Barré syndrome. The time base and polarity are identical to those of Figure 25-8. No potential rostral to the peripheral N5 is identified.

of peripheral potentials and more rostral potentials of MN-SSEP and PTN-SSEPs have also been reported (Fig. 25-13).[15,54] Similar findings have been seen in children as well.[55]

CORTICAL MAPPING

MN-SSEPs have been used to identify primary sensory and motor areas before epilepsy surgery.[56]

SUMMARY

SSEPs are a useful, reliable means of assessing somatosensory systems and gaining indirect information about motor systems in infants and children. The factors of complex maturational changes in the CNS and body growth (reviewed in Chapter 8) complicate the interpretation of SSEPs. In many clinical conditions SSEPs have been useful in diagnosis and prognosis. The full extent of the clinical applications of SSEPs is yet to be explored.

REFERENCES

1. Halliday AM, Wakefield GS: Cerebral evoked potentials in patients with dissociated sensory loss. J Neurol Neurosurg Psychiatry 1963;26:211-219.
2. Frank LM, Furgiuele TL, Etheridge JE: Prediction of chronic vegetative state in children using evoked potentials. Neurology 1985;35:931-934.
3. Lutschg J, Pfenninger J, Ludin HP, et al: Brainstem auditory evoked potentials and early somatosensory evoked potentials in neurointensively treated comatose children. Am J Dis Child 1983;137:421-426.
4. White LE, Frank LM, Furgiuele TL, et al: Prognostic value of BAEP with near- and far-field SSEP in childhood coma. Neurology 1985;35(Suppl 1):199.
5. De Meirleir LJ, Taylor MJ: The prognostic utility of SSEPs in comatose children. Pediatr Neurol 1987;3:78-82.
6. Hume AL, Cant BR: Central somatosensory conduction after head injury. Ann Neurol 1981;10:411-419.
7. Lutschg J, Hanggeli C, Huber P: The evolution of cerebral hemispheric lesions due to pre- or perinatal asphyxia (clinical and neuroradiological correlation). Helv Pediatr Acta 1983;38:245-254.
8. Gilmore RL, Lastimosa ACL: Determination of site and extent of brainstem gliomas using BAEPs and SSEPs. Electroencephalogr Clin Neurophysiol 1983;56:5P.
9. Goldie W, McMahon A: The combined use of BAEPs and SSEPs in the assessment of brainstem dysfunction in children. Electroencephalogr Clin Neurophysiol 1983; 56:35.
10. Goff WR, Shaywitz BA, Goff GD, et al: Somatic evoked potential evaluation of cerebral status in Reye syndrome. Electroencephalogr Clin Neurophysiol 1983;55:388-398.
11. Iragui VJ, Kalmijn J, Thal LJ, Grant I: Neurological dysfunction in asymptomatic HIV-1 infected men: Evidence

from evoked potentials. HNRC Group. Electroencephalogr Clin Neurophysiol 1994;92:1-10.

12. Schmitt B, Seeger J, Kreuz W, et al: Central nervous system involvement of children with HIV infection. Dev Med Child Neurol 1991;33:535-540.

13. Taylor MJ, Fagan ER: Somatosensory evoked potentials: A review of their application in paediatric neurology. *In* Gallai V (ed): Maturation of the CNS and Evoked Potentials. New York, Elsevier, 1986.

14. Fagan ER, Taylor M, Logan WJ: Somatosensory evoked potentials: II. A review of the clinical applications in pediatric neurology. Pediatr Neurol 1987;3:249-255.

15. Cracco JB, Bosch VV, Cracco RQ: Cerebral and spinal somatosensory evoked potentials in children with CNS degenerative disease. Electroencephalogr Clin Neurophysiol 1980;49:437-445.

16. Garg BP, Markand ON, DeMyer WE, Warren C: Evoked response studies in patients with adrenoleukodystrophy and heterozygous relatives. Arch Neurol 1983;40:356-359.

17. Markand O, DeMyer W, Worth R, et al: Multi-modality evoked responses in leukodystrophies. Adv Neurol 1982;32:409.

18. Rossini PM, Zarola F, Di Capu M, et al: Somatosensory evoked potentials in neurodegenerative system disorders. *In* Gallai V (ed): Maturation of the CNS and Evoked Potentials. Amsterdam, Elsevier, 1987.

19. Taylor MJ, Chan-Lui WY, Logan WJ: Longitudinal evoked potential studies in hereditary ataxias. Can J Neurol Sci 1985;12:100-105.

20. Tobimatsu S, Fukui R, Kato M, et al: Multimodality evoked potentials in patients and carriers with adrenoleukodystrophy and adrenomyeloneuropathy. Electroencephalogr Clin Neurophysiol 1985;62:18-24.

21. Fagan ER, Taylor M, Logan WJ: Somatosensory evoked potentials: I. A review of neural generators and special considerations in pediatrics. Pediatr Neurol 1987;3: 189-196.

22. Thompson PD, Bhatia KP, Brown P, et al: Cortical myoclonus in Huntington's disease. Mov Disord 1994;9:633-641.

23. Lefaucheur JP, Bachoud-Levi AC, Bourdet C, et al: Clinical relevance of electrophysiological tests in the assessment of patients with Huntington's disease. Mov Disord 2002;17:1294-1301.

24. Beniczky S, Keri S, Antal A, et al: Somatosensory evoked potentials correlate with genetics in Huntington's disease. NeuroReport 2002;13:2295-2298.

25. Caviness JN, Kurth M: Cortical Myoclonus in Huntington's disease associated with an enlarged somatosensory evoked potential. Mov Disord 1997;12:1046-1051.

26. Noth J, Engel L, Friedemann H, Lange H: Evoked potentials in patients with Huntington's disease and their offspring: I. Somatosensory evoked potentials. Electroencephalogr Clin Neurophysiol 1984;59:134-141.

27. Goldie WD, Spydell JD: Somatosensory evoked potentials following median nerve stimulation in infants: Normative and clinical studies. American EEG Society Workshop: EPs in Children 1987.

28. Cracco JB, Cracco RQ: Spinal, brainstem, and cerebral SEP in the pediatric age group. *In* Bodis-Wollner I (ed): Evoked Potentials. New York, Alan R. Liss, 1986, p 471.

29. Salamy A, Davis S, Eldredge L, et al: Neonatal status: An objective scoring method for identifying infants at risk for poor outcome. Early Hum Dev 1988;17:233-243.

30. Hrbek A, Karlberg P, Kjellmer I, et al: Clinical application of evoked electroencephalographic responses in newborn infants: I. Perinatal asphyxia. Dev Med Child Neurol 1977;19:34-44.

31. Willis J, Duncan C, Bell R: Short latency somatosensory evoked potentials in perinatal asphyxia. Pediatr Neurol 1987;3:350-355.

32. Laget P, Salbreux R, Raimbault J, et al: Relationship between changes in somesthetic evoked responses and electroencephalographic findings in the child with hemiplegia. Dev Med Child Neurol 1988;30:215-221.

33. Gorke W: Somatosensory evoked cortical potentials indicating impaired motor development in infancy. Dev Med Child Neurol 1986;28:633-641.

34. Majnemer A, Rosenblatt B, Riley P, et al: Somatosensory evoked response abnormalities in high-risk newborns. Pediatr Neurol 1987;3:350-355.

35. Klimach VJ, Cooke RW: Short-latency cortical evoked somatosensory evoked responses of preterm infants with ultrasound abnormality of the brain. Dev Med Child Neurol 1988;30:215-221.

36. Nelson FW, Goldie WD, Hecht JT, et al: Short-latency somatosensory evoked potentials in the management of patients with achondroplasia. Neurology 1984;34:1053-1058.

37. Perot PL, Vera CL: Scalp-recorded somatosensory evoked potentials to stimulation of nerves in the lower extremity in the evaluation of patients with spinal cord trauma. Ann N Y Acad Sci 1982;388:526-537.

38. Cracco JB, Cracco RQ: Spinal somatosensory evoked potentials: Maturational and clinical studies. Ann N Y Acad Sci 1982;388:526-537.

39. Emerson RG, Pavlakis SG, Carmel PC, DeVivo DC: Use of spinal somatosensory evoked potentials in the diagnosis of tethered cord. Ann Neurol 1986;20:443-444.

40. Emerson RG: The anatomic and physiologic basis of posterior tibial nerve somatosensory evoked potentials. Neurol Clin 1988;6:705-733.

41. Roy MW, Gilmore R, Walsh JW: Somatosensory evoked potentials in tethered cord syndrome. Electroencephalogr Clin Neurophysiol 1986;64:42P.

42. Yamada S, Zinke DE, Sanders D: Pathophysiology of "tethered cord syndrome." J Neurosurg 1981;54:494-503.

43. Kang JK, Kim MC, Kim DC, Song JU: Effects of tethering on regional spinal cord blood flow and sensory-evoked potentials in growing cats. Child Nerv Syst 1987;3:35-39.

44. Rotteveel JJ, Colon EJ, Hombergen G, Stoelinga GBA, Lippens R: The application of evoked potentials in the diagnosis and follow-up of children with intracranial tumors. Child Nerv Syst 1985;1:172-178.

45. Cutler JR, Aminoff JM, Brant-Zawadzki M: Evaluation of patients with multiple sclerosis by evoked potentials and

magnetic resonance imaging: A comparative study. Ann Neurol 1986;20:645-648.

46. Davis SL, Aminoff MJ, Panitch HS: Clinical correlations of serial somatosensory evoked potentials in multiple sclerosis. Neurology 1985;35:359-365.

47. Gilmore RL, Kasarskis EJ, Carr WA, Norvell E: Comparative impact of paraclinical studies in establishing the diagnosis of multiple sclerosis. Electroencephalogr Clin Neurophysiol 1989;73:433-442.

48. Gilmore RL, Kasarskis EJ, McAllister RG: Verapamil-induced changes in central conduction in patients with multiple sclerosis. J Neurol Neurosurg Psychiatry 1985;48:1140-1146.

49. Green JB, Price R, Woodbury SG: Short-latency somatosensory evoked potentials in multiple sclerosis: Comparison with auditory and visual evoked potentials. Arch Neurol 1980;37:630-633.

50. Kajer M: The value of brainstem auditory, visual, and somatosensory evoked potentials and blink reflexes in the diagnosis of multiple sclerosis. Acta Neurol Scand 1980;62:220-236.

51. Chiappa K: Evoked potentials for diagnosis of multiple sclerosis. Neurol Clin 1988;6:861-880.

52. Miller DH, Newton MR, Van der Poel JC, et al: Magnetic resonance imaging of the optic nerve in optic neuritis. Neurology 1988;38:175-179.

53. Schiff J, Cracco RQ, Rossini PM, et al: Spine and scalp somatosensory evoked potentials in normal subjects and patients with spinal cord disease: Evaluation of afferent transmission. Electroencephalogr Clin Neurophysiol 1984;59:374-387.

54. Nelson KR, Gilmore RL, Massey A: Acoustic nerve conduction abnormalities in Guillain-Barré syndrome. Neurology 1988;38:1263-1266.

55. Gilmore RL, Nelson KR: Electrodiagnosis in Guillain-Barré syndrome in children: Comparison of somatosensory evoked potentials and F-wave studies. Neurology 1986;36(Suppl 1):154.

56. Vossler DG, Wilkus RJ, Pilcher WH, Farwell JR: Epilepsy in schizencephaly: Abnormal cortical organization studied by somatosensory evoked potentials. Epilepsia 1992;33:487-494.

26

Brainstem Auditory Evoked Potentials in Pediatrics—Abnormal

Sandra L. Helmers

In Chapter 9, the anatomy, physiology, and normal developmental changes of brainstem auditory pathways and evoked potentials were discussed. Many aspects of the performance of the tests and the basis of interpretation were presented. The use of wave V threshold determinations or latency-intensity measurements in the evaluation of the peripheral auditory system was also introduced. The clinical use of brainstem auditory evoked potentials (BAEPs) is further illustrated in the evaluation of the central and peripheral auditory system. Especially in pediatrics, BAEPs are extremely useful and, in some cases, the only way to test central auditory pathways, neighboring brainstem regions, and hearing. We are now able to assess hearing in patients we were not able to assess easily 20 to 25 years ago, such as infants, uncooperative children, and comatose patients.[1-5]

When performing and interpreting BAEPs, technical factors are important, and any problems must be corrected to ensure good waveform resolution. This is particularly relevant in children who may not be cooperative. In interpreting studies from children one must be aware of the developmental changes that occur: The younger the patient, the longer the latencies and the more variable the responses. What follows are specific abnormalities one may see using BAEPs in neurologic disorders and the most common peripheral defects a neurologist will encounter.

Specific Abnormalities

The distribution of BAEP parameters is best described as Gaussian, which gives a bell-shaped curve. Therefore,

standard deviations are useful in determining the limits of normality. It is recommended that a laboratory use a range that includes at least 98% of the normal population. A standard deviation of 2.5 (98.8%) to 3.0 (99.7%) is most commonly used by most clinical neurophysiology laboratories.[6,7] Absolute latencies and interpeak latencies that fall outside 2.5 to 3 standard deviations in children are therefore considered to be abnormal.

Latency Abnormalities

The primary generator of wave I is the distal eighth nerve near the cochlea. Therefore, wave I is affected by pathology of the peripheral auditory apparatus, at or distal to this part of the nerve. This includes not only the nerve but the spiral ganglion, middle ear, and external auditory canal. When all waveforms are clearly seen but there is a prolongation of waves I, III, and V absolute latencies with normal interpeak latencies, a peripheral hearing defect is present with normal central conduction from the peripheral eighth nerve to the midbrain. A shorter than normal I-V interpeak latency with prolongation of all absolute latencies has also been described in high-frequency hearing loss. This is likely due to a differential response of the cochlea (apical vs. basal) as a result of the hearing loss, therefore changing the absolute latency of wave I to a greater extent.[7,8] If wave I is absent with a normal III-V interpeak latency, this is also usually due to a peripheral deficit. The conduction of the click stimulus is normal from the lower pons to the midbrain, but the conduction

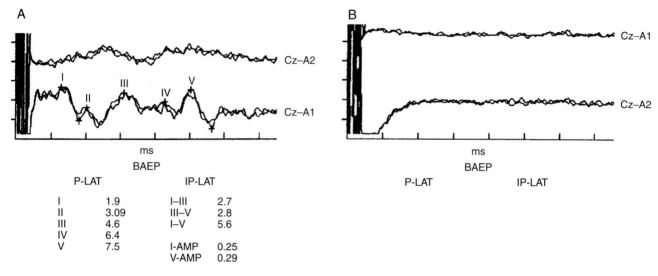

FIGURE 26–1

Bilateral brainstem auditory evoked potentials (BAEPs) in an infant with congenital absence of the right external auditory canal. A, Left ear BAEP, bottom left with well-formed waves I, III, V at normal absolute and interpeak latencies. Responses from the contralateral ear (III, V) are poorly formed or absent. B, Right ear BAEP, bottom right with absence of all waveforms. Responses from the contralateral ear (III, V) are absent.

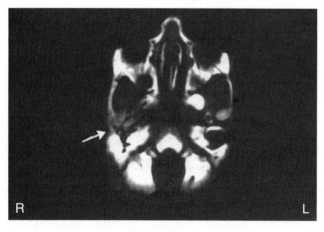

FIGURE 26–2

CT scan showing absence of the external auditory canal on the right (arrow). The patient's brainstem auditory evoked potentials are shown in Figure 26-1.

from the peripheral eighth nerve to the lower pons cannot be determined. When complete absence of responses from one or both ears occurs and is not due to technical difficulties, it suggests a severe conductive hearing loss as seen in Figure 26-1. This infant had a congenital absence of the external auditory canal as shown in the computed tomographic (CT) scan (Fig. 26-2). Severe sensorineural hearing loss or desynchronization of the conducting path-

ways that may take place in multiple sclerosis may also cause absence of all waveforms.[9,10] The conduction of the response to the click stimulus from the peripheral eighth nerve through the brainstem cannot be determined.

Prolongation of the I-III interpeak latency demonstrates a conduction defect in the brainstem auditory system between the distal eighth nerve and the lower pons. When an abnormal increase in the III-V interpeak latency occurs, the conduction defect is in the brainstem auditory system between the lower pons and midbrain.

With monaural stimulation, the responses from each ear should always be compared. If the latencies from both ears are normal, but there is an asymmetry between the sides, a conduction defect from the ear that has the relative prolongation is likely.

Amplitude Abnormalities

Absolute amplitudes are not a reliable indicator of abnormality owing to the large amount of variability. The V/I amplitude ratio is helpful but should be interpreted conservatively, especially in the pediatric population.[11] The ratio can vary with the stimulus intensity and shape of the audiogram, so the V/I amplitude ratio should only be used when the hearing threshold is normal.[7] Wave V is usually about twice the size of wave I. With a significant amplitude loss or absence of wave V, a conduction defect in the brainstem auditory system rostral to the lower pons is suggested.

Lateralization

With monaural stimulation, the brainstem pathology is most commonly ipsilateral to the ear showing the greatest abnormality.[12-14] York[15] studied a patient with a closed head injury and a unilateral brainstem lesion. The most abnormal BAEP was ipsilateral to the brainstem lesion as demonstrated by neuroimaging and pathology. Chiappa and associates[16] studied patients with multiple sclerosis and abnormal BAEPs. The authors reported that 45% of the patients had abnormalities on their BAEPs ipsilateral to their brainstem lesions. Patients with posterior fossa lesions have the most abnormal BAEP ipsilateral to the brainstem lesion.[17]

Clinical Correlation

Audiologic Testing

The BAEP can be helpful in assessing the peripheral auditory system by determining hearing thresholds and the type of hearing defect. The latency-intensity study (LIS) or wave V recognition threshold is quite useful in conjunction with the BAEP, especially in children at risk for hearing impairment.

Deafness or a significant hearing loss is quite common in the United States. Approximately 1 in 750 children have significantly impaired hearing. Screening every infant with BAEPs is impractical. However, there are several factors that can identify an infant at high risk for having a hearing deficit. The American Academy of Pediatrics Joint Committee on Infant Hearing 1994 position statement[18] identified several risk factors for neonates and infants who may develop hearing loss, with 10% to 12% of all newborns being identified and 2.5% to 5.0% of these infants having a significant hearing problem. As one can see, most of these high-risk infants will have been treated in a neonatal intensive care unit (NICU). Therefore, this population should have their hearing assessed within the first few months of life. Schulman-Galambos and colleagues[19] studied 373 high-risk infants who were graduates of the NICU. Using BAEPs, they initially identified 8 patients with a severe peripheral hearing loss while still in the NICU. In follow-up over the year following discharge, these results were confirmed. In a group of 220 normal fullterm infants, no hearing deficits were found. Other studies of high-risk NICU patients have also shown an increased incidence of hearing disabilities with a strong association between the results of the BAEPs and hearing status at 1 year of age.[20-23] These risk factors are shown in Box 26-1.

The purpose of screening this high-risk group of infants is to allow early therapeutic intervention. BAEPs in premature infants must be interpreted cautiously with awareness of the developmental changes in latency and amplitude. It is

---

BOX 26-1
RISK FACTORS ASSOCIATED WITH SENSORINEURAL AND/OR CONDUCTIVE HEARING LOSS

Birth to 28 Days
1. Family history of hereditary childhood sensorineural hearing loss
2. In utero infection, e.g., cytomegalovirus, rubella, syphilis, herpes, toxoplasmosis
3. Craniofacial anomalies including abnormalities of the pinna and ear canal
4. Birthweight < 1500 gm
5. Hyperbilirubinemia at a serum level requiring exchange transfusion
6. Ototoxic medications including but limited to medications such as multiple courses of aminoglycosides or use in combination with loop diuretics
7. Bacterial meningitis
8. Apgar scores of 0-4 at 1 minute or 0-6 at 5 minutes
9. Mechanical ventilation lasting ≥ 5 days
10. Stigmata or other findings associated with a syndrome known to include sensorineural and/or conductive hearing loss

29 Days Through 2 Years
1. Parent/caregiver concern with hearing, speech, language, and/or developmental delay
2. Bacterial meningitis or other infections associated with sensorineural hearing loss
3. Head trauma associated with loss of consciousness or skull fracture
4. Stigmata or other findings associated with a syndrome known to include a sensorineural and/or conductive hearing loss
5. Ototoxic medications including but limited to such medications as multiple courses of aminoglycosides, or use in combination with loop diuretics
6. Recurrent or persistent otitis media with effusion for at least 3 months

29 Days Through 3 Years in Those Who Require Periodic Monitoring of Hearing to Detect Delayed-Onset Sensorineural and/or Conductive Hearing Loss
1. Family history of hereditary childhood hearing loss
2. In utero infection, e.g., cytomegalovirus, rubella, syphilis, herpes, toxoplasmosis

Continued

also recommended that follow-up studies be performed in preterm infants. Other problems such as antibiotic usage,[24] middle ear effusions, serous otitis media, or meningitis[25] may also cause reversible abnormalities of the BAEPs, warranting follow-up studies. We recommend that whenever a BAEP is abnormal, a follow-up study be repeated with further audiologic testing by an audiologist. This ensures that hearing aids are not used inappropriately in the case of a reversible abnormality. Serial abnormalities on BAEPs are far more useful in determining eventual outcome than a single study. Because a hearing impairment can be globally detrimental to the development of the child, detection of a hearing deficit with early intervention is imperative.

Audiologic testing can be done with behavioral and nonbehavioral techniques. Behavioral audiometry requires cooperation of the patient that may not be possible in children. Either the patient is too young, or cannot sit still long enough for the full test battery, or will just not comply with the examiner's wishes. In these situations nonbehavioral BAEP testing using BAEPs and LISs are optimal. Using BAEPs, one is able to evaluate the peripheral and central auditory components up to the level of the midbrain. A hearing threshold can also be obtained. This can be done by behavioral and nonbehavioral techniques.[26-34]

The LIS is performed monaurally by decreasing the click stimulus intensity and measuring wave V. The rate of stimulation can be increased to 40/sec or more to allow a quicker performance without significantly attenuating wave V. With decreasing intensities, the latencies of waves I, III, and V increase while the absolute amplitudes decrease, eventually disappearing. Wave I is usually the first waveform to disappear followed by wave III. Wave V is the last wave to disappear and is therefore a good indicator of peripheral auditory activity. The intensity at which wave V disappears is the threshold of hearing. The use of a 30-dB nHL cutoff level in the screening of infants and young children seems to be a sensitive predictor of a child at high risk for hearing loss. Failure to obtain wave V with stimulation intensities above 30 dB is a worrisome finding (Fig. 26-3). The severity of the impairment can be determined by increasing the intensity of the click until a wave V is recognized.

A normal LIS is not a guarantee of normal hearing thresholds. The click is a mixed-frequency stimulus. If there is at least some part of the frequency range intact, the LIS may be normal. In addition, if wave V is poorly formed in the routine BAEP, the LIS will be difficult or impossible to perform.

There are two types of abnormality seen on the LIS.[35,36] A conductive hearing loss interferes with the effectiveness of transmission of the stimulus to the cochlea. This can delay all waves and causes a shift of the latency-intensity curve to the right (Fig. 26-4), with the shift corresponding to the amount of hearing deficit. The second pattern is seen with a cochlear or sensorineural hearing loss. The latency of wave V is normal at high intensities and rapidly increases or disappears with a decrease in the stimulus intensity (Fig. 26-5). Use of the LIS and BAEPs can help the clinician determine where the hearing loss is, possible etiologies, and more appropriate treatments.

BAEPs may be useful in ruling out abnormalities in auditory transmission through the brainstem in patients with tinnitus. Figure 26-6 demonstrates a normal BAEP in a 16-year-old girl with tinnitus.

Neurologic Testing

In children, as in adults, BAEPs are a valuable tool not only in assessing hearing but as part of a neurologic evaluation. BAEPs are helpful when a degenerative or demyelinating disease is suspected. Another more common problem in pediatrics in which BAEPs are helpful is in the diagnosis of brainstem or posterior fossa tumors. Evaluation and prognosis in encephalopathies and coma using BAEPs can also be useful. Brainstem responses can also be monitored intraoperatively during neurosurgical procedures.

BAEP IN SPECIFIC DISORDERS

In this section, disorders in which BAEP studies may be helpful are reviewed.

White Matter Disorders

Leukodystrophies

In white matter diseases the pathologic lesion is demyelination or dysmyelination, and BAEPs are often abnormal, with prolonged latencies of waveforms. As the disease progresses, there is a disappearance of waves II to V. A number of authors have found prolonged absolute and interpeak latencies in children with metachromatic leukodystrophy.[2,37,38]

Adrenoleukodystrophy frequently results in abnormal BAEPs.[37,39,40] The degree of the BAEP abnormality appears to be related to the severity and stage of the condition. Asymptomatic patients may have abnormalities.[39-41]

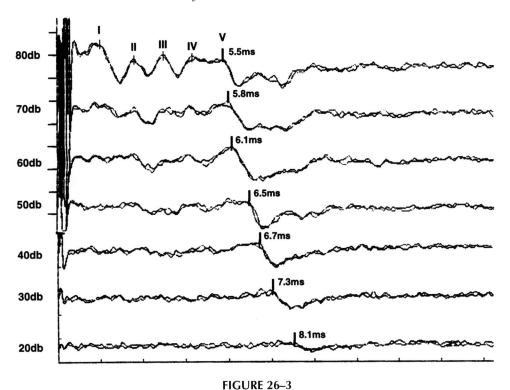

FIGURE 26–3

Latency-intensity study beginning at 80 dB, with decreasing stimulus intensity to 20 dB. Absolute latencies of waves I, III, and V increase as the stimulus intensity decreases. The amplitude decreases in all responses as the stimulus intensity decreases until waveforms disappear.

In the infantile forms of white matter disease (Krabbe's disease and Pelizaeus-Merzbacher disease), the BAEP abnormalities are severely abnormal. Typically, the early waveforms are usually the only ones seen. Ochs and associates[37] studied seven children with Pelizaeus-Merzbacher disease and found an absence of all components after wave II. Garg,[42] Hodes,[43] and their colleagues recorded BAEPs in infants with an abnormal neurologic examination with nystagmus and an extensive family history for Pelizaeus-Merzbacher disease. The BAEPs showed well-formed waves I with normal latencies and absence of waves III to V.

Multiple Sclerosis

Multiple sclerosis is another white matter disorder that can occur in children, with the BAEPs being very helpful in the neurologic workup. BAEPs can identify silent lesions in the brainstem, thus helping to solidify a diagnosis in equivocal cases. Various investigators[8,16,44] have studied adults with definite, probable, and possible multiple sclerosis using BAEPs. The percentage of patients with abnormal BAEPs was greatest in the definite group (47% to 90%). The percentages were less in the probable and possible groups (21% to 67%). There was a higher percentage of abnormalities if brainstem signs or symptoms

were present. The types of abnormalities ranged from no responses, to interwave latency prolongation, to abnormalities of the V/I amplitude ratio.

Central Pontine Myelinolysis

BAEPs have been examined in a few adults with central pontine myelinolysis. The I-V interpeak latencies were markedly prolonged at the peak of the illness. As the patient improved clinically, the BAEPs showed improvement.[45,46] There are no reports of BAEPs in children with central pontine myelinolysis.

Gray Matter Disorders

Gray matter diseases in general tend to produce abnormalities on the EEG but do not tend to affect BAEPs to a significant degree.[38] BAEPs in neuronal ceroid lipofuscinosis have been unremarkable.[47-49]

Spinocerebellar Degeneration

In Friedreich's ataxia the BAEPs are usually abnormal, although most patients have good hearing function. The abnormalities range from poorly formed responses and absence of one or more waveforms to prolonged interpeak

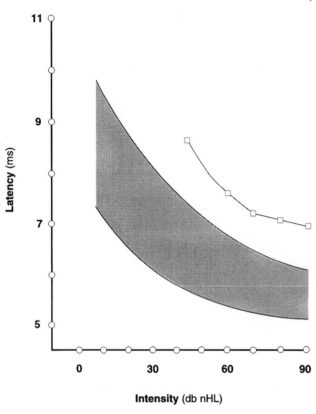

FIGURE 26–4
Latency-intensity curve in a conductive hearing loss. The curve is shifted to the right as compared with a normal latency-intensity study.

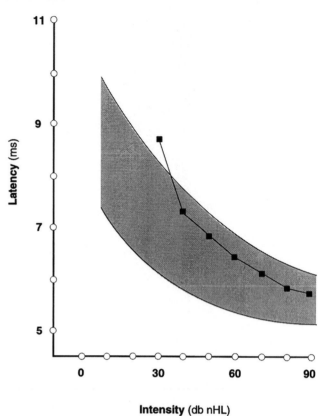

FIGURE 26–5
Latency-intensity curve in a cochlear or sensorineural hearing loss. At high intensities the curve is normal, but it rapidly shifts to the right with a decrease in the stimulus intensity.

latencies and elevated latency-intensity thresholds.[50-53] The various alterations are thought to be due to degeneration and selective damage to spinal ganglion neurons. In cases of atypical Friedreich's ataxia, cerebellar degenerations, and olivopontocerebellar atrophy, the BAEPs are usually, but not always, abnormal.[2,52,54-59]

Mucopolysaccharidoses

BAEPs have often been abnormal in patients with mucopolysaccharidoses.[60-62] A total of 15 subjects with either Hurler's (5 patients), Hunter's (7 patients), or Sanfilippo's (3 patients) disease were reported by Calogero and coworkers.[38] All 15 had a peripheral hearing deficit. In some of these cases, the BAEPs showed a shift in all absolute latencies with almost complete absence of wave I thought to be attributable to the peripheral hearing deficit. In others, there was an increase in the I-V interpeak latency. In a few of their subjects, all responses were absent, which was thought to be due to the severe degree of hearing loss.

Copper Metabolism

In Wilson's disease, BAEPs have been reported to be abnormal in patients with neurologic symptoms.[63-65] Interpeak latencies are typically prolonged. The presence or absence of BAEP abnormalities is related to clinical symptoms and signs. Patients with symptoms are more likely to have abnormal recordings than asymptomatic patients.[58] The 3 asymptomatic patients they studied had normal BAEPs. Menkes' disease, a rare disorder of copper metabolism, has been associated with abnormal BAEPs.[3]

Progressive Myoclonic Epilepsy

Patients with Lafora's disease often show progressive changes in their BAEPs as the disease progresses.[66] However, Aguglia and associates[67] studied five patients with the diagnosis of Lafora's disease who had normal BAEPs.

Kasai and colleagues[68] found that patients with dentatorubral-pallidoluysian atrophy had absent BAEPs, whereas patients with other forms of progressive myoclonic

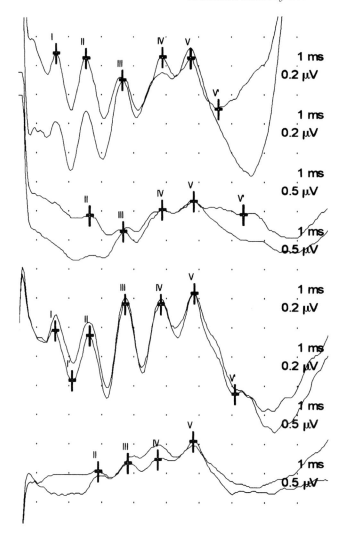

FIGURE 26–6

Normal brainstem auditory evoked potentials in a 16-year-old girl with tinnitus. The first two channels are with left ear stimulation (ipsilateral and contralateral), and the second two traces are with right ear stimulation. The stimulation frequency was 11.1 Hz at 85 dB.

epilepsy such as Unverricht-Lundborg disease had normal BAEPs. Patients with myoclonic epilepsy with ragged-red fibers (MERRF) have variable BAEPs.[69] Patients with MERRF who do have abnormal BAEPs often have a primary problem in the cochlea, although a retrocochlear lesion may be involved in some patients.

Basal Ganglia Disorders

Huntington's disease rarely begins in children. In adult patients BAEPs are usually normal.[70] Likewise, other disorders of the basal ganglia rarely alter BAEPs (Parkinson's disease, Hallervorden-Spatz disease, progressive supranuclear palsy), BAEPs are usually normal.[71]

Disorders of Amino Acid Metabolism

A number of disorders of amino acid metabolism can result in abnormal BAEPs, including maple syrup urine disease,[2] phenylketonuria,[2,38,72] homocystinuria,[38] and hyperglycinemia.[48,73] BAEPs may be useful in following the response to treatment in metabolic disorders.

Mitochondrial Disorders

Mitochondrial disorders are responsible for a variety of neurologic syndromes, some of which have progressive hearing loss. BAEPs have been useful in detecting audiologic abnormalities in children with a variety of mitochondrial encephalomyopathies,[74] including MERRF[69]: mitochondrial myopathy, encephalopathy, lactic acidosis, and strokelike episodes; Leigh's disease[2,48,75,76]; and Kearnes-Sayre syndrome.[3]

Rett's Syndrome

BAEP abnormalities are common in Rett's syndrome.[77,78] Wu and associates[77] reported on 9 girls with Rett's syndrome. Five of the 9 had BAEPs with a prolonged wave I latency and 3 had an increased threshold. In a large study of 81 girls with Rett's syndrome, sensorineural hearing loss was in 17.3% of the 162 ears tested and conductive involvement was observed in 9.9%.[78] Neither the type of hearing loss nor the presence of preserved speech seemed to be correlated with the type of mutation in methyl-CpG-binding protein 2 (*MeCP2*) gene that is associated with Rett's syndrome.

Tumors

Although neuroimaging using magnetic resonance imaging (MRI) is the most important diagnostic test in children with tumors, BAEPs can be a useful adjunct in the work-up of brainstem tumors. Intrinsic and extrinsic tumors in the posterior fossa are more common in children than in adults. BAEPs are usually abnormal with a brainstem tumor. They are easily performed; they are noninvasive; and they are usually able to indicate the level and side of the brainstem lesion. Abnormalities after wave III indicate a lesion central to the lower pons, with the lesion on the side with the more abnormal response. BAEP alterations after wave I and before wave III suggest a lesion of the auditory nerve or lower pons, again with the lesion on the side with the most abnormal responses. The BAEP alterations in brainstem tumors can range from prolonged interpeak latencies to poorly formed or absent waveforms.[3,79-81] Serial BAEPs can also be useful in assessing efficacy of treatment.

Intrinsic Brainstem Tumors

Brainstem tumors often result in BAEP abnormalities, with the type of abnormality corresponding to the location of the tumor. Pontine gliomas typically result in delayed latencies for waves III-V with reduction of amplitude or even loss of the waveforms.[12,82] Depending on the location of the tumor, responses may be asymmetrical.[81-84] In a series of 14 children with brainstem gliomas, 13 had abnormalities of the BAEPs.[81] In 1 case, the patient had a glioma of the medulla with normal BAEPs. The lesion was predominantly caudal to the eighth nerve entry zone (Fig. 26-7).

Extrinsic Brainstem Tumors

Other posterior fossa tumors may occur that are extrinsic to the brainstem such as medulloblastomas, cerebellar

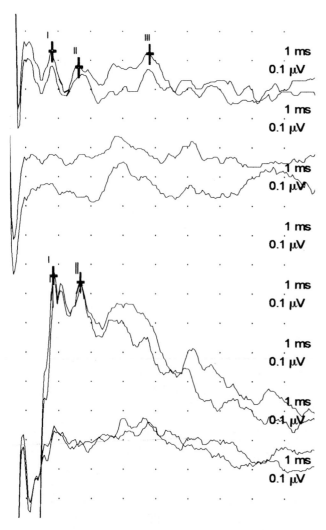

FIGURE 26–7

Brainstem auditory evoked potentials in a 7-year-old child with probable brainstem glioma. Well-defined waveforms above wave II were absent. The first two channels are left ear stimulation (ipsilateral and contralateral), and the second two channels are right ear stimulation. The stimulation frequency was 11.1 Hz at 85 dB.

astrocytomas, neurofibromas, and acoustic neuromas. In a patient complaining of vertigo, tinnitus, or hearing loss and a retrocochlear lesion is suspected, the BAEPs are helpful in screening for these lesions.[82,84-86] In disorders such as Menière's disease or other labyrinthine abnormalities, the BAEP is normal; if the BAEP is abnormal, a further evaluation may be indicated.[87]

Patients with cerebellar pontine angle tumors including neurofibromas have abnormal BAEPs.[88] The most common alteration is a unilateral prolongation of waves III-V or wave V alone. A smaller number of these patients showed a unilateral distortion or absence of waveforms. Posterior fossa masses frequently lead to abnormalities of the BAEPs due to brainstem compression.[12]

In acoustic neuromas, BAEPs are a highly sensitive screening test, comparable to enhanced CT scans and MRIs. The detection rate for BAEPs in suspected acoustic neuromas is 98%.[89] The most sensitive abnormality on the BAEP that indicates a lesion of the eighth nerve secondary to an acoustic neuroma is an ipsilateral prolonged I-III interpeak latency. Other abnormalities have been described with acoustic neuromas and include a normal wave I with poorly formed or absent later waves. All waveforms may be absent, or the III-V, I-V interpeak latencies may be prolonged (Figs. 26-8 and 26-9). Contralateral abnormalities may be superimposed on these ipsilateral alterations.[90] These abnormalities seem to be due to distortion and cross-compression of the brainstem by a large tumor. In other CPA masses, BAEPs are less sensitive owing to the fact that the eighth nerve or brainstem auditory pathways may not be involved until the mass is rather large, at which time one presents with signs and symptoms referable to other regions of the brainstem.

Brainstem Hemorrhages and Contusions

Hemorrhages and contusions that involve the pons or lower midbrain are usually associated with abnormal BAEPs. The alterations of the responses are similar to those discussed with intrinsic brainstem lesions. The abnormalities closely correspond to the location of the lesion.[12,14,82,84]

Arnold-Chiari Malformation and Other Brain Malformations

In a study of 37 asymptomatic neonates with myelomeningocele, BAEPs were done within the first days of life.[91] Twelve of these infants later developed brainstem dysfunction. Of these 12 infants, 11 had abnormal brainstem conduction on the BAEPs. Of the remaining 25 infants who did not develop brainstem problems, only 10 had abnormalities of their BAEPs. Thus, BAEPs in

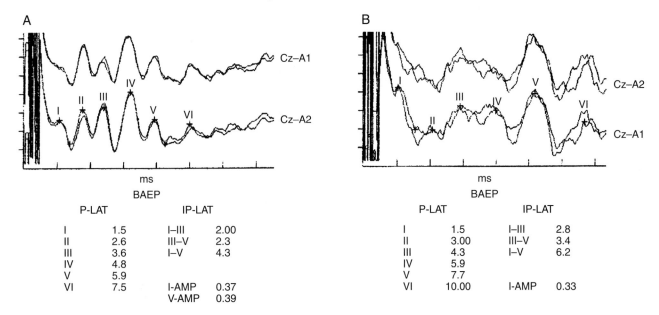

A

Cz–A1

Cz–A2

ms

BAEP

P-LAT		IP-LAT	
I	1.5	I–III	2.00
II	2.6	III–V	2.3
III	3.6	I–V	4.3
IV	4.8		
V	5.9		
VI	7.5	I-AMP	0.37
		V-AMP	0.39

B

Cz–A2

Cz–A1

ms

BAEP

P-LAT		IP-LAT	
I	1.5	I–III	2.8
II	3.00	III–V	3.4
III	4.3	I–V	6.2
IV	5.9		
V	7.7		
VI	10.00	I-AMP	0.33

FIGURE 26–8

Bilateral brainstem auditory evoked potentials (BAEPs) in a child with an acoustic neuroma. A, Right BAEP on the left, showing well-formed waves I, III, and V ipsilaterally and III and V contralaterally with normal absolute and interpeak latencies. B, Left BAEP on the right, showing poorly formed waves III, V ipsilaterally and contralaterally with prolonged absolute and interpeak latencies.

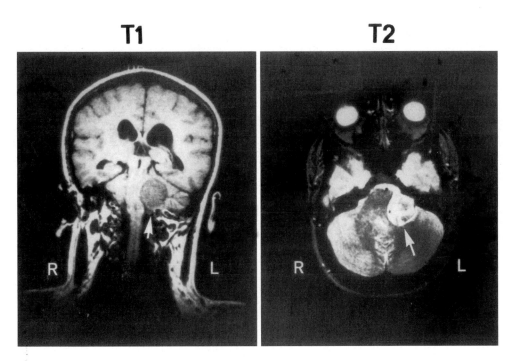

T1   **T2**

FIGURE 26–9

MRI (T1 and T2) showing an acoustic neuroma on the left (arrows).

neonates with myelomeningoceles may be able to identify infants at risk for brainstem dysfunction.[91]

BAEPs may be useful in evaluating patients for surgical management with both Chiari I and II malformations.[92-94]

BAEPs may be useful in assessing brainstem function in children with developmental brain anomalies (Fig. 26-10).

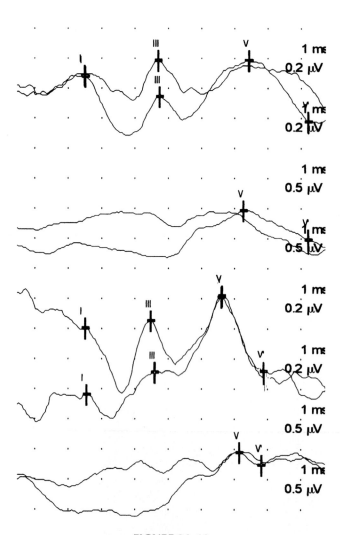

FIGURE 26–10

Brainstem auditory evoked potentials in a 1-year-old child with cerebral dysgenesis and a small brainstem on MRI scan. The first two channels are with left ear stimulation (ipsilateral and contralateral), and the second two traces are with right ear stimulation. The stimulation frequency was 11.1 Hz at 85 dB. The absolute latencies of wave I = 2.48 milliseconds left, 2.54 milliseconds right; wave III = 4.69 milliseconds left, 4.58 milliseconds right; and wave V = 7.36 milliseconds left, 6.60 milliseconds right were all above normal. The I-III interpeak latency was normal bilaterally, but the II-V interpeak latency was prolonged.

Coma and Brain Death

In general, evaluating patients in coma, the BAEPs are limited in predicting clinical outcome. Each patient must be individually considered with regard to the etiology of the coma.[95,96] Patients in coma from toxic or metabolic causes may have normal BAEPs[97] or interpeak latency prolongation.[98]

The severity of the BAEP abnormalities is correlated with outcome.[99,100] Kaga and associates[99] demonstrated that a staging classification based on BAEPs in acutely comatose patients was correlated with the neurologic outcome. Although their patients had various causes for their coma, the most common cause was head trauma. Patients with normal BAEPs had a better outcome than those with abnormal BAEPs. Similar conclusions were reached for patients who were comatose from drowning.[100] Hecox and Cone[83] reported 21 infants who suffered from asphyxia and were comatose. In comatose infants suffering from hypoxic-ischemic encephalopathy, a markedly abnormal V/I amplitude ratio was useful in determining ultimate neurologic outcome, although a normal ratio did not ensure a normal outcome.

The BAEP can be complementary to neuroimaging with MRI in severe head trauma.[100] Since BAEPs are unaffected by high doses of barbiturates, they are useful in assessing neurologic status when barbiturate coma is induced. Since BAEPs evaluate the brainstem auditory system only up to the inferior collicular region, their ability to predict neurologic outcome is only fair. BAEPs can be normal with lesions above this level.[101-107]

In brain death, BAEPs may also be helpful as a noninvasive adjunct to the physical examination.[108] Absence of waveforms central to wave I are significantly correlated with brain death.[109] Steinhart and Weiss[110] studied 23 comatose children. These children were subdivided into two groups based on physical examinations consistent with brain death or preservation of some brainstem/cortical function. BAEPs in the brain-dead group revealed only wave I or complete absence of all responses. This is in comparison with the BAEPs in the non–brain-dead children who showed at least two waveforms: wave I and usually wave V. All of the non–brain-dead children had waveforms despite the use of high-dose barbiturates for treatment of increased intracranial pressure. All of the clinically brain-dead children died, whereas only 2 of the 13 died in the second group. In the brain-dead group, the absence of all waves including wave I is thought to be related to the cessation of intracranial circulation, interfering with the blood supply to the eighth nerve. Absence of waves must be interpreted with care since a disruption of the peripheral auditory apparatus could lead to an absence of waveforms. This may occur with fractures of the temporal bone, hemotympanum, middle ear effusions, or previous sensorineural hearing loss.[82,111]

Therefore, BAEPs are a useful adjunct to the physical examination of the brain-dead patient. The use of BAEPs to predict neurologic outcome in comatose patients is more controversial, and the etiology of the coma must be taken into consideration.

Intraoperative Monitoring

BAEPs are not affected significantly by general anesthesia.[112] This makes it possible to use BAEPs intraoperatively to monitor brainstem function. The surgical procedures in which BAEPs have been used most commonly involve the eighth nerve or surrounding region and brainstem/posterior fossa surgery.

Intraoperative BAEP monitoring is useful in preventing auditory deficits due to intraoperative damage involving the eighth nerve or brainstem. If a surgical complication occurs, continuous BAEP surgical monitoring can indicate the time of injury and may localize the lesion. The type of changes seen with the intraoperative BAEPs may also help define the pathophysiology and prognosis of the lesion. For a more complete discussion of intraoperative BAEP monitoring, the reader is referred to Lüders[23] and John and coworkers.[113]

Miscellaneous

Anemia. BAEPs have been shown to be abnormal, with increased absolute and interpeak latencies, in children with a prior history of iron deficiency anemia,[114] although the abnormality may take time to develop.[115,116] BAEPs have been demonstrated to be abnormal during sickle cell crises.[117]

Toxins and Drugs. BAEPs are a sensitive indicator of lead poisoning in young children, with longer latencies in children with elevated lead levels.[118] BAEP abnormalities were seen even in children without symptoms of lead intoxication. Some antiepileptic drugs have been associated with changes in peak latencies of BAEPs, although the clinical significance of these findings is unclear.[119]

Angelman's Syndrome. In Angelman's syndrome the thresholds for wave V have been reported to be elevated along with a prolongation of wave I.[120] It has been shown that some patients with Angelman's syndrome develop deafness, but since few patients with Angelman's syndrome have had BAEPs, the significance of the described BAEP abnormalities is not clear.

Arthrogryposis Multiplex Congenita. BAEPs have been used as an adjunct to the physical examination and other testing in the evaluation of infants with arthrogryposis multiplex congenita.[121] In infants with brainstem signs, the BAEPs were helpful.

Behavioral Disorders. Abnormal BAEPs have been reported in autistic children.[122] In conjunction with other studies, it is postulated that autistic children have a diffuse brain lesion.

Bell's Palsy. BAEPs have been variable in patients with Bell's palsy; both normal[123] and abnormal results have been reported.[124] There was no significant relationship between the abnormal BAEP, stapedial reflex, or affected side.

Down Syndrome. It has been reported by several investigators that the amplitudes of all the BAEP components were significantly larger in patients with Down syndrome than in normal subjects.[125,126] Increased thresholds were also reported in Down syndrome by Widen and associates.[126]

Hereditary Motor Sensory Neuropathy. BAEPs were abnormal in several studies on people with hereditary motor sensory neuropathies (HMSN) I and II, usually showing a prolonged I-III interpeak latency or poorly formed responses. This was more commonly seen in adults with HMSN. Thus, BAEPs were useful in detecting subclinical involvement of the central nervous system.[56,59,127,128] In familial dysautonomia, the absolute latencies of waves III and V along with the I-V interpeak latency were significantly higher than control, suggesting that the mid to upper brainstem is also involved in the disease process.[129]

Hydrocephalus. Abnormal BAEPs have been reported in hydrocephalus. Wave V has also been reported to be of very low amplitude or absent, making assessment of the brainstem conduction time and midbrain neurophysiologic function difficult or impossible. This can also make the LIS impossible to perform.[4]

Hyperbilirubinemia. Elevated bilirubin level in infants is a risk factor for hearing impairment and has been associated with abnormalities of the BAEPs and thresholds.[130] The latencies of wave V and the I-V and III-V interpeak latencies can improve significantly with phototherapy.

Hypothyroidism. Hypothyroidism can be associated with altered BAEPs.[38,131] Treatment of the hypothyroidism can result in normalization or shortening of the absolute latencies.[132] Premature infants with low serum thyroxine levels were studied by Kohelet and coworkers.[133] The infants were compared to euthyroid premature infants, and no significant differences in the absolute or interpeak latencies were found.

Hysteria and Malingering. BAEPs can be helpful in evaluation of hysterical or malingering patients. An abnormal response is a reliable indicator of an organic lesion. Likewise, a normal BAEP can be useful in supporting the diagnosis of hysteria or malingering.[134]

Language Disorders

Auditory Processing. In developmentally aphasic children with receptive disorders, the absolute latencies of waves I, III, and V were found to be significantly shorter than in control children.[135]

Autism. Children with autism often have abnormal BAEPs. In 101 children with autism undergoing testing the II-V interpeak latency and the latencies of waves I and V were also significantly prolonged in both boys and girls with autism, compared with controls.[136] In this study more than half of the children had an abnormality with BAEP testing. Wong and Wong[137] performed BAEPs in 109 children with infantile autism and compared the results with BAEPs from children with autistic condition, mental retardation, and normal children. They found prolonged latencies of wave V and all interpeak measurements in the autistic children. This suggests an abnormality in brainstem function in autism (see Chapter 12).

Learning Disabilities. BAEPs have been found to be abnormal in children with learning disorders by some authors[122] but not others.[138] The causes of learning disabilities are heterogeneous, and whether BAEPs are abnormal likely depends on the cause of the learning disability. BAEPs do not assess the cortical auditory system. In disorders of auditory perception or cortical deafness, the BAEPs are normal. Therefore, these patients will not benefit from a hearing aid.

Malnutrition. BAEPs have been reported to be abnormal in severely malnourished children with kwashiorkor.[139] With treatment of the malnutrition, the abnormalities may resolve.[140]

Myotonic Dystrophy. Some patients with myotonic dystrophy have been shown to have abnormal BAEPs.[141]

Neurofibromatosis. There is a high incidence of tumors in patients with neurofibromatosis. Acoustic tumors are particularly common in patients with neurofibromatosis. BAEPs can be helpful in the evaluation of these patients, because lesions are identified fairly early and noninvasively.[142,143]

Postinfectious Illness. Brainstem alterations may occur in bacterial meningitis.[144] Abnormalities include prolonged latencies, unilateral or bilateral absent responses, and prolonged interwave intervals. These findings are most commonly due to middle and inner ear disturbances. A permanent hearing defect may occur as a consequence of the meningitis or from therapy with aminoglycosides. Brainstem responses are useful in evaluating these high-risk infants and children.[2,25] Although many of the abnormalities improve with time, children with absent responses typically have permanent damage.[144]

Sudden Infant Death Syndrome (SIDS). Patients with near-SIDS have normal BAEPs.[145,146] BAEPs appear to have no value in predicting whether an infant is at risk for SIDS.

REFERENCES

1. Barajas JJ, Olaozola F, Tapia MC, et al: Audiometric study of the neonate: Impedance audiometry—behavioural responses and brain stem audiometry. Audiology 1981;20:41-52.
2. Hecox KE, Cone B, Blaw ME: Brainstem auditory evoked response in the diagnosis of pediatric neurologic diseases. Neurology 1981;31:832-839.
3. Picton TW, Taylor MJ, Durieux-Smith A, Edwards CG: Brainstem auditory evoked potentials in pediatrics. *In* Aminoff MJ (ed): Electrodiagnosis in Clinical Neurology. New York, Churchill Livingstone, 1986, p 505.
4. Picton TW, Taylor MJ, Durieux-Smith A, Edwards CG: Brainstem auditory evoked potentials in pediatrics. *In* Aminoff MJ (ed): Electrodiagnosis in Clinical Neurology, 2nd ed. New York, Churchill Livingstone, 1992, p 537.
5. Warren MP: The auditory brainstem response in pediatrics. Otolaryngol Clin North Am 1989;22:473-500.
6. American Electroencephalographic Society: Guidelines for clinical evoked potential studies. J Clin Neurophysiol 1984;1:3-53.
7. Chiappa KH: Brainstem auditory evoked potentials: Interpretation. *In* Chiappa KH (ed): Evoked Potentials in Clinical Medicine. New York, Raven Press, 1990, p 223.
8. Tedeschi G, Allocca S, Di Costanzo A, et al: The contribution of saccadic eye movements analysis, visual and auditory evoked responses to the diagnosis of multiple sclerosis. Clin Neurol Neurosurg 1989;91:123-128.
9. Hildesheimer M, Muchnik C, Rubinstein M: Problems in interpretation of brainstem-evoked response audiometry results. Audiology 1985;24:374-379.
10. Kraus N, Özdamar Ö, Stein L, Reed N: Absent auditory brain stem response: Peripheral hearing loss or brain stem dysfunction? Laryngoscope 1984;94:400-406.
11. Psatta DM, Mate M: Incidence of brain stem auditory evoked potential amplitude disorders in oto-neurologic pathology. Rev Roum Med Neurol Psychiatry 1987;25:145-160.
12. Hashimoto I, Ishiyama Y, Tozuka G: Bilaterally recorded brain stem auditory evoked responses: Their asymmetric abnormalities and lesions of the brain stem. Arch Neurol 1979;36:161-167.
13. Musiek FE, Guerkink NA: Auditory brain stem response and central auditory test findings for patients with brainstem lesions: A preliminary report. Laryngoscope 1982;92:891-900.
14. Oh SJ, Kuba T, Aoyer A, et al: Lateralization of brainstem lesions by brainstem auditory evoked potentials. Neurology 1981;31:14-18.
15. York DH: Correlation between a unilateral midbrain-pontine lesion and abnormalities of brain-stem auditory evoked potential. Electroencephalogr Clin Neurophysiol 1986;65:282-288.
16. Chiappa KH, Harrison JL, Brooks EB, Young RR: Brainstem auditory evoked responses in 200 patients with multiple sclerosis. Ann Neurol 1980;7:135-143.

17. Brown RH, Chiappa KH, Brooks EB: Brainstem auditory evoked responses in 22 patients with intrinsic brainstem lesions: Implications for clinical interpretations. Electroencephalogr Clin Neurophysiol 1981;51:38.

18. American Academy of Pediatrics Joint Committe on Infant Hearing: Position statement 1994. Pediatrics 1994;70:496-497.

19. Schulman-Galambos C, Galambos R: Brain stem evoked audiometry in newborn hearing screening. Arch Otolaryngol 1979;105:86-90.

20. Bradford BC, Baudin J, Conway MJ, et al: Identification of sensory neural hearing loss in very preterm infants by brainstem auditory evoked potentials. Arch Dis Child 1985;60:105-109.

21. Duara S, Suter CM, Bessard KK, Gutberlet RL: Neonatal screening with auditory brainstem responses: Results of follow-up audiometry and risk factor evaluation. J Pediatr 1986;108:276-281.

22. Kramer SJ, Vertes DR, Condon M: Auditory brainstem responses and clinical follow-up of high-risk infants. Pediatrics 1989;83:385-392.

23. Lüders H: Surgical monitoring with auditory evoked potentials. J Clin Neurophysiol 1988;5:261-285.

24. Poblano A, Belmont A, Sosa J, et al: Amikacin alters auditory brainstem conduction time in newborns. J Perinat Med 2003;31:237-241.

25. Guiscafre H, Benitez-Diaz L, Martinez MC, Munoz O: Reversible hearing loss after meningitis: Prospective assessment using auditory evoked responses. Ann Otorhinolaryngol 1984;93:229-232.

26. Cox LC: The current status of auditory brainstem response testing in neonatal populations. Pediatr Res 1984;18:780-783.

27. Fria TJ: Assessment of hearing. Pediatr Clin North Am 1981;28:757-775.

28. Picton TW, Durieux-Smith A: Auditory evoked potentials in the assessment of hearing. Neurol Clin 1988;6:791-808.

29. Crowell DH, Pang-Ching G, Anderson RE, et al: Auditory screening of high-risk infants with brainstem evoked responses and impedance audiometry. Haw Med J 1980;39:277-282.

30. Pratt H, Shenhav R, Goldsher M: Applications of auditory evoked potentials to evaluate hearing disorders: Assets and limitations. Israel J Med Sci 1985;21:44-49.

31. Kileny P, Robertson MT: Neurological aspects of infant hearing assessment. J Otolaryngol 1985;14(Suppl):34-39.

32. Richmond KH, Konkle DF, Potsic WP: ABR screening of high-risk infants: Effects of ambient noise in the neonatal nursery. Otolaryngol Head Neck Surg 1986;94:552-560.

33. Robier A, Lemaire MC, Garreau B, et al: Auditory brain stem responses and cortical auditory-evoked potentials in difficult-to-test children. Audiology 1983;22:219-228.

34. Fjermedal O, Laukli E: Paediatric auditory brainstem response and pure-tone audiometry: Threshold comparisons—a study of 142 difficult-to-test children. Scand Audiol 1989;18:105-111.

35. Galambos R, Hecox KE: Clinical applications of the auditory brain stem response. Otolaryngol Clin North Am 1978;11:709-722.

36. Yamada O, Kodera K, Yagi T: Cochlear processes affecting wave V latency of the auditory evoked brain stem response. Scand Audiol 1979;96:291-299.

37. Ochs R, Markand ON, DeMyer WE: Brainstem auditory evoked responses in leukodystrophies. Neurology 1979;29:1089-1093.

38. Calogero B, Cassandro E, Sequino L: Auditory brainstem evoked potentials in syndromes linked to metabolic disorders in childhood. *In* Gallai V (ed): Maturation of the CNS and Evoked Potentials. Amsterdam, Elsevier, 1986, p 204.

39. Garg BP, Markand ON, DeMyer WE: Evoked responses in patients and carriers of adrenoleukodystrophy: Implications for carrier detection. Ann Neurol 1980;8:219.

40. Moloney JBM, Masterson JC: Detection of adrenoleukodystrophy by means of evoked potential. Lancet 1982;2:852.

41. Garg BP, Markand ON, DeMyer WE, Warren C: Evoked response studies in patients with adrenoleukodystrophy and heterozygous relatives. Arch Neurol 1983;40:356-359.

42. Garg BP, Markand ON, DeMeyer WE: Usefulness of BAER studies in the early diagnosis of Pelizaeus-Merzbacher disease. Neurology 1983;33:955-956.

43. Hodes ME, DeMyer WE, Pratt VM, et al: Girl with signs of Pelizaeus-Merzbacher disease heterozygous for a mutation in exon 2 of the proteolipid protein gene. Am J Med Genet 1995;55:397-401.

44. Rumbach L, Warter JM, Marescaux C, et al: Multiple sclerosis diagnosis: Magnetic resonance imaging compared with other paraclinical examination. Eur Neurol 1987;27:92-96.

45. Stockard JJ, Rossiter VS, Wiederholt WC, Kobayashi RM: Brain stem auditory-evoked responses in suspected central pontine myelinolysis. Arch Neurol 1976;33:726-728.

46. Ingram DA, Traub M, Kopelman PG, et al: Brain-stem auditory evoked responses in diagnosis of central pontine myelinolysis. J Neurol 1986;233:23-24.

47. Wu JM, Young C, Wang PJ, et al: Late infantile type neuronal ceroid lipofuscinosis: Report of one case. Zhonghua Min Guo Xiao Er Ke Yi Xue Hui Za Zhi 2000;37:376-380.

48. Markand ON, Ochs R, Worth RM, DeMyer WE: Brainstem auditory evoked potentials in chronic degenerative central nervous system disorders. *In* Barber C (ed): Evoked Potentials. Baltimore, University Park Press, 1980, p 367.

49. Scaioli V, Nardocci N: A pathophysiological study of neuronal ceroid lipofuscinoses in 17 patients: Critical review and methodological proposal. Neurol Sci 2000;21:S89-S92.

50. Lopez-Diaz de Leon E, Silva-Rojas A, Ysunza A, et al: Auditory neuropathy in Friedreich ataxia: A report of two cases. Int J Pediatr Otorhinolaryngol 2003;67:641-648.

51. Satya-Murti S, Cacace A, Hanson P: Auditory dysfunction in Friedreich ataxia: Result of spiral ganglion degeneration. Neurology 1980;30:1047-1053.

52. Ell J, Prasher D, Rudge P: Neuro-otological abnormalities in Friedreich's ataxia. J Neurol Neurosurg Psychiatry 1984;47:26-32.

53. Jabbari B, Schwartz DM, MacNeil DM, Coker SB: Early abnormalities of brainstem auditory evoked potentials in Friedreich's ataxia: Evidence of primary brainstem dysfunction. Neurology 1983;33:1071-1074.

54. Aiba K, Yokochi K, Ishikawa T: A case of ataxic diplegia, mental retardation, congenital nystagmus, and abnormal auditory brain stem responses showing only waves I and II. Brain Dev 1986;8:630-632.

55. Amantini A, Rossi L, De Scisciolo G, et al: Auditory evoked potentials (early, middle, late components) and audiological tests in Friedreich's ataxia. Electroencephalogr Clin Neurophysiol 1984;58:37-47.

56. Campanella G, De Falco FA, Santoro L, et al: Specific impairment of BAERs in Friedreich's ataxia: Auditory evoked responses in clinical evaluation and differential diagnosis. J Neurol Sci 1984;65:111-120.

57. Cassandro E, Mosca F, Sequino L, et al: Otoneurological findings in Friedreich's ataxia and other inherited neuropathies. Audiology 1986;25:84-91.

58. Fujita M, Hosoki M, Miyazaki M: Brainstem auditory evoked responses in spinocerebellar degeneration and Wilson disease. Ann Neurol 1981;9:42-47.

59. Rossini PM, Cracco JB: Somatosensory and brainstem auditory evoked potentials in neurodegenerative system disorders. Eur Neurol 1987;26:176-188.

60. Perretti A, Petrillo A, Pelosi L, et al: Detection of early abnormalities in the mucopolysaccharidoses by the use of visual and brainstem auditory evoked potentials. Neuropediatrics 1990;21:83-86.

61. Komura Y, Kaga K, Ogawa Y, et al: ABR and temporal bone pathology in Hurler's disease. Int J Pediatr Otorhinolaryngol 1998;43:179-188.

62. Peretti P, Raybaud C, Dravet C, et al: MRI in partial epilepsy of childhood. J Neuroradiol 1989;16:308-316.

63. Hsu YS, Chang YC, Lee WT, et al: The diagnostic value of sensory evoked potentials in pediatric Wilson disease. Pediatr Neurol 2003;29:42-45.

64. Topcu M, Topcuoglu MA, Kose G, et al: Evoked potentials in children with Wilson's disease. Brain Dev 2002;24:276-280.

65. Giagheddu M, Tamburini G, Piga M, et al: Comparison of MRI, EEG, EPs, and ECD-SPECT in Wilson's disease. Acta Neurol Scand 2001;103:71-81.

66. Kobayashi K, Iyoda K, Ohtsuka Y, et al: Longitudinal clinicoelectrophysiologic study of a case of Lafora disease proven by skin biopsy. Epilepsia 1990;31:194-201.

67. Aguglia U, Farnarier G, Tinuper P, Quattrone A: Brainstem auditory evoked responses in Lafora disease. Clin Electroencephalogr 1985;16:202-207.

68. Kasai K, Onuma T, Kato M, et al: Differences in evoked potential characteristics between DRPLA patients and patients with progressive myoclonic epilepsy: Preliminary findings indicating usefulness for differential diagnosis. Epilepsy Res 1999;37:3-11.

69. Tsutsumi T, Nishida H, Noguchi Y, et al: Audiological findings in patients with myoclonic epilepsy associated with ragged-red fibers. J Laryngol Otol 2001;115:771-781.

70. Ehle AL, Stewart RM, Lellelid NA, Leventhal NA: Evoked potentials in Huntington's disease: A comparative and longitudinal study. Arch Neurol 1984;41:379-383.

71. Pierelli F, Pozzessere G, Bianco F, et al: Brainstem auditory evoked potentials in neurodegenerative diseases. *In* Morocutti C, Rizzo PA (eds): Neurophysiological and Clinical Aspects. Amsterdam, Elsevier, 1985, p 157.

72. Leuzzi V, Cardona F, Antonozzi I, Liozzo A: Visual, auditory and somatosensorial evoked potentials in early and late treated adolescents with phenylketonuria. J Clin Neurophysiol 1994;11:602-606.

73. Scher MS, Bergman I, Ahdab-Barmada M, Fria T: Neurophysiological and anatomical correlations in neonatal nonketotic hyperglycinemia. Neuropediatrics 1986;17:137-143.

74. Zwirner P, Wilichowski E: Progressive sensorineural hearing loss in children with mitochondrial encephalomyopathies. Laryngoscope 2001;111:515-521.

75. Yoshinaga H, Ogino T, Endo F, et al: Longitudinal study of auditory brainstem response in Leigh syndrome. Neuropediatrics 2003;34:81-86.

76. Taylor MJ, Robinson BH: Evoked potentials in children with oxidative metabolic defects leading to Leigh syndrome. Pediatr Neurol 1992;8:25-29.

77. Wu X-R, Zhao D-H, Ling Q, et al: Rett syndrome in China: Report of nine patients. Pediatr Neurol 1988;4:126-127.

78. Pillion JP, Rawool VW, Bibat G, Naidu S: Prevalence of hearing loss in Rett syndrome. Dev Med Child Neurol 2003;45:338-343.

79. Maurer K, Strümpel D, Wende S: Acoustic tumor detection with early auditory evoked potentials and neuroradiological methods. J Neurol 1982;227:177-185.

80. Rotteveel JJ, Colon EJ, Hombergen G, et al: The application of evoked potentials in the diagnosis and follow-up of children with intracranial tumors. Childs Nerv Syst 1985;1:172-178.

81. Weston PF, Manson JI, Abbott KJ: Auditory brainstem-evoked response in childhood brainstem glioma. Childs Nerv Syst 1986;2:301-305.

82. Starr A, Hamilton AE: Correlation between confirmed sites of neurological lesions and abnormalities of far-field auditory brainstem responses. Electroencephalogr Clin Neurophysiol 1976;41:595-608.

83. Hecox KE, Cone B: Prognostic importance of brainstem auditory evoked responses after asphyxia. Neurology 1981;31:1429-1434.

84. Stockard JJ, Rossiter VS: Clinical and pathologic correlates of brain stem auditory response abnormalities. Neurology 1977;27:316-325.

85. Mair IWS, Okstad S, Laukli E, Anke IM: Screening for retrocochlear pathology. Scand Audiol 1988;17:163-169.

86. Wielaard R, Kemp B: Auditory brainstem evoked responses in brainstem compression due to posterior fossa tumors. Clin Neurol Neurosurg 1979;81:185-193.

87. Hausler R, Toupet M, Guidetti G, et al: Menière's disease in children. Am J Otolaryngol 1987;8:187-193.

88. Cohen M, Prasher D: The value of combining auditory brainstem responses and acoustic reflex threshold measurements in neuro-otological diagnosis. Scand Audiol 1988;17:153-162.

89. Barrs DM, Brackmann DE, Olson JE, House WF: Changing concepts of acoustic neuroma diagnosis. Arch Otolaryngol 1985;111:17-21.

90. Parker SW, Chiappa KH, Brooks EB: Brainstem auditory evoked responses (BAERs) in patients with acoustic neuromas and cerebellar-pontine angle (CPA) meningiomas. Neurology 1980;30:413-414.

91. Worley G, Erwin CW, Schuster JM, et al: BAEPs in infants with myelomeningocele and later development of Chiari II malformation-related brainstem dysfunction. Dev Med Child Neurol 1994;36:707-715.

92. Anderson RC, Dowling KC, Feldstein NA, et al: Chiari I malformation: Potential role for intraoperative electrophysiologic monitoring. J Clin Neurophysiol 2003;20:65-72.

93. Anderson RC, Emerson RG, Dowling KC, Feldstein NA: Improvement in brainstem auditory evoked potentials after suboccipital decompression in patients with Chiari I malformation. J Neurosurg 2003;98:459-464.

94. Koehler J, Schwarz M, Boor R, et al: Assessment of brainstem function in Chiari II malformation utilizing brainstem auditory evoked potentials (BAEP), blink reflex, and masseter reflex. Brain Dev 2000;22:417-420.

95. Rosenberg C, Wogensen K, Starr A: Auditory brain-stem and middle- and long-latency evoked potentials in coma. Arch Neurol 1984;45:235-244.

96. Pauranik A, Maheshwari MC, Tandon RK: Cerebral evoked responses in prognostication of hepatic encephalopathy. Indian J Med Res 1987;85:46-48.

97. Starr A, Achor LJ: Auditory brain stem responses in neurological disease. Arch Neurol 1975;32:761-768.

98. Rumpl E, Prugger M, Battista HJ, et al: Short latency somatosensory evoked potentials and brain-stem auditory evoked potentials in coma due to CNS depressant drug poisoning: Preliminary observations. Electroencephalogr Clin Neurophysiol 1988;70:482-489.

99. Kaga K, Nagai T, Takamori A, Marsh RR: Auditory short, middle, and long latency responses in acutely comatose patients. Laryngoscope 1985;95:321-325.

100. Rappaport M, Maloney JR, Ortega H, et al: Survival in young children after drowning: Brain evoked potentials as outcome predictors. Clin Electroencephalogr 1985;16:183-191.

101. Facco E, Martini A, Zuccarello M, et al: Is the auditory brain-stem response (ABR) effective in the assessment of post-traumatic coma? Electroencephalogr Clin Neurophysiol 1985;62:332-337.

102. Karmel BZ, Gardner JM, Zappulla RA, et al: Brain-stem auditory evoked responses as indicators of early brain insult. Electroencephalogr Clin Neurophysiol 1988;71:429-442.

103. Hall JW, Huang-Fu M, Gennarelli TA: Auditory function in acute severe head injury. Laryngoscope 1982;92:883-890.

104. Newlon PG, Greenberg RP: Evoked potentials in severe head injury. J Trauma 1984;24:61-66.

105. Anderson DC, Bundlie S, Rockswold GL: Multimodality evoked potentials in closed head trauma. Arch Neurol 1984;41:369-374.

106. de Weerd AW, Groeneveld C: The use of evoked potentials in the management of patients with severe cerebral trauma. Acta Neurol Scand 1985;72:489-494.

107. Facco E, Munari M, Liviero MC, et al: Serial recordings of auditory brainstem responses in severe head injury: Relationship between test timing and prognostic power. Intensive Care Med 1988;14:422-428.

108. Mejia RE, Pollack MM: Variability in brain death determination practices in children. JAMA 1995;274:1761-1762.

109. Goodwin SR, Friedman WA, Bellefleur M: Is it time to use evoked potentials to predict outcome in comatose children and adults? Crit Care Med 1991;19:518-524.

110. Steinhart CM, Weiss IP: Use of brainstem auditory evoked potentials in pediatric brain death. Crit Care Med 1985;13:560-562.

111. Goldie WD, Chiappa KH, Young RR, Brooks EB: Brainstem auditory and short-latency somatosensory evoked responses in brain death. Neurology 1981;31:248-256.

112. Sanders RA, Duncan PG, McCullough DW: Clinical experience with brain stem audiometry performed under general anesthesia. J Otolaryngol 1979;8:24-32.

113. John ER, Chabot RJ, Prichep LS, et al: Real-time intraoperative monitoring during neurosurgical and neuroradiological procedures. J Clin Neurophysiol 1989;6:125-158.

114. Algarin C, Peiranao P, Garrido M, et al: Iron deficiency anemia in infancy: Long-lasting effects on auditory and visual system functioning. Pediatr Res 2003;53:217-223.

115. Sarici SU, Serdar MA, Dundaroz MR, et al: Brainstem auditory-evoked potentials in iron-deficiency anemia. Pediatr Neurol 2001;24:205-208.

116. Cankaya H, Oner AF, Egeli E, et al: Auditory brainstem response in children with iron deficiency anemia. Acta Paediatr Taiwan 2003;44:21-24.

117. Elwany S, Kamel T: Sensorineural hearing loss in sickle cell crisis. Laryngoscope 1988;98:386-389.

118. Zou C, Zhao Z, Tang L, et al: The effect of lead on brainstem auditory evoked potentials in children. Chin Med J 2003;116:565-568.

119. Verotti A, Trotta D, Cutarella R, et al: Effects of antiepileptic drugs on evoked potentials in epileptic children. Pediatr Neurol 2000;23:397-402.

120. Sugimoto T, Yasuhara A, Ohta T, et al: Angelman syndrome in three siblings: Characteristic epileptic seizures and EEG abnormalities. Epilepsia 1982;33:1078-1082.

121. Paugh DR, Koopmann CF, Babyak JW: Arthrogryposis multiplex congenita: Otolaryngologic diagnosis and management. Int J Pediatr Otorhinolaryngol 1988;16:45-53.

122. Sohmer H, Student M: Auditory nerve and brain-stem evoked responses in normal, autistic, minimal brain dysfunction and psychomotor retarded children. Electroencephalogr Clin Neurophysiol 1978;44:380-388.

123. Hendrix RA, Melnick W: Auditory brain stem response and audiologic tests in idiopathic facial nerve paralysis. Otolaryngol Head Neck Surg 1983;91:686-690.

124. Uri N, Schuchman G, Pratt H: Auditory brain-stem evoked potentials in Bell's palsy. Arch Otolaryngol 1984;110:301-304.

125. Straumanis JJ, Shagass C, Overton DA: Auditory evoked responses in young adults with Down's syndrome and idiopathic mental retardation. Biol Psychiatry 1973;6:75-79.

126. Widen JE, Folsom RC, Thompson G, Wilson WR: Auditory brainstem responses in young adults with Down syndrome. Am J Ment Defic 1987;91:472-479.

127. Garg BP, Markand ON, Bustion PF: Brainstem auditory evoked responses in hereditary motor-sensory neuropathy: Site of origin of wave II. Neurology 1982;32:1017-1019.

128. Baiocco F, Testa D, D'Angelo A, Cocchini F: Abnormal auditory evoked potentials in Déjérine-Sottas disease: Report of two cases with central acoustic and vestibular impairment. J Neurol 1984;231:46-49.

129. Lahat E, Aladjem M, Mor A, et al: Brainstem auditory evoked potentials in familial dysautonomia. Dev Med Child Neurol 1992;34:690-693.

130. Tan KL, Skurr BA, Yip YY: Phototherapy and the brain-stem auditory evoked response in neonatal hyperbilirubinemia. J Pediatr 1992;120:306-308.

131. Chou YH, Wang PJ: Auditory brainstem evoked potentials in early-treated congenital hypothyroidism. J Child Neurol 2000;17:510-514.

132. Himelfarb MZ, Lakretz T, Gold S, Shanon E: Auditory brain stem responses in thyroid dysfunction. J Laryngol Otol 1981;95:679-686.

133. Kohelet D, Arbel E, Goldberg M, Arlazzoroff A: Transient neonatal hypothyroxinemia and the auditory brainstem evoked response. Pediatr Res 1992;32:530-531.

134. Howard JE, Dorfman LJ: Evoked potentials in hysteria and malingering. J Clin Neurophysiol 1986;3:39-49.

135. Roncagliolo M, Benitez J, Perez M: Auditory brainstem responses of children with developmental language disorders. Dev Med Child Neurol 1994;36:26-33.

136. Rosenhall U, Nordin V, Brantberg K, Gillberg C: Autism and auditory brain stem responses. Ear Hear 2003;24:206-214.

137. Wong V, Wong SN: Brainstem auditory evoked potential study in children with autistic disorder. J Autism Dev Disord 1991;21:329-340.

138. Tait CA, Rousch J, Johns J: Normal ABRs in children classified as learning disabled. J Audiol Res 1983;23:56-62.

139. Bartel PR, Robinson E, Conradie JM, Prinsloo JG: Brainstem auditory evoked potentials in severely malnourished children. Neuropediatrics 1986;17:178-182.

140. Flinn JM, Barnet AB, Lydick S, Lackner J: Infant malnutrition affects cortical auditory evoked potentials. Percept Motor Skills 1993;76:1359-1362.

141. Wright RB, Glantz RH: Hearing loss in myotonic dystrophy. Ann Neurol 1988;23:202-203.

142. Pensak ML, Keith RW, Dignan PSG, et al: Neuroaudiologic abnormalities in patients with type 1 neurofibromatosis. Laryngoscope 1989;99:702-706.

143. Jones RM, Stewart IF, House WF: Familial central neurofibromatosis. Otolaryngol Head Neck Surg 1983;91:527-531.

144. Kapoor RK, Kumar R, Misra PK, et al: Brainstem auditory evoked response (BAER) in childhood bacterial meningitis. Indian J Pediatr 2004;63:217-225.

145. Lüders H, Orlowski JP, Dinner DS, et al: Far-field auditory evoked potentials in near-miss sudden infant death syndrome. Arch Neurol 1984;41:615-617.

146. Stockard JJ: Brainstem auditory evoked potentials in adult and infant sleep apnea syndromes, including sudden infant death syndrome and near-miss for sudden infant death. Ann N Y Acad Sci 1982;388:443-467.

27

Visual Evoked Potentials in Pediatrics—Abnormal

WILLIAM D. GOLDIE

The visual evoked potential (VEP) is an objective physiologic measurement of the electrical activation of the visual pathways of the brain that has become a valuable tool in vision research and clinical medicine. Most VEP studies have been performed on the adult and have been used most effectively as a test of optic nerve function. Although the VEP has been most widely used in cases of multiple sclerosis,[1] there are numerous other clinical conditions in which VEPs provide useful information. This chapter concerns the use of the VEP in evaluating the visual system of the infant and young child. Chapter 10 reviews the basic physiology of the developing visual system, particularly as this would relate to the development of the VEP.

In this chapter observations about the manner in which the VEPs in children are obtained and interpreted are discussed, and illustrations of their usefulness in different clinical settings are provided. In the first section caveats concerning the techniques and settings used for collecting VEPs in children are given. The latter part of the chapter deals with the utility of the VEP in a variety of disorders affecting the nervous system. First, the usefulness in disorders of development of the visual pathways, in amblyopia ex anopsia, and in compressive lesions of the visual pathways is discussed. Second, the role of VEP in vascular-ischemic lesions of the visual pathways, metabolic and toxic disorders, demyelinating and dysmyelinating disorders of the developing nervous system, and hypoxic-ischemic encephalopathy of the premature infant is then reviewed. Finally, clinical issues concerning the use of the VEP in retinal lesions, in occipital infarcts, cortical malformations, and in the setting of dyslexia are discussed.

OVERVIEW

Problems with Technique

The VEP in infants and young children has limitations compared to the VEP in adults. With a cooperative child or adult the pattern reversal VEP can be readily elicited in a standardized setting with a consistent level of ambient light, a constant distance from the stimulus to the eye, and a constant level of arousal. In the infant, it is difficult to consistently maintain these features. Many infant VEPs are performed with the strobe flash[2-4] or light-emitting diode (LED) goggle technique,[5] and a few series have been studied with the pattern reversal method.[6] The strobe and LED methods have a considerable margin of variability, as mentioned in Chapter 10, and do not allow for highly consistent normative data.

For the pattern reversal VEP, a video monitor is placed in front of the child that allows a shifting checkerboard pattern to stimulate the fovea in a very consistent manner. The screen contrasts may have to be altered by the use of cartoons behind the pattern[7], and the level of arousal may be quite variable throughout the examination. Variance in each of these parameters can cause inconsistencies in the VEP waveforms.[8]

Background EEG activity, muscle artifact, and electrical noise may be several times higher in amplitude in the infant and young child than the adult. Averaging the VEP signal from the background noise using standard signal detection techniques may be much less efficient for the infant and young child than for the adult.[9] The placement of the recording electrodes on the scalp of the infant is more difficult to standardize compared to adults. The infant and young child are more prone to have muscle and electrocardiographic artifacts that contaminate the ear and occipital electrodes, whereas the eye movement and sucking artifacts may be widespread over the scalp.

Pattern reversal VEPs have been used in some infants and children.[6,10-13] Although this technique has resulted in data that are remarkably stable and consistent (see discussion in Chapter 10), this method is not easy to reproduce in a clinical neurophysiology laboratory, and it is particularly time consuming and labor intensive. Most clinical laboratories are not able to perform the pattern reversal VEP in infants in a consistent and reliable manner.

Wright and associates[14] have used pattern stimulation to record VEPs in infants and children in a busy clinical research setting using a special method of presentation of the television checkerboard to stimulate infants sedated with chloral hydrate. This has been used to monitor the degree of amblyopia in preparation for strabismus surgery.[15] Although the technique is difficult to implement, it can produce fairly consistent results.

Problems with Defining Age

It may be difficult to assess the physiologic age of infants. The electroencephalogram (EEG) appears to mature at a rate consistent with conceptional age (see Chapter 4). A 32-week premature infant who is now 8 weeks old will have similar neurophysiologic findings as a newly born term infant. When that premature infant is 6 months old, he or she should be expected to have neurophysiologic findings comparable to term infants when they are 4 months old. However, the nervous system of an infant does not mature at a constant rate nor mature on a rigid time table. Environmental factors likely affect the rate of maturation, such as infection, antibiotics, or external stimulation.

The rate of myelination of the nervous system pathways is also quite variable, and the infolding of the occipital lobes can be variable. It would be expected that the improvement in the latency and morphology of the VEP waveforms that occur with maturation would be difficult to predict. Any individual infant follows his or her own rate of maturation of pathways that does not reflect abnormal processes but rather just reflects some genetic pattern. Variations in the rate of maturation are difficult to interpret, especially if the only datum is a single VEP latency measurement at a single point in time. If an initial latency measurement is delayed compared with normative data, it may be found that "catch-up" improvement may occur over the next 3 to 6 months.

SPECIFIC DISORDERS

Developmental Defects

Defects in the development of the visual pathways can be divided into three separate types. The first involves anterior pathway defects that result from abnormal formation of the globe and retina. Malformations of the globe are usually quite obvious. Anophthalmia and micro-ophthalmia can be easily observed clinically and usually result in blindness. VEPs performed in these patients typically show absent electroretinographic (ERG) and cortical waveforms.[16,17] A rare case may demonstrate an intact ERG, and perhaps a low-amplitude and delayed VEP, but these waveforms usually disappear over time.

During development the retina and optic nerve form as a protuberance of the brain that flattens and then folds over and closes. If this folding and closure is not complete, there will be clefts that will leave wedge-shaped defects. These closure defects are referred to as *colobomata*, and they can occur in the lens, iris, choroid, retina, and/or optic nerve. Colobomata of the lens and iris usually cause no alteration in the function of the visual pathways. Colobomata of the choroid, retina, and optic nerve usually spare central vision, and remarkably intact visual function may still develop. VEPs performed in these infants are often normal, but some have waveforms that are low in amplitude and have an unusual morphology. Optic nerve hypoplasia, and atrophic processes of the retina, such as Leber's congenital optic atrophy or Rubinstein-Taybi syndrome, have very low amplitude or absent VEP waveforms, which may deteriorate over time.[18-21] If the ganglion cells of the macula are relatively spared, then the VEP may show normal waveforms. If these ganglion cells begin to degenerate, then the VEP waveform amplitude will decrease and then disappear.

The second type of developmental defect of the visual pathways involves the neocortical structures and white matter pathways. The migrational disorders of the cortex include such disorders as lissencephaly, pachygyria, and polymicrogyria. The occipital cortex layers are usually distorted, and the VEP waveforms are very poorly developed. However, the visual function may be remarkably intact at a primitive level. The visual processing at a cortical level may be highly abnormal, but this may not be reflected in the VEP. A major problem with these defects is that the background EEG may be extremely abnormal with high-voltage chaotic activity including hypsarrhythmia. Although well-developed VEPs may occur in this setting, most of these patients have markedly abnormal VEPs. Children with progressive white matter disease frequently have severely abnormal VEPs.[22-24]

The third form of developmental defect involves delays or alterations in the course of brain maturation. Some infants appear to show a relative delay in the maturation of their visual processing.[25-27] This has been studied in the setting of the neonatal intensive care unit (NICU) where the VEP has been used in the evaluation of the premature infant.[28] See Figures 27-1 through 27-7 for examples.

As noted earlier, the VEP waveforms obtained from premature infants are variable. The ill premature infant is not easy to study, and the results are often not interpretable.[29] When the premature infant is healthy enough to be discharged from the NICU, the VEP is useful in assessing the integrity and the relative state of maturation of the visual pathways.[30] What is not clear, however, is whether this information helps make clinical decisions about future

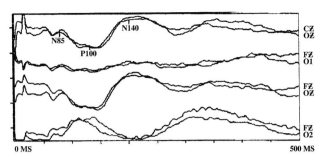

FIGURE 27–3

An infant with a stormy neonatal course with asphyxia and seizures at presumed 34 weeks gestational age, now studied at 8 months of age with possible cortical blindness. Note lateral dipole over posterior scalp. Filter setting 1.0 Hz low frequency, 100 Hz high frequency, rate 1.7 stimuli per second, summed 150 sweeps.

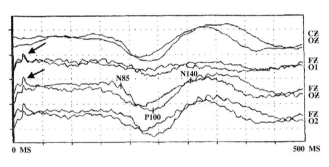

FIGURE 27–1

A normal 2-month-old infant born 1 month premature. Note the electroretinogram response (arrows) and the distribution over the posterior scalp. Filter setting 1.0 Hz low frequency, 100 Hz high frequency, rate 1.7 stimuli per second, summed 150 sweeps. Montage, top to bottom: CZ-OZ, FZ-O1, FZ-OZ, FZ-O1.

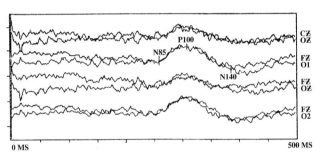

FIGURE 27–4

A premature infant born at 33 weeks gestational age with microcephaly but no definite neurologic problems who does blink to light, and the eyes are normal on examination (studied at 9 days of age). Note the inverted polarity diffusely over the posterior scalp. Filter setting 1.0 Hz low frequency, 100 Hz high frequency, rate 1.7 stimuli per second, summed 150 sweeps.

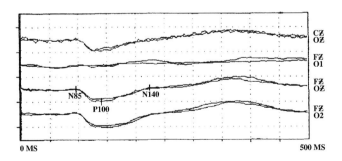

FIGURE 27–2

An asphyxiated term infant who underwent extracorporeal membrane oxygenation treatment at birth due to meconium aspiration, now studied at 3 months of age. No significant visual problems are noted. Filter setting 1.0 Hz low frequency, 100 Hz high frequency, rate 1.7 stimuli per second, summed 150 sweeps.

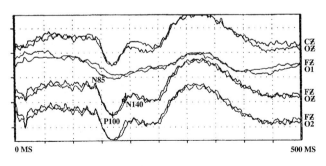

FIGURE 27–5

A hypotonic child born at home at term with significant asphyxia but otherwise healthy, now studied at 1 month of age. Note the "W" waveform with a double peak and broad waveform. Filter setting 1.0 Hz low frequency, 100 Hz high frequency, rate 1.7 stimuli per second, summed 150 sweeps.

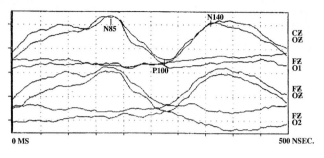

FIGURE 27–6

A premature infant with intraventricular hemorrhage and posthemorrhagic hydrocephalus, now studied at 2 months of age. There is no clinical evidence of significant pressure, and the shunt is working well. Filter setting 1.0 Hz low frequency, 100 Hz high frequency, rate 1.7 stimuli per second, summed 150 sweeps.

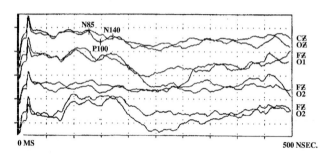

FIGURE 27–7

A normal infant at birth who developed motor deterioration and was found to have a severe form of methylmalonic acidemia (studied at 5 months of age). The infant had a poor response to diet and died 2 months later. Note that the midline lead shows nearly no response, but lateral leads show broad and possibly inverted waveform. Filter setting 1.0 Hz low frequency, 100 Hz high frequency, rate 1.7 stimuli per second, summed 150 sweeps.

visual function of the infant. The VEP does provide an objective measure of brain pathway function that can be followed on a longitudinal basis.[30-32] If the VEP waveforms are absent, there is a risk for blindness, but the VEP may be intact in infants with clinical cortical blindness.[33,34] Whatever the finding, the results must be confirmed by repeat studies at about 6 months of age and by behavioral methods when the infant's age permits adequate testing.[35]

Amblyopia ex Anopsia

When binocular vision is disturbed by strabismus, the afferent input to the cortex from one of the eyes is inhibited. If this persists for an extended period, particularly during the critical period of visual development, then that eye may progressively lose visual function. The mechanism for this loss of function is still not understood, but it is a functional process that can alter the VEP waveforms from that eye. The VEP from the "weak" eye will be of low amplitude and may be delayed relative to the stronger eye.[15] These findings can revert to normal if appropriate patching of the "good" eye is carried out or if appropriate surgery is performed.[36]

VEPs have been used to study visual function in patients with amblyopia.[37-40] The results provide an objective tool to use to complement the clinical evaluation of the child's visual function. In some cases, the clinical assessment may be invalid or too variable to use for clinical decisions, and the VEP results can help in decision making. The VEP can also be a valuable tool to monitor the effects of treatment and correction of the amblyopia.[11,15] To make the clinical decisions in a consistent and reliable manner, the VEP should be performed in specialized laboratories that perform these tests using either the pattern reversal or sinusoidal method under uniform recording protocols.

Compressive Lesions

Pressure on the axons of the nerve fibers anywhere along the visual pathways can alter the appearance of the VEP waveforms. Pressure on the visual pathway anterior to the chiasm affects unilateral VEP data, which is convenient, since the good eye can be used as the normal control.[41] Optic gliomas or retinoblastomas produce loss of amplitude and marked distortion of the VEP waveform from the involved eye.[42,43] These tumors do not result in marked latency delays but produce alteration of the VEPS and cause attenuation of the responses. The waveforms may be difficult to define.

The VEP can be a sensitive tool in the detection of intrinsic optic nerve lesions, particularly in tuberous sclerosis and neurofibromatosis, even before they become evident clinically or on routine computed tomography or magnetic resonance imaging.[44] Retinoblastomas are more difficult to assess, because they frequently may be bilateral, which makes it difficult to compare the involved eye with the good eye. Other rare tumors may also put pressure on the optic nerve, including meningiomas, rhabdomyosarcomas, osteosarcomas, granulomas, and lymphomas.[45,46] In these settings, the VEP may be helpful in identifying involvement of the optic nerve before consideration of surgical intervention. In addition, the VEP can be used to monitor the results of the surgery or subsequent radiation and/or chemotherapy.

Glaucoma, a condition in which elevation of intraocular pressure is associated with the loss of visual function, is known to produce an alteration of the VEP waveforms.[47-49] This disruption is believed to be caused by pressure on the retinal nerve fiber bundles as they course into the optic nerve. The degree of disruption appears to correlate with the intraocular pressure, and the VEP waveforms can return to normal with treatment of the glaucoma.[19,50,51] Pseudotumor cerebri, a diffuse swelling of the brain with increased intracranial pressure, produces mild delays and dispersion of the VEP waveforms that may be asymmetrical. Treatment of these conditions can be monitored by the use of the VEP, since the waveforms return to normal as the pressures are reduced. Arachnoid cysts can put pressure on the visual pathways, and dispersions of the VEP can be seen that may revert to normal when the cyst is removed or decompressed.

Tumors in the pituitary or adjacent regions frequently disrupt the VEP.[45] In adults, VEP monitoring has been performed during pituitary region surgery with some success.[52] LED goggles are typically used, and the active electrodes are over the occipital region with ear reference.

During surgery, dramatic changes in the latency of P1 and/or the amplitude of N1-P1 may indicate a disturbance in the integrity of the visual pathways in the operative field. However, other potential sources for these need to be excluded first. The anesthetic agent can cause changes in the VEP waveform (see Chapter 10). The stimulation parameters may change, as can the orientation of the eyeball and the level of anesthesia. Each of these parameters changes the appearance of the VEP waveform. If there is a recordable and reproducible waveform, then one can assume that the pathways have remained intact. If there is no recordable waveform, no specific assumptions can be drawn. It is often not possible to stop the surgery at that point, and by the time the system is thoroughly checked out, the critical period for reversible effects may have passed.

Hydrocephalus is known to alter the latency and morphology of the VEP.[53-55] This has been studied in older children as well as the term and preterm infant (Fig. 27-8).[56] The latency and morphology of the VEP waveform can be used to monitor whether a ventriculoperitoneal shunt is no longer working.[54] The presumed mechanism is that pressure is exerted on the optic radiations as they stretch around the distended ventricles. However, increased intracranial pressure can also put pressure on the optic chiasm in the region of the third ventricle, and on the optic nerves where the dural sheath extends into the optic channel. Significant increased intracranial pressure may decrease relative cerebral perfusion, and ischemic changes may occur at any or all levels of the visual pathways (Fig. 27-9). It has been shown that the changes in the VEP waveform can be reversible when the intracranial pressure is reduced.[53] However, it is not clear whether these latency changes are linear relative to increasing intracranial pressure or whether there is an abrupt change in latency once the threshold for compensation is exceeded. It is also not known whether the changes in the VEP waveforms reflect any serious deterioration in acuity or other visual performance; conversely, it is not known if the recovery of the VEP waveform back to baseline means that the risks to visual performance are alleviated. Our own experience has been that the VEP is less

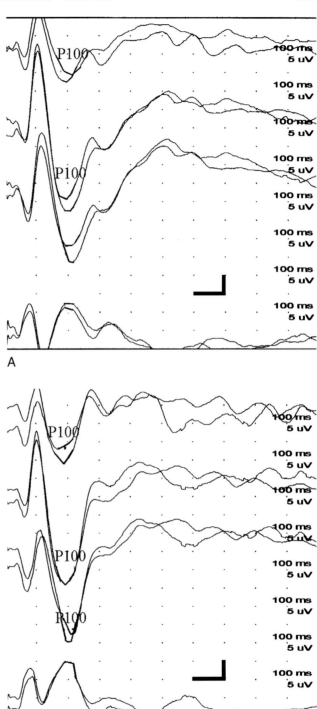

FIGURE 27–8

A 1-year-old child with hydrocephalus. A, Left eye stimulated. P100 = 178 milliseconds. B, Right eye stimulated. P100 = 198 milliseconds. Filter setting 1.0 Hz low frequency, 100 Hz high frequency, rate 0.9 stimuli per second, summed 150 sweeps. Calibration: 100 milliseconds, 5 μV.

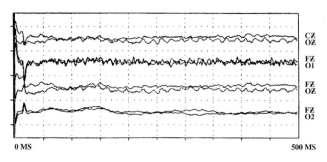

FIGURE 27–9

A 6-month-old infant presenting in deep coma with bilateral subdural hematomas and diffuse brain infarction. This is a presumed battered child who is cortically blind. Note the probable electroretinogram response. Filter setting 1.0 Hz low frequency, 100 Hz high frequency, rate 1.7 stimuli per second, summed 150 sweeps.

helpful than more established clinical parameters for determining whether a ventriculoperitoneal shunt needs to be revised.

It has been suggested that the VEP might be a valuable method to predict the development of hydrocephalus in a premature infant with intraventricular hemorrhage. However, this has not proved to be a reliable clinical tool in the management of the sick premature infant. Deterioration in VEP waveforms monitored serially in a sick premature infant may be due to a variety of causes unrelated to increasing intraventricular pressure.[57,58]

Some rare metabolic and connective tissue diseases can cause compressive lesions of the visual pathways. These include some of the mucopolysaccharidoses where the accumulated material can thicken the dural structures surrounding the optic nerves. Defects in the bone formation of the skull can affect the visual pathways as well. These include achondroplasia, Apert's disease, and Crouzon's disease. There have been adult studies from patients with sarcoidosis that demonstrate changes in the VEP waveforms, but this disorder is extremely uncommon in children.

Vascular-Ischemic Lesions

Compressive lesions of the optic pathways are difficult to separate from ischemic lesions. Pressure on the optic nerve interferes with blood perfusion, and permanent injury from pressure is probably due to ischemic damage. However, a more direct vascular process is known to occur in migraine. The visual pathways are particularly vulnerable to this disorder. Studies of VEP in migraine show variable results.[59-61] During the process of the migraine prodrome, the VEP waveforms can be distorted or disrupted. During treatment, the migraine medications may cause an alteration of the VEP.[62] However, in the nonheadache intervals the VEPs are usually normal. In severe cases of migraine the vascular-

ischemic changes may be prolonged or even permanent. It is not uncommon to see transient unilateral scotomas and homonymous hemianopsias in children with migraine. In those rare cases where the visual impairment persists, the VEP changes are consistent with ischemic stroke.

Strokes in children may be secondary to vascular malformations and cardiac disease; due to metabolic defects such as homocystinuria, or mitochondrial disorders, such as mitochondrial encephalopathy, lactic acidosis, and stroke (MELAS); or may be idiopathic. If the stroke involves visual pathways, then the VEP waveforms will be affected. Most of these lesions involve the optic tracts or radiations, with the corresponding VEP abnormalities of asymmetric field distribution of the waveforms over the occipital region.[63] This is often difficult to demonstrate unless hemifield testing is used. The results are often inconsistent or inconclusive, but, when they correlate with the known cortical lesion, they are informative and can be useful in following recovery. Arteriovenous malformations are a relatively common finding in childhood; they can result in hematomas that can involve the visual pathways. Hematomas, as a rule, do not cause ischemic damage, and the disruption of the pathways may totally recover.

The VEP may be used to effectively monitor the recovery process in the setting of vascular disease. Small-vessel ischemic lesions of the visual pathways are uncommon in children. They are seen in the collagen vascular disorders and in systemic lupus erythematosus. Children with renal disease or cardiac problems that predispose to hypertension may have vascular retinopathy as well as a risk for hypertensive stroke or hemorrhage involving the visual pathways. A rare but devastating condition can occur in cases of sudden blindness following trauma to the eye.[64] It is assumed that this is due to abrupt ischemic injury as a result of vascular spasm. Some children with juvenile-onset diabetes mellitus may have retinopathy as well as microvascular disease.[65] Abrupt infarcts of the optic nerves can occur with diabetes as well as with migraine. The VEP is not usually considered a necessary study in these conditions but may be of value in documenting the degree of functional disruption and in following the course of recovery.[66]

Metabolic and Toxic Disorders

Metabolic dysfunction can alter the effectiveness of the graded potentials at the cell membrane; interfere with effective neurotransmitter production, release, or uptake; and affect the efficiency of conduction along the axons. Any one of these changes can result in a VEP waveform that is lower in amplitude or delayed in latency compared to normal. The VEP allows an objective measurement of visual function in a child with a known metabolic disorder or who is receiving a therapeutic agent with known neurotoxicity.

The VEP could potentially identify patients at risk for visual dysfunction and can be used to monitor the disease process or treatment to provide objective evidence for worsening or improvement.

Various alterations in the VEP have been reported in disorders of vitamin B$_{12}$ and folate metabolism,[67-69] vitamin E deficiency,[70,71] diabetic ketoacidosis,[65] and phenylketonuria.[72-74] These reports of VEP changes due to metabolic disorders or toxic exposures are generally anecdotal in nature, and the cause of the VEP alteration has not been systematically studied. VEPs may be used to assess effectiveness of therapy in metabolic disorders. For example, fish oil supplementation improves VEPs in children with phenylketonuria.[75]

VEPs have been used to evaluate and monitor children with disorders of energy metabolism.[76,77] Taylor and Robinson[78] did VEPs in children with deficiencies of pyruvate dehydrogenase, complex 1, 4, and 5, and cytochrome oxidase deficiencies. The VEPs and somatosensory evoked potentials usually were abnormal in these patients, but the findings were not specific to the patient subgroups. Infantile neuraxonal dystrophy can also disrupt evoked potentials in a similar manner, and it can result in a peripheral neuropathy.[79] Other disorders, including Guillain-Barré syndrome, may cause both demyelination as well as a neuropathy with axonal injury. Visual pathways may be involved in the disorder.[80,81] The VEP waveforms are often distorted in morphology, delayed in latency, and low in amplitude.

VEP latencies may be a useful measure of central nervous system function following a variety of acute toxic insults (Figs. 27-10 and 27-11). Children can present with acute toxicity from a medication or drug that may be accompanied by dysfunction of the visual pathways. Some agents, such as solvents or insecticides, can be associated with profound effects on optic nerve function. It may not be clear whether this disruption is caused by a direct effect of the toxic agent. Therefore, it would be reasonable to monitor

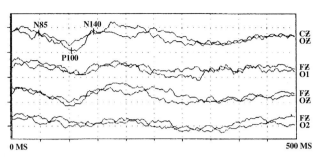

FIGURE 27–11

A 14-year-old child with definite subacute sclerosing panencephalitis with myoclonic seizures, in the end stages. Filter setting 1.0 Hz low frequency, 100 Hz high frequency, rate 1.7 stimuli per second, summed 150 sweeps.

the child's VEP on an intermittent basis to document functional recovery of the visual pathways.

Demyelinating and Dysmyelinating Diseases

An extensive literature is available that deals with the VEP findings in demyelinating diseases. Most of this literature deals with multiple sclerosis.[82] Although rare, multiple sclerosis occurs in children, and VEPs can be useful in the evaluation and monitoring of treatment in these children.[83,84]

Conduction along the white matter tracts of the brain is by saltatory conduction. This provides a highly efficient means of signal transmission that depends on the thick lipid coating of myelin and the intermediate nodes. A variety of disorders may occur that disrupts this signal transmission. The thick lipid coating of myelin may be stripped away. This occurs in multiple sclerosis as well as other disorders such as postviral processes or in autoimmune hypersensitivity reactions to vaccines. The demyelination in these processes produces delays in the VEP latencies and may also result in a dispersion pattern. This is caused by a mixture of signals being transmitted by demyelinated axons in different stages of disruption including a few remaining normal axons. The signal traveling such a pathway arrives at different times and may result in a very broad waveform or in a waveform with two or more peaks. The VEP amplitudes usually remain near normal, but the waveform components are markedly delayed in latency.

Dysmyelination can occur due to defects in the formation of the myelin structure during development or due to a defective repair process caused by a deficiency in key structural components. Adrenoleukodystrophy and metachromatic leukodystrophy are good examples of this type of disorder. Krabbe's disease and hyperglycinemia can also result in profound dysmyelination, and the VEPs in these disorders are usually severely disrupted. It is not clear to what extent the

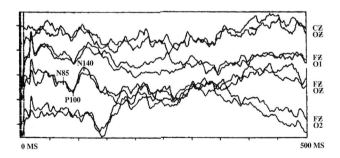

FIGURE 27–10

A 13-year-old child in coma due to metabolic encephalopathy. Note the well-formed initial waveforms, with broad and spread out later waveforms. Filter setting 1.0 Hz low frequency, 100 Hz high frequency, rate 1.7 stimuli per second, summed 150 sweeps.

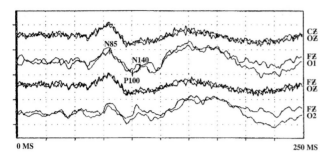

FIGURE 27–12

A 1-year-old child with a leukodystrophy. Visual function appears to be intact, but motor function is markedly impaired. Note low-voltage and complex waveform with lateral dipole over the posterior scalp. Filter setting 1.0 Hz low frequency, 100 Hz high frequency, rate 1.7 stimuli per second, summed 150 sweeps.

VEP can monitor the progression of these disorders, but it does offer an objective tool for measuring the effects of myelin deterioration. In recent cases of leukodystrophies that have been treated with bone marrow transplantation, VEPs and other evoked potentials have been used to monitor clinical improvement.[85] Figures 27-12 and 27-13 provide examples of VEPs in disorders of myelinization.

The efficiency of conduction of an electrical signal depends on the quality of the myelin sheath, the resting membrane potential, and intrinsic properties of the intermediate nodes. Each of these components is critical to the conduction of a VEP signal. A defect of any one or combination of these components disrupts or delays the VEP signal. It is not reasonable to assume that a given demyelinating or dysmyelinating disorder causes a characteristic VEP change, but a delayed or disrupted VEP waveform found in a child with an unusual degenerative process should suggest a defect in myelination. Often the process may be patchy and nonuniform, regardless of the underlying cause, and the resultant VEP change in a given patient may be unique.

Hypoxic-Ischemic Encephalopathy of Premature Infants

Over the past 10 years the term *hypoxic-ischemic encephalopathy* (HIE) has become established because it describes the changes taking place in the brains of newborn infants who are exposed to severe stress during the first few days and weeks of life. Excellent studies have provided a better understanding of cerebral dynamics in the face of hypotension, poor perfusion, and excessive demands for cerebral blood flow such as occurs during neonatal seizures. It is clear that the developing white matter pathways are especially vulnerable to injury during stress. It has been suggested that cerebral evoked potentials should be an excellent noninvasive method for assessing the integrity

of these white matter pathways.[29] Studies indicate that VEPs are valuable in predicting neurologic outcome.[4,69,86] However, these studies have not been consistent or reliable enough for important clinical decision making. There is no question that ill newborns, especially premature infants, are more likely to have absent VEP waveforms when studied during the recovery phase of their acute illness. However, the absence of the VEP is not reliable enough to predict either blindness or cerebral palsy.[33,64,87-89] Our own studies have shown that some asphyxiated infants who initially have flat VEPs can recover their VEP waveforms within 3 months and may have fairly normal outcomes (see Figs. 27-2 and 27-3).

The premature infant is especially vulnerable to cystic changes (periventricular leukomalacia) in the white matter. VEPs have proven to be accurate predictors of outcome in term infants with hypoxic-ischemic encephalopathy. Parallels between term *asphyxia* and hypoxic-ischemic injury in the preterm brain suggested the hypothesis that VEPs may predict the development of periventricular leukomalacia, and later, cerebral palsy. Ekert and associates[90] found that in 123 infants less than 32 weeks gestational age VEPs during the first 3 weeks of life (usually the 1st week) showed a statistically significant association with periventricular leukomalacia ($P < 0.04$), although false-positive recordings were twice as frequent as true-positive recordings. VEPs were not associated with grade III-IV intraventricular hemorrhage ($P = 1.0$). Unlike asphyxiated term infants, VEPs were not predictive of abnormal neurodevelopmental outcome in the preterm population.

Retinal Lesions

The VEP does not offer specific information concerning the cells of the retina. However, the integrity of the VEP does depend on the integrity of the ganglion cells. The ERG is highly specific for the receptor cells of the retina, and it may also give information about some of the intermediate cells as well as the ganglion cells. Therefore, the combined use of the two studies can offer considerable information concerning the integrity of the retina.[19,51]

Retinitis pigmentosa is a disease entity in which the rods and cones progressively degenerate. It can predispose to night blindness owing to the degeneration of the rods, which are the receptors that function in the low-level light at dusk and at night. In the early stages of this disease process, the ERG may be flat while the VEP waveforms appear normal. Patterned VEPs have been shown to be a useful method for objectively evaluating visual function in patients with retinitis pigmentosa. In retinitis pigmentosa, the ERG may be the more sensitive study to perform initially, and the VEP may still be normal even as the ERG becomes flat.[91] Similar features are described in the con-

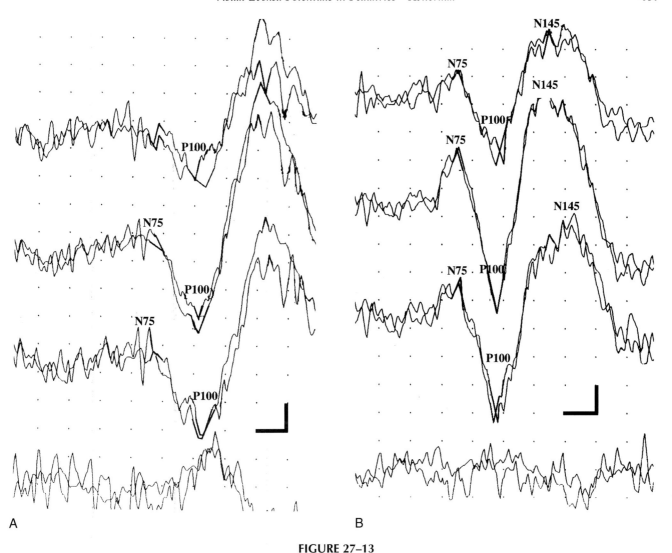

A   B

FIGURE 27–13

An 18-year-old child with left optic neuritis. A, Left eye stimulated. P100 = 114 milliseconds. B, Right eye stimulation. P100 = 103 milliseconds. Filter setting 1.0 Hz low frequency, 100 Hz high frequency, rate 1.9 stimuli per second, summed 150 sweeps. Calibration: 20 milliseconds, 2 μV.

dition of congenital stationary night blindness and in rod monochromatism.[92,93] VEPs are also frequently abnormal in patients with albinism, congenital cone dysfunction, and cone-rod dystrophy.[94,95] Patients with macular disease may have reduced amplitude of VEPs.[96]

Leber's congenital amaurosis is a familial disorder that presents with progressive blindness during the first few years of life. The combined ERG-VEP studies may demonstrate the loss of the VEP early in the disease process, even before the blindness is obvious clinically.[20]

Tay-Sachs disease is a GM_2 storage disease involving the deposition of ganglioside in various neurons including the ganglion cells of the retina. It represents the infantile amaurotic idiocies that can result in blindness and dementia in the young child. Other examples include GM_1 gangliosido-

sis, Niemann-Pick disease, and some of the mucopolysaccharidoses. In these disorders, the ganglion cells of the retina become dysfunctional even while the receptor cells remain intact. Therefore, the combined ERG-VEP studies demonstrate normal ERG waveforms but the VEP is flat. In the early stages of the disorder, the VEP waveform is low in amplitude and broad in morphology and then progressively disappears.

Antiepileptic Drugs

Vigabatin is an antiepileptic drug that acts as a selective irreversible inhibitor of gamma-aminobutyric acid transaminase. The drug has been associated with visual field constriction.[97,98]

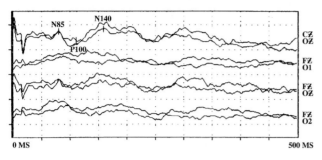

FIGURE 27–14
A 7-year-old child with severe brain malformation with encephalocele, colpocephaly, and profound retardation. There is no definite visual function. Filter setting 1.0 Hz Low frequency, 100 Hz High frequency, rate 1.7 stimuli per second, summed 150 sweeps.

Patients treated with carbamazepine and sodium valproate have been reported to have mild increases in P100 latency or reductions in N75/P100 and P100/N145 amplitudes, compared with baseline studies.[98,99]

Occipital Infarcts or Lobar Malformations

The occipital lobes of the brain provide the cortical distribution of the visual pathways. If there has been a disruption of the integrity of the visual cortex of the occipital lobes, then the scalp distribution of the VEP waveforms will be altered (Fig. 27-14).[63,100] The scalp distribution of the VEP can be paradoxically suppressed over the opposite side from a cortical lesion due to the fact that the primary visual cortex is deep in the medial aspect of the occipital lobes and the dipole field points out to the opposite scalp region. If there is dysfunction of the left occipital lobe, then the right scalp distribution of the VEP will be attenuated. However, in children this is not always the case.

The most effective method for demonstrating asymmetric occipital lobe lesions is to perform hemifield stimulation. In this manner, only one occipital lobe is stimulated at a time, and the scalp distribution can be measured separately. However, hemifield stimulation is difficult to perform in the infant and young child, particularly since it is most effective with pattern stimulation. The child must fixate consistently on a point in the middle of the screen while only half of the screen shows the pattern, or he or she may fixate on one or the other side edge of the screen so that only half of the visual field will be stimulated by the pattern.

Conversion Reactions

VEPs can be used to objectively predict visual acuity in patients with functional visual loss.[101]

Dyslexia

Numerous studies have been performed trying to find a consistent anatomic or functional abnormality in this disorder. Occasional clinical series may find a consistent abnormality in one form of study or another, but no single consistent abnormality seems to be found in all studies.[102-104] Other forms of neurophysiologic testing with event-related potentials, particularly the long latency auditory evoked potential and P300 waveforms, may give more specific information concerning cortical processing.[105]

If the VEP is to be used to investigate cortical processing of visual information, it would be of interest to look at the later components of the VEP to pattern-shift stimulation. It may be valuable to examine the VEP waveforms to formed visual images, such as words or objects that have to be identified. The diagnosis of dyslexia should be based on detailed neuropsychological and neurologic evaluations, and very careful subclassification should be followed. However, the use of evoked or event-related potentials may eventually provide a valuable method to probe into the cerebral processing in a noninvasive and reproducible manner.

CONCLUSION

The VEP is a valuable clinical test that allows the clinical neurophysiologist a probe into the functional integrity of the visual pathways of the brain. To perform the test in a reliable manner, several factors must be carefully adhered to, and the stimulus parameters must be carefully controlled. But, with conscientious attention, reliable clinical information can be obtained, even in infants and children. The VEP will never be an independent examination, but the results must be applied to the clinical setting. It is an extension of the neurologic or ophthalmologic examination that can assess the functional integrity of the visual pathways.

The VEP test itself is not harmful or painful; it is relatively inexpensive; and it can be repeated numerous times with high reliability. There is no reason that the VEP test should be scorned, nor should it be abused. Rather, the VEP should be appreciated for its limitations and its qualities.

REFERENCES

1. Neima D, Regan D: Pattern visual evoked potentials and spatial vision in retrobulbar neuritis and multiple sclerosis. Arch Neurol 1984;41:198-201.
2. Tsuneishi S, Casaer P: Effects of preterm extrauterine visual experience on the development of the human visual system: A flash VEP study. Dev Med Child Neurol 2000;42:663-668.

3. Kraemer M, Abrahamsson M, Sjostrom A: The neonatal development of the light flash visual evoked potential. Doc Ophthalmol 1999;99:21-39.

4. Pyrds O, Griesen G: Preservation of single-flash visual evoked potentials at very low cerebral oxygen delivery in preterm infants. Pediatr Neurol 1990;6:151-158.

5. Wiesel TN: Postnatal development of the visual cortex and the influence of environment. Nature 1982;299:583-591.

6. Sokol S: Measurement of infant visual acuity from pattern reversal evoked potentials. Vision Res 1978;18:33-39.

7. Shors TJ, Eriksen KJ, Wright KW: Superimposition of a cartoon program as an aid in recording pattern visual evoked potentials in children. J Pediatr Ophthalmol Strabismus 1987;24:224-227.

8. Fenwick PBC, Brown D, Hennesey J: The visual evoked response to pattern reversal in "normal" 6 to 11-year-old children. Electroencephalogr Clin Neurophysiol 1981;51:49-62.

9. Shors TJ, Ary JP, Eriksen KJ, Wright KW: P100 amplitude variability of the pattern visual evoked potential. Electroencephalogr Clin Neurophysiol 1986;65:316-319.

10. Sokol S, Jones K: Implicit time of pattern evoked potentials in infants: An index of maturation of spatial vision. Vision Res 1979;19:747-755.

11. Sokol S, Hansen V, Moskowitz A, et al: Evoked potential and preferential looking estimates of visual acuity in pediatric patients. Ophthalmology 1983;90:552-562.

12. Sokol S, Moskowitz A, Paul A: Evoked potential estimates of visual accommodation in infants. Vision Res 1983;23:851-860.

13. Sokol S, Moskowitz A, McCormack G, Augliere R: Infant grating acuity is temporally tuned. Vision Res 1988;28:1357-1366.

14. Wright KW, Eriksen KJ, Shors TJ, Ary JP: Recording pattern visual evoked potentials under chloral hydrate sedation. Arch Ophthalmol 1986;104:718-721.

15. Wright KW, Eriksen KJ, Shors TJ: Detection of amblyopia with P-VEP during chloral hydrate sedation. J Pediatr Ophthalmol Strabismus 1987;24:170-175.

16. Tormene AP, Riva C: Electroretinogram and visual-evoked potentials in children with optic nerve coloboma. Doc Ophthalmol 1998;96:347-354.

17. Parsa CF, Silva ED, Sundin OH, et al: Redefining papillorenal syndrome: An underdiagnosed cause of ocular and renal morbidity. Ophthalmology 2001;108:738-749.

18. van Genderen NM, Kind GF, Riemslag FC, Hennekam RC: Ocular features in Rubinstein-Taybi syndrome: Investigation of 24 patients and review of the literature. J Neurol 2000;84:1177-1184.

19. Celesia GG, Kaufman D: Pattern ERGs and visual evoked potentials in maculopathies and optic nerve diseases. Invest Ophthalmol Vis Sci 1985;26:726-735.

20. Dorfman LJ, Nikoskelainen E, Rosenthal AR, Sogg RL: Visual evoked potentials in Leber's hereditary optic neuropathy. Ann Neurol 1977;1:565-568.

21. Brecelj J, Stirn-Kranjc B: ERG and VEP follow-up study in children with Leber's congenital amaurosis. Eye 1999;13:47-54.

22. Markand ON, Garg BP, DeMyer WE, et al: Brain stem auditory, visual, and somatosensory evoked potentials in leukodystrophies. Electroencephalogr Clin Neurophysiol 1982;54:39-48.

23. Kristjansdottir R, Sjostrom A, Uvebrant P: Ophthalmological abnormalities in children with cerebral white matter disorders. Eur J Paediatr Neurol 2002;6:25-33.

24. Apkarian P, Koetsveld-Baart JC, Barth PG: Visual evoked potential characteristics and early diagnosis of Pelizaeus-Merzbacher disease. Arch Neurol 1993;50:981-985.

25. Lambert SR, Kriss A, Taylor D: Delayed visual maturation: A longitudinal clinical and electrophysiological assessment. Ophthalmology 1989;96:524-529.

26. Mellor DH, Fielder AR: Dissociated visual development: Electrodiagnostic studies in infants who are "slow to see." Dev Med Child Neurol 1980;22:327-335.

27. Moskowitz A, Sokol S: Developmental changes in the human visual system as reflected by the latency of the pattern reversal VEP. Electroencephalogr Clin Neurophysiol 1983;56:1-15.

28. Taylor MJ, Menzies R, MacMillan LJ, Whyte HE: VEPs in normal full-term and premature neonates: Longitudinal versus cross-sectional data. Electroencephalogr Clin Neurophysiol 1987;68:20-27.

29. Greisen G, Trojaborg W: Cerebral blood flow, $PaCO_2$ changes, and visual evoked potentials in mechanically ventilated, preterm infants. Acta Paediatr Scand 1987;76:394-400.

30. Harding GFA, Grose J, Wilton A, Bissenden JG: The pattern reversal VEP in short-gestation infants. Electroencephalogr Clin Neurophysiol 1988;70:130P.

31. Häkkinen VK, Ignatius J, Koskinen M, et al: Visual evoked potentials in high-risk infants. Neuropadiatrie 1987;18:70-74.

32. Hoyt CS, Nickel BL, Billson FA: Ophthalmological examination of the infant: Developmental aspects. Surv Ophthalmol 1982;26:177-189.

33. Kupersmith MJ, Nelson JL: Preserved visual evoked potentials in infant cortical blindness: Relationship to blindsight. Neuroophthalmol 1986;6:85-94.

34. Shefrin SL, Goodin DS, Aminoff MJ: Visual evoked potentials in the investigation of "blindsight." Neurology 1988;38:104-109.

35. Jorch G, Schneider G: Optical evoked responses (OER) and photic driving (PD) in very sick premature infants less than 33 weeks of gestational age. Pediatr Res 1987;22:241.

36. Odom JV, Hoyt CS, Marg E: Effect of natural deprivation and unilateral eye patching on visual acuity of infants and children: Evoked potential measurements. Arch Ophthalmol 1981;99:1412-1416.

37. Gwiazda JE: Detection of amblyopia and development of binocular vision in infants and children. Curr Opin Ophthalmol 1992;3:735-740.

38. Demirci H, Gezer A, Sezen F, et al: Examination of the functions of the parvocellular and magnocellular pathways

in strabismic amblyopia. J Pediatr Ophthalmol Strabismus 2002;39:215-221.

39. Davis AR, Sloper JJ, Neveu MM, et al: Electrophysiological and psychophysical differences between early- and late-onset strabismic amblyopia. Invest Ophthalmol Vis Sci 2003;44:610-617.

40. Watts PO, Neveu MM, Holder GE, Sloper JJ: Visual evoked potentials in successfully treated strabismic amblyopes and normal subjects. J AAPOS 2002;6:389-392.

41. Mahapatra AK, Bhatia R: Predictive value of visual evoked potentials in unilateral optic nerve injury. Surg Neurol 1989;31:339-342.

42. Cohen ME, Duffner PK: Visual-evoked responses in children with optic gliomas, with and without neurofibromatosis. Childs Brain 1983;10:99-111.

43. Ng YT, North KN: Visual-evoked potentials in the assessment of optic gliomas. Pediatr Neurol 2001;24:44-48.

44. Iannaccone A, McCluney RA, Brewer VR, et al: Visual evoked potentials in children with neurofibromatosis type 1. Doc Ophthalmol 2002;105:63-81.

45. Bullock P, Holder GE: Pattern visual evoked responses in the management and evaluation of pituitary tumours. J Neurol Neurosurg Psychiatry 1988;51:461.

46. Wenzel D, Brandl U, Beck JD, et al: Visual evoked potentials in tumors from orbit to occipital lobe in childhood. Neurosurgery 1988;11:279-286.

47. Graham SL, Klistorner A: The diagnostic significance of the multifocal pattern visual evoked potential in glaucoma. Curr Opin Ophthalmol 1999;10:140-146.

48. Hood DC: Objective measurement of visual function in glaucoma. Curr Opin Ophthalmol 2003;14:78-82.

49. Chen CS, Hood DC, Zhang X, et al: Repeat reliability of the multifocal visual evoked potential in normal and glaucomatous eyes. J Glaucoma 2003;12:399-408.

50. Bass SJ, Sherman J, Bodis-Wollner I, Nath S: Visual evoked potentials in macular disease. Invest Ophthalmol Vis Sci 1985;26:1071-1074.

51. Bodis-Wollner I, Feldman RG, Guillory SL, Mylin L: Delayed visual evoked potentials are independent of pattern orientation in macular disease. Electroencephalogr Clin Neurophysiol 1987;68:172-179.

52. Ducati A, Fava E, Motti EDF: Neuronal generators of the visual evoked potentials: Intracerebral recording in awake humans. Electroencephalogr Clin Neurophysiol 1988;71:89-99.

53. Coupland SG, Cochrane DD: Visual evoked potentials, intracranial pressure, and ventricular size in hydrocephalus. Doc Ophthalmol 1987;66:321-330.

54. Sklar FH, Ehle AL, Clark WK: Visual evoked potentials: A noninvasive technique to monitor patients with shunted hydrocephalus. Neurosurgery 1979;4:529-534.

55. Desch LW: Longitudinal stability of visual evoked potentials in children and adolescents with hydrocephalus. Dev Med Child Neurol 2001;43:113-117.

56. Ehle A, Sklar F: Visual evoked potentials in infants with hydrocephalus. Neurology 1979;29:1541-1544.

57. Kurtzberg D: Event-related potentials in the evaluation of high-risk infants. Ann N Y Acad Sci 1982;388:557-571.

58. Muttitt SC, Taylor MJ, Whyte HE: Serial visual evoked potentials (VEPs) and outcome in full-term birth asphyxia. Pediatr Res 1989;25:359A.

59. Marsters JB, Good PA, Martimer MJ: A diagnostic test for migraine using the visual evoked potential. Headache 1988;28:526-530.

60. Orban LC, Orban GA: A new VEP technique reveals functional disturbances in migraine. Electroencephalogr Clin Neurophysiol 1987;67:4P.

61. Polich J, Ehlers CL, Dalessio DJ: Pattern shift visual evoked responses and EEG in migraine. Headache 1986;26:451-456.

62. Diener H-C, Scholz E, Dichgans J, et al: Central effects of drugs used in migraine prophylaxis evaluated by visual evoked potentials. Ann Neurol 1989;25:125-130.

63. Maitland CG, Aminoff MJ, Kennard C, Hoyt WF: Evoked potentials in the evaluation of visual field defects due to chiasmal or retrochiasmal lesions. Neurology 1982;32:986-991.

64. Duchowny MS, Weiss IP, Majlessi H, Barnet AB: Visual evoked responses in childhood cortical blindness after head trauma and meningitis: A longitudinal study of six cases. Neurology 1974;24:933-940.

65. Comi G, Martinelli V, Galardi G, et al: Evaluation of central nervous conduction by visual evoked potentials in insulin dependent diabetic children: Metabolic and clinical correlations. Acta Diabet Lat 1987;24:157-162.

66. Khedr EM, Khedr T, Farweez HM, et al: Multimodal electroneurophysiological studies of systemic lupus erythematosus. Neuropsychobiol 2001;43:204-212.

67. Krumholz A, Weiss HD, Goldstein PJ, Harris KC: Evoked responses in vitamin B_{12} deficiency. Ann Neurol 1981;9:407-409.

68. Tomoda H, Shibasaki H, Hirata I, Oda K: Central versus peripheral nerve conduction: Before and after treatment of subacute combined degeneration. Arch Neurol 1988;45:526-529.

69. Troncoso J, Mancall EL, Schatz NJ: Visual evoked responses in pernicious anemia. Arch Neurol 1979;36:168-169.

70. Kaplan PW, Rawal K, Erwin CD, et al: Visual and somatosensory evoked potentials in vitamin E deficiency with cystic fibrosis. Electroencephalogr Clin Neurophysiol 1988;71:266-272.

71. Messenheimer JA, Greenwood RS, Tennison MB, et al: Reversible visual evoked potential abnormalities in vitamin E deficiency. Ann Neurol 1984;15:499-501.

72. Giovannini M, Valsasina R, Villani RA, et al: Pattern reversal visual evoked potentials in phenylketonuria. J Inherit Metab Dis 1988;11:416-421.

73. Korinthenberg R, Ulbrick K, Fullenkemper F: Evoked potentials and electroencephalograms in adolescents with phenylketonuria. Neuropediatrics 1988;19:175-178.

74. Landi A, Ducati A, Villani R, et al: Pattern-reversal visual evoked potentials in phenylketonuric children. Childs Nerv Syst 1987;3:278-281.

75. Beblo S, Reinhardt H, Muntau AC, et al: Fish oil supplementation improves visual evoked potentials in children with phenylketonuria. Neurology 2001;57:1488-1491.

76. Scaioli V, Antozzi C, Villani F, et al: Utility of multimodal evoked potential study and electroencephalography in mitochondrial encephalomyopathy. Ital J Neurol Sci 1998;19:291-300.

77. Finsterer J: Visual evoked potentials in respiratory chain disorders. Acta Neurol Scand 2001;104:31-35.

78. Taylor MJ, Robinson BH: Evoked potentials in children with oxidative metabolic defects leading to Leigh syndrome. Pediatr Neurol 1992;8:25-29.

79. Nardocci N, Zorzi G, Farina L, et al: Infantile neuroaxonal dystrophy: Clinical spectrum and diagnostic criteria. Neurology 1999;52:1472-1478.

80. Barbieri S, Nobile-Orazio E, Baldini L, et al: Visual evoked potentials in patients with neuropathy and macroglobulinemia. Ann Neurol 1987;22:663-666.

81. Ropper AH, Chiappa KH: Evoked potentials in Guillain-Barré syndrome. Neurology 1986;36:587-590.

82. Drislane FW: Use of evoked potentials in the diagnosis and follow-up of multiple sclerosis. Clin Neurosci 1994;2:196-201.

83. Kornek B, Bernert G, Balassy C, et al: Glatiramer acetate treatment in patients with childhood and juvenile-onset multiple sclerosis. Neuropediatrics 2003;34:120-126.

84. Miyazaki I, Adachi E, Kuroda N: Follow-up studies in pattern VECP in demyelinating diseases in children. Doc Ophthalmol 1986;63:5-12.

85. Kaleita TA, Shields WD, Feig SA, Nuwer MR: Nervous system assessment with evoked potential tests in pediatric bone marrow transplant patients. Am J Pediatr Hematol Oncol 1984;6:329-332.

86. Eken P, Toet MC, Groenendaal F, De Vries LS: Predictive value of early neuroimaging, pulsed Doppler, and neurophysiology in full-term infants with hypoxic-ischaemic encephalopathy. Arch Dis Child Fetal Neonat Ed 1995;73:F75-F80.

87. Dubowitz LMS, Mushin L, De Vries J, Arden GB: Visual function in the newborn infant: Is it cortically mediated? Lancet 1986;1:1139-1141.

88. Frank Y, Kurtzberg D, Kreuzer JA, Vaughan HG: Flash and pattern-reversal visual evoked potential abnormalities in infants and children with cerebral blindness. Ann Neurol 1988;24:325.

89. Snyder RD, Brann BS, Hata SK: Absence of cerebral hemispheres in a surviving neonate with preserved vision: Electrophysiological and MRI correlations. J Clin Exp Neurol 1987;9:276-277.

90. Ekert PG, Keenan NK, Whyte HE, et al: Visual evoked potentials for prediction of neurodevelopmental outcome in preterm infants. Biol Neonate 1997;71:148-155.

91. Paranhos FR, Katsum O, Arai M, et al: Pattern reversal visual evoked response in retinitis pigmentosa. Doc Ophthalmol 1998;96:321-331.

92. Barnes CS, Brigell MG, Alexander KR: ON-pathway dysfunction in a patient with acquired unilateral night blindness. Retina 1998;18:531-538.

93. Yankov E, Nakova A, Tzekov R: Spectral sensitivity of the visual system as revealed by evoked potentials in normal and anomalous trichomats. Acta Physiol Pharmacol Bulg 1999;24:91-100.

94. Shaw FS, Kriss A, Russel-Eggitt I, et al: Diagnosing children presenting with asymmetric pendular nystagmus. Dev Med Child Neurol 2001;43:622-627.

95. Neveu MM, Jeffrey G, Burton LC, et al: Age-related changes in the dynamics of human albino visual pathways. Eur J Neurosci 2003;18:1939-1949.

96. Negishi C, Takasoh M, Fujimoto N, et al: Visual evoked potentials in relation to visual acuity in macular disease. Acta Ophthalmol Scand 2001;79:271-276.

97. Kalviainen R, Nousiainen I: Visual field defects with vigabatrin: Epidemiology and therapeutic implications. CNS Drugs 2001;15:217-230.

98. Zgorzalewicz M, Galas-Zgorzalewicz B: Visual and auditory evoked potentials during long-term vigabatrin treatment in children and adolescents with epilepsy. Clin Neurophysiol 2000;111:2150-2154.

99. Verrotti A, Trotta D, Cutarella R, et al: Effects of antiepileptic drugs on evoked potentials in epileptic children. Pediatr Neurol 2000;23:397-402.

100. Bodis-Wollner I, Atkin A, Raab E, Wolkstein M: Visual association cortex in vision in man: Pattern evoked potentials in a blind boy. Science 1977;9:629-631.

101. Xu S, Meyer D, Yoser S, et al: Pattern visual evoked potential in the diagnosis of functional visual loss. Ophthalmology 2001;108:76-80.

102. Romani A, Conte S, Callieco R, et al: Visual evoked potential abnormalities in dyslexic children. Funct Neurol 2001;16:219-229.

103. Kuba M, Szanyi J, Gayer D, et al: Electrophysiological testing of dyslexia. Acta Med (Hradec Kralove) 2001;44:131-134.

104. Brecelj J, Strucl M, Raic V: Simultaneous pattern electroretinogram and visual evoked potential recordings in dyslexic children. Doc Ophthalmol 1997;94:355-364.

105. Habib M: The neurological basis of developmental dyslexia: An overview and working hypothesis. Brain 2000;123:2373-2399.

III

Neuromuscular Disorders

28

The Floppy Infant

Kathryn J. Swoboda and H. Royden Jones, Jr.

The floppy infant syndrome (FIS) is the most common reason for referral of infants to a pediatric electromyography (EMG) laboratory. These infants provide a major challenge to the pediatric electromyographer. Approximately 80% of such babies have a primary central nervous system etiology.[1] Peripheral motor unit disorders comprise another major diagnostic category. Central and peripheral nervous system involvement are not mutually exclusive. Examples include babies with infantile neuronal degeneration, congenital muscular dystrophy variants such as Walker-Warburg syndrome, and metabolic disorders including carbohydrate deficient glycosylation defects and mitochondrial disease. Electrophysiologic evaluation of these infants is of value in that it can often distinguish between central and peripheral causes.

When a lesion of the peripheral motor unit is ascertained, EMG allows anatomic localization of the pathologic process to the anterior horn cell, the peripheral nerve, the neuromuscular junction, or muscle.[2] The results may offer therapeutic options, support the diagnosis of a specific genetic condition or syndrome, or provide prognostic information. More readily available and sophisticated molecular testing has increasingly supplanted the need for EMG in the evaluation of some infants, such as those with suspected congenital myotonic dystrophy or spinal muscular atrophy (SMA).[3]

During a pregnancy, sometimes the mother recognizes a paucity or significant diminution of fetal muscular activity. In these instances hypotonia, muscle weakness, or contractures may be evident at birth. These infants characteristically have decreased limb movements, poor muscle tone, and a limp appearance leading to the designation *FIS*

(Fig. 28-1). Lower bulbar motor dysfunction may be manifest by a weak cry and suck, with a compromised ability to protect the airway during feedings. Such infants are predisposed to episodes of aspiration and recurrent pneumonia. Although most floppy infants have recognizable signs of hypotonia at birth, initially such findings may be subtle. Additionally, there are occasional newborns who appear normal at birth but later demonstrate delayed acquisition of motor milestones. The differential diagnosis includes a broad spectrum of infantile neuromuscular disorders (Box 28-1).

Experienced child neurologists are able to select the infants who are most likely to have a peripheral motor unit disorder that may be further defined by an EMG evaluation. In some instances, the clinical appearance is so stereotyped that the pediatric neurologist recognizes the clinical problem immediately (e.g., SMA type 1 [Werdnig-Hoffmann disease]). The advent of survival motor neuron gene deletion testing makes EMG testing unnecessary in many infants with a classic clinical presentation. However, in some instances, EMG is indicated to differentiate certain motor unit lesions, including (1) identifying disorders that may clinically mimic SMA-1, such as congenital neuropathies, or X-linked or other forms of SMA; (2) defining the level of the motor unit abnormality in the rare instance of a spinal cord lesion; or (3) facilitating an early diagnosis while awaiting the DNA analysis in an infant in whom SMA is the apparent clinical cause and who is quite ill, wherein quality of life issues may need to be addressed.[3] When the clinical phenotype is less well defined, or when there is a combination of features suggesting both brain and peripheral motor unit involvement, the EMG also provides useful differential diagnostic information.

Floppy Baby

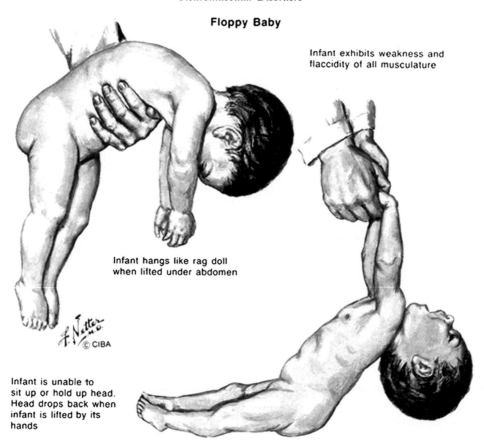

Infant exhibits weakness and flaccidity of all musculature

Infant hangs like rag doll when lifted under abdomen

Infant is unable to sit up or hold up head. Head drops back when infant is lifted by its hands

FIGURE 28–1

Primary presenting features of the floppy baby. (Copyright© 1997, Icon Learning Systems, LLC. A subsidiary of MediMedia, USA, Inc. All rights reserved.)

It is important for the electromyographer to observe whether the floppy infant has joint contractures compatible with the clinical designation of *arthrogryposis multiplex congenita* (AMC).[4] This floppy infant phenotype may result from lesions at any level of the neuraxis, including upper and lower motor neuron, peripheral nerve, neuromuscular junction, or muscle.[4-14] However, the concomitant presence of joint contractures is not specific to one disorder affecting any of the primary portions of the peripheral motor unit. AMC occurs in association with any longstanding process associated with limited intrauterine mobility. EMG is helpful in defining if a peripheral motor unit problem is the etiologic mechanism in these infants.

EMG PARAMETERS FOR EVALUATION OF THE FLOPPY INFANT

The basic techniques for nerve conduction study (NCS) and needle EMG in infants is similar to those for adults.

However, the technical evaluation and normal values for children are different. The inexperienced pediatric electromyographer may be concerned about the infant's small size. The interelectrode distances are short. Any error in measurement is amplified to the degree that erroneous conclusions may be reached. Therefore, measurement of distances must be fastidious. Infants, particularly newborns, may readily cool in the laboratory setting, and temperature must be monitored carefully. The distal skin temperature should be monitored and maintained at 31°C to 35°C.

We can carefully evaluate most FIS babies directly in the EMG laboratory. However, occasionally we need to evaluate infants when they are confined to an incubator in the neonatal intensive care unit (NICU). NICU beds, with their open exposure and continuously monitored overhead heating, provide ready access to the baby. Although motor NCSs are relatively easily performed, electrical artifacts, related to all the monitoring systems necessary in this setting, occasionally make it difficult to perform sensory NCS

BOX 28-1
FLOPPY INFANT SYNDROME: DISORDERS OF THE MOTOR UNIT

Anterior Horn Cell
Spinal muscular atrophy: 5q and X-linked forms
Poliomyelitis
Acid maltase deficiency (Pompe's disease)

Polyneuropathies
Congenital/genetic
 Hypomyelinating congenital
 Axonal congenital
 Infantile neuronal degeneration
 Carbohydrate-deficient glycosylation disorders
 Neuroaxonal dystrophy
 Leukodystrophies: Krabbe's disease
 Niemann-Pick disease
 Leigh's syndrome and other mitochondrial disorders
 Giant axonal neuropathy
Acquired
 Guillain-Barré syndrome
 Chronic inflammatory demyelinating
  polyneuropathy

Neuromuscular Junction
Presynaptic
 Acquired
  Infantile botulism
  Toxic
  Hypermagnesemia secondary to treatment of
   maternal eclampsia
  Aminoglycoside antibiotics
 Congenital
  Acetylcholine vesicle paucity
  Decreased quantal release
  Familial infantile myasthenia gravis
Postsynaptic
 Acquired
  Neonatal myasthenia gravis
 Congenital
  Acetylcholinesterase deficiency
  Slow channel
  Acetylcholine receptor deficiency

Myopathies
Congenital myopathies
 Nemaline rod
 Central core
 Centronuclear
 Congenital fiber type disproportion

Congenital muscular dystrophies (CMDs)
 Myotonic dystrophy
 Walker-Warburg syndrome
 Fukuyama type
 Muscle-eye-brain disorders
 Merosin-deficient CMDs
 Other CMD variants

Metabolic Disorders
Defects in glycogen metabolism
 Acid maltase (Pompe) (GSD-2)
 Myophosphorylase deficiency (GSD-5)
 Phosphofructokinase (GSD-7)
Other defects in energy metabolism
 Banayan-Riley-Ruvalcaba syndrome
 Fatty acid oxidation disorders
 Mitochondrial myopathies
 Carnitine transport/deficiency states

Inflammatory
 Polymyositis

and needle EMG. Better grounding and careful attention to detail while performing studies in the NICU have significantly improved these issues.

Routine Nerve Conduction Study Techniques

Multiple (at least two) motor and sensory nerves need to be studied in the routine NCS evaluation of most infants with FIS, although occasionally one study for each modality will suffice. Sensory nerve action potentials (SNAPs) are essential to consider the unusual neonatal, usually congenital, polyneuropathies that sometimes mimic more common causes of the FIS such as SMA-1 or congenital muscular dystrophy. Obtaining SNAPs in neonates and young infants may require a longer duration stimulus. Furthermore, the increased subcutaneous tissue within the calf makes obtaining sural studies a more challenging task than in the older patient. Typically in the neonate and young infant we preferentially study the median, ulnar, or even the medial plantar SNAPs rather than attempt to obtain the traditional sural responses; these are more easily obtained in the somewhat older child.

Repetitive Motor Nerve Stimulation

Occasionally the pediatric electromyographer must consider the possibility of a neuromuscular transmission defect

(NMTD) when evaluating a floppy infant, particularly when the onset is of acute character between the ages of 1 and 6 months.[15-17] A hereditary NMTD should be considered in those babies with ptosis and poor facial mobility.[15,16] Infantile botulism also requires serious consideration in any previously healthy baby who suddenly or subacutely develops generalized hypotonia.[17] Typically these babies are younger than 6 months of age, but older infants are sometimes affected. Repetitive motor nerve stimulation (RMNS) is required for diagnosis in this setting as well as the rare instance that a floppy infant may have a congenital NMTD.

In contrast, infantile autoimmune, maternally transmitted, acquired myasthenia gravis is usually a clinical diagnosis not requiring EMG. The youngest child with autoimmune-mediated primary myasthenia gravis that we have seen was 15 months of age. Hypotonia and transient respiratory depression are observed in some infants whose mothers received magnesium sulfate treatment for preeclampsia. Typically, this is short lived, on the order of several hours, but the effect can be potentiated with the use of aminoglycoside antibiotics.

Although RMNS is not routinely performed in each floppy infant, it is indicated in babies under the following clinical circumstances:

1. In the presence of ptosis, with extraocular muscle weakness or significant bulbar involvement
2. Clinical history compatible with infantile botulism (i.e., acute onset of weakness in a previously healthy infant with constipation or other autonomic feature without routine EMG evidence of an acute demyelinating neuropathy or anterior horn cell disease)
3. Repetitive compound muscle action potentials (CMAPs) after single supramaximal stimuli on routine NCS, suggesting diagnosis of either a congenital acetylcholinesterase deficiency or slow-channel syndrome[15]
4. Small motor unit potentials (MUPs) suggestive of a myopathy are present on routine needle EMG and the biopsy is nondiagnostic
5. Routine NCS and EMG are normal, yet the clinical suspicion of an NMTD remains high, such as in moderate to severe FIS with normal noninvasive testing for central nervous system disorders

Needle EMG

Needle EMG may be a challenge when evaluating a floppy infant. In contrast with the older child or adult, it is not possible to obtain an orderly assessment of the MUPs and insertional activity. Infantile MUPs are normally activated in an inconsistent, sporadic fashion. Often one gains a gestalt impression of the MUP amplitude, duration, phases, and firing pattern. Various technical maneuvers enhance the quality of MUP data. Because our aim in the evaluation of a floppy baby is not to attempt to define a specific peripheral nerve or root lesion, the evaluation of both MUPs and insertional activity in the same muscles is often not essential. This approach accurately and expeditiously provides a means to evaluate the floppy infant without fastidiously defining MUPs and insertional activity in each muscle.

There are a few helpful methods to enhance the evaluation of motor units and insertional activity in babies. The tibialis anterior and iliopsoas muscles offer the most information in the leg. Gentle stimulation of the plantar surface of the foot activates both muscles as part of the withdrawal reflex. The biceps brachii muscle is frequently active in repose; on occasion, touching the volar surface of the forearm or eliciting a grasp reflex also helps activate this muscle. Because of the spontaneous activation of MUPs in both the iliopsoas muscle and the biceps brachii, it is often difficult to evaluate insertional and abnormal forms of spontaneous activity. In contrast, the antagonists of these muscles are good muscles to evaluate for insertional activity. Sometimes in this setting the major issue is finding enough MUPs to analyze; this is particularly so in babies with SMA-1.

Insertional Activity

Historically opinions differed with respect to the type of insertion and spontaneous activity that may occur in normal newborns, particularly as to whether fibrillation potentials may "normally" be present at birth. We do not have any evidence to support the opinion that "fibrillation potentials are normally present" in the healthy newborn infant.[18] The resting membrane potential in normally innervated skeletal muscle is stable. When denervation occurs, rhythmic oscillations of the muscle membrane potential occur that trigger an action potential when the oscillations exceed a threshold voltage.[19] When firing is in a rhythmic fashion, these are fibrillation potentials. Similar findings are present in fetal muscle as well as in noninnervated muscle cells grown in culture.[19] Fibrillation potentials per se are a nonspecific finding and may be found in a number of disorders leading to FIS at each level of the motor unit (Box 28-2).

One frequently observes normal spontaneous biphasic end plate potentials during infancy. These waveforms have a typically negative initial deflection in contrast with the triphasic, initially positive, deflection of fibrillation potentials. End plates account for a greater percentage of muscle bulk in the infant as compared with adults.[20] Normal neonatal MUPs are small, and some of these units may mimic fibrillation potentials. The pediatric electromyographer needs to be able to distinguish normal end plate noise

BOX 28-2
DISORDERS ASSOCIATED WITH FIBRILLATION POTENTIALS

Neuronal
Werdnig-Hoffmann disease
Poliomyelitis
Spinal cord injury

Polyneuropathies (As noted in box 28-1)

Neuromuscular Transmission Defects
Infantile botulism

Myopathies/Dystrophies
Centronuclear (myotubular)
Congenital fiber type disproportion (rarely)
Nemaline rod (rarely)
Congenital myotonic dystrophy
Congenital muscular dystrophies/muscle-eye-brain
disease
Amyoplasia congenita

Enzymatic (glycogen storage diseases)
Type 2: Acid maltase (Pompe's disease)
Type 5: Myophosphorylase (McArdle's disease)
Type 7: Phosphofructokinase (Tarui's disease)

Inflammatory
Polymyositis

In summary, the pediatric electromyographer must be cautious when interpreting the nature and significance of insertional potentials in newborns, especially when an infant's motor units appear to be normal size with good recruitment, because the presence of such is not primarily indicative of an anterior horn cell disorder.[14,48]

Motor Unit Potentials

Normal MUP size parameters differ appreciably for infants and toddlers when compared with adults. Infantile MUP amplitudes vary between 100 and 1600 μV, with most on the lower end of the spectrum.[21,22] Normal MUPs greater than 1000 μV are much less common than in the older child or adult. Additionally the normal newborn MUP duration is shorter than in the mature child. Such characteristics sometimes challenge the pediatric electromyographer to differentiate a normal infant's MUPs from subtle myopathic changes or, on occasion, even fibrillation potentials when one cannot obtain full relaxation. The recruitment pattern is often sporadic, and the gestalt approach is often necessary to define such units and their firing patterns. To date no computerized techniques are available to provide a precise differentiation of abnormal infantile MUPs from normal, but immature, neonatal units.

Because the evaluation of MUPs is not precise, the pediatric electromyographer must be cautious to not overinterpret when reporting borderline or even normal results. Correlation studies assessing the reliability between EMG and muscle biopsy have noted that the most concordance occurs with the SMAs (Table 28-1).[22-27] Concomitantly, the referring clinician needs to be advised that a normal needle EMG does not exclude a myopathic process, especially many of the congenital myopathies. In this instance, DNA testing or a biopsy often provides the only definitive diagnostic tool.

Some motor unit disorders are unique to neonates such as SMA-1 and SMA-2, some of the unusual congenital polyneuropathies, infantile botulism, and a number of the myopathies, including the infantile forms of glycogen storage disorders. An in-depth EMG experience with infants is helpful. Reference to standard tables of normal values for

from small normal MUPs or abnormal insertional waveforms in the newborn infant. In the more vigorous infant, discomfort from the testing may cause crying, which has the potential to mask the important auditory components of the study, such as the characteristic ticking sound associated with typical fibrillation potentials. This can be particularly problematic in a noisy NICU environment.

TABLE 28–1. RESULTS OF EMG ANALYSES OF FLOPPY INFANTS: CORRELATION WITH MUSCLE/NERVE BIOPSY[27]

Year	No. of Cases	SMA, No. (% correlation)	PN, No. (% correlation)	NMTD, No. (% correlation)	Myopathy, No. (% correlation)	ND, No. (% correlation)
1982[24]	51	21 (41)	0 (0)	11 (22)	8 (16)	11 (64)
1992[26]	79	20 (40)	0 (0)	2 (4)	27 (55)	29 (10-90)
1992[26]	122	46 (43)	19 (18)	18 (16)	25 (23)	14
1994[27]	41	15 (37)	3 (7)	2 (5)	10 (24)	11 (40-93)

ND, nondiagnostic, normal, or central hypotonia; SMA, spinal muscular atrophy; NMTD, neuromuscular transmission defects; PN, peripheral neuropathy.
Adapted from David WS, Jones HR Jr: Electromyography and biopsy correlation with suggested protocol for evaluation of the floppy infant. Muscle Nerve 1994;17:424-431.

NCS and EMG in this age group provides an important foundation for neonatal EMG.[23] Unless the EMG physician's experience includes infants and toddlers on a fairly routine basis, it is often prudent to refer the baby to a major pediatric neuromuscular center. If the infant possibly has an NMTD, sedation in an outpatient day surgery center makes the testing more comfortable and often provides for a technically better study. On the other hand, sedation in the EMG laboratory is ill advised, since these infants are at greater risk for respiratory depression and aspiration.

SPECTRUM OF NEUROMUSCULAR DISEASE OBSERVED WITH EMG STUDIES OF FLOPPY INFANTS

Electromyographers evaluating the floppy infant need to consider multiple disorders affecting each motor unit level from the anterior horn to the muscle cell per se. The accuracy and spectrum of EMG findings in the evaluation of floppy infants are summarized in Table 28-1.[24-27] Two retrospective reviews studied 28 and 41 hypotonic infants, all younger than 1 year of age seen at either the Children's Hospital of Philadelphia (CHoP)[24] or our EMG laboratory at Children's Hospital Boston (CHB).[27] There was a 64% and 76% correlation, respectively, comparing EMG results with muscle biopsy[24] or with muscle and nerve biopsy, a biochemical analysis, or, rarely, microbiologic definition for infantile botulism.[27]

Motor Neuron Disorders

Until the advent of DNA diagnosis for SMA-1, SMA-1 has been the most common cause for a baby with the FIS presenting to the EMG laboratory. This diagnosis accounted for 21 (41%) of 51 infants seen at CHoP[24] and 15 (37%) of 41 infants seen at CHB.[27] EMG study provides a highly accurate means to diagnose SMA with basically no false-positive or false-negative results. This diagnosis correlated with the findings on muscle biopsy in 93% of our patients[27] similar to other studies.[25,26,28] To date, the 79 floppy infants studied at Iowa during a 20-year period were the only ones to have a greater proportion of myopathies than SMA.[26] Subsequent to the recent availability of DNA testing for SMA, most infants with classic clinical phenotypes are no longer referred for EMG evaluation. Therefore, the number of babies with SMA-1 now evaluated in an EMG laboratory constitutes a smaller percentage of the total floppy infant population.

The presence of arthrogryposis in a child with the classic SMA phenotype suggests an alternative diagnosis. Although it is atypical for infants with classic SMA to present with joint contractures,[14] such may occur and the diagnosis is identified with appropriate DNA testing.

At time the rare baby with a congenital infantile polyneuropathy may have a phenotype similar to an infant with SMA.[29] This is the reason that it is important *not* to limit NCSs to motor studies in floppy infants, particularly when such is based entirely on the clinical phenotype. We have seen infants preliminarily diagnosed by senior child neurologists as having Werdnig-Hoffman disease when these babies presented with the classic frog-legged jug-handle posture, areflexia, and tongue fasciculation. However, when we performed an NCS, the study failed to demonstrate elicitable SNAPs. Sural nerve biopsy confirmed the presence of a congenital polyneuropathy.[27] This illustrates the importance of obtaining SNAPs. If the EMG demonstrates abnormalities of sensory conduction, a sural nerve biopsy will often provide the means to diagnose arthrogryposis.[30]

Polyneuropathies

Both motor and sensory NCSs are routinely performed in the EMG analysis of floppy infants. As noted, if SNAPs are not attempted, some early-onset peripheral neuropathies may be confused with SMA-1. We routinely perform sensory NCS in every infant with FIS, and when these results are abnormal, a congenital neuropathy is readily differentiated from SMA. In our review of EMG studies among floppy infants, we identified three infants with a congenital peripheral neuropathy,[27] whereas no congenital polyneuropathies were identified in two other studies[24,26] when sensory NCSs were not reported. Sural nerve biopsy was pathologic in each of our floppy infants with abnormal sensory NCS.

Sensory NCSs are relatively easy to perform in infants, particularly the median SNAP and a medial plantar SNAP rather than a sural nerve potential. The medial plantar SNAP is readily found with either antidromic or orthodromic stimulation in the infant, when a lower extremity sensory study is needed (Kuntz NL, personal communication, 1992.) In contrast, a sural SNAP is technically difficult to obtain even in normal babies. Furthermore, in contrast with adults, in whom early signs of polyneuropathies may be limited to the lower extremities, the polyneuropathies identified among our floppy infants have had diffuse involvement.

A broad differential diagnosis exists for the uncommon polyneuropathies that present at birth or during infancy, even including Guillain-Barré syndrome (Box 28-3). When we analyzed our experience with FIS, only 6 infants were identified as having a polyneuropathy: 3 were found among a series of 80 infants with uncomplicated FIS,[27] and another 3 were present in our group of 35 floppy infants associated with AMC.[14]

BOX 28-3
INFANTILE POLYNEUROPATHIES

Congenital, Hereditary, and Metabolic
Congenital hypomyelinating
Carbohydrate-deficient glycosylation disorders
Infantile neuronal degeneration
Infantile neuroaxonal dystrophy
Infantile porphyria

Acquired
Guillain-Barré syndrome
Chronic inflammatory demyelinating polyneuropathy

BOX 28-4
DISORDERS OF THE NEUROMUSCULAR JUNCTION

Presynaptic Defects
Infantile botulism
Toxic
    Hypermagnesemia (therapy of eclampsia)
    Aminoglycoside antibiotics
Congenital
    Familial myasthenia gravis
    Acetylcholine vesicle paucity
    Acetylcholine quantal release diminished
    Miscellaneous, poorly categorized
Postsynaptic defects
Autoimmune (antibody positive)
Acquired myasthenia gravis
    Maternal
    Primary – earliest known onset age 9 months
Congenital (antibody negative)
    Acetylcholine receptor deficiency
    Acetylcholinesterase deficiencies
    Classic slow-channel syndrome

When a floppy infant is identified as having a polyneuropathy, the essential issue is to determine whether a potentially treatable condition is present.[31-35] An acquired intrauterine demyelinating neuropathy, particularly Guillain-Barré syndrome, always requires consideration. This is likely in the rare instance when the EMG findings demonstrate dispersed CMAPs and slow motor conduction velocities. Here immunotherapy, particularly intravenous immunoglobulins, may be beneficial.[33,35]

As potential therapies are developed for other forms of neonatal neuropathies, a better appreciation of their pathophysiology will be required. Possibly those associated with AMC may have longstanding developmental arrest and, therefore, are less prone to therapeutic intervention. However, infants without AMC whose EMG suggests a primary demyelinating process may respond to intravenous immunoglobulin[33] or the various other therapies used for Guillain-Barré syndrome in the older child and adult.

Disorders of Neuromuscular Transmission

Rarely, a lesion at the neuromuscular junction is identified in the context of a baby who has been floppy since birth (Box 28-4). In three reviews of the EMG experience in the evaluation of the floppy infant at major children's hospitals, no instances of either a congenital NMTD or autoimmune neonatal myasthenia gravis were recorded.[24,26,27] Although the congenital variants are exceedingly rare, we recently documented an NMTD, presumed congenital, in a 5-month-old infant with generalized hypotonia and failure to thrive. She has had a remarkable response to pyridostigmine. Infants with clinically obvious autoimmune neonatal myasthenia gravis do not require an EMG when the mother has known myasthenia gravis. Infantile botulism is the one acquired NMTD that occurs in this age group, sometimes as early as 2 to 3 weeks of age, although usually not until 3 to 4 months of age.

Presynaptic Neuromuscular Transmission Disorders

Infantile botulism is the most common acquired neuromuscular junction disorder that occurs during the first year of life (see Box 28-4). Rarely, one is confronted by an infant with a congenital presynaptic NMTD. Even less likely is the possibility of a toxic drug mechanism such as hypermagnesemia or aminoglycosides. The incidence of botulism varies greatly from one geographic region of the country to another. Infantile botulism is especially prevalent in certain areas of this country, particularly the middle Atlantic states, California, and the Rocky Mountain states where one of us (K.J.S.) has seen 14 cases in just 5 years at Salt Lake City. *Clostridium botulinum* is clearly endemic in some geographic areas more than others. Infantile botulism was present in 11 (22%) of 50 floppy infants seen at CHoP.[24] In contrast, no instances of infantile botulism were reported in the Iowa study[26] and just a single case was initially reported by us among 80 FIS evaluated in New England.[27] However, we have subsequently diagnosed 4 more cases, including one at 10 months of age. Therefore, it is important to always consider infantile botulism in the differential diagnosis when evaluating a previously healthy infant who has suddenly become hypotonic, particularly if associated with dysautonomia such as constipation and poorly reactive pupils.[17,36]

Infantile botulism has a stereotyped clinical set. This typically occurs in a previously healthy infant who develops the acute onset of hypotonia, poor feeding, and constipation.[37-44] However, the rapidity of progression and eventual severity of the illness are variable. Some infants have a relatively benign course, and others require rapid intubation with prolonged hospitalization. Rarely, there even may be a clinical relapse.[41] The differential diagnosis includes other acute disorders of the motor unit (see Box 28-1), a nonspecific encephalopathy, sepsis, or respiratory distress. Consequently, the pediatric electromyographer is sometimes asked to evaluate a broad spectrum of infants with acute hypotonia during the first 6 months of life.

A diagnosis of infantile botulism may be established by appropriate NCS, repetitive nerve stimulation and needle EMG as summarized in Box 28-5. The setting may vary from the outpatient laboratory to the NICU. Compared with Lambert-Eaton myasthenic syndrome (LEMS) in the adult, babies with infantile botulism may have just a relatively modest degree of facilitation with RMNS and often less than or not greater than 100% routinely seen with LEMS.[17,44,45] This association also was illustrated by one of the infantile botulism seen by us (H.R.J.). This baby was in respiratory distress and had a modest 23% to 65% facilitation.

BOX 28-5
EMG PROTOCOL FOR SUSPECTED PRESYNAPTIC NEUROMUSCULAR TRANSMISSION DEFECTS, PARTICULARLY INFANTILE BOTULISM

Motor/sensory NCS in one arm and leg
RMNS at 2 Hz to two distal muscles
Tetanizing stimulation at 50 Hz for 10 seconds
    followed by stimulation every 30 seconds until
    CMAP is baseline
Diagnostic features for infantile botulism
    1) CMAP < 2.0 mV in at least two muscles
    2) PTF >120% of baseline
    3) PTF prolonged >120 seconds with no PTE

NCS, nerve conduction study; RMNS, repetitive motor nerve stimulation; CMAP, compound muscle action potential; PTF, post-tetanic facilitation; PTE, post-tetanic exhaustion.
    Adapted from Gutierrez AR, Bodensteiner J, Gutmann L: Electrodiagnosis of infantile botulism. J Child Neurol 1994;9:362-365.

A more difficult question arises as to when to test other floppy babies for the presence of an NMTD. Although most hypotonic babies with either a presynaptic or postsynaptic disorder have obvious signs of bulbar involvement, we are unaware of any study that has routinely used RMNS to evaluate a broad spectrum of floppy infants. Because one needs to use 20- to 50-Hz stimulation frequencies, this is a painful procedure. Sedation under anesthesia in a surgical day-care center allows the pediatric electromyographer to accomplish the best results.

We suggest that the primary indications for RMNS studies still depend on clinical judgment. The routine use of RMNS is indicated in the floppy infant with evidence of ocular, or lower bulbar, dysfunction and those babies with intermittency of symptoms such as is seen in some of the familial NMTDs. However, there still remains the issue of the floppy baby having none of these indications but in whom no diagnosis is identified to explain the generalized hypotonia. Perhaps these infants also deserve this more extensive testing. Certainly as more colleagues begin to routinely use anesthesia for EMG for these infants, these data may become available. Similarly, as stimulated single-fiber EMG gains wider usage, this may also be an effective means to screen this population.[17]

Postsynaptic Disorders of Neuromuscular Transmission

With the exception of neonatal autoimmune maternal-acquired myasthenia gravis, it is unusual for autoimmune myasthenia gravis to present before 1 year of age. The youngest child we have seen at CHB is 15 months old. Rarely, one may be confronted with an early presentation of a postsynaptic congenital NMTD such as the slow-channel syndrome or acetylcholinesterase deficiency. These two inborn postsynaptic disorders may be suspected by the presence of repetitive or late component on the CMAP (Fig. 28-2).[46,47] These are further defined in Chapter 35.

Myopathies

There are a large number of myopathies that may present in the neonatal period as a floppy infant (Box 28-6). Normal newborn infant MUPs are shorter in duration and sometimes of lower amplitude, not unlike those identified as myopathic in adults. Pediatric electromyographers usually need to form a gestalt impression of both individual MUP parameters and firing patterns that typically occur sporadically and unpredictably.

When the FIS is secondary to a myopathy, in a number of instances this is particularly difficult to define by EMG. Ten (24%) of the 41 floppy infant cases seen at CHB were caused by a myopathy.[15] The EMG pathology correlation was good in 4 (67%) of 6 babies when the EMG

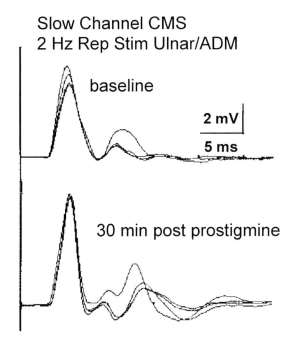

Slow Channel CMS
2 Hz Rep Stim Ulnar/ADM

baseline

2 mV

5 ms

30 min post prostigmine

FIGURE 28–2

Effect of cholinesterase inhibitor (prostigmine) on repetitive stimulation (2 Hz/4 superimposed traces) of the ulnar nerve recording over the abductor digiti minimi (ADM) muscle in slow-channel congenital myasthenic syndrome (CMS). Following administration of prostigmine, the decrement of the main compound muscle action potential (CMAP) was partially repaired and there was an increase in both the number and amplitude of repetitive CMAPs. (From Engel AC, Ohno K, Harper CM: Congenital myasthenic syndromes. In Jones HR, DeVivo DC, Darras BT [eds]: Neuromuscular Disorders of Infancy, Childhood, and Adolescence: A Clinician's Approach. Philadelphia, Butterworth-Heinemann, 2003, pp 555-574.)

> **BOX 28-6**
> **NEONATAL MYOPATHIES**
>
> ***Congenital Myopathies***
> Nemaline rod
> Centronuclear
> Central core
> Fiber-type disproportion
>
> ***Dystrophies***
> Congenital myotonic dystrophy
> Congenital muscular dystrophy variants
>
> ***Inflammatory***
> Polymyositis
>
> ***Enzymatic Myopathies***
> Carbohydrate cycle deficiencies
>   Type 2: acid maltase, some with debrancher
>   Type 5: muscle phosphorylase
>   Type 7: phosphofructokinase
> Lipid metabolism
>   Infantile carnitine palmitoyltransferase deficiency
>   Primary systemic carnitine deficiency
>   Acetyl coenzyme dehydrogenase deficiency
>
> ***Electron Transport Chain Disorders***
> Severe infantile myopathy
> Complex II deficiency
> Complex IV deficiency
>
> ***Benign Infantile Myopathy***
> Complex IV deficiency

---

demonstrated classic myopathic features. However, myopathies were also found in 2 of 3 floppy infants with "nonspecific" EMG changes and in 4 of 12 infants with normal results on EMG. Therefore, only 4 (40%) of 10 CHB infants with histologically and clinically confirmed myopathies had EMGs compatible with that diagnosis.[27] At CHoP, 8 children (16%) in a series of floppy infants had a myopathy.[24] Four (50%) of these 8 floppy infants had concordant EMG and biopsy results.

Motor Unit Parameters

The disparity between the sensitivity of EMG in the definition of neurogenic processes versus myopathic disorders in the newborn infant relates to several factors. A major issue concerns the striking diminution in the number of MUPs found in SMA-1 infants, providing an easy window and ease for one to identify these isolated, somewhat enlarged, rapidly firing MUPs. Typically these motor units have a widespread anatomic distribution in multiple nerve root supplies and extremities. In contrast, infants with myopathies challenge the electromyographer because the MUP changes herein are more subtle in character as well as more difficult to define. This is because it is often more difficult to determine if an infant's MUPs are significantly abnormally smaller or unequivocally state they are predominantly abnormal. This is particularly so because activation requires a degree of patient cooperation that cannot readily be obtained in the neonate.

In the florid neonatal myopathies, the recruitment of increased numbers of smaller MUPs is best appreciated in the iliopsoas muscle when the infant withdraws the thigh from a light stimulus to the plantar surface of the foot. However, with more subtle myopathic lesions, without much fiber destruction as occurs with the congenital myopathies, this differentiation is much more difficult, if not impossible, to define. Furthermore, one must be cautious in not overcalling a myopathic process when indeed the findings are representative of the normal immaturity of the infantile muscle fiber.

Conversely pediatric electromyographers need to also emphasize to the referring clinician that normal results on infantile EMG do not exclude a myopathic process. If a myopathy is suspected clinically, a muscle biopsy is required to define this possibility further. In contrast, when significant neurogenic changes are present supporting the diagnosis of SMA-1, a muscle biopsy is not necessary because DNA testing provides accurate diagnosis.[3]

Insertional Activity

Fibrillation potentials are a nonspecific finding, and their identification is not to be used to differentiate SMA from a myopathic process (see Box 28-2). Early in our experience, the results of the EMG in some floppy infants confused us by the finding of a few fibrillation potentials without specific changes in the MUPs.[27] We inadvertently classified these infants as having "nonspecific neurogenic changes." Later we correlated our floppy infants' EMG results with muscle biopsy findings.[27] Most babies with nonspecific needle EMG findings, such as a few fibrillation potentials but without large motor units, fortunately did not have an incipient neurogenic process, such as SMA.[27] In fact these findings usually represented a myopathic process, either a congenital myopathy or dystrophy. One sentinel study of a floppy infant illustrated this principle: this baby had diffuse fibrillation potentials and therefore was diagnosed as having SMA.[48] In retrospect, this floppy infant also had increased numbers of small MUPs, and this information should have provided the true means to clinically define this baby's difficulties. Myophosphorylase deficiency was diagnosed at age 3 months, at the time of autopsy.[48]

OVERVIEW OF EMG EVALUATION OF THE FLOPPY INFANT

An EMG protocol for the evaluation of the floppy infant is outlined in Box 28-7. Sensory NCSs are a logical initial study because they are the least uncomfortable component of pediatric EMG. In most infants with FIS, including SMA, myopathies, and the rare infantile NMTDs, the SNAPs are normal. The one exception is the diffuse sensory dysfunction present with infantile polyneuropathies. In all other instances, the initial evaluation of SNAPs permits the pediatric electromyographer to test the overall function of the peripheral nervous system as well as the integrity of the testing equipment. In general, when a normal SNAP is obtained in a floppy infant, it is rare to

---

BOX 28-7
EMG PROTOCOL FOR EVALUATION OF FLOPPY INFANT

Sensory NCS
At least one sensory nerve

Motor NCS
At least two motor nerves

Needle EMG
At least four to six muscles in one or two extremities, including distal and proximal sites

Anterior Horn Cell Disease (SMA) is a Consideration
At least two muscles innervated by different nerve roots
Nerves should be sampled in at least two extremities plus DNA testing for SMA, or three extremities

Repetitive Motor Nerve Stimulation (2 and 50 Hz) Indications
Clinical acute or subacute deterioration in motor function (infantile botulism?)
Ptosis or ophthalmoparesis
EMG stimulus-linked repetitive CMAP
Myopathy defined by EMG
EMG/NCS normal and high suspicion of peripheral motor unit lesion

EMG, electromyograph; CMAP, compound muscle action potential; SMA, spinal muscular atrophy; NCS, nerve conduction study.
Adapted from David WS, Jones HR Jr: Electromyography and biopsy correlation with suggested protocol for evaluation of the floppy infant. Muscle Nerve 1994;17:424-431.

---

gain more diagnostic information by testing of additional sensory nerves. However, when no SNAP is defined, the presence of a primary and diffuse loss of sensory function must be confirmed by evaluating at least one other sensory nerve, usually in another extremity.

Because the CMAP amplitude may be compromised by lesions at any level of the motor unit, including the anterior horn cell, peripheral nerve, neuromuscular junction, and muscle, it is important to sample the responses of at least two peripheral motor nerves, one in an arm and another in a leg. When no CMAP can be defined with standard sweep speeds, the time base should be extended to avoid failure to appreciate the prolonged latencies that may occur when a profound degree of dysmyelination is present. Similarly, as reported by Bolton and associates,[49] one has to carefully use maximal stimulation potential to identify the rare infant with a high motor threshold. In addition, particular attention must be paid to the configuration of the CMAP (Figure 28-2). The presence of a CMAP with a repetitive component provides a clue to the presence of an uncommon congenital NMTD at the postsynaptic level.[46]

The most useful EMG parameter in the evaluation of FIS is the assessment of MUPs.[24,27] In general, we test four to six muscles in the upper and lower extremity, although on occasion we confine the needle examination to just one leg,

carefully analyzing both proximal and distal muscles (Fig. 28-3). When neurogenic changes are confined to either both upper or both lower extremities one needs to exclude the unlikely instance of an isolated spinal injury. Nonarthrogrypotic infants with MUPs of increased duration and high amplitude that are recruited in decreased numbers and at an increased rate usually have SMA. This can now be confirmed with DNA testing. These findings may be sufficient for a diagnosis of SMA when the clinical context is appropriate.[27] Similar MUP changes have been noted in seven newborns with congenital neuropathy (Jones HR, unpublished data 2005), an illness that must strongly be considered when no SNAPs are present.[15]

Most newborns with low-amplitude, short-duration MUPs have a recognizable myopathy.[24,27] However, many

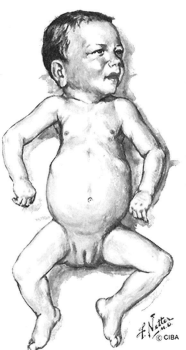

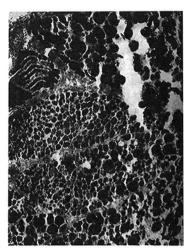

Muscle biopsy specimen showing groups of small atrophic muscle fibers and areas of normal or enlarged fibers (group atrophy). (Trichrome stain)

Infant with typical bell-shaped thorax, frog-leg posture, and "jug-handle" position of upper limbs

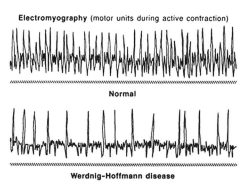

Electromyography (motor units during active contraction)

Normal

Werdnig-Hoffmann disease

FIGURE 28–3

Infant with classic body posture and needle EMG and muscle biopsy findings of spinal muscular atrophy (SMA)-1 (Werdnig-Hoffmann disease). (From Netter FH: The Ciba Collection of Medical Illustrations. Vol. 1, Nervous System: II, Neurologic and Neuromuscular Disorders. West Caldwell, NJ, Ciba-Geigy Medical Education, 1986.)

infantile myopathies may be associated with healthy-appearing MUPs.[24,,26,27] The pediatric electromyographer must always keep this in mind when dictating a clinical correlation for a floppy infant who has normal results on EMG by advising the referring physician of this particular limit of the study. Therefore, when a floppy baby shows normal results on EMG, the pediatric neurologist should be encouraged to proceed with muscle biopsy when a lesion in the peripheral motor unit is suspected clinically.

Fibrillation potentials may be associated with a disorder at any level of the motor unit, including the motor neuron, peripheral nerve, neuromuscular junction, and some myopathies (see Box 28-2). The scattered occurrence of fibrillation potentials without specific MUP abnormalities, sometimes suggesting nonspecific "neurogenic" changes, was more commonly associated with infants whose biopsy showed a myopathy, particularly congenital muscular dystrophy.[27] It is the characteristics of the MUP per se that are most accurate for defining the abnormal site of disease.[2]

To our knowledge, no study has addressed the issue of the role of routine testing for a neuromuscular junction disorder in the floppy infant. However, one must always keep this important portion of the peripheral motor unit in the differential diagnosis of a floppy newborn or any baby with an acutely acquired generalized hypotonia. The predominant clinical settings where these rare lesions need to be considered and formally tested for an NMTD are outlined earlier in this chapter.

An uncommon subset of infants are those who develop the fulminant onset of diffuse hypotonia after an initially seemingly healthy first few weeks or months of life (Box 28-8). The differential diagnosis of acute infantile hypotonia includes disorders at each level of the entire peripheral motor unit. Rarely this may involve anterior horn cell disorders; today this primarily occurs with an unrecognized case of SMA-1, usually with first-time parents who have not recognized their baby's hypotonia and the infant develops a bronchiolitis or other pulmonary problem, requires intubation, and then cannot be weaned.

Additionally some countries still have incomplete primary polio immunization, particularly in Africa and India, and there has been an increased number of wild cases. Furthermore they are primarily using live vaccines where poliomyelitis may occur after the first vaccination.[50-57] We had this experience, with phone consultations, on some acute floppy babies less than 10 years ago. These turned out to have vaccine-induced poliomyelitis.[54,55] The essential clues to the diagnosis were the low-amplitude CMAPs, normal SNAPs, and a cerebrospinal fluid pleocytosis. This is no longer an issue in the United States since the return to initially using the killed vaccine a few years ago.[57,58]

Other motor unit disorders that may lead to an acute FIS include certain polyneuropathies, primarily Guillain-

---

BOX 28-8
ACUTE-ONSET FLOPPY INFANT SYNDROME

Anterior Horn Cell
Poliomyelitis, other enteroviruses

Peripheral Nerve
Acute inflammatory demyelinating polyneuropathy
Chronic inflammatory demyelinating polyneuropathy
Tick paralysis

Neuromuscular Junction
Infantile botulism
Familial infantile myasthenia gravis

Muscle
Polymyositis
Glycogen storage disease
Muscle phosphorylase deficiency

Barré syndrome,[31] or chronic inflammatory demyelinating polyneuropathy.[35] The most common clinical cause in this country occurs at the level of the neuromuscular junction (i.e., infantile botulism[36-38]) or rarely the various familial congenital myasthenia syndromes.[46,47] It is very uncommon to have a myopathy lead to an acute loss of muscle tone in a baby. Considerations include some glycolytic enzyme deficiencies[48,59-63] and possibly infantile polymyositis.[64-67]

SUMMARY

A pediatric electromyographer with knowledge of the various clinical syndromes affecting the motor unit in infancy (see Box 28-1) can provide considerable help to the pediatric neurologist in the evaluation of floppy infants. Occasionally, examination of a parent may add specific diagnostic definition, especially for diagnosing unsuspected myotonic dystrophy. An EMG evaluation of a hypotonic baby has the potential to define a specific motor unit disorder at the anterior horn cell, peripheral nerve, neuromuscular junction, and muscle cell. These results are helpful to the pediatric neurologist, providing a useful guide to the early management of the floppy infant.

Initial results of EMG often provide encouragement to parents awaiting the muscle biopsy processing, because

SMA-1 may be virtually excluded with a carefully executed EMG.[27] In contrast, when the EMG does indicate a diffuse process affecting motor neurons, the primary child neurologist can provide support to the parents so that when results of further studies, particularly DNA testing for the survival motor neuron are available, the family may be prepared for the seriousness of their child's illness.

We have awaited the potential for computed analysis of MUPs to provide a more accurate definition of subtle myopathies that still defy EMG and/or DNA classification. Whether such will eventually become available is still unclear because various models to date have been disappointing. However, genetic definition of many of these syndromes continues to evolve rapidly and shows increasing promise. This is particularly true in a number of the congenital myasthenic syndromes that are so difficult to clinically and electrically clarify without specialized biopsy techniques available only in a few research settings.[16] As with many SMA cases, these future discoveries may eventually obviate the need for EMG in some floppy babies in the future.

REFERENCES

1. Dubowitz V: The floppy infant. Clin Dev Med 1980;2:89-94.
2. Jones HR Jr: EMG evaluation of the floppy infant: Differential diagnosis and technical aspects. Muscle Nerve 1990;13:338-347.
3. Darras BT, Jones HR: Diagnosis of neuromuscular disorders in the era of DNA analysis: The role of pediatric electromyography. Pediatr Neurol 2000;23:289-306.
4. Banker BO: Arthrogryposis multiplex congenita: Spectrum of pathologic changes. Hum Pathol 1986;17:656-672.
5. Drachman DB, Sokoloff L: The role of movement in embryonic joint development. Dev Biol 1966;14:401-420.
6. Holmes LB, Driscoll SG, Bradley WG: Contractures in a newborn infant of a mother with myasthenia gravis. J Pediatr 1980;96:1067-1069.
7. Smit LME, Barth PG: Arthrogryposis multiplex congenita due to congenital myasthenia. Dev Med Child Neurol 1980;22:371-374.
8. Banker BO: Neuropathologic aspects of arthrogryposis multiplex congenita. Clin Orthop 1985;194:30-43.
9. Smith EM, Bender LF, Stover CN: Lower motor neuron deficit in arthrogryposis: An EMG study. Arch Neurol 1963;8:97-100.
10. Amick LD, Johnson WW, Smith HL: Electromyographic and histopathologic correlation in arthrogryposis. Arch Neurol 1967;16:512-523.
11. Fisher RL, Johnstone WT, Fisher WH Jr, Goldkamp OG: Arthrogryposis multiplex congenita: A clinical investigation. J Pediatr 1970;76:255-261.
12. Bharucha EP, Pandya SS, Dastur DK: Arthrogryposis multiplex congenita: I. Clinical and electromyographic aspects. J Neurol Neurosurg Psychiatry 1972;35:425-434.
13. Strehl E, Vanasse M, Brochu P: EMG and needle muscle biopsy studies in arthrogryposis multiplex congenita. Neuropediatrics 1985;16:225-227.
14. Kang PB, Lidov HGW, Torres A, et al: Arthrogryposis multiplex congenita: A 23-year study comparing electromyography and neuropathology. Ann Neurol 2003;54:790-795.
15. Engel A: Overview of the Congenital myasthenic syndromes, 73rd ENMC International Workshop. Neuromuscul Disord 2001;11:315-321.
16. Engel AG, Ohno K, Harper CM: Congenital myasthenic syndromes. *In* Jones HR, De Vivo DC, Darras BT (eds): Neuromuscular Disorders of Infancy, Childhood, and Adolescence. Philadelphia, Butterworth-Heinemann, Elsevier, 2003, 555-574.
17. Crawford TO: Infantile botulism. *In* Jones HR, De Vivo DC, Darras BT (eds): Neuromuscular Disorders of Infancy, Childhood, and Adolescence. Philadelphia, Butterworth-Heinemann, 2003, pp 547-554.
18. Eng GD: Spontaneous potentials in premature and full term infants. Arch Phys Med Rehabil 1976;57:120-121.
19. Purves D, Sakmann B: Membrane properties underlying spontaneous activity of denervated muscle. J Physiol 1974;239:125-153.
20. Coers C, Woolf AL: The innervation of muscle: A biopsy study. Oxford, Blackwell Scientific, 1959, pp 16-17.
21. do Carmo RJ: Motor unit action potential parameters in human newborn infants. Arch Neurol 1960;3:136-140.
22. Sacco G, Buchthal F, Rosenfalck P: Motor unit potentials at different ages. Arch Neurol 1962;6:366-373.
23. Jones HR, Harmon RL, Bolton CF, Harper CM: Introduction to pediatric EMG. *In* Jones HR, Bolton CF, Harper CM (eds): Clinical Pediatric Electromyography. Philadelphia, Lippincott-Raven, 1996, pp 1-37.
24. Packer RJ, Brown MJ, Berman PH: The diagnostic value of electromyography in infantile hypotonia. Am J Dis Child 1982;136:1057-1059.
25. Papazian O, Duenas DA, Cullen RF Jr, et al: Outcome of neonatal floppy syndrome [Abstract]. Ann Neurol 1990;28:430.
26. Russell JW, Afifi AK, Ross MA: Predictive value of electromyography in diagnosis and prognosis of the hypotonic infant. J Child Neurol 1992;7:387-391.
27. David WS, Jones HR Jr: Electromyography and biopsy correlation with suggested protocol for evaluation of the floppy infant. Muscle Nerve 1994;17:424-431.
28. Cotliar R, Eng GD, Koch B, et al: Correlation of electrodiagnosis and muscle biopsy results [Abstract]. Muscle Nerve 1992;15:1197-1198.
29. Jones HR: Electromyographic evaluation of the floppy infant. *In* Jones HR, Bolton CF, Harper CM (eds): Pediatric Clinical Electromyography. Philadelphia, Lippincott-Raven, 1996, pp 37-104.

30. Seitz RJ, Wechsler W, Mosny DS, Lenard HG: Hypomyelination neuropathy in a female newborn presenting as arthrogryposis multiplex congenita. Neuropediatrics 1986;17:132-136.

31. Jones HR: Guillain-Barré syndrome perspectives with infants and children. Semin Pediatr Neurol 2000;7:91-102.

32. Jackson AH, Baquis GD, Shaw BL: Congenital Guillain-Barré syndrome. J Child Neurol 1996;5:407-410.

33. Rolfs A, Bolik A: Guillain-Barré syndrome in pregnancy: Reflections on immunopathogenesis. Acta Neurol Scand 1994;89:400-492.

34. Luijckx GJ, Vies J, de Baets M, et al: Guillain-Barré syndrome in mother and child. Lancet 1997;349:27.

35. Sladky JT, Brown MJ, Berman PH: Chronic inflammatory demyelinating polyneuropathy of infancy: A corticosteroid-responsive disorder. Ann Neurol 1986;20:76-81.

36. Cornblath DR, Sladky JT, Sumner AJ: Clinical electrophysiology of infantile botulism. Muscle Nerve 1983;6:448-452.

37. Pickett J, Berg B, Chaplin E, et al: Syndrome of botulism in infancy: Clinical and electrophysiologic study. N Engl J Med 1976;295:770-772.

38. Clay SA, Ramseyer JC, Fishman LS, Sedgwick RP: Acute infantile motor unit disorder: Infantile botulism? Arch Neurol 1977;34:236-249.

39. Hoffman RE, Pincomb BJ, Skeels MR: Type F infant botulism. Am J Dis Child 1982;136:270-271.

40. Schwartz RH, Eng G: Infant botulism: Exacerbation by aminoglycosides [Letter]. Am J Dis Child 1982;136:952.

41. Glauser TA, Maguire HC, Sladky JT: Relapse of infantile botulism [Abstract]. Ann Neurol 1989;26:449.

42. Thompson JA, Glasgow LA, Warpinski JR, Olson C: Infant botulism: Clinical spectrum and epidemiology. Pediatrics 1980;66:936-942.

43. Donley DK, Knight P, Tenorio G, Oh SJ: A patient with infant botulism, improving with edrophonium [Abstract]. Muscle Nerve 1991;41:201.

44. Gutierrez AR, Bodensteiner J, Gutmann L: Electrodiagnosis of infantile botulism. J Child Neurol 1994;9:362-365.

45. Fakadej AV, Gutmann L: Prolongation of post-tetanic facilitation in infant botulism. Muscle Nerve 1982;5:727-729.

46. Harper CM: Congenital myasthenic syndromes. *In* Brown W, Bolton CF, Aminoff M (eds): Clinical Neurophysiology and Neuromuscular Diseases. Philadelphia, WB Saunders, 2002.

47. Ohno K, Engel AG, Brengman JM, et al: The spectrum of mutations causing endplate acetylcholinesterase deficiency. Ann Neurol 2000;47:162-170.

48. DiMauro S, Hartlage PL: Fatal infantile form of muscle phosphorylase deficiency. Neurology 1978;28:1124-1129.

49. Bolton CF, Hahn AF, Hinton GG: The syndrome of high-stimulation threshold and low-conduction velocity [Abstract]. Ann Neurol 1988;24:165.

50. Moore M, Katona P, Kaplan JE, et al: Poliomyelitis in the United States, 1969-1981. J Infect Dis 1982;146:558-563.

51. Robbins FC: Eradication of polio in the Americas. JAMA 1993;270:1857-1859.

52. Bergeisen GH, Bauman RJ, Gilmore RL: Neonatal paralytic poliomyelitis: A case report. Arch Neurol 1986;43:192-194.

53. Beausoleil JL, Nordgren RE, Medlin JF: Vaccine associated paralytic poliomyelitis. J Child Neurol 1994;9:334-335.

54. David WS, Doyle JJ: Acute infantile weakness: A case of vaccine-associated poliomyelitis. Muscle Nerve 1997;20:747-749.

55. Goldstein J: Infantile poliomyelitis in a recently immunized baby seen at Yale. Personal communication, 1995.

56. CDC: Recommendations of the Advisory Committee on Immunization Practices: Revised recommendations for routine poliomyelitis vaccination. MMWR Morb Mortal Wkly Rep 1999;48:590.

57. David WS: Vaccine-associated poliomyelitis. *In* Jones HR, De Vivo DC, Darras BT (eds): Neuromuscular Disorders of Infancy, Childhood, and Adolescence. Philadelphia, Butterworth-Heinemann, 2003, pp 207-218.

58. Verity MA: Infantile Pompe's disease, lipid storage, and partial carnitine deficiency. Muscle Nerve 1991;14:435-440.

59. Hogan GR, Gutmann L, Schmidt R, Gilbert E: Pompe's disease. Neurology 1969;19:894-900.

60. Tsao CY, Boesel CP, Wright FS: A hypotonic infant with complete deficiencies of acid maltase and debrancher enzyme. J Child Neurol 1994;9:90-91.

61. Milstein JM, Herron TM, Haas JE: Fatal infantile muscle phosphorylase deficiency. J Child Neurol 1989;4:186-188.

62. Servidei S, Bonilla E, Diedrich RG, et al: Fatal infantile form of muscle phosphofructokinase deficiency. Neurology 1986;36:1465-1470.

63. Swoboda K, Specht L, Jones HR, et al: Infantile phosphofructokinase deficiency with arthrogryposis: Clinical benefit using a ketogenic diet. J Pediatr 1997;131:932-934.

64. Thompson CE: Infantile myositis. Dev Med Child Neurol 1982;24:307-313.

65. Shevell M, Rosenblatt B, Silver K, et al: Congenital inflammatory myopathy. Neurology 1990;40:1111-1114.

66. Chou SM, Miles JM: Floppy infant syndrome with "congenital infantile polymyositis" [Abstract]. Ann Neurol 1989;26:449.

67. Jones HR, Darras B: Acute care pediatric electromyography. Muscle Nerve 2000;23:S53-S62.

29

Facial and Bulbar Weakness

Francis Renault and Susana Quijano-Roy

Assessment of facial weakness, orofacial congenital malformations, and dysphagia is a challenging task, especially in newborn infants. Orofacial sensorimotor functions involve brainstem structures and cranial nerves that are not easy to assess clinically and rarely show neuroimaging abnormalities. Electrophysiology studies investigate the brainstem and paired cranial nerves using needle electromyography (EMG) of muscles of the face, tongue, and soft palate; nerve conduction studies (NCSs) of facial and hypoglossal nerves; facial compound muscle action potential (CMAP) amplitudes; and blink responses (BRs). These neurophysiologic techniques help to diagnose neurologic dysfunctions as well as to elucidate the pathogenesis. These studies provide the means to assess the degree of axonal loss, the presence or absence of demyelination, and definition of the topography and severity of the paralysis. Owing to the close anatomic and functional relationships of the cranial nerves within the brainstem structures, one must be certain that their electrophysiologic examination should not be limited to one single nerve or pathway, even in clinically isolated paralyses. Repeated EMG examinations may be required to assess the course of denervation and reinnervation, to demonstrate functional maturation, and to guide therapeutic options.

Dysfunction of cranial nerve VII is manifested by unilateral, partial, or complete paralysis of the facial musculature. In newborn babies, facial EMG and NCSs are used to evaluate perinatal trauma or anoxic-ischemic injuries as well as to identify facial defects associated with the various congenital malformation syndromes. In cases of bilateral facial weakness, facial EMG and NCSs help distinguish neuromuscular disorders, Möbius' syndrome, or apraxic diplegia. In older children, unilateral idiopathic Bell's palsy is the most common condition. Electrodiagnostic studies may be used to assess its severity as well as to diagnose other conditions by detecting a subclinical involvement of the contralateral nerve VII or other cranial nerves.

Bulbar weakness may be revealed by difficulties in sucking, swallowing, breathing, or speaking and also by aspiration events, recurrent bronchopulmonary infections, or failure to thrive. This is more frequently observed in the neonatal period as a consequence of congenital cerebral and neuromuscular disorders, but it may also occur later in life owing to acquired central or peripheral nervous system dysfunction. The earlier dysphagia is diagnosed, the greater the likelihood of preventing its respiratory and nutritional complications. Clinical, radiologic, and neurophysiologic investigations enable the severity of swallowing disorders to be evaluated and the etiologic mechanisms of dysphagia to be elucidated and thus provide a good starting point for therapeutic decisions. At any age, electrodiagnostic study can combine several techniques, including needle EMG of muscles of the face, tongue, and soft palate; facial and hypoglossal NCSs; BRs; and EMG during bottle-feeding. Results observed in different clinical conditions are useful in assessing the sucking-swallowing automatism and also in revealing functional disturbances of cranial nerve nuclei and pathways within the brainstem.

PRESENTING SYMPTOMS AND CLINICAL APPROACH

Acquired Facial Palsies

Clinical Presentation

Facial weakness may be due to any lesion involving the supranuclear structures, the brainstem, or the motor unit (Box 29-1). Although most infants present with unilateral

---

BOX 29-1
ACQUIRED FACIAL WEAKNESS IN CHILDHOOD

Idiopathic Bell's Palsy

Infection and Inflammation
Otitis media, mastoiditis, parotitis
Meningitis (viral, bacterial, tuberculosis, leukemia, trichinosis)
Guillain-Barré syndrome, polyneuritis cranialis, Miller Fisher syndrome
Epstein-Barr virus, mycoplasma, herpes zoster/varicella virus (Ramsay Hunt syndrome), herpes simplex virus, human immunodeficiency virus, echovirus
Borrelia burgdorferi (Lyme disease)
Kawasaki's disease
Vasculitis (Henoch-Schönlein purpura)
Neurosarcoidosis

Recurrent Facial Palsies
Melkersson-Rosenthal syndrome
Familial alternating Bell's palsy
Hereditary neuropathy with liability to pressure palsies

Trauma
Craniofacial trauma, penetrative injury
Iatrogenic

Mass Lesions
Brainstem glioma and other posterior fossa tumors and vascular malformations
Cholesteatoma
Osteopetrosis
Lymphoma
Histiocytosis X
Facial tumor (e.g., vascular, osseous, lymphangioma, parotid gland tumor, myofibroma, rhabdomyosarcoma)

Schwannoma of cranial nerve VII
Benign intracranial hypertension (pseudotumor cerebri)

Malformation
Chiari malformation, syringobulbia

Neuromuscular Disorders
Muscular dystrophies (facioscapulohumeral dystrophy, myotonic dystrophy, congenital muscular dystrophies)
Progressive bulbar palsy
Myasthenia gravis
Botulism

Cerebral Disorders
Neoplastic, vascular, degenerative, metabolic, inflammatory

---

and benign acquired facial palsy (AFP), other more severe conditions must be considered and excluded by history, physical examination, and, if necessary, complementary tests. History of trauma or ear infection, time interval since onset, rapidity of progression, associated symptoms, previous paralytic episodes, skin rashes or infection antecedents, exposure to tick bites, triggering factors, systemic diseases such as diabetes mellitus or human immunodeficiency virus (HIV) risk factors, and familial history should be noted.

Central paralysis, which is caused by lesion in the parietal motor cortex or the corticobulbar pathways, is usually associated with other symptoms of central nervous system (CNS) dysfunction, and has a more ominous course than peripheral palsies. Central facial paralysis mostly affects the lower face musculature and spares the forehead; emotional facial reaction remains intact, although voluntary motion may be severely affected. In such paralyses of suprabulbar origin, EMG is normal, and magnetic resonance imaging (MRI) is the preferred diagnostic tool to search for signs of CNS impairment.

Isolated AFPs typically have a peripheral origin. These are either partial or complete, but they either immediately or eventually affect both the upper and lower face musculature. Children with peripheral AFP demonstrate inability to close the eye, a flattened nasolabial fold, and deviation of the mouth to the unaffected side. A common finding is the Bell's sign, an upward and outward eye movement when blinking. Facial motion in the different branches of the facial motor nerve may be assessed by observing the response to commands for closing the eyes, elevating the eyebrows, frowning, showing the teeth, puckering the lips, and tensing the soft tissues of the neck. The neurologic examination must be directed to exclude involvement of other cranial nerves or a more widespread nervous system disorder. Progression of symptoms, including facial diplegia, strabismus, loss of gag reflex, asymmetry of the soft palate, dysphagia, and fasciculations or atrophy of the tongue, indicates involvement of bulbar structures and/or other cranial nerves. General physical examination includes evaluation of mastoid and parotid areas, visualization of the external auditory canal, and inspection of the tympanic membrane. Mass lesions, inflammation, or infection may lead to facial neuropathy; vesicles or "scabbing" may implicate a zoster virus infection. Ophthalmologic examination may reveal concomitant conjunctival or corneal complications and, rarely, funduscopic signs of increased intracranial pressure.

Certain associated clinical features often help define the specific site of cranial nerve VII lesion or its nucleus. A lesion in the pons may produce hyperacusis due to dysfunction of motor fibers to the stapedius muscle. Involvement between the pons and the geniculate ganglion may also cause hyperacusis as well as impairment of lacrimation, salivation, and taste of the anterior two thirds of the tongue. A lesion in the area from the geniculate ganglion to the stapedius nerve may be manifested by hyperacusis and impairment of salivation and taste but normal lacrimation. Impairment of salivation and taste without hyperacusis indicates involvement distal to the stapedius nerve to the chorda tympani. Finally, a lesion below the exit of the chorda tympani nerve shows isolated facial weakness.

Idiopathic Bell's palsy, local infection, and traumatic injuries combined account for at least 80% of AFP.[1-3] However, a neoplasm needs consideration in all children with AFP, especially noting that as many as 20% of documented tumors involving the facial nerve have a sudden onset clinically indistinguishable from Bell's palsy.[4] A gradual progression of paralysis beyond 3 weeks, no return of function after 6 months, ipsilateral recurrence, hemifacial spasm, associated cranial neuropathies, pain, and single-branch involvement should alert the physician to the possibility of a neoplasm.[5] Therefore, caution dictates that a close follow-up of the child with AFP is always required.

It is important to perform a follow-up examination of any child who has an acute idiopathic AFP. Such may direct one to the specific etiology. Examples include ear vesicles of Ramsay-Hunt syndrome, target rash of Lyme disease, or involvement of other cranial nerves.

Evaluation
Cerebrospinal Fluid Examination

Cerebrospinal fluid (CSF) examination is required for assessing the possibility of an infectious, inflammatory, or neoplastic meningeal involvement to allow early diagnosis and appropriate antibiotic treatment in areas in which Lyme disease is endemic. Serologic tests in serum or CSF are not

---

BOX 29-2
INDICATIONS OF NEUROIMAGING IN ACQUIRED FACIAL PALSIES IN CHILDHOOD

Trauma
Complicated otitis media
History of chronic otitis media
Mass lesion on otoscopy
Clinical suspicion of mastoiditis
Previous mastoid surgery
Atypical facial palsy
Associated other cranial nerve involvement
Gradual progression beyond 3 weeks
No improvement 6 months after onset
Recurrent ipsilateral facial paralysis
Facial hemispasm or other neurologic complications
Retrocochlear abnormalities in the brainstem auditory evoked responses

---

routinely performed, but they are occasionally useful in processes such as sarcoidosis. Although herpes viruses seem to be involved in some instances of AFP, current standard tests do not distinguish recent infection.

Neuroimaging Studies

Neuroimaging studies are indicated early on in a number of instances of facial nerve lesions (Box 29-2). MRI is currently the most accurate study method for evaluating the brain, brainstem, nerve trunk, and parotid gland. Gadolinium-enhanced MRI (Gd-MRI) is very sensitive in imaging the intratemporal facial nerve affected by inflammation.[6] High-resolution axial and coronal computed tomography (CT) provides better visualization of the facial nerve's course through the petrous portion of the temporal bone.

Middle Ear and Auditory Investigations

Several noninvasive studies provide a means to localize facial nerve lesions, search for middle ear infection or trauma, and define concomitant cranial nerve VIII involvement. These studies are particularly useful in young children predisposed to ear, nose, and throat infections with no localizing symptoms as well as in older patients with associated hearing loss or nonspecific ear complaints.

Otoscopy determines the presence or absence of outer and middle ear disease. It is complemented with impedance audiometry, which evaluates the middle ear system.

Stapedius muscle reflex thresholds assess the integrity of the reflex neural pathways, which consist of the auditory afferent pathway (the outer, middle, and inner ears); the auditory nerve; brainstem structures (the auditory nucleus, superior olivary complex, and facial nucleus); the facial nerve; and the stapedius muscle. The acoustic or stapedial reflex is easy to perform in children, even in infants, and detects the contraction of the ipsilateral stapedius muscle in response to an intensive acoustic stimulus (70 to 90 dB in a normal subject) at different testing frequencies. The results are shown as absent reflex, reflex requiring elevated thresholds (>90 dB), and normal response. Absence of stapedial reflex is expected if the lesion is proximal to the branching of the nerve to stapedius.

Pure-tone and speech audiometry can detect hearing loss in children older than 4 years of age. In infants or uncooperative children, hearing thresholds may be evaluated by transiently evoked otoacoustic emissions.

Brainstem auditory evoked responses (BAERs) are useful at any age for measuring auditory thresholds and for studying retrocochlear auditory pathways. The resultant I to V waves have electrophysiologic-anatomic correlates that allow one to diagnose conductive hearing loss, abnormalities of the auditory nerve, or brainstem disease.

Other Studies

Studies of facial nerve function such as the Schirmer lacrimation test, the salivary flow test, and electrogustometry are not frequently done because they are difficult to perform, especially in young children. Motor evoked potentials after magnetic transcranial stimulation measure proximal facial nerve conduction and can detect conduction block or axonal degeneration early, but they are less reproducible in young infants than in older children.

Congenital Facial Asymmetry or Diplegia

Clinical Presentation

In newborns and young infants, a unilateral facial paralysis presents with deviation of the mouth toward the unaffected side and a wider fissure of the eyelid with incomplete closure of the eye on the affected side (Fig. 29-1). The facial asymmetry may be evident only when the baby cries because of preservation of facial muscle tone at rest. However, careful observation during quiet sleep may reveal the ipsilateral absence of the fine nostril dilation movements that are synchronous with breathing, as well as the loss of overlapping of the eyelashes. Examination while the infant is crying reveals unilateral absence of puckering of the brow, faulty closing of the eyelids, and asymmetry of the mouth. Certain associated clinical features may suggest the origin of the congenital facial weakness (Box 29-3).

Evaluation

A combination of neurophysiologic tests and neuroimaging provides an opportunity for early diagnosis and management of congenital facial asymmetry or diplegia. CT scan is performed systematically to search for a fracture line or post-traumatic hemorrhage and a possible malformation of the skull. MRI is mainly used to rule out associated cerebral lesions but may also show an abnormal signal in the area of cranial nerve VII nucleus or hypoplasia of the nerve trunk.[7] Facial EMG provides key information to elucidate the pathogenesis of the facial weakness,

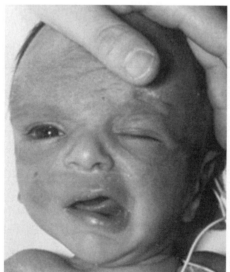 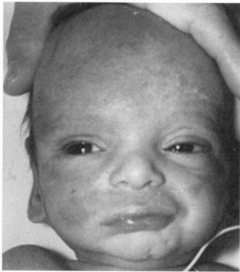

FIGURE 29–1

Congenital facial palsy in a neonate at rest (right) *and during crying* (left). (*From Renault F, Quijano-Roy S: Congenital and acquired facial palsies. In Jones HR, DeVivo DC, Darras BT [eds]: Neuromuscular Disorders of Infancy, Childhood, and Adolescence: A Clinician's Approach. Philadelphia, Butterworth Heinemann, 2003, p 283.*)

BOX 29-3
CONGENITAL FACIAL WEAKNESS

Birth Trauma
Congenital facial palsy (with or without forceps)
Hypoxic-ischemic encephalopathy (bulbar and/or
  suprabulbar)
Posterior fossa hematoma

Developmental Defect
First and second branchial arch syndromes
  (facioauriculovertebral spectrum, hemifacial
  microsomia, mandibulofacial dysostosis)
Asymmetrical crying facies (hypoplasia of the
  depressor anguli oris muscle)
CHARGE association (*c*olobomata, *h*eart disease,
  *a*tresia of the choanae, *r*etarded growth and
  development, *g*enital hypoplasia, and *e*ar
  anomalies or deafness)
Möbius' syndrome

Neuromuscular Disease
Congenital myotonic muscular dystrophy
Congenital muscular dystrophy
Facioscapulohumeral muscular dystrophy, early-onset
  type
Congenital myopathies, nemaline, myotubular,
  fiber-type disproportion
Neonatal transient myasthenia gravis

Pseudoparalysis
Mandibular hypoplasia
Intrauterine postural asymmetry

BOX 29-4
CHARACTERISTICS OF SUCKING-SWALLOWING DISORDERS OF THE NEWBORN AND INFANT

Clinical Features
Absence of sucking
Absence of swallowing
Salivary stasis
Slow sucking
Nasal reflux
Cyanosis and tachypnea during feeding
Apnea and/or bradycardia during feeding
Coughing
Noisy respiration, bronchial congestion
Recurrent bronchopulmonary infections
Poor weight gain

Predisposing Factors
Prematurity
Lethargy
Hypotonia
Poor cough reflex
Dyspnea
Prolonged tube feeding
Parenteral feeding
Tracheotomy
Family history of swallowing disorders, severe
  malaise, or unexplained sudden death

Associated Disorders
Gastroesophageal reflux
Esophageal dyskinesia
Laryngotracheomalacia
Tracheobronchial dyskinesia
Congenital heart disease
Failure to thrive

permitting distinction of neurogenic from myopathic changes. When the clinical expression of facial palsy is not evident at birth, it may be clinically difficult to distinguish a congenital from an early AFP.

Congenital Dysphagia

Clinical Presentation

Sucking-swallowing disorders of the newborn present as feeding and/or respiratory difficulties.[8,9] It is not always easy to demonstrate that a pulmonary disease is secondary to aspiration because aspiration is often silent and chest radiographs may be normal.[10] The diagnosis of dysphagia should immediately be considered in patients with major feeding difficulties, with salivary stasis, as well as in babies who are at risk because of orofacial malformations, neuromuscular

disease, or an encephalopathy. Swallowing disorders should also be sought in cases of early refractory bronchopulmonary disorders and in infants with predisposing factors or anomalies that are often associated with sucking-swallowing difficulties (Box 29-4). Sucking abnormalities can be obvious at the first attempts at feeding. These present simply as an absence of sucking, or sometimes even if a sucking reflex is present, it may not be accompanied by effective swallowing.

Aspiration is readily evident when acute asphyxia occurs with cyanosis and tachypnea during feeding. The signs of obstruction of the airways may be less severe and less specific (cyanosis, apnea, bradycardia), but their onset during a meal is indicative. Cough is also a sign that is immediately suggestive of aspiration if it is accompanied by oropharyngeal or bronchial congestion. Coughing is often wrongly attributed to viral tracheitis or bronchitis, but the parents can clarify the circumstances of onset, whether the cough is precipitated by meals, and whether it existed before any infection. However, cough may be completely absent. Feeding often appears to proceed correctly and aspiration is not noted, but repeated minor aspiration episodes lead to bronchopulmonary disorders with recurrent bronchitis associated with various degrees of dyspnea, frequent pneumonias, and chronic bronchial congestion. Certain subtle signs that may be overlooked are often present and are in keeping with the early onset of sucking-swallowing disorder, including slow sucking, retention of milk in the mouth, nasal reflux, noisy and difficult respirations, and poor weight gain. Respiratory signs are unreliable and nonspecific, including dyspnea of variable severity and duration and diffuse, persistent, or recurrent bronchial problems despite symptomatic treatments and antibiotics.

The face and oral cavity should be examined carefully to detect any minor facial malformations; facial hypotonia; oculomotor defect; mandibular ankylosis; salivary stasis; asymmetry of the tongue or soft palate; and tongue fasciculation or atrophy or both. Defective lingual motor activity, poor reflex contraction of the soft palate, and poor cough reflex should be sought. It is essential to watch the child having or being fed a meal to evaluate the quality of sucking. Any oral obstruction, escape of milk from the lips, or nasal reflux, and the occurrence of cough or noisy respiration should be noted. It is a good idea to bottle-feed the infant oneself; the hand that holds the bottle senses the force exerted on the nipple, and the hand that holds the head and the neck of the infant senses each swallow. One can also observe the flow of milk, sucking movements, and respirations.

Evaluation

Chest radiography often demonstrates focal or diffuse opacities, enhancement of bronchial images, and some degree of thoracic distention. Images often vary from one radiograph to another in the same child. In a series of 37 infants, aged younger than 3 months, with congenital dysphagia, chest radiographs were normal in 20 patients.[11] Findings most suggestive of aspiration pneumonia are predominance of anomalies on the right and the involvement of the right upper lobe, which may progress to atelectasis. Radiography of the pharynx and larynx checks for thickening of the walls of the pharynx and larynx and examines their anatomic relationships.

Videofluoroscopy is primarily used to study the pharyngeal and esophageal phases of swallowing.[12] The examination can show the entry of liquid into the trachea and reveal any mild or late aspiration at the end of the meal in the form of a narrow line. The absence of coughing indicates silent aspiration. In a series of 77 infants, younger than 1 month of age, with feeding difficulties, videofluoroscopic studies of swallowing demonstrated aspiration in 19 patients, including 10 with negative upper gastrointestinal series.[13] Videofluoroscopy can also show reflux to the nasal cavity, a leakage toward the pharynx during the oral phrase, or residual food in the pharynx after the swallow. It can also reveal esophageal disorder: cricopharyngeal achalasia, esophageal dyskinesia, malformation, tracheoesophageal fistula, or gastroesophageal reflux.

Esophageal manometry and pH monitoring can provide evidence for gastroesophageal reflux, esophageal dyskinesia, and dysfunction of the upper sphincter and aid in the evaluation of their involvement in feeding difficulties. Endoscopy can demonstrate anatomic abnormalities or functional disorders of the pharynx or larynx. At the level of the trachea and bronchi, aspiration generally leads to marked edema of the mucosa, first- and second-degree inflammatory signs, predominance of anomalies on the right, with abundant clear fluid secretions for which tests, pH, rheology, and amylase level, confirm their salivary nature. The methylene blue test verifies the absence of a tracheoesophageal fistula. Bronchoalveolar lavage can reveal alveolitis and demonstrate cell inclusions indicative of food aspiration.

Etiology

The principal causes of swallowing disorders in newborn and young infants can be divided into two groups: congenital malformations and neuromuscular disorders (Box 29-5). This usual distinction[9] should not make one forget the possible association of anatomic and neurologic factors in the genesis of swallowing disorders. An obstetric history of polyhydramnios suggests insufficient swallowing during fetal life, prematurity suggests immaturity of sucking-swallowing mechanisms, and perinatal abnormal events may indicate possible consecutive neurologic disorders. Electrodiagnostic investigations have two goals: to demonstrate the existence of swallowing disorders and to understand their pathogenesis. The results of the electrophysiologic study enable three types of disorders to be distinguished: (1) dysphagia with suprabulbar dysfunction, (2) dysphagia with lesions of paired cranial nerves, and (3) isolated dysphagia.

Acquired Dysphagia

Clinical Presentation

Swallowing disorders may occur in childhood in association with a variety of neurologic disorders; electrodiagnostic findings can often be indicative. Diagnosis of acquired dysphagia is straightforward when there is a bout of coughing or choking during swallowing, indicating leakage into the

BOX 29-5
PRINCIPAL CAUSES OF
SUCKING-SWALLOWING DISORDERS
IN THE NEWBORN AND INFANT

Malformations
Choanal atresia
Cleft palate
Microretrognathia
Pierre Robin sequence
Hypoglossia syndromes
Macroglossia
Facial microsomia
Opitz G/BBB syndrome
CHARGE association*
Esophageal atresia or stenosis
Cricopharyngeal achalasia
Abnormal arterial arc

Disorders of the Nervous System
Suprabulbar
   Prenatal encephalopathies
   Birth trauma and asphyxia
Bulbar
   Perinatal brainstem hypoxic-ischemia
   Möbius' syndrome
   Arnold-Chiari malformation
   Severe neonatal spinal muscular atrophy
   Pontocerebellar hypoplasia type I
Congenital isolated dysphagia
   Isolated dysfunction or immaturity of
      sucking-swallowing
Neuromuscular disease
   Congenital muscular dystrophy
   Congenital myopathy
   Congenital myasthenic syndrome
   Dysautonomia
   Lower cranial nerve birth trauma

Transient Dysphagia
Transient, isolated dysphagia in premature infants
Neonates born to myasthenic mothers
Lethargy, coma
Drug side effect
Acute disease with general status alteration
Stomatitis
Dyspneic bronchopulmonary disease
Recent tonsillectomy

---

*CHARGE association is a syndrome of associated defects, including *c*oloboma of the eye, *h*eart anomaly, choanal *a*tresia, *r*etarded growth and development, *g*enital hypoplasia, and *e*ar anomalies or deafness.

larynx, or nasal regurgitation due to velopharyngeal weakness. Examination demonstrates flaccidity of the soft palate and weakness or asymmetry of palatal reflex and voluntary contractions, associated with buccopharyngeal salivary congestion, sometimes with drooling. Symptoms may be more moderate, requiring attentive observation of the meal; the child may eat and drink slowly in small mouthfuls, keep food longer in the mouth, have to swallow three or four times to empty the mouth, and may avoid drinking. Or, on the contrary, the same youngster may take a sip of water after each mouthful. Flexion and extension of the neck to aid in projecting the food into the pharynx can also be seen. Auscultation should search for respiratory sounds after the ingestion of a small amount of water. Swallowing disorders may be subclinical and may be revealed only by the onset of bronchopulmonary complications (e.g., bronchitis, bronchopneumonia, and atelectasis). In principle, any pulmonary infection that develops in association with a neurologic condition should suggest a swallowing disorder.

Evaluation

Videofluoroscopy can reveal tracheal aspiration. Endoscopy shows the presence of food particles in the airways, verifies the absence of anatomic structural anomalies, and shows pharyngeal muscle tone. As in cases of congenital dysphagia, facial, lingual, and velopharyngeal EMG clarify the pathogenesis of acquired dysphagia, that is, paralysis of the soft palate, myopathic changes, or poor motor control.[14] A dynamic EMG method is now available to study the voluntary swallowing of saliva or an alimentary bolus.[15,16] Dysphagia associated with primary gastroenterologic, otorhinolaryngologic, and esophageal affections are not discussed here.

ELECTROPHYSIOLOGIC
EXAMINATION

Electrodiagnostic Studies of
Cranial Nerves

Facial Nerve Anatomy

The facial nerve (Fig. 29-2) emerges from multiple, functionally specialized, ventrolateral brainstem nuclei. The motor nucleus of cranial nerve VII originates in the caudal pons. Five groups of cells are defined corresponding to a topographic organization of motor neurons innervating different muscles. The ventral groups of cells supply the periorbital muscles, and the dorsal groups supply the perioral muscles.[17,18] Taste fibers for the anterior two thirds of the tongue and sensory fibers from the external acoustic canal project to the upper part of the nucleus of the tractus solitarius in the vicinity of the motor nucleus of the cranial

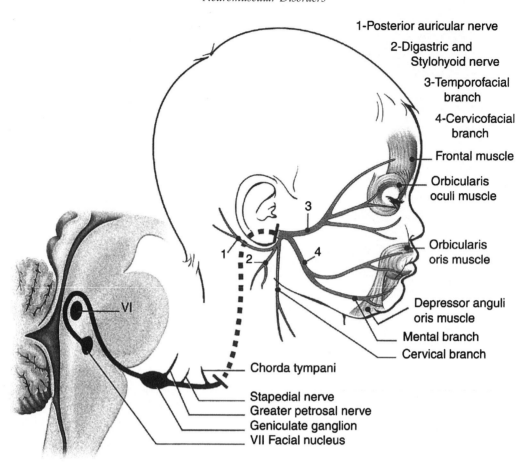

1-Posterior auricular nerve
2-Digastric and Stylohyoid nerve
3-Temporofacial branch
4-Cervicofacial branch
Frontal muscle
Orbicularis oculi muscle
Orbicularis oris muscle
Depressor anguli oris muscle
Mental branch
Cervical branch
Chorda tympani
Stapedial nerve
Greater petrosal nerve
Geniculate ganglion
VII Facial nucleus

FIGURE 29–2

Functional anatomy of the facial nerve. VI, cranial nerve VI nucleus. (From Renault F, Quijano-Roy S: Congenital and acquired facial palsies. In Jones HR, DeVivo DC, Darras BT [eds]: Neuromuscular Disorders of Infancy, Childhood, and Adolescence: A Clinician's Approach. Philadelphia, Butterworth Heinemann, 2003, p 278.)

nerve VII. The lacrimal, sublingual, and submandibular preganglionic parasympathetic fibers of the facial nerve originate at the nearby superior salivary nucleus.

The sensory and motor roots of the facial nerve emerge from the brainstem at the level of the bulbopontine sulcus between cranial nerves VI and VIII at the cerebellopontine angle. They enter the pars petrosa ossis temporalis via the internal acoustic meatus and follow a common path in the first part of the facial canal. The sensory components enter the geniculate ganglion at this level. Motor fibers of the facial nerve traverse peripherally through the internal auditory canal in the temporal bone, in company with the nervus intermedius, consisting of the sensory fibers of the cranial nerve VII as well as with cranial nerve VIII. The greater petrosal nerve arises from the labyrinthine segment of the facial nerve and carries parasympathetic fibers to the pterygopalatine ganglion where it synapses and sends fibers to the lacrimal gland. More distally, the mastoid segment of the facial nerve travels inferiorly and

lateral to the jugular fossa. Here the stapedius nerve arises to innervate the stapedius muscle. The facial nerve gives off the chorda tympani in the distal mastoid segment. The chorda tympani then passes through the middle ear to later supply afferent taste fibers for the anterior two thirds of the tongue as well as parasympathetic fibers to the submandibular and sublingual glands that synapse in the submandibular ganglion.

The primary motor bundle of the facial nerve traverses the second and third parts of the facial canal alone. The facial motor nerve emerges from the skull at the stylomastoid foramen, gives off the posterior auricular branch, and then divides into two main terminal branches in the parotid gland. The inferior cervicofacial branch passes down along the mandible to supply the muscles in the lower part of the face, giving off (1) a buccal branch to the risorius, the buccinator, and the orbicularis oris muscles; (2) a mental branch to the depressor anguli oris, the depressor labii inferioris, and the mentalis muscles; and (3) a cervical branch to the platysma. The superior temporofacial branch runs horizontally forward giving off (1) frontal branches to the frontalis and orbicularis oculi muscles; (2) suborbital branches to the levator labii superioris, zygomaticus, levator anguli oris, and dilatator naris muscles; and (3) buccal branches to the buccinator and orbicularis oris muscles. Although there is considerable diversity in its trajectory and divisions, cranial nerve VII innervates all muscles of facial expression except the levator palpebrae superioris muscle.

When one evaluates children with facial nerve lesions, several clinical anatomic relationships inherent to the complex course of the facial nerve need consideration. The close anatomic proximity of cranial nerves V, VI, VII, and VIII within the brainstem and at the cerebellopontine angle has important clinical connotations, particularly in certain congenital malformations and ischemic and compressive disorders. Multiple cranial nerves are frequently involved. Interneuronal and synaptic connections also exist within the brainstem between the trigeminal and the bilateral facial nerve nuclei, thus providing the neurophysiologic basis for the blink reflex.[19,20]

The geniculate ganglion, containing the soma of sensory facial fibers, is another important anatomic reference; it is located within the internal auditory canal. Reactivation of viral particles latent in the geniculate ganglion is believed to be involved in the pathogenesis of idiopathic and Ramsay Hunt facial palsies. Lesions of the facial nerve trunk, localized distal to the ganglion, may involve different facial nerve branches (i.e., greater superficial petrosal nerve, nerve to stapedius muscle, and chorda tympani) causing variable dysfunctions in lacrimation, salivation, taste, or hearing. Facial nerve entrapment typically occurs at the narrowest segment of its intraosseous course, the meatal foramen, where nerve and canal are of equal diameter.[21,22] Injuries to this nerve within its bony canal are also more severe because the nerve is no longer invested by the protective epineurium and perineurium that exist in more proximal segments.

Facial Nerve Conduction Studies and Electroneuronography

Neurophysiologic examination of the facial nerve can be performed as early as the first hours of life. Here one can provide a definition of the specific characteristics and severity of a facial nerve lesion. In congenital facial palsies (CFPs), these are indicated as soon as possible to date the timing of injury. Orthodromic facial NCSs assess conduction function of the distal nerve. Surface electrodes are placed over facial muscles to record the response elicited by a supramaximal (20 to 60 mA), brief (0.2 millisecond) duration, square-wave, electrical stimulus applied to the facial nerve. When performing NCSs of the cervicofacial branch, one first stimulates at a point anterior to the tragus and then stimulates at a point along the horizontal portion of the mandible while

recording from the orbicularis oris muscle. Facial nerve conduction velocity (NCV) increases markedly with age, particularly during the 1st year of life, averaging 42.8%; 11.1% in the 2nd year, 9.1% from 2 to 5 years, and 5.3% from 5 to 10 years (Table 29-1). In contrast the distal latencies induced by stimulation at the pretragal point do not show significant variation between birth and 15 years, ranging from 3.6 to 7.3 milliseconds for the orbicularis oris and from 2.3 to 4.4 milliseconds for the orbicularis oculi (Table 29-2).[14,23]

Electroneuronography (ENOG) uses surface electrodes placed along the nasolabial fold over the nasalis and perioral

TABLE 29–1. NORMAL FACIAL AND HYPOGLOSSAL NERVE CONDUCTION VELOCITIES (m/sec ± 2 SD) FROM BIRTH TO 15 YEARS

Age	No. of Subjects	Facial Nerve (Cervicofacial Branch)	Hypoglossal Nerve
0-30 days	18	19.0 ± 2.5	23.5 ± 2.2
1-2 mo	14	21.4 ± 3.4	24.1 ± 2.2
2-4 mo	12	24.5 ± 3.9	26.6 ± 2.7
4-6 mo	24	26.3 ± 2.8	28.9 ± 2.9
6-8 mo	23	29.1 ± 3.3	31.8 ± 3.4
8-10 mo	15	31.7 ± 3.7	34.3 ± 2.9
10-12 mo	14	33.3 ± 3.3	35.7 ± 3.0
12-18 mo	30	36.1 ± 3.0	37.5 ± 2.1
18 mo-2 yr	27	37.5 ± 4.7	40.6 ± 2.6
2-3 yr	34	39.5 ± 2.7	42.1 ± 3.0
3-4 yr	16	41.9 ± 4.5	43.5 ± 3.4
4-5 yr	21	43.4 ± 3.3	46.1 ± 2.5
5-6 yr	12	45.5 ± 4.8	46.5 ± 4.9
6-7 yr	12	45.8 ± 5.3	47.3 ± 2.1
7-8 yr	13	46.5 ± 4.1	48.1 ± 6.9
8-9 yr	15	48.1 ± 3.8	49.0 ± 2.6
9-11 yr	17	48.3 ± 2.8	50.2 ± 7.1
11-13 yr	12	48.7 ± 5.6	50.9 ± 6.4
13-15 yr	15	48.5 ± 2.8	50.7 ± 5.4

The distances between the two stimulation points for facial nerve are 34.6 ± 6.6 mm for up to 12 months, 48.7 ± 9.7 mm for 1 to 5 years, and 56.1 ± 6 mm for 5 to 15 years. The distances for hypoglossal nerve are 32.5 ± 9.3 mm for up to 12 months, 36.1 ± 6.5 mm for 1 to 5 years, and 38.2 ± 9.7 mm for 5 to 15 years.

TABLE 29–2. NORMAL VALUES FOR LATENCIES OF ORBICULARIS ORIS, ORBICULARIS OCULI, AND GENIOGLOSSUS MUSCLES (m/sec ± 2 SD) FROM BIRTH TO 15 YEARS

Age	No. of Subjects	Orbicularis Oris	Orbicularis Oculi	Genioglossus
0-1 yr	120	5.3 ± 1.7	3.1 ± 0.8	3.8 ± 1.0
1-3 yr	91	5.4 ± 1.6	3.3 ± 0.5	3.5 ± 1.1
3-9 yr	89	5.6 ± 1.5	3.5 ± 1.0	3.3 ± 0.9
9-15 yr	44	5.6 ± 1.7	3.5 ± 0.9	3.4 ± 0.6

Stimulation is applied to cranial nerve VII at the pretragal point and to cranial nerve XII behind the mandible.

muscles to record the response elicited by a brief supra-maximal electrical stimulus applied to the facial nerve near the stylomastoid foramen. The peak-to-peak CMAP amplitude is recorded as a percentage of the amplitude of the contralateral normal side. This percentage is presumed to correspond to the number of surviving motor neurons. Asymmetry greater than 30% is considered abnormal.[24] ENOG has shown prognostic value in complete acute non-traumatic unilateral facial paralysis in childhood.[25] In idiopathic AFP, CMAP amplitudes reach their minimum level between 7 to 14 days after the onset of weakness in most patients.[26] When performed in the neonatal period, serial facial NCSs and ENOGs help distinguish developmental from traumatic CFPs; some or complete recovery of function favors traumatic lesions.

Needle EMG of Facial Muscles

Needle EMG examination is typically performed at rest and under voluntary contraction. It can also be studied after stimulation (stimulation-detection EMG). This last technique is useful in young children or in very severe cases, since one can perform this either in the absence of cooperation or when there is no apparent voluntary recruitment of motor unit potentials (MUPs) despite the effort. Lidocaine/prilocaine cream (EMLA) is used to anesthetize the skin prior to needle insertion. We use a concentric needle electrode recording from at least one muscle innervated by the temporofacial branch (orbicularis oculi, frontalis) and another innervated by the cervicofacial branch (orbicularis oris, depressor anguli oris). It is preferable to not feed the baby for 4 hours prior to the study. This increases the likelihood of recording bursts of facial muscle activity while the baby is either crying or sucking a pacifier. In older children, voluntary contraction can be recorded by asking the child to imitate the examiner when closing the eyes, smiling, and whistling. Analysis of the recruitment pattern, amplitude, morphology, and duration of the MUPs may be manually or automatically performed.

The electrode is inserted in the external part of the orbicularis oris muscle more than 1 cm outside the labial commissure. The orbicularis oculi muscle is approached tangentially 2 cm from the lateral angle of the eye. One approaches the frontalis muscle and inserts the electrode tangentially just above the eyebrow in a medial direction. The depressor anguli oris muscle (DAOM) is approached 1.5 to 2 cm below the labial commissure (see Fig. 29-2). The normal maximal amplitude of the interference pattern of these facial muscles is 0.85 mV (range, 0.4 to 1.2 mV). In more than 50% of MUPs, the duration is 2 to 4 milliseconds. The proportion of polyphasic potentials is above 30%. The motor response has a highly polyphasic morphology with a mean duration of 8 to 12 milliseconds and amplitude from 0.4 to 1.2 mV (Fig. 29-3).

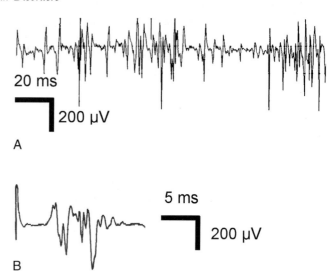

FIGURE 29–3

Needle electromyography of the orbicularis oris muscle in a fullterm newborn infant at age 6 days. A, Normal recruitment pattern on crying. B, Normal response evoked by electrical stimulation applied to cranial nerve VII before the tragus.

Blink Responses

BR is an electrodiagnostic technique that explores the blink reflex arc between the trigeminal and facial nerves. This provides information about both facial and trigeminal nerve function as well as the pathways between their respective cranial nuclei within the brainstem. This is a valuable means for predicting clinical outcome of patients with facial palsies as well as detecting brainstem dysfunction, albeit of lessened utility vis-à-vis MRI.[27,28]

The blink reflex results from the contraction of the orbicularis oculi muscle provoked by stimulation of the supraorbital branch of the trigeminal nerve at the supraorbital foramen.[29] A single electric shock is applied to elicit BRs while recording bilaterally from the orbicularis oculi muscles. Stimulation of the ipsilateral nerve V provokes a direct response with two components: R1, which is immediate and brief, and R2, which is delayed and more lasting (Fig. 29-4). Stimulation of the contralateral nerve V provokes a crossed R2 response.

The R1 component corresponds to an oligosynaptic reflex arc involving at least two and no more than three synapses in the pons between the main sensory nucleus of cranial nerve V and the motor nucleus of the ipsilateral cranial nerve VII. The R2 component follows polysynaptic medullary pathways, which are more caudal and closer to the bulbar formations. The spinal trigeminal nucleus has projections to the adjacent paramedian reticular formation and the motor nuclei of the two cranial nerves VII.[30-33]

Clinically, the respective R1 and R2 latencies provide the means to differentiate between damage within the

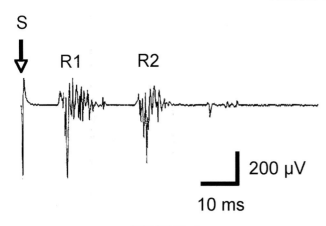

FIGURE 29–4

Blink reflex in a fullterm newborn, day 6. Needle EMG recording of the orbicularis oculi muscle, showing normal responses (R1 and R2) to electrical stimulation (S) of the ipsilateral supraorbital nerve.

trigeminal pathway (delayed/absent ipsilateral R1 and R2 responses and contralateral R2 response) and facial pathway (delayed ipsilateral R1 and R2 but normal contralateral R2). Furthermore, the R1 response investigates the pons (ipsilateral stimulus results in an abnormal R1, while the contralateral stimulus has normal R1), and R2 response on the paretic side is abnormal, either stimulating the unaffected or the affected side in lateral medullary lesions.[34]

Maturation studies of BRs demonstrate that the R1 response is always present from birth on. The latency of the R1 component rapidly matures achieving normal adult values before 44 weeks of gestational age.[35-38] In contrast, the R2 responses are more difficult to elicit, even disappearing when the stimulation rate is above 0.5 Hz. The ipsilateral R2 response can be evoked in most newborns and infants. Its latency ranges from 34 to 43 milliseconds in fullterm newborns, then increases and remains stable in early childhood, and finally decreases to adult values between 7 and 12 years. The contralateral R2 response can be obtained in 80% of fullterm newborns but may be absent up to age 8 months. Its latency is longer than the ipsilateral R2 until 2 years.

Genioglossus Muscle and Hypoglossal Nerve

Cranial nerve XII (i.e., hypoglossal) is a purely motor nerve. Its nucleus consists of a column of neurons extending for nearly the full length of the medulla oblongata with its nerve emerging near its midline base. Emerging from the skull by the anterior condylar canal, cranial nerve XII crosses the pharyngomaxillary space and curves anteriorly in the carotid groove. In the sublingual region, it sends terminal branches to the ipsilateral muscles of the tongue. In addition, cranial nerve XII carries fibers from the first two cervical roots to the geniohyoid and thyrohyoid muscles.

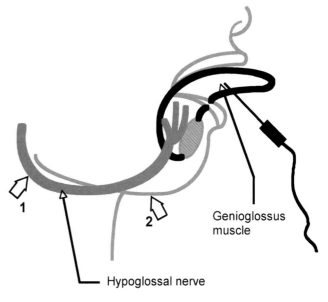

FIGURE 29–5

Genioglossus muscle needle EMG recording via endo-oral route. Hypoglossal nerve conduction study: electrical stimulation is applied proximally behind the mandible (1) and distally under the chin (2).

The genioglossus is a paired paramedian muscle of the tongue. It can be recorded by the endo-oral route: the ventral surface of the tongue is anesthetized by touching the mucosa with a solution of lidocaine; the needle electrode is inserted slightly lateral to the midline (Fig. 29-5). The genioglossus may also be reached via a transcutaneous route: lidocaine/prilocaine cream is used to anesthetize the skin of the submental area; the needle is inserted 1 cm outside the midline line (see Fig. 29-9).

The interference pattern is recorded when the infant is crying and also when sucking a nipple. In normal subjects, the maximal amplitude of the interference pattern is 0.96 mV (range, 0.41 to 1.5 mV). In more than 50% of MUPs, the duration is from 1 to 2 milliseconds. The proportion of polyphasic potentials is more than 30%.[14]

A brief (0.2 millisecond) square-wave electric shock of supramaximal intensity (30 to 70 mA) is used for hypoglossal NCSs. Cranial nerve XII is stimulated proximally behind the mandible and then more distally under the chin (see Fig. 29-5). Results in normal subjects between birth and 15 years demonstrate that hypoglossal NCV increases by 34.2 % in the 1st year, 11.2% in the 2nd year, 10.4% from 2 to 5 years, and 5.1% from 5 to 10 years (see Table 29-1). In contrast, the latencies induced by stimulation under the angle of the mandible do not show a significant change between birth and 15 years, ranging from 2.8 to 4.6 milliseconds (see Table 29-2).[14,23]

Muscles of Soft Palate and Pharyngeal Plexus

The motor fibers of cranial nerves IX and X that supply the muscles of the pharynx arise from the upper part of the nucleus ambiguus. The pharyngeal branches of cranial nerve X merge with the fibers of cranial nerve IX to constitute the pharyngeal plexus that innervates muscles of the soft palate.

We record the EMG activity of muscles that are easily accessible via the oral route. The levator veli palatini muscle spreads into the large paramedian section of the soft palate. The electrode is inserted 1 to 1.5 cm outside the median line, about 0.5 cm under the mucous membrane. The palatoglossus muscle is recorded by placing the needle in the palatoglossal arch just under the mucous membrane. Similarly, the pharyngoglossus muscle is recorded in the palatopharyngeal arch (Fig. 29-6).

The normal maximal amplitude of the interference pattern in these muscles of the soft palate is 1.3 mV (range, 0.38 to 1.8 mV). In more than 50% of MUPs, the duration is from 1 to 2 milliseconds. An additional 30% of the MUPs are polyphasic (Fig. 29-7).[14]

EMG Study of Sucking-Swallowing Function

Anatomy, Physiology, and Ontogeny

Sucking and swallowing are vital functions in the newborn, and their evaluation is essential. Any abnormality of these functions exposes infants to feeding difficulties as well as aspiration-induced pulmonary disease. Sucking and swallowing are a fundamental expression of prenatal neurologic development and reflect the ontogeny of the brainstem. These complex activities require the interaction of various anatomic and functional elements: the face, tongue, soft palate, pharynx, larynx, and esophagus. Swallowing in

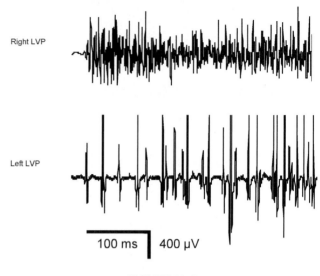

100 ms | **400 µV**

FIGURE 29–7

Needle EMG of the levator veli palatini (LVP) muscle in a 2-month-old infant with congenital dysphagia. Voluntary contraction was recorded during crying. Top, *Normal recruitment pattern in the right LVP.* Bottom, *Reduced neurogenic recruitment pattern in the left LVP.*

human newborns has been studied by manometry, cineradiography,[39-41] and, more recently, ultrasound[42-45] and videofluoroscopy; the latter is the main technique currently used in clinical practice.[12]

The first phase is oral: the combined action of lingual muscles results in compression of the nipple against the upper gums, the induction of a depression in the oral cavity, and the triggering of waves of contractions that direct the milk into the pharynx. The oral cavity is closed anteriorly by the lips and posteriorly by pressure of the tongue against the soft palate. Traversing the pharyngeal conduit constitutes the second, pharyngeal, phase. The soft palate rises, the base of the tongue projects the milk into the laryngopharynx, and the superior esophageal sphincter relaxes. Simultaneously the airways are protected by several means: raising the soft palate closes the nasal cavities, the larynx moves up and forward, the glottis closes, the aperture of the larynx is covered by the epiglottis and the base of the tongue, and the milk is directed laterally and posteriorly. Respiration resumes as soon as the bolus passes into the esophagus. These oral and pharyngeal phases are highly interlinked and are followed by the purely esophageal third phase.

Swallowing and respiration follow one another in an order that avoids aspiration. Deglutition apnea occurs simultaneously with the elevation of the soft palate, even before the closing of the glottis. Swallowing occurs during the natural pause between the end of inspiration and the onset of expiration. This apnea lasts 450 to 600 milliseconds. Thus new-

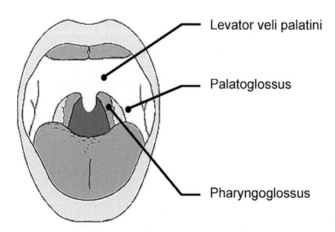

Levator veli palatini

Palatoglossus

Pharyngoglossus

FIGURE 29–6

Needle EMG recording of muscles of the soft palate.

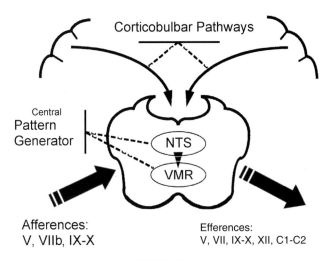

FIGURE 29–8

The central control of sucking and swallowing. C1-C2, first two cervical roots; NTS, nucleus of the tractus solitarius; VIIb, intermedius nerve; VMR, ventromedian reticular formation.

borns can feed themselves without interrupting respiration, the rate of which is governed by the sucking rhythm and returns to its previous baseline rate when the meal is finished.[43,46] At the beginning of the meal, respiration can be suspended during the first sucks, when rhythm is rapid, higher than 1.4/sec, and this can lead to prolonged deglutition apnea, which can affect blood gases.[47,48]

The regulation of sucking and swallowing involves a number of nervous system structures (Fig. 29-8). The central pattern generator for swallowing involves the nucleus of the tractus solitarius and adjacent ventromedian reticular formation.[41,49] This center receives afferent sensory fibers from the tongue, the oral cavity, the pharynx, and the larynx via the paired cranial nerves V, VIIb (intermedius nerve), IX, and X (superior laryngeal nerve). The bilateral corticobulbar pathways arising from the opercular motor zones exercise suprabulbar control.[50] Thus the generator is influenced by excitatory and inhibitory peripheral afferent pathways and by the voluntary control of the frontal cortex.[51] The efferent pathways are the paired cranial nerves V, VII, IX, X, and XII and the first two cervical roots, which send a bundle of fibers to the ansa cervicalis.

In the newborn infant the oral phase is inseparable from the sucking reflex: on contact with the nipple, rhythmic contractions of the tongue occur and the lips are pressed together. The frequency of sucking varies from 0.6 to 2/sec. The variations in frequency are not correlated with age[14,52] but depend on feeding conditions, the availability and quality of the maternal milk, or the elasticity of the nipple and the size of its opening. The progressive slowing of sucking during a meal can be attributed to fatigue and satiety.[52] The pharyn-

geal phase occurs in a reflex manner after each suck so that the organization 1 suck/1 swallow and its coordination with respiration occur in an entirely automatic sequence.

Sucking-swallowing automatism in the newborn is the result of prenatal neurologic maturation: lingual contractions appear at 7 to 9 weeks of gestational age, and sucking and swallowing start at about 12 to 14 weeks.[53] The alternating rhythmic organization 1 suck/1 swallow is normally mature at the time of birth in term infants and at 34 to 36 weeks of gestational age in premature infants.[54] In preterm infants, postmenstrual age but not postnatal age correlates with the suck rate and the duration of sucking runs.[55] The ratio of sucking to swallowing can increase from 1:1 to 2:1 or 3:1 when the flow of milk is low.[43] Suck-swallow rhythmic organization shows only little change in the first months of life in term infants.[56] This motor automatism persists as long as the newborn children continue to feed themselves at breast or bottle. The voluntary control, which results in dissociation of the oral and pharyngeal phases, inhibits the sucking-swallowing automatism without eliminating it entirely, inasmuch as it can be observed in certain pathologic conditions in adults.[57]

The coordination of sucking and swallowing with respiration is generally functional at birth, but in the premature infant and during the first few days in term infants one can sometimes observe an imperfect coordination with a series of "apneic" swallowings alternating with respiratory cycles without sucking.[45,46] The duration and number of episodes of apneic swallowing decrease regularly with maturation from 32 to 42 weeks of gestational age.[54]

In case of aspiration, the arrival of milk in the larynx leads to reflex closure of the glottis, which could account for certain apneas that occur during feeding and which can induce hypoxia.[58,59] With maturation, the cough reflex replaces apnea, but this reflex is absent during the first weeks of life in 50% of term newborns and in 75% of premature infants.[59]

EMG during Bottle-Feeding

EMG during bottle-feeding is characterized by the simultaneous recording of a muscle specific for the oral phase, the genioglossus, and of a muscle specific for the pharyngeal phase, the thyrohyoid, during a liquid bottle-feed (Fig. 29-9).[60] The genioglossus muscle is recorded via the transcutaneous submental route; the needle electrode traverses the mylohyoid, which is brought into play synchronously with the genioglossus.[61] The thyrohyoid muscle is easily accessible on the lateral face of the thyroid cartilage. Elevation of the larynx accompanies the second phase of swallowing.[62] The recording continues during the entire feed. The activity of each muscle and the timing of their activation are analyzed. This enables the coordination of the first two phases of swallowing to be evaluated.

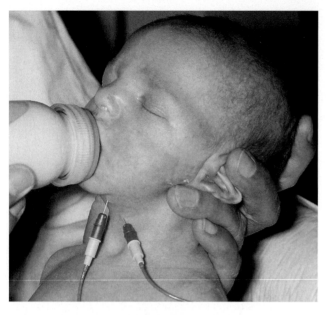

FIGURE 29–9
Dynamic EMG during bottle-feeding: two concentric needle electrodes recording the genioglossus muscle via submental route and the thyrohyoid muscle on the lateral face of the thyroid cartilage.

Normal results are established in healthy term infants aged from 3 days to 18 months.[14,63] The genioglossus and thyrohyoid muscles alternate regularly (Fig. 29-10). The EMG activity of the genioglossus muscle during suction is organized in bursts with a full interference pattern showing a rapid increase then a decrease in amplitude, giving a fusiform aspect. The bursts are separated by a quiescent period. Initial frequency of sucking ranges from 0.6 to 2 Hz (mean, 1.4 Hz). Mean duration of genioglossal bursts, calculated for the first 20 sucks, ranges from 180 to 460 milliseconds depending on the infant, without any correlation with age. The duration of the bursts and quiescent periods between sucks increases progressively (from 35% to 100%) during the course of the feeding. This probably reflects both fatigue and decreasing appetite.

EMG activity of the thyrohyoid muscle is also organized into bursts with the same fusiform shape, separated by a rest period, with identical frequency: each suck is systematically followed by a swallow. For the thyrohyoid, the mean duration of bursts calculated for the first 20 sucks is 210 to 520 milliseconds. The start of the burst varies in relation to the end of lingual activity: the onset of thyrohyoid activity ranges from 100 milliseconds before to 220 milliseconds after the end of lingual activity, depending on the infant, and is unrelated to age. The timing of the two muscle contractions varies from one child to another but varies little from one swallow to another during feeding in the same child. Abnormal sucking-swallowing results[14,64] are classified into three stages of severity: mild, where sucking is present but the alternation between sucking and swallowing is irregular; moderate, where sucking is present but the pharyngeal phase is either synchronous (Fig. 29-11) or uncertain; and severe, where the tongue does not perform rhythmic sucking activity and the pharyngeal phase is either tonic (Fig. 29-12) or inactive.

Summary

Therefore, several EMG techniques provide convergent information on some nuclei and pathways of the brainstem involved in sucking-swallowing. Needle EMG of the face, tongue, and soft palate provides information about the function of the motor units in the territory of the facial nerve, the pharyngeal plexus, and the hypoglossal nerve. BRs involve the fibers and nuclei of the cranial nerve V, the V to VII internuclear pathways, the motor nucleus of the cranial nerve VII and its temporofacial fibers. During bottle-feeding, the EMG evaluates the automatism generated and regulated in the central pattern generator for swallowing. These EMG investigations target the dis-

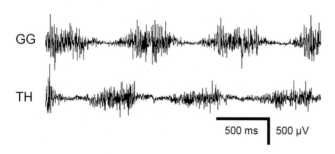

GG

TH

500 ms | 500 µV

FIGURE 29–10
*Dynamic EMG during bottle-feeding: normal **alternating pattern** of sucking and swallowing. GG, genioglossus muscle; TH, thyrohyoid muscle.*

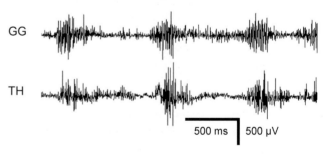

GG

TH

500 ms | 500 µV

FIGURE 29–11
*Dynamic EMG during bottle-feeding: moderate disorder. **Synchronization** of the oral and pharyngeal phases in a 27-day-old fullterm newborn infant with Pierre Robin syndrome. GG, genioglossus muscle; TH, thyrohyoid muscle.*

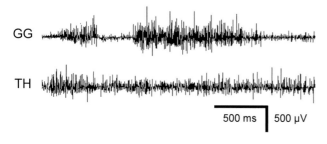

FIGURE 29–12

Dynamic EMG during bottle-feeding: severe disorder. **Absence of lingual rhythmic sucking** *activity and tonic activity of the pharyngeal phase in a 16-day-old fullterm newborn infant with Pierre Robin syndrome. GG, genioglossus muscle; TH, thyrohyoid muscle.*

turbed motor organization, assess its severity, and show whether it is isolated or associated with a lesion of the bulbar motor nuclei. Other neurophysiologic examinations, electroencephalography, BAERs, somatosensory and visual evoked responses and neuroimaging, MRI, CT, and ultrasonography can be used to assess any other anatomic or functional CNS involvement, or both.

CLINICAL NEUROPHYSIOLOGIC APPROACH TO THE DIAGNOSIS OF SPECIFIC FACIAL AND BULBAR LESIONS

Acquired Facial Palsy

Bell's Idiopathic Facial Palsy
Clinical Presentation

Bell's idiopathic facial palsy is the most frequent cause of AFP in children (see Box 29-1).[65-67] Bell's palsy may occur in the first months of life but is most frequently seen after age 8 years. Its annual age-specific incidence per 100,000 population in Rochester, Minnesota is 4.2 for children younger than 10 years of age and 15.3 for those aged 10 through 19 years, with an incidence at least twofold higher for the population group of 30 years of age and older.[68] To investigate anatomic reasons for these age-related differences, Eicher and coworkers studied 20 temporal bones from children younger than 2 years and 10 temporal bones from adults and found significant differences in the nerve/canal diameter ratios.[22] The results of this study suggest that children may be less vulnerable to facial nerve entrapment.

About one third of children with Bell's palsy have an antecedent upper airway infection. Pain in the ear or surrounding area is the initial symptom in many cases and is followed by a rapid evolution of the paralysis in just a few hours or days. This typically involves the musculature of the forehead, periocular area, cheek, and perioral area. About one half of patients lose the sensation of taste, but lacrimation is usually spared. Hyperacusis is a frequent complaint due to stapedius muscle dysfunction. Bell's palsy usually presents as an isolated mononeuropathy form. However, in some instances the presence of postauricular pain, facial numbness, abnormal BAERs, or abnormal BRs supports the hypothesis of a subtle polyneuropathy in a subgroup of subjects with Bell's palsy. No statistical difference in outcome was found when comparing the mononeuritic and polyneuritic forms.[69]

Most of Bell's palsies are unilateral and have no recurrence. Bilateral Bell's palsy is seen in less than 1% of the cases.[70] Up to 15% of patients with Bell's palsy present with recurrent episodes.[71] Familial cases have been variously estimated to be from 3% to 28%.[3,72,73] AFP with a positive family history of Bell's palsy may represent a distinct hereditary facial palsy group. This feature has been suggested by several reports of families with several cases, segregating with dominant and recessive inheritance.[74] Anatomic abnormalities in the facial nerve bony canal were found in some members of a family with multiple cases. It is not clear whether this was an innocent familial anatomic variation or a potential inherited etiologic factor.[75] A familial occurrence was the only factor found to be significantly associated with incomplete recovery in a retrospective series of 76 children with Bell's palsy.[3]

Herpes simplex virus (HSV)-1 is the most probable etiologic factor of AFP in children.[76-80] HSV-1 reactivation is widely accepted as the likely cause of Bell's palsy in most adult cases in nonendemic areas for Lyme disease.[81,82] Other viral agents have been implicated less frequently, including varicella zoster virus (VZV), Ebstein-Barr virus, echovirus, poliovirus, adenovirus, rubella, cytomegalovirus, mycoplasma, hepatitis virus, influenza A and B,[83] and HIV.[84] Some cases of acute AFP have been reported after diphtheria-pertussis-tetanus or poliomyelitis immunization.[85]

Investigation

Gd-MRI may be used to localize inflammation within the facial nerve. Contrast enhancement occurring at the labyrinthine segment and the geniculate ganglion is a common finding in patients with Bell's palsy.[5] The abnormal signal induced by inflammation persists despite clinical resolution, and its continued presence over time is of no prognostic significance.[86,87] However, gadolinium enhancement is not a specific finding and can be observed occasionally in normal controls.[6]

Lacrimal or *gustatory tests* are not expected to provide clear information about the level of the lesion because Bell's palsy is usually associated with varying degrees of conduction block and axonal degeneration changes.[88]

Stapedial reflex testing has been studied as a guide to prognosis in 22 children with Bell's palsy. All patients who had normal stapedial reflex results, when tested during the first week after clinical onset of AFP, recovered within 3 months. In contrast, recovery occurred in just 50% of patients with an abnormal stapedial reflex.[26]

Electrodiagnostic tests including facial NCSs, BRs, ENOG, and needle EMG demonstrate a wide range of changes in children with an AFP; they are particularly useful in their assessment and follow-up. These can differentiate between a primary demyelinating or axonal lesion and therefore provide significant prognostic correlations. However, electrodiagnostic studies do not enable one to distinguish an idiopathic Bell's palsy from other facial palsies having axonal loss. Needle EMG and BRs may be helpful in the first days of paralysis. Reduced interference patterns can be detected in facial muscles within hours of onset. In contrast, CMAP amplitudes cannot be relied for prognosis until potential axonal wallerian degeneration is completed; this usually occurs 5 to 12 days after onset.[89] Blink reflex findings are more useful initial information. In one series of 32 patients with idiopathic AFP, BRs on the affected versus the contralateral nonaffected side demonstrated a sensitivity of 81% and a specificity of 94%.[90]

Follow-up Correlation of Clinical and Electrodiagnostic Findings

Clinical recovery may start 2 or 3 weeks after onset if there is a primary demyelinating lesion. At times there is a "plateau," with residual facial weakness persisting for several weeks to months before recovery. A complete spontaneous recovery is the rule in children with Bell's palsy; the percentages vary in different series but are generally close to 90%.[68,91-93] Complications of faulty reinnervation such as crocodile tears and synkinesis, seen in 10% of adults, are rarely observed in children. In general, the younger the patient, the more favorable the prognosis.

Certain findings noted in the first 2 weeks of the paralysis are associated with good recovery, including incomplete paralysis, early improvement, normal salivary flow, normal taste, mild needle EMG signs of denervation, and normal BRs.[28] Percentages of complete recovery usually refer to clinical recovery as assessed by physical examination; perhaps small permanent deficits could have been demonstrated in more patients if innervations of the facial muscles were assessed by EMG.[68]

Most patients are referred to the EMG laboratory to determine whether they are among the small group who will not recover fully.[94] Early needle EMG, performed between the 5th and 15th days, is a decisive factor in the final prognosis[95]; the presence of fibrillation potentials within the first 14 days predicts an unfavorable outcome.[96] Preservation and/or return of BRs within the first 3 weeks

of a Bell's palsy is seen in cases in which recovery is complete.[97-99] In a series of 30 children with idiopathic AFP, ENOG carried out from the 1st to the 4th week after onset correlated with clinical outcome.[26] A normal motor latency during the 2nd week after onset predicted complete recovery in adults[100] as well as in children.[101] Initially if paralysis is clinically complete with abolition of BRs, recovery may be late and slow, but complete recovery may finally occur.[102,103] The presence of even a few voluntary MUPs in patients with complete clinical paralysis is consistent with a better prognosis than in those patients with none. When the paralysis remains clinically complete after the 6th week, improvement in ENOG at successive examinations is a useful predictor of a favorable outcome.[104]

Inexcitability of the facial nerve and marked decrease in CMAP amplitude correlate with a severe lesion of cranial nerve VII and indicate a poor prognosis.[100,105] When ENOG is performed from 8 to 12 days after onset and shows the functional motor deficit of the facial nerve to be from 50% to 90%, recovery is usually rapid, in 7 or 8 weeks. When the deficit in ENOG is between 90% and 98%, recovery is slower but usually is complete. When the deficit is between 98% and 100%, especially after the 3rd week of onset, there is high risk of incomplete recovery.[93,106]

Ramsay Hunt syndrome

Reactivation of latent VZV in the geniculate ganglion is the cause of the Ramsay Hunt syndrome characterized by an AFP with vesicular eruption on the auricle or the oral mucosa. It is frequently associated with vestibulocochlear dysfunction. If no eruption develops, VZV-related AFP is clinically indistinguishable from idiopathic Bell's palsy. Ramsay Hunt syndrome is relatively rare in children younger than 6 years of age, although it is becoming more frequent in developed countries.[107] In a review of facial palsies caused by VZV, Hato and coworkers reported a milder degree of facial weakness at onset and a later and less widespread eruption of vesicles in children compared to adults.[108] Half of the children showed vesicles several days after the onset of the facial palsy, whereas in about 68% of adults they were evident before or simultaneous with the facial weakness. Prognosis in Ramsay Hunt syndrome was found to be worse than in idiopathic facial palsies, because only 78% of patients showed complete recovery, compared to a recovery rate of 90% in children with idiopathic Bell's palsy. In one series of adult patients, EMG and ENOG signs of axonal loss were detected in 44% of patients with Ramsay Hunt syndrome compared with just 14% of patients with idiopathic Bell's palsy.[109] Using Gd-MRI, VZV may be suspected, even in the absence of vesicular eruption, if the enhancement is localized in the inner ear structures.[110]

Lyme Disease

Clinical Presentation

The tick-borne spirochete *Borrelia burgdorferi* is the agent responsible for Lyme disease, an endemic condition in some areas of the United States and in northeastern countries of Europe. In children, paralysis of cranial nerve VII may be the presenting sign of Lyme disease and is the most common neurologic manifestation of the disease (16% to 50%).[111,112] Great differences in the geographic distribution of the infection explain the various frequencies reported by different authors. Within endemic regions Lyme disease is the most common cause of AFP among children.[113,114] In nonendemic countries, the borreliosis does not seem to be a major cause of unilateral AFP.[115]

Patients may not have other symptoms of Lyme disease, and the signs of a recent tick bite may not be present. Headache is the single most common neurologic symptom in children with Lyme disease. It is important to ask specifically about headaches during the episode of facial weakness or in the previous days or weeks, because facial palsy is frequently associated with an occult meningitis with minimal or absent stiff neck.

The finding of a peculiar skin rash extending centrifugally around the area of the tick bite, *erythema chronicum migrans*, characterizes the first stage of the infection and has been reported in up to 90% of cases. Preceding the facial palsy there may be associated auricular pain, hemifacial edema, or erythema of the face. AFP associated with Lyme disease is rarely complete, and the outcome is usually favorable.

Presentation may be unilateral, occurring on the same side as the erythema migrans, or bilateral, typically 10 to 15 days apart, and usually lasts less than 2 months. The patient often shows signs of a meningeal syndrome. It is important to maintain a high degree of suspicion, especially in endemic areas, because a specific antibiotic treatment stops the infectious process and thus the subsequent neurologic manifestations that occur via dissemination of the infection during the second stage of the disease. Associated symptoms such as general malaise, fever, myalgia, or sometimes limb paresthesias may be present but are seen less frequently than in adults. Meningoradiculitis (Bannwarth's syndrome) and peripheral neuropathy syndromes are also rare. In contrast, a "pseudotumor cerebri" syndrome consisting of papilledema, mildly increased intracranial pressure, and slightly increased CSF protein content without pleocytosis has been found to be relatively common in the pediatric population with Lyme disease in North America.[113,116]

Diagnosis

Diagnosis rests on the history, clinical manifestations, and serologic demonstration of antibodies against *B. burgdorferi* by enzyme-linked immunosorbent assay (ELISA), and then coupled with immunoblot if the ELISA testing is positive.[117] Identifying the DNA of *B. burgdorferi* in CSF by polymerase chain reaction (PCR) is possible. Serum antibodies and, if possible, intrathecal antibody synthesis should be routinely screened in AFP patients from areas endemic for Lyme disease, especially from spring to fall. Early negative blood serologic testing does not rule out Lyme disease. The IgM response usually peaks during the 3rd to 6th weeks, and IgG antibody typically arises around the 4th weeks.[118]

In contrast with adults, most children with isolated Lyme disease-induced AFP have abnormal CSF.[119] The CSF may show pleocytosis, hyperproteinorachia, and increased IgG titers, which are more sensitive and specific than serum antibody titers alone.[120] CSF analysis should be considered in Lyme disease-induced AFP, especially in children younger than 8 years of age to decide if antibiotic therapy is needed intravenously.

Electrodiagnostic studies indicate demyelination in most cases; axonal loss has been reported to be associated with a worse prognosis in adults.[121] MRI of children with neurologic manifestations of Lyme disease may detect an abnormal, hyperintense signal on T2-weighted images of the brain.[122]

Otogenic Facial Paralysis

Although the incidence of AFP due to middle ear infection has decreased from about 2% in the preantibiotic era to 0.16%, it is still a relatively common cause.[123] A high level of suspicion should be maintained for middle ear causes of AFP, because they require active treatment. Inspection of the external meatus and tympanic membrane usually leads to the diagnosis of acute otitis media. Facial paralysis may develop quickly within the first 72 hours in association with acute otitis media, and the causative agents are similar to those implicated in uncomplicated acute otitis media: *Streptococcus pneumoniae*, *Haemophilus influenzae*, and *Moraxella (Branhamella) catarrhalis*. Acute mastoiditis is easily suspected when fever, retroauricular pain, and inflammation of the mastoid process develop. Also, if an AFP develops weeks after onset of acute otitis media, a coalescent subacute mastoiditis must be suspected. Meningitis and temporal lobe abscess are rare complications.[4]

AFP due to chronic otitis media or cholesteatoma signify an invasive process that should be suspected if onset is gradual. It is more commonly due to either a gram-negative organism or *Staphylococcus aureus*. Tuberculous mastoiditis must be kept in mind in refractory otitis media with AFP, especially in older children from regions where tuberculosis is endemic, or in patients with acquired immunodeficiency syndrome (AIDS). Simple radiographs of the temporal bone may help in some instances. CT scan permits visualization of the facial nerve through the petrous portion of the temporal bone. Neuroimaging is also useful to rule out other processes such as middle ear rhabdomyosarcoma, intracranial abscess, or histiocytosis X.

Traumatic and Iatrogenic Surgical Injury to the Facial Nerve

Paralysis of cranial nerve VII may occur as a result of temporal bone fractures, penetrating head and neck wounds, or iatrogenic injuries. The paralysis is usually evident immediately after the injury, but sometimes it appears later. Surgery of the posterior fossa; of the middle ear, especially in cases of malformation or atypical nerve course; and of tumors and malformations, often of vascular origin or localized in the parotid area, constitute the main iatrogenic causes of facial palsy. Most traumatic facial nerve injuries occur within the intratemporal course of the nerve.

Axial and coronal high-resolution CT scanning of the temporal bone is essential in delineating the bony architecture of the temporal bone. It yields particularly useful information in traumatic facial paralysis where fracture lines can be seen impinging on the fallopian canal. Longitudinal fractures are the most common type of temporal bone fracture and account for most facial nerve injuries, especially in the perigeniculate area, where the facial nerve is most susceptible to injury. Associated hearing loss is typically conductive or mixed. In transverse fractures, lesions are usually confined to the tympanic and geniculate segments of the facial nerve. The selection of the surgical approach is based on radiographic findings, audiometry testing, and neural degeneration evaluated by ENOG and needle EMG.

Recurrent Facial Palsy

Multiple episodes of recurrent ipsilateral or alternating facial paralysis occur in approximately 10% of patients with Bell's palsy.[71,124] In children with recurrent idiopathic AFP, full clinical recovery was reached in 70%.[125] Electrophysiologic studies did not provide any prognostic value.[126] In the setting of recurrent ipsilateral Bell's palsy, it is important to rule out serious predisposing conditions including intracranial or extracranial tumors; meningeal leukemia; granulomatous, infectious, inflammatory, or vascular diseases; trauma; and various malformations.

Some inherited disorders may present with recurrent episodes of transient facial weakness. Most are transmitted in either an autosomal dominant pattern or form part of a recognizable genetic syndrome; therefore, it is important to inquire about family history or other specific features of these conditions. Melkersson-Rosenthal syndrome is characterized by recurrent episodes of facial palsy that may begin in childhood.[127] It is frequently associated with swollen lips (75%) and red facial edema (50%).[128] Facial swelling may be the initial isolated manifestation. This infrequent syndrome

has a dominant inheritance with incomplete penetrance and is linked to chromosome 9p11. Patients are often of Mediterranean origin and may have fissured tongue. Because residual facial weakness could increase with repeated paralyses, some authors have recommended prophylactic surgical decompression.[129]

Osteopetrosis tarda is another hereditary condition that may cause recurrent alternating facial palsy. This is an inherited bone disorder that usually presents during childhood with either osseous fractures or neurologic complications from encroachment by bony overgrowth at the cranial nerve foramina. Radiographic studies reveal abnormally dense temporal bones.

There is also a syndrome of familial recurrent facial palsies with a dominant pattern of inheritance.[75] There is also a family with hereditary neuropathy with liability to pressure palsies (HNPP) where a 16-year-old child presented with recurrent facial palsies. HNPP was not suspected until he developed more typical symptoms.[130] This disease is due to a deletion on chromosome 17p11.2-12, and its diagnosis is confirmed by molecular genetic analysis.[131] Therefore, it is possible to also identify sporadic, atypical, and almost asymptomatic cases. NCSs in these patients may demonstrate widespread motor and sensory NCV slowing. This is more frequently found across common entrapment sites, with conduction block and prolonged distal latencies.

Facial Diplegia

Bilateral facial weakness may be associated with various inflammatory or postinfectious disorders including idiopathic Bell's palsy, Lyme disease, Guillain-Barré syndrome (GBS), Miller Fisher variant of GBS, multiple idiopathic cranial neuropathies, and brainstem encephalitis.[70] In the course of GBS, facial involvement is seen in 50% of cases, most often occurring bilaterally. Miller Fisher syndrome is characterized by ophthalmoplegia, ataxia, and areflexia.[132] One clinical variant characterized by facial diplegia is either an isolated entity or associated with a deficit of multiple lower cranial nerves (i.e., *polyneuritis cranialis*) but sparing of the extremities. Rarely in children facial diplegia is a manifestation of neurosarcoidosis associated with parotid swelling, uveitis, or less commonly, an optic neuritis (Heerfordt's syndrome). Other rare infectious etiologies likely to cause facial diplegia in adults but something to always consider in children lacking an explanation include poliomyelitis, tuberculous meningitis, Hansen's disease, and cryptococcal meningitis with AIDS.[70]

Acquired facial diplegia in childhood may also be associated with either a posterior fossa tumor or meningeal leukemia. Occasionally this is also an early manifestation of a mitochondrial disorder or a neuromuscular transmission defect such as myasthenia gravis. Occult trauma is also a consideration, especially in younger children, since the inciting traumatic antecedent is not always evident.

Electrodiagnostic studies of the cranial nerves and of the muscles and nerves of the limbs may contribute significantly to establishing the etiology of bilateral facial palsy. EMG helps to (1) differentiate axonal loss from demyelination, (2) distinguish neurogenic changes from myopathic changes, and (3) evaluate neuromuscular transmission. Recovery or persistence of BRs may be valuable for prognostic information.[133] In contrast ENOG is not a reliable technique for the evaluation of bilateral facial palsy, because amplitudes are abnormal on both sides. Because facial involvement may be a presenting sign of GBS, electrodiagnostic studies allow one to investigate the multifocal nature of the process. With the clinical variant of polyneuritis cranialis, facial NCSs can be diagnostically useful by demonstrating (1) prolonged latencies and temporal dispersion of the CMAPs, as well as the BRs, (2) slowing of facial NCV, and (3) signs of denervation of the facial muscles (Fig. 29-13).[134] With Miller Fisher syndrome, the excitability thresholds of the facial nerves and the distal latencies of the facial CMAPs may be normal. The main anomalies are prolonged F waves and/or H reflexes and sometimes reduced CMAPs of the facial muscles with reduced SNAP amplitudes in the extremities. BRs may be either normal[135] or altered in parallel with the

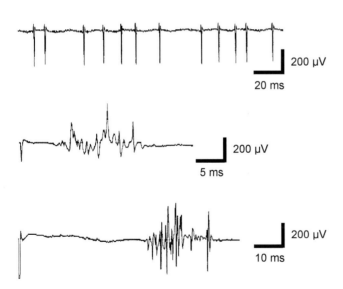

FIGURE 29–13

Needle EMG of facial muscles in a 6-year-old girl with facial diplegia due to polyneuritis cranialis on the 8th day after onset. Top, Reduced recruitment pattern in the orbicularis oris muscle. Middle, Increased-latency prolonged-duration motor response of the orbicularis oris muscle (electrical stimulation applied to cranial nerve VII before the tragus). Bottom, Increased latency (46 milliseconds) and temporal dispersion of the R1 component of the blink reflex.

decreased amplitude of the facial CMAPs and the denervation of the facial muscles.[136] A clinical study of the general course of cranial nerve dysfunction, during progression of the disease, demonstrated an overlap between polyneuritis cranialis, Miller Fisher syndrome, and classic ascending GBS in children.[137]

Congenital Unilateral Facial Weakness

Congenital Facial Palsy

CFPs have various severity and etiology. Forceps delivery, prolonged labor, birthweight above 3500 gm, and primiparity are significant risk factors for facial nerve injury.[138] MRI scans have demonstrated developmental abnormalities of the facial nucleus per se in 4 of 15 children with isolated unilateral CFP.[7] A retrospective study of 172 children with congenital facial asymmetry demonstrated that in 85 patients (67%), this asymmetry was a primary unilateral facial palsy unassociated with any congenital malformation.[139] In 48 of these 85 infants with CFP, a forceps delivery was necessary to extract the fetus. In 2 babies, a neonatal purulent otitis media was identified. No causal factor was found in the remaining 35 infants. Either a prenatal or perinatal compression of the extracranial facial nerve against the myometrium, the fetal shoulder, or the sacral prominence of the maternal pelvis may have had a possible role in these CFPs. There is often concordance between the side of CFP and that of cephalic presentation.[140]

Evaluation

Timing of Facial Nerve Injuries. When a nerve trunk injury occurs at birth, fibrillation potentials may be detected as early as the 2nd to 4th day of life.[141] Fibrillation potentials recorded in the first 24 hours may indicate a prenatal nerve injury.[142] Repeated examinations show the temporal profile for the varying changes in nerve conduction parameters, including CMAP amplitudes as well as onset of fibrillation potentials with positive waves, and the presence of voluntary MUPs, including nascent MUPs, during the process of axonal loss and muscle reinnervation. In contrast, in cases of longstanding prenatal fixed palsy, there may be no spontaneous activities, and EMG and NCSs abnormalities remain the same at repeated examinations.

Assessment of Severity of the CFP. Confirmation of the degree of hemifacial denervation by needle EMG, in addition to facial NCSs and BRs, provides a means to assess neurophysiologic signs of axonal loss as well as reinnervation and helps define the topography of the facial nerve lesion. The percentage values of facial function over time provided by serial ENOGs also correlate with prognosis.[25]

Moderate forms are distinguished where denervation is only partial affecting either the territories of the two main branches equally or predominantly the cervicofacial branch.

Progressive recovery of hemifacial motor activity may occur during the first few months. EMG may demonstrate the progress of nerve regeneration and often predicts a favorable outcome. The presence of a moderate palsy with subsequent favorable outcome was more frequent in infants delivered without forceps (71%) compared with a group delivered with forceps (54%).[139]

In severe forms of CFP, EMG demonstrates that the lesions of the temporofacial branch are complete and associated with abolition of the BRs, as well as total or partial impairment of the cervicofacial branch. Clinical and EMG monitoring of severe CFPs demonstrate that facial nerve regeneration and muscular reinnervation proceed slowly. When the palsy seems to remain clinically total, EMG may be helpful in demonstrating early signs of reinnervation indicating a more favorable prognosis by showing some nascent MUPs with the reappearance of a low-amplitude, increased latency CMAP. ENOG may be repeated to show any progress in facial nerve function. Improvement in facial motor activity and EMG parameters may continue to be evidenced as late as 2 years of age.

Asymmetric Crying Facies

Asymmetric crying facies (ACF) is characterized by a congenital facial asymmetry that is evident only when the child is crying and that is confined to the lower lip.

Regardless of the cause, this clinical presentation is characterized by a labial commissure that does not descend on the affected side, but the nasolabial folds are symmetric, as is contraction of the frontalis muscle (Fig. 29-14). ACF primarily results from hypoplasia of the DAOM.[143,144] Infrequently, this presentation represents a distal partial facial palsy.[145] The lower part of the DAOM inserts in a diffuse manner into the platysma muscle along the base of the mandible and enters as a narrow fascicle into the labial commissure, where its fibers merge with those of the orbicularis oris muscle. Its contraction draws the labial commissure and the external part of the lower lip downward and outward, producing an expression of displeasure.[146]

Electrophysiologic Tests

Electrophysiologic tests are unique and useful tools for defining the nature of ACF. We reported a series of 51 children with this clinical picture.[139] Of the 51 babies, 10 showed partial denervation of the DAOM, as well as in the depressor labii inferioris and mentalis muscles on EMG, leading to the diagnosis of partial facial palsy. This very localized nerve lesion corresponds to the territory of the mental branch of the facial nerve. This branch, arising from the cervicofacial branch, has a course that in the fetus and newborn closely follows the base of the mandible and is thus easily compressed.[147]

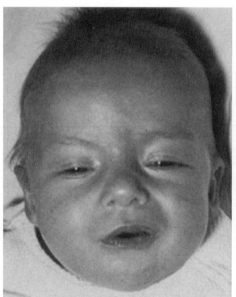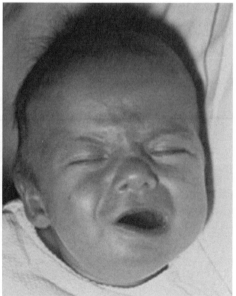

FIGURE 29–14

Asymmetric crying facies: hypoplasia of the depressor anguli oris muscle in a fullterm baby at age 20 days. The facial musculature is symmetric at rest (left); when the child is crying, the lower lip is asymmetric but the upper face and nasolabial folds remain symmetric (right). (From Renault F, Quijano-Roy S: Congenital and acquired facial palsies. In Jones HR, DeVivo DC, Darras BT [eds]: Neuromuscular Disorders of Infancy, Childhood, and Adolescence: A Clinician's Approach. Philadelphia, Butterworth Heinemann, 2003, p 286.)

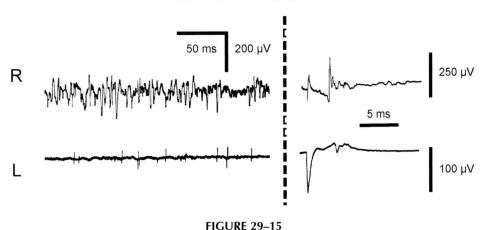

FIGURE 29–15

Asymmetric crying facies: hypoplasia of the depressor anguli oris muscle (DAOM). Needle EMG at age 20 days. Left, Two-channel recording of voluntary contraction during crying: sparse low-amplitude short-duration motor unit potentials in the left DAOM (lower tracing) compared to normal interference pattern in the right DAOM (upper tracing). Right, Response of DAOMs to facial nerve electrical stimulation before the tragus: normal-latency low-amplitude simplified-morphology response of the hypoplasic DAOM (lower tracing) compared with that of the contralateral normal muscle (upper tracing).

In the 41 other patients with ACF, electrodiagnostic studies demonstrated the absence of muscle denervation with normal facial NCSs but revealed signs of hypoplasia of the DAOM. The interference pattern on needle examination during crying was of low maximum amplitude and consisted of MUPs of brief duration and low amplitude, and the response to stimulation of the facial nerve was of low amplitude and simplified morphology (Fig. 29-15). No cases of complete muscular agenesis of the DAOM were documented; however, EMG demonstrated that hypoplasia of the depressor labii inferioris muscle was concomitantly present in 6 patients.

Associated Congenital Malformations

Associated congenital malformations were found in 5 of the 41 children with DAOM hypoplasia, including two cardiac septal defects, one complex cardiopathy, one dysmorphic syndrome, and one cleft palate. Since the Cayler cardiofacial syndrome has been described,[148-150] prospective studies of newborns with ACF have demonstrated an increased risk of visceral malformation, particularly of the heart, great vessels, and urinary apparatus.[151,152] A deletion at chromosome 22q11 is reported with ACF as a part of the cardiofacial syndrome[153] as well as isolated ACF.[154] Therefore, when an EMG diagnosis of hypoplasia of the DAOM is confirmed, this necessitates a search for an associated visceral malformation.

Pseudoparalysis

In certain cases of congenital facial asymmetry, the facial EMG does not show any sign of paralysis or muscular hypoplasia. In these cases of "pseudoparalysis," asymmetry is noted both at rest and on crying in newborns, and no apparent malformations are observed. Such pseudoparalysis may be associated with asymmetric mandibular hypoplasia, but most often it is the result of intrauterine position. A clinical feature that is characteristic of pseudoparalysis is the lack of parallelism of the gums (Fig. 29-16). Such was identified in 5 of 172 infants in our congenital facial asymmetry series.[139] The EMG was strictly normal and demonstrated the integrity of facial muscles and nerves. This functional asymmetry resolved rapidly in all 5 babies within the first 2 months.

Congenital Multiple Cranial Nerve Palsies

Hemifacial Malformations

Congenital malformations involving the tissue derivatives of the first and second branchial arches can indicate a lesion of cranial nerves V and VII (Fig. 29-17). In these patients, dysphagia and its respiratory complications can be due to anatomic malformations, central neurologic disorders, and peripheral nerve impairment. Facial paralysis has been reported in most cases of Goldenhar's syndrome (facioauriculovertebral spectrum)[155] and 22% of hemifacial microsomia.[156] CHARGE association includes *c*oloboma, *h*eart disease, *a*tresia of the choanae, *r*etarded growth and development, *g*enital hypoplasia, and *e*ar anomalies or deafness.[157] Facial paralysis is reported in 43% of patients with CHARGE association; paralysis of several cranial nerves and poor coordination of sucking-swallowing are often seen.[157,158] EMG shows denervation in the territories of the cranial nerves involved, and EMG during bottle-feeding may demonstrate sucking-swallowing incoordination.

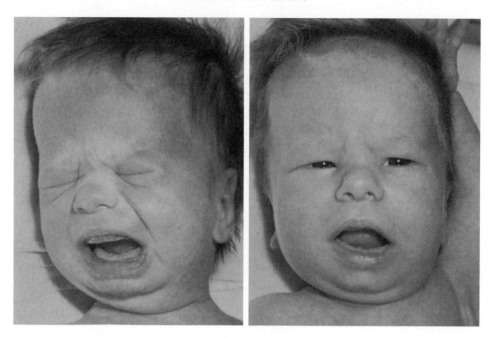

FIGURE 29–16

Left and Right, *Congenital facial asymmetry due to sustained abnormal intrauterine posture (pseudoparalysis) on the 1st day of life in a fullterm newborn baby. Note the lack of parallelism of the gums. (From Renault F, Quijano-Roy S: Congenital and acquired facial palsies. In Jones HR, DeVivo DC, Darras BT [eds]: Neuromuscular Disorders of Infancy, Childhood, and Adolescence: A Clinician's Approach. Philadelphia, Butterworth Heinemann, 2003, p 287.)*

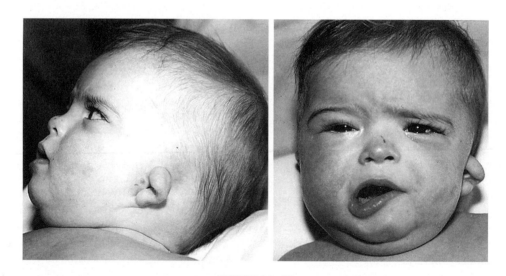

FIGURE 29–17

Left and Right, *Congenital facial palsy in facioauriculovertebral syndrome. (From Renault F, Quijano-Roy S: Congenital and acquired facial palsies. In Jones HR, DeVivo DC, Darras BT [eds]: Neuromuscular Disorders of Infancy, Childhood, and Adolescence: A Clinician's Approach. Philadelphia, Butterworth Heinemann, 2003, p 288.)*

In one series of 44 children with CHARGE association, 58% had pharyngolaryngeal anomalies (dysphagia, laryngomalacia, glossoptosis, laryngeal paralysis, cleft palate, stenosis) leading to dyspnea with altered blood gas levels.[159]

Prolonged enteral feeding was necessary in 47% of the patients and tracheotomy in 29%.

We reported facial EMG results in 33 infants with facial weakness associated with hemifacial hypoplasia and malformation of the ear.[139] Clinical diagnoses in this series included Goldenhar's syndrome,[160] Treacher-Collins-Franceschetti mandibulofacial dysostosis,[161] and CHARGE association. Facial weakness was either diffuse or localized to one side of the face. EMG activity of the facial muscles was either absent (10 cases), neurogenic (9 cases), or "myopathic" (14 cases). In facial malformations, myopathic EMG signs without denervation more probably indicate muscular hypoplasia rather than a myopathic disease. Among the 19 infants with totally inactive or partially denervated muscles, neuroimaging showed a piliferous cyst of the cerebellum in one infant and cerebellar hypoplasia in another. In contrast none of the 14 cases with myopathic EMG changes had CNS abnormalities. Thus, for babies with hemifacial congenital malformation, facial EMG and NCSs may be used to detect patients at risk for associated malformations of the CNS, in particular of the posterior fossa.[162,163]

Möbius' Syndrome

Diagnosis of Möbius' syndrome is easy in cases of total or partial facial diplegia, whether symmetric or asymmetric, when associated with bilateral paralysis of abduction of the eye (Fig. 29-18).[164] When the facial diplegia is partial, it usually involves the upper half of the face. Abducens palsy often has the appearance of esotropia.[165] Most patients with Möbius' syndrome exhibit drooling, malocclusion, velopharyngeal incompetence, dysarthria, and delayed speech.[166] A concomitant unilateral or bilateral paralysis of the hypoglossal nerve with atrophy of the tongue is present in one third of patients with Möbius' syndrome. Most patients have sucking difficulties, and lip closure is defective. Some have aspiration episodes and require tube feeding or even gastrostomy for the first months of life. They improve after a variable period and subsequently have neither feeding nor respiratory problems. Trigeminal nerve involvement with trismus is less frequent. Most cases of Möbius' syndrome are sporadic, but families with autosomal dominant inheritance are reported.[167] Talipes equinovarus, different malformations of hands or fingers, and Poland's anomaly may be associated. Additionally, six patients with Möbius' syndrome associated with an axonal neuropathy and hypogonadism had been reported. This syndrome probably constitutes a separate entity.[168]

Histologically, a heterogeneous spectrum of findings is associated with Möbius' syndrome.[169] These include hypoplasia or atrophy of cranial nerve nuclei, hypoplasia of the facial nerve, focal brainstem necrosis, brainstem hypoplasia, muscular dysplasia, and even dystrophic muscular changes.

In Möbius' syndrome, facial EMG is an important diagnostic tool and contributes to the differential diagnosis and the elucidation of its multifaceted pathogenesis. If facial EMG is difficult to interpret secondary to major muscle

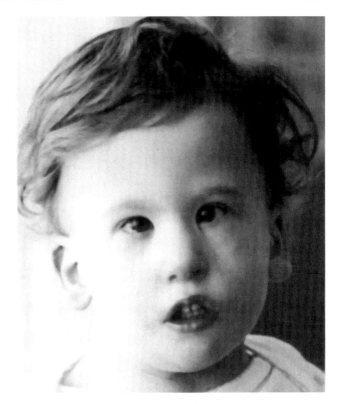

FIGURE 29–18

A child with Möbius' syndrome at age 14 months. (From Renault F, Quijano-Roy S: Congenital and acquired facial palsies. In Jones HR, DeVivo DC, Darras BT [eds]: Neuromuscular Disorders of Infancy, Childhood, and Adolescence: A Clinician's Approach. Philadelphia, Butterworth Heinemann, 2003, p 289.)

atrophy, the study of lingual and palatal muscles can be useful in demonstrating evidence of a concomitant neurogenic process in the territories of the hypoglossal nerve and pharyngeal plexus. During the neonatal period, EMG of the limbs may be necessary to differentiate Möbius' syndrome from congenital myotonic dystrophy or other myopathies. Most published EMG data confirm a neurogenic origin for the facial muscular atrophy. These data include numerous studies showing sparse motor units, increased latencies, slowed facial NCV, and sometimes altered BRs.[170] Such data support the hypothesis of a prenatal nuclear lesion of the specific cranial nerves. One study suggests that the mechanism could be ischemic.[171]

Our EMG results with 22 cases were heterogeneous but showed signs of predominant axonal loss.[172] In most of the children (17 of 22), EMG demonstrated reduced and single motor unit patterns in several but not all facial, lingual, or velopharyngeal muscles. Monophasic or biphasic MUPs with low amplitude characterized facial muscles, whereas velopharyngeal muscles showed high-amplitude, long-duration polyphasic MUPs. These results favor the hypothesis of a developmental defect of specific cranial nerve nuclei. However, spontaneous activities were not recorded in any of the 90 muscles studied. This suggests that, if axonal loss occurred, it was not in the late fetal life. In 2 of the remaining 5 children, all motor unit patterns were of full interference and of low amplitude. Motor NCSs demonstrated that all CMAPs were of low amplitude, and the latencies and conduction velocities were normal. Although a myopathy was suspected, deltoid muscle biopsy was normal. The clinical course was stable. Therefore, in Möbius' syndrome, "myopathic" EMG signs unassociated with denervation potentials in the facial muscles are not indicative of a true myopathic disorder. In the other 3 remaining children, all EMG motor unit patterns in muscles of the face, tongue, and soft palate were typically neurogenic. All three had significant history of chronic or acute fetal distress, had had severe dysphagia and respiratory complications, and might have had hypoxic-ischemic involvement of the brainstem. Therefore, electrodiagnostic studies may help to resolve the nosologic classification of patients with congenital multiple cranial nerve involvement.[173]

Hypoglossia Syndromes

In cases of hypoglossia, either isolated or associated with anomalies of the maxilla or extremities, dysphagia is severe.[174-176] The authors studied four infants with severe hypoglossia that was isolated in three patients and associated in the other one patient with upper limb malformation. Facial, lingual, and velopharyngeal EMG showed signs of bilateral denervation of the genioglossus muscles in the four infants (Fig. 29-19) and of the muscles of the soft palate in two patients, and of the face in two patients. Facial and hypoglossal NCSs were normal, and the R1 component of BRs was present with normal latency in all cases. EMG during bottle-feeding could be performed in only one infant and showed severe incoordination. The three other infants had a degree of dysphagia that precluded any attempt at oral feeding; one of them had undergone tracheotomy. These neurophysiologic findings in hypoglossia syndromes suggest involvement of the cranial nerve nuclei and can be compared with similar abnormalities seen in Möbius' syndrome, which could have the same pathogenesis.[171]

Lower Cranial Nerve Birth Trauma

Lower cranial nerve birth trauma results in dysphagia associated with dysphonia, usually with a good prognosis.[177] Congenital laryngeal paralysis is probably due to prenatal or perinatal compression: rotation and lateral flexion of the head results in stretching of the superior branch of the laryngeal nerve against the thyroid cartilage and that of the recurrent laryngeal nerve against the cricoid cartilage. More rarely, obstetric paralysis of cranial nerves IX, X, and XI has been reported,[178] and involvement of cranial nerve XII associated with obstetric paralysis of the brachial plexus.[179]

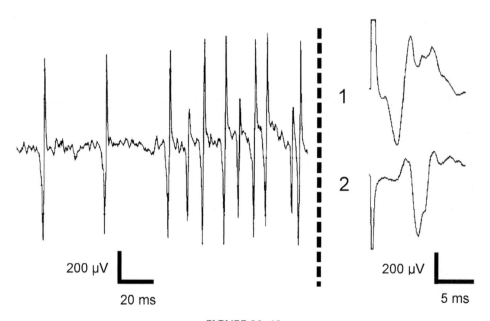

FIGURE 29–19

Hypoglossia syndrome: needle EMG of the left genioglossus muscle at age 40 days. Left, Voluntary contraction during crying, reduced neurogenic pattern. Right, Electrical stimulation of the hypoglossal nerve at distal submental point (1) and proximal retromandibular point (2): normal-latency low-amplitude simplified-morphology responses. Nerve conduction velocity, 32.4 m/sec.

Chiari Malformations

Impairment of the paired cranial nerves IX, X, and XII with paralysis of the soft palate and dysphagia may be seen in Chiari malformations, in particular the type II variant.[180] EMG study may demonstrate denervation of muscles of the soft palate.[181] In a prospective study in 22 infants with congenital Chiari II malformation, 4 infants had dysphagia and aspiration episodes resulting in respiratory complications with onset from the 3rd to the 6th month.[182]

Facial and Bulbar Weakness of Central Origin

Suprabulbar Palsies

Orofacial apraxia may be an early sign of cerebral palsy in newborn babies with prenatal or perinatal hypoxic-ischemic encephalopathy.[183,184] EMG of facial muscles, facial NCSs, and BRs are normal in these infants. Sucking-swallowing incoordination is demonstrated by the EMG during bottle-feeding, but there are no EMG signs of denervation in the muscles of the tongue and soft palate. In fact, sucking-swallowing disorders are one of the possible sequels of periventricular leukomalacia of the premature newborn, hypoxic-ischemic encephalopathy of the term newborn, and prenatal encephalopathies. These cerebral disorders lead to a suprabulbar syndrome with generalized hypotonia, lethargy, facial hypotonia with salivary incontinence, and sometimes spasm on mouth opening. Feeding difficulties and their respiratory complications reveal signs of cerebral impairment that subsequently manifest as poor axial tone, spastic hypertonia or dystonia of the limbs, and dysarthria.

When the neurophysiologic and neuroradiologic investigations show more or less diffuse bilateral anatomic and functional cerebral lesions, this can indicate eventual development of severe spastic quadriplegia. With severe encephalopathies leading to multiple disabilities, swallowing disorders are a major problem with risk of malnutrition, bronchopulmonary disease, and death due to aspiration.[185] In these severe cases aspiration of liquid foods is frequent and usually silent; tracheobronchial dyskinesia and gastroesophageal reflux with hiatal hernia are often associated findings.[186] In contrast, cerebral investigations are often normal in dystonic-athetoid forms of cerebral palsy. In relatively moderate cases, facial apraxia and dysphagia progressively improve over several months. In some children difficulties may persist, in particular during ingestion of liquids, but aspiration is rare and the dysphagia has no repercussions on bronchopulmonary status or growth.

Congenital dysphagia associated with facial diplegia and localized bilateral anterior opercular lesions constitutes the congenital type of Foix-Chavany-Marie syndrome (Fig. 29-20).[187] In addition to difficulties in swallowing and

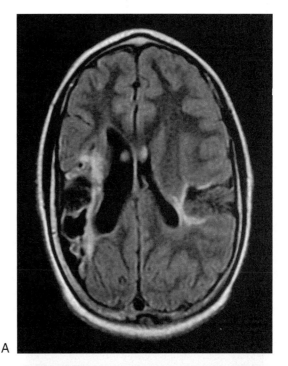

A

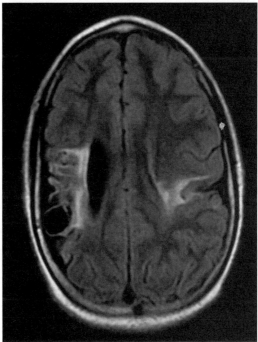

B

FIGURE 29-20

A and B, *Brain MRI of a child with Foix-Chavany-Marie syndrome at age 10 years: axial T1-weighted image; bilateral lesion of perisylvian area.*

chewing and severe dysarthria, these patients may present with psychomotor delay, cerebral palsy, epilepsy, or verbal agnosia.[188]

Feeding difficulties that necessitate tube feeding are a common feature of Prader-Willi syndrome. The generalized hypotonia is often profound, and the infant may appear motionless in the first few days of life. Dysphagia tends to resolve within the first weeks of life.[189]

Brainstem Perinatal Injury and Brainstem Dysgenesis

When the dysphagia is of bulbar origin, EMG shows signs of denervation in the territory of the cranial nerves; BRs also may be altered. Normal EEG, evoked potentials, and MRI/CT results should rule out associated cerebral lesions. We reported 12 infants with major congenital dysphagia who at birth had aspiration-induced pulmonary disease and failure to thrive that was presumed to be of bulbar origin.[190] Nasal reflux and salivary stasis were obvious in most cases. Most had facial hypotonia (Fig. 29-21), sometimes with asymmetry of the tongue or soft palate. Ten of the 12 patients subsequently had a favorable clinical course with normal mental and motor development, although their swallowing difficulties lasted from 9 to 26 months.

EMG detected neurogenic signs in the facial muscles as well as the tongue and soft palate compatible with lesions of cranial nerves VII, IX, X, and XII. The R2 component of BRs was abolished (11 of 12) with either a delayed latency (3 of 12) or abolition (3 of 12) of the R1 component. The abolition or prolongation of the latency of the R1 component of BRs associated with normal latency of the response of the orbicularis oculi muscle on stimulation of cranial nerve VII suggests an ipsilateral lesion of the pons.[30] Abolition of the R2 component suggests a more caudal location of the lesions: the spinal trigeminal nucleus and adjacent reticular formation.[31,33]

The perinatal histories of these infants suggest that both the clinical dysphagia and the electrodiagnostic findings demonstrating lesions of several cranial nerves were the consequence of perinatal hypoxic-ischemic brainstem injury (Table 29-3). Even though the brainstem and the spinal cord are less vulnerable to anoxic ischemia than the cerebral cortex, pathologic studies have shown a pattern of brainstem damage following acute asphyxia in neonatal[191] or prenatal anoxic ischemia.[192] Histologic features compatible with fetal asphyxia are described in the thalamus and brainstem in premature newborns who had respiratory failure and multiple cranial nerve palsies.[193] Hemorrhage within the brainstem and the cervical spinal cord is reported in a term newborn following meconium aspiration resulting in hypotonia, absence of sucking, lingual hemiatrophy, diaphragmatic paralysis, and EMG signs of denervation of the trapezius and sternocleidomastoid muscles.[194] The diencephalon, the pons, and the medulla oblongata are the usual sites of neuronal loss in cases of severe neonatal asphyxia such as cardiac arrest.[195] An autopsy of a child with facial diplegia, velopharyngeal incoordination, and ocular motor apraxia demonstrated neuronal depletion of cranial nerve nuclei and intact cerebral hemispheres.[173] When the anoxic-ischemic lesions or hemorrhage or a combination involve both brainstem and hemispheric structures, the dysphagia is due to the effects of both bulbar and suprabulbar dysfunction. This condition progresses to cerebral palsy.

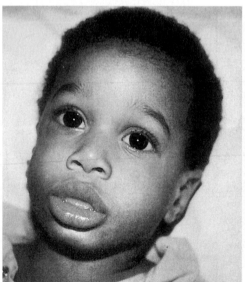 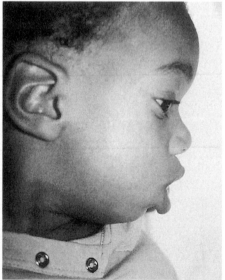

FIGURE 29–21

Left and Right, *Facial weakness in a 24-month-old child with congenital dysphagia due to birth asphyxia. (From Renault F: Neurogenic dysplasia in newborns and infants. In Jones HR, DeVivo DC, Darras BT [eds]: Neuromuscular Disorders of Infancy, Childhood, and Adolescence: A Clinician's Approach. Philadelphia, Butterworth Heinemann, 2003, p 1134.)*

TABLE 29–3. CONGENITAL DYSPHAGIA DUE TO PERINATAL BRAINSTEM INJURY: CLINICAL AND NEUROPHYSIOLOGIC FINDINGS IN 12 CASES

Characteristics	No. of Patients
Clinical Features	
Feeding difficulties	12
Aspiration pneumonia	12
Nasal reflux	10
Salivary stasis	6
Failure to thrive	9
Facial diplegia	8
Axial hypotonia	4
Soft palate asymmetry	1
Tongue asymmetry	1
EMG Data	
Reduced interference pattern	
In orbicularis oculi and/or orbicularis oris	12
In genioglossus, levator veli palatini and/or palatoglossus muscles	12
Blink responses	
R2 absent	11
R1 latency: asymmetry > 3 msec	3
R1 absent	3
Perinatal History	
Multiple gestation	2
Toxemia of pregnancy	1
Birth asphyxia	5
Premature and/or small for dates	4

Pierre Robin Syndrome

Glossoptosis, cleft palate, and retrognathia (Fig. 29-22) characterize Pierre Robin syndrome (PRS), whose origin remains obscure; in fact, it is probably heterogeneous. PRS may occur in isolation, or it may be associated with other developmental defects. About 85% of newborns with this syndrome are at risk for feeding difficulties leading to aspiration, obstruction of the airways, bronchopulmonary disease, and failure to thrive.[196-198] Careful evaluation and management of respiratory and feeding disorders have led to an improvement in both morbidity and mortality.[199,200]

We have performed polysomnography; EMG of the face, tongue, and soft palate; BRs; EMG during bottle-feeding; and BAERs in 25 infants with isolated PRS.[201] Obstructive or mixed apneas were found in all patients, including 19 of 20 patients who had no clinical signs of respiratory difficulty. The number and duration of central respiratory pauses were always normal, as well as EEG and clinical organization of sleep stages.

The EMG recruitment pattern in facial and lingual muscles, as well as BRs, were normal in all instances. However EMG recruitment pattern in the soft palate muscles was normal only in 14 of 25 children, demonstrating signs of muscular hypoplasia without denervation in 10 of 25 patients, and only showed signs of denervation in 1 of

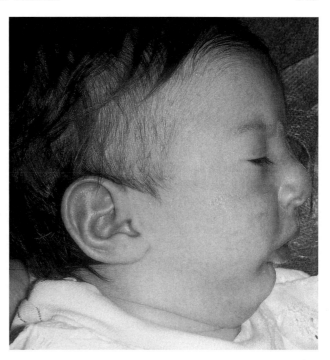

FIGURE 29–22
A 1-month-old girl with Pierre Robin syndrome.

25 patients. EMG during bottle-feeding showed sucking-swallowing disorders in 20 of 25 patients, including 4 patients without apparent feeding difficulties.

BAERs showed normal and symmetric I to III and I to V interpeak latencies in 19 of 19 cases. From a clinical viewpoint, an important finding was that polysomnography and EMG revealed a case of respiratory obstruction and lack of sucking-swallowing coordination even in the absence of a clinically apparent respiratory or feeding disorder. By establishing the presence of a sucking-swallowing disorder and its relative severity, an EMG during bottle-feeding as well as esophageal manometry can help clarify whether tube feeding is indicated.[202]

Pathophysiologically these neurophysiologic findings suggest that with an isolated PRS the main anomaly is a dysfunction of the lingual and pharyngeal motor organization, without any structural abnormality in either the brainstem nuclei or their pathways. The lingual and pharyngeal motor disorder results at birth in glossoptosis, respiratory obstruction, and dysphagia and can by itself account for other symptoms of PRS. The prenatal palate and mandibular formation results from an interaction between tissue growth processes and tongue movements. In PRS, the tongue may remain too long in its initial high position in the nasal cavity, hampering the closure of the soft and bony palate. It leaves its mark in the form of a "roman arch" in the cleft palate.[203,204] Retrognathia also can be attributed to the hypomobility and retroposition of the tongue during the fetal period.[205] This sequential and interlinked pathogenesis of the dysmorphic triad is at the origin of the term Pierre Robin Sequence.[206]

Complications of PRS should be evaluated as soon as possible after birth. When signs of respiratory distress persist after removal of pharyngeal congestion, they preclude oral feeding and necessitate transfer to an intensive care unit. Laryngoscopy and polysomnography determine obstruction of the airways and associated cardiorespiratory repercussions. An EMG performed during bottle-feeding and videofluoroscopy evaluate the coordination of the oral and pharyngeal phases and the risk of aspiration. Manometry and pH monitoring study the esophageal phase. Associated pathologies, in particular cardiac, bone, ocular, and endocrine, must be systematically sought. They can occasionally reveal the presence of a specific syndrome, such as Stickler's, DiGeorge, CATCH 22, fetal alcohol, or other syndrome.[207-210] Additionally children with PRS have a significantly higher risk of conductive hearing loss than those with isolated cleft palate.[211] Sensorineural hearing loss is reported in syndromic and isolated PRS.[212]

The *Opitz G/BBB* syndrome of dysphagia, hypertelorism, and hypospadias is an inherited disorder characterized by midline defects that can include lip-palate-laryngotracheal clefts.[213,214] Aspiration is a frequent manifestation in these infants and poses the greatest threat to life. Evaluation should include laryngeal and gastrointestinal endoscopy.[215] In a personal study of three patients with this syndrome, EMG was normal in facial, lingual, and velopharyngeal muscles, but EMG during bottle-feeding showed a severe sucking-swallowing disorder at the ages of 3, 5, and 8 weeks, respectively.

Congenital Isolated Dysphagia

Congenital isolated dysphagia exists in occasional premature and term newborns in the absence of any neuromuscular disorder, malformation syndrome, or neonatal disease. Under suitable management, the course is usually favorable after a period ranging from several weeks to 2 years. In a series of 37 newborns with congenital dysphagia,[11] the dysphagia was an isolated disorder in 10 term newborns and 9 premature infants. In each of these 19 patients, a bottle-feeding EMG showed lack of coordination between the oral and pharyngeal phases of swallowing. However, the isolated nature of the dysphagia was confirmed by the normality of all other neurophysiologic and neuroradiologic evaluations. Swallowing disorders improved progressively: normal oral feeding could be started after the 40th week of gestational age in 7 premature infants, at 6 and 10 months in the 2 other premature infants, and from 2 to 15 months in term newborns.

The classic hypothesis for congenital isolated dysphagia is that there is a transient dysfunction of the CNS organization of the sucking-swallowing automatism. It is tempting to consider the immaturity of the sucking-swallowing function as a possible mechanism, especially in cases of prematurity. However, the possibility of a specific lesion that has yet to be detected by the various current investigative modalities cannot be excluded. In fact, a history of acute fetal distress or the existence of minor abnormal neurologic findings would support the hypothesis of an unknown perinatal cerebral event.[216] In some cases videofluoroscopy revealed an abnormality mainly affecting the pharyngeal phase, suggesting defective function of the constrictor muscles of the pharynx.[217,218] However, autopsy studies failed to demonstrate any abnormality of the CNS or the cranial nerves involved in swallowing in two infants who died of tracheal aspiration at the ages 4 and 8 months.[217]

Neuromuscular Disorders

In babies with congenital disorders affecting the facial and bulbar musculature, facial diplegia is typically characterized by an expressionless face with a tent-shaped mouth (Fig. 29-23). Dysmorphology of the face may be seen; it is thought to be the sequel of the prenatal muscle weakness.

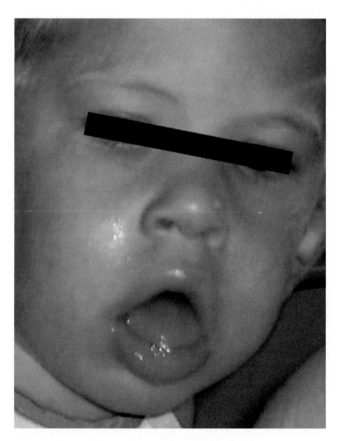

FIGURE 29–23
Facial hypotonia with open tent-shaped mouth.

Ptosis and ophthalmoplegia are also found. A weak cry and dysphagia are usually present and may be a marker of respiratory weakness. Atrophy of the muscles of mastication may provoke mandibular ankylosis.

Physical examination detects signs of generalized muscular disorder such as neck or limb weakness, poor spontaneous movements, muscle atrophy, decreased or absent muscle stretch reflexes, and joint contractures or even arthrogryposis. In the context of bulbar weakness concomitant with neonatal hypotonia, other conditions such as Prader-Willi syndrome and congenital myasthenic syndrome should also be suspected. Therefore, correct diagnosis is of important consequence to therapeutic decisions as well as to genetic counseling for future pregnancies.

Facial NCSs and BRs are normal. No neurogenic signs are detected in these infants by needle EMG of muscles of the face, tongue, and soft palate. Full interference and low-amplitude patterns may be detected in these muscles. However, one should also perform an extremity EMG to detect diffuse myopathic signs and search for myotonia. Dystrophic muscle fibers are more prone to induce myopathic activity on needle EMG than are nondystrophic lesions. Alterations in the type of fibers, in muscle fiber diameter or packing density, or in the amount of interstitial tissue are more difficult to detect with EMG unless the changes are severe.[219]

Typical myotonic discharges are rarely recorded in young infants with congenital myotonic dystrophy. In a series of 10 patients examined between birth and 4 years of age, myopathic EMG changes were obvious in two or more muscles and brief myotonic discharges were provoked by nerve stimulation in 6 infants with no clinical myotonia, including 3 newborns examined at 4, 7, and 9 days, respectively.[220] In another series, myotonia was noted as early as age 5 days; however, one infant had no myotonia noted at 3 weeks. In another infant, myotonic discharges increased in degree between the perinatal time and 17 months. Because of the profuse spontaneous activity, it was often difficult to assess MUPs satisfactorily.[221] In both series, EMG examinations of some mothers demonstrated previously unsuspected myotonia. A needle EMG examination of the mother may prove to be diagnostic of myotonic dystrophy since almost all mothers of babies born with congenital myotonic dystrophy have the disease.

Brief repetitive discharges are also reported in different types of congenital muscular dystrophy.[222]

An associated motor or sensory neuropathy may be present in cases of mitochondrial myopathies[223] as well as in cases of merosin deficiency.[222]

Facial diplegia is an important diagnostic indicator of several muscular disorders, such as congenital myotonic muscular dystrophy[224]; congenital muscular dystrophies, including merosin deficiency,[225] mutations in the *FKRP*

gene,[222] and Fukuyama type; and congenital myopathies such as nemaline, myotubular,[226] and metabolic types. Sucking and swallowing difficulties are almost constant in the severe neonatal form of nemaline myopathy, in early-onset centronuclear/myotubular myopathies, and congenital sex-linked myotubular myopathy.[90] The severity of the feeding difficulties, with their bronchopulmonary complications and persistence during growth, is particularly prominent in congenital myotonic muscular dystrophy[224] and merosin-deficient congenital muscular dystrophy.[225]

In severe spinal muscular atrophy type I, dysphagia may be present from birth, although facial muscles are not clinically affected.[189] Congenital dysphagia, generalized hypotonia, respiratory insufficiency, and joint contractures are main features of pontocerebellar hypoplasia type I.[227]

Congenital myopathies should be distinguished from Prader-Willi syndrome, which often presents in neonates who have profound generalized hypotonia and feeding difficulties necessitating tube feeding. There is facial dysmorphology with an open triangular-shaped mouth but no marked facial weakness.[189]

An infantile form of facioscapulohumeral (FSH) muscular dystrophy with early facial diplegia and a severe clinical course is also described.[228-230] The facial diplegia is obvious in the first year of life.[231] These babies have a peculiar horizontal smile, and they may be unable to close their eyes and mouth fully. In some infants, the mothers noted poor sucking and lack of facial expression at birth.[228] Sensorineural hearing loss and tortuosity of retinal arterioles also occur. Motor milestones are not delayed; however, limb and respiratory weakness worsen rapidly prior to adult age. Nevertheless the genetic, histologic, and electrophysiologic characteristics of infantile FSH muscular dystrophy are similar to late-onset FSH.[231]

Feeding difficulties and aspiration episodes may be the first signs of congenital myasthenic syndromes. Neonatal disorders of neuromuscular transmission have variable pathophysiology and clinical expression. Typical findings include feeding difficulties, respiratory dysfunction, ophthalmoparesis, ptosis, and hypotonia. Symptoms may worsen with crying and physiologic activity.[232] Repetitive motor nerve stimulation should be performed in babies who have variable muscle weakness and ptosis, ophthalmoparesis, repetitive CMAPs, or myopathic EMG signs.[233,234]

Dysphagia transient occurs in 15% of neonates born to myasthenic mothers. The incidence of neonatal transient myasthenia gravis is decreasing with improved maternal treatment. However, maternal disease may be latent, and acute choking episodes may be a presenting symptom in a floppy baby with associated bulbar weakness.[189] There is no correlation between the severity of the disease in the mother and the severity in the infant. The symptoms appear within the first few hours, and the mean disease duration is 18 days. A prenatal onset results in a severe form with hydramnios, arthrogryposis, and severe hypotonia.[235,236]

Acquired Dysphagia

Aspiration is most often a complication of a known CNS or neuromuscular deficit; when such a disorder is identified, it is important to search systematically for a swallowing disorder and to prevent sudden aspiration accidents or repetitive silent aspiration.[237] The disorder involved may be an acute or progressive dysfunction of the CNS, including coma of whatever cause, a cerebral lesion following cranial trauma,[238] ischemic stroke, acute encephalitis, a degenerative disorder with bulbar or suprabulbar involvement, or cerebral palsy.[186] The risk of aspiration is particularly high in children who have undergone tracheostomy.[59,239] Intermittent suprabulbar palsy may reveal status epilepticus of benign partial epilepsy[240] or other epileptic events associated with oromotor dyspraxia.[241]

Aspiration may occur during the course of peripheral neuromuscular disorders such as myasthenia gravis and some structural or metabolic congenital myopathies and muscular dystrophies.[225,242] Dysphagia and ophthalmoplegia may be the presenting symptoms in children with oxidative metabolic disorders who later develop more diffuse weakness.[243] Electrodiagnostic studies of the cranial nerves, and also of the upper and lower limbs, contribute to diagnosis.

One sixth of myasthenia gravis patients present with bulbar symptoms including dysphagia, nasal speech, and difficulty chewing.[244] During acute GBS as well as in severe forms of polymyositis or bulbar poliomyelitis, the occurrence of a swallowing disorder suggests a progressive clinical course associated with imminent respiratory failure. This necessitates strict surveillance and withdrawal of oral food. Oculopharyngeal muscular dystrophy begins with ptosis and dysphagia. Onset is usually in middle or late adult life; a few cases with childhood-onset dysphagia and gastrointestinal involvement are reported.[245,246]

Infantile Botulism

Infantile botulism[247,248] occurs in babies younger than 6 months of age. It is characterized by a prodromal phase of constipation with progressive development over 4 to 5 days of generalized hypotonia, areflexia, poor sucking, weak cry, ptosis, and paralysis of cranial nerves and of the limbs. Ventilatory support may be necessary. Motor NCSs reveal markedly reduced amplitude of CMAPs. High-rate (25 to 30 Hz) repetitive motor nerve stimulation provokes incremental response from 23% to 300%. The response to low-rate repetitive nerve stimulation (2 to 5 Hz) is more variable.[249] Stimulation single-fiber EMG is another useful way to demonstrate the presynaptic neuromuscular junctional transmission disorder.[250] Needle EMG may show

low-amplitude and short-duration spontaneous fibrillation potentials and reduced recruitment pattern with low-amplitude and polyphasic short-duration MUPs. Sensory NCSs are normal. Classic botulism in older children develops 12 to 36 hours after ingestion of the toxin-containing food. Early symptoms are blurred vision, diplopia, dizziness, dysarthria, and dysphagia followed by respiratory paralysis.

Diphtheria

Diphtheria is a rare disease in countries that apply systematic immunization programs. Focal neurologic complications appear 4 to 5 weeks after nasopharyngeal infection with *Corynebacterium diphtheriae*, resulting in soft palate, oculomotor, and ocular accommodation paralyses. Blurred vision and swallowing difficulties mark the onset of diphtheric neuropathy. A polyneuropathic feature mimicking GBS may appear during the subsequent weeks.[251] Segmental demyelination predominates on the posterior roots.[252] Recovery is usually complete.

Isolated Temporary Pharyngeal Paralysis

Isolated temporary pharyngeal paralysis is characterized by acute unilateral velopharyngeal paralysis provoking swallowing difficulty with nasal reflux. This rare disease is considered as idiopathic or viral neuritis of cranial nerves IX and X; a complete spontaneous recovery is usually observed after a few weeks or months.[253,254]

CNS Lesions

Rarely a velopharyngeal paralysis may be the presenting sign of a tumor of the posterior cranial fossa, Chiari malformation, bulbar poliomyelitis, or progressive bulbar paralysis. In a series of 46 patients with Chiari malformations, 15 had progressive dysphagia preceding other signs of brainstem dysfunction. All 15 had normal swallowing function before the development of dysphagic symptoms. Suboccipital craniectomy and cervical laminectomy were performed; postoperative outcome with regard to swallowing function correlated with the severity of the preoperative symptoms.[255]

Progressive Bulbar Paralysis of Childhood (Fazio-Londe Disease)

Progressive bulbar paralysis of childhood is a rare hereditary condition, with fewer than 30 children reported, including only 6 for whom an autopsy was performed.[256] The age of onset ranged from 12 months to 12 years. The most frequent presenting symptom was stridor, followed by ptosis, dysarthria, facial palsy, and dysphagia. Progressive involvement of cranial nerves and respiratory difficulties led to death in a few years. The EMG findings of reduced interference pattern with enlarged MUPs in bulbar muscles are an important diagnostic sign of the disease.

Tetanus

Salivary stasis and dysphagia associated with trismus and neck stiffness are often the first clinical manifestations of tetanus. These appear from 5 to 14 days after infection with *Clostridium tetani* introduced through an infected umbilicus in the newborn or a wound in older infants and children. The H waves are easily elicitable in distal muscles, F waves are of high amplitude, and EMG may show spontaneous high-frequency discharges.[257] Standard motor and sensory NCSs are normal. However, an EMG evaluation of 13 patients with suspected tetanus, albeit with somewhat atypical features, defined seven individuals with two findings "typical for tetanus." This was characterized by (1) spontaneous motor unit activity that could not be suppressed by voluntary activity and (2) a concomitant shortening of the silent period after a muscle stretch reflex or after electrical stimulation of the nerve. In two other patients, one of these criteria was met. Each of these 9 patients later went on to develop full-blown clinical tetanus, whereas the other 4 remained symptom free.[258] In an isolated study of single-fiber EMG, involving just one patient with cephalic tetanus, the affected frontalis muscle demonstrated increased jitter with blocking in a significant number of recorded potentials. The silent period of the masseter muscles was shortened.[259] There was no facilitation or decrement on repetitive motor nerve stimulation. An involuntary continuous firing of MUPs was also noted here. To date we are unaware of the use of stimulated single-fiber EMG in children with tetanus as has been performed with infantile botulism.

THERAPEUTIC PRINCIPLES

Facial Palsies

Birth Trauma

In birth trauma, an EMG may be helpful to determine prognosis and possible need for surgical reconstruction. The immediate issue when facial nerve palsy is present at birth is whether surgical exploration is indicated and, if so, the best time to proceed. Surgery must be avoided if it is so early that it might preclude spontaneous recovery or if there is no focal lesion for which repair is possible. In contrast, one must not fail to recognize a definitive facial nerve lesion related to a specific area of focal compression. Even if CT or MRI scans fail to define evidence of a focal cranial nerve VII lesion, surgical consideration is warranted if no signs of clinical or EMG improvement develop.

In a retrospective series,[139] surgical exploration was performed between 6 and 18 months of age in eight infants with severe CFP who had no clinical improvement. In each of them, two or three successive EMGs had demonstrated either the persistence of a major lesion of the two main facial nerve branches without any sign of recovery, or partial recovery of the cervicofacial branch but persistence of total paralysis of the temporofacial branch. In two instances the surgical investigation discovered that the facial nerve was compressed against a fracture line in the petrous temporal bone, associated in one case with chronic inflammation of the mastoid antrum. In the six other infants the facial nerve trunk was altered (pale, thin, flattened) without any obvious local cause. In another retrospective study of children with unilateral isolated CFP who had incomplete, often limited recovery by 5 years, there was no association between this poor outcome and risk factors for birth trauma to cranial nerve VII.[260]

Idiopathic Bell's Palsy

The treatment of idiopathic Bell's palsy in children remains primarily symptomatic. Protection of an exposed cornea by lubrication and eye patching during sleep is essential. In contrast to the adult population,[69,261,262] steroids and acyclovir have not improved the prognosis in children.[93,263,264] When ENOG demonstrates a 98% to 100% deficit 3 weeks after onset, there is high risk of incomplete recovery. Although surgical decompression of the facial nerve may be considered,[93,106,265] it is now performed less frequently.

However, because early detection of VZV reactivation in AFP may help in selecting patients for antiviral treatment, research is currently quite active in this field.[266] In the future, a rapid strip assay[267] in combination with the PCR method may be used to evaluate the effect of antiviral agents on the recovery of VZV reactivation-related facial palsy.

Lyme Disease

Doxycycline, 100 mg daily in children older than 8 years of age, is the treatment of choice for an isolated peripheral facial palsy. Amoxicillin, 50 to 60 mg/kg/day; penicillin, 25 to 50 mg/kg/day; or cefuroxime axetil, 20 to 30 mg/kg/day, are recommended in younger children. In case of hypersensitivity, erythromycin, 30 mg/kg/day, can be used. The duration of therapy is usually 4 weeks. In cases with disseminated infection, therapy with intravenous antibiotics is necessary for 2 to 4 weeks: ceftriaxone, 75 to 100 mg/kg/day; cefotaxime, 90 to 180 mg/kg/day; or penicillin G, 300,000 U/kg/day, in six divided doses.[114,268,269] Although prophylactic treatment is possible with two vaccines, they are not recommended in children younger than 15 years of age because the long-term safety is not certain. Both appear to be effective in 70% to 90% of adults.

Otogenic Acquired Facial Palsy

In otogenic acquired facial palsy, the prognosis is usually good if treatment is instituted early. All children with acute otitis media and facial paralysis need to be treated with intravenous antibiotics and paracentesis/surgical myringotomy.[123] Steroids may be associated to reduce inflammation. If no improvement is seen in the following days or a mastoiditis is diagnosed, a mastoidectomy may be indicated. Mastoidectomy plus decompression of the third portion of the nerve may be required for severe seromucous otitis that does not respond to paracentesis and transtympanic tubes. Cholesteatomas have to be surgically removed and require antibiotic therapy based on cultures and sensitivity testing of specimens obtained from the middle ear or mastoid. Despite surgery, a small percentage of patients with otogenic AFP may present incomplete recovery or develop synkinesias or facial hemispasm later in the course.[93]

Traumatic and Iatrogenic Injuries

The management of traumatic and iatrogenic facial nerve injuries is still controversial. Because many cases resolve spontaneously, surgical exploration is only indicated when ENOG shows greater than 90% neural degeneration and no voluntary MUPs are evident on EMG. The selection of the surgical approach is also based on radiographic findings and audiometry testing. In delayed paralysis, surgical exploration is reserved for the cases that do not show recovery after 3 weeks.[270] Postoperative paralysis requires immediate exploration not only for the psychological and forensic implications but also to achieve the best outcome. Transection requires suturing of the nerve or even placing inlay or complete interpositional grafts when end-to-end suturing is not possible.[271]

Not only in traumatic facial nerve palsy but also in AFP of other origins as well as in CFP, reconstructive surgical procedures may be performed to improve function or esthetics when deficits are fixed. For instance, eye closure may be corrected or the ability to smile enhanced by muscle transfers or microanastomosis.[272,273] Facial dyskinesia and spasms may be treated by botulinum toxin.[274]

Recurrent Facial Palsy

Surgical therapy is still controversial, and no controlled studies comparing surgical and medical interventions have been published. At this moment, it is considered in patients with recurrent facial palsies who develop residual deficits such as weakness, synkinesis, and contractures and in patients in whom the interval between episodes of palsy is decreasing.[272]

Dysphagia

Concerning both the method for maintaining a clear airway and the method of feeding, each child with dysphagia should be treated as an individual case, taking into consideration all the clinical and laboratory findings. In isolated

PRS, depending on clinical severity, therapies include nursing and postural positioning, removal of any nasopharyngeal obstruction, placement of a nasopharyngeal tube, nasogastric tube feeding, treatment of esophageal dyskinesia and gastroesophageal reflux, fitting of a palatal prosthesis, and early veloplasty.

One retrospective study demonstrated that patients with dysphagia, associated with a congenital malformation syndrome, require a higher frequency of tracheotomy and gastrostomy.[275] Once the stage of life-threatening complications has been passed, infants with PRS should be followed up closely for the first few years of life. It is important to follow the progress of feeding and growth. If gastroesophageal reflux is present, one must guard against the effects of vagal hyperreactivity. Additional parameters that need monitoring include detection and treatment of delayed speech development, monitoring of mandibular growth, and being alert to possible sleep apnea. For patients with other congenital malformation syndromes, evaluation and management of bulbar weakness are the same as described earlier for PRS.

At any age pulmonary aspiration requires respiratory physiotherapy, antibiotics, and anti-inflammatory agents. This treatment must be complemented by measures aimed at preventing recurrence of aspiration and failure to thrive, such as adaptation of feeding, dietetic review, education and stimulation of sucking and swallowing, and education of parents. The lateral decubitus position reduces the risk of aspiration of saliva. The posture must take into account any pulmonary complications and gastroesophageal reflux. If the disorder is severe and the respiratory situation precarious, oral feeding is discontinued and tube feeding becomes mandatory. Tracheotomy is indicated in cases of respiratory obstruction. Gastrostomy is sometimes necessary, in particular in major disorders persisting for several months and when associated with complicated reflux esophagitis.

During this critical period, sucking must be stimulated and maintained using a nonalimentary nipple and by tactile stimuli on the lips, gums, and tongue. This facilitates mobility, orientation, and flexibility of the tongue. It is more difficult to stimulate swallowing because each attempt may lead to aspiration. Each tube-feeding session can be preceded by oral administration of a few milliliters of water. Milk should be given only in thick form; in fact, no thin liquids should be given until recovery is complete.

Each attempt at oral feeding must be prudent and fractionated; the opening in the nipple must be sufficiently small to prevent passive flow of the meal into the oral cavity. It is often preferable to abandon use of the bottle completely, the spoon being a better tool for giving a very fractionated thick meal. To shorten the hospital stay, it is essential to ensure the early participation of the parents in this painstaking operation. Multidisciplinary care involving a pediatric nurse, speech therapist, and physiotherapist can be organized at home. Progress can be delayed by an anorexic phase, which is often seen in this clinical context, and can be due to several factors including depression due to the chronic disorder, opposition to the oral investigation, and fear of swallowing.

REFERENCES

1. Desjardins R, Guerguerian AJ, Tabchy B: [Facial paralysis in children: Study of 99 cases]. J Otolaryngol 1980;9:67-71.
2. May M, Fria TJ, Blumenthal F, et al: Facial paralysis in children: Differential diagnosis. Otolaryngol Head Neck Surg 1981;89:841-848.
3. Quijano-Roy S, Barcik U, Pascual Pascual SI, et al: Paralisis facial en la infancia: Una revision de 98 casos. Rev Neurol 1999;28:S172.
4. Grundfast KM, Guarisco JL, Thomsen JR, et al: Diverse etiologies of facial paralysis in children. Int J Pediatr Otorhinolaryngol 1990;19:223-239.
5. Jackson CG, Von Doersten PG: The facial nerve: Current trends in diagnosis, treatment, and rehabilitation. Med Clin North Am 1999;83:179-195.
6. Yetiser S, Kazkayas M, Altinok D, et al: Magnetic resonance imaging of the intratemporal facial nerve in idiopathic peripheral facial palsy. Clin Imaging 2003;27:77-81.
7. Jemec B, Grobbelaar AO, Harrison DH: The abnormal nucleus as a cause of congenital facial palsy. Arch Dis Child 2000;83:256-258.
8. Thieffry S, Job JC: [Pharyngeal deglutition disorders in infantile pathology: Clinical study, diagnosis, therapy]. Sem Hop Paris 1954;30:131-135.
9. Illingworth RS: Sucking and swallowing difficulties in infancy: Diagnostic problem of dysphagia. Arch Dis Child 1969;44:655-665.
10. Le Moing G, Raimbault J, Laget P, et al: Pneumopathies récidivantes et inhalations alimentaires liées à un déficit des structures buccopharyngées. Ann Pédiatr 1976;23:471-480.
11. Baudon JJ, Renault F, Tarhaoui L: Diagnostic et prise en charge des troubles de la déglutition chez le nouveau-né et le nourrisson de moins de 3 mois. *In* Aujard Y, Beaufils F, Chaussain JL, et al. (eds): Journées Parisiennes de Pédiatrie. Paris, Flammarion Médecine-Sciences, 1997, pp 17-22.
12. Newman LA, Cleveland RH, Blickman JG, et al: Videofluoroscopic analysis of the infant swallow. Invest Radiol 1991;26:870-872.
13. Vazquez JL, Buonomo C: Feeding difficulties in the first days of life: Findings on upper gastrointestinal series and the role of videofluoroscopic swallowing study. Pediatr Radiol 1999;29:894-896.
14. Renault F, Raimbault J: [Facial, lingual, and pharyngeal electromyography in children: A method to study sucking and swallowing disorders and their pathophysiology]. Neurophysiol Clin 1992;22:249-260.
15. Ertekin C, Pehlivan M, Aydogdu I, et al: An electrophysiological investigation of deglutition in man. Muscle Nerve 1995;18:1177-1186.
16. Ertekin C, Aydogdu I, Yüceyar N, et al: Electrodiagnostic methods for neurogenic dysphagia. Electroencephalogr Clin Neurophysiol 1998;109:331-340.
17. Courville J: The nucleus of the facial nerve: The relation between cellular groups and peripheral branches of the nerve. Brain Res 1998;1:338-354.
18. Chouard CH: Anatomie, Pathologie et Chirurgie du Nerf Facial. Paris, Masson et Cie, 1972.
19. Willer JC, Boulu B, Bratzkavski M: Electrophysiologic evidence for crossed oligosynaptic trigemino-facial connections in normal man. J Neurol Neurosurg Psychiatry 1984;47:87-90.
20. Soliven B, Meer J, Uncini A, et al: Physiologic and anatomic basis for contralateral R1 in blink reflex. Muscle Nerve 1988;11:848-851.
21. Fisch W, Esslen E: Total intratemporal exposure of the facial nerve: Pathologic findings in Bell's palsy. Arch Otolaryngol 1972;95:335-341.
22. Eicher SA, Cocker NJ, Alford BR, et al: A comparative study of the fallopian canal at the meatal foramen and labyrinthine segment in young children and adults. Arch Otolaryngol Head Neck Surg 1990;116:1030-1035.
23. Raimbault J: Les Conductions Nerveuses chez l'Enfant Normal. Paris, Expansion Scientifique Française, 1988, p 132.
24. Esslen E: Electrodiagnosis in facial palsy. *In* Miehlke A (ed): Surgery of the Facial Nerve. Philadelphia, WB Saunders, 1973, pp 45-51.
25. Shapiro NL, Cunningham MJ, Parikh SR, et al: Congenital unilateral facial paralysis. Pediatrics 1996;97:261-264.
26. Qiu WW, Shengguang S, Yin SS, et al: Neurophysiological evaluation of acute facial paralysis in children. Int J Pediatr Otorhinolaryngol 1997;39:223-236.
27. Dumitru D, Walsh NE, Porter LD: Electrophysiologic evaluation of the facial nerve in Bell's palsy: A review. Am J Phys Med Rehabil 1988;67:137-144.
28. Ghonim MR, Gavilan C: Blink reflex: Prognostic value in acute peripheral facial palsy. J Otorhinolaryngol Relat Spec 1990;52:75-79.
29. Kugelberg E: Facial reflexes. Brain 1952;75:385-396.
30. Kimura J: Alteration of the orbicularis oculi reflex by pontine lesions: Study in multiple sclerosis. Arch Neurol 1970;22:156-161.
31. Kimura J: Electrically elicited blink reflex in diagnosis of multiple sclerosis. Brain 1975;98:413-426.
32. Boulu P, Willer JC, Cambier J: [Electrophysiological study of blink reflex in man: Segmental, intersegmental, auditory and visual interactions (author's transl)]. Rev Neurol (Paris) 1981;137:523-533.
33. Kiers L, Carroll WM: Blink reflexes and magnetic resonance imaging in focal unilateral trigeminal pathway demyelination. J Neurol Neurosurg Psychiatry 1990;53:526-529.

34. Cruccu G, Deuschl G: The clinical use of brainstem reflexes and hand-muscle reflexes. Clinical Neurophysiol 2000;111:371-387.

35. Kimura J, Bodensteiner J, Yamada T: Electrically elicited blink reflex in normal neonates. Arch Neurol 1977;34:246-249.

36. Vecchierini-Blineau MF, Guiheneuc P: [Maturation of the blink reflex in infant] Eur Neurol 1984;23:449-458.

37. Kather-Boidin J, Duron B: The orbicularis oculi reflexes in healthy premature and full-term newborns. Electroencephalogr Clin Neurophysiol 1987;67:479-484.

38. Tomita Y, Schichida K, Takeshito S, et al: Maturation of blink reflex in children. Brain Dev 1989;11:389-393.

39. Ardran GM, Kemp FH, Lind J: A cineradiography of bottle feeding. Br J Radiol 1958;31:11-22.

40. Farriaux JP, Milbled G: [Physiology of deglutition: II. Suction-deglutition in the newborn infant: The nervous mechanism of deglutition] Presse Méd 1965;73:409-414.

41. Miller AJ: Deglutition. Physiol Rev 1982;62:129-184.

42. Smith WL, Erenburg A, Nowak A, et al: Physiology of sucking in the normal term infant using real-time US Radiology 1985;156:379-381.

43. Weber F, Woolridge MW, Baum JD: An ultrasonographic study of the organisation of sucking and swallowing by newborn infants. Dev Med Child Neurol 1986;28:19-24.

44. Bosma JF, Hepburn LG, Josell SD, et al: Ultrasound demonstration of tongue motions during suckle feeding. Dev Med Child Neurol 1990;32:223-229.

45. Bu'Lock F, Woolridge MW, Baum JD: Development of coordination of sucking, swallowing and breathing: Ultrasound study of term and preterm infants. Dev Med Child Neurol 1990;32:669-678.

46. Selley WG, Ellis RE, Flack FC, et al: Ultrasonographic study of sucking and swallowing by newborn infants [Letter]. Dev Med Child Neurol 1986;28:821-823.

47. Koenig JS, Davies AM, Thach BT: Coordination of breathing, sucking and swallowing during bottle feedings in human infants. J Appl Physiol 1990;69:1623-1629.

48. Thach BT: Neuromuscular control of the upper airway. In Beckerman RC, Brouillette RT, Hunt CE (eds): Respiratory Control Disorders in Infants and Children. Baltimore, Williams & Wilkins, 1992, pp 47-60.

49. Jean A: Brain stem organization of the swallowing network. Brain Behav Evol 1984;25:109-116.

50. Car A: [Cortical control of deglutition: II. Medullary impact of corticofugal swallowing pathways] J Physiol 1973;66:553-576.

51. Jean A: Control of the central swallowing program by inputs from the peripheral receptors: A review. J Autonom Nerv Syst 1984;10:225-233.

52. Bowen-Jones A, Thompson C, Drewett RF: Milk flow and sucking rates during breast feeding. Dev Med Child Neurol 1982;24:626-633.

53. Humphrey T: Function of the nervous system during prenatal life. In Stave U (ed): Perinatal Physiology. New York, Plenum, 1978, pp 651-683.

54. Hanlon MB, Tripp JH, Ellis RE, et al: Deglutition apnoeas as indicator of maturation of suckle feeding in bottle-fed preterm infants. Dev Med Child Neurol 1997;39:534-542.

55. Gewolb IH, Vice FL, Schweitzer-Kenney EL, et al: Developmental patterns of rhythmic suck and swallow in preterm infants. Dev Med Child Neurol 2001;43:22-27.

56. Gewolb IH, Bosma JF, Reynolds EW, et al: Integration of suck and swallow rhythms during feeding in preterm infants with and without bronchopulmonary dysplasia. Dev Med Child Neurol 2003;45:344-348.

57. Paulson G, Gottlieb G: Developmental reflexes: The reappearance of foetal and neonatal reflexes in aged patients. Brain 1968;91:37-52.

58. Mathew CP: Science of bottle feeding. J Pediatr 1991;119:511-519.

59. Loughlin GM, Lefton-Greif MA: Dysfunctional swallowing and respiratory disease in children. Adv Pediatr 1994;41:135-162.

60. Raimbault J, Le Moing G, Laget P: Enquête sur l'électromyographie des troubles de la déglutition chez l'enfant. Pédiatrie 1979;34:681-693.

61. Doty RW, Bosma JF: An electromyographic analysis of reflex deglutition. J Neurophysiol 1956;19:44-60.

62. Dodds WJ, Stewart ET, Logemann JA: Physiology and radiology of the normal oral and pharyngeal phases of swallowing. AJR Am J Roentgenol 1990;154:953-963.

63. Renault F: EMG during bottle feeding: A method of studying neonatal dysphagia. Muscle Nerve 1998;21:1587.

64. Renault F: EMG of the face, tongue, and pharynx in the infant: A method of studying disturbances of sucking and swallowing and studying their pathophysiology. In Improving the use of EMG in Paediatrics. London, Institute of Child Health, 1997.

65. Alberti PW, Biagioni E: Facial paralysis in children: A review of 150 cases. Laryngoscope 1972;82:1013-1020.

66. Garcin M, Magnan J, Long FX, et al: [Facial paralysis in children: Apropos of 82 cases]. J Fr Otorhinolaryngol Audiophonol Clin Maxillofac 1976;25:435-443.

67. Adour KK, Byl FM, Hilsinger RL, et al: The true nature of Bell's palsy: Analysis of 1,000 consecutive patients. Laryngoscope 1978;88:787-801.

68. Katusic SK, Beard CM, Wiederholt WC, et al: Incidence, clinical features, and prognosis in Bell's palsy, Rochester, Minnesota, 1968-1982. Ann Neurol 1986;20:622-627.

69. Adour KK, Ruboyianes JM, Von Doersten PG, et al: Bell's palsy treatment with acyclovir and prednisone compared with prednisone alone: A double-blind, randomized, controlled trial. Ann Otol Rhinol Laryngol 1996;105:371-378.

70. Keane JR: Bilateral seventh nerve palsy: Analysis of 43 cases and review of the literature. Neurology 1994;44:1198-1202.

71. English JB, Stommel EW, Bernat JL: Recurrent Bell's palsy. Neurology 1996;47:604-605.

72. Alter M: Familial aggregation of Bell's palsy. Arch Neurol 1963;8:107-114.

73. Takahashi A, Fujiwara R: Familial Bell's palsy. Clin Neurol Neurosurg 1971;11:454-461.
74. Aldrich MS, Beck RW, Albers JW: Familial recurrent Bell's palsy with ocular motor palsies. Neurology 1987;37:1369-1371.
75. Hageman G, Ippel PF, Jansen ENH, et al: Familial, alternating Bell's palsy with dominant inheritance. Eur Neurol 1990;30:310-313.
76. Adour KK, Bell DN, Hilsinger RL: Herpes simplex virus in idiopathic facial paralysis (Bell palsy). JAMA 1975;233:527-530.
77. McCormick DP: Herpes simplex virus as a cause of Bell's palsy. Lancet 1972;1:937-939.
78. Morgan M, Nathwani D: Facial palsy and infection: The unfolding history. Clin Infect Dis 1992;14:263-271.
79. Sugita T, Murakami S, Yanagihara N, et al: Facial nerve paralysis induced by herpes simplex virus in mice: An animal model of acute and transient facial paralysis. Ann Otol Rhinol Laryngol 1995;104:574-581.
80. Czornyj L, Freire C, Cisterna D, et al: Herpes virus simplex como probable factor etiologico de la paralisis facial periferica aguda idiopatica en la infancia: Estudio clinico y serologico en 169 ninos. *In* Fejerman N (ed): Neurologia Pediatrica. Buenos Aires, Ed Med Panam, 1997, pp 892-898.
81. Baringer JR: Herpes simplex virus and Bell palsy. Ann Intern Med 1996;124:63-65.
82. Schirm J, Mulkens PS: Bell's palsy and herpes simplex virus. APMIS 1997;105:815-823.
83. Mori H, Nakai Y: Bell's palsy and virus: Ten years' experience on serological examination. *In* Portmann (ed): Proceedings of the Fifth International Symposium on Facial Nerve. New York, Masson, 1984, pp 230-233.
84. Murr AH, Benecke JE: Association of facial paralysis with HIV positivity. Am J Otol 1991;12:450-451.
85. Manning JJ, Adour KK: Facial paralysis in children. Pediatrics 1972;49:102-109.
86. Jonsson L, Tien R, Engstrom M, et al: Gd-DPTA enhanced MRI in Bell's palsy and herpes zoster oticus: An overview and implications for future studies. Acta Otolaryngol 1995;115:577-584.
87. Hasuike K, Sekitani T, Imate Y: Enhanced-MRI in patients with vestibular neuronitis. Acta Otolaryngol 1995;S519:272-274.
88. Alford BR, Jerger JF, Coats AC, et al: Diagnostic tests of facial nerve function. Otolaryngol Clin North Am 1974;7:331-342.
89. Gavilan J, Gavilan C: Prognostic value of electroneurography in Bell's palsy. Eur Arch Otorhinolaryngol 1994;Dec:S57-S59.
90. Hill MD, Midroni G, Goldstein WC, et al: The spectrum of electrophysiological abnormalities in Bell's palsy. Can J Neurol Sci 2001;28:130-133.
91. Pettersen E: Natural history of Bell's palsy. *In* Graham MD, House WF (eds): Disorders of the Facial Nerve. New York, Raven Press, 1982.
92. Devriese PP: Bell's palsy in children. Acta Otorhinolaryngol Belg 1984;38:261-267.
93. Truy E, Granade G, Bensoussan J, et al: Les paralysies faciales périphériques acquises de l'enfant. Données actuelles illustrées par 66 observations personnelles récentes. Pédiatrie 1992;47:481-486.
94. Gilchrist JM, Sachs GM: Electrodiagnostic studies in the management and prognosis of neuromuscular disorders. Muscle Nerve 2004;29:165-190.
95. Guieu J, Hurtevent JF, Sandler A, et al: [Contribution of early electromyography in the prognostic assessment of facial paralysis]. Rev Laryngol Otol Rhinol (Bord) 1991;112:445-447.
96. Sittel C, Stennert E: Prognostic value of electromyography in acute peripheral facial nerve palsy. Otol Neurotol 2001;22:100-104.
97. Kimura J, Giron LT, Young SM: Electrophysiological study of Bell palsy: Electrically elicited blink reflex in assessment of prognosis. Arch Otolaryngol 1976;102:140-143.
98. Campistol Plana J, Colomer Oferil J: Application of the trigemino-facial reflex in acquired peripheral facial paralysis in childhood. An Otorrinolaringol Ibero Am 1989;16:45-56.
99. Montalt J, Barona R, Armengot M, et al: The blink reflex in the electrophysiologic exploration of Bell's palsy and its prognostic value. An Otorrinolaringol Ibero Am 1999;26:401-412.
100. Aminoff MJ: Facial neuropathies. *In* Aminoff MJ (ed): Electromyography in Clinical Practice: Clinical and Electrodiagnostic Aspects of Neuromuscular Disease. New York, Churchill Livingstone, 1998, pp 513-523.
101. Danielides V, Skevas A, Kastanioudakis I, et al: Comparative study of evoked electromyography and facial nerve latency test in the prognosis of idiopathic facial nerve palsy in childhood. Childs Nerv Syst 1994;10:122-125.
102. Wong V: Outcome of facial nerve palsy in 24 children. Brain Dev 1995;17:294-296.
103. Bouhanna S, Hagen P, Chabert R, et al: Prognostic value of electroneuronography and trigemino-facial reflex in Bell's palsy. Rev Laryngol Otol Rhinol (Bord) 1996;117:353-356.
104. Eavey RD, Herrmann BS, Joseph JM, et al: Clinical experience with electroneuronography in the pediatric patients. Arch Otolaryngol Head Neck Surg 1989;115:600-607.
105. Jenkins HA, Herzog JA, Coker NJ: Bell's palsy in children: Cases of progressive facial nerve degeneration. Ann Otol Rhinol Laryngol 1985;94:331-336.
106. Esslen E: The Acute Facial Palsies. New York, Springer-Verlag, 1977.
107. Baba K, Yabuuchi H, Takahashi M, et al: Increased incidence of herpes zoster in normal children infected with varicella zoster virus during infancy. J Pediatr 1986;108:372-377.
108. Hato N, Kisaki H, Honda N, et al: Ramsay Hunt syndrome in children. Ann Neurol 2000;48:254-256.

109. Kanzaki J: Electrodiagnostic findings in the early stages of Bell's palsy and Ramsay-Hunt syndrome. Acta Otolaryngol Suppl 1988;446:42-46.

110. Kuo MJ, Drago PC, Proops DW, et al: Early diagnosis and treatment of Ramsay Hunt syndrome: The role of magnetic resonance imaging. J Laryngol Otol 1995;109:777-780.

111. Pachner AR, Steere AC: The triad of neurological manifestations of Lyme disease: Meningitis, cranial neuritis, and radiculoneuritis. Neurology 1985;35:47-53.

112. Halperin J, Luft BJ, Volkman DJ, et al: Lyme neuroborreliosis: Peripheral nervous system manifestations. Brain 1990;113:1207-1221.

113. Belman AL, Iyer M, Coyle PK, et al: Neurologic manifestations in children with North American Lyme disease. Neurology 1993;43:2609-2614.

114. Cook SP, Macartney KK, Rose CD, et al: Lyme disease and seventh nerve paralysis in children. Am J Otolaryngol 1997;18:320-323.

115. Ruel M, Arzouni JP, Raoult D, et al: Lack of association of Bell's palsy and *Borrelia burgdorferi* antibodies. Arch Intern Med 1993;153:1725-1726.

116. Raucher HS, Kaufman DM, Goldfarb J, et al: Pseudotumor cerebri and Lyme disease: A new association. J Pediatr 1985;107:931-933.

117. Steere AC: Lyme disease. N Engl J Med 1989;321:586-596.

118. Craft JE, Grodzicki RL, Steere AC: Lyme disease: Evaluation of diagnostic tests. J Infect Dis 1984;149:789-795.

119. Albisetti M, Schaer G, Good M, et al: Diagnostic value of cerebrospinal fluid examination in children with peripheral facial palsy and suspected Lyme borreliosis. Neurology 1997;49:817-824.

120. Belman AL, Reynolds L, Preston T, et al: Cerebrospinal fluid findings in children with Lyme disease-associated facial nerve palsy. Arch Pediatr Adolesc Med 1997;151:1224-1228.

121. Angerer M, Pfadenhauer K, Stohr M: Prognosis of facial palsy in *Borrelia burgdorferi* meningopolyradiculoneuritis. J Neurol 1993;240:319-321.

122. Belman AL, Coyle PK, Roque C, et al: MRI findings in children infected by *Borrelia burgdorferi*. Pediatr Neurol 1992;8:428-431.

123. Pollac R, Brown L: Facial paralysis in otitis media. *In* Graham M , House W (eds): Disorders of the Facial Nerve: Anatomy, Diagnosis, and Management. New York, Raven Press, 1982, p 221.

124. Boddie HG: Recurrent Bell's palsy. J Laryngol Otol 1972;86:117-120.

125. Pitts DB, Adour KK, Hilsinger RL: Recurrent Bell's palsy: Analysis of 140 patients. Laryngoscope 1988;98:535-540.

126. Eidlitz-Markus T, Gilai A, Mimouni M, et al: Recurrent facial nerve palsy in paediatric patients. Eur J Pediatr 2001;160:659-663.

127. Wadlington WB, Riley HD, Lowbeer L: The Melkersson-Rosenthal syndrome. Pediatrics 1984;73:502-506.

128. Zimmer WM, Rogers RS, Reeve CM, et al: Orofacial manifestations of Melkersson-Rosenthal syndrome: A study of 42 patients and review of 220 cases from the literature. Oral Surg Oral Med Oral Pathol 1992;75:610-619.

129. Graham MD, Kemink JL: Total facial nerve decompression in recurrent facial paralysis and the Melkersson-Rosenthal syndrome: A preliminary report. Am J Otol 1986;7:34-37.

130. Poloni TE, Merlo IM, Alfonsi E, et al: Facial nerve is liable to pressure palsy. Neurology 1998;51:320-322.

131. Pareyson D, Taroni F: Deletion of the PMP22 gene and hereditary neuropathy with liability to pressure palsies. Curr Opin Neurol 1996;9:348-354.

132. Najim Al-Din AS, Anderson M, Eeg-Olofsson O: Neuro-ophthalmic manifestations of the syndrome of ophthalmoplegia, ataxia, and areflexia: Observations on 20 patients. Acta Neurol Scand 1994;89:87-94.

133. Kimura M, Nakagawa I, Niinai H, et al: Evaluation with blink reflex of bilateral facial palsy. Masui 2000;49:159-162.

134. Polo A, Manganotti P, Zanette G, et al: Polyneuritis cranialis: Clinical and electrophysiological findings. J Neurol Neurosurg Psychiatry 1992;55:398-400.

135. Sauron B, Bouche P, Cathala HP, et al: Miller Fisher syndrome: Clinical and electrophysiological evidence of peripheral origin in 10 cases. Neurology 1984;34:953-956.

136. Fross RD, Daube JR: Neuropathy in the Miller Fisher syndrome: Clinical and neurophysiological findings. Neurology 1987;37:1493-1498.

137. Ter Bruggen JP, Van der Meche FGA, De Jager AEJ, et al: Ophthalmoplegic and lower cranial nerve variants merge into each other and into classical Guillain-Barré syndrome. Muscle Nerve 1998;21:239-242.

138. Falco NA, Eriksson E: Facial nerve palsy in the newborn: Incidence and outcome. Plast Reconstr Surg 1990;85:1-4.

139. Renault F, Garabedian EN, Harpey JP: Diagnostic des paralysies et asymétries faciales congénitales. *In* Arthuis M, Beaufils F, Caille B (eds): Journées Parisiennes de Pédiatrie. Paris, Flammarion Médecine-Sciences, 1993, pp 155-161.

140. Hepner WR: Some observations on facial paresis in the newborn infant: Etiology and incidence. Pediatrics 1951;8:494-499.

141. Mancias P, Slopis JM, Yeakley JW, et al: Combined brachial plexus injury and root avulsion after complicated delivery. Muscle Nerve 1994;17:1237-1238.

142. Jones HR, Herbison GJ, Jacobs SR, et al: Intrauterine onset of a mononeuropathy: Peroneal neuropathy in a newborn with electromyographic findings at age one day compatible with prenatal onset. Muscle Nerve 1996;19:88-91.

143. McHugh HE, Sowaen KA, Levitt MN: Facial paralysis and muscle agenesis in the newborn. Arch Otolaryngol 1969;89:131-143.

144. Nelson KB, Eng GD: Congenital hypoplasia of the depressor anguli oris muscle: Differentiation from congenital facial palsy. J Pediatr 1972;81:16-20.

145. Hoefnagel D, Penry JK: Partial facial paralysis in young children. N Engl J Med 1960;262:1126-1128.

146. Duchenne de Boulogne GB: De l'Electrisation Localisée et son Application à la Pathologie et à la Thérapeutique. 2ème ed. Paris, JB Baillère et Fils, 1861.

147. Sammarco J, Ryan RF, Longenecker CG: Anatomy of the facial nerve in fetuses and stillborn infants. J Plast Reconst Surg 1966;37:556-574.

148. Cayler GG: An "epidemic" of congenital facial paresis and heart disease. Pediatrics 1967;40:666.

149. Cayler GG, Blumenfeld CM, Anderson RL: Further studies of patients with the cardiofacial syndrome. Chest 1971;60:161-165.

150. Pape KE, Pickering D: Asymmetric crying facies: An index of other congenital anomalies. J Pediatr 1972;81:21-30.

151. Perlman M, Reisner SH: Asymmetric crying facies and congenital anomalies. Arch Dis Child 1973;48:627-629.

152. Alexiou D, Manolidis C, Papaevangellou G, et al: Frequency of other malformations in congenital hypoplasia of depressor anguli oris muscle syndrome. Arch Dis Child 1976;51:891-893.

153. Giannotti A, Digilio MC, Marino B, et al: Cayler cardiofacial syndrome and del 22q11: Part of the CATCH22 phenotype. Am J Med Genet 1994;53:303-304.

154. Stewart HS, Smith JC: Two patients with asymmetric crying facies, normal cardiovascular systems, and deletion of chromosome 22q11. Clin Dysmorphol 1997;6:165-169.

155. Orobello P: Congenital and acquired facial nerve paralysis in children. Otolaryngol Clin North Am 1991;24:647-652.

156. Carvalho GJ, Song CS, Vargervik K, et al: Auditory and facial nerve dysfunction in patients with hemifacial microsomia. Arch Otolaryngol Head Neck Surg 1999;125:209-212.

157. Byerly KA, Pauli RM: Cranial nerve abnormalities in CHARGE association. Am J Med Genet 1993;45:751-757.

158. Davenport SHL, Hefner MA, Mitchell JA: The spectrum of clinical features in CHARGE syndrome. Clin Genet 1986;29:298-310.

159. Roger G, Morisseau-Durand MP, Van Den Abbeele T, et al: The CHARGE association: The role of tracheotomy. Arch Otolaryngol Head Neck Surg 1999;125:33-38.

160. Jones KL: First and second branchial arch syndrome. *In* Jones KL (ed): Smith's Recognizable Patterns of Human Malformation. Philadelphia, WB Saunders, 1997, pp 642-645.

161. Jones KL: Treacher Collins syndrome. *In* Jones KL (ed): Smith's Recognizable Patterns of Human Malformation. Philadelphia, WB Saunders, 1997, pp 250-251.

162. Couly G, Aicardi J: [Associated morphological anomalies of the face and brain infants]. Arch Fr Pediatr 1988;45:99-104.

163. Mezenes M, Coker SB: CHARGE and Joubert syndromes: Are they a single disorder? Pediatr Neurol 1990;6:428-430.

164. Sudarshan A, Goldie WD: The spectrum of congenital facial diplegia (Moebius syndrome). Pediatr Neurol 1985;1:180-184.

165. Miller MT, Stromland K: The Mobius sequence: A relook. JAAPOS 1999;3:199-208.

166. Meyerson MD, Foushee DR. Speech, language and hearing in Moebius syndrome. Dev Med Child Neurol 1978;20:357-365.

167. Verzijl HT, Van den Helm B, Veldman B, et al: A second gene for autosomal dominant Möbius syndrome is localized to chromosome 10q, in a Dutch family. Am J Hum Genet 1999;65:752-756.

168. Baraitser M, Rudge P: Moebius syndrome, and axonal neuropathy and hypogonadism. Clin Dysmorphol 1996;5:351-355.

169. Towfighi J, Marks K, Palmer E, et al: Möbius syndrome: Neuropathologic observations. Acta Neuropathol 1979;48:11-17.

170. Jaradeh S, D'Cruz ON, Howard JF, et al: Möbius syndrome: Electrophysiologic studies in seven cases. Muscle Nerve 1996;19:1148-1153.

171. Govaert P, Vanhaesebrouck P, De Praeter C, et al: Moebius sequence and prenatal brain stem ischemia. Pediatrics 1989;84:570-573.

172. Renault F: Cranial nerve studies in 22 children with Möbius syndrome. Muscle Nerve 2000;23:1631.

173. Roig M, Gratacos M, Vazquez E, et al: Brainstem dysgenesis: Report of five patients with congenital hypotonia, multiple cranial nerve involvement, and ocular motor apraxia. Dev Med Child Neurol 2003;45:489-493.

174. Nevin NC, Burrow SD, Allen G, et al: Aglossia-adactylia syndrome. J Med Genet 1975;12:89-93.

175. Chicarilli ZN, Polayes IM: Oromandibular limb hypogenesis syndromes. Plast Reconstr Surg 1985;76:13-24.

176. Jones KL: Hypoglossia-hypodactyly syndrome. *In* Jones KL (ed): Smith's Recognizable Patterns of Human Malformation. Philadelphia, WB Saunders, 1997, pp 646-648.

177. Aicardi J: Disorders of the peripheral nerves. *In* Aicardi J (ed): Diseases of the Nervous System in Childhood. London, Mac Keith Press, 1992, pp 1113-1171.

178. Greenberg SJ, Kandt RS, D'Souza BJ: Birth injury-induced glossolaryngeal paresis. Neurology 1987;37:533-535.

179. Haenggeli CA, Lacourt G: Brachial plexus injury and hypoglossal paralysis. Pediatr Neurol 1989;5:197-198.

180. Sieben RL, Ben Hamida M, Shulman K: Multiple cranial nerve deficits associated with the Arnold-Chiari malformation. Neurology 1971;21:673-681.

181. Gerard CL, Dugas M, Narcy P, et al: Chiari malformation type I in a child with velopharyngeal insufficiency. Dev Med Child Neurol 1992;34:174-176.

182. Linder A, Lindholm CE: Laryngologic management of infants with the Chiari II syndrome. Int J Pediatr Otorhinolaryngol 1997;39:187-197.

183. Worster-Drought C: Congenital suprabulbar paresis. J Laryngol 1956;70:453-462.

184. Sullivan PB, Rosenbloom L: The causes of feeding difficulties in disabled children. *In* Sullivan PB, Rosenbloom L (eds): Feeding the Disabled Child. London, Mac Keith Press, 1996, pp 23-32.

185. Reilly S, Skuse D, Poblete X: Prevalence of feeding problems and oral motor dysfunction in children with cerebral palsy: A community survey. J Paediatr 1996;129:877-880.

186. Rogers B, Arvedson J, Buck G, et al: Characteristics of dysphagia in children with cerebral palsy. Dysphagia 1994;9:69-73.

187. Graff-Radford NR, Bosch EP, Stears JC, et al: Developmental Foix-Chavany-Marie syndrome in identical twins. Ann Neurol 1986;20:632-635.

188. Christen HJ, Hanefeld F, Kruse E, et al: Foix-Chavany-Marie (anterior operculum) syndrome in childhood: A reappraisal of Worster-Drought syndrome. Dev Med Child Neurol 2000;42:122-132.

189. Dubowitz V: The floppy infant. Clin Dev Med 1980;2:158.

190. Renault F, Couvreur J: [Congenital deglutition disorder revealing cerebral stem disorders: Twelve cases with neurophysiological study]. Arch Fr Pediatr 1992;49:511-517.

191. Leech RW, Alvord EC: Anoxic-ischemic encephalopathy in the human neonatal period: The significance of brain stem involvement. Arch Neurol 1977;34:109-113.

192. Arvold EC, Shaw CM: Congenital difficulties with swallowing and breathing associated with maternal polyhydramnios: Neurocristopathy or medullary infarction? J Child Neurol 1989;4:299-306.

193. Wilson ER, Mirra SS, Schwartz JF: Congenital diencephalic and brain stem damage: Neuropathologic study of three cases. Acta Neuropathol 1982;57:70-74.

194. Blazer S, Hemli JA, Sujov PO, et al: Neonatal bilateral diaphragmatic paralysis caused by brain stem haemorrhage. Arch Dis Child 1989;64:50-52.

195. Govaert P: Cranial haemorrhage in the term newborn infant. Clin Dev Med 1993;129, 223.

196. Robin P: La chute de la langue considérée comme une nouvelle cause de gêne dans la respiration nasopharyngienne. Bull Acad Med Paris 1923;89:38-41.

197. Robin P: A fall of the base of the tongue considered as a new cause of nasopharyngeal respiratory impairment: Pierre Robin sequence, a translation. 1923. Plast Reconstr Surg 1994;93:1301-1303.

198. Cozzi F, Pierro A: Glossoptosis-apnea syndrome in infancy. Pediatrics 1985;75:836-843.

199. Bull MJ, Givan DC, Sadove AM, et al: Improved outcome in Pierre Robin sequence: Effect of multidisciplinary evaluation and management. Pediatrics 1990;86:294-301.

200. Caouette-Laberge L, Bayet B, Larocque Y: The Pierre Robin sequence: Review of 125 cases and evolution of treatment modalities. Plast Reconstr Surg 1994;93:934-942.

201. Renault F, Flores-Guevara R, Soupre V, et al: Neurophysiological brain stem investigations in isolated Pierre Robin sequence. Early Hum Dev 2000;58:141-152.

202. Baudon JJ, Renault F, Goutet JM, et al: Motor dysfunction of the upper digestive tract in Pierre Robin sequence as assessed by sucking-swallowing electromyography and esophageal manometry. J Pediatr 2002;140:719-723.

203. Veau V: Division Palatine. Paris, Masson, 1931.

204. Vanwijck R, Lengelé B, Bayet B: La langue dans la séquence de Pierre Robin. *In* Devauchelle B (ed): Langue et dysmorphie. Paris, Masson, 1996, pp 131-145.

205. Delaire J, Verdon P, Tulasne JF: [Influence of the soft palate on tongue statics and mandibular growth: Therapeutic conclusions]. Rev Stomatol 1976;77:821-834.

206. Pashayan MM, Lewis MB: Clinical experience with the Robin sequence. Cleft Palate J 1984;21:270-276.

207. Cohen MMJ: The Robin anomalad: Its nonspecificity, and associated syndromes. J Oral Surg 1976;34:587-593.

208. Cohen MMJ: Syndromology's message for craniofacial biology. J Maxillofac Surg 1979;7:89-109.

209. Sheffield LJ, Reiss JA, Strohm K, et al: A genetic follow-up study of 64 patients with the Pierre Robin complex. Am J Med Genet 1987;28:64-71.

210. Elliott MA, Studen-Pavlovich DA, Ranalli DN: Prevalence of selected pediatric conditions in children with Pierre Robin sequence. Pediatr Dent 1995;17:106-111.

211. Handzic-Cuk J, Cuk V, Risavi R, et al: Pierre Robin syndrome: Characteristics of hearing loss, effect of age on hearing level, and possibilities in therapy planning. J Laryngol Otol 1996;110:830-835.

212. Medard C, François M, Narcy P: Hearing status of Robin sequence patients. Ann Otolaryngol Chir Cervicofac 1999;116:317-321.

213. Opitz JM: G Syndrome: Perspective in 1987 and bibliography. Am J Med Genet 1987;28:275-285.

214. Quaderi NA, Schweiger S, Gaudenz K, et al: Opitz G/BBB syndrome, a defect of midline development, is due to mutations in a new RING finger gene on Xp22. Nat Genet 1997;17:285-291.

215. Bershof JF, Guyuron B, Olsen MM: G syndrome: A review of the literature and a case report. J Craniomaxillofac Surg 1992;20:24-27.

216. Renault F, Couvreur J, Ostré C, et al: [Recurrent bronchopneumopathies in the infant due to swallowing dyspraxia: Two cases]. Ann Pédiatr 1992;39:347-350.

217. Mbonda E, Claus D, Bonnier C, et al: Prolonged dysphagia caused by congenital pharyngeal dysfunction. J Pediatr 1995;126:923-927.

218. Inder TE, Volpe JJ: Recovery of congenital isolated pharyngeal dysfunction: Implications for early management. Pediatr Neurol 1998;19:222-224.

219. Harper CM: Congenital myopathies and muscular dystrophies. *In* Brown WF, Bolton CF, Aminoff MJ (eds): Neuromuscular Function and Disease. Philadelphia, WB Saunders, 2002, pp 1355-1374.

220. Renault F, Fedida A: [Early electromyographic signs in congenital myotonic dystrophy: A study of ten cases]. Neurophysiol Clin 1991;21:201-211.

221. Kuntz NL, Daube JR: Electrophysiology of congenital myotonic dystrophy. *In* Electrodiagnosis. AAEE Course E. Rochester, MN, American Association of Electrodiagnostic Medicine, 1984, p 23.

222. Quijano-Roy S, Renault F, Romero N, et al: EMG and nerve conduction studies in children with congenital muscular dystrophy. Muscle Nerve 2004;29:292-299.

223. Pascual-Pascual SI: Usefulness of neurophysiological techniques in the diagnosis of metabolic disorders. Rev Neurol (Madrid) 1999;28:24-32.

224. Aicardi J, Conti D, Goutières F: [Neonatal forms of Steinert's myotonic dystrophy]. J Neurol Sci 1974;22:149-164.

225. Philpot J, Bagnall A, King C, et al: Feeding problems in merosin-deficient congenital muscular dystrophy. Arch Dis Child 1999;80:542-547.

226. Wallgren-Pettersson C, Sainio K, Salmi T: Electromyography in congenital nemaline myopathy. Muscle Nerve 1989;12:587-593.

227. Barth PG: Pontocerebellar hypoplasia: An overview of a group of inherited neurodegenerative disorders with fetal onset. Brain Dev 1993;15:411-422.

228. Hanson PA, Rowland LP: Möbius syndrome and facioscapulohumeral muscular dystrophy. Arch Neurol 1971;24:31-39.

229. Bailey RO, Marzulo DC, Harris MB: Infantile facioscapulohumeral muscular dystrophy: New observations. Acta Neurol Scand 1986;74:51-58.

230. Yasukohchi S, Yagi Y, Akabane T, et al: Facioscapulohumeral dystrophy associated with sensorineural hearing loss, tortuosity of retinal arterioles, and an early onset and rapid progression of respiratory failure. Brain Dev 1988;10:319-324.

231. Korf BR, Bresnan MJ, Shapiro F, et al: Facioscapulohumeral dystrophy presenting in infancy with facial diplegia and sensorineural deafness. Ann Neurol 1985;17:513-516.

232. Engel AG: Congenital myasthenic syndromes. Neurol Clin 1994;12:401-437.

233. Harper CM: Neuromuscular transmission disorders in childhood. *In* Jones RH, Bolton CF, Harper CM (eds): Pediatric Clinical Electromyography. Philadelphia, Lippincott-Raven, 1996, pp 353-385.

234. Engel AG, Ohno K, Sine SM: Congenital myasthenic syndromes: Progress over the past decade. Muscle Nerve 2003;27:4-25.

235. Dinger J, Prager B: Arthrogryposis multiplex in a newborn of a myasthenic mother—case report and literature. Neuromuscul Disord 1993;3:335-339.

236. Barnes PR, Kanabar DJ, Brueton L: Recurrent congenital arthrogryposis leading to a diagnosis of myasthenia gravis in an initially asymptomatic mother. Neuromuscul Disord 1995;5:59-65.

237. Wiles CM: Neurogenic dysphagia. J Neurol Neurosurg Psychiatry 1991;54:1037-1039.

238. Schurr MJ, Ebner KA, Maser AL, et al: Formal swallowing evaluation and therapy after traumatic brain injury improves dysphagia outcomes. J Trauma 1999;46:817-821.

239. Kirshblum S, Johnston MV, Brown J, et al: Predictors of dysphagia after spinal cord injury. Arch Phys Med Rehabil 1999;80:1101-1105.

240. Fejerman N, Di Blasi AM: Status epilepticus of benign partial epilepsies in children: Report of two cases. Epilepsia 1987;28:351-355.

241. Deonna TW, Roulet E, Fontan D: Speech and oromotor deficits of epileptic origin in benign partial epilepsy of childhood with rolandic spikes. Neuropediatrics 1993;24:83-87.

242. Nowak TW, Ionasescu V, Anuras S: Gastrointestinal manifestations of the muscular dystrophy. Gastroenterology 1982;82:600-610.

243. Munnich A, Rotig A, Chretien D, et al: Clinical presentation of mitochondrial disorders in childhood. J Inherit Metab Dis 1996;19:521-527.

244. Grob D, Asura EL, Brunner NG: The course of myasthenia gravis and therapy affecting outcome. Ann N Y Acad Sci 1987;505:472-499.

245. Lacomis D, Kupsky WP, Kuban KK, et al: Childhood-onset oculopharyngeal muscular dystrophy. Pediatr Neurol 1991;7:382-384.

246. Amato AA, Jackson CE, Ridings LW, et al: Childhood-onset oculopharyngodistal myopathy with chronic intestinal pseudo-obstruction. Muscle Nerve 1995;18:842-847.

247. Thompson JA, Glasgow LA, Warpinski JR, et al: Infantile botulism: Clinical spectrum and epidemiology. Pediatrics 1980;66:936-942.

248. Schreiner MS, Field E, Ruddy R: Infantile botulism: A review of 12 years' experience at the Children's Hospital of Philadelphia. Pediatrics 1991;87:159-165.

249. Cornblath DR, Sladky JT, Summer AJ: Clinical electrophysiology of infantile botulism. Muscle Nerve 1983;6:448-452.

250. Chaudry V, Crawford TO: Stimulation single-fiber EMG in infant botulism. Muscle Nerve 1999;22:1698-1703.

251. Kurdi A, Abdul-Kader M: Clinical and electrophysiological studies in diphtheric neuritis in Jordan. J Neurol Sci 1979;42:243-250.

252. Solders G, Nennesmo I, Persson A: Diphteritic neuropathy: An analysis based on muscle and nerve biopsy and repeated neurophysiological and autonomic function tests. J Neurol Neurosurg Psychiatry 1989;52:876-880.

253. Aubergé C, Ponsot G, Gayraud P, et al: [Acquired isolated velopalatine hemiparalysis in children]. Arch Fr Pédiatr 1979;36:283-286.

254. Roberton DM, Mellor DH: Asymmetrical palatal paresis in childhood: A transient cranial mononeuropathy? Dev Med Child Neurol 1982;24:842-849.

255. Pollack IF, Pang D, Kocoshis S, et al: Neurogenic dysphagia resulting from Chiari malformations. Neurosurgery 1992;30:709-719.

256. McShane MA, Boyd S, Harding B, et al: Progressive bulbar paralysis of childhood: A reappraisal of Fazio-Londe disease. Brain 1992;115:1889-1900.

257. Khuralbet AJ, Neubauer D: A case of neonatal tetanus with characteristic neurophysiological findings. Muscle Nerve 1998;21:971-972.

258. Steinegger T, Wiederkelu M, Ludin HP, et al: Electromyography as a diagnostic aid in tetanus. Schweiz Med Wochenschr 1996;126:379-385.

259. Fernandez JM, Ferrandiz M, Larrea L, et al: Cephalic tetanus studied with single-fibre EMG. J Neurol Neurosurg Psychiatry 1983;46:862-866.

260. Laing JH, Harrison DH, Jones BM, et al: Is permanent congenital facial palsy caused by birth trauma? Arch Dis Child 1996;74:56-58.

261. Austin JR, Peskind SP, Austin SG, et al: Idiopathic facial nerve paralysis: A randomized double-blind controlled study of placebo versus prednisone. Laryngoscope 1993;103:1326-1333.

262. De Diego JI, Prim MP, De Sarria MJ, et al: Idiopathic facial paralysis: A randomized, prospective, and controlled study using single-dose prednisone versus acyclovir three times daily. Laryngoscope 1998;108:573-575.

263. Prescott CA: Idiopathic facial nerve palsy in children and the effect of treatment with steroids. Int J Pediatr Otolaryngol 1987;13:257-264.

264. Unuvar E, Oguz F, Sidal M, et al: Corticosteroid treatment of childhood Bell's palsy. Pediatr Neurol 1999;21:814-816.

265. Gantz BJ, Rubinstein JT, Gidley P, et al: Surgical management of Bell's palsy. Laryngoscope 1999;109:1177-1188.

266. Murakami S, Honda N, Mizobuchi M, et al: Rapid diagnosis of varicella zoster virus infection in acute facial palsy. Neurology 1998;51:1202-1205.

267. Ohtani F, Furuta Y, Horal P, et al: Rapid strip assay for detection of anti-herpes simplex virus antibodies: Application to prediction of varicella-zoster virus reactivation in patients with acute peripheral facial palsy. J Med Virol 2000;62:37-41.

268. Sigal LH: Current recommendations for the treatment of Lyme disease. Drugs 1992;43:683-699.

269. Eppes SC, Childs JA: Comparative study of cefuroxime axetil versus amoxicillin in children with early Lyme disease. Pediatrics 2002;109:1173-1177.

270. Cotin G, Garabedian EN, Paquelin F, et al: Acquired facial paralysis in children: Our experience apropos of 72 cases. Ann Otolaryngol Chir Cervicofac 1983;100:275-279.

271. Bauer CA, Coker NJ: Update on facial nerve disorders. Otolaryngol Clin North Am 1996;29:445-454.

272. Labbé D, Huault M: Lengthening temporalis myoplasty and lip reanimation. Plast Reconstr Surg 2000;105:1289-1297.

273. Zuker RM, Goldberg CS, Manktelow RT: Facial animation in children with Möbius syndrome after segmental gracilis muscle transplant. Plast Reconstr Surg 2000;106:1-8.

274. Angibaud G, Moreau MS, Rascol O, et al: Treatment of hemifacial spasm with botulinum toxin: Value of preinjection electromyography abnormalities for predicting postinjection lower facial paresis. Eur Neurol 1995;35:43-45.

275. Cruz MJ, Kerschner JE, Beste DJ, et al: Pierre Robin sequences: Secondary respiratory difficulties and intrinsic feeding abnormalities. Laryngoscope 1999;109:1632-1636.

30

Spinal Muscular Atrophies and Other Disorders of the Anterior Horn Cell

Thomas O. Crawford

Spinal muscular atrophy (SMA) is both the name of a specific disorder and the descriptive title for a category of disorders. The specific disorder, caused by mutation of the survival motor neuron gene (*SMN*),[1] is frequently also referred to with some combination of the descriptive labels *hereditary*, *childhood*, or *proximal* with SMA. Used as a broad categorical label, the SMA syndromes encompass a range of well to poorly defined disorders that have in common a symmetric clinical expression of weakness, the (probable) concentration of pathology within the motor neuron, and proven or probable heritable etiology.

SMN-ASSOCIATED SPINAL MUSCULAR ATROPHY

Clinical Features

In the past *SMN*-associated SMA was known by several different, more specific, labels that are now grouped together. That *Werdnig-Hoffmann disease*, *intermediate childhood SMA*, and *Kugelberg-Welander disease* describe portions of the range of a single disorder was established in the 1990s with the identification a single responsible gene, *SMN*.[1] These historic labels are now known by the categoric designations *SMA-1*, *SMA-2*, and *SMA-3*. The defining features that distinguish them are arbitrary and sometimes difficult to apply in specific single cases, but the use of these categoric descriptors as a ranking of severity continues to be of benefit for clinical care and prognosis.

SMA-1 describes those infants who are unable to maintain a sitting position when placed at any time in their course, and SMA-2 refers to those children who are unable to stand and take an independent step at any time during their development. By default, those with SMA-3 are those who have been able to walk independently for at least a short distance at some time in the course of their development. Those with SMA-1 generally first manifest weakness before 6 months of age, and those with SMA-2 in the first year. Because the age of first recognition of weakness depends on a number of medical and social factors, however, differentiation of the type of SMA by the age of onset criteria alone is the least reliable.

No matter the type, the clinical course of SMA is atypical for a neurodegenerative disease. In general, the greatest rate of decline, or departure from an advancing course associated with normal development, is at the outset, and with the passage of time the rate of degeneration slows. After the initial expression of weakness, measured muscle power can sometimes remain unchanged for decades.[2-6] Across the spectrum of the disorder, the sine qua non of SMA is symmetric weakness due to denervation. In general there is a broad caudal-to-cranial distribution of this weakness, so that legs are more affected than arms, and the limb and trunk muscles are relatively weaker than are the diaphragm, face, and bulbar muscles.[7]

The name *SMA* derives from the prominent muscle atrophy that results from abnormality within the spinal cord, that is, denervation atrophy that arises from a diminished number of functioning motor neurons. In some instances expansion of the remaining surviving motor units' territories by collateral reinnervation is evident clinically. Children with SMA-2 often manifest a fine distal tremor in outstretched fingers, termed *minipolymyoclonus*, that is caused by the coarsened baseline of contraction force that results from tonic firing of motor units that are fewer in number but larger in size.[8] Enlargement of voluntary motor units is also seen in the coarse background of routine electrocardiographic tracings.[9] Infants with severe SMA may manifest trembling of the tongue, mistakenly called *fasciculations*, that results from the diminished number of motor units. Across the range of SMA types, denervation leads to diffuse skeletal muscle weakness and atrophy. Creatin kinase values may be mildly elevated across the spectrum of disease but are most often elevated in those with milder forms.[10]

Infants with the severe SMA-1 often adopt a characteristic "frog-leg" posture while recumbent (Fig. 30-1). In the lower extremities there is often only feeble movement of the toes and ankles. The shoulders are nearly flail, while the elbow is often just strong enough to be flexed against gravity to bring the hands up to the face. The diaphragm

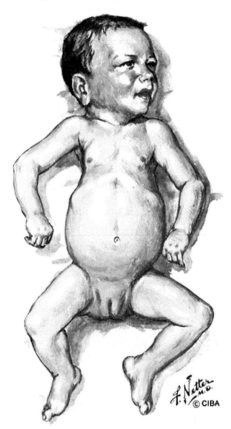

FIGURE 30–1

Infant with typical bell-shaped thorax, frog-leg posture, and "jug-handle" position of upper limbs. (Copyright© 1997, Icon Learning Systems, LLC. A subsidiary of MediMedia, USA, Inc. All rights reserved.)

is comparatively stronger than the intercostal muscles, so that with inspiration the protuberant abdomen expands while the chest collapses. The cry is poorly phonated due to diminished expiratory power. Death is due to respiratory insufficiency, sometimes precipitated by otherwise trivial upper respiratory infection. The median age of survival in SMA-1 is 8 months, with 75% mortality by the first birthday and only 5% survival to the second birthday.[11] Survival is strongly influenced by the degree of respiratory support, and with invasive or noninvasive means of ventilation survival can be extended many years or decades.[12]

Children with the intermediate SMA-2 manifest the ability to maintain an independent sitting position at some time in their development. In years past children with this form of SMA were said to survive into the school years. It is now clear that most of the progressive worsening associated with this level of SMA is associated with advancing complications of the disorder rather than to the underlying causes of the disease itself.[3] When these complications can be well managed, both prospectively and responsively, childhood mortality is much lower.

The most important factors affecting survival are respiratory function and scoliosis. Like measures of muscle power, maximum respiratory volume (vital capacity) tends not to increase commensurate with increases in body mass during development, so that the relative respiratory reserve decreases. Use of night-time non-invasive ventilation can extend respiratory function for many years or more before tracheostomy or continuous respiratory support becomes necessary.[12]

Advancing scoliosis is almost universal in children with SMA-2.[13-15] This can worsen quickly after its initial appearance, since gravity is the chief driving force in its progression. Once scoliosis is severe, compromise of internal organs can compromise vital functions that are not easily reversed. Ideal treatment for scoliosis involves anticipatory bracing at the earliest expression of curvature. Spinal fusion is often necessary. This is a major undertaking in the weak child and is best, if possible, deferred until times nearer to skeletal maturation.

Those with SMA-3 are able to walk, at least a short distance, at some time in their development. The chief problems encountered in early years are associated with orthopedic deformity of the feet. With advancing years and weakness, scoliosis and other joint restrictions are of greater concern, and many eventually require use of a motorized wheelchair for independent mobility. Respiratory compromise can become a problem late in the course.

Genetics and Genetic Diagnosis

The *SMN* gene resides in a large portion of chromosome 5 that was duplicated in the branch of primate evolution that led to chimpanzees and humans.[16] Because of this duplication, existing in an adjacent head-to-head configuration, unequal crossing over during meiosis and other large genomic rearrangements are common within this region.[17] One of these two human copies of *SMN*, *SMN2* acquired a single "wobble" mutation at the beginning of exon 7 that alters the kinetics of messenger (mRNA) processing but does not change the coded protein. Most of the *SMN2* mRNA is spliced into a truncated form that produces a nonfunctional, short-lived SMN protein, but approximately 10% of the *SMN2* message is spliced into the full-length, functional message that transcribes a normal SMN protein.[1] This instability of the *SMN* region of chromosome 5 and the partial function of *SMN2* sets up a complex and ultimately perverse interplay between the *SMN1* and *SMN2* genes that is responsible for the disorder. SMA is caused by the homozygous loss of the *SMN1* gene (Fig. 30-2).

Approximately half of the pathogenic mutations of *SMN1* are caused by deletion mutations, presumably large genomic rearrangements due to unequal crossing-over events. Most of the other half are "conversion" mutations,[18] unusual in the animal kingdom but common in plants. Conversion occurs during meiosis when the nearly identical single-strand *SMN1* and *SMN2* sequences pair up and mismatch repair systems "fix" the *SMN1* sequence to the *SMN2* configuration. This results in one fewer copy of *SMN1* and one additional copy of *SMN2* on that chromosome. Individuals

who possess only a single copy of the *SMN1* gene are carriers for SMA and manifest no weakness for a lifetime. Those with homozygous loss of the *SMN1* gene have SMA.

The clinical severity of SMA is related to the number of copies of *SMN2*, with fewer copies associated with more severe disease. Though this is not the only explanation for difference in the severity of the phenotype, it explains a substantial portion of this variation: individuals with SMA-1 most often have two copies of *SMN2* (*SMN1* deletion mutations on each chromosome); those with SMA-2 have three copies of *SMN2* (one deletion and one conversion mutation), and those with SMA-3 have four copies of *SMN2* (conversion mutations on each chromosome).[19,20] Though complex, these genetic rearrangements lend themselves to a simple and highly specific means for the diagnosis of SMA once it is suspected.[21] A polymerase chain reaction (PCR)-based assay can demonstrate the loss of the specific sequence within exons 7 and 8 of *SMN1* that distinguish it from *SMN2*. Fully 95% of individuals with *SMN*-associated SMA demonstrate this loss. For those manifesting skeletal muscle weakness, loss of the *SMN1* specific sequence in exon 7 is virtually 100% specific for the disorder.

Carrier testing for SMA is possible and reliable.[22] SMA affects some 1 in 10,000 to 6000 individuals, which corresponds to the empirically ascertained carrier rate of approximately 1 in 40. As a recessive disorder, the risk to a sibling is 25%, and affected siblings almost certainly manifest similar severity. The risk to a first cousin of an affected individual is equal to 1/2 (the risk that the parent's sibling is a carrier) times 1/40 (the risk that the spouse is a carrier) times 1/4, or 1/320. When two individuals in an extended family are both affected, however, they need not be similar in severity, since they have in common only one of their two pathogenic SMA alleles. The carrier test is not perfect, because approximately 2% of parents of children with SMA have two copies of *SMN1* and would thus appear not to be carriers.[23] Of these some are true carriers, possessing two copies of *SMN1* on one chromosome and none on the other, and the others represent true de novo mutation in the *SMN* gene.[23,24]

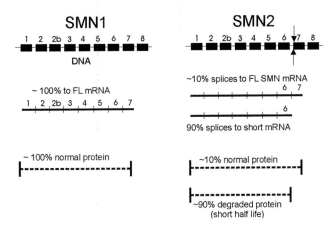

FIGURE 30–2

Alternative splicing of SMN1 and SMN2 genes. A single-point mutation at the intron 6-exon 7 boundary produces alternatively spliced SMN mRNA transcripts. The result is that SMN2 produces mostly a short-lived and dysfunctional SMN protein missing the portion coded by exon 7; a small amount of normal full-length protein is produced. FL, full length; SMN, survival motor neuron gene; mRNA, messenger RNA. (From Jones HR, DeVivo DC, Darras BT [eds]: Neuromuscular Disorders of Infancy, Childhood, and Adolescence: A Clinician's Approach. Philadelphia, Butterworth-Heinemann, 2003, p 152.)

Neurophysiology of *SMN*-Associated Spinal Muscular Atrophy

Needle EMG

The hallmark of SMA is denervation as manifested with needle electromyography (EMG). Common to all patients, and the single most specific EMG feature for denervation, is the finding of reduced recruitment of voluntary motor unit potentials. Across the spectrum of the disorder, however, loss of motor neurons may manifest with different electrophysiologic signs. The motor units of infants with severe SMA do not appear to have the capacity for abundant collateral reinnervation in the setting of neighboring denervation. As a consequence, early in the disorder abnormal spontaneous activity in the form of fibrillation and positive sharp wave potentials is common, voluntary motor unit recruitment is reduced (frequently demonstrating fast firing of only a single motor unit within any one territory), and surviving motor units may be modestly increased in amplitude but not in duration. The acute denervation EMG pattern of SMA-1 with many fibrillation potentials (Fig. 30-3) contrasts with the pattern of chronic denervation with collateral reinnervation most often seen in children and adults with SMA-2 and SMA-3. Abnormal spontaneous activity is unusual in the milder forms.

Fibrillation potentials are not sufficient by themselves to identify SMA, because they can arise from denervation from all causes or from other disorders of the motor unit as outlined in Table 30-1 and Box 30-1. The finding of reduced recruitment of voluntary motor unit potentials is of special importance to the physiologic definition of denervation. One particular entity that may have similar EMG appearance to that found in the infant with severe SMA is congenital myotonic dystrophy, where numerous fibrillation potentials in addition to atypical myotonic discharges may be found (Fig. 30-4); the latter might potentially be confused with fast-firing single motor units.

An increase in voluntary motor unit potential amplitude without increase in duration is common in infants and children with the more severe forms of SMA and may represent one or a combination of three processes separate from reinnervation by collateral sprouting. First, an increased number of innervated muscle fibers may coalesce into the space recorded by the EMG electrode because of denervation atrophy of neighboring units' muscle fibers. Second, hypertrophy of muscle fibers may increase an individual

Text continued on page 566

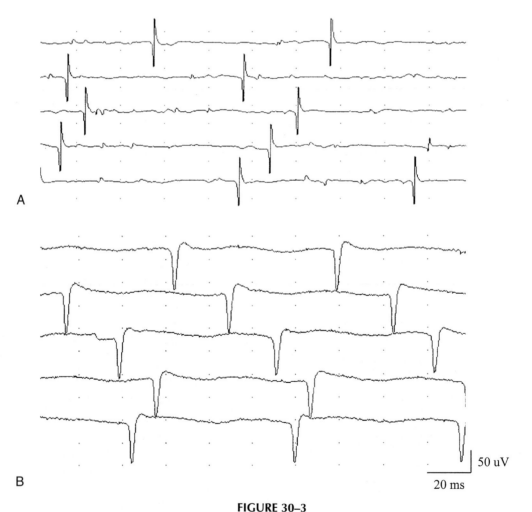

A

B

50 uV

20 ms

FIGURE 30–3

Spontaneous activity with denervation potentials. A, Fibrillations. B, Positive sharp waves in a muscle at rest. (A and B, From Jones HR, DeVivo DC, Darras BT [eds]: Neuromuscular Disorders of Infancy, Childhood, and Adolescence: A Clinician's Approach. Philadelphia, Butterworth-Heinemann, 2003, p 52.)

TABLE 30–1 SPINAL MUSCULAR ATROPHY DISORDERS AND SYNDROMES*

MIM No.	Inheritance	Title (Synonyms)	Linkage	Gene	Onset, Course	Distinguishing Features, Comments
		Confirmed Monogenic Disorders				
253300 253550 253400 271150	AR	SMA (SMA-1 to SMA-4; Werdnig-Hoffmann disease, juvenile muscular atrophy, Kugelberg-Welander disease)	5q12.2-q13.3	SMN1	SMA-1, infantile SMA-2, late infantile SMA-3, childhood through adult (also SMA-4)	Caudal-to-cranial distribution, wide range of severity
313200	X	X-linked spinal and bulbar muscular atrophy (Kennedy's disease)[88]	Xq12	Androgen receptor (CAG trinucleotide expansion)[89]	Adult, progressive	Gynecomastia, cramping, fasciculations, pain neuropathy, elevated creatine kinase
604320	AR	SMARD-1[69,70] Distal SMA-6	11q13-q21	Immunoglobulin-binding protein 2 (IGHMBP2)	Infantile, progressive	Prominent early diaphragm weakness
600794	AD	Distal SMA with upper limb predominance[114] Distal SMA-5	7p15	Glycyl tRNA synthetase (GARS) (same gene also causes CMT-2D)	Late teens, slowly progressive	Radial aspect of hand spread to distal lower extremities[67] Pyramidal features[115] suggest ASL/SPG syndrome
600794	AD	Distal SMA with upper limb predominance[115] Distal SMA-5 (same gene also causes hereditary SPG-17, Silver's syndrome)	11q13	BSCL2	Late teens, slowly progressive	Radial aspect of hand spread to distal lower extremities[68] Pyramidal features[115] suggest ALG/SPG syndrome
		Presumed Monogenic Disorders (with distinctive semiology)				
301830	X	Distal X-linked arthrogryposis (infantile X-linked SMA)[91]	Xp11.3-q11.2[92]		Congenital, progressive	Frequent congenital joint deformity, frequent fractures
158580	AD	Distal SMA with vocal cord paralysis (distal SMA-7, hereditary distal motor neuronopathy type 7)[73]	2q14[116]		Juvenile to adult, progressive	Two families link to this loci Clinically, similar to CMT 2C
607088	AR	Recessive distal SMA	11q13		Childhood, slowly progressive	Similar phenotype to SMARD-1 but older onset and slower progression; IGHMBP2 mutations not yet found
		Syndromes of Less Certain Nosology Diffuse or caudal-to-cranial weakness				
158600	AD	Dominant proximal SMA (juvenile SMA)[117,118]			Childhood, slowly progressive	AD, otherwise similar to SMN-associated SMA (multigenerational kindreds may be SMN-SMA with pseudodominant inheritance[119]) Kindreds with overlap with 182980 exist[120]

(Continued)

TABLE 30–1 *Cont'd*

MIM No.	Inheritance	Title (Synonyms)	Linkage	Gene	Onset, Course	Distinguishing Features, Comments
182980	AD	Dominant adult-onset SMA Finkel type[121]			Adult onset, slowly progressive	Frequent fasciculations Kindreds with overlap of 158600 exist[120]
271200	AR	SMA, Ryukyuan type Non-*SMN* recessive SMA	Heterogeneous		Infantile, progressive	In Ryukuyu islands of Japan, form demonstrates lower more than upper extremities, fasciculations, kyphoscoliosis, pes cavus; other scattered cases of non-*SMN* AR SMA reported[122]
						Distal SMA syndromes
271120	AR	Distal SMA (distal SMA-3, SMA-4)			Childhood	Distally predominant denervation and weakness
182960	AD	Distal SMA-1 Distal hereditary motor neuropathy			Early adulthood	Distally predominant denervation and weakness, some with hearing loss[123]
158590	AD	Distal SMA-2 SMA-4 (this term also used by some for adult-onset *SMN*-associated SMA)	Heterogeneous, 12q24.3 (one slowly progressive kindred)[72]		Adult, rapidly progressive	Distally predominant denervation and weakness; rapidly progressive in some (not yet linked)[124] in these phenotype similar to sporadic progressive muscular atrophy form of ALS (600175 and 181405 linked to same locus)
600175	AD	Congenital nonprogressive SMA of lower limbs (congenital distal SMA)[125,126]	Heterogeneous, some kindreds to 12q23-q24[127]		Congenital, nonprogressive	Lower extremities only, nonprogressive arthrogryposis with neurogenic features (158590 and 181405 linked to same locus)
605726	AR	SMA, Jerash type[128]	9p21.1-p12		Childhood, progressive	With pyramidal signs (could also be considered a form of ALS)
						Regional spinal syndromes
	AR	Cervical SMA[85]			Infancy, progressive	Cranial-to-caudal distribution, prominent head ptosis, respiratory insufficiency
	Sporadic	Congenital cervical SMA[86,96,129]			Infancy, nonprogressive	Arthrogryposis of upper extremities; may be segmental developmental defect of cervical spinal cord[96]
158650	AR	Malignant neurogenic muscular atrophy			Adult, rapidly progressive	Indistinguishable from sporadic progressive muscular atrophy form of ALS
182970	AR	SMA, fascioscapulohumeral type			Early adult, progressive	Whether distinct from FSH muscular dystrophy (158900) not clear
181405	AD	Neurogenic scapuloperoneal amyotrophy[130]	Single kindred described, linked 12q24.1-q24.31[131]		Progressive	Also congenital absence of muscles, laryngeal palsy, progressive scapuloperoneal and distal atrophy (158590 and 600175 linked to same locus)

Bulbar and cranial nerve syndromes

MIM	Disease	Inheritance	Locus	Onset/course	Features
271220	SMA with scapuloperoneal distribution	AR		Childhood	
211500	Progressive bulbar palsy of childhood (Fazio-Londe disease)	AR (AD)[74]		Childhood, progressive	Cranial-to-caudal, sparing EOMs Original case of Fazio-Londe disease had AR inheritance
157900	Möbius syndrome (MBS-1)	AD	13q12.2-q13,[81,82] sporadic	Congenital, nonprogressive	Symmetric neurogenic cranial nerves VII, VI ± XII dysfunction, often with distal finger contractures or other distal musculoskeletal anomalies
601471	Möbius syndrome (MBS-2)	AD	3q21-q22,[83] sporadic	Congenital, nonprogressive	Asymmetric weakness of facial muscles, neurogenic
211530	Progressive bulbar palsy with deafness (Vialetto-van Laere syndrome, or Madras-type motor neuron disease)[132]	Both AR and AD kindreds	50% sporadic	Juvenile, progressive	Early progressive deafness; bulbar weakness spreading caudally

*For entries with a MIM designation number, extensive reference listing can be obtained at *http://www3.ncbi.nlm.nih.gov/omim/.* SMA, spinal muscular atrophy; AR, autosomal recessive; AD, autosomal dominant; tRNA, transfer RNA; CMT, Charcot-Marie-Tooth; ALS, amyotrophic lateral sclerosis; FSH, facioscapulohumeral; EOM, extraocular movement; SMARD, SMA with respiratory distress.

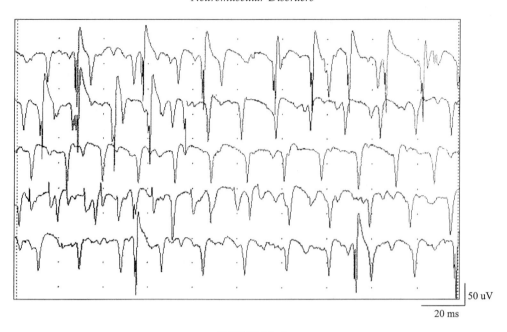

50 uV

20 ms

FIGURE 30–4

Myotonic discharges from a 10-year-old boy with congenital myotonia. The discharges were found in all examined skeletal muscles. (From Jones HR, DeVivo DC, Darras BT [eds]: Neuromuscular Disorders of Infancy, Childhood, and Adolescence: A Clinician's Approach. Philadelphia, Butterworth-Heinemann, 2003, p 53.)

muscle fiber's potential contribution to the motor unit potential. Third, units may be lost in a random manner from across the recruitment spectrum, leaving behind some of the larger amplitude motor units not ordinarily seen in the early recruitment of muscle activation.[25]

Older children with SMA, whether surviving from an early onset or first manifesting weakness at later ages, frequently manifest voluntary motor units of both increased amplitude and increased duration. This is similar to the pattern seen in patients long after recovering from paralytic polio and likely represents reinnervation by collateral sprouting with expansion of the motor unit territory by the surviving motor units.[26-28] The capacity for substantial collateral reinnervation does not appear to be universal for all surviving motor units. Instead, a few expand greatly, increasing the mean motor unit size substantially more than the median.[29] Whether this variability in capacity for expansion is a specific feature of chronic SMA, or instead a general phenomenon with longstanding severe chronic denervation, is unknown.

Fasciculation potentials are rarely seen in *SMN*-associated SMA, and, if present, argue against the disease.[30] In the older literature, however, there is much discussion and speculation about a curious rhythmic spontaneous motor unit activity that arises during sleep.[26,30-33] Within these published articles there is disagreement about frequency of discharge and the patient groups in which this spontaneous activity is most likely to be observed. This abnormality has not been

the subject of much recent investigation, and its reliability as a clinical sign, specificity to *SMN*-associated SMA, and importance as a clue to underlying pathophysiology of SMA, remains unknown.

Nerve Conduction Studies

For the most part, nerve conduction studies are normal and in those with milder forms of the disorder sensory nerve response amplitudes should also be normal. Among the youngest, most severely affected, the neuropathology of SMA includes changes in more widespread neuronal populations including the thalamus and dorsal root ganglion. In these circumstances, sensory responses may be absent.[34,35] Motor nerve conduction velocity (NCV) is generally normal, although there is some controversy on this point. Very low evoked motor amplitude may decrease the measured conduction velocity, possibly as a result of loss of the largest, fastest conducting motor units. Though wallerian-like degeneration is common in motor roots and mixed nerves, demyelination is not seen, suggesting that technical factors may also have a role in those reports describing slowing of conduction. The alternative explanation for slowing has been the presence of nerve immaturity (presumably with diminished axonal caliber), thinning of the myelin sheath, and shortening of internodal length. This alternative hypothesis has not been studied systematically. Some of the papers describing prominent conduction slowing predate the discovery of *SMN*, concentrating on the study of patients in outlying patient groups, or both, suggesting the reported findings may not be from a homogeneous group of *SMN*-associated SMA.[33,35-42]

Motor Unit Number Estimation

Recent application of advanced techniques of investigation has produced useful information about the disorder. Motor unit number estimation, using the multipoint stimulation technique in the ulnar nerve, has shown that motor unit numbers are within the normal range in presymptomatic infants with SMA-1, with a rapid decline of numbers during the early phase of acquired weakness. Thereafter the residual number of motor neurons is much more stable.[43] In a population of older, more mildly affected individuals, mean jitter was increased, suggesting that the very large motor units within this group may have some degree of junctional instability.[44]

Role of EMG in Diagnosis

For some infants and children, the manifestations of typical clinical features of SMA are sufficiently specific to warrant proceeding directly to the *SMN* gene test. In many instances, however, clinical features alone are less probative, and EMG testing can enhance efficient diagnosis and minimizing error, unnecessary testing, patient discomfort, time, and patient and family anxiety. The major differential diagnosis for infants and children with hypotonia and gross motor difficulty is reviewed in Chapter 28. In cases where SMA is considered possible but not necessarily likely, a limited study demonstrating normal NCV in a single motor nerve and clear neuropathic recruitment in a weak muscle is sufficient to justify obtaining the *SMN* gene test. Some pediatric electromyographers also attempt to obtain at least one sensory nerve conduction study to be certain that the unlikely possibility of a congenital polyneuropathy is not present.[45] A limited EMG/NCV study enhances the efficiency of the diagnostic process, by eliminating cases with obvious features of a polyneuropathy or a myopathy, or a normal EMG that suggests a central etiology. The specificity of the *SMN* gene test vastly surpasses the specificity obtainable from extensive neurophysiologic testing and biopsy combined. In this manner a limited and minimally invasive EMG study can minimize the cost, time, anxiety, and potential for errant diagnosis associated with a more "shotgun" approach to diagnosis with extensive testing. In most cases of SMA the *SMN* gene test should precede muscle biopsy in the diagnostic process, and hence biopsy should not be necessary. Moreover, in the very young infant, EMG testing is definitely more sensitive than muscle biopsy in predicting an abnormal *SMN* gene test.[45,46]

In approximately 5% of cases of bone fide *SMN*-associated SMA, the DNA test is falsely normal.[47-49] Since

the PCR based test evaluates only the presence of the unique sequences within exon 7 and 8 that identify the *SMN1* gene as opposed to the *SMN2* gene, other disabling small mutations within the *SMN1* gene will not be detected. At present, identifying these mutations by sequencing DNA is problematic, because it is not easy to know if any sequence abnormalities found in the PCR products amplified from other regions of the gene belong to the *SMN1* gene or the *SMN2* gene. These rare cases can be diagnostically challenging. More extensive EMG and NCV testing is clearly warranted, looking for evidence of significant asymmetry of denervation between sides or disproportionately greater affection of upper more than lower extremities, either of which would be unusual in *SMN*-associated SMA. Special testing to evaluate for a congenital myasthenic syndrome (see Chapter 33) should be performed. Muscle biopsy is indicated. Should all of these tests demonstrate features consistent with the diagnosis of SMA, further DNA diagnostic testing, evaluating the copy number of *SMN1*, will be of additional value[50-52] by a Bayesian probability approach.

The reasoning of this method begins with the understanding that 1 in 40 individuals is an asymptomatic carrier for SMA, having but one copy of the *SMN1* gene. The 5% of individuals with true *SMN*-associated SMA who have a normal conventional *SMN1* gene test almost all (in the absence of parental consanguinity) have a compound heterozygous genotype: one *SMN1* allele is disrupted by a conversion or deletion mutation, and the other allele is disrupted by a nondetectable small mutation. These patients have only a single copy of *SMN1* detected on the "carrier" test that measures *SMN1* gene copy number. Use of this carrier test indiscriminately in the evaluation of all floppy infants and children would lead to many errors: 1 in 40 would be falsely suspected of having *SMN*-associated SMA. However, once the prior possibility of SMA is well established by highly characteristic EMG and biopsy features, the result of the *SMN* carrier gene test then possesses substantial additional predictive diagnostic value. In this setting, the finding of two copies of *SMN1* weighs heavily against the diagnosis of *SMN*-associated SMA, whereas the finding of a single copy validates the high likelihood of the diagnosis that was established by the more conventional physiologic and pathologic means of testing.

OTHER SPINAL MUSCULAR ATROPHY DISORDERS AND SYNDROMES

SMA also designates a broad category of heritable disorders and syndromes of widely varying nosology. Some are well characterized to the level of a specific gene, whereas others are defined only by semiology.[53] Use of "SMA" in a title implies a symmetric, heritable disorder concentrated chiefly in the motor neurons. Not surprisingly, classification of the SMA disorders and syndromes—the SMAs—is not easy. The various features, such as age of onset, regional vulnerability, associated characteristics, mode of inheritance, genetic linkage, or identified gene defect, that might be used for a classification are applicable to some but not all of these variant SMAs. Moreover, the diagnosis itself has widely varying value. For some of the SMA disorders diagnosis contributes meaningfully to an understanding of prognosis amd genetics or potentially for therapy, but for others diagnosis supplies little more than a descriptive label. A summary of the various SMAs, identifying first the well-defined disorders known to be caused by mutation of an identified gene, then those intermediate defined disorders with at least one family demonstrating genetic linkage, followed by semiographic-defined syndromes is found in Table 30-1. Those disorders in which motor neuronopathy is only a part of a larger neurodegeneration are summarized in Table 30-2.

TABLE 30–2 LOWER MOTOR NEURON DISORDERS AS PART OF A LARGER NEUROLOGIC DISORDER*

MIM No.	Inheritance	Title (Synonyms)	Linkage	Gene	Onset, Course	Distinguishing Features, Comments
			Juvenile ALS Disorders			
205100	AR	Juvenile ALS-2 (juvenile ALS, juvenile PLS)	2q33	Alsin[133,134]	1st decade	Distal amyotrophy
602433	AR	Juvenile ALS-4[112,135] (same gene also causes ataxia, oculomotor apraxia 2)	9q34[136]	Senataxin	2nd decade, slowly progressive, normal survival	Distal amyotrophy, no or minimal spasticity, increased DTRs
105400	AD	Familial ALS-1	21q22.1	SODI	Single case of 6-yr-old onset[113]	Mostly adult onset, variable expression
605726	AR	SMA, Jerash type[128]	9p21.1-p12		Childhood, progressive	With pyramidal signs
	AR (?)	Infantile progressive SMA with ophthalmoplegia and pyramidal symptoms[135-137]			Infantile, progressive	Single family of affected siblings, also deafness
			Defined Disorders with Prominent Motor Neuron Degeneration			
272800	AR	Hexosaminidase A deficiency Tay-Sachs disease variant[62]	15q23-q24	HEXA	Juvenile or adult, progressive	Often with dementia, spinocerebellar ataxia <10% serum hexosaminidase A activity
308300	X dominant	Incontinentia pigmenti type 2 (Block-Sulzberger syndrome)[138,139]	Xq28	NEMO	Infantile	Females only (males presumed embryonic lethal) SMA sporadic
208900	AR	Ataxia telangiectasia[140]	11q2.3	ATM	Childhood, progressive	Motor neuronopathy reported in late stages
210200 210210	AR	3-Methylcrotonyl-CoA carboxylase deficiency (1 and 2)	3q25-127 5q12-q13	MCCA MCCB	Infancy, childhood; heterogeneous	Hypotonia, seizures, acidosis; widely heterogeneous
188250	AR	Mitochondrial DNA depletion[141,142]	16q22	Thymidine kinase type 2	Childhood, progressive	Elevated lactate; Mutations of this gene usually present with myopathy
220110	AR	Cytochrome C oxidase deficiency[143,144]	22q13	Heterogeneous SCO2	Infancy, progressive	Cardiomyopathy, elevated lactate, cyclooxygenase-negative fibers on muscle biopsy

TABLE 30–2 *Cont'd*

MIM No.	Inheritance	Title (Synonyms)	Linkage	Gene	Onset, Course	Distinguishing Features, Comments
			SMA with Other Distinctive Features			
271110 271109	AR	SMA with mental subnormality ± microcephaly[145-147]	Likely heterogeneous			
607596	AR	SMA with pontocerebellar hypoplasia type 1[104,148-150]	not 5q21		Congenital or infantile, progressive	Severe cerebellar malformation; often more widespread neuropathology Phenotype may vary within kindreds
208100	AR	Neurogenic arthrogryposis multiplex congenita[151-154]	Heterogeneous, 5q35 (one kindred)		Congenital, nonprogressive	Deformity of elbows, knees, and feet
217225	AR	Infantile SMA with congenital fractures[150-152]	Likely heterogeneous			
	AR	SMA with myoclonic epilepsy[155]	Heterogeneous		Childhood and adult forms	Heterogeneous, some kindreds associated with spasticity, mental retardation, deafness, or cerebellar findings

*For entries with a MIM designation number, extensive reference listing can be obtained at *http://www3.ncbi.nlm.nih.gov/omim/*.

SMA, spinal muscular atrophy; AR, autosomal recessive; AD, autosomal dominant; ALS, amyotrophic lateral sclerosis; PLS, progressive lateral sclerosis; DTR, deep tendon reflex.

Because *SMA* refers to a disorder of the (lower) motor neuron, certain features are common to all of the SMAs. Weakness due to muscle denervation is a required characteristic, although early slow loss of motor neurons can be masked by residual motor unit expansion through axonal sprouting and muscle fiber hypertrophy. Certain specific features that imply more widespread neuropathology, particularly of the sensory neuron or nerve or upper motor neurons, weigh against use of SMA as a label. Thus, those disorders in which sensory deficit or abnormal testing of sensory nerve function is prominent would tend to be described as a hereditary motor and sensory neuropathy or neuronopathy.

Prominent upper motor neuron signs of spasticity, enhanced tendon reflexes, or extensor toe responses suggest a form of amyotrophic lateral sclerosis (ALS). (The term *motor neuron disease*, which otherwise certainly should include the SMAs, has in some cases been coopted by those needing a broad label for the various forms of ALS.) When symmetric spasticity of the lower more than upper extremities is the most remarkable feature, the applied label may be familial spastic paraplegia, hereditary spastic paraplegia, or simply spastic paraplegia. Prominent cerebellar findings suggest the diagnosis of a spinocerebellar degeneration. Having noted these broad defining categories, some disorders may

have acquired the SMA label early in their exegesis and now maintain that label even though clinical or genetic evidence may suggest a different category is more appropriate. The future of SMA nosology almost certainly will be even more messy, as our simple categoric ideas confront the realities of genetic and phenotypic heterogeneity.

Diagnostic Evaluation

EMG and NCV studies constitute the single most important investigation in the evaluation of a suspected non-*SMN* SMA. EMG must demonstrate reduced recruitment of voluntary motor unit potentials (MUPs) with or without features of chronic collateral reinnervation. Spontaneous fibrillation and positive sharp wave potentials may or may not be present, depending on the amount of denervation and the timing of loss. They are also a nonspecific finding (Box 30-1).[54] Motor NCV must be in the normal range or only modestly reduced when continuous muscle action potential (CMAP) amplitude is substantially reduced. If there is any suggestion of regional involvement that could be explained by multiple mononeuropathies, particularly when EMG shows minimal abnormal spontaneous activity despite severe weakness, the presence of possible multiple motor nerve conduction block should be sought and specifically excluded. Most important, normal sensory nerve studies are required for the diagnosis.

Other disorders of the motor unit should be considered in the differential diagnosis. A symmetric and diffuse polyradiculopathy (see Chapter 31) can produce a similar distribution of weakness with abnormalities on conventional EMG and NCV demonstrating mostly motor involvement, but most such patients have a different clinical course, with acute or subacute onset after a lifetime of normal function. One can also rarely see a newborn who is either floppy at birth or who becomes that a few days later and is identified as having a potentially treatable demyelinating disorder such as infantile Guillain-Barré syndrome.[55-58] In the older child a polyneuropathy (see Chapter 31), particularly the chronic inflammatory demyelinating type, is much more common than all the non-*SMN* SMAs combined. In most cases clinical and neurophysiologic evidence of sensory involvement distinguishes these from the children with SMA.

Heritable and acquired disorders of the neuromuscular junction (see Chapter 33) are rarely confused with motor neuronopathy and usually also can be differentiated by appropriate electrophysiologic studies. Various forms of myopathy (see Chapter 34) may superficially appear similar to motor neuron disorders but are usually easily distinguished by electrophysiologic and pathologic features. A central disorder that disturbs motor activation can sometimes produce profound hypotonia in infants (see Chapter 28). Early on, these babies may manifest weakness rivaling that seen in SMA-1. Here the absence of EMG and NCV abnormalities can be quite useful.

Specific genetic testing is possible for only three of the SMAs: *SMN*-associated SMA, SMA with respiratory distress (SMARD-1), and X-linked spinal and bulbar muscular atrophy (Kennedy's disease), a disorder whose initial symptoms may appear during adolescence. This will likely change quickly, and the reader is advised to consult the National Library of Medicine-supported Online Mendelian Inheritance of Man catalog, OMIM (*http://www3.ncbi.nlm.nih.gov/omim/*), for up-to-date information on the state of the genetics of the emerging SMAs. Because *SMN*-associated SMA is relatively common, testing for *SMN1* deletion is frequently warranted early in the course of differential investigation.

Enzymatic testing of hexosaminidase activity may be of value because its deficiency can have protean manifestations, particularly for those with psychiatric symptoms.[60-62] All unexplained cases manifesting an SMA syndrome should have an assessment of soluble metabolism, particularly with review of the profile of excreted organic acids or the profile of acylcarnitine species. A careful G-banded karyotype with fluorescent in situ hybridization studies for subtelomeric chromosomal rearrangements[63,64] may identify novel chromosomal breaks and translocations that may be worthwhile in targeting new areas for potential linkage.

The diagnostic process for the SMAs best follows the basic path established for all of neurology: first localize the process in space and time, then evaluate the resulting shorter list of possibilities with more specific investigations. In the case of the non-*SMN* SMAs, the process of localization involved first identification of the lower motor neuron as the primary cause of weakness. The more specific groups of the SMAs are clustered on the pattern of weakness, with supplemental information from the pattern of progression, age of onset, and, when possible, the pattern of inheritance.

Defined Genetic Non-*SMN* SMA Disorders and Syndromes

Selective regional involvement of other areas has permitted isolation of many of the SMA syndromes. In some cases this has led to identification of a gene or chromosomal location, whereas in others the eponymous or descriptive labeling affords little extra predictive value regarding genetic risk, prognosis, or therapy.

Distal SMA

A prominent group of non-*SMN* SMAs is identified by the common expression of weakness in distal muscles of the legs and arms. So-called distal SMA is clearly a heterogeneous group, but one population survey suggested it may comprise 10% of the prevalence of SMA (with *SMN*-associated SMA responsible for virtually all of the remainder).[65] The essential common feature of these disorders—the predominance of weakness and amyotrophy in distal muscles of the extremities—suggests that the critical pathophysiologic vulnerability of motor neuron is related to the length of its axon. Against this hypothesis, however, is the finding that some of the disorders within this group affect distal muscles of the upper more than lower extremities, or the phrenic or recurrent laryngeal nerve relatively early, or muscles of the tibial more than peroneal distributions, so that length-dependent vulnerability itself cannot be the sole explanation for all members of this group. Whether these disorders are truly an SMA, that is, with the predominant pathology concentrated in the neuronal perikarya or instead a distal motor neuropathy, is presently not defined. This question itself may turn out to be hopelessly naive, because the cellular physiology of both axon and perikaryon are certainly intimately intertwined.

Harding identified seven types of distal SMA on the basis of clinical features and inheritance pattern,[66] a classification that persists although it is not clear that the numbered disorder that is now associated with a chromosomal locus or gene is the same disorder as that she originally described. Nonetheless, four distal SMA disorders have proved sufficiently distinctive and common that clustering of unrelated patients—or the opportunity afforded by the presence of a single large multiply affected kindred—has permitted characterization of genetic linkage and thus established a distinctive entity. Of these, a dominant form (distal SMA-5) associated with upper more than lower extremity involvement has been associated with two different genes: *GARS*[67] (mutation of which is also associated with a motor sensory neuropathy affecting the arms more than the legs) and *BSCL2*[68] (mutation of which is also associated Silver's syndrome/spastic paraplegia 17, a similar disorder with spasticity in the lower extremities and upper more than lower extremity distal amyotrophy). This one syndrome shows how difficult nosology will likely be, because it manifests both phenotypic and genotypic heterogeneity.

Another form (distal SMA-6) is recognized by rapidly progressive degeneration in infancy with prominent diaphragmatic weakness, early foot deformity, and neuropathy.[69,70] In most but not all cases it is caused by mutation of *IGHMBP2*, which was identified as a candidate for the disorder because of a previously described motor neuron disorder in the syntenic mouse gene.[71] A dominantly inherited adult-onset disorder with rapid progression after presentation, which

Harding described under the label "distal SMA type 2," has been linked to 12q24 in one kindred.[72] But a more rapidly progressive form with the same distribution of weakness, beginning in adult years, and hence easily confused with ALS, remains unlinked. Another Harding phenotype, "distal SMA type 7," describes a dominantly inherited adult-onset disorder with prominent early vocal cord paralysis. One kindred manifesting this disorder is linked to 5q31.[73] A dominantly inherited disorder with similar appearance but with the addition of sensorineural hearing loss is also described; this may either be an extended phenotype or a different, overlapping disorder.[74] Unfortunately, without the advantage of a positive family history, none of the distal SMA disorders are sufficiently distinctive on clinical grounds alone to permit genetic counseling on the basis of linkage to the identified chromosomal region.

Fazio-Londe Disease

Fazio-Londe disease is a progressive disorder of children affecting first the mid to lower brainstem myotomes, while sparing the extraocular muscles. Typically these children develop drooling, respiratory stridor, dysphagia, nasal regurgitation of liquids, and dysarthria. Bifacial, diaphragmatic, and proximal limb weakness may subsequently develop. Most cases are sporadic, but a few sibling pairs are known, and one mother-daughter kindred suggests the possibility of a dominantly inherited disorder.[75] Onset is in childhood and the course is generally progressive. An important treatable differential for this disorder is myasthenia gravis,[76] particularly "seronegative"[77,78] myasthenia gravis associated with anti-muscle-specific kinase antibodies, which appears to have special predilection for bulbar muscles. In some cases this can be particularly difficult to sort out, as bulbar muscle atrophy can be present, and the response to cholinesterase inhibitors and the results of conventional repetitive stimulation studies are equivocal. Affected individuals as young as 1 to 6 years have been reported.[79,80]

Möbius' Syndrome

Möbius' syndrome is classically thought of as a congenital, symmetric, nonprogressive motor neuronopathy of the facial and abducens nuclei, with possible involvement of bulbar motor nuclei as well. Most cases are sporadic, but dominant inheritance has been reported in a few cases that also have isolated aplasia of muscles, leading to an assigned chromosomal location.[81,82] The incidence of the disorder is too low to know whether these sporadic cases have a new dominant mutation, a possible genetic disorder with a different inheritance pattern, or a nongenetic disorder of brainstem development. More recently the title *Möbius syndrome* has been appropriated for two additional disorders: (1) MBS2 is characterized by isolated asymmetric facial weakness that can be distinguished from congenital facial nerve dysgenesis (congenital Bell's palsy) only by the dominant inheritance pattern in the family[83]; and (2) MBS3 is characterized by asymmetric facial weakness and frequent deafness. This syndrome is also known to manifest with dominant inheritance in some kindreds, but with incomplete penetrance of the mutant gene.[84] For Möbius syndrome as well, precise counseling about genetic risk for first-degree relatives of an isolated case is problematic.

Cervical Spinal Muscular Atrophy

Cervical spinal muscular atrophy is another selective regional SMA. Cervical SMA is rare and frequently progressive.[85] Most cases are sporadic, and the potential for other nongenetic localized spinal cord disorders, including syringomyelia, vasculitis or vascular malformation, transverse myelitis (which frequently affects lower motor neurons at the site of involvement), or other localized progressive etiologies should be pursued vigorously. A rare nonprogressive amyotrophy of cervical myotomes is also described. Whether this is a genetic or acquired disorder of the cervical cord is unknown.[86]

Kennedy's Disease

Kennedy's disease, also known as *hereditary spinobulbar muscular atrophy*, is an X-linked disorder in males. It is the best characterized form of non-*SMN* SMA.[87] Symptoms of muscle pain, cramps, and a sense of exhaustion with a modest elevation of creatine kinase appear during adolescence, well before the first manifestation of bulbar signs or weakness. This disorder is difficult to clinically identify in this age group but with the easy availability of the DNA testing, perhaps some teenagers will be identified much earlier before its more typical recognition during their 3rd decade or later. At that time symptoms of weakness develop concentrating in bulbar muscles, face, and proximal muscles of the limbs. Gynecomastia is a frequent early sign.[88] By middle age there is often a characteristic appearance of fasciculations around the lower face, longitudinal furrowing of an atrophic tongue with relatively mild and variable dysarthria and dysphagia, distal upper extremity fine postural and action tremor, cramping, and muscle fatigue.

This disorder was the first of an increasing number of neurodegenerative disorders in which a novel form of mutation was identified.[89] Within the responsible gene, in this case a gene on the X chromosome coding for the androgen receptor, there is a repetitive series of codons (CAG) coding for the amino acid glutamine. Normally there are less than 21 repeated glutamines in this sequence. In Kennedy's disease, however, this trinucleotide repeat region is expanded to more than 40 glutamine codons in a row. The protein containing an expanded polyglutamine region possesses toxic properties within the cell in which it is synthesized. The mechanism of this toxicity is the subject of intense

scrutiny because the polyglutamine repeat mutation is also responsible for Huntington's disease and numerous dominantly inherited spinocerebellar degenerations.[90] The reason for specific motor neuron vulnerability is, in part, likely related to expression of the androgen receptor, but other factors appear to be necessary as well.

X-Linked Arthrogryposis

X-linked arthrogryposis, an X-linked genetic mimic of infantile SMA, is often associated with congenital contractures and fractures.[91] It is associated with a poor prognosis, although milder forms with survival into school years have been reported. Multiple kindreds manifesting X-linkage have been linked to the same region, indicating genetic homogeneity for the syndrome and the high probability that the responsible gene will soon be identified.[92]

Nongenetic Mimics of SMA

The various signs and symptoms that suggest the possibility of a genetic disorder such as a non-*SMN* SMA also have various nongenetic causes, the course of which may be influenced by effective or partially effective specific therapy. These include disorders that affect every level of the neuraxis, including brain, spinal cord, plexus, nerve, neuromuscular junction, and muscle.[93] A categoric summary of these is provided in Table 30-3, and specific entities not covered elsewhere in this book are discussed further here.

Cerebral Causes

Profound hypotonia on a central basis can be indistinguishable from a neuromuscular disorder emanating from disruption of the motor unit. In some cases, after extensive investigation the relative contribution of the motor unit, or the central nervous system (CNS), to hypotonia and weakness is difficult to know in the short run. In these cases the clinical course may be essential to a better understanding of the underlying level of dysfunction. Two well-defined disorders, Prader-Willi syndrome and congenital myotonic dystrophy, have marked central hypotonia that improves with time; the relative contribution of motor unit dysfunction to the early weakness is unknown. Other degenerative disorders of gray and white matter may present initially with hypotonia. In many of these instances, proximal hypotonia is mixed with increases in tone more distally, including abnormal increased passive resistance to thumb abduction, forearm supination, or ankle dorsiflexion. Such a mixture of decreased and increased tone is almost never associated with an SMA syndrome, and along with other signs and symptoms of abnormal brain function such as enhanced or depressed mental status, cognitive changes, or seizures, should strongly direct attention to the CNS in the search for a primary cause.

TABLE 30–3 POTENTIAL MIMICS OF SPINAL MUSCULAR ATROPHY*

Anatomic Entity	Disorders that Mimic SMA
Brain	Degenerative disease
	Hypotonic cerebral palsy
	Congenital myotonic dystrophy
	Prader-Willi syndrome, other genetic disorders
Spinal cord and spinal column	Trauma*
	Structural disorders, e.g., syringomyelia, tethered cord*
	Vascular disorders*
	Tumor*
	Acute transverse myelitis*
	Epidermal abscess*
	Monomelic amyotrophy
Other motor neuron disorders	Poliomyelitis syndrome due to poliovirus, other enteroviruses, or West Nile virus*
	Following severe acute asthma attack (Hopkins' syndrome)
	Associated with other features (see Table 30-2)
Root	Polyradiculitis*
	Leukemia/lymphoma*
Plexus	Chronic lumbar or brachial plexitis*
Nerve	Progressive axonal polyneuropathy
	Multifocal motor neuropathy*
	Chronic inflammatory demyelinating polyneuropathy*
	Toxic polyneuropathy*
Neuromuscular junction	Myasthenia gravis*
	Botulism*
	Tic paralysis*
	Drug-induced neuromuscular blockade or AChE inhibitor*
Muscle	Myopathy*

*Denotes entities with potential specific therapy.
AChE, acetylcholinesterase.

Spinal Cord Lesions

Spinal Trauma

In some settings spinal shock after an acute cervical spinal injury may have the appearance of SMA, particularly in that there is flaccid quadriparesis with preservation of active facial expression.[94,95] This may partially simulate the caudal-to-rostral distribution of classic infantile *SMN*-associated SMA. Occasional newborn infants manifest quadriparesis as a complication of unsuspected spinal cord injury. Obvious spasticity may not be apparent for weeks, but there is usually mixed tone, combining increased plantar flexion tone with decreased tone elsewhere in the leg, much earlier. Because of small size, magnetic resonance imaging (MRI) or contrast-enhanced computed tomographic myelography have the best chance of demonstrating a lesion, but in some cases even these studies are normal. EMG can easily distinguish these spinal injury syndromes from SMA. However, other myelopathies also directly affect the anterior horn cells and thus are indistinguishable from SMA by EMG.

Spinal Infarction

Occlusion of the anterior spinal artery injures anterior horn cells, but generally this also affects the adjacent spinothalamic tracts, producing associated sensory changes. Infants with severe hypoxic ischemic encephalopathy at birth manifest electrophysiologic features of acute denervation and ischemic myelopathy in postmortem specimens, indicating that motor neurons may be affected along with the more diffuse and dramatic cerebral injury. Hypotension can produce a border zone infarction of the T4-T6 region with associated sensory and motor deficits and denervation of paraspinal muscles at the level of the lesion. MRI and somatosensory evoked potentials offer a means to distinguish these lesions.

Cervical Syringomyelia

Cervical syringomyelia is a disorder that can selectively affect motor neurons of the anterior horn of the myotomes at the level of the syrinx swelling. Patients with a syrinx manifest segmental weakness, amyotrophy, and usually also have a demonstrable suspended or cape distribution sensory deficit to pin and temperature. The last relates to the decussation of spinothalamic sensory fibers immediately anterior to the expanding fluid cavity that ruptures out of the central canal. Syringomyelia often occurs at the cervicothoracic junction, producing selective hand weakness that mimics distal SMA of the upper extremity. EMG of the lower cervical paraspinal muscles should be abnormal, because of the location of their respective motor neurons, immediately adjacent to the expanding cavity. Other chronic progressive or nonprogressive spinal cord disorders also may be mistaken for SMA.[86,96-98]

Other Nongenetic Causes that Might Mimic Spinal Muscular Atrophy

Poliomyelitis

Poliomyelitis, thankfully, is now a very uncommon illness. Because of its importance to public health, however, it must be considered early in the setting of a relatively quick appearance of weakness, particularly if focal or asymmetric in nature.[99] It is important to ascertain the child's poliomyelitis vaccination history as well as geographic origin. Poliovirus-associated poliomyelitis is now almost eliminated worldwide, though surveillance for polio, and thus final elimination of it from the world, is made more difficult by the fact that relatively few who harbor a poliovirus enteritis suffer from classic poliomyelitis. In the developed world, the rare cases of classic poliomyelitis that now exist are now more likely a complication of live oral virus (Sabin) vaccination where it is still used without prior administration of the killed (Salk) vaccine as advocated by Centers for Disease Control and Prevention. Other enteroviruses have a low propensity for infecting the nervous system in a similar fashion as poliovirus and are likely responsible for the bulk of those rare patients with a poliovirus syndrome in countries where the killed vaccine is widely used. West Nile virus has also produced a poliomyelitis syndrome in adults, and there is no reason to believe it might not also affect children similarly. To date there is no immunization for this newly emerging pathologic virus. Polio itself clinically presents as a gastroenteritis and evolves into a flaccid encephalitis out of which the classic asymmetric weakness emerges during recovery.

Neurophysiologic testing of children with a poliomyelitis syndrome, from whatever cause, demonstrates low-amplitude CMAPs, relatively normal motor conduction velocity, and normal sensory nerve studies. There is a marked diminution in the number of functioning motor units. When recovered, individual motor unit potentials in weak and recovered muscles can be remarkably enlarged in amplitude and duration. Classic poliomyelitis has a distinctive appearance even long after the recovery phase. The persistence of significant weakness (or EMG changes) in functionally related muscles of a limb that do not share a common root or nerve, with normal or near-normal findings in other muscles that share the same roots and nerves, argues for the diagnosis of old poliomyelitis. This distribution suggests that virus spreads regionally between adjacent neuronal perikarya, which are functionally organized, once it is established within a segmental region of the spinal cord's anterior horn. Since adjacent motor neuron columns within the spinal cord share common function even while their axonal processes course through different pathways, the pattern of vulnerability often follows related motor functions more than anything else.

Asthma-Precipitated Weakness

Rarely an acute flaccid asymmetric weakness is reported having developed in children who suffered from a severe acute asthmatic attack 4 to 7 days earlier. This occurs even though the child had been normally vaccinated against poliomyelitis.[100,101] Like poliomyelitis, this can be associated with a mild cerebrospinal fluid pleocytosis. Nerve conduction studies and needle EMG demonstrate normal compound sensory nerve action potentials (SNAPs) and signs of a severe primary axonal motor neuropathy. That this disorder is caused by a denervating disorder extending well up the innervating motor axon to very proximal levels is suggested by the finding on EMG of some of respiratory muscle-biceps synkinesis that occurs with aberrant regrowth of phrenic nerve axons into the brachial plexus.[102] This syndrome is to

be distinguished from that of critical illness myopathy in the child who cannot be weaned from a ventilator following severe respiratory compromise. EMG can be quite helpful in this differential.[103]

Hexosaminidase Deficiency

Deficiency of hexosaminidase A has been reported in association with a wide range of features including dementia, ataxia, psychiatric abnormalities, and retinal cherry red spot, extending the clinical expression of Tay-Sachs disease to young adults. The associated features may be sufficiently subtle that determination of hexosaminidase A activity should be a part of the evaluation of any patient beyond early childhood years with an otherwise unexplained symmetric progressive motor neuron degeneration.

Spinal Muscular Atrophy with Posterior Anomaly of the Posterior Fossa

A progressive motor neuronopathy has been associated with severe pontocerebellar hypoplasia in a number of recessive and sporadic kindreds. Prognosis is poor, with progressive weakness and often substantial mental subnormality associated with widespread neuropathology. Pontocerebellar hypoplasia with associated SMA (type 1 pontocerebellar hypoplasia), may yet be a mixture of heterogeneous disorders.[104,105]

Monomelic Amyotrophy

There exists in teenagers and young adults an overlapping progressive disorder that is known under many different titles including *monomelic amyotrophy*, *segmental cervical SMA*, *juvenile muscular atrophy of the distal upper extremity*, or, most recently, *Hirayama flexion myelopathy*.[106-108] This was originally described in Japan, where it is relatively common, but it is now recognized but with lower incidence worldwide. This is a sporadic disorder that generally occurs in males between the ages of 15 and 25 years. Most develop slowly progressive asymmetric weakness that usually remains unilateral, though the opposite side may be affected to a variable degree in up to 10% of cases. Slow, progressive weakness stabilizes after several years.

EMG demonstrates signs of both active and chronic denervation in an asymmetric C7-T1 distribution. This involves median-, ulnar-, and radial-innervated muscles without sensory symptoms or neurophysiologic SNAP impairment.

The routine MRI is normal, though ipsilateral or bilateral anteroposterior thinning of the mid cervical cord is common, as are abnormalities of cord and dural sac position with neck flexion. Important considerations in the differential diagnosis include juvenile ALS, poliomyelitis, cervical disc disease, and syringomyelia. The prognosis is relatively benign after stabilization, though acquired deficits are significant and permanent.

Sporadic ALS

Sporadic ALS is rare in children, adolescents, and young adults, but it can and does occur.[109] At its inception it can mimic various plexopathies or mononeuropathies with the exception that there is absolutely no history of pain or paresthesia. The EMG is particularly important to the diagnosis. Motor NCS may fail to elicit CMAPs in the affected extremity while the SNAPS are normal. Needle EMG demonstrates a predominant loss of motor unit potentials, with those few remaining having the typical signs of reinnervation (i.e., high amplitude, long duration, and rapid recruitment). In the most severely affected regions, no motor unit potentials may be recruited, and all one may find are profuse fibrillation potentials.

In most cases ALS remains an idiopathic disorder, although evidence to date suggests that there are a variety of genetic and environmental contributions to disease initiation with a common pathophysiology once the disease process is established. Family studies suggest that as many as 10% of cases of adult ALS may be significantly related to abnormality in a single gene. Clinical experience[110] and plausibility arguments suggest that ALS, like *SMN*-related SMA, affect a broader range of neurologic systems when it affects the very young.[111] The presence of an ALS syndrome in a child raises increased suspicion that the primary underlying cause is genetic, whether or not the gene has yet been identified. Each of the three genes so far identified was found with the advantage of a different fortuitous opportunity that is unlikely to be available for finding the genes responsible for the rare single cases most often seen.

Two of the three identified familial forms of ALS primarily cause a juvenile-onset disorder, but, as is increasingly common in genetics, the association between the gene and the disease is not straightforward. The opportunity to identify the gene *Alsin* was provided by the presence of a large consanguineous kindred. Homozygous mutations of *Alsin* are associated with two recessive disorders: a form of juvenile onset ALS and a pure upper motor neuron degeneration, termed *progressive lateral sclerosis*. The opportunity to find the second was afforded by its very mild and slow progression, thus permitting the identification and collection of DNA samples from a single large extended family with multiple affected members.

Recessive mutation of *Senataxin* was previously found to cause a quite different neurodegenerative disorder, ataxia oculomotor apraxia 2. The *Senataxin*-associated juvenile ALS is slowly progressive with mostly lower motor neuron features, minimal or no spasticity, but increased tendon reflexes.[112] The third identified cause of familial ALS was found by a massive gene search among kindreds with multiply affected adults. Mutation of *SOD1* has so far been associated with ALS in only one child of 6 years; otherwise it is generally a disease of middle age and older.[113]

Prominent progressive degeneration of motor neurons is part of a number of neurodegenerative disorders (see Tables 30-2 and 30-3). Specific identification can generally be made by the associated characteristics. Deficiency of hexosaminidase A has been reported in association with a wide range of features including dementia, ataxia, psychiatric abnormalities, and retinal cherry red spot, extending the clinical expression of Tay-Sachs disease to young adults. The associated features may be sufficiently subtle that determination of hexosaminidase A activity should be a part of the evaluation of any patient beyond early childhood years with an otherwise unexplained symmetric, progressive motor neuron degeneration.

REFERENCES

1. Lefebvre S, Bürglen L, Reboullet S, et al: Identification and characterization of a spinal muscular atrophy-determining gene. Cell 1995;80:155-165.
2. Dubowitz V: Infantile muscular atrophy: A prospective study with particular reference to a slowly progressive variety. Brain 1964;87:707-718.
3. Crawford TO, Pardo CA: The neurobiology of childhood spinal muscular atrophy. Neurobiol Dis 1996;3:97-110.
4. Iannaccone ST, Russman BS, Brown RH, et al: Prospective analysis of strength in spinal muscular atrophy. J Child Neurol 2000;15:97-101.
5. Merlini L, Estournet-Mathiaud B, Iannaccone S, et al: 90th ENMC international workshop: European Spinal Muscular Atrophy Randomised Trial (EuroSMART) 9-10 February 2001, Naarden, The Netherlands. Neuromuscul Disord 2002;12:201-210.
6. Carter GT, Abresch RT, Fowler WM, et al: Profiles of neuromuscular diseases: Spinal muscular atrophy. Am J Phys Med Rehabil 1995;74(Suppl):S150-S159.
7. Dubowitz V: Muscle Disorders in Childhood, 2nd ed. Philadelphia, WB Saunders, 1995.
8. Moosa A, Dubowitz V: Spinal muscular atrophy in childhood: Two clues to clinical diagnosis. Arch Dis Child 1973;48:386-388.
9. Russman BS, Fredericks EJ: Use of the ECG in the diagnosis of childhood spinal muscular atrophy. Arch Neurol 1979;36:317-318.
10. Rudnik-Schöneborn S, Lutzenrath S, Borkowska J, et al: Analysis of creatine kinase activity in 504 patients with proximal spinal muscular atrophy types I-III from the point of view of progression and severity. Eur Neurol 1998;39:154-162.
11. Thomas NH, Dubowitz V: The natural history of type I (severe) spinal muscular atrophy. Neuromuscul Disord 1994;4:497-502.
12. Bach JR, Baird JS, Plosky D, et al: Spinal muscular atrophy type 1: Management and outcomes. Pediatr Pulmonol 2002;34:16-22.

13. Phillips DP, Roye DP Jr, Farcy JP, et al: Surgical treatment of scoliosis in a spinal muscular atrophy population. Spine 1990;15:942-945.

14. Rodillo E, Marini ML, Heckmatt JZ, Dubowitz V: Scoliosis in spinal muscular atrophy: Review of 63 cases. J Child Neurol 1989;4:118-123.

15. Granata C, Merlini L, Magni E, et al: Spinal muscular atrophy: Natural history and orthopaedic treatment of scoliosis. Spine 1989;14:760-762.

16. Rochette CF, Gilchrist JM, Simard L: *SMN* gene duplication and the emergence of the *SMN2* gene occurred in distinct hominids: *SMN2* is unique to *Homo sapiens*. Hum Genet 2001;108:255-266.

17. Crawford TO: From enigmatic to problematic: The new molecular genetics of childhood spinal muscular atrophy. Neurology 1996;46:335-340.

18. Burghes AHM: When is a deletion not a deletion? When it is converted. Am J Hum Genet 1997;61:9-15.

19. Mailman MD, Heinz JW, Papp AC, et al: Molecular analysis of spinal muscular atrophy and modification of the phenotype by *SMN2*. Genet Med 2002;4:20-26.

20. Feldkötter M, Schwarzer V, Wirth R, et al: Quantitative analyses of *SMN1* and *SMN2* based on real-time light Cycler PCR: Fast and highly reliable carrier testing and prediction of severity of spinal muscular atrophy. Am J Hum Genet 2002;70:358-368.

21. van der Steege G, Grootscholten PM, van der Vlies P, et al: PCR-based DNA test to confirm clinical diagnosis of autosomal recessive spinal muscular atrophy. Lancet 1995;345:985-986.

22. McAndrew PE, Parsons DW, Simard LR, et al: Identification of proximal spinal muscular atrophy carriers and patients by analysis of *SMNt* and *SMNc* gene copy number. Am J Hum Genet 1997;60:1411-1422.

23. Chen KL, Wang YL, Rennert H, et al: Duplications and de novo deletions of the *SMNt* gene demonstrated by fluorescence-based carrier testing for spinal muscular atrophy. Am J Med Genet 1999;85:463-469.

24. Mailman MD, Hemingway T, Darsey RL, et al: Hybrids monosomal for human chromosome 5 reveal the presence of a spinal muscular atrophy (SMA) carrier with two *SMN1* copies on one chromosome. Hum Genet 2001;108:109-115.

25. Crawford TO, Chaudhry V, Sladky JT: Lack of reinnervation in severe infantile spinal muscular atrophy [Abstract]. Ann Neurol 1995;38:539.

26. Hausmanowa-Petrusewicz I, Karwanska A: Electromyographic findings in different forms of infantile and juvenile proximal spinal muscular atrophy. Muscle Nerve 1986;9:37-46.

27. Emeryk-Szajewska B, Kopec J, Karwanska A: The reorganisation of motor units in different motor neuron disorders. Electromyogr Clin Neurophysiol 2003;43:23-31.

28. Ramaekers VT, Disselhorst-Klug C, Schneider J, et al: Clinical application of a noninvasive multi-electrode array EMG for the recording of single motor unit activity. Neuropediatrics 1993;24:134-138.

29. Galea V, Fehlings D, Kirsch S, McComas A: Depletion and sizes of motor units in spinal muscular atrophy. Muscle Nerve 2001;24:1168-1172.

30. Hausmanowa-Petrusewicz I: Electrophysiological findings in childhood spinal muscular atrophies. Rev Neurol (Paris) 1988;144:716-720.

31. Buchthal F, Olsen PZ: Electromyography and muscle biopsy in infantile spinal muscular atrophy. Brain 1970;93:15-30.

32. Buchthal F: Spontaneous electrical activity: An overview. Muscle Nerve 1982;5:S52-S59.

33. Hausmanowa-Petrusewicz I: [Bioelectric characteristics of spinal muscular atrophy]. Neurol Neurochir Pol 1983;17:171-176.

34. Kuo AA, Pulst SM, Eliashiv DS, Adams CR: Electrical inexcitability of nerves and muscles in severe infantile spinal muscular atrophy. J Neurol Neurosurg Psychiatry 1999;67:122.

35. Schwartz MS, Moosa A: Sensory nerve conduction in the spinal muscular atrophies. Dev Med Child Neurol 1977;19:50-53.

36. Echenne B, Georgesco M, Dapres G: [Motor nerve conduction velocity in early forms of infantile spinal amyotrophy: Diagnostic problems]. Rev Electroencephalogr Neurophysiol Clin 1984;13:329-335.

37. Iijima M, Arasaki K, Iwamoto H, Nakanishi T: Maximal and minimal motor nerve conduction velocities in patients with motor neuron diseases: Correlation with age of onset and duration of illness. Muscle Nerve 1991;14:1110-1115.

38. Krajewska G, Hausmanowa-Petrusewicz I: Abnormal nerve conduction velocity as a marker of immaturity in childhood muscle spinal atrophy. Folia Neuropathol 2002;40:67-74.

39. Miyanomae Y, Takeuchi Y, Nishimura A, et al: Motor nerve conduction studies on children with spinal muscular atrophy. Acta Paediatr Jpn 1996;38:576-579.

40. Renault F, Raimbault J, Praud JP, Laget P: [Electromyographic study of 50 cases of Werdnig-Hoffmann disease]. Rev Electroencephalogr Neurophysiol Clin 1983;13:301-305.

41. Ryniewicz B: Motor and sensory conduction velocity in spinal muscular atrophy: Follow-up study. Electromyogr Clin Neurophysiol 1977;17:385-391.

42. Ryniewicz B: [Conduction velocity in peripheral nerves in healthy and sick children]. Neurol Neurochir Pol 1975;9:701-704.

43. Bromberg MB, Swoboda KJ: Motor unit number estimation in infants and children with spinal muscular atrophy. Muscle Nerve 2002;25:445-447.

44. Bartousek J, Hlustik P, Grenarova O, Beranova M: Advanced EMG techniques in diagnostics of spinal muscular atrophies and motor neuron disease—magnetic stimulation, single-fiber EMG, and macro EMG. Acta Univ Palacki Olomuc Fac Med 1993;136:37-39.

45. David WS, Jones HR: Electromyography and biopsy correlation with suggested protocol for evaluation of the floppy infant. Muscle Nerve 1994;17:424-430.

46. Renault F, Chartier JP, Harpey JP: [Contribution of the electromyogram in the diagnosis of infantile spinal muscular atrophy in the neonatal period]. Arch Pediatr 1996;3:319-323.

47. Ogino S, Leonard DG, Rennert H, et al: Genetic risk assessment in carrier testing for spinal muscular atrophy. Am J Med Genet 2002;110:301-307.

48. Rudnik-Schöneborn S, Forkert R, Hahnen E, et al: Clinical spectrum and diagnostic criteria of infantile spinal muscular atrophy: Further delineation on the basis of *SMN* gene deletion findings. Neuropediatrics 1996;27:8-15.

49. Brahe C, Bertini E: Spinal muscular atrophies: Recent insights and impact on molecular diagnosis. J Mol Med 1996;74:555-562.

50. Rochette CF, Surh L, Ray PN, et al: Molecular diagnosis of non-deletion SMA patients using quantitative PCR of SMN exon 7. Neurogenetics 1997;1:141-147.

51. Parsons DW, McAndrew PE, Allinson PS, et al: Diagnosis of spinal muscular atrophy in an *SMN* non-deletion patient using a quantitative PCR screen and mutation analysis. J Med Genet 1998;35:674-676.

52. Martin Y, Valero A, del Castillo E, et al: Genetic study of SMA patients without homozygous *SMN1* deletions: Identification of compound heterozygotes and characterisation of novel intragenic *SMN1* mutations. Hum Genet 2002;110:257-263.

53. Zerres K, Rudnik-Schöneborn S: 93rd ENMC international workshop: Non-5q-spinal muscular atrophies (SMA)—clinical picture (6-8 April 2001, Naarden, The Netherlands). Neuromuscul Disord 2003;13:179-183.

54. Jones HR: EMG evaluation of the floppy infant: Differential diagnosis and technical aspects. Muscle Nerve 1990;13:338-347.

55. Al-Qudah AA: Immunoglobulins in the treatment of Guillain-Barré syndrome in early childhood. J Child Neurol 1994;9:178-180.

56. Rolfs A, Bolik A: Guillain-Barré syndrome in pregnancy: Reflections on immunopathogenesis. Acta Neurol Scand 1994;89:400-402.

57. Jackson AH, Baquis GD, Shaw BL: Congenital Guillain-Barré syndrome. J Child Neurol 1996;5:407-410.

58. Luijckx GJ, Vies J, de Baets M, et al: Guillain-Barré syndrome in mother and child. Lancet 1997;349:27.

59. Reference deleted.

60. Navon R, Khosravi R, Korczyn T, et al: A new mutation in the *HEXA* gene associated with a spinal muscular atrophy phenotype. Neurology 1995;45:539-543.

61. Parnes S, Karpati G, Carpenter S, et al: Hexosaminidase-A deficiency presenting as atypical juvenile-onset spinal muscular atrophy. Arch Neurol 1985;42:1176-1180.

62. Johnson WG, Wigger HJ, Glaubiger LM, Rowland LP: Juvenile spinal muscular atrophy: A new hexosaminidase deficiency phenotype. Ann Neurol 1982;11:11-16.

63. Horsley SW, Knight SJ, Nixon J, et al: Del(18p) shown to be a cryptic translocation using a multiprobe FISH assay for subtelomeric chromosome rearrangements. J Med Genet 1998;35:722-726.

64. Tolksdorf M, Kunze J, Gross-Selbeck G, et al: Familial trisomy 9p and spinal muscular atrophy: Clinical, cytogenetic, and embryological findings. Eur J Pediatr 1977;126:13-27.

65. Pearn JH, Hudgson P: Distal spinal muscular atrophy—a clinical and genetic study of eight kindreds. J Neurol Sci 1979;43:183.

66. Harding AE: Inherited neuronal atrophy and degeneration predominantly of lower motor neurons. *In* Dyck PJ, Thomas PK, Griffin JW (eds): Peripheral Neuropathy, 3rd ed. Philadephia, WB Saunders, 1993, pp 1051-1064.

67. Antonellis A, Ellsworth RE, Sambuughin N, et al: Glycyl tRNA synthetase mutations in Charcot-Marie-Tooth disease type 2D and distal spinal muscular atrophy type V. Am J Hum Genet 2003;72:1293-1299.

68. Windpassinger C, Auer-Grumbach M, Irobi J, et al: Heterozygous missense mutations in *BSCL2* are associated with distal hereditary motor neuropathy and Silver syndrome. Nat Genet 2004;36:271-276.

69. Pitt M, Houlden H, Jacobs J, et al: Severe infantile neuropathy with diaphragmatic weakness and its relationship to SMARD-1. Brain 2003;126:2682-2692.

70. Grohmann K, Varon R, Stolz P, et al: Infantile spinal muscular atrophy with respiratory distress type 1 (*SMARD1*). Ann Neurol 2003;54:719-724.

71. Cox GA, Mahaffey CL, Frankel WN: Identification of the mouse neuromuscular degeneration gene and mapping of a second site suppressor allele. Neuron 1998;21:1327-1337.

72. Timmerman V, De Jonghe P, Simokovic S, et al: Distal hereditary motor neuropathy type II (distal *HMNII*): Mapping of a locus to 12q24. Hum Mol Genet 1996;5:1065-1069.

73. McEntagart M, Spurlock G, Jackson C, et al: Distal spinal muscular atrophy with vocal cord paralysis (dSMA-VII) is not linked to the *MPD2* locus on chromosome 5q31. J Med Genet 2000;37:E14.

74. Boltshauser E, Lang W, Spillmann T, Hof E: Hereditary distal muscular atrophy with vocal cord paralysis and sensorineural hearing loss: A dominant form of spinal muscular atrophy? J Med Genet 1989;26:105-108.

75. Gomez MR, Clermont V, Bernstein J: Progressive bulbar paralysis in childhood (Fazio-Londe's disease). Arch Neurol 1962;6:323.

76. Albers JW, Zimnowodzki S, Lowrey CM, Miller B: Juvenile progressive bulbar palsy. Arch Neurol 1983;40:351-353.

77. Alexander MP, Emery ES, Koerner FC: Progressive bulbar paresis in childhood. Arch Neurol 1976;33:66-68.

78. Benjamins D: Progressive bulbar palsy of childhood in siblings. Ann Neurol 1980;8:203.

79. Jones HR: Personal communication (A 15-month-old child seen at CHB with antibody-positive myasthenia gravis), 1990.

80. Evoli A, Tonali PA, Padua L, et al: Clinical correlates with anti-MuSK antibodies in generalized seronegative myasthenia gravis. Brain 2003;126:2304-2311.

81. Ziter FA, Wiser WC, Robinson A: Three-generation pedigree of a Möbius syndrome variant with chromosome translocation. Arch Neurol 1977;34:437-442.

82. Slee JJ, Smart RD, Viljoen DL: Deletion of chromosome 13 in Moebius syndrome. J Med Genet 1991;28:413-414.

83. Kremer H, Kuyt LP, van der Helm B, et al: Localization of a gene for Möbius syndrome to chromosome 3q by linkage analysis in a Dutch family. Hum Mol Genet 1996;5:1367-1371.

84. Verzijl HT, van den Helm B, Veldman B, et al: A second gene for autosomal dominant Möbius syndrome is localized to chromosome 10q, in a Dutch family. Am J Hum Genet 1999;65:752-756.

85. Tandan R, Sharma KR, Bradley WG, et al: Chronic segmental spinal muscular atrophy of upper extremities in identical twins. Neurology 1990;40:236-239.

86. Ebinger F, Boor R, Brühl K, Reitter B: Cervical spinal cord atrophy in the atraumatically born neonate: One form of prenatal or perinatal ischaemic insult? Neuropediatrics 2003;34:45-51.

87. Kennedy WR, Alter M, Sung JH: Progressive proximal spinal and bulbar muscular atrophy of late onset. Neurology 1968;18:671-680.

88. Sperfeld AD, Karitzky J, Brummer D, et al: X-linked bulbospinal neuronopathy: Kennedy disease. Arch Neurol 2002;59:1921-1926.

89. La Spada AR, Wilson EM, Lubahn DB, et al: Androgen receptor gene mutations in X-linked spinal and bulbar muscular atrophy. Nature 1991;352:77-79.

90. Jana NR, Nukina N: Recent advances in understanding the pathogenesis of polyglutamine diseases: Involvement of molecular chaperones and ubiquitin-proteasome pathway. J Chem Neuroanat 2003;26:95-101.

91. Greenberg F, Fenolio KR, Hejtmancik JF, et al: X-linked infantile spinal muscular atrophy. Am J Dis Child 1988;142:217-219.

92. Kobayashi H, Baumbach L, Matise TC, et al: A gene for a severe lethal form of X-linked arthrogryposis (X-linked infantile spinal muscular atrophy) maps to human chromosome Xp11.3-q11.2. Hum Mol Genet 1995;4:1213-1216.

93. Visser J, van den Berg-Vos RM, Franssen H, et al: Mimic syndromes in sporadic cases of progressive spinal muscular atrophy. Neurology 2002;58:1593-1596.

94. Beevor CE: A case of congenital spinal muscular atrophy (family type), and a case of hæmorrhage into the spinal cord at birth, giving similar symptoms. Brain 1902;25:85-108.

95. Rousseau S, Metral S, Lacroix C, et al: Anterior spinal artery syndrome mimicking infantile spinal muscular atrophy. Am J Perinatol 1993;10:316-318.

96. Darwish H, Sarnat H, Archer C, et al: Congenital cervical spinal atrophy. Muscle Nerve 1981;4:106-110.

97. Aysun S, Cinbis M, Özcan OE: Intramedullary astrocytoma presenting as spinal muscular atrophy. J Child Neurol 1993;8:354-356.

98. Narbona J, Mestre M, Beguiristain JL, Martinez-Lage JM: Intramedullary telangiectasis causing congenital cervical spinal atrophy [Letter]. Muscle Nerve 1982;5:256.

99. Bergeisen GH, Bauman RJ, Gilmore RL: Neonatal paralytic poliomyelitis. Arch Neurol 1986;43:192-194.

100. Hopkins IJ: A new syndrome: poliomyelitis-like illness associated with acute asthma in childhood. Aust Paediatr J 1974;10:273-276.

101. Nihei K, Naitoh H, Ikeda K: Poliomyelitis-like syndrome following asthmatic attack (Hopkins syndrome). Pediatr Neurol 1987;3:166-168.

102. Wheeler SD, Ochoa J: Poliomyelitis-like syndrome associated with asthma: A case report and review of the literature. Arch Neurol 1980;37:52-53.

103. Lacomis D, Zochodne DW, Bird SJ, et al: Critical illness myopathy. Muscle Nerve 2000;23:1785-1788.

104. Barth PG: Pontocerebellar hypoplasias: An overview of a group of inherited neurodegenerative disorders with fetal onset. Brain Dev 1993;15:411-422.

105. Rudnik-Schöneborn S, Sztriha L, Aithala GR, et al: Extended phenotype of pontocerebellar hypoplasia with infantile spinal muscular atrophy [Abstract]. Am J Med Genet 2003;117A:10-17.

106. Sobue I, Saito N, Iida M, Ando K: Juvenile type of distal and segmental muscular atrophy of upper extremities. Ann Neurol 1978;3:429-432.

107. Chaine P, Bouche P, Leger JM, et al: [Progressive muscular atrophy localized in the hand: Monomelic form of motor neuron disease?] Rev Neurol (Paris) 1988;144:759-763.

108. Chen CJ, Hsu HL, Tseng YC, et al: Hirayama flexion myelopathy: Neutral-position MR imaging findings—importance of loss of attachment. Radiology 2004;231:39-44.

109. Nelson JS, Prensky AL: Sporadic juvenile amyotrophic lateral sclerosis: A clinicopathological study of a case with neuronal cytoplasmic inclusions containing RNA. Arch Neurol 1972;27:300-306.

110. Otero Siliceo E, Arriada-Mendicoa N, Balderrama J: Juvenile familial amyotrophic lateral sclerosis: Four cases with long survival. Dev Med Child Neurol 1998;40:425-428.

111. Grunnet ML, Donaldson JO: Juvenile multisystem degeneration with motor neuron involvement and eosinophilic intracytoplasmic inclusions. Arch Neurol 1985;42:1114-1116.

112. Rabin BA, Griffin JW, Crain BJ, et al: Autosomal dominant juvenile amyotrophic lateral sclerosis. Brain 1999;122:1539-1550.

113. Ikeda M, Abe K, Aoki M, et al: Variable clinical symptoms in familial amyotrophic lateral sclerosis with a novel point mutation in the Cu/Zn superoxide dismutase gene. Neurology 1995;45:2038-2042.

114. Auer-Grumbach M, Loscher WN, Wagner K, et al: Phenotypic and genotypic heterogeneity in hereditary motor neuronopathy type V: A clinical, electrophysiological and genetic study. Brain 2000;123:1612-1623.

115. van Gent EM, Hoogland RA, Jennekens FG: Distal amyotrophy of predominantly the upper limbs with

pyramidal features in a large kinship. J Neurol Neurosurg Psychiatry 1985;48:266-269.

116. McEntagart M, Norton N, Williams H, et al: Localization of the gene for distal hereditary motor neuronopathy (dHMN-VII) to chromosome 2q14. Am J Hum Genet 2001;68:1270-1276.

117. Rudnik-Schöneborn S, Wirth B, Zerres K: Evidence of autosomal dominant mutations in childhood-onset proximal spinal muscular atrophy. Am J Hum Genet 1994;55:112-119.

118. Cao A, Cainchetti C, Calisti L, Tangheroni W: A family of juvenile proximal spinal muscular atrophy with dominant inheritance. J Med Genet 1976;13:131-135.

119. Rudnik-Schöneborn S, Zerres K, Hahnen E, et al: Apparent autosomal recessive inheritance in families with proximal spinal muscular atrophy affecting individuals in two generations. Am J Hum Genet 1996;59:1163-1165.

120. Rietschel M, Rudnik-Schöneborn S, Zerres K: Clinical variability of autosomal dominant spinal muscular atrophy. J Neurol Sci 1992;107:65-73.

121. Richieri-Costa A, Rogatko A, Levisky R, et al: Autosomal dominant late adult spinal muscular atrophy, type Finkel. Am J Med Genet 1981;9:119-128.

122. Cobben JM, Scheffer H, de Visser M, et al: Apparent *SMAI* unlinked to 5q. J Med Genet 1994;31:242-244.

123. De Angelis MV, Gatta V, Stuppia L, et al: Autosomal dominant distal spinal muscular atrophy: An Italian family not linked to 12q24 and 7p14. Neuromuscul Disord 2002;12:26-30.

124. van den Berg-Vos RM, van den Berg LH, Jansen GH, et al: Hereditary pure lower motor neuron disease with adult onset and rapid progression. J Neurol 2001; 248:290-296.

125. Fleury P, Hageman G: A dominantly inherited lower motor neuron disorder presenting at birth with associated arthrogryposis. J Neurol Neurosurg Psychiatry 1985;48:1037-1048.

126. Frijns CJ, Van Deutekom J, Frants RR, Jennekens FG: Dominant congenital benign spinal muscular atrophy. Muscle Nerve 1994;17:192-197.

127. van der Vleuten AJ, Ravenswaaij-Arts CM, Frijns CJ, et al: Localisation of the gene for a dominant congenital spinal muscular atrophy predominantly affecting the lower limbs to chromosome 12q23-q24. Eur J Hum Genet 1998;6:376-382.

128. Christodoulou K, Zamba E, Tsingis M, et al: A novel form of distal hereditary motor neuronopathy maps to chromosome 9p21.1-p12. Ann Neurol 2000;48:877-884.

129. Hageman G, Ramaekers VT, Hilhorst BG, Rozeboom AR: Congenital cervical spinal muscular atrophy: A non-familial, non progressive condition of the upper limbs. J Neurol Neurosurg Psychiatry 1993;56:365-368.

130. DeLong R, Siddique T: A large New England kindred with autosomal dominant neurogenic scapuloperoneal amyotrophy with unique features. Arch Neurol 1992;49:905-908.

131. Isozumi K, DeLong R, Kaplan J, et al: Linkage of scapuloperoneal spinal muscular atrophy to chromosome 12q24.1-q24.31. Hum Mol Genet 1996;5:1377-1382.

132. Summers BA, Swash M, Schwartz MS, Ingram DA: Juvenile-onset bulbospinal muscular atrophy with deafness: Vialetta-van Laere syndrome or Madras-type motor neuron disease? J Neurol 1987;234:440-442.

133. Yang Y, Hentati A, Deng HX, et al: The gene encoding alsin, a protein with three guanine-nucleotide exchange factor domains, is mutated in a form of recessive amyotrophic lateral sclerosis. Nat Genet 2001;29:160-165.

134. Hadano S, Hand CK, Osuga H, et al: A gene encoding a putative GTPase regulator is mutated in familial amyotrophic lateral sclerosis 2. Nat Genet 2001;29:166-173.

135. De Jonghe P, Auer-Grumbach M, Irobi J, et al: Autosomal dominant juvenile amyotrophic lateral sclerosis and distal hereditary motor neuronopathy with pyramidal tract signs: Synonyms for the same disorder? Brain 2002;125:1320-1325.

136. Chance PF, Rabin BA, Ryan SG, et al: Linkage of the gene for an autosomal dominant form of juvenile amyotrophic lateral sclerosis to chromosome 9q34. Am J Hum Genet 1998;62:633-640.

137. Hamano K, Tsukamoto H, Yazawa T, et al: Infantile progressive spinal muscular atrophy with ophthalmplegia and pyramidal symptoms. Pediatr Neurol 1994;10:320-324.

138. Larsen R, Ashwal S, Peckham N: Incontinentia pigmenti: Association with anterior horn cell degeneration. Neurology 1987;37:446-450.

139. Pascual-Castroviejo I, Roche C, Martinez-Bermejo A, et al: Hypomelanosis of ITO: A study of 76 infantile cases. Brain Dev 1998;20:36-43.

140. Goodman WN, Cooper WC, Kessler GB, et al: Ataxia-telangiectasia: A report of two cases in siblings presenting a picture of progressive spinal muscular atrophy. Bull Los Angeles Neurol Soc 1969;34:1-22.

141. Mancuso M, Salviati L, Sacconi S, et al: Mitochondrial DNA depletion: Mutations in thymidine kinase gene with myopathy and SMA. Neurology 2002;59:1197-1202.

142. Pons R, Andreetta F, Wang CH, et al: Mitochondrial myopathy simulating spinal muscular atrophy. Pediatr Neurol 1996;15:153-158.

143. Rubio-Gozalbo ME, Smeitink JA, Ruitenbeek W, et al: Spinal muscular atrophy-like picture, cardiomyopathy, and cytochrome c oxidase deficiency. Neurology 1999;52:383-386.

144. Salviati L, Sacconi S, Rasalan MM, et al: Cytochrome c oxidase deficiency due to a novel *SCO2* mutation mimics Werdnig-Hoffmann disease. Arch Neurol 2002;59:862-865.

145. Halperin JJ, Williams RS, Kolodny EH: Microcephaly vera, progressive motor neuron disease, and nigral degeneration. Neurology 1982;32:317-320.

146. Spiro AJ, Fogelson MH, Goldberg AC: Microcephaly and mental subnormality in chronic progressive spinal muscular atrophy of childhood. Dev Med Child Neurol 1967;9:594-601.

147. Staal A, Went LN, Busch HF: An unusual form of spinal muscular atrophy with mental retardation occurring in an inbred population. J Neurol Sci 1975;25:57-64.

148. Görgen-Pauly U, Sperner J, Reiss I, et al: Familial pontocerebellar hypoplasia type I with anterior horn cell disease. Eur J Paediatr Neurol 1999;3:33-38.

149. Muntoni F, Goodwin F, Sewry C, et al: Clinical spectrum and diagnostic difficulties of infantile ponto-cerebellar hypoplasia type 1. Neuropediatrics 1999;30:243-248.

150. Ryan MM, Cooke-Yarborough CM, Procopis PG, Ouvrier RA: Anterior horn cell disease and olivopontocerebellar hypoplasia. Pediatr Neurol 2000;23:180-184.

151. Adams C, Becker LE, Murphy EG: Neurogenic arthrogryposis multiplex congenita: Clinical and muscle biopsy findings. Pediatr Neurosci 1988;14:97-102.

152. Courtens W, Johansson AB, Dachy B, et al: Infantile spinal muscular atrophy variant with congenital fractures in a female neonate: Evidence for autosomal recessive inheritance. J Med Genet 2002;39:74-77.

153. Kelly TE, Amoroso K, Ferre M, et al: Spinal muscular atrophy variant with congenital fractures. Am J Med Genet 1999;87:65-68.

154. Van Toorn R, Davies J, Wilmshurst JM: Spinal muscular atrophy with congenital fractures: Postmortem analysis. J Child Neurol 2002;17:721-723.

155. Haliloglu G, Chattopadhyay A, Skorodis L, et al: Spinal muscular atrophy with progressive myoclonic epilepsy: Report of new cases and review of the literature. Neuropediatrics 2002;33:314-319.

31

Plexopathies and Nerve Root Lesions

Thomas A. Miller and H. Royden Jones, Jr.

Overview

Children much more commonly experience disorders of the brachial plexus (BP) than either a femoral-lumbosacral plexus disorder or, rarely, a cervical or lumbosacral radiculopathy (LSR). The superficial nature of the BP makes it a common site for injury subsequent to many types of neonatal, childhood, or adolescent trauma, including child abuse. Other less common mechanisms include various inflammatory, autoimmune, neoplastic, and iatrogenic sources. The importance of electrodiagnostic testing and its relationship to clinical neurophysiology are emphasized in this chapter. This section discusses the relevant anatomy and diagnostic procedures to provide an understanding and emphasis on the electrodiagnostic assessment of preganglionic and postganglionic pathology.

Anatomy

The electromyographer's ability to appreciate the intricacies of the BP anatomy determines how successful she or he may be in finding an answer to what are sometimes relatively subtle diagnostic challenges. This is particularly important when evaluating children because the opportunity to examine multiple nerves and muscles is obviously more limited than in adults. Pediatric electromyographers are often well served by reviewing the intricacies of the plexus anatomy prior to commencing an electromyogram (EMG) for a presumed plexopathy. A more precise understanding of these anatomic details increases the opportunities to solve the child's clinical problem. A series of five anatomic plates are included here for that purpose (Figs. 31-1 to 31-5).

Nerve Roots

There are a total of 31 nerve root pairs: 8 in the cervical region with just seven vertebrae, 12 thoracic, 5 lumbar, and 5 sacral. In the cervical spine each nerve root exits above the cervical vertebral body, with the exception being that the 8th root exists below C7 and above T1. Subsequently, all nerve roots exit below their numbered vertebra.

At each level there is an anterior (ventral) and a posterior (dorsal) root (see Fig. 31-1). The anterior (somatic motor) and posterior (sensory) roots join at the intervertebral foramen to form the spinal nerve. As is shown in Figure 31-1 the anterior horn cells of the spinal level provide the cells of origin of the anterior somatic motor root contribution to the spinal nerve. Just distal to the intervertebral foramen, the spinal nerve bifurcates into the anterior and posterior primary rami. The **anterior primary rami** innervate the muscles in the extremities (**myotomes**), whereas the posterior primary rami innervate the paraspinal musculature. In contrast, the sensory component relates to the **posterior dorsal root**, providing the source for the sensation to the skin (**dermatome**). The posterior primary rami innervate the paraspinal muscles as well as the skin of the neck, trunk, and back. The primary sensory neurons originate in the dorsal root ganglion at the level of the intervertebral foramina. This anatomic feature is crucial in understanding the EMG findings when making the differentiation between a preganglionic and a postganglionic lesion (see Fig. 31-2).

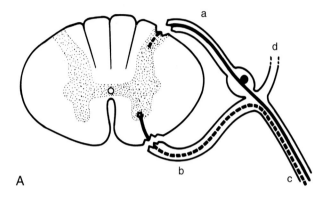

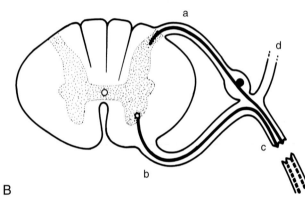

FIGURE 31–1

Configuration of vertebrae and nerve root. A, *Preganglionic lesion.* B, *Postganglionic lesion.* a, dorsal root; b, ventral root; c, anterior primary ramus; d, posterior primary ramus. (A and B, From Jones HR Jr: Radiculopathies and plexopathies. In Jones HR Jr, De Vivo DC, Darras BT [eds]: Neuromuscular Disorders of Infancy, Childhood, and Adolescence: A Clinician's Approach. Philadelphia, Butterworth Heinemann Health, 2003, p 234.)*

At or very near its origin, the anterior primary ramus receives a contribution, the gray ramus communicans, from the corresponding sympathetic trunk ganglion. In addition, the first thoracic anterior primary ramus contributes preganglionic sympathetic fibers to the inferior cervical (stellate) ganglion via a white ramus communicans.

Injury to these fibers produces Horner's syndrome (unilateral miosis, ptosis, enophthalmos, and facial anhidrosis). It is crucial to look for evidence of Horner's syndrome in any child with a BP lesion because, unfortunately, this is consistent with the poor prognosis of an avulsion of the preganglionic spinal root and nerve entry zone at the T1 level. The relative EMG characteristics of a preganglionic lesion are outlined in Figure 31-5.

Brachial Plexus

The nerve supply to the entire upper extremity and most of the shoulder girdle originates in the BP and its contiguous nerve roots C5 to T1. This consists of the following components:

1. Five roots (C5 to T1)
2. Three trunks (upper, middle, and lower)
3. Two divisions (consisting of six elements in all)
4. Three cords (lateral, posterior, and medial)
5. Various terminal nerves particularly the axillary, musculocutaneous, radial, median, and ulnar (see Fig. 31-3)

The following clinically significant peripheral nerves originate supraclavicularly or very proximal in the BP:

1. The *dorsal scapular nerve* arises from the C5 anterior primary ramus, near the intervertebral foramen, and innervates the rhomboid muscle. Denervation in the

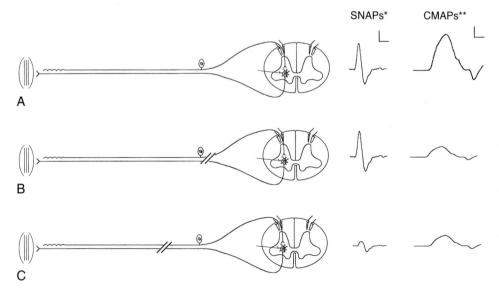

FIGURE 31–2

Sensory and motor potentials in axonal lesions distal and proximal to the dorsal root ganglion. A, *Normal.* B, *Lesion proximal to the dorsal root ganglion.* C, *Lesion distal to the dorsal root ganglion.* *Sensory nerve action potentials (SNAPs), **Compound motor action potentials (CMAPs) (A to C, From Preston DC, Shapiro BE: Electromyography and Neuromuscular Disorders: Clinical-Electrophysiologic Correlations. Woburn, MA, Butterworth, 1998, p 419.)*

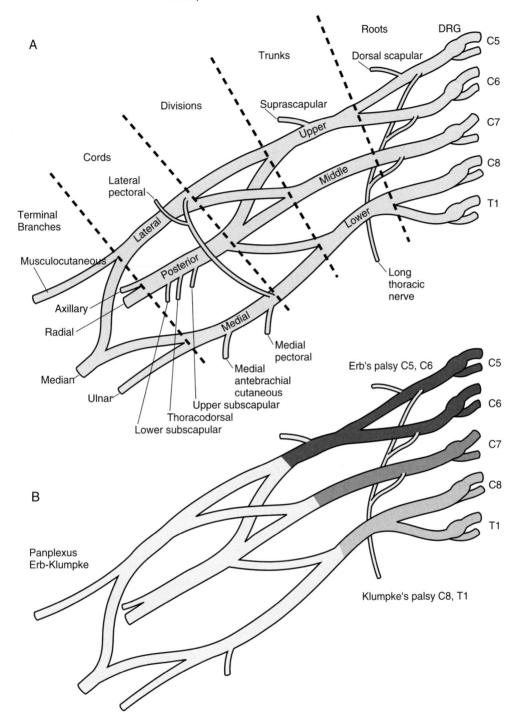

FIGURE 31–3

A, Schematic representation of the brachial plexus with its terminal branches. B, The most common pediatric plexus injury is the C5-6 *palsy also known as Erb's palsy; occasionally,* C7 *is also affected. The second most common palsy is a pan-plexus injury (Erb-Klumpke). A rare isolated palsy of the C8-T1 segment is commonly referred to as Klumpke's palsy. (A and B, From Brown WF, Bolton CF, Aminoff MJ [eds]: Neuromuscular Function and Disease. Philadelphia, WB Saunders, 2002, p 1603.)*

SENSORY   **MOTOR**

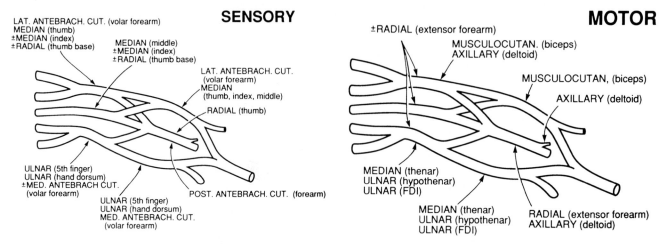

FIGURE 31–4

The primary sensory and motor components of the brachial plexus and their specific peripheral nerve derivatives. (From Wilbourn AJ: Brachial plexus disorders. In Dyck PJ, Thomas PK, Griffin JW, et al [eds]: Peripheral Neuropathy, 3rd ed. Philadelphia, WB Saunders, 1993, p 922.)

rhomboids is often a poor prognostic sign for a child with a BP lesion. This finding suggests a proximal lesion, particularly including the possibility of C5 root avulsion.

2. The *long thoracic nerve* originates from the C5, C6, and C7 anterior primary rami. It primarily innervates the serratus anterior muscle. Scapula winging is the usual manifestation of weakness of this muscle secondary to long thoracic nerve injury. This is often difficult to recognize in newborns but, again, is associated with a proximal lesion.

3. The *suprascapular nerve* innervates both the supraspinatus and infraspinatus muscles and is the only nerve derived from the upper trunk. No nerves are derived from the middle or lower trunks nor any of the primary divisions.

The three major BP cords each provide the primary source for the various individual nerves of the arm with the exception of the conjoint origin of the median nerve from both the lateral and medial cords. The lateral cord (C5-C6 source) of the BP is the origin for the *musculocutaneous nerve*, the *lateral head of the median nerve*, and the *lateral pectoral nerves*. The *ulnar* and *medial head of the median nerves* as well as the *medial pectoral, medial brachial*, and *antebrachial cutaneous nerves* are each derived from the medial cord (C8-T1 source) of this plexus. Finally, the posterior cord (C6-C7 source) gives rise to the *subscapular, thoracodorsal, axillary*, and *radial nerves* (see Fig. 31-3). Thus, the predominant terminal branches of the three BP cords are the axillary, musculocutaneous, radial, median, and ulnar nerves.

Lumbosacral Plexus

Although the generic term *lumbosacral plexus* (LSP) is used as a means of logical organization, on occasion the clinical lesion may predominate in either the lumbar or sacral plexus (Fig. 31-6). This is more clearly defined in adults than in children, where these LSP variants sometimes appear to be almost separate anatomic structures. However, in pediatric patients, a significant overlap is seen, probably the result of the relatively small body size. This emphasizes the contiguous nature of this plexus of nerves in the infant and young child.

The *femoral* nerve is the predominant nerve to arise from the lumbar portion of the LSP primarily innervating the iliopsoas, quadriceps femoris, and sartorius muscles. The obturator is the other major nerve derived from the lumbar portion of this plexus. It innervates the proximal 80% of the adductor magnus. The latter muscle also receives some distal innervation from the sciatic nerve. This mixed innervation of the adductor is particularly important when evaluating potential sciatic nerve lesions. One must not be misled by signs of denervation in the distal adductor, as well as other primary sciatic innervated muscles, and then falsely conclude that a plexus lesion is present.

The sacral portion of the LSP innervates the remainder of the leg, including the posterior thigh and buttocks muscles as well as the entire leg below the knee. These nerves include the superior and inferior gluteal nerves, which innervate the gluteus medius, and minimus and gluteus maximus, respectively. The medial and lateral hamstrings are supplied by the sciatic nerve (with its respective peroneal and tibial divisions). It functionally divides into the peroneal and tibial nerves, and most of its remaining motor

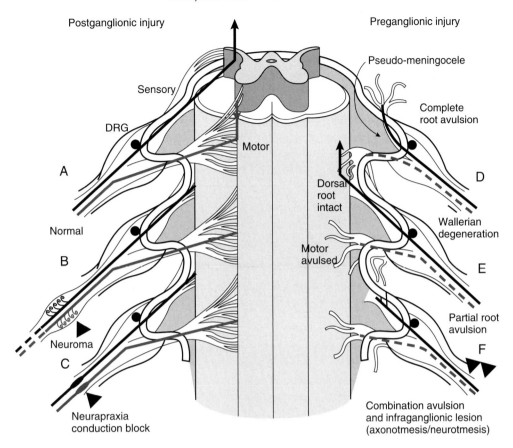

FIGURE 31-5

Schematic representation of the normal anatomy of and injuries to the roots of plexus, demonstrating the typical preganglionic and postganglionic abnormalities that are possible. A, Normal ventral (motor) rootlets and dorsal (sensory) rootlets. B, Postganglionic injury (axonotmesis or neurotmesis) with neuroma formation and partial or complete disconnection of neural elements. Continuity can be determined only by intraoperative neurophysiology across damaged segments. The compound muscle action potentials (CMAPs) and sensory nerve action potentials (SNAPs) from the corresponding territory will be abnormal (amplitude decreased owing to axonal loss). C, A neurapraxic lesion resulting in abnormal sensation and weakness but normal SNAPs and CMAPs distal to the area of focal conduction block. Conduction intraoperatively across the segment may be blocked. D, Preganglionic injury with complete avulsion and traumatic pseudomeningocele seen on imaging. The cell body of the sensory neuron is intact (dorsal root ganglion); therefore, a normal SNAP is recorded in an asensate territory. CMAPs will be absent or nonrecordable. E, Partial root avulsion with dorsal root intact and ventral (motor) root avulsed. This produces weakness and normal sensation and a normal SNAP with absent or abnormal CMAPs in respective segmental distribution. F, Combination of a preganglionic and postganglionic lesion, which often can be determined only intraoperatively and correlated with imaging. The roots (motor and sensory) have been avulsed, but the infraganglionic component is also abnormal (axonotmesis-neurotmesis), similar to B. Therefore, the SNAPs and CMAPs are absent or abnormal. This can mislead electromyographers into thinking that the lesion is infraganglionic, and they might miss the preganglionic injury. (A to F, From Brown WF, Bolton CF, Aminoff MJ [eds]: Neuromuscular Function and Disease. Philadelphia, WB Saunders, 2002, p 1604.)

innervation is below the knee, with the exception of the short head of the biceps femoris. The short head of biceps is a useful muscle electromyographicaly because it is innervated by the peroneal nerve (lateral portion of the sciatic nerve) proximal to the knee.

This nerve then proceeds to bifurcate at the knee into the superficial and the deep peroneal nerves. These two branches of the peroneal nerves supply all of the anterior compartment of the lower leg. In contrast, the tibial nerve, the other primary derivative of the sciatic nerve, supplies the posterior compartment. The primary superficial sensory nerves derived from the peroneal and tibial, respectively, are the superficial peroneal and the sural and plantar nerves.

Histologically the LSP is similar to that of other peripheral nerves.[1,2] The epineurium occupies approximately 45% to 65% of the total cross-sectional area of the nerve

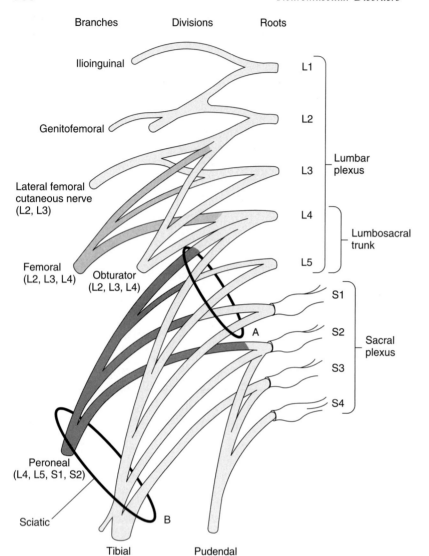

Branches   Divisions   Roots

FIGURE 31–6

The lumbosacral plexus (A). *The most common sites affected include femoral and the lumbosacral trunk* (B). *(From Brown WF, Bolton CF, Aminoff MJ [eds]: Neuromuscular Function and Disease. Philadelphia, WB Saunders, 2002, p 1623.)*

roots of the LSP and is more condensed toward the periphery.[3] The relatively higher connective tissue content in the L5 and S1 roots as well as the lumbosacral trunk may contribute to their inherent strength. These factors provide a cushion against any untoward deforming forces. The relatively higher incidence of injury to L5, the lumbosacral trunk, and the S1 trunk is not likely due to any microscopic differences but rather to their close proximity to the sacrum and sacroiliac joint.[3]

PRINCIPLES OF EMG EVALUATION

The importance of electrodiagnostic testing and its relationship to clinical assessment, imaging, rehabilitation, and surgical options are emphasized. We highlight the

---

BOX 31-1
EMG GOALS WITH BRACHIAL PLEXUS PALSY OF THE NEWBORN

Determine level and extent of involvement of individual components.
Differentiate a preganglionic lesion and/or root avulsion.
Define the nature of the lesion (see Box 31-2).

---

various clinical challenges in the assessment and treatment of neonatal plexus lesions. In the evaluation of an infant with a possible BP lesion, the goals are similar to those in the adult population. These are outlined in Box 31-1.

BOX 31-2
TYPES OF PERIPHERAL NERVE LESIONS

Neurapraxia: demyelination, but intact axons
Axonotmesis: axonal injury, but intact nerve sheath
Neurotmesis: transection of entire nerve

Adapted from Sunderland S: The anatomy and physiology of nerve injury. Muscle Nerve 1990;13:771-784.

The nature and pathophysiologic response to nerve injury are outlined in Box 31-2; appropriate use of these results provides information allowing the electromyographer to form a prognostic opinion (see Fig. 31-5).

One of the most useful EMG criteria for differentiation between a nerve root (i.e., preganglionic) and postganglionic plexus lesion is often technically impossible in the pediatric population, especially newborns. Traditionally, nerve root avulsion or preganglionic lesions are suggested by the preservation of sensory nerve action potentials (SNAPs) in an asensate area and/or in the area of a significant clinical loss of sensory function. However, the determination of sensory loss on clinical examination of infants and toddlers, is possible. It is also more common for neonatal plexus lesions to have conjoint preganglionic and postganglionic components. Therefore, an avulsion, with its inherently poor prognosis, may be present despite the absence of SNAPs in the appropriate segment. This makes it impossible to provide an absolute EMG opinion as to whether or not a root avulsion is present (see Fig. 31-5E).[4]

Furthermore, the use of paraspinal needle EMG examination (NEE) is almost always technically impossible in the neonate because of the baby's inherent inability to relax these muscles, and the same applies to a lesser degree in older children. In most instances it is at best challenging, and usually not technically feasible, for an electromyographer to provide a definitive opinion about the presence of denervation potentials in this setting. Finally, even in the ideal case, one cannot comment on the specific cervical level owing to the significant segmental overlap within the paravertebral musculature.

Magnetic resonance imaging (MRI) of the cervical spinal cord and the BP provides excellent imaging possibilities. This is helpful for defining the presence of avulsed nerve roots, particularly in those babies who have combined preganglionic and postganglionic lesions (Fig. 31-7).

The technical challenges of recording CMAPs and SNAPs are described in Chapter 6. The recording of motor and sensory conduction studies from the median and ulnar nerves allows a comment on the lower trunk and medial cord. Radial motor and sensory studies provide

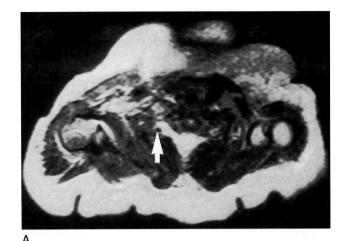

A

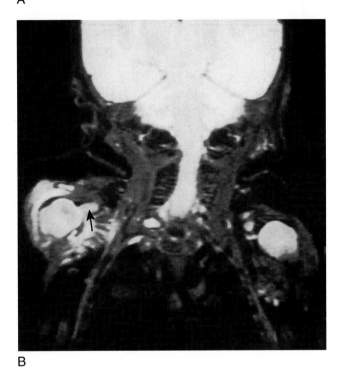

B

FIGURE 31–7

A, *Coronal STIR fat-suppression MRI scan indicative of a pseudomeningocele secondary to nerve root avulsion on the right side* (arrow). B, *Axial T2-weighted MRI shows the pseudomeningocele from the nerve root avulsion* (arrow). (A and B, From Mancias P, Slopis JM, Yeakley JW, Vriesendorp FJ: Combined brachial plexus injury and root avulsion after complicated delivery [Letter]. Muscle Nerve 1994;17:1237-1238.)

information on the posterior cord and stimulation at Erb's point recording from the musculocutaneous innervated biceps muscle can allow comment on the continuity of the upper trunk and specifically that of the lateral cord. Wilbourn has emphasized the value of using the thumb to record median sensory fibers from the upper trunk. He noted that this provides an equally effective evaluation as the lateral antebrachial cutaneous nerve from the volar aspect of the radial forearm.[5,6] This is sometimes technically difficult with neonates to 1 year of age because of the limited size of the thumb. However, in the toddler (18 to 24 months) it is generally our experience that the thumb provides an excellent site to evaluate sensory function of this portion of the BP. Sensory function of the median nerve, recording from the middle finger (a digit that is large enough to permit the use of two electrodes at sufficient distance for a technically adequate response), is a good starting point. A comparative study between the involved and uninvolved contralateral limb often provides the most accurate information. Volume conduction and issues of impedance are other technical factors that require careful attention.

Because of the wide range of normal compound muscle action potential (CMAP) and SNAP amplitudes, as well as nerve conduction values, depending on age and maturation (as outlined in the Chapter 6 appendices) the precise definition of an abnormality in an individual baby is sometimes difficult to determine. There are limited data available about the use of long-latency waves in children, particularly with BP palsies of the newborn (BPPNs). However, H reflexes have recently been added to the assessment of these lesions by recording them from the brachioradialis muscle.[7] Parenthetically H reflexes are normally found only in the upper extremities during early life, generally disappearing at ages 6 to 12 months. Comparison with the apparently normal opposite side is sometimes potentially helpful; however, the electromyographer is usually pressed to complete the detailed analysis of the affected extremity. Therefore one generally needs to reach a clinical conclusion based on the relevant and available EMG data.

The use of nerve action potentials (NAPs) from the median and ulnar nerves potentially provides a more definitive technique than do digital SNAP recordings in small infants.[8-10] Supramaximal stimulation is used to obtain a mixed NAP, providing a more definite means for comparison of amplitudes (i.e., axonal loss) with the contralateral limb. This is potentially a good complementary technique for determining axonal continuity in the neonatal period.[8] It also correlates well with outcome.[11] One of the writers of this chapter (H.R.J.) has not had personal experience with this technique to date. One can ask whether, considering the need for maximal strength stimuli, and thus for unequivocal sedation, there is a role for NAP when we have the complementary MRI available. As one attempts to better define the prognostic value of EMG and MRI in these relatively uncommon settings, it will be a challenge to gain enough information to make more specific recommendations.

An appreciation of the precise temporal profile of the neurogenic insult and its consequent effect on the BP is crucial for understanding the specific pathophysiologic characteristics of nerve damage (i.e., whether one is dealing with neurapraxia, axonotmesis, or neurotmesis). Although standards are set after acute neurotmesis in adults as to the temporal profile for the loss of CMAPs and SNAPs and the appearance of fibrillation potentials, a similar set of findings for these acute nerve conduction studies (NCSs) and needle EMG changes has not been carefully defined in children and infants. This is not because of our own lack of interest. Rather this relates to both the relative rarity of these lesions as well as our inability to choose the timing of the study, let alone our own as well as the parents' resistance to performing multiple studies on these babies. In adults CMAP responses usually disappear within 4 or 5 days and definitely within a week of complete axonal disruption.[5] The temporal relationship for the loss of SNAPs is longer, about 10 days, in adults.[12]

As with the adult who has sustained a brachial plexopathy, the needle electrodiagnostic examination (NEE) is of the utmost importance for defining the degree of BP injury. When studying infants and children, the examiner needs to be both careful and economical in the performance of the study. Concomitantly, it is important to be thorough enough to provide the referring clinician with an adequate study. Ideally the EMG will provide both anatomic and functional information as to the presence or absence of axonal damage. To do so accurately, one needs to know the precise timing for the onset of positive waves and fibrillation potentials in the infant. For the older child this is assumed to be similar to that of the adult, namely 10 to 14 days.[5,6,13] However, in the neonate and young infant, few studies have attempted to define the first appearance of EMG signs of denervation with sequential NEE. The timing of the onset of denervation depends on both the severity of nerve lesion and the length of nerve between muscle and the site of injury. The short distances and smaller diameter axons makes the cross-section in infants 2.5 times less. Compared with the 10- to 14-day adult period until appearance of denervation activity, a period of 1 to 2 days or even less may be expected in infants.[14,15]

In a single case, Mancias and colleagues documented the results of such an evaluation in a 4-day-old infant.[16] This baby had both an avulsion and concomitant plexus damage as defined by an MRI (see Fig. 31-7). Mancias and colleagues' results suggest that positive waves are seen in the newborn as early as the fourth postinjury day. In addition, Gerald Herbison, MD, a colleague of one author (H.R.J.), evaluated a newborn with what was most likely an intrauterine onset of a peroneal neuropathy. This baby had lost both his peroneal CMAP and had active denervation identified at age 18 hours, both believed to be indicative of a prenatal lesion.[17] A few other authors have demonstrated signs of very early denervation and EMG patterns consistent with a "prenatally" occurring lesion.[18-20] Thus, when confronted with a baby younger than 4 days old who has both lost her or his CMAPs and has fibrillation potentials present, one cannot exclude the possibility that this lesion had an intrauterine onset even though the early onset of fibrillation potentials have been reproduced in an animal model. Gonik and colleagues demonstrated denervation at 24 hours after transection in a newborn pig. They also found a proximal-to-distal gradient and correlation with nerve length.[21] Therefore two possible mechanisms may account for the earlier appearance of denervation potentials in the neonate. These include short distances from the site of the injury and an immature peripheral nervous system.

BRACHIAL PLEXUS PALSIES OF THE NEWBORN

Typically obstetricians are cited as being responsible for so-called obstetrical palsies when there is a newborn with a BP lesion. This is presumably because of their having placed lateral traction on the baby's head to facilitate the delivery of the shoulder. Much of the literature refers to these as *obstetric palsy*, a term coined by Duchenne de Boulogne in 1872.[22] This terminology unfortunately also has been adopted by lawyers and now inappropriately suggests one (i.e., the obstetrician) is guilty until proven innocent of medical malfeasance when a baby is born with such a lesion. Most likely an occasional obstetric misadventure may account for some BPPNs, especially in the setting of a macrosomic infant whose vaginal delivery is complicated by shoulder dystocia. We suggest that one needs to treat these disorders as any other BP lesion, exploring all diagnostic possibilities without prejudice.

Therefore, we believe that the term *obstetric palsy* should be retired. It has caused undue bias for more than 100 years. The physician must retain an absolutely open diagnostic mind when looking into the primary etiologic aspects of every infant with a BPPN.

The definition of alternative in utero etiologies for a mononeuropathy,[17,20,23] as well as those babies whose Erb's palsy occurred concomitant with a cesarean section, serves to provide consideration of alternative mechanisms in some instances rather than direct obstetrician-induced injury.[19,24-28] Recognizing that autoimmune Guillain-Barré syndrome is well documented to occur in newborns,[29-32] one has to ask whether indeed another autoimmune peripheral nerve lesion can occur in utero, namely a Parsonage-Turner syndrome–type brachial plexopathy.[33] Similarly, if a neonate can develop a streptococcal-induced

BP lesion as early as age 10 to 20 days, it may be possible that other infectious processes could account for an occasional intrauterine-onset plexopathy in a newborn.[34]

To better understand these clinical neurophysiologic challenges, we suggest that obstetricians and pediatricians in the future request sequential EMG recordings beginning within 24 hours of birth of an infant with a brachial plexopathy. Until we gain more information as to what the possibilities are, one must be cautious in assessing etiology. The EMG laboratory will not only be able to further define the timing of onset of signs of denervation in these neonates but also provide a means to accurately provide a clinical correlation as to whether a baby's Erb's palsy is truly a birth-related versus a potentially intrauterine antenatal process. When enough of these data are compiled, these findings will allow us to provide a more accurate comment regarding the natural history of neonatal BPs. It is clear that multiple factors, including the medicolegal implications of these EMG observations, regarding the temporal profile of the onset of fibrillation potentials and loss of CMAPs, occurring in neonates less than age 1 week with a BP injury, merits further study.

There is a potential discrepancy between the clinical examination and the EMG findings, as the EMG presage clinical improvement. These discrepancies further add to the controversial opinions in the literature with regard to the benefit of open repair. For example, the presence of motor unit action potentials (MUAPs) in a clinically paralyzed muscle suggests to the electromyographer an incomplete lesion or signs of reinnervation.

If the presence of MUAPs at 3 months of age indicates a functional contact with axons, why is this not always associated with clinically observable movements? Box 31-3 is a summary of the excellent review by Van Dijk and colleagues.[14,15]

Clinical Aspects of Brachial Plexus Palsies of the Newborn

Historical

Brachial palsies occurring at birth were first described by Smellie in 1768 citing a case of bilateral arm paralysis at birth that rapidly resolved in a matter of days. Duchenne de Boulogne in 1872 described four neonates with the typical unilateral BPPN palsy, attributing the injury to traction on the arm.[35,36] Erb, in 1874, reported electrical stimulation of the BP in both normal individuals, and BPPN. He described the typical upper root palsy localizing the lesion to the junction of the C5-C6 roots with the upper trunk of the BP. Erb acknowledged Duchenne's prior description and cited his own neonatal cases attributing them to pressure on the plexus during delivery. Thus, the classic upper BP palsy, first described by

BOX 31-3
EXPLANATIONS FOR APPARENT CLINICAL INACTIVITY OF MUPs IN BIRTH-RELATED BPs

Overly pessimistic clinical examination (inadequacy of clinical examination)

Overestimation of the number of MUAPs, per se.

Luxury innervation (i.e., muscle fibers are equipped with more than one neuromuscular synapse during early stages of fetal development)

Central motor disorders concept of apraxia

Abnormal nerve branching and misdirection

MUAP, motor unit action potential; BP, brachial plexus.
Adapted from van Dijk JG, Pondaag W, Malessy MJ: Obstetric lesions of the brachial plexus. Muscle Nerve 2001;24:1451-1461.

Duchenne, bears the name *Erb's palsy*, although some still more appropriately refer to this entity as an Erb-Duchenne palsy. In 1885, Klumpke described the lower root C8-T1 BP paralysis associated with concomitant sympathetic fiber involvement manifested by Horner's syndrome.[35] When the entire plexus is affected (i.e., a pan-plexus injury) it is referred to as an *Erb-Klumpke paralysis* (Fig. 31-8).

Incidence

BPPNs have an incidence varying from 0.9 to 2.3 per 1000 live births.[15,37-40] In New York there was a decreasing BPPN incidence between 1938 (1.56 per 1000 live births) to 1963 (0.38 per 1000 live births).[41] In a 1973 American report an "anterospective" collective perinatal study from 12 centers primarily caring for low-income families demonstrated a 1.89 instance per 1000 live births. These pregnancies were associated with a markedly increased incidence of antepartum complications. Later studies estimated that neonatal brachial plexopathies occur much less frequently (0.4 and 0.67, respectively, per 1000 births).[27,28,42] However, as recently as 1999 the BPPN incidence in California was 1.5 in 1000.[43] The incidence of plexopathies, relating to birthweights, was almost three times more common (2.6 in 1000) for newborns who weighed more than 4500 gm.[44]

Classification of BPPNs

These lesions are best classified on an anatomic neurologic basis at 2 to 3 weeks of age.[45,46] (Box 31-4). Paralysis of the upper roots—group I (Erb's palsy)—and complete paralysis—group IV (Erb-Klumpke paralysis)—are the predominant two types (see Fig. 31-8), whereas Klumpke's palsy is an exceedingly rare (0.6%) form of all BPPNs.[47] The incidence of the classic Erb's palsy (upper trunk and lateral cord) versus the other types of BP injuries ranges from 81.5% to 99.8%.[37,42,47,48]

Risk Factors

The large baby (>4000 gm) who has had a vertex delivery with an associated shoulder dystocia presents the most common setting for a BPPN.[47,49] Other major risk factors are summarized in Box 31-5. These are detailed earlier.[36,43,44,49-53] Less commonly a BPPN occurs in some low-birthweight babies born in a breech position.[47,54,55]

The knowledge of risk factors would be most useful if it were to provide a means to prevent a BPPN. To date prenatal prediction of the risk of shoulder dystocia in large-birthweight fetuses is difficult and imprecise. Kay stated that "it seems unlikely that we are any nearer preventative strategies for this rare complication."[44,55,57,58] Although a 52-fold increased rate of BPPN occurs in macrosomic newborns of diabetic mothers, delivered by instrumentation, 92% of these babies were delivered vaginally without complications.[59] Furthermore, and possibly paradoxically, a BPPN occasionally occurs after caesarean section.[60] Rarely, fetal positioning and intrauterine amniotic bands may contribute to the presence of a BPPN.[9,61] Engineering force analysis demonstrates that, in the presence of a shoulder dystocia, endogenous forces (i.e., uterine and maternal expulsive efforts) are four to nine times greater when contrasted with exogenous forces such as clinically applied traction to the fetal head.[62]

Clinical Examination

The evaluation of a baby with a BPPN is often difficult and imprecise. A baby with classic Erb's palsy lies with the affected arm limp at her or his side with the shoulder adducted, internally rotated, elbow extended, forearm pronated, fingers and wrists flexed—a characteristic posture referred to as "porter's tip." The shoulder is adducted secondary to paralysis of the deltoid, teres minor, infraspinatus, and supraspinatus muscles. Shoulder internal rotation occurs due to the unopposed contraction of the pectoralis, latissimus dorsi as well as the subscapularis muscles. Elbow extension results from the effect of gravity as well as paralysis of the elbow flexors (biceps, brachialis, and brachioradialis [C5-C6]). Paralysis of the supinator and biceps leads to forearm pronation (C5-C6). The flexed wrist and fingers occur because the wrist extensors are weakened also (C5-C6) (Fig. 31-9). A number of authors have suggested a more global assessment of upper limb function, allowing a predictive as well as prognostic clinical tool. One refinement designed to study recovery com-

Brachial Plexus and/or Cervical Nerve Root Injuries at Birth

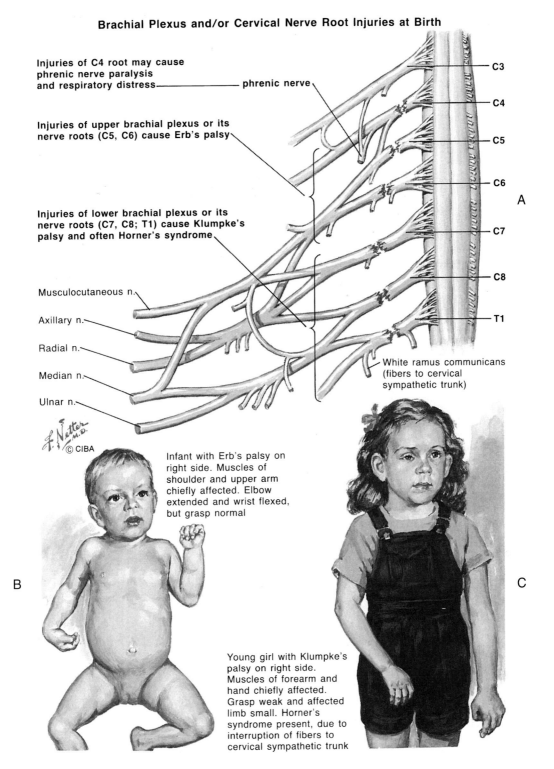

Injuries of C4 root may cause phrenic nerve paralysis and respiratory distress——— phrenic nerve

Injuries of upper brachial plexus or its nerve roots (C5, C6) cause Erb's palsy

Injuries of lower brachial plexus or its nerve roots (C7, C8; T1) cause Klumpke's palsy and often Horner's syndrome

Musculocutaneous n.

Axillary n.

Radial n.

Median n.

Ulnar n.

C3
C4
C5
C6
C7
C8
T1

A

White ramus communicans (fibers to cervical sympathetic trunk)

Infant with Erb's palsy on right side. Muscles of shoulder and upper arm chiefly affected. Elbow extended and wrist flexed, but grasp normal

B

C

Young girl with Klumpke's palsy on right side. Muscles of forearm and hand chiefly affected. Grasp weak and affected limb small. Horner's syndrome present, due to interruption of fibers to cervical sympathetic trunk

FIGURE 31–8

A, Brachial plexus anatomy after a severe stretch injury, with major roots being avulsed from the spinal cord. Note that the anterior primary ramus of each nerve root receives a contribution from the corresponding sympathetic trunk ganglion, the gray ramus communicans. In addition, the first thoracic anterior primary ramus contributes preganglionic sympathetic fibers to the inferior cervical (stellate) ganglion via a white ramus communicans. B, Classic "waiter's tip" posture of an infant with neonatal brachial plexopathy. C, An older child with associated Horner's syndrome. (A to C, Copyright ©1987, Icon Learning Systems, LLC. A subsidiary of MediMedia, USA, Inc. All rights reserved.)

BOX 31-4
CLASSIFICATION OF OBSTETRIC BRACHIAL PLEXUS PALSY

Group I (C5-C6): paralysis of the shoulder and biceps
Group II (C5-C7): paralysis of the shoulder biceps and forearm extensors
Group III (C5-T1): complete paralysis of the limb
Group IV (C5-T1): complete paralysis of the limb with Horner's syndrome

From Brown WF, Bolton CF, Aminoff MJ (eds): Neuromuscular Function and Disease. Philadelphia, WB Saunders, 2002, p 1606.

BOX 31-5
BPPN RISK FACTORS

Shoulder dystocia
Large birthweight (>4 kg)
Maternal diabetes
Multiparity
Second-stage labor > 60 min
Assisted delivery (e.g., use of forceps, vacuum extraction)
Previous child with BPPN
Intrauterine torticollis

BPPN, brachial plexus palsy of the newborn.

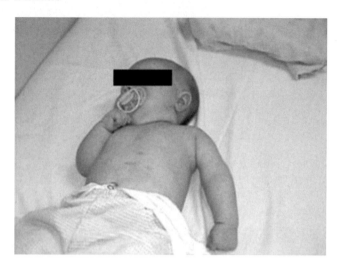

FIGURE 31–9
The classic posture of an infant with Erb's palsy (upper trunk C5-C6). A large macrosomic baby (>4200 gm) at 6 weeks of age. The extremity is held adducted, in internal rotation and pronated, and extended at the elbow. The wrist, fingers, and thumb are flexed. (From Brown WF, Bolton CF, Aminoff MJ [eds]: Neuromuscular Function and Disease. Philadelphia, WB Saunders, 2002, p 1607.)

bines a measurement of active limb movements and compares them with the normal side.[63]

Prognostic Factors

Significant recovery is usually seen with an Erb's BPPN, excluding the relatively rare, unfortunate infant with rupture and avulsion of each affected nerve root (Table 31-1 and Box 31-6). However, there is extensive debate vis-à-vis the timing and degree of effective reinnervation. The incidence of complete recovery varies enormously because of differing populations selected at different stages of reinnervation with varied criteria for the diagnosis of full or complete recovery.

A pan-plexus injury with either a Horner's sign or an associated phrenic nerve palsy has an especially poor prognosis with greater than 50% developing little or no clinical function.[46,54,56,64-66] Although a concurrent

TABLE 31–1. PROGNOSTIC FACTORS: NEONATAL BRACHIAL PLEXOPATHIES

Prognosis	Factors
Poor	Completely flail upper limb with Horner's syndrome (Narakas[46] group IV)
	Horner's syndrome
	Phrenic nerve paralysis
	No recovery of biceps function (elbow flexion) by 3-4 mo
	Score of < 3.5 at 3 mo (HSCT scale)
	Root avulsion; pseudomeningocele (nerve rootlets absent)
Good	Recovery of elbow flexion by 2 mo
	Antigravity strength of elbow flexion by 3 mo
	No EMG evidence of axonal loss
	Scores of > 3.5 at 3 mo (HSCT scale)
	No root avulsion; no pseudomeningoceles with MRI imaging
Unknown/ indeterminate	Motor unit recovery MUAPs volitional in biceps at 4/12 but not antigravity elbow flexion
	Clavicular fracture
	Narakas group II (C5-C7)
	Early recovery of elbow flexion but less than antigravity (by age 4 mo) and then plateau

HSCT, Hospital for Sick Children Toronto; MUAP, motor unit action potential.

BOX 31-6
UNFAVORABLE PROGNOSTIC
SIGNS OF BPPN

Lower plexus lesions
Erb-Klumpke lesion lacking some improvement
   within 1st wk
No appreciable recovery by age 6 mo
Nature of injury (avulsion or rupture)
Horner's syndrome
Associated fracture of ribs, clavicle, and humerus

BPPN, brachial plexus palsy of the newborn.

clavicular fracture in a newborn supports a traumatic process, when this is associated with a BPPN, it surprisingly holds no prognostic value in predicting spontaneous recovery.[64,67]

Natural History

Prognosis is clearly the best for infants with BP lesions confined to the upper trunk and lateral cord. Overall, 70% to 92% of infants with neonatal brachial plexopathy have a good to excellent result when followed over a long-term period.[42,68,69] Close to 15% of infants with BPPN experience significant permanent disability.[56,69-71] In contradistinction other clinical researchers are somewhat less optimistic. A Swedish study showed that complete recovery occurred in only 49% and severe impairment in 22%.[40]

Neurophysiologic Prediction of Outcome

Most centers today combine clinical assessment and neurophysiology to improve accuracy in evaluating the severity. In general, the items in Table 31-2 provide a good guideline vis-à-vis the neural lesion.

The extent of the lesion is evaluated by the features at presentation, whereas the type of nerve injury is determined by the clinical improvement over time. Neurophysiologic findings enhance their predictive value.[10,11] The predictive outcome was particularly good for nerves innervated by the C6-C7 roots. The lower predictive value for C5 likely reflects the fact that it is not possible to record CMAPs from C5-innervated muscles. Because of some of the EMG limitations in the newborn population as described earlier in this chapter, at times there is significant difficulty attempting to define the presence of root avulsion utilizing this methodology. This highlights the need for appropriate complementary imaging of the plexus, particularly MRI, or computed tomographic (CT) myelography for evaluation of BPPN.

The Role of Neuroimaging

Avulsion of ventral or dorsal nerve rootlets from the spinal cord results in preganglionic nerve root injury with no potential for nerve regeneration (see Fig. 31-5D-F). The diagnosis of nerve root avulsion is based on showing deformity of the subarachnoid space or a pseudomeningocele. Unfortunately this is not a precise technique because a significant percentage of avulsions show no evidence of pseudomeningocele, and pseudomeningoceles do occur without root avulsion.[72-74]

Root avulsions are best defined by identifying the absence of rootlets in the pseudomeningocele.[49,75] This absence on

TABLE 31-2. THE NEUROPHYSIOLOGIC GRADING SYSTEM

Type	CMAP	EMG	Lesion*
A: Generally quite good	Normal	No spontaneous activity Reduced number of normal MUPs Increased firing rates Decreased recruitment	Conduction block Neurapraxia (Sunderland 1)
B: Favorable	Normal or >50% of uninjured side	Relatively good MUP recruitment Mixture of normal MUPs with polyphasic MUPs suggesting collateral reinnervation	Mild axonal lesion Axonotmesis (Sunderland 2 and 3)
B: Unfavorable	Absent or <50% of uninjured side	Few or absent MUPs	Significant axonal lesion (Sunderland 3)
C: Very unfavorable	Absent	Spontaneous activity Poor or absent recruitment	Severe axonal lesion Neurotmesis Root avulsion (Sunderland 4 or 5)

*Nerve injury adapted from classification of Seddon and Sunderland (see Box 31-2).

N, normal; NAP, nerve action potential (comparison between sides from stimulation at the wrist recording from the elbow over the median and ulnar nerves [averaged response]); MUP, motor unit potential; CMAP, compound muscle action potential.

Adapted from Smith SJ: The role of neurophysiological investigation in traumatic brachial plexus lesions in adults and children. J Hand Surg [Br] 1996;21:145-147.

CT myelography may be used to suggest an extraforaminal nerve root avulsion due to its high specificity (r = .98) but corresponding very low sensitivity. In other words, the sensitivity or proportion of root avulsions correctly associated with a pseudomeningocele varies between 63% and 37%, respectively (absence of rootlets vs. presence of rootlets in the pseudomeningocele). As a predictor for root avulsion the presence of a pseudomeningocele on CT myelogram (thin slices < 1.5 mm) and concomitant absence of rootlets are far more important than the presence of pseudomeningoceles alone.[73,76]

MRI is noninvasive, providing better anatomic definition of the spinal cord, excellent depiction of pseudomeningoceles, identification of cord displacement or deformity, as well as the peripheral soft tissue surrounding the BP (see Fig. 31-9). To date there are no specific reports comparing MR imaging with CT myelography vis-à-vis BPPN.[4,72,77-83]

One "anterospective" study comparing the respective value of the clinical assessment, MRI, and EMG in the evaluation of 13 BPPN infants, ages 7 to 41 days and again at age 3 months, emphasized the complementary nature of clinical, neurophysiologic, and imaging studies to best define a prognosis.[4] This descriptive study evaluated MRI with electromyography (the first between age 27 to 50 days and the second at age 3 months) and the muscle scoring system of Hospital for Sick Children at ages 3, 6, and 9 months (Table 31-3). The existence of MRI defined pseudomeningocele in the first days after birth is predictive of a poor prognosis.

EMG evidence of root avulsion was found in three babies; it correlated with the poor clinical outcome and the MRI in two of the three (Box 31-7). If the EMG findings are suspicious for root avulsion.

With this combination of findings a poor outcome is suggested; however, it is still wise to obtain complementary

TABLE 31–3. HOSPITAL FOR SICK CHILDREN MUSCLE GRADING SYSTEM

Motion	Score	Muscle Grade Score
Gravity Eliminated		
No contraction	0	0
Contraction, no motion	0.3	1
Motion ≤ $\frac{1}{2}$ range	0.3	2
Motion ≥ $\frac{1}{2}$ range	0.6	3
Full motion	0.6	4
Against Gravity		
Motion ≤ $\frac{1}{2}$ range	0.6	5
Motion ≥ $\frac{1}{2}$ range	1.3	6
Full motion	2	7

The scores for elbow flexion, together with elbow, wrist, thumb and finger extension at 3-13 months of age are then added (maximum 10). If the score was less than 3.5, of a possible 10 at 3 months, poor recovery could be expected.[70]

BOX 31-7
EMG FINDINGS OF ROOT AVULSION

Profuse fibrillation potentials
Nonrecordable or "scanty" MUAPs
No CMAPs
Normal sensory conduction studies
No improvement at the second EMG

MUAP, motor unit action potential; CMAP, compound muscle action potential.

MRI imaging before diagnosing root avulsion with its inherent poor prognosis.[4]

Ultrasound

Ultrasound is a technique that provides a valuable tool to assess the congruency of the humeral head in chronic BPPN. Ultrasound is important to identify the all too often unrecognized medial rotation contracture and/or posterior shoulder dislocation. This common orthopedic lesion often mars neurologic recovery; it can lead the unwary clinician into incorrectly predicting results of surgical outcome.[84-86]

Surgical Exploration and Operative Intervention

Currently the primary challenge lies in identifying those babies predestined to have an excellent spontaneous recovery while concomitantly selecting those infants who may benefit from early nerve repair surgery to aid their progress. When one considers this therapeutic option for BPPN, the typically good prognosis for the common Erb's palsy suggests that at least 6 months of clinical observation is certainly the baseline standard.[42,56,68,69,87]

Surgical treatment of a BPPN consists of neurotization or microsurgical reinnervation of the distal portion of the plexus by nerve transfer from the spinal accessory, cervical plexus, or intercostal nerves.[56,87-90] Currently there are two reasonably accepted surgical indications (Box 31-8). These include (1) a total BPPN with a flail arm and Horner's syndrome and (2) a complete C5-C6 BPPN without any clinical muscle contraction in the C5-C6–innervated muscles at age 6 months with an EMG demonstrating a significant axonal lesion, that is, profuse denervation with no recordable MUAPs.[91]

Some centers or surgeons do not utilize EMG findings. Here the surgical decision is strictly based on clinical assessment. Some surgical investigators conclude that if the recovery in the muscles innervated by C5-C6 is delayed beyond 3 months, then root disruption is likely, and one should consider exploration immediately.

BOX 31-8
INDICATIONS FOR SURGICAL EXPLORATION OF BPPN

Upper trunk lesion that does not improve at > age 6 mo

Total plexus (Erb-Klumpke) lesion, particularly with Horner's syndrome*

Avulsion suggested by an Erb's palsy with no change > 3 mo[†]

Upper trunk lesion with phrenic nerve lesion[†]

*The Swedish study[93] found no value for surgery here.
[†]Indication has been advocated by surgeons and it is primarily based on clinical and not EMG findings.
BPPN, brachial plexus palsy of the newborn.

Furthermore, surgical colleagues believe that an upper BP lesion combined with a phrenic nerve palsy represents an indication for early exploration, as does the presence of a phrenic nerve palsy following breech delivery.[56] This continues to be a controversial area, with still no well-defined, absolutely agreed on indications. This was reviewed in detail by Jones and associates in 2003.[92]

Certain favorable neurophysiologic findings, particularly ones including demonstration of neurapraxia, often lessen the urgency to explore the plexus. Even when EMG findings suggest an unfavorable prognosis, it is wise to delay exploration of the plexus for 2 to 6 months while clinical evolution is monitored. If clinical features still do not improve and continue to be concordant with the neurophysiologic findings, surgical exploration is indicated, ideally at about 6 months of age.[10]

A detailed report from the Karolinska Institute in Stockholm merits careful consideration for those committed to a better understanding of BPPN.[93] A nonoperative approach was compared to microneurosurgical sural or nerve root graft. This study is unique in that it studied the children's "functional outcome." (A detailed analysis of these data is provided in Reference 94.) In summary, all children who achieved complete recovery by 5 years of age had already gained some recovery by 2 months of age, and all children with Erb-type lesions achieved normal hand and wrist movement. However, functional outcome monitored by the "pick-up" test was somewhat limited (among those operated on, 50% of 8 performed well; among those not operated on, 77% of 15 performed well; and in the early recovery group, 91% of 32 performed well).

Note, however, that our Swedish colleagues' analyses do not include the abilities of the 67 of 135 children who had complete resolution at age 6 months. Retrospectively, most of these infants were recovered at age 6 months. Nonoperated children who experienced a late recovery had higher grip strength and bimanual activity than those who were operated among the Erb-plus (C5-C7) group. In those infants with a BPPN who had early intervention and were operated before 6 months, such an approach was *no more effective* than those who later had surgery.

Surgery provided no advantage in those with Erb-Klumpke type lesions, even though this has been listed as a standard indication for intervention.[94] The finding that 67 of 135 children who had the most common Erb-type BPPN lesion, who achieved full recovery by age 6 months, were not included in this evaluation, as well as relatively small operative numbers (32 of 214 of C5-C6 or C5-C7 lesions), significantly *biases* their study's opening discussion comment that "a better shoulder movement is apparent in C5-C6 palsies that have been operated on."[93,95]

It is clear that new approaches are needed to both treat and analyze the value of various therapeutic interventions for BPPN that occurs in about 2 of 1000 births, or 40 times annually, in Sweden.[93]

Newer Therapies

What with the relatively poor results to date of various therapeutic approaches, it is apparent that new clinical and research approaches are indicated if there is going to be any type of reasonable progress in the care of these infants. The reader is referred to the thoughtful papers of Korak and coworkers[22] in 2004 and Strombeck and Fernell in 2003.[95] These consider the role of central nervous system plasticity after injury and the eventual outcome. If progress is to be made, these authors and their colleagues may be leading us into a more fruitful albeit extremely challenging pathway for success.

POSTNEONATAL BRACHIAL PLEXOPATHIES

With the exception of BPPN, these are generally uncommon occurrences among neonates and infants with the one exception of a rare form of occult osteomyelitis affecting the humeral head and extending to the adjacent plexus.[96-98] This pathologic process contrasts with the precipitous onset of root avulsion and plexus injury at birth.[16] Beyond the immediate perinatal period there are various hereditary, postinflammatory, and traumatic mechanisms, particularly including child abuse, that require diagnostic consideration. The differential diagnosis of BP palsy also includes rare other congenital motor unit lesions such as segmental anterior horn cell processes at the cervical spinal cord, amyoplasia, and a pseudoparesis.[99]

Osteomyelitis-Related Brachial Plexopathy

Osteomyelitis-related brachial plexopathy is an unusual BP with an acute onset in the immediate postneonatal period. Failure to consider this lesion in the differential diagnosis of an acutely acquired infantile BP in a previously healthy baby may lead to a serious plexus insult because of a delay in instituting appropriate antibiotic therapy. Criteria for differentiating this idiopathic BP are summarized in Box 31-9.[34,100]

We have recognized one instance in a 19-day-old girl with a 5-day history of fever and rhinorrhea with diminished movement in one arm over the prior 24 hours. An EMG performed at Children's Hospital Boston (CHB) 3 weeks after onset of arm weakness demonstrated normal motor and sensory conduction studies.[98] However, there was a markedly diminished number of MUAPs with many fibrillation potentials confined to the affected deltoid and biceps muscles. This was compatible with an upper cord BP lesion. She was successfully treated with penicillin G. Repeat bone scan on the 5th day of admission demonstrated a proximal right humerus osteomyelitis near the shoulder (Fig. 31-10). Later Clay reported a similar illness in a 9-week-old infant with 2-week history of an occult osteomyelitis. Initial EMG at 14 days was unremarkable; however, EMG findings demonstrated active denervation at 6 days later.[34] Full recovery did not occur for 8 months.

Both children had very elevated erythrocyte sedimentation rates (ESRs) of 90 and 81 mm/hr; modest leukocytosis; and positive cultures for group B beta-hemolytic streptococci, one from blood culture and the other on shoulder tap after blood culture was negative. Bone scan may be diagnostic for a proximal *humeral osteomyelitis;* however, a delay in onset of a specific change should not dissuade one from making the clinical diagnosis. The pathophysiology of this relationship awaits elucidation. An

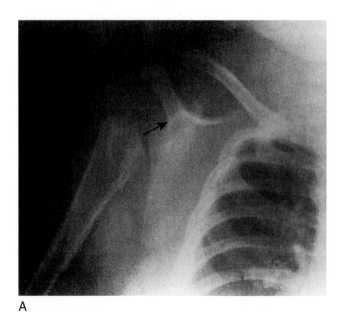

A

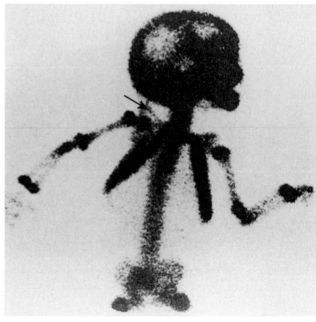

B

FIGURE 31–10

Osteomyelitis of the proximal humerus as a cause of brachial plexus neuropathy. Routine radiograph of the humerus (A) *and bone scan* (B) *both demonstrate osteomyelitis* (arrows). (A *and* B, *From Clay SA: Osteomyelitis as a cause of brachial plexus neuropathy. Am J Dis Child 1982;136:1054-1056.*)

unusual case of pyogenic *Staphylococcus aureus* cervical osteomyelitis with paraspinal abscess and resulting. Erb's palsy is reported from Oman.[101]

Hereditary Brachial Plexus Neuropathies

Hereditary Neuralgic Amyotrophy

Hereditary BP neuropathy (HBPN) is also known as *hereditary neuralgic amyotrophy*. Typically these children have intermittent episodes of shoulder and arm pain, weakness, and atrophy initially presenting before age 5 years. One of three children also experienced an isolated phrenic nerve paralysis at age 7 weeks.[96] A characteristic Modigliani physiognomy of slender-faced youth characterized by close-set eyes (hypotelorism), long nasal bridge, and facial asymmetry is characteristic (Figs. 31-11 and 31-12).[96,102] Except for their recurrent nature, these *painful* BPs mimic idiopathic BP neuropathy (IBPN), that is, neuralgic amyotrophy.

This contrasts with the exclusively *painless presentation* of another hereditary neuropathic process sometimes hav-

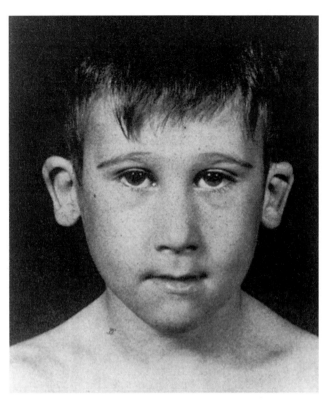

FIGURE 31–12
Child with heredofamilial brachial plexopathy. (From Dunn HG, Daube JR, Gomez MR: Heredofamilial brachial plexus neuropathy [hereditary neuralgic amyotrophy with brachial predilection] in childhood. Dev Med Child Neurol 1978;20:28-46.)

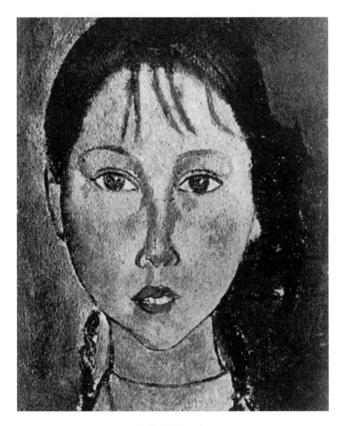

FIGURE 31–11
Modigliani portrait with hypotelorism and a slender facies. (From Dunn HG, Daube JR, Gomez MR: Heredofamilial brachial plexus neuropathy [hereditary neuralgic amyotrophy with brachial predilection] in childhood. Dev Med Child Neurol 1978;20:28-46.)

ing a recurrent course. It is known as *hereditary neuropathy with liability to pressure palsy* (HNPP). Recovery was often incomplete.[97,103,104] This must also be differentiated from both HBPN and IBPN.[96,97,103,105,106]

Children with HBPN have an autosomal dominant inheritance pattern. The primary genetic site involved is non-neuronal, perhaps related to connective tissue.[102] Thus genes coding for connective tissue could lead to a BP neuropathy due to direct pressure, diminished blood supply, or an immune mechanism.[104] The tissue inhibitor of metalloproteinase 2 (*TIMP2*) is another intriguing gene on chromosome 17. Matrix metalloproteinases are involved in the pathogenesis of experimental autoimmune neuritis (an animal model of immune mediated neuropathies).[104] Certain characteristics may guide one in ordering DNA testing when seeing children with their first BP (Box 31-10).

There are just a few reports of NCS in HBPN, not enough to establish a specific pattern. A predominant median and radial sensory fiber involvement with low-amplitude SNAPs was noted.[96] Motor conduction velocity was usually normal or only mildly slowed. Fibrillation potentials in the affected

BP, brachial plexus; IBPN, idiopathic BP neuropathy;
HBPN, hereditary BP neuropathy.

muscles are compatible with an axonal process in some children with HBPN.

Hereditary Neuropathy with Liability to Pressure Palsy

About 10% of patients with HNPP have BP involvement.[107] This often can be differentiated from HBPN, usually associated with pain similar to IBPN, by the fact that HNPP is usually painless. The generic locus for HNPP is located on 17p11.2 differing from HBPN at 17q25.[102] This locus is similar to Charcot-Marie Tooth (type 1A) hereditary motor sensory neuropathy. The genetic abnormality is a duplication at 17p11.2 with HNPP in contrast to the deletion located at 17p11.2. with Charcot-Marie Tooth.[108] This interstitial deletion causes the complete loss of one allele of the peripheral myelin protein 22 (*PMP22* gene).

Current molecular genetic tests and clinical guidelines provide for improved diagnosis and counseling for patients with HNPP. In general, these families experience isolated mononeuropathies, particularly to nerves sensitive to compression (i.e., median, radial, and peroneal). Occasionally, some HNPP children have a painless brachial plexopathy or even a monomelic mononeuritis multiplex picture. One 16-year-old child developed a paresis of the posterior and lateral portions of the BP after sleeping with his arm tucked under his head.[109]

Idiopathic Brachial Plexus Neuropathy (Neuralgic Amyotrophy)

Idiopathic, likely autoimmune, acute BP neuropathy has multiple terminologies, including *Parsonage-Turner*

syndrome, neuralgic amyotrophy, and *idiopathic brachial neuritis*. The nonspecific term *IBPN* is most appropriate because no etiologic or pathophysiologic implications are inherent in this designation. Others suggest that neuralgic amyotrophy is the most appropriate name because pain is often the first symptom subsequently followed by shoulder girdle weakness.[33,110-112] This is much more commonly recognized in the adult. However, the Mayo Clinic experience included 7 of 99 patients younger than 20 years of age, the youngest presenting at age 3 months.[33] Typically IBPN affects nerves innervating the shoulder girdle muscles; however, some other portions of this plexus and its terminal branches, such as the anterior interosseous nerve, are occasionally involved.[113] Bilateral but asymmetric involvement is noted in about one third of patients.[5,33]

IBPN is a diagnosis of exclusion; therefore, one needs to search for other pathophysiologic mechanisms. Two reports of childhood IBPN include at least three nonfamilial instances, with onset between the ages of 16 months and 9 years. The youngest child had a painless, diffuse brachial plexitis with flaccid weakness of the entire arm and weak grasp 4 days after a febrile illness.[114] Eight months later this infant had a poor recovery in comparison with the excellent recovery at 6 months in the 3.5-year-old child whose IBPN was confined to the proximal arm.[114]

Brachial Plexus Pressure Palsies

Two areas of potential compressive injuries to the BP are defined in children. They are relatively uncommon.[115,116] With the wise introduction of mandatory automobile infant safety seats to prevent free-flight injuries of the unrestrained baby, one might consider that the potential for a compressive injury to the BP may be more frequent. However, to date, that has not been our experience.

There is one interesting notation of a previously healthy 9-month-old infant who was confined in a rear-facing infant restraint seat with a self-retracting shoulder harness during a 7-day, 2500-mile journey. This baby was never confined to the seat for more than 4 hours. On the last leg of the trip, the infant lost function in the left arm. Neurologic examination documented weakness in the distribution of the BP lateral and posterior cords. There were no other possible etiologic mechanisms. Unfortunately DNA testing for HNPP was not yet available; one would wonder whether the infant or parents had the same findings. No EMG was performed. This baby had a full recovery, suggesting neurapraxic injury secondary to the harness.[117]

Despite the increasing use of backpacks by school-aged children, an increased incidence of previously described rucksack palsies, initially noted in children participating in scouting,[118] has yet to be experienced. In Japan, 15 of 16 sports-related BPs were secondary to mountain climbing with packs as heavy as 40 kg. It is suggested that these lesions occurred secondary to axillary nerve compression. None of these injuries was further defined by EMG.[119] However, again the possibility of HNPP and/or HBPN would deserve consideration today.

Traumatic Brachial Plexopathies

The older child and adolescent, in particular, are exposed to a number of potential traumatic mechanisms. These include motorcycle injuries, other accidental sports trauma, various war wounds, hunting injuries, other gunshot wounds, and surgery.[119-128]

Sports injuries frequently cause BP injuries among adolescents.[129-138] Typically these occur in football, lacrosse, and/or rugby where these are referred to as a "burner" or "stinger." Their exact pathophysiology is unclear.

There are two major proposed etiologies: (1) traction of the C5-C6 cervical nerve roots and/or (2) a mild stretch injury to the upper trunk of the BP. Anatomically, based on the location of the "weak link" at the root level (because of the lack of supporting connective tissue structures), a number of authors suggest that the nerve root is a prime consideration for the lesion.[121] Neither injury has any long-term sequela.

Only a few nondefinitive EMG studies are available.[5,121,133,134] Needle EMG was the most sensitive, sometimes noting neurogenic changes in the upper trunk muscles, although in most cases the EMG was normal or only suggestive of a decreased recruitment and interference pattern compatible with neuropraxia. EMG is primarily valuable for individuals who sustain more than a period of episodic pain and weakness or are unable to "shake it off."[129] A normal NEE, particularly in supraspinatus and infraspinatus muscles, when the patient reports feelings of weakness in the shoulder girdle alerts the clinician to consider certain musculoskeletal causes. These include a rotator cuff tear and/or fracture.

Neoplasms

It is extremely rare for a child to have a brachial plexopathy as the presentation of a tumor. This contrasts with the adult experience. Important features that distinguish these children with a tumor from idiopathic BP are outlined in Box 31-11.[100]

Thoracic Outlet Syndrome

Thoracic outlet syndrome (TOS) is a rare condition, in our experience, if one follows the strict electrodiagnostic criteria for a neurologic TOS as defined by Gilliatt and

---

BOX 31-11
FEATURES OF A CHILDHOOD BP SUGGESTING A TUMOR

History of normal delivery and birthweight
Onset after the neonatal period
Progressive course
Scratch marks on a weak arm
Supraclavicular mass in area with no radiographic clavicular fracture

BP, brachial plexus.
Adapted from Alfonso I, Alfonso DT, Papazian O: Focal upper extremity neuropathy in neonates. Semin Pediatr Neurol 2000;7:4-14.

BOX 31-12
MODIFIED GILLIATT[139,141,144] NCS EMG CRITERIA FOR THORACIC OUTLET SYNDROME

Ulnar SNAP 5th finger low amplitude to absent*
Medial antebrachial cutaneous SNAP absent*
Median innervated thenar CMAP low amplitude*
Median II digit SNAP normal
Ulnar-innervated hypothenar CMAP normal to low amplitude
Motor NCV, DL preserved
F waves slight to moderately prolonged, median more than ulnar
Active and chronic denervation in ulnar and median intrinsics, flexor carpi ulnaris, and extensor indicis proprius

*Essential for diagnosis.
NCS, nerve conduction study; SNAP, sensory nerve action potential; CMAP, compound motor action potential; NCV, nerve conduction velocity; DL, distal latency.

---

associates[139] (Box 31-12). The incidence of this condition has been estimated to be 1 in 1 million.[140] However, it is important to recognize because its sequelae can become quite disabling.[141] In general TOS primarily occurs in young women who undergo strenuous activities of the upper extremities or have bad working postures.[141]

Most of Gilliatt's patients presented with hand weakness and/or atrophy affecting median more than the ulnar intrinsics. Pain and paresthesia, primarily on the medial aspect of the arm, forearm, and occasionally the hand, was present in 12 of 14 patients; however, it was usually mild and the primary complaint in only 5 patients. The cause was either a cervical rib or increased length of the C7 transverse process.[139] Usually these patients have sharp fibrous bands extending from the rudimentary rib or the tip of the C7 transverse process. The C8 and T1 anterior primary rami or the lower trunk of the BP become stretched and compressed while passing over these bands.[5,142,143]

This is almost always a unilateral process clinically, although there is a recent well-documented instance of a bilaterally significant TOS beginning at age 17 years in a girl shortly after she commenced work as a hairdresser.[141] This teenager had profound atrophy of both hands. Axial CT confirmed the chest radiograph presence of rudimentary C7 cervical ribs. There are multiple reports of bilateral cervical ribs, but this was the first one found to have clinically significant findings on examination and EMG.

At surgery the cervical ribs and thick fibrous bands were removed by a transaxillary approach. Within a short time her pain and paresthesia disappeared. There was no follow-up after 1 month when repeat EMG was unchanged.

Gilliatt and associates in 1978[139] proposed the major EMG criteria for diagnosis of TOS, and in general these have been reliable. They have since been modified somewhat by Wilbourn and coworkers[144] in 1999 and Tilki in 2004.[141] (See the items identified as "essential for diagnosis" in Box 31-12.) The absent ulnar and medial antebrachial cutaneous SNAP, in keeping with the low-amplitude median CMAP, primarily T1 fibers, is classic for a medial plexus/lower trunk lesion. This is the only area where these respective fibers are contiguous.

Wilbourn[144] advised utilizing the medial antebrachial cutaneous nerve of the forearm in patients with "true" or neurogenic TOS. He provided an excellent discussion of TOS, including its controversial nature and clinical findings.

Ouvrier and associates[145] reported a 4-year-old child with thenar atrophy and weakness who, on cervical spine radiography, demonstrated a congenital Klippel-Feil anomaly associated with *small* cervical ribs. The ipsilateral median SNAP amplitude was low to normal, but still only 50% of the opposite unaffected side. The ipsilateral ulnar SNAPs from the nerve were of low amplitude. Needle EMG demonstrated chronic denervation in thenar muscles. An elongated C7 transverse process articulating with the first rib was found at surgery. There was only a little improvement over the next 5 years. One of us (H.R.J.), in 26 years at CHB, has also seen just one TOS case. He refused surgery and was lost to follow-up after 1 year.

Rare Brachial Plexopathies

There are a few other unusual causes for a pediatric BP. These include neonatal hemangiomatosis,[146,147] neck compression,[112] and an exostosis of the first rib.[100] A brachial plexopathy is also described following therapy for childhood acute lymphoblastic leukemia.[148-150]

Pseudoparesis

It is sometimes a diagnostic challenge when dealing with a youngster who complains of limb pain or deformity and feels the arm is weak or numb. Often the neurologic examination as well as EMG are normal. Many of these individuals are splinting their extremities because the pain is exacerbated by movement and they thus interpret this as "weakness." Conditions such as complex regional pain syndrome, also known as reflex sympathies dystrophy or causalgia, are a significant consideration, particularly if there has been a history of minor trauma. In this setting the EMG is always normal. To better understand this condition, the reader is referred to a recent excellent review.[151]

It is always wise to follow such patients longitudinally rather than to suggest at first pass that the normal evaluation must thus suggest a diagnosis of a somatoform disorder. At times the subtle early signs of a peripheral motor unit lesion, at most any level, will declare themselves later on as new clinical findings evolve to point to the correct diagnosis. Repeat EMG may be helpful in this regard. On other occasions conditions such as juvenile rheumatoid arthritis and soft tissue, bony, or spinal cord tumors may emerge as the clinical course evolves.

LUMBOSACRAL PLEXOPATHIES

Lesions of the LSP are the most uncommon peripheral nerve problems seen in our pediatric EMG laboratories. Most occur secondary to trauma including motor vehicle accidents, pelvic fracture, and gunshot wounds.[122,152-163] LSPs are also linked to more subtle trauma associated with an underlying predisposing factor including hereditary liability to pressure palsy and Ehlers-Danlos syndrome.[164,165]

Some LSPs are most probably related to an immune-related postviral plexitis.[153,166,167] Tumors are another rare cause and can be a malignant one such as a lymphoma (H.R.J., personal experience at CHB) or benign (lipoma).[168] Additionally, and rarely, iatrogenic etiologies occur.[168-172]

General Principles of EMG Evaluation for Pediatric Lumbosacral Plexopathies

With the exception of the femoral nerve, none of the other nerves originating in the lumbar plexus lend themselves to direct stimulation for conventional NCS. This is especially true in children; in fact, for emotional sensitivities we do not even attempt to stimulate the femoral nerve in any child. Therefore, one is dependent on the results of needle EMG to assess function of the femoral and obturator nerves. In contrast, the sacral sciatic-derived peroneal and tibial nerve components are available for routine NCS. Occasionally, a child does not tolerate stimulation in the popliteal fossa, and we are often content to study only the distal component. In the infant, sural stimulation is sometimes technically difficult.[173]

As in the cervical spine, a normal SNAP amplitude in an area of abnormal sensation (peripheral nerve and/or dermatome) may suggest a preganglionic lesion and help differentiate a root or intraspinal (i.e., preganglionic) lesion from a plexus abnormality (see Fig. 31-5). To further differentiate a plexus lesion, especially from the more common proximal sciatic nerve defect, multiple muscles require examination, occasionally including the gluteae medius and maximus. Additionally, one must exclude an intraspinal or nerve root process by examining the paraspinal muscles. These investigations are demanding in children. It is also difficult to obtain appropriate relaxation here, especially with infants and young children. Therefore, when there is a possible LSP diagnosis (see Fig. 31-6), one may best perform the EMG with anesthetic help in the outpatient surgical center.

Neuroimaging

MRI provides excellent detail. When there is a reasonable clinical suspicion of a plexopathy, an MRI is the study of choice. The new 3.0 Tesla MRIs will be particularly helpful.

Lumbosacral Plexus Lesions

Neonatal Lumbosacral Plexopathies

Trauma to the LSP is rare in newborns.[174,175] Eng[176] summarized her experience with three neonates during a 7-year period. These babies sustained lumbosacral "traction" injuries after breech delivery. She emphasized the importance of differentiating these lesions from an asymmetric myelomeningocele, infantile poliomyelitis, parenteral injection injury, or a central nervous system process. Unfortunately no precise details of the clinical or EMG findings were described. None of these three infants had a complete recovery; however, the length of follow-up time is not reported.[176]

Another infant is reported who had a precise EMG performed after a precipitous double-footed breech delivery.[175] At birth, this infant was unable to extend the knee or to rotate it internally. A follow-up evaluation at 4 months of age demonstrated inability to extend the knee or internally rotate the leg, atrophy and hypotonia of the quadriceps muscle, mild flexion contracture at the knee, and an absent quadriceps muscle stretch reflex. Radi-

ographic examination of the lumbar spine and hip were normal. No pelvic or paravertebral masses were found on ultrasonography of the pelvis and spine.

An EMG demonstrated denervation confined to the quadriceps and adductor magnus muscles. Excessive birth traction was suggested as a possible cause for the injury to the lumbar plexus; however, an isolated injury to the L2-L4 nerve roots was not excluded. Volpe described one similar infant who had a good recovery.[177]

Idiopathic Lumbosacral Plexopathy

Primary LSP rarely occurs, particularly in children. It has been reported in six children from ages 2 to 16 years. It presents with a rapid onset of pain, weakness, and muscle atrophy. A viral illness preceded the LSP onset by 3 to 10 days in five of these six children. The lumbar plexus was predominantly involved.

The LSP diagnosis was confirmed by EMG; however, details of these studies were not reported. Four children recovered within 3 months, and two had mild residual weakness.[153,178,179]

Evans[166] reported a 15-year-old girl who presented with sudden, sharp inguinal pain associated with mid-thigh paresthesias. Weakness of the iliopsoas, quadriceps, and adductor muscles occurred 1 day later. EMG demonstrated denervation in both the femoral and obturator innervated muscles with a normal paraspinal evaluation. Significant recovery occurred in 3 months. They likened this condition to the well-described counterpart of IBPN known as *neuralgic amyotrophy*.[166]

Traumatic Lumbosacral Plexopathies

Infants are susceptible to stretch injuries at the LSP similar to the BP. Traumatic lumbosacral nerve root avulsion rarely occurs.[177,180] It is variously associated with flexion-abduction injury to the hip, hyperextension of the thigh with pelvic fracture,[181] posterior dislocation of the hip, and sacral fractures.[182,183] According to pathologic studies at a postmortem study,[184] the L3-S3 roots rupture proximal to the spinal ganglion but distal to their origin at the cord. This contrasts with the more common root avulsion that occurs directly from the spinal cord in the cervical spine.[181] However, both have the same effects on the outcome of an EMG with preservation of SNAPs because the dorsal root ganglia remain intact.

Stretch injuries to the LSP are more common than root avulsion but are still relatively rare.[152,155,185] The sciatic is the predominant nerve involved. This is reported subsequent to pelvic-sacral fractures and hip dislocations.[158,186,187] Potentially serious lumbosacral plexopathies may result from unusual, seemingly innocent activities of children, particularly babies, as illustrated by one Raggedy Ann-like case seen at CHB.[17] There, a 4-month-old infant's sister playfully but vigorously pulled him across the floor by his leg. Later that day, his leg was limp, lacked spontaneous motion, and was cool. Examination demonstrated a flaccid leg with no muscle stretch reflexes. Orthopedic evaluation, including appropriate radiographs, was normal.

NCS demonstrated a low-amplitude posterior tibial CMAP but normal tibial NCV and distal latencies with normal peroneal nerve function. The EMG study demonstrated fibrillation potentials in the tibialis anterior and medial gastrocnemius, with diminished number of MUAP in these muscles and the vastus lateralis. Seven months later, proximal strength was normal; however, there was some residual distal weakness.

Lumbosacral Injuries Related to Abdominal Trauma

Infants rarely sustain crush injuries that result in pressure-induced lumbosacral plexopathies. One 13-month-old developed a flaccid leg, with the exception of preserved iliopsoas function. This was secondary to an acute abdominal crush injury.[156] During the next few days, loss of function ensued in the opposite leg with iliopsoas and quadriceps being the only muscles with preserved strength. Muscle stretch reflexes were absent bilaterally. An MRI of the lumbosacral spine was normal. EMG performed 72 hours after injury demonstrated bilaterally absent peroneal F waves and tibial H-reflexes but otherwise normal peroneal motor NCS. No MUAP were activated; however, no signs of denervation were demonstrated in the leg and the lumbosacral paraspinal muscles. Within 1 month the child had clinically recovered. Repeat EMG demonstrated normal MUPs in the previously silent muscles. The only signs of axonal damage were noted in the tibialis anterior muscles. F waves returned 3 months after injury. The clinical and EMG courses were thought to be primarily compatible with a neurapraxic injury.[156] Other traumatic mechanisms include knife injuries, gunshot wounds, and motor vehicle accidents.[122,154]

HEMORRHAGIC COMPLICATIONS

Iliopsoas hemorrhage can result in a femoral neuropathy, especially in the context of a bleeding diathesis. This occurred in a 15-year-old boy with hemophilia.[188] Similar to that in adults receiving anticoagulant medication, the lesion is related to hemorrhage within the iliopsoas muscle.

Neoplasms

When the onset of weakness is more insidious, the possibility of a retroperitoneal mass also needs consideration. Imaging (MRI) and EMG are helpful in localizing the lesion. Cancer, metastatic disease, and primary tumor affecting the LSP are rare conditions in children.[148]

Pyriformis Syndrome

It has been suggested that the pyriformis muscle entraps the sciatic nerve as it passes through this muscle palsy. This is an often disputed entity, and if it does occur it must be an exceedingly rare condition. We have never seen such. However, this was postulated to have occurred as a complication of posterior fossa surgery performed in the seated position in a 10-year-old boy.[189]

The most common differential is a sciatic nerve palsy (see discussion of mononeuropathies in Chapter 30).

Miscellaneous Lumbosacral Plexopathy

There are a few other rare etiologies to consider in the differential diagnosis of sudden leg weakness in children. Fortunately, poliomyelitis is no longer a problem in North America. In the mid 1990s when the live vaccine was the primary form of immunization, there were at least three cases of postimmunization infantile poliomyelitis for which one of our authors (H.R.J.) was consulted.[190-192] However, one must still keep the possibility of poliomyelitis in the differential diagnosis of any child with acute leg weakness, usually with pain and fever just before embarkation from their native land and who has recently arrived from endemic areas of the world particularly Africa, Egypt, and India. The EMG demonstrates a primary motor lesion with acute denervation and preserved sensory function.

PEDIATRIC NERVE ROOT LESIONS: OVERVIEW OF NEUROPHYSIOLOGIC AND MRI TESTING MODALITIES

Cervical or lumbosacral radiculopathies or LSRs caused by disorders of bones and/or supporting structures (intervertebral disks) surrounding the spinal cord and cauda equina are rare disorders in children, although such has been documented in the lumbosacral region as early as age 27 months.[193] It is occasionally difficult to make a differential diagnosis between the more common mononeuropathies, or brachial plexopathies, and the rare case of cervical root damage while performing a pediatric EMG. As nerve root avulsions and BP injury often occur concomitantly particularly in children, the presence of EMG findings compatible with a primary plexus lesion does not exclude damage at the nerve root level. Because it is much more difficult to obtain cervical paraspinal muscle relaxation in kids, this essential EMG differential diagnostic technique is usually a problem in the unrelaxed child.

Most children do not require operative intervention. From a structural (anatomic) standpoint, an MRI is the study of choice for any child with a suspected nerve root lesion. The question of a radiculopathy is an unusual reason for referral to a pediatric EMG laboratory. Nevertheless, it is important to consider the rare possibility of a nerve root process in the differential diagnosis of any child with cervical or lumbosacral pain, especially those with a radicular component.

EMG

General Principles of EMG Diagnosis in Nerve Root Disorders

In the uncommon instance of a child presenting with a radiculopathy, the MRI is the study of choice. *If the MRI is diagnostic, there is absolutely no need to proceed with an EMG.*

The nerve root responds to a focal lesion by undergoing axonal loss, focal demyelination, or both. There are no reports of EMG findings in asymptomatic healthy children. In adults these also are limited except with regard to paraspinal muscles. Haig has found a false-positive rate in the order of 5% in adults.[194]

The understanding of the difference between a preganglionic injury and a postganglionic lesion is crucial in the electrodiagnostic assessment of neck and arm or back and leg pain (see Fig. 31-2). Compressive radiculopathies occur so proximally that a potential conduction block in a preganglionic locus cannot be evaluated by routine NCSs. Given that the dorsal root ganglion is outside (distal to the intervertebral foramen), the corresponding SNAP will not be impaired. However, the corresponding motor component measured by CMAP amplitude can be affected if the lesion produces axonal loss. Thus CMAP amplitude will be reduced.

Recent adult studies demonstrate that EMG and MRI findings agree in the majority (60%) of patients with a clinical history compatible with cervical or lumbosacral radiculopathy (LSR). EMG provides the best information in those instances when the MRI is normal and there is need to establish a diagnosis, particularly when the clinical picture strongly suggests a radiculopathy.

Sensitivity, Specificity, and Limitation of EMG

Before commencing the EMG study, it is important to appreciate the limiting factors of EMG in the assessment and diagnosis of radiculopathies. These are mainly related to the location and nature of the lesion as just noted. Furthermore, there is an important dependence on the timing of the original lesion and thereby the duration of the pathology. Even when all "new" techniques are included, electrodiagnosis does not detect "all" compressive radiculopathies. EMG findings can therefore never be used to exclude a radiculopathy. In the context of the clinical presentation and findings, one of the most important values of EMG testing is that it can help distinguish other causes of pain, numbness, and/or neurogenic phenomena in the affected extremity.

Nerve Conduction Studies

The presence of normal SNAPs when the patient has clinically verified sensory loss is one of the essential criteria for a diagnosis of a nerve root lesion. The finding of normal median and ulnar SNAPs lends support to the diagnosis of a C7-C8 intraspinal lesion. When one attempts to differentiate lesions at C6 from those involving the BP, normal median SNAPs recorded from the thumb or lateral antebrachial cutaneous SNAPs provide a useful means to localize lesions to the C6 roots especially when paraspinal muscle EMG is unreliable.[5,195] The converse does not apply, that is, the absence of SNAPS, implying a postganglionic plexus lesion does not exclude a concomitant nerve root lesion.[16]

In most radiculopathies, because of dual root innervation to most muscles, there is little significant effect on CMAP amplitude. However, the L5 root primarily innervates the extensor digitorum brevis, and it may atrophy quite rapidly with an acute root lesion. Thus the peroneal CMAP may be diminished in this setting. Such is a nonspecific finding until the electromyographer also finds a retained superficial peroneal SNAP compatible with a preganglionic nerve root lesion (see Fig. 31-1).

Although both types of late responses (F waves and H reflexes) may be abnormal when there is a nerve root lesion, these are relatively nonspecific findings. The value of H reflexes in the assessment of children with radiculopathies has not been studied. From the practical viewpoint, stimulation in the popliteal fossa is relatively uncomfortable and the tolerance of children is quite limited when one has to perform the repetitive testing necessary to confirm the true absence of this response if indeed there is a pathology present impacting on the H reflex. Thus, at CHB we rarely use this study.

Needle EMG Examination

Needle EMG is the most important and useful procedure of the various electrodiagnostic methods available to assess patients with a suspected radiculopathy.[196] The presence of fibrillation potentials and neurogenic MUPs within specific myotomes, primarily the C5-C8 or L4-S1 distribution, are dependent on the severity of the lesion. Although needle EMG is essential, it requires fairly extensive assessment. Unfortunately, many children are unable to tolerate the careful evaluation that adult electromyographers typically pursue in search of a subtle nerve root lesion. Furthermore, needle EMG assesses only motor fibers and can only primarily detect the effects of motor axonal loss. If the clinical

BOX 31-13
CLASSIC NEEDLE EMG NEUROPATHIC CHANGES

Membrane instability, positive sharp waves and fibrillation potentials

Other signs of membrane instability and ectopic motor discharge, including CRDs, fasciculations

Large MUAP amplitude, increased percentage of polyphasic MUAP potentials

Decreased MUAP recruitment and interference pattern

MUAP, motor unit potential; CRD, complex repetitive discharge.

picture is primarily one of a sensory radiculopathy, without damage to the ventral or dorsal primary motor rami, needle EMG, is by definition, going to be normal. However, when the motor nerve root does sustain axonal damage, one can often find fibrillation potentials and other insertional abnormalities as well as neurogenic MUPs of large size that fire rapidly (Box 31-13). This offers confirmation of a chronic radiculopathy if the findings are confined to the distribution of a single root.

Generally abnormalities within the myotome in question need to be demonstrated in at least two or more muscles receiving innervation from the same root and preferably via different peripheral nerves and/or the paraspinal muscles (see Chapter 6 for myotome charts appendix). The sensitivity of needle EMG is dependent on the severity of the axonal loss and the duration of symptoms. Studies may be falsely negative if they are performed either too early or too late in the course of a radiculopathy.

One cannot exclude a radiculopathy with a normal EMG.

MRI and CT in the Diagnosis of Radiculopathies

Clinical correlation with MRI and/or CT myelography and surgery has been demonstrated (sensitivity and correlation coefficients of 70% to 95%) in adults.[196] However, no similar studies are known in children. Nevertheless an MRI is the study of choice for children with possible radiculopathies. At times one will initially be evaluating a child with an EMG for a possible mononeuropathy or plexus lesion when the findings do not support such a diagnosis, and one should move on to exclude the unusual childhood radiculopathy. It is here where a combined utilization of EMG and MRI may provide the diagnosis.

Somatosensory Evoked Potentials

Somatosensory evoked potentials (SSEPs) theoretically should help in the evaluation of patients with suspected root lesions. However, extensive evaluation has shown that they are not helpful in the assessment of patients with radicular pathology.[197] Furthermore, recent studies in children with brachial plexopathies show extensive somatosensory innervation, further limiting their clinical applicability.[198] In summary, somatosensory potentials evoked by nerve trunk stimulation are diagnostically unhelpful, whereas both cutaneous and dermatomal SSEPs are insensitive in patients with chronically unequivocal root lesions, making it unlikely that they will be of any clinical use when the diagnosis is less clear.[197] These are primarily of value in the assessment of spinal cord involvement.

Magnetic Stimulation

The spinal roots and the proximal portions of peripheral nerves can be stimulated by a rapidly changing magnetic field. However, from a practical clinical viewpoint it is not clear whether magnetic stimulation has any advantage over electrical stimulation and their clinical applicability requires further research.[199]

PEDIATRIC ROOT DISORDERS

It is often difficult to make a differential diagnosis between the more common mononeuropathies, or brachial plexopathies, and the rare case of cervical root damage while performing a pediatric EMG. As nerve root avulsions and BP injury often occur concomitantly, particularly in children, the presence of EMG findings compatible with a primary plexus lesion does not exclude damage at the nerve root level. Because it is much more difficult to obtain cervical paraspinal muscle relaxation in kids, this EMG differential diagnosis is sometimes a problem in the setting of a possible traumatic mechanism. The finding of normal median and ulnar SNAPs lends support to the diagnosis of a C7-C8 intraspinal lesion. When one attempts to differentiate lesions at C6 from those involving the BP, normal median SNAPs recorded from the thumb or lateral antebrachial cutaneous SNAPs provide a useful means to localize lesions to the C6 roots especially when paraspinal muscle EMG is unreliable.[5,192] The converse does not apply, that is, the absence of SNAPS, implying a postganglionic plexus lesion does not exclude a concomitant nerve root lesion.[15]

CERVICAL RADICULOPATHY

Children rarely have primary cervical nerve root lesions. In a review of 561 Mayo Clinic patients with a cervical radiculopathy, only 41 individuals (7%) were 15 to 29 years old.[200] No more specific breakdown of the adolescents included in this report is available. The study excluded one 13-year-old girl with a cervical radiculopathy. This exclusion further supports the rarity of this lesion in children and adolescents.[200]

Clinical Profile

Cervical radiculopathies do occur in adolescents but are exceedingly rare in younger children. We are unaware of any instance in a preschool-aged child in contrast with one instance of LSR.[193] In general we have not seen the typical case of a classic C6 or C7 radiculopathy among children or adolescents as is so common in adults. Although uncommon, this most likely relates to the excellent diagnostic accuracy of MRI for these lesions. However, occasionally one performs an EMG on a teenager who is referred with a query of a cervical radiculopathy who primarily has painless arm weakness and not any symptoms of pain or paresthesia. This should raise a question of other disorders, including congenital spinal stenosis, or some primary intramedullary lesions, including Hirayama's disorder, or, rarely, early motor neuron disease.

EMG testing in both congenital spinal stenosis and Hirayama flexion myelopathy demonstrates a primary active neurogenic process in the affected extremity. In addition, each of these entities has modest chronic neurogenic changes in the clinically silent, or less affected, contralateral extremity.

HNPP is another rare entity that also requires consideration in the presentation of painless arm weakness (see Chapter 32).[201] There is a similar, also genetically linked, process of an acute, recurrent, painful brachial plexopathy that may also mimic a nerve root lesion, as noted earlier in this chapter.[202]

Differential Diagnosis of Pediatric Cervical Root Lesions

Congenital Cervical Stenosis

Although our experience has not included any typical cervical radiculopathies secondary to disk or uncovertebral (osteophyte-induced foraminal stenosis) mechanisms,[200] two children with congenital cervical spine lesions have been studied at CHB. One was a 13-year-old child with a short history of pain in the right shoulder and arm exacerbated by swimming. EMG demonstrated C7-T1 denervation. Cervical spine radiography demonstrated anomalous hypoplastic vertebral bodies with incompletely developed interspaces.

Another case, a 16-year-old boy with a 3-month history of progressive painless arm weakness first apparent when he played basketball, had not had any paresthesias or other sensory symptoms to suggest spinal root involvement. Prior to his EMG the clinical diagnosis had been a possible BP lesion. Weakness predominantly affected the infraspinatus, supraspinatus, serratus anterior, deltoid, and possibly the opposite deltoid muscles. Muscle stretch reflexes were normal, and no sensory loss was detected.

Motor and sensory NCSs were normal. Needle EMG demonstrated active denervation in C5 to C8 dermatomes; contralateral changes were confined to C5. We were unable to obtain total relaxation of the cervical paraspinal muscles. Cervical spine radiography demonstrated en bloc C2-C3 vertebrae with diminished diameter of the spinal canal from C4 to C7. Myelography demonstrated spinal stenosis from C2 to C7. Decompressive cervical laminectomy was performed. His outcome was unknown, because he was lost to follow-up review shortly after the operation.

Juvenile Muscular Atrophy of Distal Upper Extremity; Hirayama Flexion Myelopathy

Juvenile muscular atrophy of distal upper extremity is another rare cause for painless arm weakness in an adolescent.[203] Initially this affects hand function and is confused with a C8 radiculopathy, medial brachial plexopathy, or an ulnar neuropathy. However, these patients have no pain or paresthesia making these more common mechanisms unlikely. Initially this is reminiscent of amyotrophic lateral sclerosis, something even more rare in this age group. Fortunately, amyotrophic lateral sclerosis has been seen just once in a teenager during one of our authors' career (H.R.J.).

Hirayama's disease generally affects adolescent boys of eastern Pacific rim heritage. However, we have seen a total of four similar cases among caucasians at CHB and Lahey. Typically this insidiously progressive disorder has a self-limiting course usually not progressing for more than 5 years. It predominantly affects just one upper extremity and to a much lesser extent its contralateral homologue.[204] The cervical spinal cord is the primary site of pathology. It is now thought that this is related to a flexion myelopathy.[205]

Grisel's Syndrome

Grisel's syndrome is an uncommon infectious process that primarily produces subluxation of the atlantoaxial joint. It is found in both children and adults.[206,207] Typically these patients present with unrelenting neck and/or throat pain. This is often followed by torticollis and sometimes subluxation at this spinal joint. Typically there is a preceding history of a flulike illness, otitis, tonsillitis, or pharyngitis. Subsequently an insidious onset of a progressively severe and localized unremitting spinal pain develops. About 15% of patients develop a cervical radiculopathy radiating into the shoulder. Some have a relatively precipitous onset of a torticollis and/or greater occipital nerve paresthesia. A myelopathy may follow characterized by transient or fixed quadriparesis and rarely death.[206,207]

Despite the infectious nature of this illness, it is uncommon for these children to appear highly septic. Spinal percussion tenderness and restriction of neck movement, including torticollis are the primary findings with physical examination. No EMG studies are mentioned in this review. However, their report points to the importance of considering this potentially serious illness in the rare instance of a child referred to the EMG laboratory with severe neck pain and symptoms of a cervical radiculopathy.

LUMBOSACRAL ROOT (LSR) DISEASE

On the rare occasions that herniation of the nucleus pulposus occurs in children, it usually occurs in the lumbosacral area. At the Mayo Clinic an orthopedic report evaluated 1368 pediatric cases 16 years or younger for back, disk, or sciatic pain between 1950 and 1975.[208] In many patients, a diagnosis of lumbar disk herniation was considered a possibility, and most of these responded well to conservative, nonoperative forms of therapy. However, 50 (3.7%) required surgical removal of one or more disks. These children with lumbar disk procedures represented 0.5% of lumbar laminectomies performed at the Mayo Clinic during that time span.[208] In a later surgically proven series of LSRs seen at Mayo Clinic, the estimated pediatric prevalence was 0.8% and 3.2%.[209] Another U.S. university hospital experience reported 10 adolescents with LSR seen during a 30-year epoch.[210] Thus they saw one instance every 3 years! There may be a significantly higher incidence of juvenile disk LSR in Japan. One Japanese study reported 70 patients, age 9 to 19 years. This represented 15.4% of 456 patients having LSR surgery from 1951 to 1977.[211] Fifty-five of 70 were boys; 21 were younger than 15 years of age. The youngest reported case is a 27-month-old child who fell from his cradle and over 2 weeks developed back pain, irritability, and gait difficulty. MRI demonstrated the LSR abnormality, and surgery was successful.[188]

Clinical Presentation

Back pain or sciatica, or both, is the typical clinical presentation. Although all children had sciatica, 12 (17%) in Japan[211] and 17 (34%) at Mayo Clinic had sciatica without back pain.[208] Trauma related to athletic injuries, lifting, falls, or back injury occurring at work accounted for at least half of the cases in two series.[210,211] In the Mayo study where there was a 36% incidence of trauma, the athletic injuries occurred in a variety of sports, including football, basketball, baseball, soccer, cheerleading, tennis, and running.[208]

Clinical examination demonstrated relatively subtle neurologic deficits. Although focal weakness primarily involving the tibialis anterior and/or toe extensors was detected in some, in one series no footdrop was noted in any child. Recognizable sensory loss was identifiable in 10% (lateral foot 8% and medial foot 2%) to 58% of these adolescents. Severe paravertebral muscle spasm was also present along with limited spinal motion, cough-sneeze exacerbation in many (76%), or a positive Lasègue sign in up to 86% of children.[208] Bowel and urinary tract disturbance occurred just once among the 155 children reported in four studies of adolescent LSRs. This was a 14-year-old boy with a cauda equina syndrome secondary to lumbar disk disease that required surgical repair.[208-211]

Imaging Studies

MRI is the diagnostic study of choice. Eleven of 20 patients in a 37-year retrospective study at CHB had an MRI performed for disk disease. In 1996 this senior neurosurgeon still believed that CT imaging was the best modality because it was simple, briefer, and kinder to the child. It gave a clear differentiation between bone, disk, ligaments, and ossified ligament.[212] Myelography was the primary means of diagnosis in the earlier studies.

Standard spinal radiography demonstrated a 30% incidence of congenital bony abnormalities.[208] These included spina bifida occulta in 16%, sacralization of the last lumbar vertebra in 14%, and an extra lumbar vertebra in 10%. In another study routine spine radiographs were diagnostic in 18 (58%) of the 32 children with a specific final diagnosis.[213] The value of a combined diagnostic approach including lumbosacral radiographs, CT, or MRI, along with EMG, is suggested for LSRs in teenage children.[214]

EMG

It is now unusual to evaluate children with back and/or sciatic pain in our CHB EMG laboratory. When we do, these are atypical clinical circumstances not infrequently having a significant suggestion of a complex regional pain syndrome such as reflex sympathetic dystrophy and causalgia after a relatively minor injury. There are few data on this subject from other institutions. EMGs were positive in five instances, including one child with normal results on myelography.[214] In this one instance with

TABLE 31–4. DIFFERENTIAL DIAGNOSIS OF BACK PAIN IN CHILDREN

Age < 10 Years	*Age ≥ 10 Years*
Infectious	Infectious
Vertebral osteomyelitis	Spondylolysis, spondylolisthesis
Diskitis	Scheuermann's disease
Tumor	Herniated nucleus pulposus
	Tumors

negative myelography, CT suggested superior facet entrapment. This was confirmed surgically. No data are included as to whether more than 5 EMGs were performed and, if so, what the false-negative rate was with this procedure.

Differential Diagnosis

Because pediatric lumbosacral disk disease is uncommon, unusual mechanisms need to be considered in children with lumbar nerve root symptoms (Table 31-4). One 6-year Orthopaedic Surgery Department review from Royal Manchester Children's Hospital in the United Kingdom evaluated their low back pain experience in children 15 years of age or younger. This represented 2% of nontrauma referrals to this clinic.[213] They were able to define a specific diagnosis in 32 of these 61 children. The variety of pathologic mechanisms included various infections (*n* = 5); tumors (*n* = 4); spondylosis, including spondylolisthesis (*n* = 8); Scheuermann's disease (*n* = 9); and miscellaneous processes (*n* = 2).

Inflammatory

Diskitis. Disk protrusion may sometimes be secondary to diskitis.[211] This same diagnosis was also considered in one 3-year-old boy who was seen because of acute severe low back pain, fever, and refusal to walk, sit, or stand.[215] The neurologic examination was difficult to perform because he kept his legs tightly flexed on his abdomen. Straight-leg testing was markedly positive bilaterally. The right patellar muscle stretch reflex was absent. No other focal signs were detected. He was managed conservatively, but no improvement occurred.

Myelography demonstrated a protruded L4-L5 disk. Surgery failed to identify any unusual mechanism for the nerve root lesion. He had an excellent surgical result. The fever subsided spontaneously, and no cause for it was identified. Today, MRI helps exclude spontaneous disk space infections because these lesions have a presentation similar to that of classic disk disease.[216,217]

Ankylosing Spondylitis. In older children, especially adolescents, the possibility of early ankylosing spondylitis always deserves consideration in the differential diagnosis of sciatica particularly with adolescent boys who present with classic sciatica. Routine radiographs and/or bony CT of the sacroiliac joints is often the diagnostic tool of choice in these young men, especially one with a positive human leukocyte antigen (HLA) B27 study.

The electromyographer needs to be alert to this possibility in any adolescent male presenting to the laboratory with sciatica because ankylosing spondylitis is eventually crippling if not recognized early on. Often these patients have a concomitant history of early morning stiffness and "jelling" associated with diminished chest excursion on examination.

Neoplasms

Schwannoma. Nerve root tumors, although quite uncommon, always require consideration in the differential diagnosis of lumbosacral disk disease. A 16-year-old high school wrestler experienced 1 year of pain in the left buttock radiating into the thigh and calf. CT of the lumbosacral spine demonstrated a mass at L5-S1; at laminectomy this was an S1 schwannoma.[218] EMG was not performed.

Osteoblastoma. In another instance, a 13-year-old girl presented with a 6-month history of vague low back pain precipitated in gymnasium class. She had hypoesthesia in the L3 dermatome, weakness of the quadriceps, and absent knee jerk. EMG demonstrated an L3 radiculopathy. Simple palpation detected a paravertebral mass that proved to be an osteoblastoma.[219]

Congenital Spinal Tumors. Occasionally lipomas, often associated with a tethered cord, need to be considered in the differential diagnosis of lumbar radiculopathies presenting with footdrop or foot deformities. In the two instances we evaluated (one at Lahey and the other at CHB), there was no associated back pain.

One was a 13-year-old boy with 2 years of progressive footdrop. He had 3/5 weakness of the tibialis anterior, 0.5-cm calf atrophy, and pes cavus. Peroneal and tibial NCS and sural SNAPs were normal. EMG demonstrated findings of S1 > L5 nerve root involvement including abnormal insertional activity in the lumbar paraspinal muscles. The normal SNAPs suggested a preganglionic lesion excluding a much more common evolving peroneal or peroneal division sciatic nerve lesion in this youngster with no back pain. This case emphasizes the need for a thorough EMG especially when the findings do not fit the usual pattern. Spinal MRI demonstrated a tethered cord and congenital tumor. MRI is the diagnostic study of choice.

Sacral Bone Tumors. Primary sacral bone tumors may present with radicular pain, paresthesias, progressive weakness, and later paresis of the extremity.[220] MRI and CT are the best diagnostic studies. Standard spinal radiographs often demonstrate normal results in the early stages of these lesions. In Kozlowski and coworkers' review[220] of 16 children, 13 had Ewing's sarcoma, and the other 3 each had an osteoblastoma, hemangiopericytoma, and a chordoma, respectively.

Scoliosis

Primary spinal scoliosis surgery also predisposes to the occurrence of pediatric LSRs. A 29% incidence of postoperative LSRs was reported.[221] EMG signs of myotomal weakness (not otherwise defined) were found in 4 of 14 children (mean age, 16 years). Fifty percent of these lesions were related to direct surgical trauma. The remaining LSRs occurred secondary to traction within the lumbosacral area.

Pediatric Gynecologic Lesion Mimicking an LSR

A 12-year-old girl who had not begun to menstruate presented with symptoms mimicking an LSR characterized by 8 months of intermittent, low back and right sacroiliac pain. She then had 6- to 8-week symptom-free intervals only to once again have a recurrence. This interfered with sleeping and sitting but was relieved by bending forward or lying on the side.

Examination demonstrated typical findings of an L5 radiculopathy. Additionally, a gynecologic evaluation demonstrated no vaginal opening. Pelvic ultrasonography showed a 13×10 cm mid-pelvic mass. At surgery this proved to be a congenital absence of the lower one third of the vagina. A vaginoplasty released 750 mL of menstrual fluids. Her low back pain was relieved immediately. Six months later, all signs of an L5 radiculopathy disappeared.[222] The dilated imperforate vagina with the hematometra was thought to have compressed the LSP, mimicking a nerve root lesion.

Noting that only about half of the referrals to an orthopedic children's hospital outpatient clinic proved to have spinal disease and that no diagnosis was reached in the other children, Deathe[222] suggested that pelvic ultrasonography needs to be part of the evaluation of indeterminate back pain and lumbar radiculopathy, especially in adolescent girls. This is especially pertinent noting that the incidence of this type of congenital anomaly is about 1 in 5000 phenotype females.

Therapy

Conservative management is usually quite successful for the treatment of adolescents and children with LSRs. At Mayo fewer than 1 in 25 children who had lumbar disk disease required surgery.[208] In contrast, a significantly higher percentage of Australian adolescents with disk disease (30 [35%] of 87) required surgery.[223] Only 40% of Japanese children initially improved with conservative therapy; however, even then their symptoms tended to recur on return to school.[211] Although results of LSR disk

surgery in children and adolescents were good, a reoperation was required in 10% to 25% of cases.[208,211]

SUMMARY AND OVERVIEW

In the adolescent population lumbosacral disk disorders are relatively uncommon.[212] The presentation in children is often different from that in the adult. It is important for the clinician to always add this diagnosis to the differential and to consider the possibility of LSR and/or one of the more unusual conditions that may mimic a radiculopathy.

Summary points include the following:
- MRI provides an excellent anatomic correlation.
- EMG cannot exclude a radiculopathy.
- Back and leg pain in children and adolescents is most likely related to an LSR. However, one must always exclude a primary vertebral or disk space infection, spinal or nerve root tumor, other intraspinal pathology, or, in adolescent girls, an imperforate vagina.

REFERENCES

1. Sunderland S: Anatomical features of nerve trunks in relation to nerve injury and nerve repair. Clin Neurosurg 1970;17:38-62.
2. Sunderland S: The anatomy and physiology of nerve injury. Muscle Nerve 1990;13:771-784.
3. Ebraheim NA, Lu J, Yang H, et al: Lumbosacral plexus: A histological study. Acta Anat (Basel) 1997;158:274-278.
4. Yilmaz K, Caliskan M, Oge E, et al: Clinical assessment, MRI, and EMG in congenital brachial plexus palsy. Pediatr Neurol 1999;21:705-710.
5. Wilbourn AJ: Brachial plexus disorders. *In* Dyck PJ, Thomas PK, Griffin JW, et al (eds): Peripheral Neuropathy. Philadelphia, WB Saunders, 1993, pp 911-950.
6. Wilbourn AJ: The electrodiagnostic examination with peripheral nerve injuries. Clin Plast Surg 2003;30:139-154.
7. Kao JT, Sharma S, Curtis CG, Clarke HM: The role of the brachioradialis H reflex in the management and prognosis of obstetrical brachial plexus palsy. Handchir Mikrochir Plast Chir 2003;35:106-111.
8. Smith SJ: The role of neurophysiological investigation in traumatic brachial plexus lesions in adults and children. J Hand Surg [Br] 1996;21:145-147.
9. Pollack RN, Buchman AS, Yaffe H, Divon MY: Obstetrical brachial palsy: Pathogenesis, risk factors, and prevention. Clin Obstet Gynecol 2000;43:236-246.
10. Bisinella GL, Birch R, Smith SJ: Neurophysiological prediction of outcome in obstetric lesions of the brachial plexus. J Hand Surg [Br] 2003;28:148-152.
11. Bisinella GL, Birch R: Obstetric brachial plexus lesions: A study of 74 children registered with the British Paediatric Surveillance Unit (March 1998-March 1999). J Hand Surg [Br] 2003;28:40-45.

12. Chaudhry V, Cornblath DR: Wallerian degeneration in human nerves: Serial electrophysiological studies. Muscle Nerve 1992;15:687-693.

13. Luco JV, Eyzaguirre C: Fibrillation and hypersensitivity to ACh in denervated muscle: Effect of length of degenerating nerve fibers. J Neurophysiol 1955;18:65-73.

14. van Dijk JG, Malessy MJ, Stegeman DF: Why is the electromyogram in obstetric brachial plexus lesions overly optimistic? Muscle Nerve 1998;21:260-261.

15. van Dijk JG, Pondaag W, Malessy MJ: Obstetric lesions of the brachial plexus. Muscle Nerve 2001;24:1451-1461.

16. Mancias P, Slopis JM, Yeakley JW, Vriesendorp FJ: Combined brachial plexus injury and root avulsion after complicated delivery. Muscle Nerve 1994;17:1237-1238.

17. Jones HR Jr, Herbison GJ, Jacob SR, et al: Intrauterine onset of a mononeuropathy: Peroneal neuropathy in a newborn. Muscle Nerve 1996;19:88-91.

18. Koenigsberger MR: Brachial plexus palsy at birth: Intrauterine or due to delivery trauma? Ann Neurol 1980;8:228.

19. Ouzounian JG, Korst LM, Phelan JP: Permanent Erb palsy: A traction-related injury? Obstet Gynecol 1997;89:139-141.

20. Paradiso G, Granana N, Maza E: Prenatal brachial plexus paralysis. Neurology 1997;49:261-262.

21. Gonik B, McCormick EM, Verweij BH, et al: The timing of congenital brachial plexus injury: A study of electromyography findings in the newborn piglet. Am J Obstet Gynecol 1998;178:688-695.

22. Korak KJ, Tam SL, Gordon T, et al: Changes in spinal cord architecture after brachial plexus injury in the newborn. Brain 2004;127:1488-1495.

23. Ross D, Jones R, Fisher J, Konkol RJ: Isolated radial nerve lesion in the newborn. Neurology 1983;33:1354-1356.

24. Allen RH: Brachial plexus palsy: An in utero injury? Am J Obstet Gynecol 1999;181:1271-1272.

25. Dunn DW, Engle WA: Brachial plexus palsy: Intrauterine onset. Pediatr Neurol 1985;1:367.

26. Gherman RB, Ouzounian JG, Goodwin TM: Brachial plexus palsy: an in utero injury? Am J Obstet Gynecol 1999;180:1303-1307.

27. Jennett RJ, Tarby TJ, Kreinick CJ: Brachial plexus palsy: An old problem revisited. Am J Obstet Gynecol 1992;166:1673-1676.

28. Jennett RJ, Tarby TJ: Brachial plexus palsy: An old problem revisited again: II. Cases in point. Am J Obstet Gynecol 1997;176:1354-1356.

29. Al-Qudah AA, Shahar E, Logan WJ, Murphy EG: Neonatal Guillain-Barré syndrome. Pediatr Neurol 1988;4:255-256.

30. Jackson AH, Baquis GD, Shaw BL: Congenital Guillain-Barré syndrome. J Child Neurol 1996;5:407-410.

31. Luijckx GJ, Vles J, de Baets M, et al: Guillain-Barré syndrome in mother and child. Lancet 1997;349:27.

32. Rolfs A, Bolik A: Guillain-Barré syndrome in pregnancy: Reflections on immunopathogenesis. Acta Neurol Scand 1994;89:400-492.

33. Tsairis P, Dyck PJ, Mulder DW: Natural history of brachial plexus neuropathy: Report on 99 patients. Arch Neurol 1972;27:109-117.

34. Clay SA: Osteomyelitis as a cause of brachial plexus neuropathy. Am J Dis Child 1982;136:1054-1056.

35. Robotti E, Longhi P, Verna G, Bocchiotti G: Brachial plexus surgery: An historical perspective. Hand Clin 1995;11:517-533.

36. Miller TA, Jones HR Jr: Disorders of plexus and nerve root. *In* Brown WF, Bolton CF, Aminoff MJ (eds): Neuromuscular Function and Disease: Basic, Clinical, and Electrodiagnostic Aspects. Philadelphia, WB Saunders, 2002, pp 1601-1634.

37. Gordon M, Rich H, Deutschberger J, Green M: The immediate and long-term outcome of obstetric birth trauma: I. Brachial plexus paralysis. Am J Obstet Gynecol 1973;117:51-56.

38. Hardy AE: Birth injuries of the brachial plexus: Incidence and prognosis. J Bone Joint Surg Br 1981;63-B:98-101.

39. Sjoberg I, Erichs K, Bjerre I: Cause and effect of obstetric (neonatal) brachial plexus palsy. Acta Paediatr Scand 1988;77:357-364.

40. Bager B: Perinatally acquired brachial plexus palsy: A persisting challenge. Acta Paediatr 1997;86:1214-1219.

41. Adler JB, Patterson RL Jr: Erb's palsy: Long-term results of treatment in eighty-eight cases. J Bone Joint Surg Am 1967;49:1052-1064.

42. Eng GD, Koch B, Smokvia M: Brachial plexus palsy in neonates and children. Arch Phys Med Rehabil 1978;59:458.

43. Gilbert WM, Nesbitt TS, Danielsen B: Associated factors in 1611 cases of brachial plexus injury. Obstet Gynecol 1999;93:536-540.

44. Rouse DJ, Owen J, Goldenberg RL, Cliver SP: The effectiveness and costs of elective cesarean delivery for fetal macrosomia diagnosed by ultrasound. JAMA 1996;276:1480-1486.

45. Egloff DV, Raffoul W, Bonnard C, Stalder J: Palliative surgical procedures to restore shoulder function in obstetric brachial palsy: Critical analysis of Narakas' series. Hand Clin 1995;11:597-606.

46. Narakas AO: Obstetrical Brachial Plexus Injuries: The Paralysed Hand. Edinburgh, Churchill Livingstone, 1987, pp 116-135.

47. Al Qattan MM, Clarke HM, Curtis CG: Klumpke's birth palsy: Does it really exist? J Hand Surg [Br] 1995;20:19-23.

48. Vassalos E, Prevedourakis C, Paraschopoulou-Prevedourakis P: Brachial plexus paralysis in the newborn: An analysis of 169 cases. Am J Obstet Gynecol 1968;101:554-556.

49. Laurent JP, Lee RT: Birth-related upper brachial plexus injuries in infants: Operative and nonoperative approaches. J Child Neurol 1994;9:111-117.

50. Ballock RT, Song KM: The prevalence of nonmuscular causes of torticollis in children. J Pediatr Orthop 1996;16:500-504.

51. Benjamin B, Khan MR: Pattern of external birth trauma in southwestern Saudi Arabia. J Trauma 1993;35:737-741.

52. Dodds SD, Wolfe SW: Perinatal brachial plexus palsy. Curr Opin Pediatr 2000;12:40-47.

53. Ubachs JM, Slooff AC, Peeters LL: Obstetric antecedents of surgically treated obstetric brachial plexus injuries. Br J Obstet Gynaecol 1995;102:813-817.

54. Al Qattan MM: Obstetric brachial plexus palsy associated with breech delivery. Ann Plast Surg 2003;51:257-264.

55. Kay SP: Obstetrical brachial palsy. Br J Plast Surg 1998;51:43-50.

56. Geutjens G, Gilbert A, Helsen K: Obstetric brachial plexus associated with breech delivery. J Bone Joint Surg 1996;78:303-306.

57. Ecker JL, Greenberg JA, Norwitz ER, et al: Birth weight as a predictor of brachial plexus injury. Obstet Gynecol 1997;89:643-647.

58. Bryant DR, Leonardi MR, Landwehr JB, Bottoms SF: Limited usefulness of fetal weight in predicting neonatal brachial plexus injuries. Am J Obstet Gynecol 1998;179:686-689.

59. McFarland MB, Langer O, Piper JM, Berkus MD: Perinatal outcome and the type and number of maneuvers in shoulder dystocia. Int J Gynaecol Obstet 1996;55:219-224.

60. Al Qattan MM, el Sayed AA, al Kharfy TM, al Jurayyan NA: Obstetrical brachial plexus injury in newborn babies delivered by caesarean section. J Hand Surg [Br] 1996;21:263-265.

61. Iffy L, Mcardle JJ: The role of medico-legal reviews in medical research. Med Law 1996;15:399-406.

62. Gonik B, Walker A, Grimm M: Mathematic modeling of forces associated with shoulder dystocia: A comparison of endogenous and exogenous sources. Am J Obstet Gynecol 2000;182:689-691.

63. Basheer H, Zelic V, Rabia F: Functional scoring system for obstetric brachial plexus palsy. J Hand Surg [Br] 2000;25:41-45.

64. Al Qattan MM, Clarke HM, Curtis CG: The prognostic value of concurrent clavicular fractures in newborns with obstetric brachial plexus palsy. J Hand Surg [Br] 1994;19:729-730.

65. Al Qattan MM, Clarke HM, Curtis CG: The prognostic value of concurrent Horner's syndrome in total obstetric brachial plexus injury. J Hand Surg [Br] 2000;25:166-167.

66. Jeffery AR, Ellis FJ, Repka MX, Buncic JR: Pediatric Horner syndrome. J AAPOS 1998;2:159-167.

67. Oppenheim WL, Davis A, Growdon WA, et al: Clavicle fractures in the newborn. Clin Orthop 1990;250:176-180.

68. Eng GD: Brachial plexus palsy in newborn infants. Pediatrics 1971;48:18.

69. Eng GD, Binder H, Getson P, O'Donnell R: Obstetrical brachial plexus palsy (OBPP) outcome with conservative management. Muscle Nerve 1996;19:884-891.

70. Michelow BJ, Clarke HM, Curtis CG, et al: The natural history of obstetrical brachial plexus palsy. Plast Reconstr Surg 1994;93:675-680.

71. Rust RS: Congenital brachial plexus palsy: Where have we been and where are we now? Semin Pediatr Neurol 2000;7:58-63.

72. Birchansky S, Altman N: Imaging the brachial plexus and peripheral nerves in infants and children. Semin Pediatr Neurol 2000;7:15-25.

73. Hashimoto T, Mitomo M, Hirabuki N, et al: Nerve root avulsion of birth palsy: Comparison of myelography with CT. Radiology 1991;178:841-845.

74. Trojaborg W: Clinical, electrophysiological, and myelographic studies of 9 patients with cervical spinal root avulsions: Discrepancies between EMG and x-ray findings. Muscle Nerve 1994;17:913-922.

75. Chow BC, Blaser S, Clarke HM: Predictive value of computed tomographic myelography in obstetrical brachial plexus palsy. Plast Reconstr Surg 2000;106:971-977.

76. van Ouwerkerk WJ, van der Sluijs JA, Nollet F, et al: Management of obstetric brachial plexus lesions: State of the art and future developments. Childs Nerv Syst 2000;16:638-644.

77. Azouz EM, Oudjhane K: Disorders of the upper extremity in children. Magn Reson Imaging Clin North Am 1998;6:677-695.

78. Francel PC, Koby M, Park TS, et al: Fast spin-echo magnetic resonance imaging for radiological assessment of neonatal brachial plexus injury. J Neurosurg 1995;83:461-466.

79. Gomez-Anson B: MR imaging of the brachial plexus. J Neurol Neurosurg Psychiatry 2000;68:801.

80. Hems TEJ, Birch R, Carlstedt T: The role of magnetic resonance imaging in the management of traction injuries to the adult brachial plexus. J Hand Surg 1999;24B:550-555.

81. Miller SF, Glasier CM, Griebel ML, Boop FA: Brachial plexopathy in infants after traumatic delivery: Evaluation with MR imaging. Radiology 1993;189:481-484.

82. Nakamura T, Yabe Y, Takayama S: Magnetic resonance myelography in brachial plexus injury. J Bone Joint Surg Br 1997;79-B:764-769.

83. Uetani M, Hayashi K, Hashmi R, et al: Traction injuries of the brachial plexus: Signal intensity changes of the posterior cervical paraspinal muscles on MRI. J Comput Assist Tomogr 1997;21:790-795.

84. Birch R: Obstetric brachial plexus palsy. J Hand Surg [Br] 2002;27:3-8.

85. Bisinella GL, Birch R, Smith SJ: Neurophysiological prediction of outcome in obstetric lesions of the brachial plexus. J Hand Surg [Br] 2003;28:148-152.

86. Saifuddin A, Heffernan G, Birch R: Ultrasound diagnosis of shoulder congruity in chronic obstetric brachial plexus palsy. J Bone Joint Surg Br 2002;84-B:100-103.

87. Grossman JA: Early operative intervention for birth injuries to the brachial plexus. Semin Pediatr Neurol 2000;7:36-43.

88. Laurent JP, Lee R, Shenaq S, et al: Neurosurgical correction of upper brachial plexus birth injuries. J Neurosurg 1993;79:197-203.

89. Terzis JK, Papakonstantinou KC: Management of obstetric brachial plexus palsy. Hand Clin 1999;15:717-736.

90. Terzis JK, Vekris MD, Okajima S, Soucacos PN: Shoulder deformities in obstetric brachial plexus paralysis: a

computed tomography study. J Pediatr Orthop 2003;23(2):254-260.

91. Gilbert A, Razaboni R, Amar-Khodja S: Indications and results of brachial plexus surgery in obstetrical palsy. Orthop Clin North Am 1988;19:91-105.

92. Jones HR, Miller TA, Wilbourn A: Brachial and lumbosacral plexus lesions. *In* Jones HR, De Vivo D, Darras B (eds): Neuromuscular Disorders of Infancy, Childhood, and Adolescence: A Clinician's Approach. Philadelphia, Butterworth-Heinemann, 2003, pp 245-277.

93. Strombeck C, Krumlinde-Sundholm L, Forssberg H. Functional outcome at 5 years in children with obstetrical brachial plexus palsy with and without microsurgical reconstruction. Dev Med Child Neurol 2000;42:148-157.

94. Jones HR, Miller TA, Wilbourn A: Brachial and lumbosacral plexus lesions. *In* Jones HR, De Vivo D, Darras B (eds): Neuromuscular Disorders of Infancy, Childhood, and Adolescence: A Clinician's Approach. Philadelphia, Butterworth Heinemann Health, 2003, p 261.

95. Strombeck C, Fernell E: Aspects of activities and participation in daily life related to body structure and function in adolescents with obstetrical brachial plexus palsy: A descriptive follow-up study. Acta Paediatr 2003;92:740-746.

96. Dunn HG, Daube JR, Gomez MR: Heredofamilial branchial plexus neuropathy (hereditary neuralgic amyotrophy with branchial predilection) in childhood. Dev Med Child Neurol 1978;20:28-46.

97. Gouider R, LeGuern E, Emile J, et al: Hereditary neuralgic amyotrophy and hereditary neuropathy with liability to pressure palsies: Two distinct clinical, electrophysiologic, and genetic entities. Neurology 1994;44:2250-2252.

98. Jones HR, Herbison GJ, Jacob SR, et al: Intrauterine onset of mononeuropathy: Peroneal neuropathy in the newborn Muscle Nerve 1996;19:88-91.

99. Agboatwalla M, Kirmani SR, Sonawalla A, Akram DS: Nerve conduction studies and its importance in diagnosis of acute poliomyelitis. Indian J Pediatr 1993;60:265-268.

100. Alfonso I, Alfonso DT, Papazian O: Focal upper extremity neuropathy in neonates. Semin Pediatr Neurol 2000;7:4-14.

101. Sharma RR, Sethu AU, Mahapatra AK, et al: Neonatal cervical osteomyelitis with paraspinal abscess and Erb's palsy: A case report and brief review of the literature. Pediatr Neurosurg 2000;32:230-233.

102. Pellegrino JE, George RA, Biegel J, et al: Hereditary neuralgic amyotrophy: Evidence for genetic homogeneity and mapping to chromosome 17q25. Hum Genet 1997;101:277-283.

103. Chance PF, Lensch MW, Lipe H, et al: Hereditary neuralgic amyotrophy and hereditary neuropathy with liability to pressure palsies: Two distinct genetic disorders. Neurology 1994;44:2253-2257.

104. Stogbauer F, Young P, Kuhlenbaumer G, et al: Hereditary recurrent focal neuropathies: Clinical and molecular features. Neurology 2000;54:546-551.

105. Bradley WG, Madrid R, Thrush DC, Campbell MJ: Recurrent brachial plexus neuropathy. Brain 1975;98:381-398.

106. Geiger LR, Mancall EL, Penn AS, Tucker SH: Familial neuralgic amyotrophy: Report of three families with review of the literature. Brain 1974;97:87-102.

107. Verhagen WI, Gabreels-Festen AA, van Wensen PJ, et al: Hereditary neuropathy with liability to pressure palsies: A clinical, electroneurophysiological, and morphological study. J Neurol Sci 1993;116:176-184.

108. Chance PF, Escolar DM, Redmond A, Pasquali L, Ouvrier R Hereditary Neuropathies in: Late Childhood and Adolescence. *In* Jones HR, De Vivo DC and Darras (eds): Neuromuscular Disorders of Infancy, Childhood, and Adolescence: A Clinician's Approach. Philadelphia, Butterworth-Heinemann, 2003, pp 389-406.

109. Behse F, Buchthal F, Carlsen F, Knappeis GG: Hereditary neuropathy with liability to pressure palsies: Electrophysiological and histopathological aspects. Brain 1972;95:777-794.

110. Parsonage MJ, Turner JWA: Neuralgic amyotrophy: The shoulder-girdle syndrome. Lancet 1948;1:973-978.

111. To WC, Traquina DN: Neuralgic amyotrophy presenting with bilateral vocal cord paralysis in a child: A case report. Int J Pediatr Otorhinolaryngol 1999;48:251-254.

112. Turner JWA, Parsonage MJ: Neuralgic amyotrophy (paralytic brachial neuritis), with special reference to prognosis. Lancet 1957;2:209-212.

113. England JD, Sumner AJ: Neuralgic amyotrophy: An increasingly diverse entity. Muscle Nerve 1987;10:60-68.

114. Bale JF Jr, Thompson JA, Petajan JH, Ziter FA: Childhood brachial plexus neuropathy. J Pediatr 1979;95:741-742.

115. Piatt JH, Hudson AR, Hoffman HJ: Preliminary experiences with brachial plexus exploration in children: Birth injury and vehicular trauma. Neurosurgery 1988;22:715-723.

116. Piatt JH: Neurosurgical management of birth injuries of the brachial plexus. Neurosurg Clin North Am 1991;2:175-185.

117. Peterson CR, Peterson CM: Brachial-plexus injury in an infant from a car safety seat. N Engl J Med 1991;325:1587-1588.

118. Rothner AD, Wilbourn A, Mercer RD: Rucksack palsy. Pediatrics 1975;56:822-824.

119. Hirasawa Y, Sakakida K: Sports and peripheral nerve injury. Am J Sports Med 1983;11:420-426.

120. Barisic N, Mitrovic Z, et al: Electrophysiological assessment of children with peripheral nerve injury due to war or accident. Pediatr Neurol 1994;11:180.

120a. Barisic N, Perovic D, Mitrovic Z, et al: Assessment of war and accidental nerve injuries in children. Pediatr Neurol 1999; 21:451-455.

121. Dumitru D: Brachial Plexopathies and Proximal Mononeuropathies: Electrodiagnostic Medicine. Philadelphia, Hanley & Belfus, 1995, pp 585-642.

122. Kline DG: Operative management of major nerve lesions of the lower extremity. Surg Clin North Am 1972;52:1247-1265.

123. Kline DG, Judice DJ: Operative management of selected brachial plexus lesions. J Neurosurg 1983;58: 631-649.

124. Kline DG: Civilian gunshot wounds to the brachial plexus. J Neurosurg 1989;70:166-174.

125. Kline DG, Hudson AR: Diagnosis of root avulsions. J Neurosurg 1997;87:483-484.

126. Mehlman CT, Scott KA, Koch BL, Garcia VF: Orthopaedic injuries in children secondary to airbag deployment. J Bone Joint Surg Am 2000;82-A:895-898.

127. Menegaux F, Keeffe EB, Andrews BT, et al: Neurological complications of liver transplantation in adult versus pediatric patients. Transplantation 1994;58:447-450.

128. Schwartz DM, Drummond DS, Hahn M, et al: Prevention of positional brachial plexopathy during surgical correction of scoliosis. J Spinal Disord 2000;13:178-182.

129. Chrisman OD, Snook GA, Stanitis JM, et al: Lateral flexion neck injuries in athletic competition. JAMA 1965;192:613-615.

130. Clancy WG, Brand RL, Bergfield JA: Upper trunk brachial plexus injuries in contact sports. Am J Sports Med 1977;5:209-216.

131. Clancy WG: Brachial plexus and upper extremity peripheral nerve injuries. *In* Torg JS (ed): Athletic Injuries to the Head, Neck, and Face. Philadelphia, Lea & Febiger, 1982, pp 215-220.

132. Di Benedetto M, Markey K: Electrodiagnostic localization of traumatic upper trunk brachial plexopathy. Arch Phys Med Rehabil 1984;65:15-17.

133. Poindexter DP, Johnson EW: Football shoulder and neck injury: A study of the "stinger." Arch Phys Med Rehabil 1984;65:601-602.

134. Robertson WC, Eichman PL, Clancy WG: Upper trunk brachial plexopathy in football players. JAMA 1979;241:1480-1482.

135. Rockett FX: Observations on the "burner:" Traumatic cervical radiculopathy. Clin Orthop 1982;164:18-19.

136. Watkins RG: Nerve injuries in football players. Clin Sports Med 1986;5:215-246.

137. Wilbourn AJ: Electrodiagnostic testing of neurologic injuries in athletes. Clin Sports Med 1990;9:229-245.

138. Wroble RR, Albright JP: Neck and low back injuries in wrestling. Clin Sports Med 1986;5:295-325.

139. Gilliatt RW, Willison RG, Dietz V, Williams IR: Peripheral nerve conduction in patients with a cervical rib and band. Ann Neurol 1978;4:124-129.

140. Wulff CH, Gilliatt RW: F waves in patients with hand wasting caused by a cervical rib and band. Muscle Nerve. 1979;2(6):452-457.

141. Tilki HE, Stalberg E, Incesu L, Basoglu A: Bilateral neurogenic thoracic outlet syndrome. Muscle Nerve 2004;29(1):147-150.

142. Roos DB: Thoracic outlet syndrome is underdiagnosed. Muscle Nerve 1999;22:126-129.

143. Wilbourn AJ: The thoracic outlet syndrome is overdiagnosed. Arch Neurol 1990;47:328-330.

144. Wilbourn AJ: Thoracic outlet syndrome is overdiagnosed. Muscle Nerve 1999;22:130-136.

145. Ouvrier RA, McLeod JG, Pollard JD: Peripheral Neuropathy in Childhood. New York, Mac Keith, 1990.

146. Lucas JW, Holden KR, Purohit DM, Cure JK: Neonatal hemangiomatosis associated with brachial plexus palsy. J Child Neurol 1995;10:411-413.

147. Sadleir LG, Connolly MB: Acquired brachial plexus neuropathy in the neonate: A rare presentation of late-onset group-B streptococcal osteomyelitis. Dev Med Child Neurol 1998;40:496-499.

148. Harila-Saari AH, Vainionpaa LK, Kovala TT, et al: Nerve lesions after therapy for childhood acute lymphoblastic leukemia. Cancer 1998;82:200-207.

149. Alessandri AJ, Pritchard SL, Massing BG, et al: Misleading leads: Bone pain caused by isolated paraspinal extramedullary relapse of childhood acute lymphoblastic leukemia. Med Pediatr Oncol 1999;33:113-115.

150. Inoue M, Kawano T, Matsumura H, et al: Solitary benign schwannoma of the brachial plexus. Surg Neurol 1983;20:103-108.

151. Sethna NF: Complex regional pain syndromes I and II (reflex sympathetic dystrophy). *In* Jones HR, De Vivo D, Darras B (eds): Neuromuscular Disorders of Infancy, Childhood, and Adolescence. Philadelphia, Butterworth Heinemann Health, 2003, pp 1185-1197.

152. Barquet A: Traumatic anterior dislocation of the hip in childhood. Injury 1982;13:435-440.

153. Chad DA, Bradley WG: Lumbosacral plexopathy. Semin Neurol 1987;7:97-107.

154. Chiou-Tan FY, Kemp K, Elfenbaum M, et al: Lumbosacral plexopathy in gunshot wounds and motor vehicle accidents: Comparison of electrophysiologic findings. Am J Phys Med Rehabil 2001;80:280-285.

155. Christie J, Jamieson EW: Traction lesion of the lumbosacral plexus. J R Coll Surg Edinb 1974;19:384-385.

156. Egel RT, Cueva JP, Adair RL: Posttraumatic childhood lumbosacral plexus neuropathy. Pediatr Neurol 1995;12:62-64.

157. Jellis JE, Helal B: Childhood sciatic palsies: Congenital and traumatic. Proc R Soc Med 1970;63:655-656.

158. Kline DG, Kim D, Midha R, et al: Management and results of sciatic nerve injuries: A 24-year experience. J Neurosurg 1998;89:13-23.

159. Kim DH, Murovic JA, Tiel R, Kline DG: Management and outcomes in 353 surgically treated sciatic nerve lesions. J Neurosurg 2004;101(1):8-17.

160. Marra TA: Recurrent lumbosacral and brachial plexopathy associated with schistosomiasis. Arch Neurol 1983;40:586-587.

161. Rai SK, Far RF, Ghovanlou B: Neurologic deficits associated with sacral wing fractures. Orthopedics 1990;13:1363-1366.

162. Switzer JA, Nork SE, Routt ML: Comminuted fractures of the iliac wing. J Orthop Trauma 2000;14:270-276.

163. Stoehr M: Traumatic and postoperative lesions of the lumbosacral plexus. Arch Neurol 1978;35:757-760.

164. Gabreels-Festen AA, Gabreels FJ, Joosten EM, et al: Hereditary neuropathy with liability to pressure palsies in childhood. Neuropediatrics 1992;23:138-143.

165. Galan E, Kousseff BG: Peripheral neuropathy in Ehlers-Danlos syndrome. Pediatr Neurol 1995;12:242-245.

166. Evans BA, Stevens JC, Dyck PJ: Lumbosacral plexus neuropathy. Neurology 1981;31:1327-1330.

167. Thomson AJ: Idiopathic lumbosacral plexus neuropathy in two children. Dev Med Child Neurol 1993;35:258-261.

168. Pasternak JF, Volpe JJ: Lumbosacral lipoma with acute deterioration during infancy. Pediatrics 1980;66:125-128.

169. MacDonald NE, Marcuse EK: Neurologic injury after vaccination: Buttocks as injection site. Can Med Assoc J 1994;150:326.

170. MacDonald NE: Does immunization in the buttocks cause sciatic nerve injury? Pediatrics 1994;93:351.

171. Marin R, Bryant PR, Eng GD: Lumbosacral plexopathy temporally related to vaccination. Clin Pediatr 1994;33:175-177.

172. Villarejo FJ, Pascual AM: Injection injury of the sciatic nerve (370 cases). Childs Nerv Syst 1993;9:229-232.

173. Bye A, Fagan E: Nerve conduction studies of the sural nerve in childhood. J Child Neurol 1988;3:94-99.

174. Dumitru D: Lumbosacral Plexopathies and Proximal Mononeuropathies: Electrodiagnostic Medicine. Philadelphia, Hanley & Belfus, 1995, pp 643-688.

175. Hope EE, Bodensteiner JB, Thong N: Neonatal lumbar plexus injury. Arch Neurol 1985;42:94-95.

176. Eng GD: Neuromuscular disease. *In* Avery GB, Fletcher MA, Macdonald MG (eds): Neonatology: Pathophysiology and Management of the Newborn. Philadelphia, WB Saunders, 1981, pp 989-992.

177. Volpe JJ: Injuries of extracranial, cranial, intracranial, spinal cord, and peripheral nervous system structures. *In* Neurology of the Newborn. Philadelphia, JB Lippincott, 1987, pp 638-658.

178. Awerbuch G, Levin GR, Dabrowski E: Lumbosacral plexus neuropathy of children. Ann Neurol 1989;26:452.

179. Awerbuch GI, Nigro MA, Dabrowski E, Levin JR: Childhood lumbosacral plexus neuropathy. Pediatr Neurol 1989;5:314-316.

180. Chin CH, Chew KC: Lumbosacral nerve root avulsion. Injury 1997;28:674-678.

181. Verstraete KL, Martens F, Smeets P, et al: Traumatic lumbosacral nerve root meningoceles: The value of myelography in the assessment of nerve root. Neuroradiology 1989;31:425-429.

182. Barnett HG, Connolly ES: Lumbosacral nerve root avulsion: Report of a case and review of the literature. J Trauma 1975;15:532-535.

183. Kolawole TM, Hawass ND, Shaheen MA, et al: Lumbosacral plexus avulsion injury: Clinical, myelographic, and computerized features. J Trauma 1988;28:861-865.

184. Huittinen VM: Lumbosacral nerve injury in fracture of the pelvis: A postmortem radiographic and patho-anatomical study. Acta Chir Scand Suppl 1972;429:3-43.

185. Young NL, Davis RJ, Bell DF, Redmond DM: Electromyographic and nerve conduction changes after tibial lengthening by the Ilizarov method. J Pediatr Orthop 1993;13:473-477.

186. Jones HR, Gianturco LE, Gross PT, Buchhalter J: Sciatic neuropathies in childhood: A report of ten cases and review of the literature. J Child Neurol 1988;3:193-199.

187. Yuen EC, Olney RK, So YT: Sciatic neuropathy: Clinical and prognostic features in 73 patients. Neurology 1994;44:1669-1674.

188. Gertzbein SD, Evans DC: Femoral nerve neuropathy complicating iliopsoas haemorrhage in patients. J Bone Joint Surg Br 1972;54-B:149-151.

189. Brown JA, Braun MA, Namey TC: Pyriformis syndrome in a 10-year-old boy as a complication of operation with the patient in the sitting position. Neurosurgery 1988;23:117-119.

190. Beausoleil JL, Nordgren RE, Modlin JF: Vaccine-associated paralytic poliomyelitis. J Child Neurol 1994;9:334-335.

191. David W, Doyle J: Acute Infantile Weakness: A case of vaccine associated poliomyelitis. Muscle Nerve 1997;20:747-749.

192. Goldstein J: Infantile poliomyelitis in a recently immunized baby seen at Yale. Personal Communication, 1995.

193. Revuelta R, De Juambelz PP, Fernandez B, Flores JA: Lumbar disc herniation in a 27-month-old child: Case report. J Neurosurg 2000;92:98-100.

194. Haig AJ: The prevalence of lumbar paraspinal spontaneous activity in asymptomatic subjects. Muscle Nerve 1996;19:1503-1504.

195. Wilbourn AJ: Electrodiagnosis of plexopathies. Neurol Clin 1985;3:511-529.

196. Wilbourn AJ, Aminoff MJ: AAEM minimonograph 32: The electrodiagnostic examination in patients with radiculopathies. American Association of Electrodiagnostic Medicine. Muscle Nerve 1998;21:1612-1631.

197. Eisen A: The utility of proximal nerve conduction in radiculopathies: The cons. Electroencephalogr Clin Neurophysiol 1991;78:171-172.

198. Colon AJ, Vredeveld JW, Blaauw G, et al: Extensive somatosensory innervation in infants with obstetric brachial palsy. Clin Anat 2003;16:25-29.

199. Burke D, Adams RW, Skuse NF: The effects of voluntary contraction on the H reflex of human limb muscles. Brain 1989;112:417-433.

200. Radhakrishnan K, Litchy WJ, O'Fallon WM, Kurland LT: Epidemiology of cervical radiculopathy: A population-based study from Rochester, Minnesota, 1976 through 1990. Brain 1994;117:325-335.

201. Infante J, Garcia A, Combarros O, et al: Diagnostic strategy for familial and sporadic cases of neuropathy associated with 17p11.2 deletion. Muscle Nerve 2001;24:1149-1155.

202. Stogbauer F, Young P, Kerschensteiner M, et al: Recurrent brachial plexus palsies as the only clinical expression of

hereditary neuropathy with liability to pressure palsies associated with a de novo deletion of the peripheral myeline protein-22 gene. Muscle Nerve 1998;21:1199-1201.

203. Kikuchi S, Tashiro K: Juvenile Muscular Atrophy of Distal Upper Extremity Hirayama Disease. *In* Jones HR, De Vivo D, Darras BT: Neuromuscular Disorders of Infancy, Childhoods and Adolescence: A Clinician's Approach. Philadelphia, Butterworth-Heinemann, 2003.

204. Hirayama K, Tsubaki T, Toyokura Y, et al: Juvenile muscular atrophy of unilateral upper extremity. Neurology (Minneapolis) 1963;13:373-380.

205. Chen CJ, Hsu HL, Tseng YC, et al: Hirayama flexion myelopathy: neutral-position MR imaging findings— importance of loss of attachment. Radiology 2004;231(1):39-44.

206. Mathern GW, Batzdorf U: Grisel's syndrome: Cervical spine clinical, pathologic, and neurologic manifestations. Clin Orthop 1989;244:131-146.

207. Fernandez Cornejo VJ, Martinez-Lage JF, Piqueras C, et al: Inflammatory atlanto-axial subluxation (Grisel's syndrome) in children: clinical diagnosis and management. Childs Nerv Syst 2003;19(5-6):342-347.

208. DeOrio JK, Bianco AJ Jr: Lumbar disc excision in children and adolescents. J Bone Joint Surg Am 1982;64-A:991-996.

209. Weinert AM Jr, Rizzo TD Jr: Nonoperative management of multilevel lumbar disk herniations in an adolescent athlete. Mayo Clin Proc 1992;67:137-141.

210. Fisher RG, Saunders RL: Lumbar disc protrusion in children. J Neurosurg 1981;54:480-483.

211. Kurihara A, Kataoka O: Lumbar disc herniation in children and adolescents: A review of 70 operated cases and their minimum 5-year follow-up studies. Spine 1980;5:443-451.

212. Shillito J Jr: Pediatric lumbar disc surgery: Twenty patients under 15 years of age. Surg Neurol 1996;46:14-18.

213. Turner PG, Green JH, Galasko CSB: Back pain in childhood. Spine 1989;14:812-814.

214. Epstein JA, Epstein NE, Marc J, Rosenthal AD, Lavine LS: Lumbar intervertebral disk herniation in teenage children: recognition and management of associated anomalies. Spine 1984;9:427-432.

215. King AB: Surgical removal of a ruptured intervertebral disc in early childhood. J Pediatr 1959;55:57-62.

216. Garcia FF, Semba CP, Sartoris DJ: Diagnostic imaging of childhood spinal infection. Orthop Rev 1993;22:321-327.

217. Conforti R, Scuotto A, Muras I, et al: Les hernies discales de adolescents. [Herniated disk adolescents.] J Neuroradiol 1993;20:60-69.

218. Lahat E, Rothman AS, Aron AM: Schwannoma presenting as lumbar disc disease in an adolescent girl. Spine 1984;9:695-701.

219. Rothschild EJ, Savitz MH, Chang T, et al: Primary vertebral tumor in an adolescent girl. Spine 1984;9:695-701.

220. Kozlowski K, Barylak A, Campbell J, et al: Primary sacral bone tumours in children (report of 16 cases with a short literature review). Aust Radiol 1990;34:142-149.

221. Dunne JW, Silbert PL, Wren M: A prospective study of acute radiculopathy after scoliosis surgery. Clin Exp Neurol 1991;28:180-190.

222. Deathe AB: Hematometra as a cause of lumbar radiculopathy: a case report. Spine 1993;18:1920-1921.

223. Ghabriel YAE, Tarrant MJ: Adolescent lumbar disc prolapse. Acta Orthop Scand 1989;60:174-176.

32

Focal Neuropathies in Children

KEVIN J. FELICE AND H. ROYDEN JONES, JR.

Mononeuropathies in children are uncommon, accounting for less than 10% of pediatric referrals for electroneuromyography testing.[1-3] This is in contrast to mononeuropathies in adults, which account for about 30% of electromyogram (EMG) referrals. The particular nerve involvement also distinguishes focal neuropathies in children from those in adults. In children, nerve involvement is nearly equal in distribution among the median, ulnar, radial, peroneal, and sciatic nerves, whereas in adults, median mononeuropathies, mainly due to carpal tunnel syndrome (CTS), account for 65% of focal neuropathies (Fig 32-1). The major reason for this is the much lower incidence of CTS in children.

The mechanisms of nerve injury are another major difference between focal neuropathies in children and adults. Trauma is the most common injury type in children, accounting for 37% to 76% of cases. Traumatic injuries due to fractures and lacerations are a major cause of mononeuropathies in children, and many are related to sports injuries. Compression injuries are the second most common cause of pediatric mononeuropathies, whereas nerve entrapment injuries are relatively uncommon. In distinction, entrapment and compression injuries account for the majority of injuries in adults. The following sections discuss the diagnosis and management of focal neuropathies in children. The reader should also supplement this material by referring to larger texts dedicated to the topics of pediatric EMG and focal neuropathies.[3,4]

MEDIAN NERVE

Anatomy

The median nerve is formed in the axilla by branches of the lateral and medial cords of the brachial plexus (Fig. 32-2).[4] In the forearm, the median nerve innervates the pronator teres (C6-7), flexor carpi radialis (C6-7), palmaris longus (C7-T1) and flexor digitorum superficialis (C7-8). The anterior interosseous nerve, a primarily motor nerve, separates from the main trunk of the median nerve in the upper forearm and travels distally to innervate the lateral head of the flexor digitorum profundus (C7-8), flexor pollicis longus (C7-8), and pronator quadratus (C7-8). In the lower forearm, the median nerve gives off the palmar cutaneous branch. The main trunk then enters the wrist and travels through the carpal tunnel. Distal to the carpal tunnel, the median nerve divides into sensory and motor terminal branches. The motor branch supplies the first and second lumbricals (C8-T1) in the palm; in addition, a recurrent thenar motor branch supplies the abductor pollicis brevis (C8-T1), opponens pollicis (C8-T1), and superficial head of the flexor pollicis brevis (C8-T1). The terminal sensory branches supply sensation to the thumb, index and middle fingers, and the lateral aspect of the ring finger. Proximal median nerve injuries are associated with weakness and sensory loss in the entire distribution of the nerve, whereas distal injuries (e.g., CTS) usually cause restricted

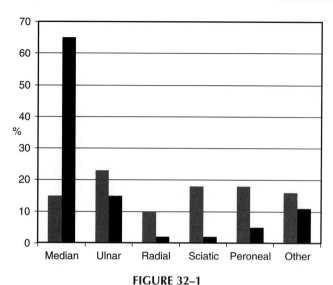

FIGURE 32–1

Distribution of mononeuropathies in 113 pediatric and 712 adult patients. The solid bar represents pediatric patients.

involvement in the distribution of the terminal motor and sensory nerves.

Etiology

Distal Median Mononeuropathies

Carpal Tunnel Syndrome. The causes of distal median mononeuropathies are shown in Box 32-1. In young children, CTS is uncommon and, when present, is usually associated with an underlying disorder. In a recent large epidemiologic study of CTS in the general population over a 2-year period in Marshfield, Wisconsin, the diagnosis of probable or definite CTS was made in 309 patients.[5] Of these, seven (2.3%) were children, younger than 17 years of age, establishing an incidence rate of 0.26 per 1000 person-years. The specific pediatric ages in this large study were not reported. However, case reports have documented CTS in infants with a positive family history of the disorder[6] and in children as young as age 2 years with mucopolysaccharidosis type IV.[7]

Idiopathic CTS is more common in older children and teens.[3,8] The symptoms of CTS in older children are similar to those of adults and include bilateral hand pain and numbness, occasional radiating pain into the upper arm and shoulder, nocturnal tingling in the fingers, morning hand paresthesia, and worsening of symptoms with certain activities (e.g., skiing, computer games).[3] Clinical signs may be absent or range in severity from mild sensory loss in the distribution of the median nerve (usually sparing the palm) to thenar muscle weakness and atrophy. In infants and small children with CTS, the signs may include reduced movements of the fingers and insensitivity to pain.[3,6]

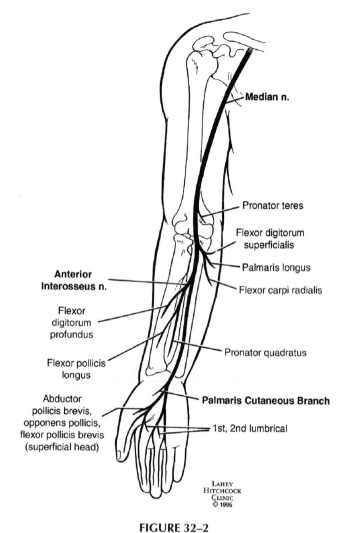

FIGURE 32–2

Diagram of the median nerve and the muscles that it supplies. (Courtesy of Lahey Clinic, Burlington, MA.)

Predisposing factors in pediatric CTS include congenital canal stenosis (e.g., familial CTS),[6,9-12] wrist trauma or injuries,[3,13,14] thickening of the flexor retinaculum (e.g., mucopolysaccharidoses, mucolipidoses, trigger finger),[7,15-19] repetitive hand and wrist movements (e.g., sports related, work related, cerebral palsy with dystonic hand movements),[3,13,15,20,21] tenosynovitis (e.g., scleroderma, rubella),[3,22] Schwartz-Jampel syndrome,[23] hereditary neuropathy with liability to pressure palsies (HNPP),[24] pyogenic infections,[25] and juvenile chronic arthritis.[26] CTS has also been associated with Poland's syndrome.[27] In addition to CTS, distal median mononeuropathies may result from congenital constriction bands,[28] hematoma from blood gas determination,[29] compression from a cast,[13] compression from a calcified flexor digitorum tendon,[30] and secondary to burns at the wrist.[31]

BOX 32-1
CAUSES OF DISTAL MEDIAN MONONEUROPATHIES

Carpal tunnel syndrome
  Idiopathic
  Activity related (e.g., skiing, bicycling, golfing, computer games)
  Trauma
  Inborn errors of metabolism
    (e.g., mucopolysaccharidoses, mucolipidoses)
  Scleroderma
  Poland's syndrome
  Cerebral palsy with dystonic hand movements
  Schwartz-Jampel syndrome
  Trigger finger
  Lipofibromatous hamartoma
  Rubella
  Hereditary neuropathy with liability to
    pressure palsies
  Familial carpal tunnel syndrome
Other distal median mononeuropathies
  Hematoma (e.g., radial artery puncture)
  Constriction bands
  Compression from cast

BOX 32-2
CAUSES OF PROXIMAL MEDIAN MONONEUROPATHIES

Trauma
  Fractures
  Blunt nerve trauma
  Lacerations
  Trauma following arterial or venous puncture
Entrapment
  Ligament of Struthers
  Fibromuscular bands
  Pronator syndrome
  Bicipital aponeurosis
Tumors
  Lipofibromas
  Hamartomas
  Neurofibromas
  Hemangiomas
Other
  Osteoid osteoma
  Juvenile cutaneous mucinosis
  Abscess
  Idiopathic
  Calcified flexor digitorum superficialis tendon

Thenar Atrophy. Thenar atrophy is an unusual manifestation of CTS in children. Rare cases of thenar atrophy have been associated with inborn errors of metabolism, pseudoneuroma of the median nerve, congenital constriction bands, foreshortened index finger, and trigger finger.[3] In the latter two conditions, the median nerve appears to be compressed by idiopathic thickening of the flexor retinaculum. These conditions are usually associated with concomitant involvement of the median sensory fibers. In distinction, Cavanaugh's syndrome, a hypoplastic disorder of the thenar muscles and hand bones, is not associated with median nerve compression or sensory fiber involvement.[32]

Proximal Median Mononeuropathies

Overview. The causes of proximal median mononeuropathies are shown in Box 32-2. Trauma is the most common cause of proximal median nerve injuries in children. In the Children's Hospital Boston (CHB) series of 17 patients, 10 (59%) developed median mononeuropathies as a direct result of limb trauma.[13] Bone fractures seem to be the most common cause of nerve trauma. Median nerve compression, entrapment, or laceration injuries have resulted from traumatic fractures of the supracondylar humerus, midradius, and radioulnar joint. Most of these injuries involve

the main trunk of the median nerve; however, the anterior interosseous nerve may also be traumatized in isolation as the result of a supracondylar fracture.[33] Traumatic median nerve injuries have also resulted from elbow dislocations, lacerations, blunt nerve trauma from athletic activities, and trauma inflicted by arterial or venous puncture.[3,29,34,35]

Entrapment. Rarely, the median nerve may be entrapped by an osteoid osteoma,[13] the ligament of Struthers,[16] congenital fibromuscular bands,[27,35-37] pronator teres,[38,39] and bicipital aponeurosis.[40] The ligament of Struthers, a fibrous band extending from a small supracondylar spur to the medial epicondyle of the humerus, forms the roof of a tunnel through which the median nerve and brachial artery pass. Despite the common occurrence of the spur, visible on plain radiograph in about 2% of the population, the ligament of Struthers is a rare cause of median nerve entrapment.[4]

In pronator syndrome, the median nerve is entrapped by the hypertrophied heads or thickened tendinous bands of the pronator teres muscle. Given that involvement is distal to the motor branch innervating the pronator teres, this muscle is usually not involved; this is in distinction to more proximal median lesions (e.g., ligament of Struthers entrapment). Congenital constriction bands may cause proximal median nerve entrapment injuries, occasionally with concurrent involvement of the radial and ulnar nerves.[28]

Miscellaneous Median Nerve Lesions

The proximal and distal segments of the median nerve have also been damaged secondary to contiguous lipofibromas,[41,42] hamartomas,[43] neurofibromas,[44] and hemangiomas.[45] Other causes of median nerve pediatric median mononeuropathy include juvenile cutaneous mucinosis,[3] calcified flexor digitorum superficialis tendon,[30] and abscess.[25]

Anterior interosseous neuropathy has been reported in several children, either of spontaneous onset due to probable brachial neuritis[33,46] or associated with supracondylar fractures of the humerus.[46,47]

Evaluation

EMG

Our EMG evaluation of the median nerve in infants and small children includes a sensory nerve action potential (SNAP) from either the index or middle finger, compound muscle action potential (CMAP) from the thenar muscles, median motor conduction velocity across the forearm segment, comparative ulnar sensory and motor conduction studies, and needle examination of the minimal number of necessary muscles. In older children with mild symptoms, the examination should also include median and ulnar mixed nerve action potentials (MNAPs), or "palmar" studies.

Distal Median Nerve Lesions. In cases of mild CTS, one may expect to find prolonged peak latencies of the median MNAP and SNAP. Prolongation of the median CMAP distal latency and attenuation of the SNAP amplitude indicate more moderate disease. Severe CTS is associated with an absent or attenuated thenar CMAP and needle examination abnormalities indicating both active (e.g., fibrillations, positive sharp waves) and chronic (e.g., large and polyphasic motor unit action potentials) changes of denervation and reinnervation in the abductor pollicis brevis.

Proximal Median Nerve Lesions. The distal latencies are usually normal although mild prolongation of the median SNAP latency is occasionally reported in some of these lesions.[13] In contrast, conduction velocities across the forearm segment may be reduced with demyelinating injuries. Needle examination abnormalities often extend into median-innervated forearm muscles with axonal or mixed injuries.

Congenital Thenar Hypoplasia (Cavanaugh's Syndrome). The CMAP is of low amplitude or absent, whereas the median SNAP amplitude and peak latency are normal. Thenar motor unit action potentials are reduced in number without associated denervation potentials.

Other Studies

The clinical findings and EMG results may dictate the need for additional studies in the evaluation of median mononeuropathies. Magnetic resonance imaging (MRI) may offer more precise anatomic assessment of suspected soft tissue infiltrative or compressive lesions, especially with symptoms of slowly progressive dysfunction or with signs of palpable focal tenderness or fullness.[3,4] Plain roentgenograms of the hand may be indicated in suspected cases of congenital thenar hypotrophy to assess for hypoplastic changes of hand bones.[32] In suspected cases of ligament of Struthers entrapment, radiographs of the distal humerus are useful to identify the bony spur often seen in that disorder. Metabolic studies for the mucopolysaccharidoses and mucolipidoses are indicated in suspected cases of CTS associated with dysmorphic features, organomegaly, and other system disease.

Treatment and Prognosis

Traumatic mononeuropathies require prompt attention. EMG studies are usually employed initially following trauma to assess for nerve continuity, characterize the injury type (e.g., axonal, demyelinating, or mixed), and predict a prognosis for recovery.

Within 9 to 11 days following acute axonal injury, wallerian degeneration is complete,[48] and EMG studies are recommended at this point in cases with severe dysfunction or when nerve function cannot be assessed clinically due to other factors related to the trauma (e.g., immobilization, casting).[49] In *neuropraxia* (focal demyelinating injury), the distal median SNAP and CMAP are preserved; however, stimulation proximal to the site of injury evokes an attenuated or absent response, that is, a partial or complete conduction block.

With mild or moderate *axonotmesis* (axonal injury), the distal SNAP and CMAP are attenuated or absent. Two to 3 weeks following an axonal injury, the needle examination reveals fibrillations and positive sharp waves in median-innervated muscles distal to the site of injury. In severe axonotmesis or when there is total lack of continuity of the peripheral nerve, *neurotmesis* occurs. In this setting the distal median SNAP and CMAP are absent.

Because nerve continuity may be uncertain in some of these cases, early surgical exploration and, if necessary, repair is usually recommended. Quite often, EMG findings indicate both demyelinating and axonal features (mixed nerve injury) in traumatic nerve injuries. In cases with preserved continuity and slow return of function, periodic EMG evaluation may be helpful in understanding the dynamics of nerve regeneration, collateral sprouting, and muscle reinnervation.

Treatment in mild idiopathic and activity-related CTS should be focused on conservative measures and avoidance of compromising hand positions and activities such as occurred with a high school ski racer whose symptoms cleared by changing the manner in which he held his ski poles. Median nerve decompression surgery should be reserved for patients with continued or progressive symptoms refractory to conservative measures or when the EMG study indicates axon–loss. Surgical decompression is indicated in distal median mononeuropathies associated with the inborn errors of metabolism, pseudoneuroma, trigger finger, and congenital constriction bands. Distal mononeuropathies related to trauma or activity may improve with conservative therapy only. Surgical decompression usually affords some improvement in symptoms and function, with ultimate recovery related to the degree of axonal loss.

In general, children with median mononeuropathies tend to have a good prognosis. Of 17 CHB patients with various types of pediatric median mononeuropathies, 12 (70%) had documented improvement at follow-up.[13] Improvement was noted with traumatic, compressive, and entrapment injuries. Poor prognosis was documented in 4 children, 2 with entrapment due to supracondylar fractures and 2 with CTS.[13]

CASE STUDY 1.

A 6-year-old boy with Hunter's syndrome (mucopolysaccharidosis type II) was noted to have weak thumb opposition and hand weakness. The neurologic examination was remarkable for reduced thumb movements and generalized hyporeflexia. Nerve conduction studies were remarkable for absent median SNAPs, low-amplitude median CMAPs, and prolonged median CMAP distal latencies on both sides (Fig. 32-3). The ulnar and sural sensory and ulnar and peroneal motor nerve conduction studies were normal. Needle EMG of the abductor pollicis brevis showed reduced insertional activity, no fibrillations or positive sharp waves, and absent recruitment of motor unit action potentials. It was unclear whether the absence of motor unit recruitment was due to poor recruitment from chronic denervation or poor activation due to discomfort.

Comments
The EMG findings showed evidence of severe bilateral median mononeuropathies, localized at the wrist/palm segments, and were consistent CTS. The association between CTS and the mucopolysaccharidoses is well known. Thickening of the flexor retinaculum causes compression of the median nerve within the narrow confines of the

carpal tunnel. Such cases should be considered for surgical treatment.

CASE STUDY 2.

A 12-year-old girl developed left hand weakness and numbness following a left supracondylar elbow fracture 2 months prior to the EMG study. The neurologic examination revealed marked weakness and atrophy of the thenar muscles; weakness of the flexor digitorum profundus of digit 2 and flexor pollicis longus; and light touch sensory loss along the palmar aspect of the lateral hand, thumb, and index and middle fingers. Nerve conduction studies revealed an absent left median SNAP and low-amplitude median CMAP (i.e., 0.6 mV) from the thenar muscles. The median motor conduction velocity across the forearm segment was preserved at 50 m/sec. Other nerve conduction studies including left ulnar and radial sensory, and right median and left ulnar motor were normal. Needle examination showed increased insertional activity, sustained fibrillations and positive sharp waves, and absent recruitment of motor unit action potentials from the left abductor pollicis brevis and flexor pollicis longus. Needle examination of the left pronator teres, first dorsal interosseous, and extensor indicis was normal.

Comments
The EMG findings showed evidence of a severe axon-loss median mononeuropathy, localized proximal to the innervation of the flexor pollicis longus (forearm segment), consistent with a traumatic nerve injury. The preserved, albeit low-amplitude, median CMAP was evidence for nerve continuity. Based on these findings, the referring physician opted for conservative therapy and follow-up clinical assessments.

ULNAR NERVE

Anatomy

The ulnar nerve is derived from the medial cord of the brachial plexus (C8-T1) (Fig. 32-4).[4] In the forearm, the ulnar nerve innervates the flexor carpi ulnaris (C8-T1) and the medial head of flexor digitorum profundus (C8-T1). Prior to reaching the hand, the ulnar nerve gives off the palmar and dorsal cutaneous branches in the lower forearm. At the wrist, the nerve enters Guyon canal and then bifurcates into the superficial and deep branches. The superficial branch innervates the palmaris brevis muscle (C8-T1) and then becomes the terminal sensory nerves, which supply

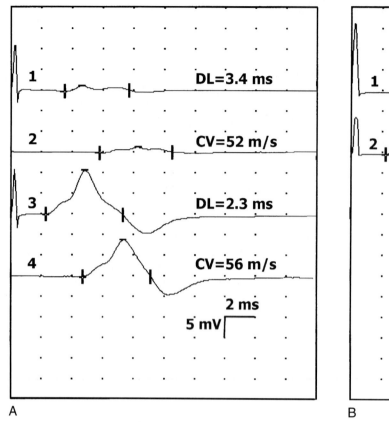

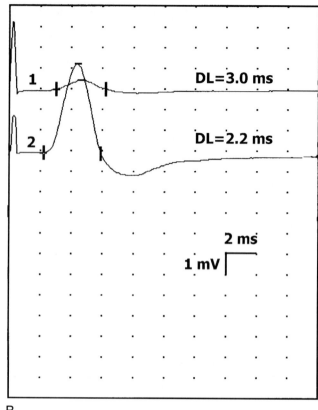

A   B

FIGURE 32–3

Nerve conduction studies for Case Study 1. A, The median motor nerve conduction study with stimulation at the wrist (waveform 1) and elbow (waveform 2) is compared to the ulnar study with stimulation at the wrist (waveform 3) and below elbow segment (waveform 4). Note the low-amplitude median compound muscle action potentials and prolonged median distal latency. B, The median to second lumbrical motor nerve conduction study is compared to the ulnar to interosseous study. For both, stimulation is at the wrist at a fixed distance of 70 mm. Note the comparative distal latency difference of 0.8 mm (normal, < 0.5 mm). DL, distal latency; CV, conduction velocity.

sensation to the fifth digit and medial aspect of the ring finger. The deep branch supplies the hypothenar muscles (C8-T1), including the abductor digiti minimi, opponens digiti minimi, and flexor digiti minimi, then curves along the palm providing motor branches to the third and fourth lumbricals (C8-T1), the four dorsal and three palmar interossei (C8-T1), adductor pollicis (C8-T1), and the deep head of the flexor pollicis brevis (C8-T1).

Etiology

Trauma

The most common cause of ulnar mononeuropathy in children is trauma (Box 32-3). Of the 21 CHB pediatric ulnar mononeuropathy cases described in 1996, 11 (52%) resulted directly from nerve trauma.[50] Proximal ulnar mononeuropathies due to trauma resulted from supracondylar fracture, medial epicondylar fracture, forearm

fracture, elbow laceration, stab wound, and an elbow puncture wound. Distal radial fractures are a cause of ulnar mononeuropathies at the wrist. Fractures and dislocations may cause nerve damage via blunt injury, entrapment, compression, or laceration.[51] The ulnar nerve may also be damaged as the result of surgery to repair an elbow or forearm fracture. Delayed or "tardy" ulnar nerve palsy is described in children following elbow trauma, presumably due to post-traumatic bony changes and fibrosis.[8]

Entrapment

The *cubital tunnel syndrome* was a surgically documented cause of entrapment in two children in our series.[50] A third case of presumed cubital tunnel syndrome occurred in an 18-year-old hockey goalie during one season when he carried heavy goalie pads with his arm in flexion; the symptoms improved at the end of the season. Other causes of ulnar nerve entrapment include a persist-

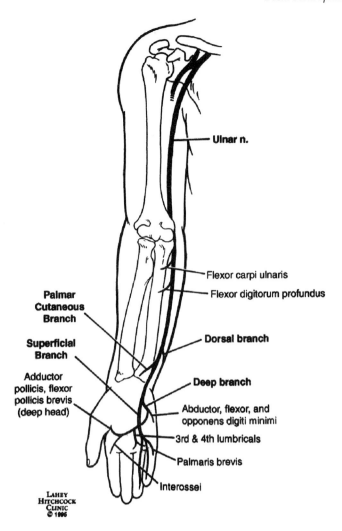

FIGURE 32–4
Diagram of the ulnar nerve and the muscles that it supplies. (Courtesy of Lahey Clinic, Burlington, MA.)

Trauma
  Fractures—supracondylar, medial epicondylar,
    forearm, distal radial
  Lacerations, puncture and stab wounds
  Blunt trauma
  Superficial burns
  Repetitive throwing movements
  Nerve ischemia
Entrapment
  Cubital tunnel syndrome
  Persistent epitrochleoanconeus muscle
  Congenital constriction bands
Compression
  Surgical compression
  Wheelchair arm rests
  Bicycle hand rests
  Weightlifting bar
  Hemorrhage related to hemophilia
  Infiltration of intravenous fluids
  Compartment syndrome
  Following fracture or dislocation
Tumors
  Hamartomas
  Neurofibromas
  Neurilemomas
Other
  Leprosy
  Focal hypertrophic neuropathy
  Recurrent dislocation
  Hereditary neuropathy with liability to pressure
    palsies

---

ent epitrochleoanconeus muscle[52] and congenital constriction bands.[28]

Compression

Five children at CHB suffered from compressive ulnar mononeuropathies.[50] Of these, two had compressive mononeuropathies at the elbow during surgical procedures, one developed a transient sleep palsy restricted to the dorsal cutaneous branch, one had bilateral compressive mononeuropathies at the forearm or elbow due to wheelchair rests, and one had compression at the wrist from bicycle hand rests. The ulnar nerve may be compressed from a weightlifting bar[53] and bicycle hand rests.[54]

Miscellaneous Mechanisms

Other causes of ulnar mononeuropathies include leprosy,[55] hemorrhage in hemophilia,[56] extravasation of intravenous fluids with subsequent compartment syndrome,[57] focal hypertrophic neuropathy,[58] burns,[59] repetitive throwing injuries in baseball pitchers,[60] tumors,[61] and hamartomas.[62]

EMG Evaluation

Our EMG evaluation of the ulnar nerve includes an ulnar SNAP from the small finger; ulnar motor nerve conduction studies from the hypothenar muscles; motor conduction velocities across the forearm and elbow segments; comparative median sensory and motor nerve conduction studies; and needle examination of the first dorsal interosseous, abductor digiti minimi, and flexor carpi ulnaris muscles. Occasionally, ulnar motor nerve conduction studies recorded from the first dorsal interosseous provide additional information as to the degree of conduction abnormalities at the wrist or elbow segments.[63] The addition of the dorsal ulnar cutaneous SNAP may help in differentiating between ulnar lesions at the wrist and elbow. Also, the medial antebrachial cutaneous SNAP may help exclude brachial plexus involvement in selected cases.

Ulnar mononeuropathies localized at the **wrist** or hand may involve the terminal motor branch, proximal or distal to the innervation of the hypothenar muscles, the terminal sensory branch, or both. These lesions spare the dorsal ulnar cutaneous SNAP and are associated with preserved motor conduction velocities across the **elbow** segment.

Demyelinating ulnar mononeuropathies at the elbow segment are associated with focal motor conduction block or conduction slowing; axonal mononeuropathies with absent or attenuated distal SNAP and CMAP amplitudes, and evidence of variable changes of denervation and reinnervation on needle examination of ulnar hand and forearm muscles; and mixed injuries with combination of demyelinating and axonal features.

Treatment and Prognosis

EMG is useful for deciding on the appropriate management of pediatric ulnar mononeuropathies. This includes nerve decompression and repair of fractures following trauma, surgical nerve repair and grafting following nerve lacerations and severe traumatic injuries, resection of compressive masses and tumors, nerve decompression in cubital tunnel syndrome, and nerve transposition and decompression with progressive lesions localized at the elbow segment. Twelve surgical procedures were performed at CHB among 21 children with ulnar mononeuropathy: five to repair acute fractures and lacerations, two to decompress the nerve in cubital tunnel, one to decompress the nerve following a medial epicondylar fracture, one transposition surgery, two resections of neuromas, and one nerve graft procedure following a laceration.[50]

In the CHB series of 21 children with pediatric ulnar mononeuropathy, 15 (71%) were seen in follow-up (range 2 months to 6 years) after the initial evaluation.[50] Follow-up examinations found that only 56% of children with traumatic versus 83% with nontraumatic ulnar mononeuropathies had a favorable outcome. Two children with cubital tunnel syndrome improved following ulnar nerve decompression and anterior transposition surgeries.

CASE STUDY 3.

An 18-year-old high school senior complained of painless right hand weakness (i.e., inability to spread or fan his fingers).[53] The symptoms began abruptly 2 weeks prior to the

EMG study, following weightlifting exercises. The exercises consisted of several sets of bench presses with a heavy bar held in the palms. There was no pain or sensory loss. The neurologic examination was remarkable for moderate weakness without atrophy of the right palmar and dorsal interossei, lumbrical of fingers 4 and 5, and adductor pollicis; mild weakness of right hypothenar muscles; normal thenar, forearm, and upper arm muscle strength; normal and symmetric reflexes; and a normal sensory examination. The right median, ulnar, and medial antebrachial cutaneous SNAPs were normal. The right median motor nerve conduction studies were normal. The right ulnar CMAPs from the hypothenar and first dorsal interosseous muscles showed prolonged distal latencies and reduced amplitudes. Ulnar motor conduction velocities across the elbow segment were normal. Stimulation of the right ulnar nerve at the palm and wrist sites, distal and proximal to the suspected injury, revealed severe partial conduction block of 85% and conduction velocity slowing across the wrist/palm segment (Fig. 32-5). Needle EMG of the abductor

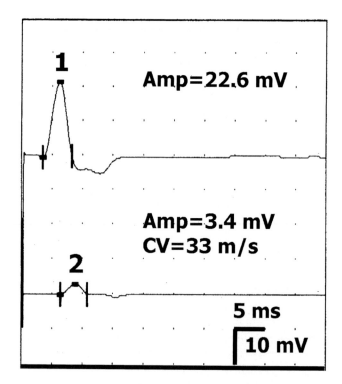

FIGURE 32–5

Nerve conduction studies for Case Study 3. The right ulnar nerve is stimulated at the palm (waveform 1) and wrist (waveform 2) sites, distal and proximal to the suspected injury, with a recording electrode on the first dorsal interosseous muscle. Note the severe partial conduction block of 85% and conduction velocity slowing of 33 m/sec across the wrist/palm segment. Amp, amplitude; CV, conduction velocity.

digiti minimi and first dorsal interosseous revealed markedly reduced recruitment of normal-appearing and faster-frequency motor unit action potentials. Fibrillations and positive sharp waves were not present.

Comments

The EMG findings were consistent with a severe demyelinating injury to the terminal motor branch of the right ulnar nerve, proximal to the innervation of the hypothenar muscles. We recommended that the patient discontinue weightlifting, and within 3 months his right hand strength returned to normal and the motor conduction block had completely resolved.[53] This is the typical response to removal of an acute or recurrent source of nerve compression. This type of injury has been previously described with other types of activities, including long distance bicycling.

CASE STUDY 4.

A 17-year-old girl complained of right hand numbness for the 2 months prior to the EMG study. The symptoms began soon after starting a part-time telemarketing job. During her work, she would lean on her right elbow for prolonged periods. She denied weakness or pain. The neurologic examination was remarkable for reduced light touch sensation along the medial right hand (dorsal and palmar surfaces), and fourth and fifth fingers. Muscle bulk, strength, and reflexes were normal. Bilateral ulnar and right median SNAPs and motor nerve conduction studies were normal. Right ulnar sensory nerve conduction studies showed conduction slowing and probable partial sensory conduction block across the elbow segment (Fig. 32-6). Needle examination of right ulnar-innervated hand muscles was normal.

Comments

The EMG findings showed evidence of an ulnar mononeuropathy at the elbow segment due to a mild demyelinating injury to sensory fibers. The clinical and EMG findings suggested mild recurrent nerve compression from poor elbow positioning during her work. The symptoms completely resolved over the next several weeks following adjustments to her arm and elbow during subsequent telemarketing work.

RADIAL NERVE

Anatomy

The radial nerve is derived from the posterior cord of the brachial plexus (C5-8) (Fig. 32-7).[4] It descends in the

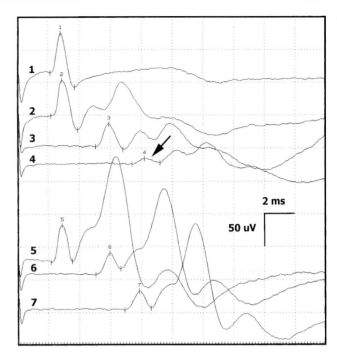

FIGURE 32–6

Nerve conduction studies for Case Study 4. Right median (waveform 1), right ulnar (waveforms 2 to 4), and left ulnar (waveforms 5 to 7) sensory nerve action potentials (SNAPs) are shown. The ulnar SNAPs are recorded from the small finger with stimulation at the wrist (waveforms 2 and 5), below-elbow (waveforms 3 and 6), and above-elbow (waveforms 4 and 7) sites. Note the low-amplitude ulnar SNAP (arrow) with stimulation above the right elbow (waveform 4) as compared to the contralateral SNAP (waveform 7). The sensory conduction velocity across the right elbow segment is 47 m/sec (normal, > 53 m/sec).

upper arm between the long and medial heads of the triceps, posterior to the axillary artery. Proximal to the spiral groove, the radial nerve gives off the *posterior cutaneous nerve of the arm, motor branches* to the triceps (C6-8) and anconeus (C6-8), and *posterior cutaneous nerve of the forearm*. At the spiral groove, the nerve travels from the medial to the posterolateral aspect of the lower arm. Distal to the groove, the radial nerve innervates the brachioradialis (C5-6) and extensor carpi radialis longus (C5-6).

Here this nerve bifurcates into superficial and deep branches. The *superficial branch* descends in the forearm under the brachioradialis prior to emerging in the distal forearm as the superficial sensory branch, supplying sensation to the posteromedial hand and first web space.

The *deep branch* continues as the *posterior interosseous nerve* and enters the supinator muscle through an opening termed the *arcade of Fröhse*. Within the extensor compartment of the forearm, the posterior interosseous nerve innervates the supinator (C6-7), extensor carpi radialis

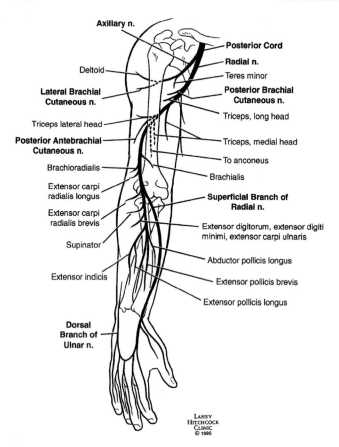

FIGURE 32–7
Diagram of the radial and axillary nerves and the muscles that they supply. (Courtesy of Lahey Clinic, Burlington, MA.)

brevis (C5-7), extensor digitorum (C7-8), extensor digiti minimi (C7-8), extensor carpi ulnaris (C7-8), abductor pollicis longus (C7-8), extensor pollicis longus (C7-8), extensor pollicis brevis (C7-8), and extensor indicis (C7-8).

Etiology (Box 32-4)

At CHB 8 (53%) of 15 children with radial mononeuropathies had traumatic injuries, 5 due to fractures and 3 due to lacerations.[64] All of these were axon-loss injuries, 4 involving the main trunk of the radial nerve distal to the spiral groove and 1 involving the posterior interosseous nerve fibers only due to a supracondylar fracture. Of the lacerations, 2 involved the upper arm and the other involved the forearm. All were axon-loss injuries, including isolated posterior interosseous neuropathies in 2 cases and a distal radial neuropathy in the other. Others report radial nerve trauma due to injection injuries and arthroscopic elbow surgery.[65]

Compression Injuries

In children the radial nerve is most susceptible to compression injury at the spiral groove segment. Compression

---

BOX 32-4
CAUSES OF RADIAL MONONEUROPATHIES

Trauma
   Fractures—Monteggia, supracondylar, lateral
      condylar
   Lacerations
   Injection injuries
   Arthroscopic elbow surgery
Compression
   Neonatal
   Perioperative
   Compartment syndrome
   Sleep palsy
   Crutch palsy
Tumors
   Lipomas
   Ganglia
   Fibromas
   Neuromas
   Hemangiomas
Other
   Multiple septal entrapment
   Hereditary neuropathy with liability to pressure
      palsies

---

injuries of the radial nerve were documented in 6 (40%) of 15 children, including 2 neonatal and 4 postnatal injuries.[64] Two of the 4 postnatal injuries were localized at the spiral groove segment, one a conduction block injury due to nerve compression sustained during surgery, and the other a mixed injury due to a sleep palsy. The other 2 postnatal compression injuries included a demyelinating posterior interosseous injury due to an acute compartment syndrome from infiltration of intravenously administered chemotherapy in a child with Hodgkin's disease and bilateral axon-loss proximal trunk radial mononeuropathies due to improper use of crutches.

Neonatal Radial Mononeuropathy

Neonatal radial mononeuropathies occur with intrauterine compression by uterine contraction rings,[66,67] prolonged labor,[3] subcutaneous fat necrosis,[68] and subcutaneous abscess or hematoma.[69] At birth, the radial nerve may be injured by a humeral fracture, hematoma, blood pressure monitoring,[70] and prolonged birth-related external compression.[71]

In HNPP, radial mononeuropathies may be the presenting feature. Up to 3% of HNPP patients younger than 10 years of age, including infants, have radial nerve involvement in the spiral groove of the humerus.[72]

Entrapment

One of our 15 children with radial nerve palsy, a 3-year-old girl, developed a progressive radial distribution weakness over the first 3 years of life.[64] At surgical exploration the nerve resembled a string of sausages with multiple areas of tight compression. However, the microscopic specimen consisted of scar tissue related to entrapment within the interfascial septum and did not represent a tomaculous neuropathy. Entrapment of the radial nerve within the triceps muscle has also been reported.[73,74]

Miscellaneous

The radial nerve may also be affected by benign tumors and other compressive lesions. These have included lipomas, ganglia, fibromas, neuromas, and hemangiomas.[3]

Evaluation

Our EMG evaluation of the radial nerve includes a radial SNAP from the affected limb, comparative radial SNAP from the unaffected limb (or ipsilateral median SNAP if both limbs are affected), and needle EMG of upper arm (e.g., triceps) and forearm (e.g., brachioradialis) radial-innervated muscles, and a muscle innervated by the posterior interosseous nerve (e.g., extensor indicis). Radial motor nerve conduction studies are technically difficult in neonates and small children. In older children, we find the radial motor study, recorded from the extensor indicis and stimulated at three sites (forearm, below and above spiral groove), to be relatively easy to perform and reliable in demonstrating conduction abnormalities across the spiral groove segment.

Pure demyelinating injuries at the spiral groove segment are associated with motor conduction block, slowing or both; normal distal radial SNAPs and CMAPs; and reduced recruitment of motor unit action potentials without abnormal spontaneous activity in affected muscles. Axonal injuries are associated with absent or attenuated radial SNAPs and CMAPs and reduced recruitment of motor unit action potentials with fibrillations and positive sharp waves in affected muscles. Posterior interosseous neuropathies are associated with a normal radial SNAP, a low-amplitude or absent CMAP from the extensor indicis, and needle examination abnormalities limited to radial-innervated muscles distal to the supinator.

Treatment and Prognosis

Traumatic Injuries

Traumatic injuries related to fractures require prompt surgical repair. Early EMG studies are indicated with lacerations and fractures to assess for nerve continuity. An absent radial SNAP and CMAP distal to the site of injury at 9 to 11 days post-trauma indicates severe axonotmesis or neu-rotmesis, raises the possibility of a radial nerve laceration or severe disruption, and warrants surgical exploration and, if necessary, nerve repair. Seven (88%) of the eight children with traumatic radial mononeuropathies at CHB improved or completely recovered within 7 to 17 months.[64] A 6-year-old boy with a severe axon-loss posterior interosseous nerve injury following a supracondylar fracture showed no clinical improvement after 4 years.

Compression Injuries

Acute compression injuries at the spiral groove segment, usually associated with demyelinating or mixed nerve injuries, afford a more favorable prognosis for full recovery. All six cases of neonatal and postnatal radial mononeuropathies due to nerve compression injuries had complete recoveries at follow-up. Slowly progressive radial or posterior interosseous nerve dysfunction may require MRI studies and surgical exploration to search for possible tumors, fascial bands, or other sources of nerve compression or entrapment.

CASE STUDY 5.

A 17-year-old boy awakened with a right wrist drop about 1 month prior to the EMG study. He denied prior medical or neurologic problems, neck or arm injuries, or pain. The neurologic examination revealed severe weakness without atrophy of the right brachioradialis, wrist extensors, and finger extensors. Triceps muscle bulk and strength were normal. There was reduced light touch and pinprick sensation along the dorsal aspect of the first web space between the right thumb and index finger. Nerve conduction studies revealed symmetrically normal radial SNAP amplitudes in the 24 to 28 µV range. The right radial to extensor indicis motor nerve conduction study showed partial conduction block and conduction velocity slowing across the upper arm (spiral groove) segment (Fig. 32-8). The right median, right ulnar, and left radial motor nerve conduction studies were normal. Needle examination was remarkable for slightly increased insertional activity, rare fibrillations and positive sharp waves, and markedly reduced recruitment of normal-appearing and faster frequency motor unit action potentials restricted to the right extensor indicis, extensor digitorum communis, and brachioradialis muscles. Needle examination of the triceps was normal.

Comments

The EMG findings were consistent with a right radial mononeuropathy, localized at the spiral groove segment, due to a demyelinating nerve injury. Despite the severity of the clinical findings, the EMG results predicted a complete recovery of function and, in fact, the follow-up examination

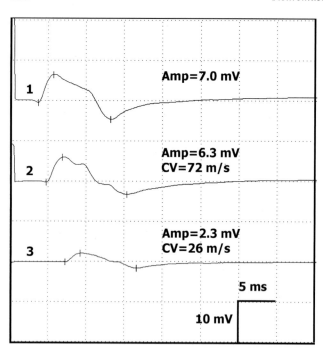

FIGURE 32–8
Nerve conduction studies for Case Study 5. With a recording electrode over the extensor indicis muscle, the right radial nerve is stimulated at the forearm (waveform 1), below-spiral groove (waveform 2), and above-spiral groove (waveform 3) sites. Note the partial conduction block and conduction velocity slowing across the spiral groove segment. Amp, amplitude; CV, conduction velocity.

3 months later was normal. The cause of the injury was presumed to be nerve compression during sleep (sleep palsy).

OTHER UPPER EXTREMITY NERVES

Axillary Nerve

Along with the radial nerve, the axillary nerve is the other major derivation of the posterior cord of the brachial plexus and lies in close proximity to the surgical neck of the humerus (see Fig. 32-7).[4] The major branches of the axillary nerve include motor branches to the deltoid and teres minor muscles (C5-6) and the lateral cutaneous nerve of the arm.

Axillary nerve injuries cause weakness of arm abduction, deltoid muscle atrophy with severe axonal injuries, and sensory loss along the upper lateral arm. In children, axillary mononeuropathies are reported in sports-related shoulder trauma and exostosis of the humerus (Box 32-5).[3,75]

EMG evaluation of axillary mononeuropathies in children is usually limited to the needle examination of the deltoid muscle.

BOX 32-5
CAUSES OF OTHER UPPER EXTREMITY MONONEUROPATHIES

Axillary nerve
    Exostosis of the humerus
    Sports-related injuries
    Trauma
Long thoracic nerve
    Milwaukee brace
    Trauma
    Sports-related injuries
    Idiopathic
Musculocutaneous nerve
    Body cast
    Hereditary neuropathy with liability to pressure
        palsies
    Idiopathic
Suprascapular nerve
    Entrapment within transverse ligament at
        suprascapular notch
    Compression by ganglion
    Trauma
Thoracodorsal nerve
    Thoracotomy and chest tube insertion
Spinal accessory nerve
    Surgical injury
    Hereditary neuropathy with liability to pressure
        palsies
    Idiopathic

Long Thoracic Nerve

The long thoracic nerve originates from the C5-7 roots and descends in the axilla, posterior to the brachial plexus, to innervate the serratus anterior muscle, which anchors the scapula to the chest wall.[4] Injuries to the long thoracic nerve cause winging of the scapula, especially with the arms in anterior abduction.

Reported causes of long thoracic mononeuropathies (see Box 32-5) in children include sports-related injuries (e.g., tennis, weightlifting), shoulder trauma, compression from a Milwaukee brace, and idiopathic lesions.[3,76,77]

EMG evaluation is usually limited to the needle examination of the serratus anterior at its digitations over the ribs at the mid-axillary line.

Musculocutaneous Nerve

The musculocutaneous nerve is derived from the lateral cord of the brachial plexus; innervates the biceps brachii,

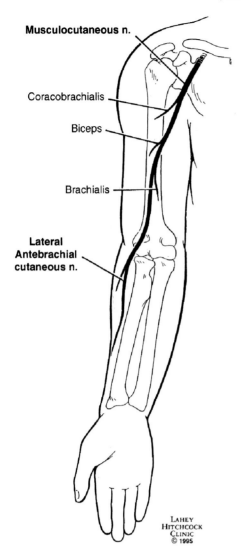

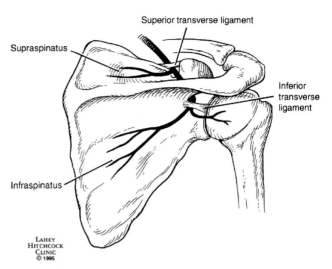

FIGURE 32–10

Diagram of the suprascapular nerve and the muscles that it supplies. (Courtesy of Lahey Clinic, Burlington, MA.)

FIGURE 32–9

Diagram of the musculocutaneous nerve and the muscles that it supplies. (Courtesy of Lahey Clinic, Burlington, MA.)

brachialis, and coracobrachialis muscles (C5-6); and terminates as the lateral cutaneous nerve of the forearm (Fig. 32-9).[4] Injuries to the musculocutaneous nerve are associated with weakness of arm flexion and sensory loss along the lateral forearm.

Three cases reported in 1986 included a child with compression of the nerve by a body cast, another child with an idiopathic lesion causing biceps muscle atrophy, and a third child with isolated involvement of lateral antebrachial cutaneous nerve (see Box 32-5).[71]

One 16-year-old boy with painless right biceps weakness and atrophy was found to have a musculocutaneous mononeuropathy superimposed on a diffuse demyelinating sensorimotor polyneuropathy.[24] The diagnosis of HNPP was later confirmed with DNA studies. The cause of the muscu-

locutaneous mononeuropathy was not previously identified since no known injury could be identified.

The EMG evaluation of the musculocutaneous nerve may include the lateral antebrachial cutaneous SNAP, a biceps brachii CMAP, and needle examination of the biceps brachii and coracobrachialis.

Suprascapular Nerve

The suprascapular nerve originates from the upper trunk of the brachial plexus and innervates the supraspinatus and infraspinatus (C5-6) muscles (Fig. 32-10).[4] Injuries to this nerve cause shoulder abduction and external rotation weakness. Lesions to this nerve usually result from entrapment injuries or trauma (see Box 32-5).

A 14-year-old girl sustained a blow to her shoulder as she stumbled in gymnastics and was later found to have entrapment of the nerve by the transverse ligament in the suprascapular notch.[78] Other identified mechanisms of pediatric suprascapular mononeuropathies include sports-related injuries and compression by a ganglion cyst.[79,80]

The EMG evaluation includes needle EMG of the supraspinatus and infraspinatus muscles. In a cooperative child, one may consider obtaining CMAPs from both muscles with needle recording electrodes.

Thoracodorsal Nerve

The thoracodorsal nerve is derived from the posterior cord of the brachial plexus and innervates the latissimus dorsi (C6-8).[4] One of us (K.J.F.) recently evaluated an 8-year-old girl who developed right latissimus dorsi atrophy following insertion of a chest tube with subsequent development of a chest wall empyema (see Case Study 7). The authors have not seen other reported cases of thoracodorsal mononeuropathy in children.

Spinal Accessory Nerve

The spinal accessory nerve is derived from two populations of motor neurons: cranial fibers from the nucleus ambiguus and spinal fibers from upper cervical motor neurons. The nerve exits the skull via the jugular foramen. The cranial fibers are destined to innervate the laryngeal muscles while the spinal fibers innervate the sternocleidomastoid and trapezius muscles.

Injury to the spinal accessory nerve occurs rarely and usually results as a complication of surgical procedures involving the posterior triangle of the neck (see Box 32-5).[3] One of us (K.J.F.) has evaluated two children with isolated spinal accessory mononeuropathy. One was a 16-year-old girl with an idiopathic spinal accessory mononeuropathy. The other was a 13-year-old girl who was found to have a droopy left shoulder during a school scoliosis screening evaluation.[24] The examination was remarkable for left trapezius weakness and atrophy, mild left scapular winging, diffusely hypoactive reflexes, and pes cavus foot deformities.

The EMG study documented a left spinal accessory mononeuropathy superimposed on a diffuse sensorimotor polyneuropathy. Subsequent DNA studies confirmed the diagnosis of HNPP. The EMG evaluation of spinal accessory mononeuropathies includes obtaining a CMAP from the trapezius, and needle examination of the trapezius and sternocleidomastoid.

CASE STUDY 6.

A 17-year-old boy noted right arm weakness following right shoulder surgery 3 weeks prior to the EMG study. The surgery was indicated to repair a torn labrum. The neurologic examination was remarkable for marked weakness of right arm flexion, an absent right biceps brachii reflex, and reduced light touch sensation along the lateral aspect of the right forearm. Nerve conduction studies showed an absent right musculocutaneous SNAP. The right median, right radial, and left musculocutaneous SNAPs were normal. The right musculocutaneous CMAP amplitude was markedly reduced at 0.2 mV as compared to the left response of 4.2 mV. The right median motor nerve conduction study and F-wave latency were normal. Needle examination revealed increased insertional activity, sustained fibrillations and positive sharp waves, and absent recruitment of motor unit action potentials from the right

biceps brachii and coracobrachialis muscles. Needle examination of the right deltoid and triceps was normal.

Comments

The EMG findings were consistent with a severe axon-loss right musculocutaneous mononeuropathy, probably resulting from compression or trauma of the nerve incurred during the shoulder surgery. The preservation of the right musculocutaneous CMAP suggested some degree of nerve continuity. Given the absence of clinical and EMG improvement 3 months later, the patient underwent nerve grafting microsurgery. Two years following surgery, he reported partial improvement in arm flexion strength.

CASE STUDY 7.

A 15-month-old girl was referred to the EMG laboratory to assess for left shoulder weakness and mild scapular winging. The weakness was noted soon after a complicated birth that resulted in a left thoracotomy and chest tube insertion for a chest wall empyema. The neurologic examination revealed atrophy of the left latissimus dorsi and mild left scapular winging. The left median sensory and motor nerve conduction studies were normal. Needle examination revealed reduced recruitment of motor unit action potentials from the left latissimus dorsi. The motor unit action potentials from this muscle were of increased amplitude and duration, showed increased phases and turns, and fired at faster than normal frequencies. No fibrillations or positive sharp waves were observed. Needle examination of the left trapezius, serratus anterior, and rhomboids was normal.

Comments

The EMG findings were consistent with a chronic axon-loss injury to the left thoracodorsal nerve or motor branch innervating the latissimus dorsi muscle. The injury probably resulted from the thoracotomy, chest tube insertion, or both.

CASE STUDY 8.

A 16-year-old girl was referred to the EMG laboratory to assess her left shoulder weakness. The weakness was first noticed during a routine physical examination by her pediatrician 3 years earlier. There was no known injury, and she denied neck, shoulder, or arm pain. The neurologic examination was remarkable for atrophy and weakness of the upper left trapezius muscle and mild scapular winging, especially prominent with the arm in lateral abduction.

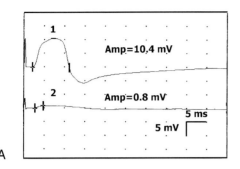

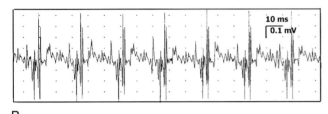

A

B

FIGURE 32–11

Nerve conduction studies and needle electromyography for Case Study 8. A, Comparative studies of the right (waveform 1) and left (waveform 2) spinal accessory compound muscle action potentials (CMAPs). The spinal accessory nerve is stimulated just posterior to the sternocleidomastoid muscle with recording electrodes over the upper trapezius. Note the low-amplitude CMAP on the left side. B, Example of complex repetitive discharge recorded from the left trapezius muscle. Amp, amplitude.

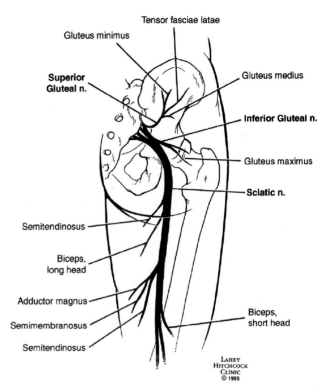

FIGURE 32–12

Diagram of the sciatic nerve and the muscles that it supplies. (Courtesy of Lahey Clinic, Burlington, MA.)

Otherwise, left shoulder and limb muscles were of normal bulk and strength. The left sternocleidomastoid muscle was also of normal bulk and strength. Nerve conduction studies were remarkable for a markedly reduced left spinal accessory CMAP, recorded from the upper trapezius (Fig. 32-11). The left upper extremity SNAPs, left median and ulnar motor nerve conduction studies, and right spinal accessory CMAP were normal. Needle examination was remarkable for reduced insertional activity, abundant complex repetitive discharges, and markedly reduced recruitment of motor unit action potentials from the left trapezius muscle (see Fig. 32-11). Motor unit action potentials were of increased amplitude and duration and fired at faster than normal frequencies. Needle examination of selected left arm muscles, left serratus anterior, left sternocleidomastoid, and right trapezius was normal.

Comments

The EMG findings were consistent with a chronic axon-loss left spinal accessory mononeuropathy, localized distal to the branch innervating the sternocleidomastoid muscle. This was called an idiopathic spinal accessory mononeuropathy; however, it is possible that the neuropathy was due to a prior nerve injury in the neck (e.g., compression from backpack) or partial form of brachial neuritis.

SCIATIC NERVE

Anatomy

The sciatic nerve is derived from the lower lumbar (L4-5) and upper sacral (S1-2) roots, emerges from the lumbosacral plexus, exits the pelvis through the infrapiriform foramen, and descends in the posterior thigh to innervate the semitendinosus (L4-S2), semimembranosus (L4-S2), biceps femoris (L4-S2), and distal part of the adductor magnus (Fig. 32-12).[4] The sciatic nerve consists of two well-defined nerve bundles including the lateral or peroneal division and medial or tibial division.

The lateral division innervates the short head of biceps femoris while the medial division supplies the other hamstring muscles. At the apex of the popliteal fossa, the sciatic nerve bifurcates into its two terminal branches: the common peroneal and tibial nerves.

Etiology (Box 32-6)

Sciatic mononeuropathies account for more than 20% of pediatric mononeuropathies.[2] Pediatric sciatic mononeuropathies can affect all age groups, from neonates to

BOX 32-6
CAUSES OF SCIATIC MONONEUROPATHIES

Neonatal trauma
  Breech deliveries
  Intragluteal injections
  Umbilical artery injections and catheterizations
Other trauma
  Lacerations
  Crush injuries
  Hip dislocations
  Surgery
Compression
  Hard surfaces
  Orthopedic appliances
Entrapment
  Myofascial bands
  Iliac bony exostoses
Systemic disease
  Vasculitis
  Purpura fulminans
Tumors
  Lymphoma
  Chloroma
  Neurofibromas
Localized hypertrophic neuropathy
Idiopathic progressive mononeuropathy

adolescents, and the location of nerve injuries is similar to those occurring in adults. The nerve can be injured in the pelvis, the sciatic notch, or in the thigh with an acute, subacute, or chronic clinical course. Sciatic mononeuropathies manifest with weakness of knee flexion and weakness and sensory loss in the distributions of the common peroneal and tibial nerves.

Sciatic Compression Neuropathies

Compression is one of the primary causes for a child's sciatic mononeuropathy. In a retrospective review of sciatic mononeuropathies seen at CHB, 21 cases were diagnosed in a 14-year period.[81] A nontraumatic mechanism was present in 85% and, of these, 33% were due to compressive injuries.

At CHB sciatic compression neuropathies have included multiple mechanisms such as long leg and body casts, prolonged pressure on the nerve in a newborn, and heel compression in a child who slept with the leg tucked under his buttock.[81] Other causes of sciatic mononeuropathy include external compression by sitting on hard surfaces,[82] nerve injury in the setting of severe weight loss,[83] after a prolonged sitting position during surgery,[84-87] and prolonged pressure

in critically ill patients in the intensive care unit.[87-89] A lithotomy position is frequently reported as a cause of adult sciatic mononeuropathies, and we have also seen this in children.[81,90,91] Sitting in the lotus position has also caused compressive sciatic mononeuropathy.[92] The mechanism of injury is unclear and is postulated to be due to ischemia, stretch, or external compression.[93,94] Endometriosis[95] and persistent sciatic artery at the pelvic notch may predispose to sciatic nerve compression mononeuropathy.[96]

Hematomas

Six of 36 sciatic nerve injuries described in one report were due to compression by hematomas in patients with hemophilia.[97] Sciatic mononeuropathy due to an occult hematocolpos was reported in an adolescent girl who had longstanding back pain and leg weakness.[98]

Tumors

Benign and malignant tumors should be considered in any child with a progressive sciatic mononeuropathy. A Mayo Clinic review identified 35 cases of sciatic mononeuropathies in patients ranging in age from 5 to 72 years, with various tumors including neurilemomas, neurofibromas, and neurofibrosarcomas.[99] Most of these patients present with pain and progressive weakness in the affected limb. Painless footdrop or progressive foot deformities are other presenting features of sciatic nerve tumors.[99,100] Tumor compression of the sciatic nerve is reported with neurofibromas,[101] primary lymphomas,[3,81,102] pelvic neuroblastomas,[81,103] and chloromas.[104]

Trauma

Traumatic injuries to the sciatic nerve occur less commonly than traumatic injuries to other lower and upper extremity nerves.[1-3,81] At the CHB traumatic sciatic mononeuropathies resulted from laceration, crush injury, and a hip dislocation.[81] Other traumatic sciatic mononeuropathies include fracture-dislocation of the hip,[105] stretch injuries,[106] and crush injuries during natural catastrophies.[107] The nerve can be acutely lacerated, stretched, or compressed or later entrapped in heterotopic ossification. This is the mechanism involved in sciatic mononeuropathies in athletes[108] and during hip surgery in children with juvenile rheumatoid arthritis.[105]

Infants. Babies are also subject to experiencing a traumatic sciatic mononeuropathy. Mechanisms include breech deliveries,[3,109] intragluteal injections,[110-112] toxic injuries during umbilical vessel injections,[113-115] and idiopathic neonatal sciatic mononeuropathy.[116,117] Prenatal compression of the sciatic and other nerves has been documented clinically and electromyographically.[81,118,119] Prenatal injuries are usually secondary to external compression due to reduced fetal activity, especially with decreased amniotic fluid, abnormal uterine contractions during prolonged labor, amniotic fluid bands, or uterine abnormalities.[119] Such an infant may have a necrotic ischemic lesion (eschar) at the site of compression as evidence of intrauterine onset.[119] EMG performed in the first days of life becomes important to document the prenatal onset of the nerve injury.[118]

Miscellaneous

Other causes of sciatic mononeuropathies include nerve entrapment by myofascial bands or congenital iliac anomalies,[120-123] nerve ischemia from hypereosinophilic vasculitis,[124] and idiopathic injuries.[125,126]

Evaluation

Our EMG evaluation of the sciatic nerve includes the sural and superficial peroneal SNAPs, peroneal and tibial motor nerve conduction studies, F-wave and H-reflex studies, and needle examination of selected muscles innervated by the medial and lateral division of the sciatic nerve (e.g., short and long head of biceps femoris, medial gastrocnemius, anterior tibialis). Needle examination of gluteal muscles may be necessary for differentiation between sciatic and lumbosacral plexus injuries. Lumbosacral root lesions can usually be differentiated from sciatic mononeuropathies by the preservation of the sural and superficial peroneal SNAPs in the former; however, these are rare in children.

Nerve imaging studies including MRI and magnetic resonance neurography may be helpful in disclosing nerve enlargement or compression by a mass or tumor.[127-134] The large size of the sciatic nerve is conducive to imaging study diagnosis; however, some lesions including myofascial bands and perineuromas are not yet readily visible by MRI and may require magnetic resonance neurography, ultrasonography, or surgical exploration.[135-137]

Surgical Exploration

Surgery proved to be diagnostic and curable in one instance when a fibrous band was identified entrapping the sciatic nerve in the posterior thigh.[125] At CHB we had a negative exploration but were disappointed with the limited degree of exploration.

Treatment and Prognosis

At CHB the degree of recovery for sciatic mononeuropathies could not necessarily be predicted by the EMG findings or mechanism of nerve injury.[81] Seven (44%) of 16 children with long-term follow up did not improve, including those who underwent exploratory surgery and nerve repair.[81] In a much larger series of sciatic mononeuropathies, including both adults as well as children, surgical repair was performed only in those individuals with persistent deficits in the peroneal or tibial distribution.[137] Management was guided by nerve action potential recordings, which indicated whether neurolysis or resection of the lesion was required. Useful peroneal function was achieved when the nerve action potential was recorded distal to the lesion, but overall improvement was only 36%. The tibial division had a much better recovery, regardless of the level or mechanism of injury.[137]

CASE STUDY 9.

A 2-year-old boy developed a right leg limp soon after receiving a right intragluteal injection of an antipyretic medication while visiting his African home 3 months prior to the EMG study. The past medical history was otherwise unremarkable. The examination was remarkable for weakness of right foot plantar flexion while ambulant, weakness of toe flexion and extension, atrophy of right intrinsic foot muscles, and absent right ankle jerk. The nerve conduction studies showed absent right sural and superficial peroneal SNAPs, absent right tibial CMAP from the adductor hallucis muscle, and markedly attenuated right peroneal CMAP from the extensor digitorum brevis muscle. The left sural SNAP and left peroneal motor nerve conduction studies were normal. The needle examination showed increased insertional activity; sustained fibrillations and positive sharp waves; and reduced recruitment of motor unit action potentials from the right medial gastrocnemius, biceps femoris, and anterior tibialis. No motor unit action potentials were recorded from the medial gastrocnemius. Motor unit action potential were of slightly increased amplitude and duration and fired at faster than normal frequencies from the biceps femoris and anterior tibialis. Needle examination of the vastus lateralis and gluteus maximus was normal.

Comments

The EMG findings were consistent with a subacute to early chronic axon-loss right sciatic mononeuropathy. Fortunately, intragluteal injection injuries are no longer a commonly reported cause of sciatic mononeuropathies in children. Education and proper knowledge of how to perform intramuscular injections by health care providers have undoubtedly reduced the incidence of this type of nerve injury.

PERONEAL NERVE

Anatomy

The common peroneal or lateral popliteal nerve derives from the sciatic nerve in the popliteal fossa (Fig. 32-13).[4]

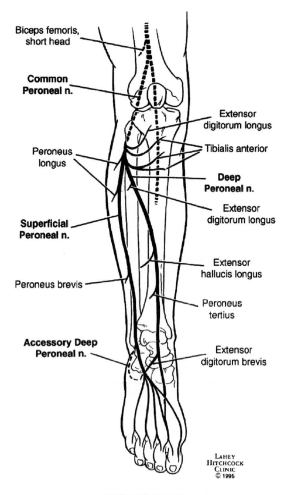

FIGURE 32–13

Diagram of the peroneal nerve and the muscles that it supplies. (Courtesy of Lahey Clinic, Burlington, MA.)

In the popliteal fossa, the common peroneal nerve gives off two sensory branches, the lateral sural cutaneous nerve, and the lateral cutaneous nerve of the calf. After rounding the head of the fibula, the common peroneal nerve bifurcates into its two terminal branches: the deep and superficial peroneal nerves.

The deep peroneal nerve innervates the tibialis anterior (L4-5), extensor hallucis longus (L5-S1), extensor digitorum longus and brevis (L5-S1), and the peroneus tertius (L5-S1) muscles. After supplying the extensor digitorum brevis on the dorsum of the foot, the deep peroneal nerve terminates as a small sensory branch, innervating the dorsal skin between the first and second toes.

The superficial peroneal nerve innervates the peroneus longus and brevis (L5-S1) muscles and then terminates as a sensory branch that innervates the skin of the lateral lower foreleg and dorsum of the foot and toes. An important anomaly in up to 20% of subjects is the accessory peroneal

nerve, a motor branch of the superficial peroneal nerve, which provides partial innervation of the extensor digitorum brevis muscle.

Etiology

Children with peroneal mononeuropathies typically present with a footdrop and, less commonly, with pain and paresthesia on the dorsum of the foot. The site of involvement in pediatric peroneal mononeuropathies is similar to that of adults,[138] being at the fibular head in 94% and at the ankle in 6% at CHB.[139] The common peroneal nerve was affected in 59% of the cases, deep peroneal nerve in 12%, and superficial peroneal nerve in 6%. In the remaining 23%, a precise localization was limited by technical factors.[139] Causes of peroneal mononeuropathy are shown in Box 32-7.

Compression

Compression was the primary mechanism for pediatric peroneal mononeuropathies, 10 (59%) of 17, in our experience.[138] The mode of onset was acute in 4 patients and indeterminate in the other 6. Half of the compressive peroneal mononeuropathies were iatrogenic, caused by casts, Buck's traction, Velcro straps, and intravenous footboard tape in a newborn. Three girls with anorexia nervosa had compression at the fibular head due to severe weight loss and chronic leg crossing.[139] This is similar to "slimmer's palsy" seen in adolescents, as well as adults.[140-143]

There are other rather unique causes of peroneal nerve compression in children. These include prolonged compression during water skiing on a knee board,[144,145] with anterior tibial compartment syndrome,[146] and from complications of anaphylactoid purpura[147] and critical illness.[148]

Newborns are also subject to iatrogenic compression injuries to the peroneal nerve. Mechanisms include intravenous fluid infiltration[149] and compression by tape used to secure a footboard.[139,150]

Entrapment

Less commonly, common or deep peroneal mononeuropathies present with a chronic progressive footdrop, repeated ankle sprains secondary to peroneal muscle weakness, or a cavus foot deformity due to entrapment of the peroneal nerve. Childhood causes of entrapment include at the division of the common peroneal nerve near the tendinous origin of the peroneus longus muscle at the fibula head.[139,151] Bony exostoses at the fibular head or talotibial exostosis deriving from osteochondromas have provided another proximal entrapment site.[152,153]

Isolated *superficial peroneal mononeuropathy* can result from entrapment by scarring due to repetitive ankle sprain.[154] MRI can assist in the diagnosis, and limited fasciec-

BOX 32-7
CAUSES OF PERONEAL
MONONEUROPATHIES

Newborn
    Intrauterine
    Idiopathic
    Intravenous fluid infiltration
    Footboards
    Birth trauma with popliteal fossa hematomas
Compression
    Orthopedic appliance
    Anorexia and chronic leg crossing
    Weight reduction
    Anaphylactoid purpura
Entrapment
    Bony exostoses
    Fibrotendinous bands
    Hemangioma
    Synovial cyst
    Ganglia
Trauma
    Lacerations
    Martial arts injuries
    Blunt trauma
    Traction stretch injury
    Burns
Tumors
    Schwannoma
    Hemangioma
    Osteochondroma
Systemic
    Diabetes mellitus
    Hereditary neuropathy with liability to pressure
      palsies

tomy often helps alleviate the symptoms.[154,155] This nerve may also be entrapped where it exits the lateral compartment.[156]

Mass Lesions: Cysts, Schwannomas, and Hemangiomas

Various cystic lesions can affect the peroneal nerve in children including synovial cysts, intraneural ganglion cysts, and a ganglion in the anterior compartment.[133,157-162] Occult nerve tumors can involve either the common, superficial, or deep peroneal nerves and often present with protracted symptoms. A child with a schwannoma of the superficial peroneal nerve presented with chronic paresthesia of the calf and toes for 1 year; the diagnosis was established dur-

ing surgical exploration.[139] Hemangioma is another rare cause of peroneal mononeuropathy.[163]

Localized hypertrophic neuropathy or intraneural perineuromas also lead to pediatric peroneal mononeuropathy.[135,164] This benign condition was difficult to diagnose in the past, usually requiring surgical exploration.[139] However, magnetic resonance neurography has improved the diagnosis of nerve tumors and has allowed for preoperative localization.[134,135,137,165]

Trauma

Trauma to the peroneal nerve occurs relatively infrequently, accounting for just 17% of our CHB experience.[139] Laceration of the deep peroneal nerve at the fibula head occurred in one child,[139] and a similar injury in an adolescent who lacerated the nerve with a skate blade.[166] Another child suffered a traumatic peroneal mononeuropathy during a motor vehicle accident, and a third child during repetitive blunt trauma in martial arts.[139] Surfing trauma is also reported in adolescents.[167]

Newborn

Newborns may also develop peroneal mononeuropathies; one had an antenatal onset.[118,168-170] The etiology in these is unclear, but the rapid and complete recovery in most cases points to a neuropraxic lesion. Two of the infants had abnormal intrauterine positions with a breech presentation and a stretching mechanism was postulated.[168-170] In others, uterine contraction rings might have caused a compressive lesion with axonal injury. One infant had fibrillation potentials present just 18 hours after delivery.[118]

Miscellaneous

Diffuse polyneuropathies may rarely underlie some childhood peroneal mononeuropathy including diabetes mellitus,[171-173] leprosy,[174] and HNPP.[175-178] In some children, the etiology of a progressive peroneal mononeuropathy remains elusive despite surgical exploration and pathologic analysis of the nerve.[125]

Evaluation

EMG evaluation of the peroneal nerve includes the superficial peroneal SNAP, peroneal motor nerve conduction studies from the extensor digitorum brevis and the tibialis anterior muscles, and needle examination of peroneal-innervated muscles.[179] The sural SNAP, tibial motor nerve conduction studies, and contralateral peroneal nerve studies may be indicated sometimes in children when isolated primary etiology is not apparent. Motor conduction studies below and above the fibular head are required to assess for conduction block or slowing across this segment. Occasionally, peroneal motor nerve conduction studies with recording electrodes on the tibialis anterior or peroneus longus may be required. The preservation of the superficial peroneal SNAP in a child with footdrop usually points to either a pure conduction block injury at the fibular head or to another process (i.e., L5 radiculopathy). Nerve conduction studies in most instances of peroneal compression show conduction block at the fibular head; the degree of conduction block correlates with clinical weakness.[139,141]

Sciatic mononeuropathies presenting with footdrop usually show EMG evidence of more diffuse and proximal abnormalities, including absent or attenuated sural and tibial motor responses, and needle examination abnormalities of the short head of biceps femoris. Needle examination of the lumbosacral paraspinal muscles can assist in differentiating peroneal mononeuropathies from the uncommon L5 root lesions leading to pediatric footdrop.

Imaging studies, particularly MRI or computed tomography (CT), may be helpful in localization and diagnosis, especially in patients presenting with a slowing progressive deficit that warrants consideration of chronic nerve compression or focal entrapment from a synovial cyst nerve tumor or osteochondromas.[152]

DNA Testing

The presence of conduction block superimposed on a diffuse polyneuropathy with pronounced segmental demyelinating features at common sites of compression and entrapment should also raise the question of HNPP. Specific DNA testing for the deletion on chromosome 17 can be diagnostic in this instance. If the parents have normal nerve conduction studies, this suggests a de novo mutation in the *PMP22* gene.

Surgical Exploration

On occasion, surgical exploration may be indicated with progressive lesions. In our CHB experience this approach defined a peroneal nerve entrapment at the knee from the peroneus longus tendon. In another instance a schwannoma at the fibular head was demonstrated.[139]

Treatment and Prognosis

Childhood peroneal mononeuropathies have a variable but often good prognosis. EMG results might provide useful prognostic information, since an absent or low-amplitude CMAP has been related to an unfavorable outcome.[139] At CHB 13 (76%) of 17 patients had complete or significant improvement.[139] The 4 patients with a poor recovery included 2 with blunt trauma, 1 a perioperative lesion, and 1 an entrapment lesion where surgical release was delayed.[139] The best prognosis was for children with demonstrable conduction block at the fibular head.[139]

Skillful primary repair of peripheral nerves in children is often followed by significant recovery.[180] Near nerve intraoperative recordings can help detect early nerve injury and avoid more severe damage during surgery.[181] If a childhood peroneal mononeuropathy fails to improve within 3 to 4 months, it is best to perform reparative surgery early on.[182,183] When improvement is not achieved despite surgical release or decompression of the nerve, tendon transfer operation can re-establish functional foot dorsiflexion and improve ambulation.[184]

CASE STUDY 10.

A 5-year-old girl developed insidiously progressive right footdrop over a 3-month period. There was no known antecedent injury, and she denied back or leg pain. The neurologic examination was remarkable for severe weakness of the right foot and toe extensors, moderate weakness of right foot evertors, atrophy of the right anterolateral foreleg muscles and extensor digitorum brevis, and reduced light touch sensation along the dorsum of the right foot. The ankle jerks were symmetrically normal. Nerve conduction studies revealed an absent right superficial peroneal SNAP and absent peroneal CMAPs recorded from the extensor digitorum brevis, tibialis anterior, and peroneus longus. The right sural SNAP, right tibial motor nerve conduction study, left superficial peroneal SNAP, and left peroneal motor nerve conduction study were normal. Needle examination revealed slightly increased insertional activity and reduced recruitment of motor unit action potentials from the right peroneus longus and anterior tibialis. The motor unit action potentials were of increased amplitude and duration and fired at faster than normal frequencies. No sustained fibrillations or positive sharp waves were observed. Needle examination of the right posterior tibialis and short head of biceps femoris was normal. Plain radiographs of the right leg revealed a large mass in the area of the proximal fibula. Surgical resection and biopsy disclosed a benign osteochondroma. Follow-up clinical and EMG examinations 1 year later showed no improvement.

Comments

The EMG findings were consistent with a chronic axon-loss right common peroneal mononeuropathy, localized distal to the innervation of the short head of biceps femoris. The insidiously progressive clinical course and EMG findings prompted imaging studies of the right knee and proximal foreleg. Benign tumors including osteochondromas should be considered in such cases of slowly progressive footdrop in an otherwise healthy child.

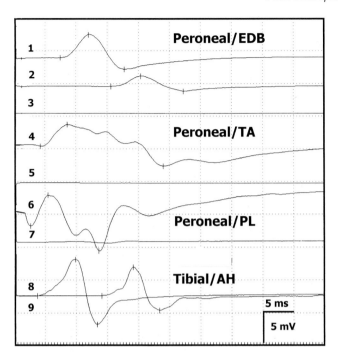

FIGURE 32–14

Motor nerve conduction studies for Case Study 11. The left peroneal to the extensor digitorum brevis (EDB) (waveforms 1 to 3), peroneal to the tibialis anterior (TA) (waveforms 4 and 5), peroneal to peroneus longus (PL) (waveforms 6 and 7), and tibial to adductor hallucis (AH) (waveforms 8 and 9) compound muscle action potentials are shown. For the peroneal motor nerves, stimulation is at the ankle (waveform 1), below-fibular head (waveforms 2, 4, and 6), and above-fibular head (waveforms 3, 5, and 7) sites. Note the complete motor conduction block (waveforms 3, 5, and 7). Also of note is the prolonged peroneal to extensor digitorum brevis distal latency of 7.5 milliseconds (normal, < 6.1 milliseconds), a common finding in hereditary neuropathy with liability to pressure palsies.

CASE STUDY 11.

A 12-year-old girl awoke with left footdrop about 5 weeks prior to the EMG study. She complained of severe weakness and sensory symptoms but denied back or limb pain. There was no personal or family history of neurologic or medical problems. The neurologic examination revealed complete weakness of the left foot and toe extensors and left foot evertors. Light touch sensation was reduced along the lateral foreleg and dorsum of the foot on the left side. The ankle jerks were symmetrically normal. Nerve conduction studies showed a low-amplitude left superficial peroneal SNAP and complete left peroneal motor conduction block across the fibular head (Fig. 32-14). Diffuse

nerve conduction abnormalities were also present and included low-amplitude SNAPs, prolonged median SNAP peak latency, prolonged peroneal and median CMAP distal latencies, and reduced motor conduction velocities across the fibular head for the right peroneal nerve and across the elbow segment for the left ulnar nerve. Needle examination of the left anterior tibialis revealed increased insertional activity, sustained fibrillations and positive sharp waves, and absent recruitment of motor unit action potentials. The results of nerve conduction studies prompted clinical and EMG evaluations of her parents and DNA testing for HNPP. Nerve conduction studies on her parents were normal. DNA studies on the patient were positive for the 1.5 Mb deletion mutation of the peripheral myelin protein 22 (*PMP22*) gene on 17p11.2.

Comments

The EMG findings were consistent with a left common peroneal mononeuropathy due to a severe conduction block injury (mild concurrent axonal injury as well) at the fibular head, superimposed on a diffuse polyneuropathy with pronounced, segmentally demyelinating features at common sites of compression and entrapment. The features of the polyneuropathy strongly raised the possibility of HNPP; subsequent DNA testing in this patient confirmed this diagnosis. The normal nerve conduction studies in her parents suggested a de novo mutation in the *PMP22* gene; however, this was not confirmed with DNA testing of her parents. HNPPs should be considered in any child with recurrent mononeuropathies or diffuse sensorimotor polyneuropathy with segmentally demyelinating features at common sites of nerve compression and entrapment.

FEMORAL NERVE

Anatomy

The femoral nerve derives from the posterior rami of the L2-4 segments and roots, innervates and passes through the psoas muscle (L2-3), runs along the iliacus muscle (L2-3) that it also innervates, descends beneath the inguinal ligament to enter the thigh, and then bifurcates into the anterior and posterior divisions (Fig. 32-15).[4] The *anterior division* divides into a muscular branch to the sartorius (L2-3) and a sensory branch, the medial cutaneous nerve of the thigh. The *posterior division* divides into the muscular branches that innervate the pectineus (L2-3) and quadriceps (L2-4) muscles, and the saphenous nerve that provides sensation to the skin over the medial aspect of the foreleg.

Femoral nerve lesions proximal to the innervation of the psoas and iliacus are associated with weakness of hip flexion

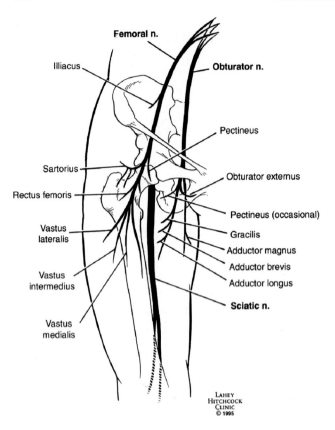

Femoral n.

Illiacus

Obturator n.

Pectineus

Sartorius

Rectus femoris

Obturator externus

Pectineus (occasional)

Gracilis

Vastus
lateralis

Adductor magnus

Adductor brevis

Adductor longus

Vastus
intermedius

Sciatic n.

Vastus
medialis

LAHEY
HITCHCOCK
CLINIC
© 1995

FIGURE 32–15

*Diagram of the femoral and obturator nerves and the muscles
that they supply. (Courtesy of Lahey Clinic, Burlington, MA.)*

and knee extension and sensory loss along anteromedial
thigh and medial foreleg. Lesions localized distal to this site
but proximal to the femoral triangle cause similar clinical
findings, with the exception that hip flexion is preserved.

Etiology

Femoral mononeuropathies are extremely rare in children (Box 32-8). One of us (K.J.F.) has evaluated three children with femoral mononeuropathies over a 10-year period.
The first child developed a severe femoral mononeuropathy
with involvement of hip flexors following renal transplant
surgery. Follow-up evaluation 1 year later showed minimal
improvement in function. The second child developed thigh
weakness and numbness following a spontaneous iliacus
hematoma resulting from hemophilia. In our third child, the
cause of the mild femoral mononeuropathy was not determined. Other reported causes of femoral mononeuropathy
include surgical injury, stretch injuries, perineuromas, intraneural hemorrhage or iliopsoas hematomas, neurofibromas,
and idiopathic injuries.[2,3,97,125,135,185-187]

BOX 32-8
**CAUSES OF OTHER LOWER EXTREMITY
MONONEUROPATHIES**

Femoral nerve
  Postsurgical
  Perineuromas
  Intraneural and iliopsoas hematomas in
    hemophilia
  Neurofibromas
  Idiopathic
Lateral femoral cutaneous nerve
  Orthopedic appliance
  Blunt trauma
  Idiopathic (meralgia paresthetica)
Sural nerve
  Ankle jewelry
Tibial nerve
  Trauma in popliteal fossa
  Tarsal tunnel syndrome
Obturator nerve
  Birth-related trauma

Evaluation

The EMG evaluation of a femoral mononeuropathy in a
child does not routinely include femoral motor nerve conduction studies because these studies are uncomfortable,
somewhat emotionally disconcerting to the natural shyness
in children, and do not seem to add much to the overall
EMG evaluation per se. However, we do obtain a saphenous
SNAP.

Needle examination of muscles innervated by the
femoral nerve generally includes the iliacus and vastus lateralis, and on occasion the vastus medialis, rectus femoris,
and sartorius muscles. Needle examination of the adductor
longus and lumbar paraspinal muscles is usually performed
as well to differentiate between isolated femoral mononeuropathies and more proximal lesions.

Imaging studies including MRI and CT scans are recommended in cases with slowly progressive symptoms or
when a nerve tumor is suspected.

Treatment and Prognosis

Femoral nerve lesions are too uncommon to make any
form of generalization. However, as with the previously
discussed mononeuropathies, the amount of axonal damage determines the timing to recovery and its eventual outcome. It is difficult to generalize with children because

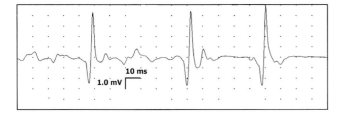

FIGURE 32–16
Needle electromyography for Case Study 12. Note the large motor unit action potentials from the left vastus lateralis, a finding consistent with chronic reinnervation via collateral sprouting.

they often have more potential for a more significant functional return than do adults with a "similar" lesion.

CASE STUDY 12.

A 13-year-old boy developed left thigh weakness, atrophy, and sensory symptoms following a motor vehicle accident about 5 years prior to the EMG test. The injury involved some upper thigh and back trauma but no fractures or dislocations. There was no prior history of neurologic disease. The neurologic examination revealed moderate weakness and atrophy of the left quadriceps muscles, mild left hip flexor weakness, and an absent left ankle jerk. Nerve conduction studies showed an absent left saphenous SNAP. The right saphenous and left sural, superficial peroneal, and median SNAPs were normal. The left peroneal, tibial, and ulnar motor nerve conduction studies and F-wave latencies were normal. The left tibial H-reflex study was normal. Needle examination revealed reduced recruitment of motor unit action potentials from the left vastus lateralis and iliacus. Motor unit action potentials were of increased amplitude and duration, showed increased phases and turns, and fired at faster than normal frequencies (Fig. 32-16). No fibrillations or positive sharp waves were observed. Needle examination of other left leg muscles including the adductor longus, left lumbosacral paraspinal muscles, and right vastus lateralis muscle was normal.

Comments
The EMG findings were consistent with a chronic axonloss left femoral mononeuropathy, localized proximal to the innervation of the iliacus muscle. Although the cause of injury was not certain, it was suspected that the proximal femoral nerve was injured directly by trauma or from a compressive hematoma.

OTHER LOWER EXTREMITY NERVES

Lateral Femoral Cutaneous Nerve

The lateral femoral cutaneous nerve is a pure sensory nerve that derives from the second and third lumbar segments and supplies sensation to the skin along the anterolateral thigh.[4]

Its clinical manifestations are similar to adults with numbness and pain along the lateral thigh. An extremely rare neuropathy in children, it has been observed as an idiopathic lesion,[3] caused by compression with an orthopedic harness[8] and by sport injuries, either by direct blunt trauma to the thigh in high-energy sports,[108] or in girl gymnasts due to the repetitive impact on the thigh by the bars (see Box 32-8).[188]

Although, previously the lateral femoral cutaneous SNAP was thought to be difficult to obtain with routine nerve conduction study in normal subjects the technology has improved and we should consider using this study in the occasional child where there is clinical indication. In general the diagnosis of meralgia paresthetica is usually based on clinical findings.

Sural Nerve

The sural nerve is another primary sensory nerve. It derives from the medial sural cutaneous (branch of tibial) and lateral sural cutaneous (branch of common peroneal) nerves in the distal popliteal fossa. It supplies sensation to the lateral ankle and foot.[4]

A compressive sural mononeuropathy caused by a tight ankle bracelet was reported in a young girl (see Box 32-8).[189]

Tibial Nerve

The tibial nerve derives from the sciatic nerve in the popliteal fossa and courses down the back of the leg to the medial ankle (Fig. 32-17).[4] In the popliteal fossa, it gives off the medial sural cutaneous nerve. In the back of the leg it gives off the motor branches to the medial and lateral gastrocnemius (S1-2), soleus (S1-2), tibialis posterior (L4-5), flexor digitorum longus (L5-S2), and flexor hallucis longus (S1-2). The nerve then passes along the medial malleolus, through the tarsal tunnel, and terminates into the medial plantar, lateral plantar, and calcaneal nerves (S1-2).

Tibial mononeuropathies in children are extremely rare and often occur concomitantly with peroneal nerve injuries in the popliteal fossa (see Box 32-8).[3] One report of "tarsal tunnel syndrome" in children noted improvement in symptoms following decompression surgery; however, none of the cases were confirmed by EMG studies.[190]

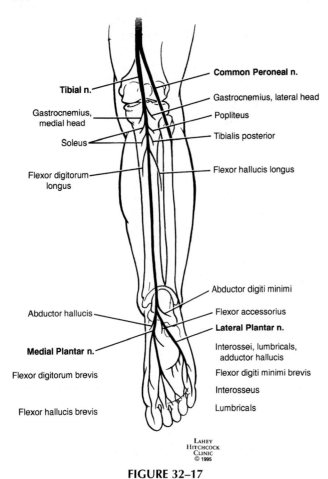

Tibial n.

Gastrocnemius, medial head

Soleus

Flexor digitorum longus

Abductor hallucis

Medial Plantar n.

Flexor digitorum brevis

Flexor hallucis brevis

Common Peroneal n.

Gastrocnemius, lateral head

Popliteus

Tibialis posterior

Flexor hallucis longus

Abductor digiti minimi

Flexor accessorius

Lateral Plantar n.

Interossei, lumbricals, adductor hallucis

Flexor digiti minimi brevis

Interosseus

Lumbricals

LAHEY
HITCHCOCK
CLINIC
© 1995

FIGURE 32–17
Diagram of the tibial nerve and the muscles that it supplies. (Courtesy of Lahey Clinic, Burlington, MA.)

Obturator Nerve

The obturator nerve derives from the lumbar plexus and L2-4 roots, courses along the pelvis, and enters the obturator canal. It then descends into the medial thigh as the anterior and posterior branches (see Fig. 32-15).[4] The anterior branch supplies the pectineus, adductor longus, adductor brevis, and gracilis muscles. It then terminates in a sensory branch that supplies the skin along the medial thigh. The posterior branch supplies the obturator externus, adductor magnus, and adductor brevis muscles.

Two instances of "obturator mononeuropathy" due to birth-related injuries have been reported. However, neither was confirmed with EMG studies (see Box 32-8).[191,192] Obturator mononeuropathies are exceedingly rare in children, and we have not documented such an injury in our EMG laboratories.

REFERENCES

1. Felice KJ, Jones HR: Upper extremity mononeuropathies. *In* Jones HR, De Vivo DC, Darras BT (eds): Neuromuscular Disorders of Infancy, Childhood, and Adolescence: A Clinician's Approach. Philadelphia, Butterworth-Heinemann, 2003, pp 301-319.
2. Escolar DM, Ryan MM, Jones HR: Lower extremity mononeuropathies. *In* Jones HR, De Vivo DC, Darras BT (eds): Neuromuscular Disorders of Infancy, Childhood, and Adolescence: A Clinician's Approach. Philadelphia, Butterworth-Heinemann, 2003, pp 321-338.
3. Jones HR: Mononeuropathies. *In* Jones HR, Bolton CF, Harper CM (eds): Pediatric Clinical Electromyography. Philadelphia, Lippincott-Raven, 1996, pp 171-250.
4. Stewart JD: Focal Peripheral Neuropathies. Philadelphia, Lippincott Williams & Wilkins, 2000.
5. Nordstrom DL, DeStefano F, Vierkant RA, Layde PM: Incidence of diagnosed carpal tunnel syndrome in a general population. Epidemiology 1998;9:342-345.
6. Swoboda KJ, Engle EC, Scheindlin B, et al: Mutilating hand syndrome in an infant with familial carpal tunnel syndrome. Muscle Nerve 1998;21:104-111.
7. Haddad FS, Jones DHA, Vellodi A, et al: Carpal tunnel syndrome in the mucopolysaccharidoses. J Bone Joint Surg Br 1997;79-B:576-582.
8. Ouvrier RA, Shield L: Focal lesions of peripheral nerves. *In* Ouvrier RA, McLeod JG, Pollard JD (eds): Peripheral Neuropathy in Childhood, 2nd ed. London, Mac Keith, 1999, pp 244-264.
9. Danta G: Familial carpal tunnel syndrome with onset in childhood. J Neurol Neurosurg Psychiatry 1975;38:350-355.
10. De Smet L, Fabry G: Carpal tunnel syndrome: Familial occurrence presenting in childhood. J Pediatr Orthop 1999;8:127-128.
11. McDonnell JM, Makley JT, Horwitz SJ: Familial carpal tunnel syndrome presenting in childhood: Report of two cases. J Bone Joint Surg Am 1987;69-A:928-930.
12. Stoll C, Maitrot D: Autosomal dominant carpal tunnel syndrome. Clin Genet 1998;54:345-348.
13. Deymeer F, Jones HR: Pediatric median mononeuropathies: A clinical and electromyographic study. Muscle Nerve 1994;17:755-762.
14. Koenigsberger MR, Moessinger AC: Iatrogenic carpal tunnel syndrome in the newborn infant. J Pediatr 1977;91:443-445.
15. Cruz Martinez A, Arpa J: Carpal tunnel syndrome in childhood: Study of six cases. Electroencephal Clin Neurophysiol 1998;109:304-308.
16. MacDougal B, Weeks PM, Wray RC Jr: Median nerve compression and trigger finger in the mucopolysaccharidosis and related disorders. Plast Reconstr Surg 1977;59:260-263.
17. McArthur RG, Hayles AB, Gomez MR, Bianco AJ Jr: Carpal tunnel syndrome and trigger finger in childhood. Am J Dis Child 1969;117:463-469.
18. Miner ME, Schimke RN: Carpal tunnel syndrome in pediatric mucopolysaccharidoses: Report of four cases. J Neurosurg 1975;43:102-103.

19. Starreveld E, Ashenhurst EM: Bilateral carpal tunnel syndrome in childhood: A report of two sisters with mucolipidosis III (pseudo-Hurler polydystrophy). Neurology 1975;25:234-238.

20. Alvarez N, Larkin C, Roxborough J: Carpal tunnel syndrome in athetoid-dystonic cerebral palsy. Arch Neurol 1982;39:311-312.

21. Senveli ME, Turker A, Arda MN, Altinors MN: Bilateral carpal tunnel syndrome in a young carpet weaver. Clin Neurol Neurosurg 1987;89:281-282.

22. Blennow G, Bekassy AN, Eriksson M, Rosendahl R: Transient carpal tunnel syndrome accompanying rubella infection. Acta Paediatr Scand 1982;71:1025-1028.

23. Cruz Martinez A, Arpa J, Perez Conde MC, Ferrer MT: Bilateral carpal tunnel in childhood associated with Schwartz-Jampel syndrome. Muscle Nerve 1984;7:66-72.

24. Felice KJ, Leicher CR, DiMario FJ: Hereditary neuropathy with liability to pressure palsies in children. Pediatr Neurol 1999;21:818-821.

25. Williams LF, Greer T: Acute carpal tunnel syndrome secondary to pyogenic infection of the forearm. JAMA 1963;185:409-410.

26. Unal O, Ozcakar L, Cetin A, Kaymak B: Severe bilateral carpal tunnel syndrome in juvenile arthritis. Pediatr Neurol 2003;29:345-348.

27. Harpf C, Schwabegger A, Hussl H: Carpal median nerve entrapment in a child with Poland's syndrome [Letter]. Ann Plastic Surg 1999;42:458-459.

28. Weeks PM: Radial, median, and ulnar nerve dysfunction associated with a congenital constricting band of the arm. Plast Reconstr Surg 1982;69:333-336.

29. Pape KE, Armstrong DL, Fitzhardinge PM: Peripheral median nerve damage secondary to brachial arterial blood gas sampling. J Pediatr 1978;93:852-856.

30. Hotta T, Kanbara H, Soto S, et al: Case of carpal tunnel syndrome due to calcification of the flexor digitorum sublimis II in a child. Orthop Surg (Tokyo) 1970;21:948-950.

31. Fissette J, Onkelinx A, Fandi N: Carpal and Guyon tunnel syndrome in burns at the wrist. J Hand Surg 1981;6:13-15.

32. Cavanagh NPC, Yates DAH, Sutcliffe J: Thenar hypoplasia with associated radiologic abnormalities. Muscle Nerve 1979;2:431-436.

33. Fearn CB, Goodfellow JW: Anterior interosseous nerve palsy. J Bone Joint Surg 1965;47:91-93.

34. Floyd WE III, Gebhardt MC, Emans JB: Intra-articular entrapment of the median nerve after elbow dislocation in children. J Hand Surg Am 1987;12-A:704-707.

35. Sumner JM, Khuri SM: Entrapment of the median nerve and flexor pollicis longus tendon in an epiphyseal fracture-dislocation of the distal radioulnar joint: A case report. J Hand Surg Am 1984;9-A:711-714.

36. Marlow N, Jarratt J, Hosking G: Congenital ring constrictions with entrapment neuropathies. J Neurol Neurosurg Psychiatry 1981;44:247-249.

37. Uchida Y, Sugioka Y: Peripheral nerve palsy associated with congenital constriction band syndrome. J Hand Surg Br 1991;16-B:109-112.

38. Danielsson LG: Iatrogenic pronator syndrome. Scand J Plast Reconstr Surg 1980;14:201-203.

39. Hartz CR, Linscheid RL, Gramse RR, Daube JR: The pronator syndrome: Compressive neuropathy of the median nerve. J Bone Joint Surg 1981;63:885-890.

40. Gessini L, Jandolo B, Pietrangeli A: Entrapment neuropathies of the median nerve at the elbow. Surg Neurol 1983;19:112-116.

41. Amadio PC, Reiman HM, Dobyns JH: Lipofibromatous hamartoma of nerve. J Hand Surg Am 1988;13-A:67-75.

42. Louis DS, Hankin FM, Greene TL, Dick HM: Lipofibromas of the median nerve: Long-term follow-up of four cases. J Hand Surg Am 1985;10-A:403-408.

43. Callison JR, Thomas OJ, White WL: Fibrofatty proliferation of the median nerve. Plast Reconstr Surg 1968;42:403-413.

44. Barfred T, Zachariae L: Neurofibroma in the median nerve treated with resection and free nerve transplantation: Case reports. Scand J Plast Reconstr Surg 1975;9:245-248.

45. Patel CB, Tsai T-M, Kleinert HE: Hemangioma of the median nerve: A report of two cases. J Hand Surg Am 1986;11-A:76-79.

46. Nakano KK, Lundergran C, Okihiro MM: Anterior interosseous nerve syndromes: Diagnostic methods and alternative treatments. Arch Neurol 1977;34:477-480.

47. Spinner M, Schreiber SN: Anterior interosseous nerve paralysis as a complication of supracondylar fractures in children. J Bone Joint Surg 1969;51:1584-1590.

48. Chaudhry V, Cornblath DR: Wallerian degeneration in human nerves: Serial electrophysiologic studies. Muscle Nerve 1992;15:687-693.

49. Robinson LR: Traumatic injury to peripheral nerves. Muscle Nerve 2000;23:863-873.

50. Felice KJ, Jones HR: Pediatric ulnar mononeuropathy: Report of 21 electromyography-documented cases and review of the literature. J Child Neurol 1996;11:116-120.

51. Uchida Y, Sugioka Y: Ulnar nerve palsy after supracondylar humerus fracture. Acta Orthop Scand 1990;61:118-119.

52. Gessini L, Jandolo B, Pietrangeli A, Occhipinti E: Ulnar nerve entrapment at the elbow by persistent epitrochleoanconeus muscle: Case report. J Neurosurg 1981;55:830-831.

53. Montoya L, Felice KJ: Recovery from distal ulnar motor conduction block injury: Serial EMG studies. Muscle Nerve 2002;26:145-149.

54. Noth J, Dietz V, Mauritz KH: Cyclist's palsy: Neurological and EMG study in four cases with distal ulnar lesions. J Neurol Sci 1980;47:111-116.

55. Saxena U, Ramesh V, Misra RS, Mukherjee A: Giant nerve abscesses in leprosy. Clin Exp Dermatol 1990;15:349-351.

56. Cordingley FT, Crawford GP: Ulnar nerve palsy in a haemophiliac due to intraneural haemorrhage. BMJ 1984;289:18-19.

57. Dunn D, Wilensky M: Median and ulnar nerve palsies after infiltration of intravenous fluid [Letter]. South Med J 1984;77:1345.

58. Phillips LH II, Persing JA, Vandenberg SR: Electrophysiological findings in localized hypertrophic mononeuropathy. Muscle Nerve 1991;14:335-341.

59. Marquez S, Turley JJE, Peters WJ: Neuropathy in burns patients. Brain 1993;116:471-483.

60. Godshall RW, Hansen CA: Traumatic ulnar neuropathy in adolescent baseball pitchers. J Bone Joint Surg Am 1971;53-A:359-361.

61. Cavanagh NPC, Pincott JR: Ulnar nerve tumours of the hand in childhood. J Neurol Neurosurg Psychiatry 1977;40:795-800.

62. Drut R: Ossifying fibrolipomatous hamartoma of the ulnar nerve. Pediatr Pathol 1988;8:179-184.

63. Kothari MJ, Heistand M, Rutkove S: Three ulnar motor conduction studies in patients with ulnar neuropathy at the elbow. Arch Phys Med Rehabil 1998;79:87-89.

64. Escolar DM, Jones HR: Pediatric radial mononeuropathies: A clinical and electromyographic study of sixteen children with review of the literature. Muscle Nerve 1996;19:876-883.

65. Papilion JD, Neff RS, Shall LM: Compression neuropathy of the radial nerve as a complication of elbow arthroscopy: A case report and review of the literature. Arthroscopy 1988;4:284-286.

66. Feldman GV: Radial nerve palsies in the newborn. Arch Dis Child 1957;32:469-471.

67. Morgan L: Radial nerve paralysis in the newborn. Arch Dis Child 1948;23:137-139.

68. Lightwood R: Radial nerve palsy associated with localized subcutaneous fat necrosis in the newborn. Arch Dis Child 1951;26:436-437.

69. Ross D, Jones HR Jr, Fisher J, Konkol RJ: Isolated radial nerve lesion in the newborn. Neurology 1983;33:1354-1356.

70. Tollner U, Bechinger D, Pohlandt F: Radial nerve palsy in a premature infant following long-term measurement of blood pressure. J Pediatr 1980;96:921-922.

71. Jones HR: Compressive neuropathy in childhood: A report of 14 cases. Muscle Nerve 1986;9:720-723.

72. Meier C, Moll C: Hereditary neuropathy with liability to pressure palsies: Report of two families and review of the literature. J Neurol 1982;228:73-95.

73. Lotem M, Fried A, Levy M: Radial nerve palsy following muscular effort: A nerve compression syndrome possibly related to a fibrous arch of the lateral head of the triceps. J Bone Joint Surg Br 1971;53-B:500-506.

74. Manske PR: Compression of the radial nerve by the triceps muscle: a case report. J Bone Joint Surg Am 1977;59-A:835-836.

75. Witthout J, Steffens KJ, Koob E: Intermittent axillary nerve palsy caused by humeral exostosis. J Hand Surg Br 1994;19-B:422-423.

76. Foo CL, Swann M: Isolated paralysis of the serratus anterior: A report of 20 cases. J Bone Joint Surg Br 1983;65-B:552-556.

77. Gregg JR, Labosky D, Harty M, et al: Serratus anterior paralysis in the young athlete. J Bone Joint Surg Am 1979;61-A:825-832.

78. Laulund T, Fedders O, Sogaard I, Kornum M: Suprascapular nerve compression syndrome. Surg Neurol 1984;22:308-312.

79. Montagna P, Colonna S: Suprascapular neuropathy restricted to the infraspinatus muscle in volleyball players. Acta Neurol Scand 1993;87:248-250.

80. Okino T, Minami A, Kato H, et al: Entrapment neuropathy of the suprascapular nerve by a ganglion. J Bone Joint Surg Am 1991;73-A:141-147.

81. Escolar DM, Jones HR: Pediatric sciatic mononeuropathies: A clinical and electromyographic analysis [Abstract]. Muscle Nerve 1994;17:108.

82. Deverell WF, Ferguson JH: An unusual case of sciatic nerve paralysis. JAMA 1968;205:699-700.

83. Lee R, Fann AV, Sobus K: Bilateral sciatic nerve entrapment due to weight loss. J Ark Med Soc 1998;95:153-155.

84. Brown JA, Braun MA, Namey TC: Pyriformis syndrome in a 10-year-old boy as a complication of operation with the patient in the sitting position. Neurosurgery 1988;23:117-119.

85. Gozal Y, Pomeranz S: Sciatic nerve palsy as a complication after acoustic neurinoma resection in the sitting position. J Neurosurg Anesthesiol 1994;6:40-42.

86. Yuen EC, So YT: Sciatic neuropathy. Neurol Clin 1999;17:617-631.

87. Yuen EC, So YT, Olney RK: The electrophysiologic features of sciatic neuropathy in 100 patients. Muscle Nerve 1995;18:414-420.

88. Goh KJ, Tan CB, Tjia HT: Sciatic neuropathies: A retrospective review of electrodiagnostic features in 29 patients. Ann Acad Med Singapore 1996;25:566-569.

89. Yuen EC, Olney RK, So YT: Sciatic neuropathy: Clinical and prognostic features in 73 patients. Neurology 1994;44:1669-1674.

90. Kubiak R, Wilcox DT, Spitz L, Kiely EM: Neurovascular morbidity from the lithotomy position. J Pediatr Surg 1998;33:1808-1810.

91. Warner MA, Warner DO, Harper CM, et al: Lower extremity neuropathies associated with lithotomy positions. Anesthesiology 2000;93:938-942.

92. Vogel CM, Albin R, Alberts JW. Lotus footdrop: Sciatic neuropathy in the thigh. Neurology 1991;41:605-606.

93. Romfh JH, Currier RD: Sciatic neuropathy induced by the lithotomy position. Arch Neurol 1983;40:127.

94. Burkhart F, Daly J: Sciatic and peroneal nerve injury: A complication of vaginal operations. Obstet Gynecol 1996;28:99-102.

95. Dhote R, Tudoret L, Bachmeyer C, et al: Cyclic sciatica—a manifestation of compression of the sciatic nerve by endometriosis: A case report. Spine 1996;21:2277-2279.

96. Gasecki AP, Ebers GC, Vellet AD, Buchan A: Sciatic neuropathy associated with persistent sciatic artery. Arch Neurol 1992;49:967-968.

97. Ehrmann L, Lechner K, Mamoli B, et al: Peripheral nerve lesions in haemophilia. J Neurol 1981;225:175-182.

98. London N, Sefton G: Hematocolpos: An unusual cause of sciatica in an adolescent girl. Spine 1996;21:1381-1382.

99. Thomas JE, Piepgras DG, Scheithauer B, et al: Neurogenic tumors of the sciatic nerve. A clinicopathologic study of 35 cases. Mayo Clin Proc 1983;58:640-647.

100. Katirji MB, Wilbourn AJ: High sciatic lesion mimicking peroneal neuropathy at the fibular head. J Neurol Sci 1994;121:172-175.

101. Hruban RH, Shiu MH, Senie RT, Woodruff JM: Malignant peripheral nerve sheath tumors of the buttock and lower extremity: A study of 43 cases. Cancer 1990;66:1253-1265.

102. Misdraji J, Ino Y, Louis DN, et al: Primary lymphoma of peripheral nerve: Report of four cases. Am J Surg Pathol 2000;24:1257-1265.

103. Cruccetti A, Kiely EM, Spitz L, et al: Pelvic neuroblastoma: Low mortality and high morbidity. J Pediatr Surg 2000;35:724-728.

104. Stillman MJ, Christensen W, Payne R, Foley KM: Leukemic relapse presenting as sciatic nerve involvement by chloroma (granulocytic sarcoma). Cancer 1988;62:2047-2050.

105. Cornwall R, Radomisli TE: Nerve injury in traumatic dislocation of the hip. Clin Orthop 2000;377:84-91.

106. Cullen MC, Roy DR, Crawford AH, et al: Open fracture of the tibia in children. J Bone Joint Surg Am 1996;78-A:1039-1047.

107. Yoshida T, Tada K, Uemura K, Yonenobu K: Peripheral nerve palsies in victims of the Hanshin-Awaji earthquake. Clin Orthop 1999;362:208-217.

108. Lorei MP, Hershman EB: Peripheral nerve injuries in athletes: Treatment and prevention. Sports Med 1993;16:130-147.

109. Sriram K, Sakthivel A: Sciatic nerve palsy in the newborn. Ann Acad Med Singapore 1981;10:472-475.

110. Clark K, Williams PE, Willis W, McGavran WL: Injection injury of the sciatic nerve. Clin Neurosurg 1970;17:111-125.

111. Combes M, Clark W: Sciatic nerve injury following intragluteal injection: Pathogenesis and prevention. Am J Dis Child 1960;100:579.

112. MacDonald NE, Marcuse EK: Neurologic injury after vaccination: Buttocks as injection site. Can Med Assoc J 1994;150:326.

113. de Sanctis N, Cardillo G, Nunziata Rega A: Gluteoperineal gangrene and sciatic nerve palsy after umbilical vessel injection. Clin Orthop 1995;316:180-184.

114. Fok TF, Ha MH, Leung KW, Wong W: Sciatic nerve palsy complicating umbilical arterial catheterization. Eur J Pediatr 1986;145:308-309.

115. Goven'ko FS, Babin AV: Lesions of the sciatic nerve in newborn infants after administration of various drugs into the umbilical arteries. Akush Ginekol (Mosk) 1990;61-63.

116. Ramos-Fernandez JM, Oliete-Garcia FM, Roldan-Aparicio S, et al: Neonatal sciatic palsy: Etiology and outcome of 21 cases. Rev Neurol 1998;26:752-755.

117. Sharrard WJ: Neonatal sciatic paralysis (two cases). Proc R Soc Med 1973;66:218-219.

118. Jones HR, Herbison GJ, Jacobs SR, et al: Intrauterine onset of a mononeuropathy: Peroneal neuropathy in a newborn with electromyographic findings at age one day compatible with prenatal onset. Muscle Nerve 1996;19:88-91.

119. Sheth D, Gutmann L, Blumenthal DT, et al: Compressive sciatic neuropathy due to uterine abnormality. Muscle Nerve 1994;17:1486-1488.

120. Sayson SC, Ducey JP, Maybrey JB, et al: Sciatic entrapment neuropathy associated with an anomalous piriformis muscle. Pain 1994;59:149-152.

121. Sogaard I: Sciatic nerve entrapment: Case report. J Neurosurg 1983;58:275-276.

122. Tada K, Yonenobu K, Swanson AB: Congenital constriction band syndrome. J Pediatr Orthop 1984;4:726-730.

123. Venna N, Bielawski M, Spatz EM: Sciatic nerve entrapment in a child: Case report. J Neurosurg 1991;75:652-654.

124. Jones HR, Gianturco LE, Gross PT, Buchhalter J: Sciatic neuropathies in childhood: A report of ten cases and review of the literature. J Child Neurol 1988;3:193-199.

125. Engstrom JW, Layzer RB, Olney RK, Edwards MB: Idiopathic progressive mononeuropathy in young people. Arch Neurol 1993;50:20-23.

126. Sawaya RA: Idiopathic sciatic mononeuropathy. Clin Neurol Neurosurg 1999;101:256-259.

127. Aagaard BD, Maravilla KR, Kliot M: MR neurography: MR imaging of peripheral nerves. Magn Reson Imaging Clin North Am 1998;6:179-194.

128. Almanza MY, Poon-Chue A, Terk MR: Dual oblique MR method for imaging the sciatic nerve. J Comput Assist Tomogr 1999;23:138-140.

129. Filler AG, Kliot M, Howe FA, et al: Application of magnetic resonance neurography in the evaluation of patients with peripheral nerve pathology. J Neurosurg 1996;85:299-309.

130. Kuntz C, Blake CL, Britz G, et al: Magnetic resonance neurography of peripheral nerve lesions in the lower extremity. Neurosurgery 1996;39:750-757.

131. Marom EM, Helms CA: Fibrolipomatous hamartoma: Pathognomonic on MR imaging. Skeletal Radiol 1999;28:260-264.

132. Tachi N, Kozuka N, Ohya K, et al: MRI of peripheral nerves and pathology of sural nerves in hereditary motor and sensory neuropathy type III. Neuroradiology 1995;37:496-499.

133. Uetani M, Hashmi R, Hayashi K, et al: Peripheral nerve intraneural ganglion cyst: MR findings in three cases. J Comput Assist Tomogr 1998;22:629-632.

134. Weig SG, Waite RJ, McAvoy K: MRI in unexplained mononeuropathy. Pediatr Neurol 2000;22:314-317.

135. Emory TS, Scheithauer BW, Hirose T, et al: Intraneural perineurioma: A clonal neoplasm associated with abnormalities of chromosome 22. Am J Clin Pathol 1995;103:696-704.

136. Martinoli C, Bianchi S, Derchi L: Ultrasonography of peripheral nerves. Semin Ultrasound CT MR 2000;21:205-213.

137. Kline DG, Kim D, Midha R, et al: Management and results of sciatic nerve injuries: A 24-year experience. J Neurosurg 1998;89:13-23.

138. Katirji MB, Wilbourn AJ: Common peroneal mononeuropathy: A clinical and electrophysiologic study of 116 lesions. Neurology 1988;38:1723-1728.

139. Jones HR, Felice KJ, Gross PT: Pediatric peroneal mononeuropathy: A clinical and electromyographic study. Muscle Nerve 1993;16:1167-1173.

140. Constanty A, Vodoff MV, Gilbert B, et al: Peroneal nerve palsy in anorexia nervosa: Three cases. Arch Pediatr 2000;7:316-317.

141. Cruz Martinez A: Slimmer's paralysis: Electrophysiological evidence of compressive lesion. Eur Neurol 1987;26:189-192.

142. Sotaniemi KA: Slimmer's paralysis: Peroneal neuropathy during weight reduction. J Neurol Neurosurg Psychiatry 1984;47:564-566.

143. Streib E: Weight loss and foot drop. Iowa Med 1993;83:224-225.

144. Wilbourn A, Levin K, Sweeney P: Peroneal neuropathies in children and adolescents [Abstract]. Can J Neurol Sci 1990;17:227.

145. Vaccaro AR, Ludwig SC, Klein GR, et al: Bilateral peroneal nerve palsy secondary to a knee board: Report of two cases. Am J Orthop 1998;27:746-748.

146. Sloane AE, Vajsar J, Laxer RM, et al: Spontaneous non-traumatic anterior compartment syndrome with peroneal neuropathy and favorable outcome. Neuropediatrics 1994;25:268-270.

147. Ritter FJ, Seay AR, Lahey ME: Peripheral mononeuropathy complicating anaphylactoid purpura. J Pediatr 1983;103:77-78.

148. Tan MJ, Kandler R, Baxter PS: Focal neuropathy in children with critical illness. Neuropediatrics 2003;34:149-151.

149. Kreusser KL, Volpe JJ: Peroneal palsy produced by intravenous fluid infiltration in a newborn. Dev Med Child Neurol 1984;26:522-524.

150. Fischer AQ, Strasburger J: Footdrop in the neonate secondary to use of footboards. J Pediatr 1982;101:1003-1004.

151. Sidi J: Weak ankles: A study of common peroneal entrapment neuropathy. BMJ 1969;3:623-626.

152. Levin KH, Wilbourn AJ, Jones HR: Childhood peroneal neuropathy from bone tumors. Pediatr Neurol 1991;7:308-309.

153. Edlich HS, Fariss BL, Phillips VA, et al: Talotibial exostoses with entrapment of the deep peroneal nerve. J Emerg Med 1987;5:109-113.

154. Daghino W, Pasquali M, Faletti C: Superficial peroneal nerve entrapment in a young athlete: The diagnostic contribution of magnetic resonance imaging. J Foot Ankle Surg 1997;36:170-172.

155. Styf J, Morberg P: The superficial peroneal tunnel syndrome: Results of treatment by decompression. J Bone Joint Surg Br 1997;79-B:801-803.

156. McAuliffe T, Fiddian N, Browett J: Entrapment neuropathy of the superficial peroneal nerve: A bilateral case. J Bone Joint Surg Am 1985;67-A:62-63.

157. Antonini G, Bastianello S, Nucci F, et al: Ganglion of deep peroneal nerve: Electrophysiology and CT scan in the diagnosis. Electromyogr Clin Neurophysiol 1991;31:9-13.

158. Gayet LE, Morand F, Goujon JM, et al: Compression of the peroneal nerve by a cyst in a seven-year-old child. Eur J Pediatr Surg 1998;8:61-63.

159. Gurdjian ES, Larsen RD, Lindner DW: Intraneural cyst of the peroneal and ulnar nerves: Report of two cases. J Neurosurg 1965;23:76-78.

160. Martins RS, Martinez J, de Aguiar PH, et al: Intraneural synovial cyst of the peroneal nerve: Case report. Arq Neuropsiquiatr 1997;55:831-833.

161. Nucci F, Artico M, Santoro A, et al: Intraneural synovial cyst of the peroneal nerve: Report of two cases and review of the literature. Neurosurgery 1990;26:339-344.

162. Beck TD, Miller KE, Kruse RW: An unusual presentation of intoeing in a child. J Am Osteopath Assoc 1998;98:48-50.

163. Bilge T, Kaya A, Alatli M, et al: Hemangioma of the peroneal nerve: Case report and review of the literature. Neurosurgery 1989;25:649-652.

164. Johnson PC, Kline DG: Localized hypertrophic neuropathy: Possible focal perineurial barrier defect. Acta Neuropathol 1989;77:514-518.

165. Houshian S, Freund KG: Gigantic benign schwannoma in the lateral peroneal nerve. Am J Knee Surg 1999;12:41-42.

166. Shevell MI, Stewart JD: Laceration of the common peroneal nerve by a skate blade. Can Med Assoc J 1988;139:311-312.

167. Watemberg N, Amsel S, Sadeh M, Lerman-Sagie T: Common peroneal neuropathy due to surfing. J Child Neurol 2000;15:420-421.

168. Crumrine PK, Koenigsberger MR, Chutorian AM: Footdrop in the neonate with neurologic and electrophysiologic data. J Pediatr 1975;86:779-780.

169. Godley DR: Neonatal peroneal neurapraxia: A report of two cases and review of the literature. Am J Orthop 1998;27:803-804.

170. Yilmaz Y, Oge AE, Yilmaz-Degpirmenci S, Say A: Peroneal nerve palsy: The role of early electromyography. Europ J Paediatr Neurol 2000;4:239-242.

171. Barkai L, Kempler P, Vamosi I, et al: Peripheral sensory nerve dysfunction in children and adolescents with type 1 diabetes mellitus. Diabet Med 1998;15:228-233.

172. el Bahri-Ben M, Gouider FR, Fredj M, et al: Childhood diabetic neuropathy: A clinical and electrophysiological study. Funct Neurol 2000;15:35-40.

173. Lawrence D, Locke S: Neuropathy in children with diabetes mellitus. BMJ 1963;5333:784-785.

174. Choe W: Leprosy presenting as unilateral foot drop in an immigrant boy. Postgrad Med J 1994;70:111-112.

175. Cruz-Martinez A, Arpa J, Palau F: Peroneal neuropathy after weight loss. J Peripher Nerv Syst 2000;5:101-105.

176. Mouton P, Tardieu S, Gouider R, et al: Spectrum of clinical and electrophysiologic features in HNPP patients with the 17p11.2 deletion. Neurology 1999;52:1440-1446.

177. Gabreels-Festen AA, Gabreels FJ, Joosten EM, et al: Hereditary neuropathy with liability to pressure palsies in childhood. Neuropediatrics 1992;23:138-143.

178. Pareyson D, Solari A, Taroni F, et al: Detection of hereditary neuropathy with liability to pressure palsies among patients with acute painless mononeuropathy or plexopathy. Muscle Nerve 1998;21:1686-1691.

179. Sourkes M, Stewart JD: Common peroneal neuropathy: A study of selective motor and sensory involvement. Neurology 1991;41:1029-1033.

180. Birch R, Achan P: Peripheral nerve repairs and their results in children. Hand Clin 2000;16:579-595.

181. Wexler I, Paley D, Herzenberg JE, Herbert A: Detection of nerve entrapment during limb lengthening by means of near-nerve recording. Electromyogr Clin Neurophysiol 1998;38:161-167.

182. Fabre T, Piton C, Andre D, et al: Peroneal nerve entrapment. J Bone Joint Surg Am 1998;80-A:47-53.

183. Piton C, Fabre T, Lasseur E, et al: Common fibular nerve lesions—etiology and treatment: Apropos of 146 cases with surgical treatment. Rev Chir Orthop Reparatrice Appar Mot 1997;83:515-521.

184. Breukink SO, Spronk CA, Dijkstra PU, et al: Transposition of the tendon of M. tibialis posterior an effective treatment of drop foot: Retrospective study with follow-up in 12 patients. Ned Tijdschr Geneeskd 2000;144:604-608.

185. Carter GT, McDonald CM, Chan TT, Margherita AJ: Isolated femoral mononeuropathy to the vastus lateralis: EMG and MRI findings. Muscle Nerve 1995;18:341-344.

186. Takao M, Fukuuchi Y, Koto A, et al: Localized hypertrophic mononeuropathy involving the femoral nerve. Neurology 1999;52:389-392.

187. Sharma S, Ray R: Femoral pain of solitary neurofibromatous origin. Ind Pediatr 1988;25:1221-1223.

188. Macgregor J, Moncur JA: Meralgia paraesthetica: A sports lesion in girl gymnasts. Br J Sports Med 1977;11:16-19.

189. Reisin R, Pardal A, Ruggieri V, Gold L: Sural neuropathy due to external pressure: Report of three cases. Neurology 1994;44:2408-2409.

190. Albrektsson B, Rydholm A, Rydholm U: The tarsal tunnel syndrome in children. J Bone Joint Surg Br 1982;64-B:215-217.

191. Craig WS, Clark JMP: Obturator palsy in the newly born. Arch Dis Child 1962;37:661-662.

192. Craig WS, Clark JMP: Of peripheral nerve palsies in the newborn. J Obstet Gynecol Br Empire 1958;65:229-237.

33

Clinical Neurophysiology of Pediatric Polyneuropathies

TED M. BURNS, DEBORAH Y. BRADSHAW, NANCY L. KUNTZ,
AND H. ROYDEN JONES, JR.

OVERVIEW TO THE ELECTRODIAGNOSTIC EVALUATION OF PEDIATRIC POLYNEUROPATHIES

Epidemiology

The epidemiology of polyneuropathy in children differs significantly from that in adults. Awareness of these differences allows rational design, modification, and interpretation of the electrodiagnostic study in children. Four key principles should be kept in mind. First, genetically determined polyneuropathies are much more common than acquired neuropathies in children.[1-5] It is estimated that two thirds to three quarters of pediatric neuropathies are inherited.[4,6] Second, under the genetically determined rubric, all types of Charcot-Marie-Tooth (CMT) (hereditary motor and sensory neuropathy) predominate. The prevalence of CMT has been estimated at 1 per 2500 to 10,000, which makes it far and away the single most common cause of polyneuropathy in the pediatric population.[7,8] Third, of acquired polyneuropathies, acute and chronic inflammatory demyelinating polyradiculoneuropathies (CIDPs) make up the majority of cases. Guillain-Barré syndrome (GBS) has an estimated incidence of 1 per 100,000 in the pediatric population. The incidence of childhood CIDP is probably one tenth that of childhood GBS, whereas the prevalence of childhood CIDP, a chronic disorder, is estimated at less than 1 per 100,000.[9-16] Fourth, a striking difference between the adult and pediatric populations is that polyneuropathies associated with systemic diseases such as diabetes mellitus, malignancy, paraproteinemia, chronic alcohol use, collagen vascular disease, vitamin deficiencies, and chronic renal disease are rare in childhood.

Large case series of pediatric polyneuropathy are limited by referral and selection bias, as well as by variable classification of the inherited neuropathies. Thus, they often do not mirror epidemiologic studies. Nonetheless, they provide insight into the etiologies and frequency of the pediatric polyneuropathies seen at neuromuscular clinics. A series of 61 children with polyneuropathy admitted to the Vanderbilt Medical Center from 1971 to 1977 included 17 cases of GBS (28%), 11 cases of CMT (18%), 5 cases of spinocerebellar degeneration (8%), 5 polyneuropathies associated with systemic disease (8%) and 16 idiopathic cases (26%).[2] Hereditary motor and sensory neuropathies (CMT) made up only 42% of cases in a series of 249 pediatric polyneuropathies seen at Children's Hospital of Philadelphia over a 12-year period.[17] An inflammatory demyelinating polyradiculoneuropathy was diagnosed in 41% of children; a referral bias may have contributed to this higher frequency of acquired demyelinating polyneuropathies in this series. Polyneuropathies associated with collagen vascular disease, metabolic disorders, and toxins were much less common.

An Australian series based on sural nerve analysis in children with subacute or chronic polyneuropathies found that at least 71% of cases were inherited.[18] CMT-1 was the most common diagnosis, followed by CMT-2. CIDP was diagnosed in 11% of patients. Cases of GBS were excluded. Other studies confirm that CMT-1 is much more common than CMT-2, especially in the pediatric population.[18-25]

Of a pooled European pediatric series of 287 inherited peripheral neuropathies, 51% had CMT-1.[23] CMT-2 was identified in 21% of children. CMT-3 (Dejerine-Sottas disease [DSD]), defined in this series as autosomal recessive congenital demyelinating neuropathy, was diagnosed in 12% of cases. Many DSD cases are now known to be due to de novo mutations in the same genes that cause CMT-1.[22,25,26] The X-linked form of CMT (CMT-X), now identified as the second most common form of CMT, was not recognized at the time of this series. Hereditary sensory neuropathies were diagnosed in only 3% of cases.

Clinical History

The clinical history is a most important guide for the child electrodiagnostician. The age of onset and temporal evolution of the polyneuropathy provide important clues that must influence the design of the electrodiagnostic study. Although inherited polyneuropathies are more common than acquired etiologies at all ages of the pediatric population, inherited polyneuropathies are increasingly likely the earlier the onset of polyneuropathy. Age of onset is also helpful because individual inherited polyneuropathies tend to present at ages typical for those disorders. For example, CMT is not usually clinically apparent until the 2nd decade, although if an EMG is performed early in the 1st decade it is usually abnormal[27] but not invariably so.[28] Age of onset may be difficult to determine in younger children. This is especially true of the inherited polyneuropathies in which clinical deficits manifest insidiously. In fact, patient or parent uncertainty about the time of onset suggests that the polyneuropathy has a genetic basis. Physicians should ask specific questions about the child's present and past activities, milestones, and motor skills. A temporal profile characterized by an unequivocal loss of skills or milestones points away from a CMT diagnosis and is in keeping with an acquired etiology such as GBS or, in the chronic setting, CIDP. However, a loss of motor milestones per se does not exclude certain other inherited neuropathies, particularly those caused by inborn errors of metabolism. The loss of skills in GBS or CIDP is limited to motor functions, whereas inborn neurometabolic errors impact the child's development globally (i.e., also includes cognition, personality, and so forth).

Given the likelihood that a child presenting with polyneuropathy has a hereditary disorder, the family history should receive special attention. Parents should be questioned carefully about the family history. This may, by itself, reveal the diagnosis. In addition, parents and siblings should be examined. Any living family member with suspicious symptoms should be interviewed and examined, if at all possible. In many instances, focused electrodiagnostic testing on family members should be considered.

Neurologic Examination

Clues to etiology are often present in the general examination. Pes cavus and hammertoe deformities are complications of longstanding neuropathies such as CMT. Pes planus and valgus angulation of the forefoot are less common.[19-21,29,30] Pes cavus is not, however, a sine qua non of a hereditary polyneuropathy. At the Children's Hospital, Boston (CHB), only 50% of children seen in the electrodiagnostic laboratory for evaluation of such orthopedic abnormalities have had nerve conduction studies (NCSs) compatible with a hereditary polyneuropathy.[31] Enlarged peripheral nerves may be present in longstanding hereditary or acquired demyelinating and remyelinating (hypertrophic) polyneuropathies, including CMT-1 and CIDP. The general physical examination may offer further diagnostic clues, particularly in the form of dermatologic and ophthalmologic abnormalities associated with specific childhood polyneuropathies.

The examiner should assess whether the motor findings have a predominantly distal, generalized, or proximal distribution. Most polyneuropathies have a distal predominance. Predominantly proximal weakness is occasionally seen, usually in the lower extremities, and suggests an acquired inflammatory demyelinating polyradiculoneuropathy. Almost all childhood peripheral neuropathies are bilaterally symmetric. Rarely, asymmetric findings compatible with the diagnosis of mononeuritis multiplex are seen in adolescents with acquired neuropathies.[32] When asymmetry or multifocality is suspected, bilateral electrodiagnostic testing should be performed. In general, a 50% or greater reduction in motor or sensory nerve action potential amplitude or area relative to the contralateral response is considered significant.

ELECTROMYOGRAPHY

The role of electromyographic (EMG) testing is to confirm the presence of a polyneuropathy and to elucidate the underlying pathophysiology. NCSs provide the best noninvasive means of differentiating a demyelinating process from that with predominantly axonal pathology. Information on the distribution, severity, and temporal course of neuropathy can also be obtained from the electrodiagnostic assessment.

Parents accompanying their child to the electrodiagnostic laboratory are often uninformed or misinformed about the purpose and clinical value of electrodiagnosis. It is helpful for the electromyographer to speak with parents at the time the appointment is scheduled, if possible. If not, there should be a detailed discussion of the purpose and nature of the procedure when the child and parents arrive in the EMG laboratory. An understanding of the test alleviates any anxiety and guilt the parent may feel about putting their child through a painful procedure. Parents are more willing to assist in comforting the child during the study if they understand its aims and potential benefits.

Various technical approaches are used by skillful pediatric electromyographers to obtain both competent and empathetically successful studies. Techniques of pediatric EMG are discussed in detail in dedicated texts.[33,34] Dr. Kuntz's approach at the Mayo Clinic is detailed in Chapter 6. All colleagues attempt to put the child and their parents at ease by finding a means to involve the patient in the procedure. At CHB the child is encouraged to watch the recording screen "building mountains" as the motor or sensory action potentials appear or by identifying the sound of the motor unit potentials as "rain" or a "motorcycle."[33] When the youngster does have difficulty tolerating the EMG, it is preferable to reschedule this procedure at a later date under sedation, with nitrous oxide or propofol anesthesia. The major disadvantage of this approach is the diminished opportunity to carefully examine motor unit potentials under voluntary control, but one can usually gain a reasonable sense of motor unit potential characteristics under light anesthesia by reflex stimulation of the extremity, such as by tickling the sole of the foot to observe activation of the tibialis anterior or iliopsoas.

The appropriate interpretation of pediatric electrodiagnostic studies depends on appreciation of the normal neurophysiologic maturational changes of infancy and early childhood. Nerve conduction parameters and motor unit potentials evolve from less than 50% of adult values in neonates to reach adult values between ages 3 and 5 years in parallel with the maturation of peripheral nerve myelin.[35-44] The normal range of nerve conduction parameters for infants and children is annotated in Chapter 7, Tables 7:1-16.

Characterizing a polyneuropathy as demyelinating or axonal is helpful to the diagnostic process. With this in mind, this chapter categorizes the various polyneuropathies as either predominantly demyelinating or predominantly axonal. This dichotomous characterization is useful for polyneuropathies that clearly fit in one category, for example, the demyelinating CMT polyneuropathies. In many cases, however, there are electrodiagnostic featuresof a mixed demyelinating and axonal polyneuropathy. In fact, most polyneuropathies have neurophysiologic and histopathologic evidence of both myelin and axon pathology, although either myelin or axon pathology may predominate. This often means, however, that the polyneuropathies encountered in clinical practice do not conform perfectly to one category or the other. Nonetheless, because of the

significant diagnostic value obtained by making the distinction when possible, this chapter considers predominantly demyelinating and predominantly axonal polyneuropathies separately. However, the reader should keep in mind the limitations of this paradigm.

PRIMARILY DEMYELINATING POLYNEUROPATHIES: ELECTRODIAGNOSTIC FEATURES

Whenever possible, an EMG performed to evaluate polyneuropathies should characterize the polyneuropathy as either demyelinating or axonal. The identification of a primarily demyelinating polyneuropathy is critically important because the differential diagnosis for demyelinating polyneuropathies is much more limited than that of axonal polyneuropathies. The demyelinating polyneuropathies include CMT, GBS, CIDP, and, much less commonly, an inborn error of metabolism such as a leukodystrophy (e.g., globoid cell leukodystrophy, metachromatic leukodystrophy).

An important physiologic consequence of demyelination is conduction slowing, whereby motor and sensory conduction velocities (CVs) are reduced and distal motor and F-wave minimal latencies are prolonged. It is important that a polyneuropathy be considered primarily demyelinating only when the conduction is sufficiently slow. It is generally accepted that to be deemed primarily demyelinating, CV of motor nerves must be less than 80% of the lower limit of normal (LLN) if the amplitude is greater than 80% LLN, or less than 70% LLN if amplitude is less than 80% LLN. Distal latencies must be greater than 125% of upper limit of normal (ULN) if amplitude is greater than 80% of LLN, or greater than 150% of ULN if amplitude is less than 80% of LLN. F-wave latencies must be greater than 120% of ULN if amplitude is greater than 80% of LLN, or greater than 150% of ULN if amplitude is less than 80% of LLN.[45] These indices of demyelination are particularly useful for most forms of inherited demyelinating polyneuropathies where severe conduction slowing should be evident in all motor nerves and all nerve segments studied (see later). In contrast, acquired demyelinating polyneuropathies demonstrate multifocal, nonuniform slowing such that conduction slowing is not anticipated in every nerve but should be present in more than one nerve. Various research criteria for the diagnosis of CIDP reflect this fact.[46-48] Criteria adapted from the recent European Neuromuscular Center consortium on CIDP International Workshop entitled "Childhood Chronic Inflammatory Demyelinating Polyneuropathy" are listed in Box 33-1.[48]

Electromyography can help distinguish between hereditary and acquired demyelinating polyneuropathies. Most hereditary demyelinating neuropathies demonstrate uniform

BOX 33-1
CLINICAL AND ELECTROPHYSIOLOGIC CRITERIA FOR CHILDHOOD CHRONIC INFLAMMATORY DEMYELINATING POLYRADICULONEUROPATHY (CIDP)

Mandatory Clinical Criteria
Progression of muscle weakness in proximal and distal muscles of upper and lower extremities over at least 4 wk *or*

Rapid progression (Guillain-Barré-like presentation) followed by relapsing or protracted course (>1 yr)

Areflexia or hyporeflexia

Major Laboratory Features
Electrophysiologic Criteria
Must demonstrate at least three of the following four major abnormalities in motor nerves (or two of the major plus two of the supportive criteria)

A. Major
  1. Conduction block or abnormal temporal dispersion* in one or more motor nerves at sites not prone to compression
     a. Conduction block: at least 50% drop in negative peak area or peak-to-peak amplitude of proximal compound muscle action potential (CMAP) if duration of negative peak of proximal CMAP is < 130% of distal CMAP duration
     b. Temporal dispersion: abnormal if duration of negative peak of proximal CMAP is > 130% of distal CMAP duration°
  2. Reduction in conduction velocity (CV) in two or more nerves: < 75% of mean CV value for age minus 2 SD
  3. Prolonged distal latency (DL) in two or more nerves: >130% of mean DL value for age plus 2 SD
  4. Absent F waves or prolonged F-wave minimal latency (ML) in two or more nerves: > 130% of mean F-wave ML for age plus 2 SD
B. Supportive
When conduction block is absent, the following abnormal electrophysiologic parameters are indicative of nonuniform slowing and thus of an acquired neuropathy:
  1. Abnormal median sensory nerve action potential (SNAP) while the sural nerve SNAP is normal
  2. Abnormally low terminal latency index[94,97,99]: distal conduction distance (mm)/(conduction velocity [m/sec] ÷ distal motor latency [msec])

  3. Side-to-side comparison of motor CVs showing a difference of > 10 m/sec between nerves

Cerebrospinal Fluid (CSF) Criteria
Protein > 45 mg/dL
Cell count < 10 cells/mm³

Nerve Biopsy Features
Predominant features of demyelination

Exclusion Criteria
A. Clinical features or history of a hereditary neuropathy, other disease, or exposure to drugs or toxins known to cause peripheral neuropathy
B. Laboratory findings (including nerve biopsy or genetic testing) that show evidence of a cause other than CIDP
C. Electrodiagnostic features of abnormal neuromuscular transmission, myopathy, or anterior horn cell disease

Diagnostic Criteria (must meet all exclusion criteria)
A. Confirmed CIDP
  1. Mandatory clinical features
  2. Electrodiagnostic and CSF features
B. Possible CIDP
  1. Mandatory clinical features
  2. One of the three laboratory findings

---

*Conduction block and temporal dispersion can be assessed only in nerves where the amplitude of the distal CMAP is > 1 mV.
From Nevo Y, Topaloglu H: 88th ENMC International Workshop: Childhood chronic inflammatory demyelinating polyneuropathy (including revised diagnostic criteria), Naarden, The Netherlands, December 8-10, 2002. Neuromuscul Disord 12:195-200, 2002.

---

slowing along all segments of individual nerves and affect all nerves to the same degree. In contrast, acquired demyelinating neuropathies affect nerves in a multifocal or nonuniform fashion. This difference is readily explained by the fact that hereditary neuropathies are genetically determined disorders of myelin formation and thus all myelin is incorrectly formed. Acquired demyelinating disorders such as GBS or CIDP demonstrate nonuniformity of slowing because of the patchy nature of immune attack. Wilbourn, and later Lewis and Sumner, pointed out these important differences between acquired and inherited demyelinating neuropathies.[49,50] Lewis and Sumner compared the electrophysiologic studies of nerves in the upper extremities of 40 patients with acquired demyelinating neuropathy to 18 patients with CMT-1. All but 4 of the 40 patients with acquired demyelinating neuropathy showed at least one feature of differential slowing. Significant differences in slowing were observed between the ulnar and median motor nerves and between proximal and distal segments of the median motor nerve in the acquired demyelinating form, whereas slowing was uniform in CMT-1. Nineteen of 35 in the acquired neuropathy group had CVs of median motor nerves that differed from ulnar motor CVs by at least 5 m/sec; 8 of 35 had differences greater than 10 m/sec. This was not observed in CMT-1. A study of 127 CMT-1 patients found that motor CVs were almost identical when comparing ulnar nerve to median nerve, or when comparing median, ulnar, or peroneal nerves side to side. The same uniformity applied to proximal versus distal segments of the same nerve, to median versus ulnar F-wave minimal latencies, and even to median motor nerve versus peroneal motor nerve.[51] However, some exceptions to this general rule of uniformity in genetically determined polyneuropathies are occasionally noted; such has been seen in both CMT-X[28] and metrachromatic leukodystrophy.[52]

To establish whether nerve conduction is slowed uniformly or differentially, a number of motor nerves must be studied. Side-to-side comparisons of the same nerve are particularly helpful. Comparing motor nerve CVs (NCVs) of different nerves in the same limb is also useful. In general, the difference in CV between nerves does not exceed 10 m/sec in the inherited demyelinating polyneuropathies. If comparing CVs of upper to lower motor nerves, a difference up to 15 m/sec is allowable for "uniform" slowing.

Analyzing the characteristics of conduction along a particular nerve also aids in the determination of uniformity or nonuniformity of conduction. For example, conduction slowing should be similar along the entire length of the nerve in an inherited demyelinating polyneuropathy, whereas in an acquired case differential slowing is common. Differential slowing may manifest as an unusually prolonged F wave or distal latency in the setting of a normal or near-normal forelimb CV.[49,50,53,54]

In acquired demyelinating polyneuropathies, demyelination may affect individual axons or groups of axons within a nerve to differing degrees, so that some fibers conduct much more slowly than others. This results in the electrophysiologic phenomenon of abnormal temporal dispersion (Fig. 33-1). Abnormal temporal dispersion at sites not prone to entrapment is a common feature of acquired demyelinating polyneuropathies and is not typically seen in inherited demyelinating polyneuropathies. Abnormal temporal dispersion can be defined as a prolongation of compound muscle action potential (CMAP) duration of greater than 20% for the peroneal, median, and ulnar motor nerves and a greater than 30% prolongation for the tibial nerve, when comparing distal stimulation to proximal stimulation of the nerve.[55] Lewis and Sumner found that in patients with CMT-1, no patient had an increased CMAP duration of greater than 25% with proximal versus wrist stimulation. In contrast, two thirds of patients with acquired demyelinating neuropathies had an increased duration of greater than 40%, frequently with temporal dispersion of 100% or more.[49]

Another physiologic consequence of segmental demyelination is conduction block, defined as the failure of nerve fibers to transmit electrical impulses across a demyelinated segment. Thus, stimulation distal to a demyelinated segment elicits a larger CMAP amplitude than stimulation proximal to the area of demyelination (Fig. 33-2). Conduction block may be complete, in which case the impulse fails to conduct across any myelinated nerve fibers and results in an unelicitable CMAP. More commonly, partial conduction block is observed, manifested as a significant reduction in motor nerve action potential (CMAP) amplitude and area with proximal versus distal stimulation. Criteria for the diagnosis of conduction block include proper technique and the absence of significant temporal dispersion.[56] To suggest an acquired demyelinating neuropathy, the conduction block must occur at anatomic sites not prone to entrapment. For example, the conduction block may be present in the peroneal nerve between the ankle and below the fibular head, median nerve between the wrist and elbow, and/or the ulnar nerve between the wrist and below the elbow.

Proposed criteria for definite, partial, and probable partial conduction block for different motor nerves with different degrees of temporal dispersion have been published.[57] In general, conduction block is defined as a reduction in CMAP amplitude or area of greater than 40% to 50% in the absence of significant temporal dispersion. Conduction block is less commonly observed in inherited demyelinating polyneuropathies.[53] A series of 127 CMT-1 patients found that only 19 (5.3%) of 360 nerve segments studied showed a reduction of greater than 50% amplitude on proximal versus distal stimulation.[51] It is noteworthy, however, that in 13 of these 19 cases, the distal CMAP amplitude was reduced (including 6 cases with CMAP amplitude less than 50% of LLN), suggesting that interphase cancellation may have contributed. This illustrates that caution must be used in interpreting conduction block when the distal CMAP is already low (Fig. 33-3). In the 6 cases in which the distal CMAP was not reduced, the apparent conduction block was observed at common sites of entrapment, such as the fibular head in 5 cases. However, other authors have reported the presence of conduction block on NCS of patients with CMT-1,[58,59] but in one such case series the authors questioned whether supramaximal stimulation was attained. These authors found that when 3 patients were re-examined with higher stimulation, only one of three clearly displayed conduction block. This case series illustrates the importance of delivering supramaximal stimulation, especially since stronger stimuli are often required to obtain a response for some inherited demyelinating polyneuropathies.

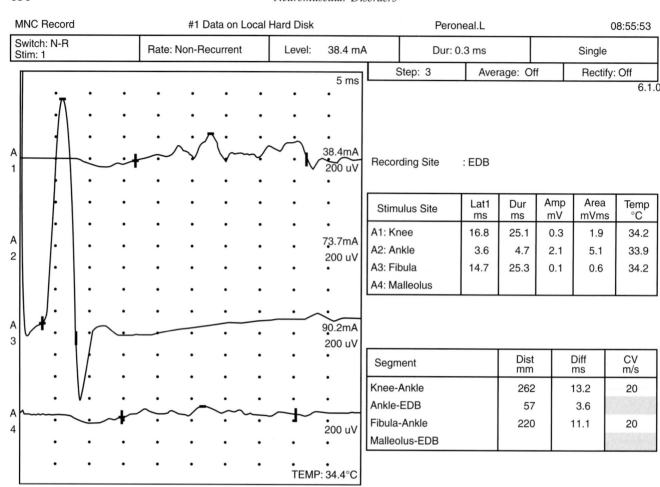

MNC Record		#1 Data on Local Hard Disk		Peroneal.L		08:55:53

Switch: N-R Stim: 1	Rate: Non-Recurrent	Level: 38.4 mA	Dur: 0.3 ms	Single

Step: 3	Average: Off	Rectify: Off

6.1.0

Recording Site : EDB

Stimulus Site	Lat1 ms	Dur ms	Amp mV	Area mVms	Temp °C
A1: Knee	16.8	25.1	0.3	1.9	34.2
A2: Ankle	3.6	4.7	2.1	5.1	33.9
A3: Fibula	14.7	25.3	0.1	0.6	34.2
A4: Malleolus					

Segment	Dist mm	Diff ms	CV m/s
Knee-Ankle	262	13.2	20
Ankle-EDB	57	3.6	
Fibula-Ankle	220	11.1	20
Malleolus-EDB			

FIGURE 33–1

Temporal dispersion of the peroneal motor nerve on nerve conduction study in a 3(1/2)-year-old girl with chronic inflammatory demyelinating polyradiculoneuropathy for 18 months. EDB, extensor digitorum brevis; CV, conduction velocity. (From Burns TM, Dyck PJ, Darras BT, Jones HR Jr: Chronic inflammatory demyelinating polyradiculoneuropathy. In Jones HR, De Vivo DC, Darras BT [eds]: Neuromuscular Disorders of Infancy, Childhood, and Adolescence: A Clinician's Approach. Philadelphia, Butterworth Heinemann Health, 2003, pp 445-468.)

Bolton characterized an unusual group of five children seen during a 15-year period with congenital or inherited polyneuropathies as having the *high-low syndrome*.[60] Typically when performing NCSs on infants, one only needs an electrical stimulus of 0.05 or 0.1 millisecond duration to easily evoke a motor or sensory response. In contrast, rarely one finds a child requiring maximal voltage and a stimulus duration of 0.5 milliseconds (Fig. 33-4). Because such stimuli are inherently uncomfortable, one needs to perform this type of study under analgesic medication. Once a CMAP was obtained, each child had remarkably low CVs; thus *high* stimulus, *low* CV syndrome. Four of these children required stimuli of 0.2 millisecond and the last a 0.5 millisecond stimulus to obtain a motor CMAP; each was of very low amplitude 0.2 mV for the three

infants, and the other two ranged from 0.5 to 1.5 mV. The one floppy infant requiring 0.5 millisecond stimulus only demonstrated a CMAP on one of three motor nerves tested. CVs in all instances were 3 to 8 m/sec with the exception of 10 to 13 m/sec for metachromatic leukodystrophy. Distal latencies were similarly very prolonged, generally ranging from 10 to 33 milliseconds.

These children had varied clinical presentations primarily as a floppy infant, or a persistent hypotonia in three, who later on evidenced developmental motor delay, gait ataxia, and clumsy limbs with relatively preserved muscle bulk. The peripheral nerves were normal to palpation in each child; none had palpably enlarged nerves. Each of these babies eventually were proved to have a variety of CMT, such as DSD (CMT-3). One of the other two chil-

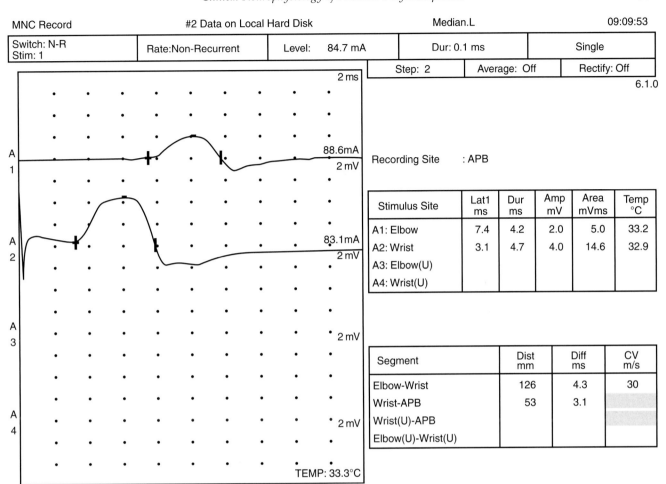

MNC Record	#2 Data on Local Hard Disk	Median.L	09:09:53

Switch: N-R Stim: 1	Rate:Non-Recurrent	Level: 84.7 mA	Dur: 0.1 ms	Single

		Step: 2	Average: Off	Rectify: Off

6.1.0

Recording Site   : APB

Stimulus Site	Lat1 ms	Dur ms	Amp mV	Area mVms	Temp °C
A1: Elbow	7.4	4.2	2.0	5.0	33.2
A2: Wrist	3.1	4.7	4.0	14.6	32.9
A3: Elbow(U)					
A4: Wrist(U)					

Segment	Dist mm	Diff ms	CV m/s
Elbow-Wrist	126	4.3	30
Wrist-APB	53	3.1	
Wrist(U)-APB			
Elbow(U)-Wrist(U)			

FIGURE 33–2

Partial conduction block of the median motor nerve in a 3{1/2}-year-old girl with chronic inflammatory demyelinating polyradiculoneuropathy. APB, abductor pollicis brevis; CV, conduction velocity. (From Burns TM, Dyck PJ, Darras BT, Jones HR Jr: Chronic inflammatory demyelinating polyradiculoneuropathy. In Jones HR, De Vivo DC, Darras BT [eds]: Neuromuscular Disorders of Infancy, Childhood, and Adolescence: A Clinician's Approach. Philadelphia, Butterworth Heinemann Health, 2003, pp 445-468.)

dren had a progressive polyneuropathy later defined as a component of metachromatic leukodystrophy, whereas the other proved to have a remitting relapsing polyneuropathy of the CIDP type.[60]

There are exceptions to the general rule that inherited demyelinating polyneuropathies display uniform conduction slowing. CMT-X[61] and hereditary neuropathy with liability to pressure palsies (HNPP) are two inherited polyneuropathies that often exhibit multifocality or nonuniformity of slowing on electrodiagnostic testing, and this may occasionally make it difficult to distinguish CIDP from these inherited disorders. HNPP and CMT-X, discussed in more detail later, more typically present in adults and less commonly in adolescents. Refsum's disease and adrenomyeloneuropathy (AMN) are rare inherited disorders in which NCS may reveal multifocal demyelination. In Refsum's disease, motor CVs usually are

markedly slow in the primarily demyelinating range and may show multifocal slowing. NCS in AMN are less abnormal and suggest a mixed neuropathic pattern of multifocal demyelination and axonal loss.[62,63] We have also observed that CMAP dispersion is a common finding on electrodiagnostic testing of children with metachromatic leukodystrophy.[52]

The CVs of normal children increase during the first 3 to 5 years from values in the 20 to 30 m/sec range to normal adult values in the 40 to 50 m/sec range. In contrast, in children with CMT-1, CVs may begin in either a similar range but often decrease slightly during this period before leveling off.[64,65] Thus, it may be difficult to conclusively determine slowing of CV during the first 2 or 3 years of life, and abnormal slowing may become much more evident in both inherited and acquired demyelinating neuropathy after the first few years. For example, in a child with

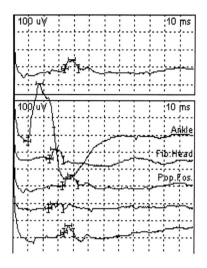

Peroneal Nerve

Rec Site: EDB	Lat (ms)	Amp (mV)	Dist (mm)	C.V. (m/s)
Stim Site:				
Ankle	10.0	0.333	75	
Fib.Head	24.7	0.053	230	15.7
Pop.Fos.	33.0	0.063	110	13.2

FIGURE 33–3

Peroneal motor nerve conduction studies in a 12-year-old boy with a 1-year history of relapsing-remitting chronic inflammatory demyelinating polyradiculoneuropathy partially responsive to intravenous immunoglobulin, plasmapheresis, or prednisone. Distal latencies are prolonged, and conduction velocities (CVs) are low. The peroneal distal compound muscle action potential (CMAP) is less than 50% of the lower limit of normal for age. Clinicians must be cautious when interpreting conduction block if the distal CMAP is already low. The clinical history and response to immunotherapy were critical in making the diagnosis. (From Burns TM, Dyck PJ, Darras BT, Jones HR Jr: Chronic inflammatory demyelinating polyradiculoneuropathy. In Jones HR, De Vivo DC, Darras BT [eds]: Neuromuscular Disorders of Infancy, Childhood, and Adolescence: A Clinician's Approach. Philadelphia, Butterworth Heinemann Health, 2003, pp 445-468.)

CMT-1, motor NCVs may be in the mid-20s (m/sec) during the first year of life—therefore in the normal range for age—then remain in the mid-20s throughout childhood and adulthood—thereby falling below the age-adjusted normal range.

ACUTE DEMYELINATING POLYNEUROPATHIES

The demyelinating form of GBS is the only acute demyelinating neuropathy seen with significant frequency. GBS is a clinical syndrome characterized by generalized weakness

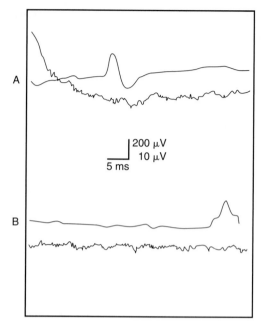

FIGURE 33–4

Median nerve conduction study. Strong stimuli (maximum voltage, 0.2-millisecond duration) at the wrist (A) and elbow (B) evoked no sensory responses from the digital nerves (lower traces in A and B) and low-amplitude compound thenar muscle action potentials of greatly prolonged latencies (upper traces in A and B). Conduction velocity was 6 m/sec between elbow and wrist, and the distal latency was 15 milliseconds. Note the prominent shock artifact on wrist stimulation. (A and B, From Bolton CF: Polyneuropathies. In Jones HR Jr, Bolton CF, Harper CM Jr: Pediatric Clinical Electromyography. Philadelphia, Lippincott-Raven, 1996, pp 251-352.)

evolving over days to a maximum of 4 weeks. Weakness and depressed or absent muscle stretch reflexes are the two features required for diagnosis.[66] Cytoalbuminologic dissociation in the cerebrospinal fluid (CSF) (elevated protein with normal cell count) also occurs in most patients.

GBS has several pathophysiologic subtypes: acute inflammatory demyelinating polyradiculoneuropathy (AIDP), acute motor axonal neuropathy (AMAN), acute motor sensory axonal neuropathy (AMSAN) and Miller-Fisher syndrome (MFS). AIDP, the demyelinating form of GBS, predominates in Western Europe, the United States, and Australia. All forms but MFS have a similar presentation. They can be readily differentiated only by electrodiagnosis, the axonal forms having a poorer prognosis than the demyelinating form. For a discussion of AMAN and AMSAN, see the section on acute axonal neuropathies.

GBS (all types) affects patients of all ages, but incidence increases throughout life, so that children are affected much less frequently than adults. Incidence in patients younger than 15 years of age is approximately 0.8 to 1.5 per 100,000.[16,67-69] Detailed data on frequency at different ages during childhood are scarce. However, a study of more than 10,000 GBS-related hospital discharges in the United States conducted by the Centers for Disease Control and Prevention found similar incidences of GBS in children of all ages, except for a particularly low incidence during infancy (0.38 per 100,000).[69] In Paraguay, GBS was more common in children aged 4 years or younger than in older children[16] and Delanoe and associates found a predominance of cases younger than 3 years of age.[70] A German study of 175 children found a bimodal age distribution with peaks at 4 and 12 years.[71]

Infantile Guillain-Barré Syndrome

Although rare, GBS does occur in infancy. It presents with acute hypotonia and weakness, which may be associated with respiratory distress and feeding difficulties. Even less commonly, GBS develops in utero or in the neonatal period.[72-75] Diagnosis is apparent when a diagnosis of acute inflammatory demyelinating polyneuropathy has already been made in the affected mother[72,74] but is more difficult where there is no maternal history of weakness or sensory loss.[73,75] Electrodiagnosis in such cases is suggestive of acquired demyelinating polyneuropathy. Findings include slowed nerve conduction, temporal dispersion, conduction block, and evidence on the needle examination of acute denervation.[73,75] The electrodiagnostic examination is useful for differentiation of infantile GBS from other causes of acquired infantile hypotonia, such as poliomyelitis, infantile botulism, and myasthenia gravis.[76] CSF protein is usually elevated; CSF cell count should be normal. In most cases recovery has been spontaneous and complete, although occasional infants subsequently developed CIDP.[77,78] There is a single report of a rapid recovery after intravenous immunoglobulin therapy in a 2-week-old infant with GBS.[72]

Childhood Guillain-Barré Syndrome

Clinical Features

GBS is the most common cause of acute flaccid paralysis in childhood.[2,79] A gastroenteritis or respiratory infection is often seen 2 to 4 weeks before the development of GBS.[71,79-81] The primary features of GBS are rapidly progressive limb weakness with lost or diminished muscle stretch reflexes. Other findings such as distal paresthesia, facial weakness, and dysautonomia often prove helpful in the early diagnosis of individual cases.[79-81] Weakness is usually symmetric in pediatric GBS and more marked in the lower extremities. Affected children have difficulty

climbing stairs, squatting, and rising. Proximal weakness is not uncommon. By definition, GBS has a rapid course, reaching a maximal deficit usually within 10 to 14 days in 80% of children but occasionally not for 4 weeks.[79]

Pain is often prominent in childhood GBS[70,82,83] and may confound the initial diagnosis, particularly in younger children. Pain was the presenting symptom in 47% of children with GBS in one large clinical series.[70] The pain typically involves the back, neck, and legs. Children may refuse to bear weight and resist passive limb movement. It is commonly associated with marked irritability and may be accompanied by vomiting and headache.[82] This "pseudomeningoencephalopathic" presentation may be associated with other signs of meningeal irritation including stiff neck and Kernig's and Brudzinski's signs. Creatine kinase may occasionally be elevated, causing confusion with an acute myopathy.

Childhood GBS may also present with an acute sensory ataxia, especially in toddlers.[84,85] The differential diagnosis of such cases also includes the Fisher variant of GBS (ophthalmoplegia, ataxia, and areflexia).[85] Cranial nerve palsies, usually of the facial or oculomotor nerves, are an uncommon presenting sign of pediatric GBS.[79,86] Respiratory insufficiency is a rare but important initial presentation of pediatric GBS.[87] In one report the development of respiratory failure was associated with rapid evolution of complete flaccid paralysis and loss of all brainstem reflexes, including pupillary responses mimicking brain death.[88] Internal ophthalmoplegia is rare in AIDP and should prompt consideration of diphtheria, tick paralysis, and botulism.[88] Transient dysautonomia sometimes occurs and may be the major risk factor for the rare occurrence of a pediatric fatal outcome. Urinary sphincter dysfunction occurs concomitantly but almost always recedes within 24 hours. When it does not, a spinal cord lesion requires immediate consideration. Occasionally, GBS is accompanied by symptomatic central nervous system (CNS) demyelination.[89-91]

Children with GBS should be admitted to hospital for monitoring. Although weakness and hypotonia may be relatively mild at onset, the potential for sudden, sometimes fatal, respiratory or autonomic compromise should always be anticipated.[79] The importance of zealous cardiovascular and autonomic monitoring in all cases of GBS must be emphasized.[92] Mortality in children with GBS is fortunately a rare occurrence (< 1% in the United States[69] and probably < 5% worldwide).[16,93] Deaths are due to potentially preventable respiratory complications. Autonomic instability is a predictor of fatal cardiac arrhythmias in GBS.[92]

Children with mild GBS who are able to ambulate unassisted are usually monitored and given supportive care, such as physical therapy and analgesics. Those unable to walk unassisted or with respiratory compromise should be treated with either intravenous immunoglobulin, a more practical therapy for childhood GBS because of its ease of administration, or plasma exchange. Retrospective studies suggest that either treatment hastens recovery of independent ambulation in GBS.[71,80,94-100] Clinical responses to intravenous immunoglobulin may be dramatic.[101,102] A total dose of 2 gm/kg of intravenous immunoglobulin is given over 2 to 5 days and is generally well tolerated at all ages.[84]

Cerebrospinal Fluid Analysis

CSF analysis usually demonstrates the classic albuminocytologic dissociation with protein values between 80 and 200 mg/dL. The presence of more than 50 leukocytes per milliliter is atypical of pediatric GBS and should prompt consideration of poliomyelitis,[103,104] West Nile virus,[105] CNS lymphoma,[106] and Lyme infection. In contrast with adults, we are unaware of any cases of children developing GBS as the presenting sign of human immunodeficiency virus (HIV).[107]

Magnetic Resonance Imaging

Magnetic resonance imaging (MRI) demonstrates hypertrophic and gadolinium-enhancing cauda equina, and lumbar roots have been demonstrated in children with GBS[83,108] and the distribution of nerve root enhancement appears to correlate with the distribution of pain.[83] Nerve root enhancement is nonspecific, however, and may also be seen in CIDP, sarcoidosis, lymphoma, and leptomeningeal carcinoma.

Subtle nerve root enhancement has been reported in severe CMT-1; thus, enhancement per se cannot rule out inherited demyelinating radiculoneuropathies.[109] MRI is an important testing modality to exclude cord lesions, including both mass lesions and transverse myelitis in those children in whom GBS is associated with sphincter dysfunction.

Electrodiagnosis in Demyelinating GBS

The typical EMG findings of childhood GBS include slowing of CVs to less than two thirds normal, prolongation of distal latencies, and loss or prolongation of F waves and H reflexes.[79] Slowing of motor nerve conduction is more profound in younger children.[79,86] However, this result does not correlate with the child's clinical features or prognosis. In those rare instances where the only neurophysiologic abnormality is the loss of F waves from affected extremities, the alternative diagnosis of transverse myelitis also requires consideration (Fig. 33-5).

Delanoe and associates, using established criteria for demyelination, examined the temporal evolution of nerve conduction abnormalities in 43 children with demyelinating GBS.[70] During week 1 of illness, the most common abnormalities in descending order of frequency were a prolonged or absent F wave (88%), prolonged distal latency (75%), and conduction block (58%). Slowing of motor CV was noted in 50% of children during the first week. Sensory conduction abnormalities were infrequent.

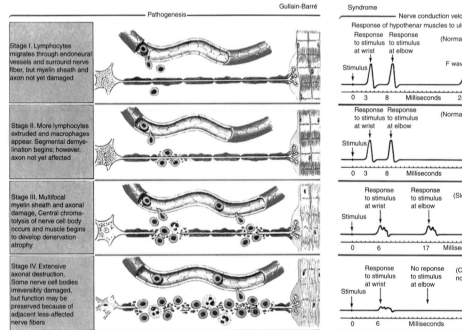
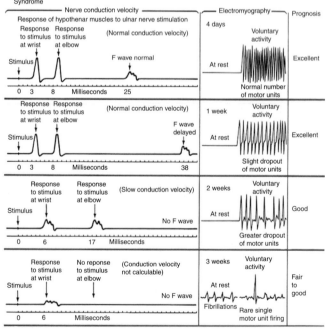

FIGURE 33–5

Pathogenesis and progression of Guillain-Barré syndrome. (Modified from Jones HR Jr: Collection of Medical Illustrations, Vol. I, part II. West Caldwell, NJ, Ciba, 1986, pp 218-219. Copyright©Ciba.)

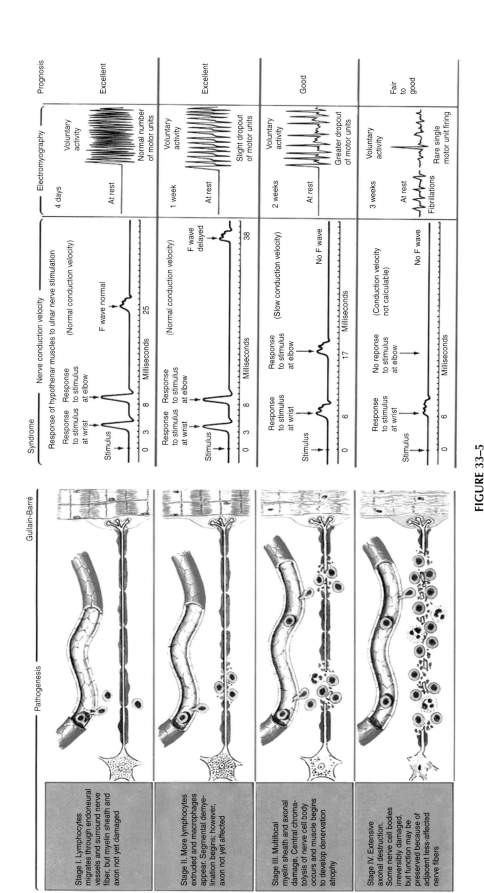

FIGURE 33–5

Pathogenesis and progression of Guillain-Barré syndrome. (Modified from Jones HR Jr: Collection of Medical Illustrations, Vol. I, part II. West Caldwell, NJ, Ciba, 1986, pp 218-219. Copyright©Ciba.)

During week 2, reduced CMAP amplitude was universal. Prolonged distal latency was present in 92% and slowed motor CV in 84%. Conduction block and/or temporal dispersion were observed in 61%. The frequency of conduction block and/or temporal dispersion declined thereafter. CMAP amplitude reduction was maximal during week 3, whereas abnormalities of CV (distal latencies, F waves) were maximally abnormal during week 5. Compared with similar data in adults,[110] children showed slower evolution of conduction slowing and much more rapid recovery of CMAP amplitudes. This group proposed diagnostic criteria for demyelinating GBS in children, which they assert would permit a tentative diagnosis in 90% of children in the first week and a definite diagnosis during week 2. Sensory conduction abnormalities were less frequent than motor and the most common abnormality was the now classic feature of GBS, abnormal median sensory with sparing of the sural response.

In adults with GBS, a mean CMAP amplitude of less than 20% of the LLN is predictive of slow and incomplete recovery.[111] Pediatric GBS series comprising patients with the AIDP form have shown good recovery despite low mean CMAP amplitudes.[79,112,113] Ammache and colleagues[113] found that the only electrophysiologic predictor of outcome in a small group of children with GBS was the presence of conduction block. This correlated with a good outcome. Some children do have slow and incomplete recovery, however.[114,115] These children probably have an axonal form of GBS, either AMAN or AMSAN (see section on acute axonal neuropathies for a full discussion).

Differential Diagnosis of Childhood Gullain-Barré Syndrome. (Box 33-2)

Both spinal cord tumors and transverse myelitis may produce a rapidly progressive paralysis, *hyporeflexia* or *areflexia*, back pain, and sphincter dysfunction.[116] Sphincter dysfunction is common with spinal cord lesions but rare and usually quite transient in GBS.[117] Transverse myelitis may be associated with marked elevation of the CSF protein and with significant CSF pleocytosis.[116] Poliomyelitis and disorders of neuromuscular transmission such as infantile botulism also require careful consideration.

West Nile virus infection occurs in the Western hemisphere. Neurologic complications are much more common in the elderly, but several cases of meningoencephalitis have been reported in children.[105,118] Adults may manifest a poliomyelitis-like syndrome of limb pain, multifocal weakness, preserved sensation, and a CSF pleocytosis. Electrophysiology shows reduced CMAP amplitudes and fibrillations with normal sensory responses. Similar cases can be anticipated in children in the future, and this diagnosis should be considered in the febrile child with limb weakness. Asymmetry, absence of sensory involve-

---

BOX 33-2
DIFFERENTIAL DIAGNOSIS IN GUILLAIN-BARRÉ SYNDROME

Pseudoencephalopathy
  Meningitis
  Meningoencephalitis
Cerebellar syndrome
  Postinfectious cerebellar ataxia
  Structural lesion
Myelopathy
  Spinal cord compression
  Transverse myelitis
  Acute disseminated encephalomyelitis
  Anterior spinal artery distribution infarction
Anterior horn cells
  Enteroviral infection
  Poliomyelitis
Peripheral nerve
  Tick paralysis
  Diphtheria
  Lyme disease
  Toxins and drugs
  Porphyria
  Critical illness polyneuropathy
  Mitochondrial disease
Neuromuscular junction
  Botulism
  Myasthenia gravis
  Neuromuscular blockade
  Pseudocholinesterase deficiency
Muscle disorders
  Acute myositis
    Infectious
    Autoimmune
  Metabolic myopathy
    Glycogen metabolism disorders and others
  Periodic paralysis
  Critical care myopathy

From Sladky JT: Guillain-Barré syndrome. *In* Jones HR, De Vivo DC, Darras BT (eds): Neuromuscular Disorders of Infancy, Childhood, and Adolescence: A Clinician's Approach. Philadelphia, Butterworth Heinemann Health, 2003, pp 407-424.

---

ment, CSF pleocytosis, and a motor axonal pattern distinguish it from demyelinating GBS. Moreover, weakness appears concurrent with fever in West Nile virus but occurs in the postinfectious period in GBS.

HIV has occasionally been associated with GBS,[107] although to our knowledge GBS has not been the presenting illness of pediatric HIV infection. Toxins, including heavy metals, glue sniffing, buckthorn wild cherry, and fish toxins may also warrant consideration in the diagnosis of GBS.[117] Although uncommon, tick paralysis is potentially fatal without specific treatment and should be considered in all children with acute flaccid paralysis. Early pupillary involvement is common in tick paralysis but only rarely observed in GBS.[119] Typical EMG findings in tick paralysis include markedly diminished CMAP amplitudes, with preserved motor CVs, motor distal latencies, and SNAPs.[119-121]

Tick paralysis can be difficult to distinguish from the axonal forms of GBS, but it does not demonstrate the multifocal demyelination characteristic of classic GBS. All children with acute generalized weakness should be examined carefully for ticks, with special attention to the scalp. Removal of ticks results in dramatic improvement.[119,120]

Diphtheria still needs consideration in children with recent pharyngitis, fever, and acute peripheral neuropathy with associated bulbar palsy. The immunization history is of importance in this clinical setting.[122] One of the authors has seen seven instances of diphtheria during his career, all of whom had incomplete immunization, and two developed neurologic problems; one a generalized polyneuropathy and the other a severe bulbar palsy (Jones HR, personal communication, 2005.) Hepatic porphyria and hereditary tyrosinemia are discussed later and should be considered in the appropriate setting. Vincristine toxicity may present as an acute polyneuropathy in children with underlying CMT disease.[123] Critical illness polyneuropathy should also be considered in the appropriate setting (Box 33-3).[124] However, in our experience a critical illness myopathy is more common in children.[125]

A few rare inborn metabolic errors, including tyrosinemia, porphyria, or Leigh's disease,[126] may also have a precipitous onset of symptoms resembling childhood GBS. Hypokalemic paralysis, presenting as a manifestation of proximal renal tubular acidosis, has mimicked GBS in a 14-year-old girl with paraplegia and areflexia.[127] Barium carbonate poisoning, severe vomiting and diarrhea, and clay ingestions have also presented with a similar clinical picture. One 18-year-old boy presented with 5 hours of numbness and quadriplegia, with hypokalemia (K$^+$ of 2.11 mEq/mL). In retrospect, he had consumed barium containing rat poison on a suicide attempt just an hour before the onset of his muscle weakness.[128] Children with overwhelming sepsis or status asthmaticus may develop a critical illness neuromuscular syndrome, either a myopathy or a polyneuropathy, mimicking GBS.[129] In the rare instance of a recurrence of GBS, before one assumes that an immunologically mediated CIDP is present,[130] some of these metabolic, toxic, and possibly hereditary neuropathies also need consideration.[131-133]

With the frequency of severe pain in childhood GBS,[134] the possible diagnosis of an inflammatory myopathy is sometimes the initial diagnostic consideration. Acute childhood myositis, in contrast with dermatomyositis, is the most likely diagnosis in this scenario. Most often these children have severe pain localized to the calves, preventing them from walking. Additionally, there is not a significant weakness. Dermatomyositis and periodic paralysis may also sometimes have subacute or acute onsets of paralysis mimicking GBS. The sometimes subtle rash distinguishes the former, whereas a careful family history may help differentiate the latter.

Prognosis of Guillain-Barré Syndrome in Children

Generally, the prognosis of GBS in childhood is good.[70,79,80] Most children have minimal residual impairment by 1 to 4 months from onset.[70,79,80,86,96,97,101,102] Children have a shorter clinical course and more complete recovery than is typical of adult GBS.[71,79,80] Clinical predictors of slower recovery include severe weakness, rapid progression of weakness, cranial nerve deficits, and the need for assisted ventilation.[71,113] Children with the axonal forms of GBS, AMAN, and AMSAN have slower and less complete recovery than children with AIDP.

A small percentage of infants and children presenting with acute GBS later develop chronic inflammatory polyneuropathy.[77,135,136]

Guillain-Barré Variants

AMAN, a variant of GBS, is predominantly seen in children and young adults in northern China but has also been noted in children in many other parts of the world (e.g.,

---

BOX 33-3
DIFFERENTIAL DIAGNOSIS OF CRITICAL ILLNESS POLYNEUROPATHY

Spinal cord lesions
Prolonged neuromuscular blockade
Steroid or relaxant-induced myopathy
Acute necrotizing myopathy
Hypophosphatemia
Toxic and thiamine-deficiency neuropathies
Asthma-amyotrophy (Hopkins) syndrome
Guillain-Barré syndrome

From Ouvrier RA: Neuropathies secondary to systemic disorders. *In* Jones HR, De Vivo DC, Darras BT (eds): Neuromuscular Disorders of Infancy, Childhood, and Adolescence: A Clinician's Approach. Philadelphia, Butterworth Heinemann Health, 2003, pp 493-503.

Argentina, Canada, Mexico, Spain, as well as the United States). AMAN occurs more commonly among younger children in rural environments with poor sanitation.[137] CMAPs are reduced in amplitude; however, motor and sensory CVs are often normal and the EMG shows early denervation. In children with AMAN, weakness, along with EMG evidence of denervation, progressed more rapidly, evolved to a greater severity, resolved more slowly, and led to greater disability at 12-month follow-up, compared with children with AIDP.[138,138a]

CHRONIC GENETICALLY DETERMINED DEMYELINATING POLYNEUROPATHIES

Most requests for neuromuscular evaluation of infants are prompted by the recognition of generalized hypotonia. Polyneuropathy is an uncommon cause of the "floppy infant" syndrome, which is due in approximately three quarters of cases to disorders of the CNS.[139-141] In those children who ultimately prove to have neuromuscular disorders, infantile spinal muscular atrophy (SMA), congenital myopathies, and neuromuscular junction disorders are more common than polyneuropathy (Box 33-4).[139-142] The absence of SNAPs, if not due to technical difficulties, is perhaps the most important electrodiagnostic clue to the diagnosis of neonatal polyneuropathies.

BOX 33-4
CONGENITAL AND EARLY INFANTILE NEUROPATHIES

Peripheral neuropathies with no associated CNS component
   Hereditary motor and sensory neuropathies (Charcot-Marie-Tooth)
   Hereditary motor neuronopathies
   Hereditary sensory and autonomic neuropathies
Peripheral neuropathies as part of metabolic or hereditary degenerative CNS disorders
Immunologically mediated neuropathies

CNS, central nervous system.
From Gabreëls-Festen A, Gabreëls F: Congenital and early infantile neuropathies. *In* Jones HR, De Vivo DC, Darras BT (eds): Neuromuscular Disorders of Infancy, Childhood, and Adolescence: A Clinician's Approach. Philadelphia, Butterworth Heinemann Health, 2003, pp 361-388.

Infantile-Onset Polyneuropathies

Classically, these inherited demyelinating and hypomyelinating polyneuropathies have been typically known as either Dejerine-Sottas disease (DSD) or congenital hypomyelinating neuropathy (CHN).[25,26,143,144] Both CHN and DSD were formerly believed to be of autosomal recessive inheritance, but today most instances are recognized to have new dominant point mutations of *MPZ*, *EGR2*, or *PMP22*.[22,25,26,145,146] However, genetic analysis is still unrevealing in a significant proportion of infantile onset polyneuropathies (see Box 33-4).[26]

Affected infants have nonprogressive weakness, severe hypotonia, areflexia, and respiratory failure. At times some of these babies have the phenotypical appearance of Werdnig-Hoffmann disease (SMA-1) with the generalized hypotonia, a bell-shaped chest and abdomen, paradoxical respirations, and even tongue fasciculations. The pulmonary compromise may lead to a fatal outcome within the first few months.

Sensory nerve action potentials are not elicitable. This finding per se is the primary distinguishing feature separating these neuropathies from SMA. Motor nerve conductions are extremely slow from birth, in the range of 3 to 10 m/sec, even more so than the axonal changes of SMA. Fibrillation potentials, positive waves, and reduced recruitment of motor unit potentials are seen on the needle examination. The CSF protein level is sometimes markedly elevated. Sural nerve biopsy generally demonstrates a severe hypomyelinating neuropathy, with or without onion bulb formation. Rarely, a primary axonal polyneuropathy is the underlying mechanism.

When confronted with any floppy infant one always needs to consider a broad spectrum of motor unit disorders. In general 80% of these babies have a primary CNS mechanism and the remainder a lesion in the peripheral motor unit. This is summarized in Box 33-5.

Autosomal recessive CMT (ARCMT, CMT-4) often presents during infancy. Mutations for demyelinating ARCMT have been identified in at least five genes: *GDAP1*, *MTMR2*, *NDRG1*, *PRX*, and *EGR2* and additional loci are identified on chromosomes 5q and 11p15. ARCMT may present as a demyelinating or axonal polyneuropathy. An updated listing of mutations for CMT can be found at *http://www.molgen.ua.ac.be/CMTMutations/default.cfm*.

Charcot-Marie-Tooth (Hereditary Motor and Sensory Neuropathy)

CMT disease, the most common inherited polyneuropathy, is a genetically heterogeneous group of sensorimotor polyneuropathies sharing a similar clinical phenotype.[19-21,29,30] The frequency of CMT is estimated to be 1 per 2500 to 10,000, making it the most common inherited neuromuscular disorder.[3,7,8] Characteristic findings include weakness and wasting of the distal limb muscles (especially the peroneal compartments), skeletal deformities such as pes cavus, absent or decreased muscle stretch reflexes, and distal sensory loss.[19-21,29,30]

Classification systems for CMT have historically been based on clinical features, mode of inheritance, NCSs, and neuropathologic findings.[19-21,29] Two major subgroups of autosomal dominant CMT were initially identified on the basis of electrophysiologic and neuropathologic criteria. Parenthetically one needs to note that for almost a quarter of a century these two common hereditary polyneuropathies were referred to as *hereditary motor sensory neuropathies* (HMSN), types I to IV. Recently, there has been a return to an acronym terminology historically recognizing CMT.

Electrophysiologic criteria are still the practical key to making the major clinical differentiation. CMT-1 patients have uniform slowing of nerve conduction, with hypertrophic nerves related to the characteristic abnormal myelination. In contrast with CMT-2, NCVs are normal, CMAP amplitudes low, and the associated pathologic changes include neuronal degeneration and axon loss.[19-21,29] CMT-2 is discussed further in the section "Genetically Determined Chronic Axonal Polyneuropathies of Infancy and Childhood."

CMT-1 usually manifests during the first or second decade of life.[19-21,29,30] Many genetic mutations have been discovered for CMT, especially for the demyelinating forms. As mentioned earlier, an updated list of mutations can be found online at *http://www.molgen.ua.ac.be/CMTMutations/default.cfm*. DNA testing is commercially available for a number of these mutations, most commonly for those causing CMT-1, DSD, and CMT-X.

The demyelinating form of autosomal dominant CMT usually presents clinically in the very late first or second decade of life. Its most frequent initial signs include difficulty walking, foot deformity (pes cavus or cavus varus, clawing of toes, atrophy of intrinsic foot muscles), lower limb areflexia, and palpable nerve enlargement (Fig. 33-6).[147,148]

NCSs reveal a uniform, demyelinating sensorimotor polyneuropathy (discussed in detail earlier in this chapter within the section discussing the electrodiagnostic features of demyelinating polyneuropathies).

The recent, rapid evolution in the application of genetic DNA technology to the clinical arena is well illustrated by the study of hereditary polyneuropathies. *PMP22* mutations characterize 60% to 80% of cases of CMT-1.[5,30,145,149-156] In almost all cases of CMT-1A, duplication of the 1.5-megabase chromosomal region containing *PMP22* results in overexpression of PMP22 protein.[25,157] Only rarely ("1% of CMT-1 cases"), point mutations of the *PMP22* gene cause CMT-1A.[24,25,158]

In contrast, deletion of the same 1.5-megabase chromosomal region results in HNPP.[159-163] HNPP is due most often to a deletion of the 17p11.2 region. This rare neuropathy characteristically results in nonuniform slowing, especially distally and at sites of compression.[164-166] Entrapment neuropathies are common in HNPP; they clinically present as classic mononeuropathies at sites of entrapment. In addition, a "distally accentuated myelinopathy" is often observed in which conduction slowing of motor and sensory fibers is more pronounced distally.[166-169] Nonuniform slowing may be seen in asymptomatic HNPP patients, including 5- and 6-year-old children.[165,166] Conduction block also may be observed in HNPP. Uncini and coworkers reported that conduction block was found in 25% of HNPP patients using a greater than 20% drop in area or amplitude as criteria and in 6% of patients using a greater than 50% drop as criteria.[165]

CMT-X is the second most common cause of a hereditary demyelinating polyneuropathy. This is caused by mutations in the Connexin 32 gene, and more than 200 different genetic mutations are identified.[54,170,171] Both males and females may be affected by this X-linked disorder. Males typically are more clinically affected and have slower NCVs than females.[172-176] The presentation of CMT-X is one of a distal sensorimotor polyneuropathy, which may be primarily demyelinating or axonal. Occasionally with CMT-1, electrophysiologic findings of slowing are nonuniform and consequently can be suggestive of an acquired (i.e., CIDP) rather than inherited disorder.[177] The nonuniformity may be more obvious in CMT-X females, but it is also observed in males.[177]

Metabolic Demyelinating Disorders

See Tables 33-1 and 33-2.

Lysosomal Storage Diseases: Sphingolipidoses
Globoid Cell Leukodystrophy and Metachromatic Leukodystrophy. These are rare autosomal recessive lyso-

Hereditary Motor-Sensory Neuropathy Type I

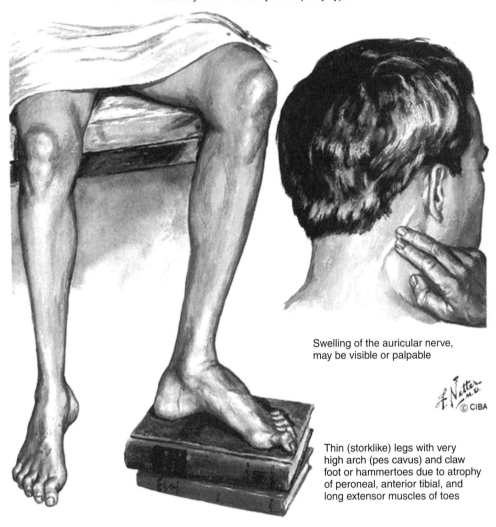

Swelling of the auricular nerve, may be visible or palpable

Thin (storklike) legs with very high arch (pes cavus) and claw foot or hammertoes due to atrophy of peroneal, anterior tibial, and long extensor muscles of toes

FIGURE 33–6

Clinical presentations of Charcot-Marie-Tooth neuropathy type 1. (Copyright©1997, Icon Learning Systems, LLC. A subsidiary of MediMedia, USA, Inc. All rights reserved.)

somal storage disorders. Typically these disorders present during infancy or early childhood with features of both progressive central and peripheral demyelination.[178,179] Both globoid cell leukodystrophy and metachromatic leukodystrophy have devastating consequences without treatment, and thus prompt diagnosis is becoming increasingly important as novel therapies are further refined. Concomitant CNS manifestations usually serve to alert the clinician that the infant's polyneuropathy is due to a more systemic disorder (i.e., globoid cell leukodystrophy and metachromatic leukodystrophy) rather than one confined to the peripheral nervous system. However, the polyneuropathy may be the presenting manifestation of either disorder, particularly metachromatic leukodystrophy; the CNS manifestations

may be subtle or do not become evident for a few more months.

Globoid cell leukodystrophy is caused by a deficiency of the enzyme galactosylceramidase present in its classic Krabbe form. The first symptoms usually become evident between 3 and 8 months of age with motor retardation, episodic tonic rigidity with opisthotic posturing, seizures, and extreme behavioral irritability.[180] These clinical features usually overshadow the associated demyelinating polyneuropathy, although occasional instances with acute-onset or clinically prominent polyneuropathy are reported in infancy and childhood.[180-182] Although nerve biopsy reveals segmental demyelination and cytoplasmic inclusions,[183] this diagnostic modality is rarely necessary given the recent availability of

TABLE 33–1. PERIPHERAL NEUROPATHY IN INHERITED METABOLIC DISEASES

Category	Disease	Stored Material	Biochemical Defect	Mechanical Defect	Chromosome
Lysosomal storage diseases: Sphingolipidoses	Krabbe's disease	Galactosylceramide	Galactosylceramide β-galactosidase	*GLAC*	14q25-31
	Metachromatic leukodystrophy	Sulfatide	Sulfatide sulfatase (arylsulfatase A)	*ARSA*	22q13.31-ter
	Fabry's disease	Trihexosylceramide	Trihexosylceramide α-galactosidase	*GLA*	Xq22.1
Peroxisomal diseases	Adrenomyeloneuropathy	VLCFA	VLCFA CoA synthetase	*ALDP*	X128
	Refsum's disease	Phytanic acid	Phytanic acid oxidase	*PHYH*	10p
	Hyperoxaluria	Calcium oxalates	Alanine-glyoxylate aminotransferase	*AGT*	2q36-37
Lipids	Cerebrotendinous xanthomatosis	Cholestanol	Cholesterol 27-hydroxylase	*CTX*	
	Tangier's disease	Cholesterol esters	Unknown	Unknown	Unknown
	Abetalipoproteinemia		Unknown	Unknown	Unknown
Mitochondrial diseases	LCHAD	3-Hydroxy dicarboxylic aciduria	Trifunctional protein and long-chain 3-hydroxy-acyl-CoA dehydrogenase	*MTP/LCHAD*	Unknown
	Leigh's disease	Lactate/pyruvate		Multiple enzymes	Multiple nucleotide 8993 (mtDNA)
	NARP	Lactate/pyruvate		ATP synthase subunit 6	
Amino acids	Tyrosinemia type 1	Tyrosine/succinyl-acetone	Fumarylacetoacetate hydrolase	*FAH*	15

CoA, coenzyme A; LCHAD, long-chain 3-hydroxyacyl-CoA dehydrogenase; NARP, neuropathy, ataxia, retinitis pigmentosa; VLCFA, very long-chain fatty acid; ATP, adenosine triphosphate; mtDNA, mitochondrial DNA.

From Moser HW, Percy AK: Peripheral neuropathy in inherited metabolic disease. *In* Jones HR, De Vivo DC, Darras BT (eds): Neuromuscular Disorders of Infancy, Childhood, and Adolescence: A Clinician's Approach. Philadelphia, Butterworth Heinemann Health, 2003, pp 469-492.

genetic testing. Bone marrow transplantation may be beneficial in the rare juvenile variant when performed early in the disease course. Unfortunately to date this modality has not been successful in the therapy of the more common (1 per 100,000) infantile form of globoid cell leukodystrophy.[184,185]

Metachromatic Leukodystrophy. This autosomal recessive disorder develops when there is a deficiency of arylsulfatase A or its activator protein.[186] This sulfatide lipidosis usually presents in infancy with rapid motor regression and the development of spasticity, dysarthria, dementia, and ataxia.[187,188] Peripheral neuropathy is invariable; occasionally this is the predominant presenting clinical feature.[187,188] At times both the late infantile and juvenile variants may mimic CMT. In one of the infants evaluated at CHB and who had a prior CMT diagnosis, the presence of Babinski signs were an important clinical indicator of concomitant CNS dysfunction.[189] On another instance a previously healthy child presented with a CIDP-like illness over a 4-week period. NCS demonstrated diffuse NCV slowing (30m/sec); the CSF had a protein 10 times the ULN. When the child only had a modest response to immunosuppressive therapy, biochemical analysis was carried out. This documented a partial arylsulfatase deficiency.[190]

NCVs in children with metachromatic leukodystrophy are in the primarily demyelinating range.[181,191] Typically motor NCVs show uniform slowing without temporal dispersion or conduction block.[54] Occasional cases are, however, associated with dispersed CMAPs that mimic CIDP.[189] Although sural nerve biopsy is no longer necessary, given the availability of DNA testing, it demonstrates metachromatic deposits within peripheral nerves. Bone marrow transplantation should be considered for treatment of presymptomatic siblings of children having infantile or the early stages of juvenile metachromatic leukodystrophy. This modality can diminish or stabilize the CNS manifestations, although it has not been helpful for the peripheral components of this disorder.[185,192]

Peroxisomal Storage Disorders
Refsum's Disease

Refsum's disease is a rare autosomal recessive disorder of lipid metabolism caused by a deficiency of phytanoyl-CoA hydroxylase.[193] Classic findings of Refsum's disease include retinitis pigmentosa with impaired night vision, cerebellar ataxia, a demyelinating peripheral neuropathy, and elevated CSF protein by age 20 years.[194] The peripheral neuropathy

TABLE 33–2. PERIPHERAL NEUROPATHIC FEATURES OF INHERITED METABOLIC DISEASES

Category	Disease	Neuropathic and EMG Features
Lysosomal storage diseases: Sphingolipidoses	Krabbe's disease	Schwann cell inclusions Segmental demyelination
	Metachromatic leukodystrophy	Schwann cell sulfatide (metachromatic) accumulation Segmental demyelination
	Fabry's disease	Lamellar inclusions in perineurial cells Axonal loss
Peroxisomal diseases	Adrenomyeloneuropathy	Schwann cell inclusions Segmental demyelination
	Refsum's disease	Schwann cell inclusions Onion bulb formation Segmental demyelination
	Hyperoxaluria	Axonal degeneration Segmental demyelination
Lipids	Cerebrotendinous xanthomatosis	Schwann cell vacuoles Axonal loss
	Tangier's disease	Schwann cell vacuoles Axonal loss
	Abetalipoproteinemia	Axonal degeneration Segmental demyelination
Mitochondrial diseases	LCHAD	Axonal loss Segmental demyelination
	Leigh's disease	Segmental demyelination
	NARP	Segmental demyelination
Amino acids	Tyrosinemia type 1	Axonal loss Segmental demyelination
Other	Acute intermittent porphyria	Axonal degeneration Segmental demyelination

LCHAD, long-chain 3-hydroxyacyl-coenzyme A dehydrogenase; NARP, neuropathy; ataxia, retinitis pigmentosa.
From Moser HW, Percy AK: Peripheral neuropathy in inherited metabolic disease. *In* Jones HR, De Vivo DC, Darras BT (eds): Neuromuscular Disorders of Infancy, Childhood, and Adolescence: A Clinician's Approach. Philadelphia, Butterworth Heinemann Health, 2003, pp 469-492.

of Refsum's disease may develop late in the disease course and is of variable severity.

Motor NCVs are usually markedly reduced into the primarily demyelinating range. Diagnosis is by assay of serum levels of phytanic acid. Treatment is by avoidance of foods that contain phytanic acid, including dairy products and beef.[195]

Adrenoleukodystrophy and Adrenomyeloneuropathy

The childhood cerebral form of adrenoleukodystrophy (CCALD) causes progressive cerebral white matter degeneration, leading to blindness, ataxia, quadriparesis, dementia, and death by the second decade of life. Peripheral nerve abnormalities are minimal relative to the CNS manifestations of CCALD.

AMN is a phenotypic variant. It usually presents as a slowly progressive myelopathy beginning in the third or fourth decade for men and the fourth or fifth decade for women.[62,196,197] However, it is occasionally seen in childhood.[198]

The typical EMG features of AMN are multifocal slowing of motor CVs, low-amplitude CMAPs, and low or absent SNAPs. In a case series of 99 men with AMN and 38 heterozygous women, 26 patients had at least one nerve variable value in the demyelinating range.[62] However, overall, NCSs in patients with AMN suggest a mixture of axonal loss and multifocal demyelination.[62,63,197,198]

Analysis of plasma saturated very long-chain fatty acids (VLCFA) is the most frequently used diagnostic assay.[199] The principal biochemical abnormality is the accumulation of VLCFA in tissues and also in the plasma. The defective gene maps to Xq28. It codes for a peroxisomal membrane protein referred to as ALDP or ABCD1. More than 300 mutations have been identified and are updated in the website *www.x-ald.nl*.

Hyperoxaluria

Hyperoxaluria is an interesting, rare disorder that occurs either as a primary genetic metabolic mechanism or develops secondary to dietary factors or coincident renal disease.[200] The inborn metabolic form of hyperoxaluria has its primary biochemical basis related to a deficiency of the liver peroxisomal enzyme, alanine glyoxylate aminotransferase (AGT), or the cytosolic enzyme, D-glycerate dehydrogenase/

glyoxylate reductase (DGDH/GR). These two disorders are classified as primary hyperoxaluria (PH)-1 due to AGT deficiency or PH-2 due to DGDH/GR deficiency. PH-1 becomes clinically apparent before 5 years of age, usually presenting with either hematuria or renal colic secondary to calcium oxalate urolithiasis whose accumulation leads to chronic renal insufficiency.

A peripheral neuropathy is one feature of the PH-1 form of hyperoxaluria. Although painful paresthesia and muscle weakness do occur, clinical manifestations of peripheral neuropathy tend to be relatively minor. This neuropathy includes features of both axonal degeneration and segmental demyelination.[201-204]

Lipid Disorder Polyneuropathies

Tangier's disease, abetalipoproteinemia, and cerebrotendinous xanthomatosis (cholestanol lipidosis) are three of the most uncommon childhood polyneuropathies. Because of the predominance of axonal pathology in this subclass of pediatric neuropathies, the first two are detailed in a later section.

Cholestanol Lipidosis (Cerebrotendinous Xanthomatosis)

Cholestanol lipidosis is also an uncommon autosomal recessive disorder; although peripheral nerve pathology is common, clinical signs are mild. More typically, initial manifestations begin in late childhood or adolescence consisting of cataracts; xanthomas over extensor tendons, especially the Achilles tendon; and slowly progressive spasticity, cerebellar ataxia, and dementia.[178] These xanthomas, containing cholesterol and cholestanol, also develop within brain white matter, particularly in the cerebellum. Psychiatric disturbance (hallucinations, delusions, or other manifestations of schizophrenia) may precede other neurologic features.

NCVs are variably reduced often in the demyelinating range. In one instance motor NCVs of peroneal and tibial nerves were 12 to 34 m/sec and 38 to 40 m/sec in median nerves.[205] The SNAPs were absent in the legs, were of low amplitude in the arms, whereas sensory NCVs were slow in the arms. Needle EMG was normal.

Sural nerve biopsy demonstrated segmental demyelination, remyelination, and axonal degeneration. When this diagnosis is detected early on, and appropriate treatment modalities with cholic acid initiated, its morbidity appears relatively benign. Treatment normalizes MCVs as well as EEG and evoked response abnormalities.

The biochemical abnormalities are characterized by defective cholesterol 27-hydroxylase activity.[206] As a consequence, cholesterol is converted via a side reaction to cholestanol (dihydrocholesterol). MRI demonstrates dif-fuse low-density white matter lesion.[207] Serum cholesterol levels are normal, but cholestanol levels in serum, CSF, and red blood cells are increased.[208] Cholesterol 27-hydroxylase activity is deficient. Several mutations have been identified in the gene for cerebrotendinous xanthomatosis.[209]

Xeroderma Pigmentosum

Xeroderma pigmentosum is a rare autosomal recessive disorder that is associated with photosensitivity, telangiectasia, predisposition to cutaneous malignancies, and ataxia. NCSs and sural nerve biopsies demonstrate mixed demyelination and axon loss.[210]

Amino Acid Disorders

Tyrosinemia is primarily discussed in the subsequent axonal polyneuropathy section, although there is a demyelinating component.

Glycoproteinoses

Sialidosis type 1 is a lysosomal storage disorder of neuraminidase function. It is characterized by myoclonus and development of nonpigmentary macular degeneration (a "cherry-red spot"). An associated demyelinating neuropathy has been rarely reported.[211]

Chediak-Higashi Syndrome

Chediak-Higashi syndrome is an autosomal recessive disorder that is associated with defective pigmentation and susceptibility to infection and to lymphoreticular malignancies. Affected children may develop a demyelinating neuropathy with conduction block.[212]

Mitochondrial Polyneuropathies

Mitochondrial polyneuropathies may be either demyelinating or axonal. Hence, they are also discussed in the chronic axonal polyneuropathy section of this chapter. The polyneuropathy is almost always chronic, although exceptions are recorded.[213] For example, Leigh's disease also presents with a pediatric Guillain-Barré-like syndrome.

Leigh's Disease (Subacute Necrotizing Encephalopathy)

Leigh's disease typically presents in early infancy or childhood. Because of its propensity for having multisystem neurologic manifestations, the clinician is continually challenged to consider a diagnosis of Leigh's disease. Symptomatology may include an encephalopathic component with lethargy or coma, particularly during infancy. Other manifestations include a peripheral neuropathy, ataxia and intention tremor, involuntary movements, external ophthalmoplegia, loss of vision, impaired hearing, vascular-type headaches, seizures, swallowing-feeding difficulties, and hypotonia.[214] Brainstem dysfunction is virtually always present; the clinical picture is dominated by lethargy or coma, feeding and swallowing difficulties, and hypotonia. Lactic acidosis may be significant. Death occurs within 6 to 24 months of onset.

Those children who initially become symptomatic during their preschool period evidence growth failure, external ophthalmoplegia, movement disorders (dystonia, choreoathetosis, or myoclonus)[215]; ataxia and intention tremor as well as vascular-type headaches are more prominent. Lactic acidosis may sometimes be documented. An older-age onset is associated with a 5- to 10-year survival. Because of the multisystem predominance, peripheral neuropathic signs may be obscured. NCVs are significantly reduced to the demyelinating range. Brainstem auditory evoked responses are affected.[216]

The typical enzyme deficiencies involve mutations of nuclear or mitochondrial DNA.[178] The inheritance pattern of Leigh's disease is heterogeneous, involving both X-linked and autosomal recessive mendelian as well as mitochondrial mechanisms.[215–217] Brain MRI most frequently demonstrates abnormalities in the thalamus, basal ganglia, and brainstem.[215] Involvement of the putamen is virtually uniform.

There is no effective therapy; however, certain supportive modalities, including home ventilator programs, may be helpful.

Mitochondrial Neurogastrointestinal Encephalomyopathy (MNGIE)

Mitochondrial neurogastrointestinal encephalomyopathy (MNGIE) is an autosomal recessive disorder due to mutations in thymidine phosphorylase.[218,219] Mutations in thymidine phosphorylase prevent normal catabolism of thymidine. The accumulation of thymidine likely impairs mitochondrial DNA replication and repair, leading to mitochondrial dysfunction.

Clinical onset ranges from ages 5 months to adulthood, with an average of 18 years. Children with MNGIE develop a polyneuropathy associated with gastrointestinal dysfunction, ophthalmoparesis, ptosis, cachexia, and hearing loss. The polyneuropathy is demyelinating in approximately half of MNGIE patients and has mixed axonal and demyelinating electrodiagnostic features in the remainder.[218] Brain MRI demonstrates evidence of a leukoencephalopathy.

CHRONIC INFLAMMATORY DEMYELINATING POLYRADICULONEUROPATHY

It is estimated that childhood CIDP may account for up to 10% of cases of all childhood polyneuropathies.[10,11,17,18]

Rarely, CIDP presents during infancy.[77,78] This neuropathy occurs more commonly during the preschool years[136,220]; however, an onset in later childhood is more typical. Generally childhood CIDP presents subacutely, although its onset may be relatively rapid and indistinguishable from GBS.[135,136,221]

The cardinal clinical features of CIDP include generalized weakness and reduced or absent muscle stretch reflexes, often associated with symmetric sensory symptoms or signs. Most children present because of gait abnormalities.[11,135,136,220–224] Muscle weakness is often both proximal and distal due to patchy immune attack along the length of the peripheral nerves and nerve roots. The presence of proximal weakness serves to differentiate this disorder from the hereditary demyelinating neuropathies where distal weakness predominates. Less commonly the upper extremities are equally or more affected.[136,220–222,224]

Paresthesia and distal sensory loss are often difficult to identify in children.[136,220–223] The cranial nerves are occasionally involved in CIDP. Facial weakness, dysarthria, and dysphagia may occur.[136,220,221,223] Significant involvement of the respiratory muscles is rare but occasionally reported.[225]

Elevation of the CSF protein (>35 mg/dL) without pleocytosis (<10 cells/mm³) occurs in 90% to 100% of pediatric CIDP patients.[220,221,223,224] If there are more than 10 white blood cells/mm³, an alternative diagnosis such as Lyme polyradiculoneuropathy must be considered.

Various electrodiagnostic clinical research criteria are proposed for CIDP (see Table 33-1).[48,226] The essential diagnostic EMG findings include nonuniform slowing of motor and sensory conduction, with prolongation of distal CMAPs and F-wave latencies, temporal dispersion of the CMAPs, as well as conduction blocks at sites not prone to entrapment. Conduction block is demonstrated in only a few children with CIDP, possibly because patient distress often limits extensive testing of young children.[220,221] The evolution of neurophysiologic changes in CIDP, in general, collates with the clinical course. Progressive worsening of CVs, distal latencies, and F-wave latencies may be observed in untreated children or patients with clinical deterioration. In some cases, however, clinical improvement may be apparent even with static or worsening neurophysiologic abnormalities.[221]

However, not all children with CIDP fulfill these strict research criteria, which are best used as broad guidelines for diagnosis. The diagnosis of the chronic demyelinating polyneuropathies differentiating CIDP vis a vis the various inherited demyelinating polyneuropathies appears in earlier publications discussing the electrodiagnostic features of demyelinating polyneuropathies.[49,52,226,227]

Oral corticosteroids, intravenous immunoglobulin, and plasmapheresis are the mainstay of therapy for childhood

CIDP.[179] Long-term maintenance therapy is often required. The eventual outcome is generally very good. Most CIDP children eventually achieve a sustained clinical remission.[135,221-223,225] However, occasionally some children with CIDP have significant persisting weakness.[220]

AXONAL POLYNEUROPATHIES

Overview: Electrophysiology

Both acute and chronic axonal neuropathies are less common than demyelinating polyneuropathies in children. Their electrophysiologic profile is relatively nonspecific and, as such, does not contribute greatly to developing specific neuropathy diagnoses. When both motor and sensory fibers are affected, reduced CMAP and SNAP amplitudes are observed. Distal latencies, CVs and F-wave/H-reflex latencies are usually normal to mildly prolonged. When there is severe axon loss, CVs may approach the demyelinating range, sometimes creating diagnostic confusion as noted in the earlier discussion of demyelinating polyneuropathies. However, even with severe axon loss, CVs should not be less than 70% of the LLN and distal latencies, and F-waves and H-reflex latencies should not exceed 150% of the ULN. When the CMAP amplitudes are severely reduced, F waves are commonly absent using standard techniques; it is important not to misinterpret such findings as evidence of proximal conduction block and a demyelinating process. Conduction block and temporal dispersion are never seen in axonal neuropathies, except at common entrapment sites where they indicate superimposed entrapment neuropathies.

Sensory NCSs are a more sensitive means of detecting axon loss than are motor conduction studies. CMAP amplitudes are a relatively sensitive measure of motor axon loss with an acutely evolving axonal polyneuropathy. In contrast with chronic polyneuropathies, the surface-recorded CMAP amplitude is often maintained within the normal range due to muscle fiber reinnervation.

Needle EMG is more sensitive to axon loss in chronic neuropathies, particularly detecting the enlarged motor unit potentials indicative of muscle fiber denervation and reinnervation. In some instances fibrillation potentials may be seen in distal intrinsic foot muscles. These findings support the important role for the needle EMG in identifying chronic denervation/reinnervation, especially when CMAPs are preserved.

The role of needle EMG is otherwise quite limited in polyneuropathies, particularly in children, where it is poorly tolerated. Some goals of needle EMG in this setting are (1) to establish a distal-to-proximal gradient of denervation as is commonly seen in dying-back polyneuropathies; (2) to identify active denervation (fibrillation potentials and positive sharp waves) that, when present, signify an ongoing and aggressive denervating neuropathy; and (3) to exclude a coexisting myopathy.

Acute Acquired Axonal Polyneuropathies

AMAN/AMSAN

The most common acute axonal neuropathies of childhood are the relatively rare axonal forms of GBS. For many years GBS was presumed to be a demyelinating disorder. However, in 1986 Feasby and associates[228] reported five cases of severe GBS with inexcitable nerves and proposed the existence of an axonal form of GBS. Concomitantly, reports emerged of annual epidemics of GBS among children and young adults in northern China.[229] An extensive American-Chinese research collaboration led to detailed electrodiagnostic and pathologic studies confirming the occurrence of an axonal GBS. These results advanced our understanding of GBS pathophysiology, leading to a fundamental change in the nosology of GBS.[230]

Clinical Aspects

Axonal forms of GBS are either purely motor (AMAN) or sensorimotor (AMSAN). AMSAN is believed to be simply a more severe form of AMAN.[231] Although initially reported in China, AMAN is now recognized to have a worldwide distribution[86,232] and occasionally we also see it at CHB. AMAN and AMSAN are clinically similar to demyelinating GBS (as noted in the preceding section on acute demyelinating polyneuropathy).

Clinically these children present with a weakness and hyporeflexia evolving over several days to several weeks, not unlike typical demyelinating GBS, and usually after a preceding infection. Back pain, limb pain, and meningismus are also frequent. AMAN is, by definition, a purely motor axonal neuropathy, and this distinguishes it from the classic demyelinating form of GBS. Because sensory symptoms are difficult to define in children, the distinction between a demyelinating and axonal GBS depends on EMG examination. Certain clinical features that suggest AMAN or AMSAN are the rapid evolution of weakness in concert with a recent infectious diarrhea caused by *Campylobacter jejuni*. At its extreme AMSAN can mimic brain death with combined quadriplegia, a total bulbar palsy, and a loss of all reflexes including loss of pupillary responses.[88] The CSF evaluation demonstrates the classic cytoalbuminologic dissociation.

Electrodiagnostic Features of AMAN

Typical findings include low CMAP amplitudes, minimal to no slowing of conduction, and normal sensory responses.

Electromyography demonstrates active denervation after the appropriate interval. AMSAN has a similar EMG profile with the added important finding of a reduction in SNAP amplitudes. In severe cases, electrically inexcitable nerves are found. However, a severe demyelinating GBS can also result in electrically inexcitable nerves, presumably due to distal conduction block. Therefore, when no CMAPs or SNAPs are elicitable, a pure demyelinating GBS and primary axonal GBS (i.e., AMSAN) cannot be differentiated early on in their course.[233]

Pathologic Correlation

There is a clear relationship between these various axonal GBS subtypes. Sural nerve biopsy in AMAN is normal or shows sparse degenerating fibers, whereas AMSAN demonstrates extensive sural nerve fiber degeneration. Lymphocytic infiltration is sparse in both entities.[234] Likewise, AMAN shows prominent wallerian-like degeneration of the ventral but not dorsal spinal roots, whereas AMSAN demonstrates degeneration of both ventral and dorsal roots.[230] Interestingly, using electron microscopy, Griffin and colleagues[230] demonstrated macrophages within the periaxonal space, surrounded by an intact myelin sheath in both AMAN and AMSAN. These findings contrast with demyelinating GBS where an intense lymphocytic infiltration is present while macrophages are demonstrated stripping the myelin sheath.[230]

Pathophysiology

All forms appear to be antibody mediated, involving complement activation.[235,236] The dominant theory of GBS pathogenesis is that of "molecular mimicry," wherein surface antigens on infecting organisms mimic epitopes on nerve fibers or Schwann cells and thereby precipitate autoimmune attack. Presumably, AMAN and AMSAN involve epitopes on the axolemma of motor and/or sensory fibers, whereas AIDP involves Schwann cell epitopes.

Differential Diagnosis

When considering a variety of conditions in the differential diagnosis, similar EMG findings may be seen in botulism, where CMAP amplitudes are reduced and fibrillations may be prominent (Chapter 35). Tick paralysis is an important consideration. The clinical picture is nearly identical to that of AMAN, and electrophysiology is consistent with an axon-loss process. CMAP amplitudes are reduced and, though generally still normal, sensory amplitudes increase after tick removal, indicating a relative depression of sensory amplitudes during tick attachment.[120,121] The only means of distinguishing tick paralysis from GBS is via a careful search of the skin and scalp. More than one tick may be present. Removal produces rapid recovery in most North American cases but there is a delayed recovery in the Australian variant.[119]

Other diagnostic considerations include periodic paralysis, marine toxin ingestion, acute myositis, poliomyelitis, West Nile virus infection, porphyria, and buckthorn intoxication.[13,237]

Prognosis

In some children the prognosis of AMAN and AMSAN is less favorable than that of AIDP. Clinical series of AIDP in children report an excellent prognosis.[70,79,80] Smaller reports of children with significant axon loss GBS,[114,115] though not labeled as AMAN or AMSAN at the time, record poorer outcomes with residual disability. Paradiso and coworkers observed a more severe illness and poorer outcome in those pediatric GBS patients demonstrating an AMAN pattern.[86] Korinthenberg and Mounting noted a similar slower recovery in children with axonal rather than demyelinating features; nevertheless, all children in their study eventually walked independently.[71]

Toxic Polyneuropathies

Most toxins have a primary axonal effect when they lead to damage of the peripheral nervous system. In children medications rarely lead to an acute polyneuropathy.

Vincristine

Although vincristine is a vinca alkaloid antineoplastic agent that is usually associated with the gradual evolution of a primary sensory polyneuropathy, children who have hereditary CMT-1 and concomitantly are treated with vincristine may develop an acute motor and sensory neuropathy suggesting GBS.[238] Pediatricians must be alert to this possibility when they consider using vincristine; therefore, one is encouraged to query as to any personal or family history of CMT-1 before initiating this medication. Because the clinical expression of CMT may be occult, clues to this diagnosis include the child with high arches, weak feet, and diminished or absent muscle stretch reflexes.

Diagnosis initially rests on a careful family history; this is a particularly important marker. Either an EMG, looking for an occult demyelinating polyneuropathy, or obtaining DNA testing for the gene having 17p11.2-12 duplication are the appropriate means to recognize this disorder in any child with these clinical findings or one who has a possible familial neuropathy.[239]

Miscellaneous Toxins

Heavy metals, glue sniffing, buckthorn wild cherry intoxication, or fish toxins always need consideration when considering the diagnosis of GBS.[13] Children in agricultural communities are at risk for organophosphate pesticide poisoning.[240] In Paraguay there was a 30% incidence of organophosphate pesticide exposure in children with an otherwise typical GBS presentation.[16]

Genetically Determined Chronic Axonal Polyneuropathies of Infancy and Childhood

Most pediatric axonal polyneuropathies have a genetic basis similar to their primary demyelinating counterparts.[241] This is in striking contrast with adults as the axonal polyneuropathies related to various systemic disorders, including diabetes mellitus, are exceedingly rare in children. Although congenital axonal polyneuropathies uncommonly occur during infancy, a few sporadic and familial cases are documented. An autosomal recessive inheritance is suspected in many instances.[242-244] Mutations of *LMNA* gene cause one form of axonal ARCMT.[245]

Charcot-Marie-Tooth Type 2

CMT-2 is the neuronal or axonal form of autosomal dominant CMT. It is clinically and genetically heterogeneous.[25,246] CMT-2 commonly presents after the age of 20 years but may occasionally first manifest during the second decade of life.[19,247,248] NCVs are normal, and CMAP amplitudes are low in CMT-2. Pathologic abnormalities include both neuronal degeneration and axon loss.[19-21,29]

Genetically, this neuropathy is less well characterized, although in recent years certain mutations have identified several causative genes, including neurofilament-light (*NFL*),[241] *KIF1B*,[249] and *GDAP1*.[250,251] The CMT-2 phenotype is also occasionally seen in patients with connexin 32 or *MPZ* mutations, for which genetic testing is commercially available.[158,252,253]

CMT-2C is a variant that may present in infancy with stridor and intermittent breathing difficulties.[254] Weakness of laryngeal muscles is responsible for the respiratory stridor in infants, and a hoarse voice may be a manifestation of vocal cord paralysis in infants, older children, and adolescents. Respiratory muscle weakness due to intercostal muscle and diaphragmatic involvement also occurs in children with CMT-2C. Sensory loss is usually mild but, when detectable clinically and/or electrodiagnostically, it helps distinguish CMT-2C from distal SMA with vocal cord paralysis (distal SMA-7 or hereditary distal motor neuronopathy type 7) and SMA with respiratory distress. The gene for CMT-2C maps to chromosome 12q23-24[255] and distal SMA-7 links to a locus on chromosome 2q14.[256]

Children who have an associated diaphragmatic weakness may fit within the clinical spectrum of SMA with respiratory distress (i.e., hereditary distal motor neuropathy type 6).[243,244,257] At least a few such cases are caused by mutations in the gene for immunoglobulin μ-binding protein 2 (*IGHMBP2*).[258] Such cases must be distinguished from infantile SMA.[259]

Hereditary Metabolically Related Axonal Polyneuropathies

Sphingolipidoses

Fabry's Disease. This is a rare X-linked disorder caused by deficiency of alpha-galactosidase A that results in accumulation of globotriaosylceramide and other glycosphingolipids in vascular endothelium; smooth muscle cells; and cells of the kidneys, heart, eyes, and nerves.[260,261] Fabry's disease primarily causes a chronic polyneuropathy although one needs to consider it within the group of acute polyneuropathies because attacks of painful neuropathy are typical early on. The clinical hallmarks of Fabry's disease are attacks of neuropathic pain, angiokeratomas of the skin, and progressive kidney disease. Onset is typically in childhood or adolescence.[262]

The classic angiokeratomas appear before the end of the first decade as blood-filled papules over the umbilical area, loins, and genitalia. Other complications include renal failure, cardiac conduction disturbances, and stroke. Heterozygous females may suffer the same symptoms and complications as affected males.

Fabry's polyneuropathy is a predominantly small-fiber sensory polyneuropathy, and consequently NCSs of large myelinated nerve fibers may be normal.[263,264] When NCSs are abnormal, typically only one or two nerves reveals abnormality, and it usually takes the form of mild slowing of CV or prolonged distal latency. Nerve biopsy demonstrates loss of small myelinated fibers,[265] whereas postmortem studies show a sensory ganglionopathy.[263]

Diagnosis is by assay of alpha-galactosidase A activity in leukocytes or plasma. Fabrazyme (agalsidase beta) has been recently approved for enzyme replacement therapy for Fabry's disease.[260]

Lipid Disorder Polyneuropathies

Tangier's Disease. This is one of the most rare autosomal recessive peripheral nerve disorders. Tangier's disease is characterized by deficiency of serum high-density lipoproteins and their constituent apolipoproteins A-I and A-II. It may have been defined in no more than 50 individuals.[178] Clinical hallmarks of Tangier's disease include a primary sensory polyneuropathy in 50% of patients, enlarged orange or yellow-gray tonsils, splenomegaly, and corneal deposits.[266] The molecular defect in Tangier's disease is a mutation in the ATP-binding cassette (ABC) transporter 1 gene (*ABC1*); its malfunction leads to an accumulation of cholesterol esters in the liver, spleen, lymph nodes, cornea, and peripheral nerves.

The polyneuropathy usually presents as one of two age-dependent syndromes. During the first 2 decades of life, multifocal mononeuropathies will occur. This is in contrast to the typical syringomyelia-like syndrome having an onset in adulthood.[266,267] The multifocal mononeuropathies typically follow a relapsing-remitting course not unlike that seen with HNPP.

EMG studies in such cases reveal multifocal slowing of motor and sensory nerves. Sural nerve biopsy demonstrates prominent demyelination and remyelination.

Abetalipoproteinemia (Bassen-Kornzweig Disease). This is an autosomal recessive disorder due to deficiency of microsomal triglyceride transfer protein, which is necessary for the assembly of very low-density lipoprotein (VLDL) particles.[268] Fewer than 100 individuals have been described with this intriguing autosomal recessive disorder.[178] Clinical involvement may be present from birth characterized by poor feeding, failure to gain weight with nausea, vomiting, abdominal distention, and fatty stools secondary to fat malabsorption. During childhood, a sensory neuropathy may develop. This involves all sensory modalities and includes reduced or absent muscle stretch reflexes. Concomitantly, widespread neurologic signs emerge reflecting involvement of spinal cord posterior columns, spinocerebellar pathways, and a retinopathy with night blindness.[269]

The presence of acanthocytes (spiked red blood cells) detected in blood smears already in the newborn may herald the diagnosis. Abetalipoproteinemia is characterized by absence of plasma apolipoprotein B and low levels of plasma cholesterol, triglycerides, and fat-soluble vitamins, particularly vitamin E as well as absence of plasma VLDL, low-density lipoprotein, and chylomicrons.[270]

SNAPs are quite prolonged or absent; however, motor NCVs are largely preserved.[271] The most typical electrodiagnostic finding is diminution or absence of SNAPs. Slowing of CV is mild and more marked distally than proximally. The needle EMG reveals chronic partial denervation in distal muscles.[272] The overall picture is that of a mixed axonal and demyelinating polyneuropathy. Peripheral nerve histology demonstrates both axonal degeneration and demyelination, although the primary pathology appears to be axonal loss.[272] Vitamin E deficiency is the likely pathogenetic mechanism in abetalipoproteinemia. Affected patients should be treated with vitamins E, A, and K supplementation.[195,273] Familial hypobetalipoproteinemia is genetically separate but clinically indistinguishable from abetalipoproteinemia.[274]

Peroxisomal Disorders

PH-1. This results from deficiency of hepatic alanine glyoxylate aminotransferase, presenting in childhood with nephrolithiasis and obstructive uropathy. Other complications include peripheral neuropathy, myopathy, and arthritis.

Nerve involvement may be subclinical or may result in painful paresthesia and distal weakness. NCSs suggest an axonal pathology.[201,275] Definitive diagnosis requires liver biopsy. Treatment of advanced PH usually necessitates combined liver-kidney transplantation, which may substantially alleviate neuropathic symptoms.[275]

Mitochondrial Polyneuropathies

The reported incidence of clinical or subclinical peripheral neuropathy in mitochondrial disease is near 25%.[213,276] Polyneuropathy is a common feature of a number of mitochondrial syndromes, including mitochondrial encephalomyopathy, lactic acidosis, and strokelike episodes, myoclonus epilepsy with ragged-red fibers, and Kearns-Sayre and Leigh's syndromes.[126,277,278] The polyneuropathy may be axonal or demyelinating.

Chronic demyelinating mitochondrial polyneuropathies are clinically predominant findings in neuropathy, ataxia, and retinitis pigmentosa (NARP), sensory ataxic neuropathy, and mitochondrial neuropathy gastrointestinal encephalomyopathy (MNGIE).[213]

Amino Acid Disorders

Hereditary Tyrosinemia. This is a rare cause of an acute, sometimes recurrent infantile polyneuropathy.[279,280] Affected children experience crises of neuropathy, weakness, axial and extensor hypertonia (sometimes opisthotonic posturing), pain, fever, and hypertension. Typically there is associated renal and liver dysfunction[279] presenting in early infancy as liver dysfunction or failure, in which case rapid progression to death may occur.[281] Tyrosinemia is caused by a defect of fumarylacetate hydrolase.[279,280]

Primary clinical features include failure to thrive, vomiting, diarrhea, and hepatosplenomegaly. Liver failure is associated with generalized edema, gastrointestinal bleeding, and ascites. Cirrhosis and hepatocellular carcinoma are common, with the latter occurring as early as 1 year of age.[178] Renal tubular dysfunction occurs with generalized aminoaciduria, glucosuria, proteinuria, and excessive excretion of tyrosine. Vitamin D-resistant renal rickets is a constant feature. The precise mechanism for hepatorenal toxicity is unknown at present.

The principal neurologic manifestation of tyrosinemia type 1 consists of painful peripheral neuropathic crises resembling those of acute intermittent porphyria (AIP) as subsequently noted. As with the hepatorenal toxicity, succinylacetone appears to be the responsible agent. Succinylacetone inhibits δ-aminolevulinic acid (ALA) hydratase leading to accumulation of δ-ALA. ALA is the likely neurotoxin of AIP. Psychomotor impairments are variable, most likely secondary to acute hepatic encephalopathy.

Treatment includes restriction of dietary tyrosine and phenylalanine and therapy with oral hematin and 2-nitro-4-trifluoro-methyl-benzoyl-1,3-cyclohexanedione (NTBC).[280,282] Liver transplantation is occasionally required.[279]

Other Metabolic Disorders

Hepatic Porphyria. AIP, unlike the other metabolic disorders in this section, is inherited in an autosomal dominant fashion.[283] AIP has its onset after puberty in most instances. Nevertheless, onset in childhood is well documented.[284-286] Episodes of the dominantly inherited hepatic porphyrias occur rarely and, when present, do so acutely similar to tyrosinemia; these are often provoked by infection or medications.

Clinical features include various combinations of a polyneuropathy, abdominal pain, constipation, vomiting, mental status changes, and autonomic disturbances. The recurrent episodes of pain are primarily visceral but may include peripheral neuropathic signs in the form of pain and subsequent weakness. The associated polyneuropathy is one of painful dysesthesia, predominantly axonal, but clinically motor findings often predominate. Weakness is typically proximal and paradoxically greater in the upper extremities; occasionally involving facial muscles and lower bulbar musculature.

The recurrent crises of porphyria resemble those of hereditary tyrosinemia, but only occasionally does AIP occur during the first decade of life; it is more common in the second to fourth decades. In contrast, hereditary tyrosinemia typically presents during infancy.[278,279]

Nerve conduction findings in AIP demonstrate segmental demyelination and axonal degeneration, but these findings are typically seen only in individuals with recurrent clinical events.[286,289,290] Bolton (personal communication, 1992) performed NCS on a child with porphyria and noted a pure axonal motor neuropathy. The results were similar to the NCS and EMG findings reported by Albers and colleagues, who demonstrated a similar neuropathy in eight patients with quadriparesis caused by acute porphyria.[291] An autonomic neuropathy typically occurs only during exacerbations. It includes hypertension[292] and postural hypotension,[293] as well as tachycardia and gastrointestinal and bladder dysfunction.

A CNS component sometimes occurs. It is characterized by severe anxiety, insomnia, hallucinations, and aggressive or violent behavior. Seizures are also occasionally witnessed.

AIP is due to deficiency of porphobilinogen deaminase, a key enzyme in porphyrin synthesis. The acute attacks, which typify AIP, are often precipitated by alcohol, barbiturates, phenytoin, carbamazepine, valproic acid, the succinimides, sulfonamides, and chloroquine.[283] Infection, inadequate nutrition, and sex hormones may trigger attacks as well.

These various medications or alcohol either induce δ-ALA synthetase or inhibit porphobilinogen deaminase.

Diagnosis is established by measuring porphobilinogen deaminase activity in erythrocytes, leukocytes, or cultured skin fibroblasts.[283,294]

Treatment is based largely on good nutrition concomitant with prevention of exposure to exogenous agents known to provoke acute attacks. Acute attack therapy includes high-carbohydrate oral intake and parenteral dextrose infusion in critical settings. Hematin or haemarginate can suppress ALA and porphobilinogen excretion.[283]

HEREDITARY SENSORY NEUROPATHIES

Hereditary Sensory Neuropathy Type 1

Hereditary sensory neuropathy (HSN)-1 (or hereditary sensory and autonomic neuropathy [HSAN]) presents in the first or second decade with impairment of pain and temperature sensation, distal muscle wasting, and weakness. Individuals are insensate to pain, and, consequently, repetitive trauma can lead to painless ulceration, cellulitis, and osteomyelitis.[295]

NCSs demonstrate that SNAPs are characteristically absent. Motor NCS may be normal, whereas needle EMG may reflect changes of distal chronic reinnervation. In vitro nerve potential studies demonstrate predominant loss of C fibers, with less marked loss of A delta and A alpha fibers.

HSN-1 is caused by dominant mutations of the gene serine palmitoyltransferase, long-chain base subunit-1 (*SPTLC1*) on chromosome 9q22.[296,297]

Hereditary Sensory Neuropathy Type 2

HSN-2 (or HSAN-2) is an autosomal recessive congenital sensory neuropathy with onset in infancy or early childhood.[298] In HSN-2 touch-pressure sensation is more affected than pain and temperature sensation. Pressure and touch sensation are defective secondary to predominant A-alpha fibers involvement. A distal acropathy, stress fractures, and digital infections are common. The muscle stretch reflexes are absent in the lower extremities and reduced in the upper extremities. Myelinated fibers are more affected than unmyelinated fibers.[298]

NCS demonstrate absent SNAPs with normally present CMAPs. The needle examination may reveal occasional fibrillation potentials and neurogenic motor unit potentials in distal muscles.

Familial Dysautonomia (Hereditary Sensory and Autonomic Neuropathy Type 3 or Riley-Day Syndrome)

Familial dysautonomia (HSAN-3 or Riley-Day syndrome) is a rare autosomal recessive illness that usually presents during infancy or early childhood till 5 years of age, with poor feeding, recurrent pulmonary infections, and autonomic dysfunction. The last is characterized by defective lacrimation, excessive perspiration, skin blotching, recurrent otherwise unexplained fevers, and labile blood pressure. It typically occurs in infants having Ashkenazi ancestry.[299] Physical examination reveals loss of pain sensation and fungiform papillae, areflexia, and absent corneal reflexes.[299,300]

SNAPs may be absent, whereas motor NCV may be slightly reduced or normal.[299,300] Familial dysautonomia is caused by mutations in the gene encoding IkappaB kinase complex-associated protein (IKAP).[283]

Hereditary Sensory and Autonomic Neuropathy Types 4 and 5 (Congenital Insensitivity to Pain)

HSAN-4 and HSAN-5 are phenotypically similar autosomal recessive disorders characterized by loss of pain sensation, impaired or absent sweating, and recurrent fevers. HSAN-4 is the dominantly inherited variant of congenital indifference to pain. Muscle strength as well as muscle stretch reflexes are preserved.[301] Onset of symptoms is usually in the first few years of life. A mutilating acropathy, neurogenic arthropathy, and ulcers may develop.[301] Anhidrosis is apparent in HSAN-4, whereas sweating is reduced but not absent in HSAN-5.

EMG demonstrates that these children have normal motor and sensory NCS. This presages the morphologic findings suggesting that the small unmyelinated or thinly myelinated pain fibers must be damaged.

Sural nerve biopsies demonstrate absence of unmyelinated fibers in HSAN-4. However, the myelinated nerve fibers are morphometrically normal. In contrast, HSAN-5 has a selective loss of small myelinated fibers.[301-303] Both HSAN-4 and HSAN-5 may be caused by mutations in the gene for the high-affinity nerve growth factor receptor, TrkA (*NTRKA*).[304] It is proposed that the *NTRK1* is inactivated in HSAN-4 and functionally impaired in HSAN-5.[305]

SPINOCEREBELLAR ATAXIAS

Friedreich's Ataxia

The estimated prevalence of Friedreich's ataxia is 1 per 50,000.[306] It is the most common spinocerebellar ataxia of childhood, accounting for three fourths of all hereditary ataxia presenting in this age group.[307] It has an autosomal recessive inheritance pattern.

Cardinal features of Friedreich's ataxia include progressive gait and appendicular ataxia, sensory loss (especially vibration sense), dysarthria, lower limb areflexia, and pyramidal tract signs.[308] Cardiomyopathy, impaired glucose tolerance, optic nerve atrophy, and skeletal abnormalities such as pes cavus and scoliosis are also common (Fig. 33-7).[308,309] Clinical onset is in the first or second decade, usually between the ages of 5 and 15 years.[308]

SNAPS are absent or of low amplitude, whereas motor NCSs are normal or only slightly affected.[308,310,311] Needle EMG reveals subtle changes of distal denervation. These findings clearly differentiate an early Friedreich's ataxia from CIDP that may also have an ataxia as its presenting feature.

Sural nerve biopsy is rarely necessary but, when performed, demonstrates considerable reduction in the percentage of large myelinated fibers.[311] The pathologic changes of Friedreich's ataxia localize to the posterior columns, lateral columns, dorsal spinocerebellar tracts, and peripheral sensory nerves.

Friedreich's ataxia is caused by GAA trinucleotide expansion in the frataxin gene on chromosome 9q13. GAA expansion in Friedreich's ataxia ranges from 90 to 1700, normal persons having 6 to 36 GAA repeats on each allele.[306,309,312] Most individuals with Friedreich's ataxia have homozygous repeat expansions, but heterozygous expansion combined with point mutations on the other allele also causes Friedreich's ataxia.[313] Patients with smaller repeat expansions have milder disease, with clinical phenotypes including late-onset Friedreich's ataxia and Friedreich's ataxia with retained reflexes.[309,312,314] DNA testing is commercially available.

Other Hereditary Ataxias

Ataxia-Telangiectasia

Ataxia-telangiectasia is an autosomal recessive disorder that is associated with progressive ataxia, oculocutaneous telangiectasia, recurrent sinopulmonary infections, and a predisposition to malignancy.[315] Involvement of the peripheral nerves is common but rarely clinically predominant.[262] Serum IgA and IgE are often absent, and the serum alpha-fetoprotein is usually elevated.

NCSs demonstrate slowing of motor CVs and a decrease in SNAP amplitude.[316] Somatosensory, auditory, and visual evoked responses are prolonged as well as dispersed.[307] Numerous genetic mutations are identified in the *ATM* gene on chromosome 11q22-23.[317]

Carbohydrate-Deficient Glycoprotein (CDG) Syndrome

Carbohydrate-deficient glycoprotein (CDG) *syndrome* refers to a spectrum of peptide hormone glycosylation disorders that is characterized by congenital hypotonia and dysmorphism with subsequent severe developmental delay and failure to thrive. Ataxia and strokelike episodes are seen in childhood. Neuroradiologic studies typically demonstrate cerebellar hypoplasia and brainstem atrophy.

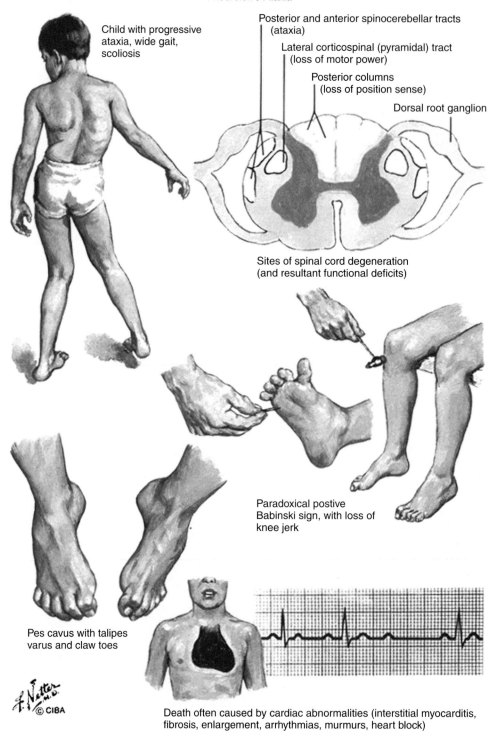

Friedreich's Ataxia

Child with progressive ataxia, wide gait, scoliosis

Posterior and anterior spinocerebellar tracts (ataxia)

Lateral corticospinal (pyramidal) tract (loss of motor power)

Posterior columns (loss of position sense)

Dorsal root ganglion

Sites of spinal cord degeneration (and resultant functional deficits)

Paradoxical postive Babinski sign, with loss of knee jerk

Pes cavus with talipes varus and claw toes

Death often caused by cardiac abnormalities (interstitial myocarditis, fibrosis, enlargement, arrhythmias, murmurs, heart block)

FIGURE 33–7

Friedreich's ataxia. (Copyright©1997, Icon Learning Systems, LLC. A subsidiary of MediMedia, USA, Inc. All rights reserved.)

Peripheral neuropathy is seen in the most common form of this disorder, CDG-1, which is caused by phosphomannomutase deficiency. The various forms of CDG syndrome are diagnosed on the basis of abnormal isoelectrophoretic patterns of serum glycoprotein isoforms.

NCSs demonstrate a slowly progressive neuropathy with mild slowing of motor nerve conduction.[318,319] Nerve biopsies demonstrate decreased myelin and microvacuolar inclusions within Schwann cells in CDG-1.

Other Spinocerebellar Ataxias

A number of other spinocerebellar ataxias occasionally present in the pediatric population. Inheritance may be autosomal dominant, autosomal recessive, or X linked. DNA testing is commercially available for many of the autosomal dominant spinal cerebellar ataxia disorders.

Autosomal Dominant Spinal Cerebellar Ataxias

Certain autosomal dominant spinal cerebellar ataxias have an associated peripheral neuropathy (especially sensory) as one of their presenting features. These are clearly reviewed by Yoo and Zoghbe.[320]

Marinesco-Sjögren Syndrome

Marinesco-Sjögren syndrome is an example of a recessive spinocerebellar disorder. It is characterized by ataxia, mental retardation, and congenital cataracts. However, in contrast to most of the spinocerebellar syndromes, the associated neuropathy is primarily of demyelinating character.[321] A recessive infantile spinal cerebellar ataxia is also described in a Finnish population.[322]

Ataxia with Vitamin E Deficiency

Ataxia with vitamin E deficiency (AVED) is due to an alpha-tocopherol transfer protein (TTP1) gene mutation.[323] It usually manifests between 4 and 18 years of age. Vitamin E deficiency is associated with cystic fibrosis, chronic malabsorption, or chronic liver disease. AVED is arrested or reversed by dietary vitamin E supplementation.[324,325]

Although AVED usually has no abnormalities defined with EMG, later in its course some children may have abnormalities of sensory conduction.[326] Somatosensory conduction abnormalities are much more common. AVED is important to recognize because of its potential for treatment.

SYSTEMIC DISORDERS AS A MECHANISM FOR CHILDHOOD NEUROPATHIES

See Table 33-3 and Box 33-6.

Connective Tissue Disorders

Polyneuropathy associated with connective tissue diseases is rare in children. Systemic lupus erythematosus (SLE) has occasionally been associated with a distal, axonal, symmetrical polyneuropathy in childhood. Less commonly an axonal mononeuritis multiplex occurs with SLE.[2,32,323,327-331,340] Systemic lupus erythematosus has also been associated with childhood CIDP.[333-335]

Focal slowing may be seen on NCSs of children with juvenile rheumatoid arthritis but is generally clinically silent.[335,336] There is a single report of progressive polyneuropathy in an adolescent with a long history of juvenile rheumatoid arthritis.[2] Other connective tissue diseases rarely associated with an axonal sensorimotor polyneuropathy in children include microscopic polyangiitis,[336,337] polyarteritis nodosa,[338,339] Wegener's granulomatosis,[339,340] Churg-Strauss syndrome,[341] and Henoch-Schönlein purpura.[342]

Infectious and Peri-infectious Disorders

Worldwide, the most common infectious cause of neuropathy is leprosy, although symptomatic pediatric cases are relatively uncommon.[343,344] Neurosarcoidosis has a peak incidence in the third and fourth decades and, rarely, causes facial palsies, hearing loss, and polyneuropathy in childhood.[337,345,346] Lyme disease has a similar predilection for the cranial nerves but is occasionally complicated in childhood by an acute inflammatory demyelinating polyneuropathy.[347,348]

Diabetes Mellitus

Symptomatic polyneuropathy in juvenile diabetics is uncommon. In contrast to the adults polyneuropathy is not a presenting sign of juvenile diabetes mellitus. Although screening neurophysiologic studies in juvenile diabetes identify subclinical, mild slowing of motor nerve conduction in as many as 72% of patients,[349-354] most children have no or minimal symptoms of neuropathy.[351,352] In the (rare) patient with significant symptoms, polyneuropathy may be reversed by improved glycemic control.[354] There is a single rather brief report implicating diabetic ketoacidosis in the pathogenesis of an axonal mononeuritis multiplex in childhood; however, a review of the data by one of us (H.R.J.) made us question the preciseness of this data.[355]

Chronic Renal Failure

Chronic renal failure is an uncommon cause of childhood axonal polyneuropathy. Neurophysiologic abnormalities tend to correlate with the severity of renal impairment

TABLE 33–3. PERIPHERAL NEUROPATHY ASSOCIATED WITH SYSTEMIC DISEASES

Systemic Disease	Predominant Type of Neuropathy	Onset and Course	Pathology
Connective Tissue Disorders			
Rheumatoid arthritis*	Sensory, mononeuritis	Chronic, acute	SD, AD
Polyarteritis nodosa*	Mononeuritis, sensory	Acute, chronic	AD, SD
Systemic lupus erythematosus*	Sensory, motor, mononeuritis	Chronic, acute	AD, SD
Metabolic Disorders			
Uremia* ±	Sensory (sensorimotor), motor	Chronic (acute)	AD, SD
Diabetes mellitus ±*	Sensory, motor	Chronic	AD, SD
Inflammatory/Infectious Disorders			
Sarcoidosis*	Sensorimotor, sensory or motor	Acute or chronic	AD
Lyme disease*	Sensory, motor	Acute or chronic	AD
Deficiency States			
Vitamin E*	Sensory	Chronic	AD
Primary			
Celiac disease			
Vitamin B$_{12}$*	Sensory	Chronic	AD
Thiamine*	Sensorimotor	Chronic	AD
Toxins			
Glue, gasoline sniffing	Sensorimotor/mononeuritis multiplex	Subacute	AD
Buckthorn wild cherry			
Fish toxins			
Organophosphate pesticide			
Heavy metals			
Medications/Iatrogenic			
Vincristine Cytosine arabinoside	Sensory	Chronic	AD
Thalidomide Cisplatin			
Paclitaxel			

*Reported in childhood.
 Words in parentheses indicate less common types.
 AD, axonal degeneration; SD, segmental demyelination.
 ±, Equivocal symptoms involvement.

BOX 33-6
DIFFERENTIAL DIAGNOSIS OF ICU PARALYSIS: FAILURE TO WEAN

Spinal cord lesions
Prolonged neuromuscular blockade
Steroid and/or relaxant-induced myopathy
Acute necrotizing myopathy
Hypophosphatemia
Toxic and thiamine deficiency neuropathies
Asthma-amyotrophy (Hopkins) syndrome
Guillain-Barré syndrome

ICU, intensive care unit.

and may be reversible after renal transplantation.[356] Most patients have no or minimal clinical symptoms.[356,357]

Toxins, Drugs, Vitamin Deficiencies, and Systemic Metabolic Diseases

Toxins, drugs, vitamin deficiencies, and systemic metabolic diseases are rarely associated with polyneuropathy in pediatric patients. The neuropathy associated with glue- or gasoline-sniffing neuropathy is probably caused by inhalation of *n*-hexane, an aromatic hydrocarbon.[358,359] Glue and gasoline sniffing are most commonly used by adolescents for their euphoric effect. The polyneuropathy is predominantly axonal. Adolescent mononeuritis multiplex has also been linked to a systemic necrotizing angiitis caused by amphetamine abuse.[360] Other causes of toxic neuropathy, including alcohol, heavy metals, and exposure to organophosphorous esters, are exceedingly rare in children.[361] Mercury and lead poisoning in children usually cause encephalopathy rather than polyneuropathy but on rare occasions may warrant diagnostic consideration.[362]

Iatrogenic Causes

Iatrogenic causes of neuropathy are relatively uncommon in pediatrics. Chemotherapy is the most common cause of drug-related neuropathy in childhood. Common causative agents including the vinca alkaloids, cytosine arabinoside, paclitaxel, thalidomide, and cisplatin. Vincristine classically leads to a chronic primary sensory polyneuropathy. It frequently causes an axonal sensorimotor and autonomic neuropathy. It may develop acutely and cause severe weakness in children with undiagnosed CMT.[363,364] Thalidomide was withdrawn from the market in 1961 because of teratogenic effects but has been reintroduced for its antiangiogenic and immunomodulatory properties.[365] Thalidomide neuropathy is a motor sensory axonal polyneuropathy.[366] Four children ages 10–15 treated with thalidomide developed NCS abnormalities as well as active EMG changes. Only one was initially symptomatic. A second child developed paresthesiae only after the treatment was stopped because of the EMG changes.[367]

Nutritional Deficiencies

Nutritional deficiencies should be considered in infants and children with malabsorptive syndromes or as a complication of maternal dietary restriction in breastfed infants. Vitamin B_{12} deficiency is an uncommon cause of pediatric polyneuropathy.[368,369] Breastfed infants are at risk of vitamin B_{12} deficiency where there is history of maternal pernicious anemia or strict vegetarianism.[369] Autoimmune pernicious anemia is extremely rare in childhood.

Vitamin B_1 (thiamine) deficiency is rare in Western civilization, although beriberi neuropathy can occur in breastfed infants of thiamine-deficient mothers. Typical clinical characteristics include dependent edema, neck stiffness, dyspnea, and acute axonal polyneuropathy, possibly associated with aphonia due to laryngeal nerve involvement.[370] Vitamin E deficiency associated with cystic fibrosis, other malabsorptive syndromes, or isolated defects of vitamin E absorption causes posterior column and dorsal root ganglia degeneration resulting in ataxia and impaired joint position and vibration sensation.[324,371-373] Other signs include gaze paresis, nystagmus, and retinitis pigmentosa. An axonal polyneuropathy, possibly related to nutritional deficiencies, has also been described in pediatric celiac disease.[374]

MISCELLANEOUS DISORDERS

Giant Axonal Neuropathy

Giant axonal neuropathy is yet another uncommon autosomal recessive disorder that presents with gait difficulties in late infancy or early childhood.[375-382] A characteristic clinical feature is tightly curled, kinky hair, although several cases with normal hair have been described.[379] Progressive weakness, ataxia, dysarthria, and sensory loss follow, and death usually occurs by the third decade.[380] CNS involvement, including mental retardation and seizures, is common.[377,380] Neurologic examination reveals generalized weakness, areflexia, Babinski signs, impaired sensation (particularly vibration and joint position), and dysarthria. Scoliosis is often present by the end of the first decade of life.

EMG demonstrates that SNAPs are usually absent and motor NCVs are typically normal or mildly decreased. Mild neurogenic changes may be seen on needle EMG. Sural nerve biopsy reveals the striking classic giant axonal swellings. These consist of densely packed accumulations of disorganized neurofilaments, predominantly intermediate filaments.[378,381] Giant axonal swellings of neurofilaments are also observed in the CNS. Causative point mutations have been identified in the gigaxonin gene.[382]

Infantile Neuroaxonal Dystrophy

Infantile neuroaxonal dystrophy is a recessively inherited disorder that presents between 6 months and 2 years of age with progressive intellectual deterioration, initial hypotonia with later spasticity, and early visual disturbances. Despite increased muscle tone, the muscle stretch reflexes are diminished or absent.

NCSs may be normal, although evidence of ongoing denervation is sometimes noted on needle EMG.[383,384] Biopsies of brain, muscle, nerve, conjunctiva, or skin demonstrate archetypical axonal spheroids within myelinated and unmyelinated axons.[385]

REFERENCES

1. Gamstorp I: Polyneuropathy in childhood. Acta Paediatr Scand 1968;57:230-238.
2. Evans OB: Polyneuropathy in childhood. Pediatrics 1979;64:96-105.
3. Hagberg B, Westerberg B: The nosology of genetic peripheral neuropathies in Swedish children. Dev Med Child Neurol 1983;25:3-18.
4. Ouvrier RA, McLeod JG: Chronic peripheral neuropathy in childhood: An overview. Aust Paediatr J 1988;24(Suppl):80-82.
5. Gabreels-Festen AA, Hoogendijk JE, Meijerink PH, et al: Two divergent types of nerve pathology in patients with different P0 mutations in Charcot-Marie-Tooth disease. Neurology 1996 Sep;47(3):761-765.
6. Ouvrier RA, Wilmshurst JM: Overview of the neuropathies: *In* Jones HR, De Vivo DC, Darras BT (eds): Neuromuscular Disorders of Infancy, Childhood, and Adolescence: A Clinician's Approach. Philadelphia, Butterworth Heinemann Health, 2003, pp 339-360.
7. Emery AH: Population frequencies of inherited neuromuscular diseases: A world survey. Neuromusc Disord 199;1:19-29.
8. Skre H: Genetic and clinical aspects of Charcot-Marie-Tooth disease. Clin Genet 1974;6:98-118.
9. McLeod JG, Pollard JD, Macaskill P, et al: Prevalence of chronic inflammatory demyelinating polyneuropathy in New South Wales, Australia. Ann Neurol 1999;46:910-913.

10. Ryan MM, Grattan-Smith PJ, Procopis PG, et al: Childhood chronic inflammatory demyelinating polyneuropathy: clinical course and long-term outcome. Neuromuscul Disord 2000; Aug;10(6):398-406.

11. Burns TM, Dyck PJ, Darras BT, Jones HR: Chronic inflammatory demyelinating polyradiculoneuropathy. *In* Jones HR, De Vivo DC, Darras BT (eds): Neuromuscular Disorders of Infancy, Childhood, and Adolescence: A Clinician's Approach. Philadelphia, Butterworth Heinemann Health, 2003, pp 445-468.

12. Sladky JT: Guillain-Barré syndrome. *In* Jones HR, De Vivo DC, Darras BT (eds): Neuromuscular Disorders of Infancy, Childhood, and Adolescence: A Clinician's Approach. Philadelphia, Butterworth Heinemann Health, 2003, pp 407-424.

13. Jones HR: Guillain-Barré syndrome: Perspectives with infants and children. Semin Pediatr Neurol 2000;7:91-102.

14. Jones HR: Guillain-Barré syndrome in children. Curr Opin Pediatr 1995;7:663-668.

15. Beghi E, Kurland LT, Mulder DW, et al: Guillain-Barré syndrome: Clinicoepidemiologic features and effect of influenza vaccine. Arch Neurol 1985;42:1053-1057.

16. Hart DE, Rojas LA, Rosariio JA, et al: Childhood Guillain-Barré syndrome in Paraguay, 1990 to 1991. Ann Neurol 1994;36:859-863.

17. Sladky JT: Immune neuropathies in childhood. Baillieres Clin Neurol 1996;5:233-243.

18. Ouvrier RA: Update on acute and chronic inflammatory polyneuropathy. J Child Neurol 1999;14:53-57.

19. Harding AE, Thomas PK: The clinical features of hereditary motor and sensory neuropathy types I and II. Brain 1980;103:259-280.

20. Dyck PJ, Lambert EH: Lower motor and primary sensory neuron diseases with peroneal muscular atrophy: I. Neurologic, genetic, and electrophysiologic findings in hereditary polyneuropathies. Arch Neurol 1968;18:603-618.

21. Dyck PJ, Lambert EH: Lower motor and primary sensory neuron diseases with peroneal muscular atrophy. II. Neurologic, genetic, and electrophysiologic findings in various neuronal degenerations. Arch Neurol 1968;18:619-625.

22. Boerkoel CF, Takshima H, Garcia CA, et al: Charcot-Marie-Tooth disease and related neuropathies: Mutation distribution and genotype-phenotype correlation. Ann Neurol 2002;51:190-201.

23. Hagberg B: Polyneuropathies in paediatrics. Eur J Pediatr 1990 Feb;149(5):296-305.

24. Parman Y, Battaloglu E, Baris I, et al: Clinicopathological and genetic study of early-onset demyelinating neuropathy. Brain 2004 Nov;127(Pt 11):2540-2550.

25. Pareyson D: Charcot-Marie-Tooth disease and related neuropathies: Molecular basis for distinction and diagnosis. Muscle Nerve 1999;22:1498-1509.

26. Plante-Bordeneuve V, Said G: Dejerine-Sottas disease and hereditary demyelinating polyneuropathy of infancy. Muscle Nerve 2002;26:608-621.

27. Gutmann L, Fakedj A, Riggs JE: Evolution of nerve conduction abnormalities in children with dominant hypertrophic neuropathy of the Charcot-Marie-Tooth type. Muscle Nerve 1983;6:515-519.

28. Ryan MM, Jones HR Jr: CMTX mimicking childhood chronic inflammatory demyelinating neuropathy with tremor. Muscle Nerve 2005 Apr;31(4):528-530.

29. Buchthal F, Behse F: Peroneal muscular atrophy (PMA) and related disorders: I. Clinical manifestations as related to biopsy findings, nerve conduction, and electromyography. Brain 1977;100:41-66.

30. Thomas PK, Marques W Jr, Davis MB, et al: The phenotypic manifestations of chromosome 17p11.2 duplication. Brain 1997;120:465-478.

31. Hsu P, Jones HR: Pes cavus as the presenting sign of childhood neuropathies: EMG evaluation in 23 otherwise asymptomatic children. Abstract presented at the American Association of Electrodiagnostic Medicine, San Diego, 1997. Muscle Nerve 1997;20:1070.

32. Ryan MM, Tilton A, De Girolami U, et al: Paediatric mononeuritis multiplex: A report of three cases and review of the literature. Neuromusc Disord 2003; 13:751-756.

33. Jones HR, Harmon RL, Bolton CF, Harper CM: An approach to pediatric electromyography. *In* Jones HR, Bolton CF, Harper CM (eds): Pediatric Clinical Electromyography. Philadelphia, Lippincott-Raven, 1996, pp 1-36.

34. Swoboda KJ, Edelbol-Eeg-Olofsson K, Harmon RL, et al: Pediatric electromyography. *In* Jones HR, De Vivo DC, Darras BT (eds): Neuromuscular Disorders of Infancy, Childhood, and Adolescence: A Clinician's Approach. Philadelphia, Butterworth Heinemann Health, 2003, pp 35-74.

35. Miller RG, Kuntz NL: Nerve conduction studies in infants and children. J Child Neurol 1986;1:19-26.

36. Gamstorp I: Normal conduction velocity of ulnar, median, and peroneal nerves in infancy, childhood, and adolescence. Acta Paediatr Scand 1963;146:68-76.

37. Baer RD, Johnson EW: Motor nerve conduction velocities in normal children. Arch Phys Med Rehabil 1965;46:698-704.

38. Wagner AL, Buchthal F: Motor and sensory conduction in infancy and childhood: Reappraisal. Dev Med Child Neurol 1972;14:189-216.

39. Cai F, Zhang J: Study of nerve conduction and late responses in normal Chinese infants, children, and adults. J Child Neurol 1997;12:13-18.

40. Sacco G, Buchthal F, Rosenfalck P: Motor unit potentials at different ages. Arch Neurol 1962;6:44-51.

41. Parano E, Uncini A, De Vivo DC, Lovelace RE: Electrophysiologic correlates of peripheral nervous system maturation in infancy and childhood. J Child Neurol 1993;8:336-338.

42. Cerra D, Johnson EW: Motor nerve conduction velocity in premature infants. Arch Phys Med Rehabil 1962;43:160-164.

43. Vecchierinin-Blineau MR, Guiheneuc P: Electrophysiological study of the peripheral nervous system in children. J Neurol Neurosurg Psychiatry 1979;42:753-759.

44. Lang HA, Puusa A, Hynninen P, et al: Evolution of nerve conduction velocity in later children and adolescence. Muscle Nerve 1985;8:38-43.

45. Kimura J: Nerve conduction and electromyography. *In* Dyck PJ and Thomas PK: Peripheral Neuropathy, 4th edition, Philadelphia, WB Saunders, Elsevier 2005:899-961.

46. Bromberg MB: Comparison of electrodiagnostic criteria for primary demyelination in chronic polyneuropathy. Muscle Nerve 1991;14:968-976.

47. Ad Hoc Subcommittee of the American Academy of Neurology AIDS Task Force: Research criteria for diagnosis of chronic inflammatory demyelinating polyneuropathy (CIDP). Neurology 1991;41:617-618.

48. Nevo Y, Topaloglu H: 88th ENMC international workshop: Childhood chronic inflammatory demyelinating polyneuropathy (including revised diagnostic criteria), Naarden, The Netherlands, December 8-10, 2000. Neuromusc Disord 2002;12:195-200.

49. Lewis RA, Sumner AJ: The electrodiagnostic distinctions between chronic familial and acquired demyelinative neuropathies. Neurology 1982;32:592-596.

50. Wilbourn AJ: Differentiating acquired from familial segmental demyelinating neuropathies by EMG. Electroencephalogr Clin Neurophysiol 1977;43:616.

51. Kaku DA, Parry GJ, Malamut R, et al: Uniform slowing of conduction velocities in Charcot-Marie-Tooth polyneuropathy type 1. Neurology 1993 Dec;43(12):2664-2667.

52. Cameron C, Kang PB, Burns TM, et al: Multifocal slowing of nerve conduction in metachromatic leukodystrophy. Muscle Nerve 2004;29:531-536.

53. Miller RG: Hereditary and acquired polyneuropathies: Electrophysiologic aspects. Neurol Clin 1985;3:543-557.

54. Lewis RA, Sumner AJ, Shy ME: Electrophysiological features of inherited demyelinating neuropathies: A reappraisal in the era of molecular diagnosis. Muscle Nerve 2000;23:1472-1487.

55. Albers JW, Kelly JJ Jr: Acquired inflammatory demyelinating polyneuropathies: clinical and electrodiagnostic features. Muscle Nerve 1989 June;12(6):435-451.

56. Olney RK, Lewis RA, Putnam TD, Campellone JV Jr: American Association of Electrodiagnostic Medicine. Consensus criteria for the diagnosis of multifocal motor neuropathy. Muscle Nerve 2003 Jan;27(1):117-121.

57. Latov N: Diagnosis of CIDP. Neurology 2002 Dec 24;59(12 Suppl 6):S2-S6.

58. Tankisi H, Pugdahl K, Fuglsang-Frederiksen A, et al: Pathophysiology inferred from electrodiagnostic nerve tests and classification of polyneuropathies. Suggested guidelines. Clin Neurophysiol 2005 Jul;116(7):1571-1580.

59. Hoogendijk JE, de Visser M, Bour LJ, et al: Conduction block in hereditary motor and sensory neuropathy type I. Muscle Nerve 1992;15(4):520-521.

60. Bolton CF: Polyneuropathies. *In* Jones HR, Bolton CF, Harper CM (eds): Pediatric Clinical Electromyography. Philadelphia, Lippincott-Raven, 1996, pp 251-353.

61. Ryan MM, Jones HR Jr: CMTX mimicking childhood chronic inflammatory demyelinating neuropathy with tremor. Muscle Nerve 2005 Apr;31(4):528-530.

62. Chaudhry V, Moser HW, Cornblath DR: Nerve conduction studies in adrenomyeloneuropathy. J Neurol Neurosurg Psychiatry 1996;61:181-185.

63. Van Geel BM, Koelman JHTM, Barth PG, et al: Peripheral nerve abnormalities in adrenomyeloneuropathy: A clinical and electrodiagnostic study. Neurology 1996;46:112-118.

64. Gutman L, Fakadej A, Riggs JE: Evolution of nerve conduction abnormalities in children with dominant hypertrophic neuropathy of the Charcot-Marie-Tooth type. Muscle Nerve 1983 Sep;6(7):515-519.

65. Ryan MM, Jones HR Jr: Delayed expression of neurophysiologic changes in CMT1a (Letter). Muscle Nerve 2004;30:123-125.

66. Asbury AK, Cornblath DR: Assessment of current diagnostic criteria for Guillain-Barré syndrome. Ann Neurol 1990;27(Suppl):S21-S24.

67. Alter M: The epidemiology of Guillain-Barré syndrome. Ann Neurol 1990;27 Suppl:S7-S12.

68. Jones HR: Guillain-Barré syndrome: perspectives with infants and children. Seminars in Pediatric Neurology 2000;7:91-102.

69. Prevots DR, Sutter RW: Assessment of Guillain-Barré syndrome mortality and morbidity in the United States: Implications for acute flaccid paralysis surveillance. J Infect Dis 1997;175(Suppl 1):S151-S155.

70. Delanoe C, Sebire G, Landrieu P, et al: Acute inflammatory demyelinating polyradiculopathy in children: Clinical and electrodiagnostic studies. Ann Neurol 1998;44:350-356.

71. Korinthenberg R, Monting JS: Natural history and treatment effects in Guillain-Barré syndrome: A multicenter study. Arch Dis Childhood 1996;74:281-287.

72. Rolfs A, Bolik A: Guillain-Barré syndrome in pregnancy: Reflections on immunopathogenesis. Acta Neurol Scand 1994;89:400-402.

73. Jackson AH, Baquis GD, Shaw BL: Congenital Guillain-Barré syndrome. J Child Neurol 1996; 5:407-410.

74. Luijckx GJ, Vies J, de Baets M, et al: Guillain-Barré syndrome in mother and child. Lancet 1997;349:27.

75. Al-Qudah AA, Shahar E, Logan WJ, Murphy EG: Neonatal Guillain-Barré syndrome. Pediatr Neurol 1988;4:255-256.

76. Jones HR, Darras BT: Acute care pediatric electromyography. Muscle Nerve 2000;23(Suppl 9):S53-S62.

77. Pasternak JF, Fulling K, Nelson J, Prensky AL: An infant with chronic relapsing polyneuropathy responsive to steroids. Dev Med Child Neurol 1982;24:505-524.

78. Sladky JT, Brown MJ, Berman PH: Chronic inflammatory demyelinating polyneuropathy of infancy: A corticosteroid-responsive disorder. Ann Neurol 1986;20:76-81.

79. Bradshaw DY, Jones HR Jr: Guillain-Barré syndrome in children: Clinical course, electrodiagnosis, and prognosis. Muscle Nerve 1992;15:500-506.

80. Epstein MA, Sladky JT: The role of plasmapheresis in childhood Guillain-Barré syndrome. Ann Neurol 1990;28:65-69.

81. Hahn AF: Guillain-Barré syndrome. Lancet 1998;352:635-641.

82. Bradshaw DY, Jones HR: "Pseudo-meningo-encephalopathic" presentation of pediatric Guillain-Barré syndrome. Neurology 1997;47:287A.

83. Wilmshurst JM, Thomas NH, Robinson RO, et al: Lower limb and back pain in Guillain-Barré syndrome and associated contrast enhancement in MRI of the cauda equina. Acta Paediatr 2001;90:691-703.

84. Jones HR: Childhood Guillain-Barré syndrome—a review: Clinical presentation, diagnosis, and therapy. J Child Neurol 1996;11:4-12.

85. Gieron-Korthals MA, Westberry KR, Emmanuel PJ: Acute childhood ataxia: Ten-year experience. J Child Neurol 1994;9:381-384.

86. Paradiso G, Tripoli J, Galicchio S, Fejerman N: Epidemiological, clinical, and electrodiagnostic findings in childhood Guillain-Barré syndrome: A reappraisal. Ann Neurol 1999;46:701-707.

87. Larsen A, Tobias JD: Landry-Guillain-Barré syndrome presenting with symptoms of upper airway obstruction. Pediatr Emerg Care 1994;10:347-348.

88. Bakshi N, Maselli R, Gospe SM, et al: Fulminating demyelinating neuropathy mimicking cerebral death. Muscle Nerve 1997;20:1595-1597.

89. Gamstorp I: Encephalo-myelo-radiculo-neuropathy: Involvement of the CNS in children with Guillain-Barré-Strohl. Dev Med Child Neurol 1974;16:654-658.

90. Amit R, Shapira Y, Blank, A, Aker M: Acute severe central and peripheral nervous system combined demyelination. Pediatr Neurol 1986;2:47-50.

91. Okumura A, Ushida H, Maruyama K, et al: Guillain-Barré syndrome associated with central nervous system lesions. Arch Dis Child 2002;86:304-306.

92. Ropper AH: The Guillain-Barré syndrome. N Engl J Med 1992;326:1130-1136.

93. McKhann GM, Cornblath DR, Ho T, et al: Clinical and electrophysiologic aspects of acute paralytic disease of children and young adults in northern China. Lancet 1991;338:593-597.

94. Lamont PJ, Johnston HM, Berdoukas VA: Plasmapheresis in children with Guillain-Barré syndrome. Neurology 1991;41:1928-1931.

95. Niparko N, Goldie WD, Mitchell W, et al: The use of plasmapheresis in the management of Guillain-Barré syndrome in pediatric patients [Abstract]. Ann Neurol 1989;26:448-449.

96. Khatri BO, Flamini JR, Baruah JK, et al: Plasmapheresis with acute inflammatory polyneuropathy. Pediatr Neurol 1990;6:17-19.

97. Jansen PW, Perkin RM, Ashwal S: Guillain-Barré syndrome in childhood: Natural course and efficacy of plasmapheresis. Pediatr Neurol 1993;9:16-20.

98. Griesemer DA, Johnson MI: Guillain-Barré syndrome and plasmapheresis in childhood. Ann Neurol 1991;29:688.

99. Jones HR Jr, Bradshaw DY: Guillain-Barré syndrome and plasmapheresis in childhood [Letter]. Ann Neurol 1991;29:688-689.

100. Yoshioka M, Kuroki S, Mizue H: Plasmapheresis in the treatment of Guillain-Barré syndrome in childhood. Pediatr Neurol 1985;1:329-334.

101. Al-Qudah AA: Immunoglobulins in the treatment of Guillain-Barré syndrome in early childhood. J Child Neurol 1994;9:178-180.

102. Abd-Allah SA, Jansen PW, Ashwal S, Perkin RM: Intravenous immunoglobulin as therapy for pediatric Guillain-Barré syndrome. J Child Neurol 1997;12:376-380.

103. Beausoleil JL, Nordgren RE, Modlin JF: Vaccine-associated paralytic poliomyelitis. J Child Neurol 1994;9:334-335.

104. David WS, Doyle JJ: Acute infantile weakness: A case of vaccine associated poliomyelitis. Muscle Nerve 1997;20:747-749.

105. Weinstein M: Atypical West Nile virus infection in a child. Pediatr Infect Dis J 2003;22:842-844.

106. Gucuyener K, Keskil S, Baykaner MK, et al: Co-incidence of Guillain-Barré syndrome and spinal cord compression in non-Hodgkins lymphoma. Neuropediatrics 1994;24:36-38.

107. Price L, Raphael SA, Lischner HW, et al: Inflammatory, demyelinating polyneuropathy in a child with symptomatic human immunodeficiency virus infection. J Pediatr 1991;118:242-245.

108. Crino PB, Zimmerman R, Laskowitz D, et al: Magnetic resonance imaging of the cauda equina in Guillain-Barré syndrome. Neurology 1994:44:1334-1336.

109. Pareyson D, Testa D, Morbin M, et al: Does *CMT1* homozygosity cause more severe disease with root hypertrophy and higher CSF proteins? Neurology 2003;60:1721-1722.

110. Albers JW, Kelly JJ Jr: Acquired inflammatory demyelinating polyneuropathies: clinical and electrodiagnostic features. Muscle Nerve 1989;12(6):435–451.

111. Alam TA, Chaudhry V, Cornblath DR: Electrophysiological studies in the Guillain-Barré syndrome: distinguishing subtypes by published criteria. Muscle Nerve 1998 Oct;21(10):1275–1279.

112. Delanoe C, Sebire G, Landrieu P, Huault G, Metral S: Acute inflammatory demyelinating polyradiculopathy in children: clinical and electrodiagnostic studies. Ann Neurol 1998;44:350-356.

113. Ammache Z, Afifi AK, Brown CK, Kimura J: Childhood Guillain-Barré syndrome: Clinical and electrophysiologic features predictive of outcome. J Child Neurol 2001;16:477-483.

114. Reisin RC, Pociecha J, Rodriguez E, et al. Severe Guillain-Barré syndrome in childhood treated with human immune globulin. Pediatric Neurol 1996;14:308-312.

115. Currie DM, Nelson MR, Buck BC: Guillain-Barré syndrome in children: Evidence of axonal degeneration and long-term follow-up. Arch Phys Med Rehabil 1990;71:244-247.

116. Knebusch M, Strassburg HM, Reiners K: Acute transverse myelitis in childhood: Nine cases and review of the literature. Dev Med Child Neurol 1998;40:631-639.

117. Jones HR: Childhood Guillain-Barré syndrome: A review: clinical presentation, diagnosis and therapy. J Child Neurol 1996;11:4-12.

118. Horga M-A, Fine A: West Nile virus. Pediatr Infect Dis J 2001;20:801-802.

119. Grattan-Smith PJ, Morris JG, Johnston HM, et al: Clinical and neurophysiological features of tick paralysis. Brain 1997;120:1975-1987.

120. Swift TR, Ignacio OJ: Tick paralysis: Electrophysiologic studies. Neurology 1975;25:1130-1133.

121. Vedanarayanan VV, Evans OB, Subramony SH: Tick paralysis in children: Electrophysiology and possibility of misdiagnosis. Neurology 2002;59:1088-1090.

122. Logina I, Donaghy M: Diphtheritic polyneuropathy: A clinical study and comparison with Guillain-Barré syndrome. J Neurol Neurosurg Psychiatry 1999;67:433-438.

123. McGuire SA, Gospe SM Jr, Dahl G: Acute vincristine neurotoxicity in the presence of hereditary motor and sensory neuropathy type I. Med Pediatr Oncol 1989;17:520-523.

124. Bolton CF, Laverty DA, Brown JD, et al: Critically ill polyneuropathy: Electrophysiological studies and differentiation from Guillain-Barré syndrome. J Neurol Neurosurg Psychiatry 1986;49:563-573.

125. Lacomis D, Zochodne DW, Bird SJ: Critical illness myopathy. Muscle Nerve 2000;23:1785-1788.

126. Coker SB: Leigh disease presenting as Guillain-Barré syndrome. Pediatr Neurol 1993;9:61-69.

127. Deda G, Ekim M, Karagol U, Tumer N: Hypopotassemic paralysis: A rare presentation of proximal renal tubular acidosis. J Child Neurol 2001;16:770-771.

128. Koley TK, Goyal AK, Gupta MD: Barium carbonate poisoning mimicking Guillain-Barré syndrome. J Assoc Physicians India 2001;49:656-657.

129. Sheth RD, Pryse-Phillips WEM, Riggs JE, Bodensteiner JB: Critical illness neuromuscular disease in children manifested as ventilatory dependence. J Pediatr 1995;126:259-261.

130. Lip GY, McColl KE, Moore MR: The acute porphyrias. Br J Clin Pract 1993;47:38-43.

131. Barohn RJ, Sanchez JA, Anderson KE: Acute peripheral neuropathy due to hereditary coproporphyria. Muscle Nerve 1994;17:793-799.

132. Jenkins T: The South African malady. Nature Genetics 1996;13:7-9.

133. Coker SB: Leigh disease presenting as Guillain-Barré syndrome. Pediatr Neurol 1993;9:61-63.

134. Bradshaw DY, Jones HR: Pseudo-meningo-encephalopathic presentation of pediatric Guillain-Barré syndrome. J Child Neurol 2001;16:505-508.

135. Quijano-Roy S, Burns TM, Darras BT, Jones HR: Childhood CIDP: The Children's Hospital of Boston experience. J Periph Nerv Sys 2001;6:171.

136. Simmons Z, Wald JJ, Albers JW: Chronic inflammatory demyelinating polyradiculoneuropathy in children: I. Presentation, electrodiagnostic studies, and initial clinical course, with comparison to adults. Muscle Nerve 1997;20:1008-1015.

137. Hafer-Macko C, Hsieh ST, Li CY, et al: Acute motor axonal neuropathy: an antibody-mediated attack on axolemma. Ann Neurol 1996;40:635-644.

138. Tekgul H, Serdaroglu G, Tutuncuoglu S: Outcome of axonal and demyelinating forms of Guillain-Barré syndrome in children. Pediatr Neurol 2003 Apr; 28(4):295-299.

138a. Massaro ME, Arroyo HA, Rodriguez E, et al: Nerve biopsy in severe Guillain-Barré syndrome and inexcitable motor nerves (abstract). Pediatr Neurol 1994;11:146.

139. Paine RS: The future of the "floppy infant": A follow-up study of 133 patients. Dev Med Child Neurol 1963;5:115-124.

140. Richer LP, Shevell MI, Miller SP: Diagnostic profile of neonatal hypotonia: An 11-year study. Pediatr Neurol 2001;25:32-37.

141. Jones HR: EMG evaluation of the floppy infant: Differential diagnosis and technical aspects. Muscle Nerve 1990;13:338-347.

142. Packer RJ, Brown MJ, Berman PH: The diagnostic value of electromyography in infantile hypotonia. Am J Dis Child 1982;136:1057-1059.

143. Kennedy WR, Sung JH, Berry JF: A case of congenital hypomyelinating neuropathy: Clinical, morphological, and chemical studies. Arch Neurol 1977;34:337-345.

144. Kasman M, Bernstein L, Schulman S: Chronic polyradiculoneuropathy of infancy. Neurology 1976;26:565-573.

145. De Jonghe P, Timmerman V, Nelis E, et al: Charcot-Marie-Tooth disease and related peripheral neuropathies. J Periph Nerv Syst 1997;2:370-387.

146. Warner LE, Mancias P, Butler IJ, et al: Mutations in the early growth response 2 (*EGR2*) gene are associated with hereditary myelinopathies. Nat Genet 1998; 18:382-384.

147. Berciano J, García A, Combarros O: Initial semeiology in children with Charcot-Marie-Tooth disease 1A duplication. Muscle Nerve 2003;27:34-39.

148. Dyck PJ, Lambert EH: Lower motor and primary sensory neuron diseases with peroneal muscular atrophy. I. Neurologic, genetic and electrophysiologic findings in hereditary polyneuropathies. Arch Neurol 1968;18:603-618.

149. Birouk N, Gouider R, LeGuern E, et al: Charcot-Marie-Tooth disease type 1A with 17p11.2 duplication: Clinical and electrophysiological phenotype study and factors influencing disease severity in 119 cases. Brain 1997;120:813-823.

150. Chance PF, Escolar D, Redmond A, et al: Hereditary neuropathies in late childhood and adolescence: clinical manifestations, molecular characteristics and treatment. *In* Jones HR, De Vivo DC, and Darras DT: Neuromuscular disorders of infancy, childhood, and adolescence. Philadelphia, Butterworth-Heinemann, Elsevier 2003:389-406.

151. Watts GD, Chance PF: Molecular basis of hereditary neuropathies. Adv Neurol 2002;88:133-146.

152. Ionasescu VV: Charcot-Marie-Tooth neuropathies: From clinical description to molecular genetics. Muscle Nerve 1995;18:267-275.

153. Wise CA, Garcia CA, Davis SN, et al: Molecular analyses of unrelated Charcot-Marie-Tooth (CMT) disease patients suggest a high frequency of the CMTIA duplication. Am J Hum Genet 1993 Oct;53(4):853-863.

154. Vance JM, Nicholson GA, Yamaoka LH, et al: Linkage of Charcot-Marie-Tooth neuropathy type 1a to chromosome 17. Exp Neurol 1989 May;104(2):186-189.

155. Vallat JM, Tazir M, Magdelaine C, et al: Autosomal-recessive Charcot-Marie-Tooth diseases. J Neuropathol Exp Neurol 2005 May;64(5):363-370.

156. Meggouh F, de Visser M, Arts WF, et al: Early onset neuropathy in a compound form of Charcot-Marie-Tooth disease. Ann Neurol 2005;57:589-591.

157. Carvalho AA, Vital A, Ferrer X, et al: Charcot-Marie-Tooth disease type 1A: clinicopathological correlations in 24 patients. J Peripher Nerv Syst 2005;10:85-92.

158. De Jonghe P, Timmerman V, Ceuterick C, et al: The Thr124Met mutation in the peripheral myelin protein zero *(MPZ)* gene is associated with a clinically distinct Charcot-Marie-Tooth phenotype. Brain 1999;122:281-290.

159. Kleopa KA, Georgiou DM, Nicolaou P, et al: A novel PMP22 mutation Ser22Phe in a family with hereditary neuropathy with liability to pressure palsies and CMT1A phenotypes. Neurogenetics 2004;5:171-175.

160. Li J, Krajewski K, Lewis RA, Shy ME: Loss-of-function phenotype of hereditary neuropathy with liability to pressure palsies. Muscle Nerve 2004;29:205-210.

161. Lonnqvist T, Pihko H: Hereditary neuropathy with liability to pressure palsies (HNPP) in a toddler presenting with toe-walking, pain and stiffness. Neuromuscul Disord 2003;13:827-829.

162. Chance PF, Alderson MK, Leppig KA, et al: DNA deletion associated with hereditary neuropathy with liability to pressure palsies. Cell 1993;72:143-151.

163. Tyson J, Malcolm S, Thomas PK, Harding AE: Deletions of chromosome 17p11.2 in multifocal neuropathies. Ann Neurol 1996;39:180-186.

164. Behse F, Buchthal F, Carlsen F, Knappeis GG: Hereditary neuropathy with liability to pressure palsies: Electrophysiological and histopathological aspects. Brain 1972;95:777-794.

165. Uncini A, Di Guglielmo G, Di Muzio A, et al: Differential electrophysiological features of neuropathies associated with 17p11.2 deletion and duplication. Muscle Nerve 1995;18:625-635.

166. Amato AA, Gronseth GS, Callerme KJ, et al: Tomaculous neuropathy: A clinical and electrophysiological study in patients with and without 1.5-Mb deletions in chromosome 17p11.2. Muscle Nerve 1996;19:16-22.

167. Hong YH, Kim M, Kim HJ, et al: Clinical and electrophysiologic features of HNPP patients with 17p11.2 deletion. Acta Neurol Scand 2003 Nov;108(5):352–358.

168. Gouider R, LeGuren E, Gugenheim M, et al: Clinical, electrophysiologic, and molecular correlations in 13 families with hereditary neuropathy with liability to pressure palsies and a chromosome 17p11.2 deletion. Neurology 1995;45:2018-2023.

169. Goikhman I, Meer J, Zelnik N: Hereditary neuropathy with liability to pressure palsies in infancy. Pediatr Neurol 2003 Apr;28(4):307-309.

170. De Jonghe P, Timmerman V, Nelis E, et al: Charcot-Marie-Tooth disease and related peripheral neuropathies. J Peripher Nerv Syst 1997;2(4):370-387.

171. Di Iorio G, Cappa V, Ciccodicola A, et al: A new de novo mutation of the connexin-32 gene in a patient with X-linked Charcot-Marie-Tooth type 1 disease. Neurol Sci 2002;2:109-112.

172. Hahn AF, Bolton CF, White CM, et al: Genotype/phenotype correlations in X-linked dominant Charcot-Marie-Tooth disease. Ann N Y Acad Sci 1999 Sep 14;883:366-382.

173. Senderek J, Hermanns B, Bergmann C, et al: X-linked dominant Charcot-Marie-Tooth neuropathy: clinical, electrophysiological, and morphological phenotype in four families with different connexin32 mutation(1). J Neurol Sci 1999 Aug 15;167(2):90-101.

174. Tabaraud F, Lagrange E, Sindou P, et al: Demyelinating X-linked Charcot-Marie-Tooth disease: unusual electrophysiological findings. Muscle Nerve 1999 Oct;22(10):1442-1447.

175. Cochrane S, Bergoffen J, Fairweather ND, et al: X-linked Charcot-Marie-Tooth disease (CMTX1): a study of 15 families with 12 highly informative polymorphisms. J Med Genet 1994 Mar;31(3):193-196.

176. Ionasescu VV, Trofatter J, Haines JL, et al: X-linked recessive Charcot-Marie-Tooth neuropathy: clinical and genetic study. Muscle Nerve 1992 Mar;15(3):368-373.

177. Ryan MM, Jones HR Jr: X-linked CMT presenting as chronic inflammatory demyelinating neuropathy. Muscle Nerve 2005;31:528-530.

178. Moser HW, Percy AK: Peripheral neuropathy in inherited metabolic disease. *In* Jones HR, De Vivo DC, Darras BT (eds): Neuromuscular Disorders of Infancy, Childhood, and Adolescence: A Clinician's Approach. Philadelphia, Butterworth Heinemann Health, 2003, pp 468-492.

179. Burns TM, Darras BT, Jones HR: Evaluation of Chronic Treatable Polyneuropathies in Childhood. Mayo Clinic Proceedings 2003;78:858-868.

180. Hagberg B: Krabbe's disease: Clinical presentation of neurological variants. Neuropediatrics 1984;15(Suppl): S11-S15.

181. Marks HG, Scavina MT, Kolodny EH, et al: Krabbe's disease presenting as a peripheral neuropathy. Muscle Nerve 1997;20:1024-1028.

182. Korn-Libutzki I, Dor-Wollman T, Soffer D, et al: Early peripheral nervous system manifestations in infantile Krabbe diseases. Pediatr Neurol 2003;28:115-118.

183. Dunn HG, Lake BD, Dolman CL, Wilson J: The neuropathy of Krabbe's infantile cerebral sclerosis (globoid cell leucodystrophy). Brain 1969;2:329-344.

184. Krivit W, Shapiro EG, Peters C, et al: Hematopoietic stem cell transplantation in globoid cell leukodystrophy. N Engl J Med 1998;338:1119-1126.

185. Krivit W, Peters C, Shapiro EG: Bone marrow transplantation as effective treatment of central nervous system disease in globoid cell leukodystrophy, metachromatic leukodystrophy, adrenoleukodystrophy, mannosidosis, fucosidosis, aspartylglucosaminuria, Hurler, Maroteaux-Lamy, and Sly syndromes, and Gaucher disease type III. Curr Opin Neurol 1999;12:167-176.

186. Gieselmann A, Polten J, Kreysing J, von Figura K: Molecular genetics of metachromatic leukodystrophy. J Inherit Metab Dis 1994;17:500-509.

187. Hagberg B: The clinical diagnosis of Krabbe's infantile leucodystrophy. Acta Paediatr Scand 1963;52:213.

188. MacFaul R, Cavanagh N, Lake BD, et al: Metachromatic leukodystrophy: Review of 38 cases. Arch Dis Child 1982;57:168-175.

189. Cameron C, Kang PB, Burns TM, et al: Multifocal slowing of nerve conduction in metachromatic leukodystrophy. Muscle Nerve 2004;29:531-536.

190. Ouvrier RA, McLeod JG, Pollard JD: Neuropathies in metabolic and degenerative disorders. *In* Ouvrier RA, McLeod JG, Pollard JD (eds): Peripheral Neuropathy in Childhood, 2nd ed. London, Mac Keith, 1999, p 176.

191. Yudell A, Gomez MR, Lambert EH, Dockerty MB: The neuropathy of sulfatide lipidosis (metachromatic leukodystrophy). Neurology 1967;17:103-111.

192. Shapiro EG, Lipton ME: White matter dysfunction and its neurophysiological correlates: A longitudinal study of a case of metachromatic leukodystrophy by bone marrow transplantation. J Clin Exp Neuropsychol 1992;14:610-624.

193. Jansen GA, Ofman R, Ferdinandusse S, et al: Refsum disease is caused by mutations in the phytanoyl-CoA hydroxylase gene. Nat Genet 1997;17:190-193.

194. Skjeldal OH, Stokke O, Refsum S, et al: Clinical and biochemical heterogeneity in conditions with phytanic acid accumulations. J Neurol Sci 1987;77:87-96.

195. Burns TM, Darras BT, Jones HR: Evaluation of Chronic Treatable Polyneuropathies in Childhood. Mayo Clinic Proceedingss 2003;78:858-868.

196. Moser HW, Naidu S, Kumar AJ, Rosenbaum AE: The adrenoleukodystrophies. Crit Rev Neurobiol 1987;3:29-88.

197. Griffin JW, Goern E, Schaumburg H, et al: Adrenomyeloneuropathy: A probable variant of adrenoleukodystrophy: I. Clinical and endocrinologic aspects. Neurology 1977;27:1107-1113.

198. Rosen NL, Lechtenberg R, Wisniewski K, et al: Adrenomyeloneuropathy with onset in early childhood. Ann Neurol 1985;17:311-312.

199. Moser H, Percy A: Peripheral neuropathy in inherited metabolic disease. *In* Jones HR, De Vivo DC, and Darras DT: Neuromuscular disorders of infancy, childhood, and adolescence. Philadelphia, Butterworth-Heinemann, Elsevier, 2003, pp 468-492.

200. Hoppe B, Langman CB: A United States survey on diagnosis, treatment, and outcome of primary hyperoxaluria. Pediatr Nephrol 2003;18:986-991.

201. Moorhead PJ, Cooper DJ, Timperley WR: Progressive peripheral neuropathy in patient with primary hyperoxaluria. BMJ 1975;2:312-313.

202. Furby A, Mourtada R, Charasse C, et al: Polyradiculoneuropathy in an adult with primitive hyperoxaluria. Rev Neurol (Paris) 2000 Jan;156(1):62-64.

203. Galloway G, Giuliani MJ, Burns DK, Lacomis D: Neuropathy associated with hyperoxaluria: improvement after combined renal and liver transplantations. Brain Pathol 1998 Apr;8(2):247-251.

204. Hall BM, Walsh JC, Horvath JS, Lytton DG: Peripheral neuropathy complicating primary hyperoxaluria. J Neurol Sci 1976 Oct;29(2-4):343-349.

205. Argov Z, Soffer D, Eisenberg S, Zimmerman Y: Chronic demyelinating peripheral neuropathy in cerebrotendinous xanthomatosis. Ann Neurol 1986 Jul;20(1):89-91.

206. Bretillon L, Siden A, Wahlund LO, et al: Plasma levels of 24S-hydroxycholesterol in patients with neurological diseases. Neurosci Lett 2000 Oct 27;293(2):87-90.

207. Berginer VM, Berginer J, Korczyn AD, Tadmor R: Magnetic resonance imaging in cerebrotendinous xanthomatosis: a prospective clinical and neuroradiological study. Journal of the Neurological Sciences 1994;122:102-108.

208. Federico A, Dotti MT: Cerebrotendinous xanthomatosis: clinical manifestations, diagnostic criteria, pathogenesis, and therapy. J Clin Neurol 2003 Sep;18(9):633-638.

209. Moghadaisan MH: Cerebrotendinous xanthomatosis: clinical course, genotypes and metabolic backgrounds. Clin Invest Med 2004;27(1):42-50.

210. Kanda T, Oda M, Yonezawa M, et al: Peripheral neuropathy in xeroderma pigmentosum. Brain 1990;113:1025-1044.

211. Steinman L, Tharp BR, Dorfman LJ, et al: Peripheral neuropathy in the cherry-red spot-myoclonus syndrome (sialidosis type I). Ann Neurol 1980;7:450-456.

212. Lockman LA, Kennedy WR, White JG: The Chediak-Higashi syndrome: Electrophysiological and electron microscopic observations on the peripheral neuropathy. J Pediatr 1967;70:942-951.

213. Nardin RA, Johns DR: Mitochondrial dysfunction and neuromuscular disease. Muscle Nerve 2001;24:170-191.

214. Stickler DE, Carney PR, Valenstein ER: Juvenile-onset Leigh syndrome with an acute polyneuropathy at presentation. J Child Neurol 2003 Aug;18(8):574-576.

215. DiMauro S, Andreu AL, De Vivo DC: Mitochondrial disorders. J Child Neurol 2002 Dec;17 Suppl 3:S35-S45; discussion 3S46-7.

216. Bernier FP, Boneh A, Dennett X, et al: Diagnostic criteria for respiratory chain disorders in adults and children. Neurology 2002 Nov 12;59(9):1406-1411.

217. Gropman AL: Diagnosis and treatment of childhood mitochondrial diseases. Curr Neurol Neurosci Rep 2001 Mar;1(2):185-194.

218. Nishino I, Spinazzola A, Papadimitriou A, et al: Mitochondrial neurogastrointestinal encephalomyopathy: An autosomal recessive disorder due to thymidine phosphorylase mutations. Ann Neurol 2000;47:792-800.

219. Teitelbaum JE, Berde CV, Nurko S, et al: Diagnosis and management of MNGIE syndrome in children: Case report and review of the literature. J Pediatr Gastroenterol Nutr 2002;35:377-383.

220. Nevo U, Pestronk A, Kornberg AJ, et al: Childhood chronic inflammatory demyelinating neuropathies: Clinical course and long-term follow-up. Neurology 1996;47:98-102.

221. Ryan MM, Grattan-Smith PJ, Procopis PG, et al: Childhood chronic inflammatory demyelinating polyneuropathy: Clinical course and long-term outcome. Neuromusc Disord 2000;10:398-406.

222. Colan RV, Snead OC III, Oh SJ, Benton JW: Steroid-responsive polyneuropathy with subacute onset in childhood. J Pediatr 1980;97:374-377.

223. Korinthenberg R: Chronic inflammatory demyelinating polyradiculoneuropathy in children and their response to treatment. Neuropediatrics 1999;30:190-196.

224. Hattori N, Ichimura M, Aoki A, et al: Clinicopathological features of chronic inflammatory demyelinating polyradiculoneuropathy in childhood. J Neurol Sci 1998;154:66-71.

225. Simmons Z, Wald JJ, Albers JW: Chronic inflammatory demyelinating polyradiculoneuropathy in children: II. Long-term follow-up, with comparison to adults. Muscle Nerve 1997;20:1569-1575.

226. Burns TM, Dyck PJ, Darras BT, Jones HR: Chronic demyelinating polyneuropathy in childhood. In Jones, De Vivo, and Darras: Neuromuscular disorders of infancy, childhood, and adolescence. Philadelphia, Butterworth-Heinemann, Elsevier, 2003, 445-469.

227. Lewis RA, Sumner AJ, Shy ME: Electrophysiological features of inherited demyelinating neuropathies: A reappraisal in the era of molecular diagnosis. Muscle Nerve 2000 Oct;23(10):1472-1487.

228. Feasby TE, Gilbert JJ, Brown WF, et al: An acute axonal form of Guillain-Barré polyneuropathy. Brain 1986;109:1115-1126.

229. Zhang ZL, Li TN: Acute polyradiculoneuritis: Clinical analysis of 514 cases. Chin J Psychiatry Neurol 1979;12:17-21.

230. Griffin JW, Li CY, Ho TW, et al: Guillain-Barré syndrome in northern China. Brain 1995;118:577-595.

231. Griffin JW, Li CY, Ho TW, et al: Pathology of the motor-sensory axonal Guillain-Barré syndrome. Ann Neurol 1996;39:17-28.

232. Nagdyman N, Behse F, Schulke M: A rare variant of Guillain-Barré syndrome with acute motor axonal neuropathy (AMAN) in a Caucasian boy. Neuropediatrics 2000 Jun;31(3):162-163.

233. Massaro ME, Rodriguez EC, Pociecha J, et al: Nerve biopsy in children with severe Guillain-Barré syndrome and inexcitable motor nerves. Neurology 1998 Aug; 51(2):394-398.

234. Lu JL, Sheikh KA, Wu HS, et al: Physiologic-pathologic correlation in Guillain-Barré syndrome in children. Neurology 2000;54:33-44.

235. Hafer-Macko C, Hsieh ST, Li CY, et al: Acute motor axonal neuropathy: An antibody-mediated attack on the axolemma. Ann Neurol 1996;40:635-644.

236. Hafer-Macko CE, Sheikh KA, Li CY, et al: Immune attack on the Schwann cell surface in acute inflammatory demyelinating polyneuropathy. Ann Neurol 1996;39:625-635.

237. Schaumberg HH, Herskovitz S: The weak child—a cautionary tale. N Engl J Med 2000;342:127-129.

238. Graf WD, Chance PF, Lensch W, et al: Severe vincristine neuropathy in Charcot-Marie-Tooth disease type 1A. Cancer 1996;77:1356-1362.

239. Pleasure D, Jones HR: Toxic polyneuropathies. In Jones HR, De Vivo DC, Darras BT (eds): Neuromuscular Disorders of Infancy, Childhood, and Adolescence: A Clinician's Approach. Philadelphia, Butterworth Heinemann Health, 2003, pp 519-528.

240. Aygun D, Onar MK, Altintop BL: The clinical and electrophysiological features of a delayed polyneuropathy developing subsequently after acute organophosphate poisoning and its correlation with the serum acetylcholinesterase. Electromyogr Clin Neurophysiol 2003 Oct-Nov;43(7):421-427.

241. Gabreels-Festen AA, Gabreels FJ: Congenital and early infantile neuropathies. In Jones HR, De Vivo DC, Darras BT (eds): Neuromuscular Disorders of Infancy, Childhood, and Adolescence: A Clinician's Approach. Philadelphia, Butterworth Heinemann Health, 2003, pp 361-388.

242. Vedanarayanan VV, Smith S, Subramony SH, et al: Lethal neonatal autosomal recessive axonal sensorimotor polyneuropathy. Muscle Nerve 1998;21:1473-1477.

243. Mohan U, Misra VP, Britto J, et al: Inherited early-onset severe axonal polyneuropathy with respiratory failure and autonomic involvement. Neuromusc Disord 2001;11:395-399.

244. Wilmshurst JM, Bye A, Rittey C, et al: Severe infantile axonal neuropathy with respiratory failure. Muscle Nerve 2001;24:760-768.

245. De Sandre-Giovannoli A, Chaouch M, Kozlov S, et al: Homozygous defects in LMNA, encoding lamin A/C nuclear-envelope proteins, cause autosomal recessive axonal neuropathy in human (Charcot-Marie-Tooth disorder type 2) and mouse. Am J Hum Genet 2002;70:726-736.

246. Nagamatsu M, Jenkins RB, Schaid DJ, et al: Hereditary motor and sensory neuropathy type 2C is genetically distinct from types 2B and 2D. Arch Neurol 2000;57:669-672.

247. Gemignani F, Marbini A: Charcot-Marie-Tooth disease (CMT): distinctive phenotypic and genotypic features in CMT type 2. J Neurol Sci 2001 Feb 15;184(1):1-9.

248. Mersiyanova IV, Perepelov AV, Polyakov AV, et al: A new variant of Charcot-Marie-Tooth type 2 is probably the result of a mutation in the neurofilament-light gene. Am J Hum Gen 2000;67:37-46.

249. Zhao C, Takita J, Tanaka Y, et al: Charcot-Marie-Tooth type 2A caused by mutation in a microtubule motor KIF1Bβ. Cell 2001;105:587-597.

250. Baxter RV, Ben Othmane K, Rochelle JM, et al: Ganglioside-induced differentiation-associated protein-α is mutant in Charcot-Marie-Tooth disease type 4A/8q21. Nat Genet 2002;30:21-22.

251. Cuesta A, Pedrola L, Sevilla T, et al: The gene encoding ganglioside-induced differentiation-associated protein 1 is mutated in axonal Charcot-Marie-Tooth type 4A disease. Nat Genet 2002;30:22-25.

252. Birouk N, LeGuern E, Maisonobe T, et al: X-linked Charcot-Marie-Tooth disease with connexin 32 mutations: Clinical and electrophysiologic study. Neurology 1998;50:1074-1082.

253. Marrosu MG, Vaccargiu S, Marrosu G, et al: Charcot-Marie-Tooth disease type 2 associated with mutation of myelin protein zero gene. Neurology 1998;50:1397-1401.

254. Dyck PJ, Litchy WJ, Minnerath S, et al: Hereditary motor and sensory neuropathy with diaphragm and vocal cord paresis. Ann Neurol 1994;35:608-615.

255. Klein CJ, Cunningham JM, Atkinson EJ, et al: The gene for HMSN2C maps to 12q23-24: A region of neuromuscular disorders. Neurology 2003;60:1151-1156.

256. McEntagart M, Norton N, Williams H, et al: Localisation of the gene for distal hereditary motor neuronopathy-VII to chromosome 2q14. Am J Hum Genet 2001; 68:1270-1276.

257. Appleton R, Riordan A, Tedman B, et al: Congenital peripheral neuropathy presenting as apnoea and respiratory insufficiency. Dev Med Child Neurol 1994;36:545-553.

258. Grohmann K, Schuelke M, Diers A, et al: Mutations in the gene encoding immunoglobulin mu-binding protein 2 cause spinal muscular atrophy with respiratory distress type 1. Nat Genet 2001;29:75-77.

259. Korinthenberg R, Sauer M, Ketelsen UP, et al: Congenital axonal neuropathy caused by deletions in the spinal muscular atrophy region. Ann Neurol 1997;42:364-368.

260. Eng CM, Guffon N, Wilcox WR, et al, for the International Collaborative Fabry Disease Study Group: Safety and efficacy of recombinant human alpha galactosidase A replacement therapy in Fabry's disease. N Engl J Med 2001;345:9-16.

261. Scott LJC, Griffin JW, Luciano C, et al: Quantitative analysis of epidermal innervation in Fabry disease. Neurology 1999;52:1249-1254.

262. Pleasure D: New treatments for denervating diseases. J Child Neurol 2005 Mar;20(3):258-262.

263. Ohnishi A, Dyck PJ: Loss of small peripheral sensory neurons in Fabry disease. Arch Neurol 1974;31:120-127.

264. Sheth KJ, Swick HM: Peripheral nerve conduction in Fabry disease. Ann Neurol 1980;7:319-323.

265. Brady RO, Schiffman R: Fabry's Disease. *In* Dyck PJ and Thomas PK: Peripheral Neuropathy, 4th edition, Philadelphia WB Saunders. Elsevier 2005; pp 1893-1904.

266. Pollock M, Nukada H, Frith RW, et al: Peripheral neuropathy in Tangier disease. Brain 1983;106:911-928.

267. Pietrini V, Rizzuto N, Vergani C, et al: Neuropathy in Tangier disease: A clinicopathologic study and review of the literature. Acta Neurol Scand 1985;72:495-505.

268. Sharp D, Blinderman L, Combs KA, et al: Cloning and gene defects in microsomal triglyceride transfer protein associated with abetalipoproteinemia. Nature 1993;365:65-69.

269. Refsum S: Heredopathia atactica polyneuritiformis. Acta Psychiatr Scand 1946;38:1-303.

270. Skjeldal OH: Heredopathia Atactica Polyneuritiformis, Refsum Disease. In Moser H, Editor, *Handbook of Clinical Neurology*, Amsterdam, Elsevier 1996:485-503.

271. Torvik A, Torp S, Kase BF, et al: Infantile Refsum's disease: a generalized peroxisomal disorder. Case report with postmortem examination. J Neurol Sci 1988;85:39-53.

272. Wichman A, Buchthal F, Pezeshkpour GH, Gregg RE: Peripheral neuropathy is abetalipoproteinemia. Neurology 1985;35:1279-1289.

273. Muller DPR, Lloyd JK, Bird AC: Long-term management of abetalipoproteinemia: Possible role for vitamin E. Arch Dis Child 1977;52:209-214.

274. Young SG, Hubl ST, Smith RS, et al: Familial hypobetalipoproteinemia caused by a mutation in the apolipoprotein B gene that results in a truncated species of apolipoprotein B (B-31). J Clin Invest 1990;85:993-942.

275. Galloway G, Giuliani MJ, Burns DK, Lacomis D: Neuropathy associated with hyperoxaluria: Improvement after combined renal and liver transplantations. Brain Pathol 1998;8:247-251.

276. Eymard B, Penicaud A, Leger JM, et al: Peripheral nerve in mitochondrial disease: Clinical and electrophysiological data—a study of 28 cases. Rev Neurol 1991;147:508-512.

277. Pezeshkpour G, Krarup C, Buchtal F, et al: Peripheral neuropathy in mitochondrial disease. J Neurol Sci 1987;77:285-304.

278. Peyronnard JM, Charron L, Bellavance A, Marchand L: Neuropathy and mitochondrial myopathy. Ann Neurol 1980;7:262-268.

279. Mitchell G, Larochelle J, Lambert M, et al: Neurologic crises in hereditary tyrosinemia. N Engl J Med 1990;322:432-437.

280. Gibbs TC, Payan J, Brett EM, et al: Peripheral neuropathy as the presenting feature of tyrosinaemia type I and effectively treated with an inhibitor of 4-hydroxyphenylpyruvate dioxygenase. J Neurol Neurosurg Psychiatry 1993;56:1129-1132.

281. Mitchell GA, Lambert M, Tanguay RM: Hypertyrosinemia. *In* Scriver CR, Beaudet AL, Sly WS, Valle D (eds): The Metabolic and Molecular Bases of Inherited Disease. New York, McGraw-Hill, 2001,pp 1777-1805.

282. Rank JM, Pascual-Leone A, Payne W, et al: Hematin therapy for the neurologic crisis of tyrosinemia. J Pediatr 1991;118:136-139.

283. Anderson SL, Coli R, Daly IW, et al: Familial dysautonomia is caused by mutations of the IKAP gene. Am J Hum Genet 2001;68:753-758.

284. Ford FR: Diseases of the Nervous System in Infancy, Childhood. and Adolescence. 5th ed. Springfield, IL, Charles C Thomas, 1966, pp 765-767.

285. Barclay N: Acute intermittent porphyria in childhood: A neglected diagnosis? Arch Dis Child 1974;49:404-406.

286. Becker DM, Kramer S: The neurological manifestations of porphyria: A review. Medicine (Baltimore) 1977; 56:411-423.

287. Elder GH: Hepatic porphyrias in children. J Inherit Metab Dis 1997;20:237-246.

288. Doss M, Schneider J, Von Tiepermann R, Brandt A: New type of acute porphyria with porphobilinogen synthase (delta-aminolevulinic acid dehydratase) defect in the homozygous state. Clin Biochem 1982;15:52-55.

289. Sorensen AW, With TK: Persistent pareses after porphyric attacks. S Afr Med J 1971;Sep 25:101-103.

290. Poser CM, Edwards K: Transient monoparesis in acute intermittent porphyria [Letter]. Arch Neurol 1978;35:550.

291. Albers JW, Robertson WC Jr, Daube JR: Electrodiagnostic findings in acute porphyric neuropathy. Muscle Nerve 1978;1:292-296.

292. Sim M, Hudon R: Acute intermittent porphyria associated with postural hypotension [letter]. Can Med Assoc J 1979;121:845-846.

293. Allen SC, Rees GA: A previous history of acute intermittent porphyria as a complication of obstetric anaesthesia. Br J Anaesth 1980;52:835-838.

294. Moser H, Percy A: Peripheral neuropathy in inherited metabolic disease...porphyria. *In* Jones HR, De Vivo DC, and Darras DT: Neuromuscular disorders of infancy, childhood, and adolescence. Philadelphia, Butterworth-Heinemann, Elsevier, 2003; pp 486-487.

295. Thomas PK: Hereditary sensory neuropathies. Brain Pathol 1993;3:157-163.

296. Dawkins JL, Hulme DJ, Brahmbhatt SB, et al: Mutations in *SPTLC1*, encoding serine palmitoyltransferase, long chain base subunit-1, cause hereditary sensory neuropathy type 1. Nat Genet 2001;27:309-312.

297. Bejaoui K, Wu C, Scheffler MD, et al: *SPTLC1* is mutated in hereditary sensory neuropathy, type 1. Nat Genet 2001;27:261-262.

298. Ohta M, Ellefson RD, Lambert EH, Dyck PJ: Hereditary sensory neuropathy, type II: Clinical, electrophysiologic, histologic, and biochemical studies of a Quebec kinship. Arch Neurol 1973;29:23-37.

299. Aguayo AJ, Nair CPV, Bray GM: Peripheral nerve abnormalities in the Riley-Day syndrome. Arch Neurol 1971;24:106-116.

300. Brown JC, Johns RJ: Nerve conduction in familial dysautonomia (Riley-Day) syndrome. JAMA 1967;201:200-203.

301. Dyck PJ, Mellinger JF, Reagan TJ, et al: Not "indifference to pain" but varieties of hereditary sensory and autonomic neuropathy. Brain 1983;106:373-390.

302. Low PA, Burke WJ, McLeod JG: Congenital sensory neuropathy with selective loss of small myelinated fibers. Ann Neurol 1978;3:179-182.

303. Goebel HH, Veit S, Dyck PJ: Confirmation of virtual unmyelinated fiber absence in hereditary sensory neuropathy type IV. J Neuropath Exp Neurol 1980; 39:670-675.

304. Indo Y, Tsuruta M, Hayashida Y, et al: Mutations in the *TRKA/NGF* receptor gene in patients with congenital insensitivity to pain with anhidrosis. Nat Genet 1996;13:485-488.

305. Indo Y: Molecular basis of congenital insensitivity to pain with anhidrosis (CIPA): Mutations and polymorphisms in *TRKA (NTRK1)* gene encoding the receptor tyrosine kinase for nerve growth factor. Hum Mutat 2001; 18:462-471.

306. Cossée M, Schmitt M, Campuzano V, et al: Evolution of the Friedreich's ataxia trinucleotide repeat expansion: Founder effect and premutations. Proc Natl Acad Sci U S A 1997;94:7452-7457.

307. Pandolfo M: Friedreich's ataxia. *In* Jones HR, De Vivo DC, Darras BT (eds): Neuromuscular Disorders of Infancy, Childhood, and Adolescence: A Clinician's Approach. Philadelphia, Butterworth Heinemann Health, 2003, pp 1141-1163.

308. Harding AE: Friedreich's ataxia: A clinical and genetic study of 90 families with an analysis of early diagnosis criteria and intrafamilial clustering of clinical features. Brain 1981;104:589-620.

309. Durr A, Cossee M, Agid Y, et al: Clinical and genetic abnormalities in patients with Friedreich's ataxia. N Engl J Med 1996;335:1169-1175.

310. Salih MA, Ahlstern G, Stålberg E, et al: Friedreich's ataxia in 13 children: Presentation and evolution with electrophysiologic, electrocardiographic, and echocardiographic feature. J Child Neurol 1990;5:321-326.

311. Hart PE, Lodi R, Rajagopalan B, et al: Antioxidant treatment of patients with Friedreich ataxia: four-year follow-up. Arch Neurol 2005 Apr;62(4):621-626.

312. Montermini L, Richter A, Morgan K, et al: Phenotypic variability in Friedreich ataxia: Role of the associated GAA triplet repeat expansion. Ann Neurol 1997;41:675-682.

313. Cossée M, Dürr A, Schmitt M, et al: Friedreich's ataxia: Point mutations and clinical presentations of compound heterozygotes. Ann Neurol 1999;45:200-206.

314. Filla A, De Michele G, Cavalcanti F, et al: The relationship between trinucleotide (GAA) repeat length and clinical features in Friedreich ataxia. Am J Hum Genet 1996;59:554-560.

315. Boder E, Sedgwick P: Ataxia telangiectasia: A review of 101 cases. Dev Med 1963;8:110-118.

316. Dunn HG: Nerve conduction studies in children with Friedreich's ataxia and ataxia-telangiectasia. Dev Med Child Neurol 1973;15:324-337.

317. Savitsky K, Bar-Shira A, Gilad S, et al: A single ataxia telangiectasia gene with a product similar to PI-3 kinase. Science 1995;268:1749-1753.

318. Hagberg BA, Blennow G, Kristiansson B, Stibler H: Carbohydrate-deficient glycoprotein syndromes: Peculiar group of new disorders. Pediatr Neurol 1993;9:255-262.

319. Veneselli E, Biancheri R, Di Rocco M, Tortorelli S: Neurophysiological findings in a case of carbohydrate-deficient glycoproteins (CDG) syndrome type I with phosphomannomutase deficiency. Eur J Paed Neurol 1998;2:239-244.

320. Yoo S-Y, Zoghbe HY: Dominantly inherited spinocerebellar syndromes. *In* Jones HR, De Vivo DC, Darras BT (eds): Neuromuscular Disorders of Infancy, Childhood, and Adolescence: A Clinician's Approach. Philadelphia, Butterworth Heinemann Health, 2003, pp 1165-1183.

321. Alexianu M, Christodorescu D, Vasilescu C, et al: Sensorimotor neuropathy in a patient with Marinesco-Sjögren syndrome. Eur Neurol 1983; 22:222-226.

322. Nikali K, Koskinen T, Suomalainen A, et al: Infantile onset spinocerebellar ataxia represents an allelic disease distinct from other hereditary ataxias. Pediatr Res 1994;36:607-612.

323. Ouvrier RA: Neuropathies secondary to systemic disorders. *In* Jones HR, De Vivo DC, Darras BT (eds): Neuromuscular Disorders of Infancy, Childhood, and Adolescence: A Clinician's Approach. Philadelphia, Butterworth Heinemann Health, 2003, pp 493-503.

324. Harding AE, Matthews S, Jones S, et al: Spinocerebellar degeneration associated with a selective defect of vitamin E absorption. N Engl J Med 1985;313:32-35.

325. Yokota T, Shiojiri T, Gotoda T, et al: Friedreich-like ataxia with retinitis pigmentosa caused by the His101Gln mutation of the alpha-tocopherol transfer protein gene. Ann Neurol 1997;41:826-832.

326. Jackson CE, Amato AA, Barohn RJ: Isolated vitamin E deficiency. Muscle Nerve 1996;19:1161-1165.

327. Scheinberg L: Polyneuritis in systemic lupus erythematosus. N Engl J Med 1956;255:41-42.

328. Gold AP, Yahr MD: Childhood lupus erythematosus. Trans Am Neurol Assoc 1960;85:96-102.

329. Steinlin MI, Blaser SI, Gilday DL, et al: Neurologic manifestations of pediatric systemic lupus erythematosus. Pediatr Neurol 1995;13:191-197.

330. Parikh S, Swaiman KF, Kim Y: Neurologic characteristics of childhood lupus erythematosus. Pediatr Neurol 1995;13:198-201.

331. Harel L, Mukamel M, Brik R, et al: Peripheral neuropathy in pediatric systemic lupus erythematosus. Pediatr Neurol 2002;27:53-56.

332. Ryan MM, Tilton A, De Girolami U, et al: Pediatric mononeuritis multiplex, a report of three cases and review of the literature. Neuromuscular Disorders 2003; 13:751-756.

333. McCombe PA, Pollard JD, McLeod JG: Chronic inflammatory demyelinating polyradiculoneuropathy: A clinical and electrophysiological study of 92 cases. Brain 1987;110:1617-1630.

334. Goldberg M, Chitanondh H: Polyneuritis with albuminocytologic dissociation in the spinal fluid in systemic lupus erythematosus: Report of a case, with review of pertinent literature. Am J Med 1959;27:342-350.

335. Bailey AA, Sayre GP, Clark EC: Neuritis associated with systemic lupus erythematosus. Arch Neurol Psychiatry 1956;75:251-259.

336. Puusa A, Lang HA, Mäkelä A-L: Nerve conduction velocity in juvenile rheumatoid arthritis. Acta Neurol Scand 1986;73:145-150.

337. Peñas PF, Porras JI, Fraga J, et al: Microscopic polyangiitis: A systemic vasculitis with positive P-ANCA. Br J Dermatol 1996;134:542-547.

338. Ford FR: Diseases of the Nervous System in Infancy, Childhood, and Adolescence, 5th ed. Springfield, IL, Charles C Thomas, 1966, pp 825-829.

339. Draaisma JM, Fiselier TJ, Mullaart RA: Mononeuritis multiplex in a child with cutaneous polyarteritis. Neuropediatrics 1992;23:28-29.

340. Rottem M, Fauci AS, Hallahan CW, et al: Wegener granulomatosis in children and adolescents: Clinical presentation and outcome. J Pediatr 1993;122:26-31.

341. Guillevin L, Cohen P, Gayraud M, et al: Churg-Strauss syndrome: Clinical study and long-term follow-up of 96 patients. Medicine 1999;78:26-37.

342. Belman AL, Leicher CR, Moshe SL, Mezey AP: Neurologic manifestations of Schönlein-Henoch purpura: Report of three cases and review of the literature. Pediatrics 1985;75:687-692.

343. Sabin TD, Swift TR, Jacobson RR: Leprosy. *In* Dyck PJ, Thomas PK (eds): Peripheral Neuropathy, 3rd ed. Philadelphia, WB Saunders, 1993, pp 1354-1379.

344. Solbrig MV, Mozaffar T, Kim RC: Hansen's disease (leprosy). *In* Jones HR, De Vivo DC, Darras BT (eds): Neuromuscular Disorders of Infancy, Childhood, and Adolescence: A Clinician's Approach. Philadelphia, Butterworth Heinemann Health, 2003, pp 505-519.

345. McGovern JP, Merritt DH: Sarcoidosis in childhood. Adv Pediatr 1956;8:97-135.

346. Le Luyer B, Devaux AM, Dailly R, Ensel P: Polyradiculoneuritis as a manifestation of childhood sarcoidosis. Arch Fr Pediatr 1983;40:175-178.

347. Williams CL, Strobino B, Lee A, et al: Lyme disease in childhood: Clinical and epidemiologic features of ninety cases. Pediatr Infect Dis J 1990;9:10-14.

348. Belman AL, Iyer M, Coyle PK, Dattwyler R: Neurologic manifestations in children with North American Lyme disease. Neurology 1993;43:2609-2614.

349. Eeg-Olofsson O, Peterson I: Childhood diabetic neuropathy: A clinical and neurophysiological study. Acta Paediatr Scand 1966;55:163-176.

350. Gamstorp I, Shelburne SA Jr, Engleson G, et al: Peripheral neuropathy in juvenile diabetics. Diabetes 1966;15:411-416.

351. Hoffman WH, Hart ZH, Frank RN: Correlates of delayed motor nerve conduction and retinopathy in juvenile-onset diabetes mellitus. J Pediatr 1983;102:351-356.

352. Lawrence DG, Locke S: Neuropathy in children with diabetes mellitus. BMJ 1963;1:784-785.

353. Gallai V, Firenze C, Mazzota G, Del Gatto F: Neuropathy in children and adolescents with diabetes mellitus. Acta Neurol Scand 1988;78:136-140.

354. White NH, Waltman SR, Krupin T, Santiago JV: Reversal of neuropathic and gastrointestinal complications related to diabetes mellitus in adolescents with improved metabolic control. J Pediatr 1981;99:41-45.

355. Atkin SL, Coady AM, Horton D, et al: Multiple cerebral haematomata and peripheral nerve palsies associated with a case of juvenile diabetic ketoacidosis. Diabet Med 1995;12:267-270.

356. Arbus GS, Barnor NA, Hsu AC, et al: Effect of chronic renal failure, dialysis, and transplantation on motor nerve conduction velocity in children. Can Med Assoc J 1975;113:517-520.

357. Alderson K, Seay A, Brewer E, Petajan J: Neuropathies in children with chronic renal failure treated by hemodialysis. Neurology 1985;35(Suppl 1):94.

358. Kuwabara S, Nakajima M, Tsuboi Y, Hirayama K: Multifocal conduction block in *n*-hexane neuropathy. Muscle Nerve 1993;16:1416-1417.

359. Burns TM, Shneker BF, Juel VC: Gasoline sniffing multifocal neuropathy. Pediatr Neurol 2001;25:419-421.

360. Stafford CR, Bogdanoff BM, Green L, Spector HB: Mononeuropathy multiplex as a complication of amphetamine angiitis. Neurology 1975 Jun;25(6):570-572.

361. Ouvrier RA, McLeod JG, Pollard JD: Toxic neuropathies. *In* Ouvrier RA, McLeod JG, Pollard JD: Peripheral Neuropathy in Childhood, 2nd ed. London, Mac Keith, 1999, pp 201-210.

362. Swaiman KF, Flagler DG: Mercury poisoning with central and peripheral nervous system involvement treated with penicillamine. Pediatrics 1971;48:639-641.

363. Hildebrandt G, Holler E, Woenkhaus M, et al: Acute deterioration of Charcot-Marie-Tooth disease IA (CMT IA) following 2 mg of vincristine chemotherapy. Ann Oncol 2000;11:743-747.

364. Igarashi M, Thompson EI, Rivera GK: Vincristine neuropathy in type I and type II Charcot-Marie-Tooth disease (hereditary motor sensory neuropathy). Med Pediatr Oncol 1995;25:113-116.

365. Chaudhry V, Chaudhry M, Crawford TO, et al: Toxic neuropathy in patients with pre-existing neuropathy. Neurology 2003;60:337-340.

366. Giannini F, Volpi N, Rossi S, et al: Thalidomide-induced neuropathy: A ganglionopathy? Neurology 2003; 60:877-878.

367. Fleming FJ, Vytopil M, Chaitow J, et al: Thalidomide neuropathy in childhood. Neuromuscular Disorders 2005;15:172-176.

368. MacLean WC, Graham GG: Vegetarianism in children. Am J Dis Child 1980;134:513-519.

369. Kühne T, Bubl R, Baumgartner R: Maternal vegan diet causing a serious infantile neurological disorder due to vitamin B_{12} deficiency. Eur J Pediatr 1991;150:205-208.

370. Yabuki S, Nakaya K, Sugimura T, et al: Juvenile polyneuropathy due to vitamin B_1 deficiency—clinical observations and pathogenetic analysis of 24 cases. Folia Psychiatr Neurol 1976;30:517-529.

371. Elias E, Muller DPR, Scott J: Association of spinocerebellar disorders with cystic fibrosis or chronic childhood cholestasis and very low serum vitamin E. Lancet 1981;2:1319-1321.

372. Werlin SL, Harb JM, Swick H, Blank E: Neuromuscular dysfunction and ultrastructural pathology in children with chronic cholestasis and vitamin E deficiency. Ann Neurol 1983;13:291-296.

373. Rosenblum JL, Keating JP, Prensky AL, Nelson JS: A progressive neurologic syndrome in children with chronic liver disease. N Engl J Med 1981;304:503-508.

374. Simonati A, Battistella PA, Guariso G, et al: Coeliac disease associated with peripheral neuropathy in a child: A case report. Neuropediatrics 1998;29:155-158.

375. Asbury AK, Gale MK, Cox SC, et al: Giant axonal neuropathy: A unique case with segmental neurofilamentous masses. Acta Neuropathol 1972;20:237-247.

376. Berg BO, Rosenberg SH, Asbury AK: Giant axonal neuropathy. Pediatrics 1972;49:894-899.

377. Igisu H, Ohta M, Tabira T, et al: Giant axonal neuropathy: A clinical entity affecting the central as well as the peripheral nervous system. Neurology 1975;25:717-721.

378. Gambarelli D, Hassoun J, Pellissier JF, et al: Giant axonal neuropathy: Involvement of peripheral nerve, myenteric plexus, and extraneuronal area. Acta Neuropathol 1977;39:261-269.

379. Kuhlenbaumer G, Young P, Oberwittler C, et al: Giant axonal neuropathy (GAN): case report and two novel mutations in the gigaxonin gene. Neurology 2002 Apr 23;58(8):1273-1276. Erratum in: Neurology 2002 May 14;58(9):1444.

380. Ouvrier RA: Giant axonal neuropathy: A review. Brain Dev 1989;11:207-214.

381. Bruno C, Bertini E, Federico A, et al: Clinical and molecular findings in patients with giant axonal neuropathy (GAN). Neurology 2004 Jan 13; 62(1):13-16.

382. Bomont P, Cavalier L, Blondeau F, et al: The gene encoding gigaxonin, a new member of the cytoskeletal BTB/kelch repeat family, is mutated in giant axonal neuropathy. Nat Genet 2000;26:370-374.

383. Aicardi J, Castelein P: Infantile neuroaxonal dystrophy. Brain 1979;102:727-748.

384. Wakai S, Asanuma H, Tachi N, et al: Infantile neuroaxonal dystrophy: Axonal changes in biopsied muscle tissue. Pediatr Neurol 1993;9:309-311.

385. Ramaekers VT, Lake BD, Harding B, et al: Diagnostic difficulties in infantile neuroaxonal dystrophy: A clinicopathological study of eight cases. Neuropediatrics 1987;18:170-175.

386. Kóbor J, Javaid A, Omojola M: Cerebellar hypoperfusion in infantile neuroaxonal dystrophy. Pediatric Neurology 2005;32:137-139.

SUGGESTED READINGS

Burns TM, Ryan MR, Darras BT, Jones HR: Current therapeutic strategies for patients with polyneuropathies secondary to inherited metabolic disorders. Mayo Clin Proc 2003;78:858-868.

Chance PF, Lensch MW, Lipe H, et al: Hereditary neuralgic amyotrophy and hereditary neuropathy with liability to pressure palsies: Two distinct genetic disorders. Neurology 1994;44:2253-2257.

Darras BT, Jones HR: Diagnosis of pediatric neuromuscular disorders in the era of DNA analysis. Pediatr Neurol 2000;23:289-300.

De Vivo DC, Engel WK: Remarkable recovery of a steroid-responsive recurrent polyneuropathy. J Neurol Neurosurg Psychiatry 1970;33:62-69.

Duarte J, Cruz Martinez A, Rodriguez F, et al: Hypertrophy of multiple cranial nerves and spinal roots in chronic inflammatory demyelinating neuropathy. J Neurol Neurosurg Psychiatry 1999;67:685-687.

Dyck PJ, Karnes JL, Lambert EH: Longitudinal study of neuropathic deficit and nerve conduction abnormalities in hereditary motor and sensory neuropathy type 1. Neurology 1989;39:1302-1308.

Dyck PJ, Lais AC, Ohta M, et al: Chronic inflammatory polyradiculoneuropathy. Mayo Clin Proc 1975;50:621-637.

Elder GH, Hift RJ: Treatment of acute porphyria. Hosp Med 2001;62:422-425.

Escolar DM, Jones HR: Pediatric radial mononeuropathies: A clinical and electromyographic study of sixteen children with review of the literature. Muscle Nerve 1996;19:876-883.

Evidente VGH, Gwinn-Hardy KA, Cavinees JN, Gilman S: Hereditary ataxias. Mayo Clin Proc 2000;75:475-490.

Gabreels-Festen AA, Gabreels FJ, Joosten EM, et al: Hereditary neuropathy with liability to pressure palsies in childhood. Neuropediatrics 1992;23:138-143.

Hagberg B, Sourander P, Thoren L: Peripheral nerve changes in the diagnosis of metachromatic leucodystrophy. Acta Paediatr 1962;51(Suppl 135):63-71.

Hahn AF, Bolton CF, White CM, et al: Genotype-phenotype correlations in X-linked dominant Charcot-Marie-Tooth disease. Ann N Y Acad Sci 1999;883:366-382.

Herskowitz A, Ishii N, Schaumburg H: n-Hexane neuropathy: A syndrome occurring as a result of industrial exposure. N Engl J Med 1971;285:82-85.

Jones HR: Mononeuropathies. In Jones HR, Bolton CF, Harper CM (eds): Pediatric Clinical Electromyography. Philadelphia, Lippincott-Raven, 1996, pp 171-250.

Jones HR Jr: Pediatric case studies. American Association of Electrodiagnostic Medicine (AAEM) Plenary Session: New Developments in Pediatric Neuromuscular Disease, Rochester, MN, AAEM, 1993, pp 51-60.

Jones HR, Hsu P: Pes cavus as the presenting sign of childhood neuropathies: EMG evaluation in 23 otherwise asymptomatic children [Abstract]. Muscle Nerve 1997;20:1070.

Katz DA, Scheinberg L, Horoupian DS, Salen G: Peripheral neuropathy in cerebrotendinous xanthomatosis. Arch Neurol 1984;42:1008-1010.

Kay SP: Obstetrical brachial palsy. Br J Plast Surg 1998;51:43-50.

King PJ, Morris JG, Pollard JD: Glue-sniffing neuropathy. Aust N Z J Med 1985;15:293-299.

Kline DG, Kim D, Midha R, et al: Management and results of sciatic nerve injuries: A 24-year experience. J Neurosurg 1998;89:13-23.

Kuritzky A, Berginer VM, Korczyn AD: Peripheral neuropathy in cerebrotendinous xanthomatosis. Neurology 1979;29:880-881.

Nance MA, Berry SA: Cockayne syndrome: Review of 140 cases. Am J Med Genet 1992;42:68-84.

Nass R, Chutorian A: Dysaesthesias and dysautonomia: A self-limited syndrome of painful dysaesthesias and autonomic dysfunction in childhood. J Neurol Neurosurg Psychiatry 1982;45:162-165.

Ohashi K, Ishibashi S, Osuga J, et al: Novel mutations in the microsomal triglyceride transfer protein gene causing abetalipoproteinemia. J Lipid Res 2000;41:1199-1204.

Orlowski JP, Clough JD, Dyment PG: Wegener's granulomatosis in the pediatric age group. Pediatrics 1978;61:83-90.

Ouvrier RA, McLeod JG, Morgan GJ, et al: Hereditary motor and sensory neuropathy of neuronal type with onset in early childhood. J Neurol Sci 1981;51:181-197.

Pellegrino JE, George RA, Biegel J, et al: Hereditary neuralgic amyotrophy: Evidence for genetic homogeneity and mapping to chromosome 17q25. Hum Genet 1997;101:277-283.

Prineas JW, McLeod JD: Chronic relapsing polyneuritis. J Neurol Sci 1976;27:247-258.

Prineas JW, Ouvrier RA, Wright RG, et al: Giant axonal neuropathy: A generalized disorder of cytoplasmic filament formation. J Neuropathol Exp Neurol 1976;35:458-470.

Roy EP, Gutmann L, Riggs JE: Longitudinal conduction studies in hereditary motor and sensory neuropathy type 1. Muscle Nerve 1989;12:52-55.

Rutkove SB: Effects of temperature on neuromuscular electrophysiology. Muscle Nerve 2001;24:867-882.

Wilbourn AJ: Electrodiagnostic testing of neurologic injuries in athletes. Clin Sports Med 1990;9:229-245.

Young RJ, Ewing DJ, Clarke BF: Nerve function and metabolic control in teenage diabetics. Diabetes 1983;32:142-147.

Young SG, Fielding CJ: The ABCs of cholesterol efflux. Nat Genet 1999;22:316-318.

Zerras K, Rudnik-Schöneborn S: Natural history in proximal spinal muscular atrophy. Arch Neurol 1995;52:518-523.

34

Autonomic Testing in Childhood

Monique M. Ryan, Ted M. Burns, and Nancy L. Kuntz

Although overt autonomic failure is rarely encountered in pediatric practice, a variety of inherited and acquired neuropathic processes cause autonomic dysfunction in infancy, childhood, and adolescence. In recent years the increasing availability of reproducible, noninvasive tests of autonomic function has enabled earlier detection and improved characterization of the autonomic neuropathies of adulthood. The remarkable expansion in our understanding of these disorders that has followed is due, in no small part, to the efforts of the pioneers in this field, including most notably Low and his colleagues from the Mayo Clinic. Pediatric autonomic disorders are much less well understood. Norms for pediatric subgroups and characteristic patterns of autonomic dysfunction in childhood remain relatively poorly characterized but are an area of great clinical and research interest.

ANATOMY

Central Autonomic System

The autonomic nervous system is an integral part of both the central and peripheral nervous systems. The central autonomic system includes the insula amygdala, medial prefrontal cortex, hypothalamus, ventrolateral medulla, nucleus of the tractus solitarius, nucleus parabrachialis, periaqueductal gray, and circumventricular organs. The central autonomic network mediates cardiovascular tone and visceral sensorimotor processing and integrates the autonomic and neuroendocrine systems.

Peripheral Autonomic System

The peripheral autonomic system has two major functional divisions: sympathetic and parasympathetic. In both, the preganglionic cell body of origin is sited in the central nervous system. Efferent axons exit the brainstem or spinal cord within the cranial nerve or ventral roots and then synapse within a peripheral autonomic ganglion. The body of the postsynaptic neuron is within the ganglion. The major axon projection of the postganglionic neuron terminates on smooth or cardiac muscle or on endocrine or exocrine gland.

The cell bodies of sympathetic preganglionic nerve fibers are located within the intermediolateral cell column of the thoracic and upper lumbar spinal cord (T1-L3): the *thoracolumbar system*. Fibers arising in the intermediolateral column are small, relatively short myelinated fibers: the *white rami communicantes*. These fibers exit the spinal cord then enter the sympathetic chain and may pass a number of segments up or down the chain before synapsing in a paravertebral ganglion.

Unmyelinated postganglionic fibers pass out of the sympathetic chain as the *gray rami communicantes*, subsequently entering spinal nerves or specialized autonomic nerves. A small subpopulation of preganglionic sympathetic fibers passes through the ganglion without synapsing. These fibers form synapses more distally, within the celiac, superior or inferior mesenteric ganglia, or directly innervate the adrenal medulla. The sympathetic nervous system is relatively diffuse and has the capacity to generate systemic responses through its innervation of the adrenal medulla and its high postganglionic-to-preganglionic fiber ratio.

Parasympathetic preganglionic cell bodies are sited within the brainstem cranial nuclei III, VII, IX, and X and the intermediolateral columns of the sacral (S2-4) regions: the *craniosacral system*. Preganglionic parasympathetic fibers are long, their ganglia lying relatively close to the target organs; therefore, the postganglionic fibers are quite short. This, and the relatively low parasympathetic postganglionic-to-preganglionic fiber ratio, renders the parasympathetic response relatively selective.

Preganglionic sympathetic and parasympathetic fibers are generally small myelinated B fibers, with a diameter of approximately 3 μm and conduction velocities of 3 to 15 m/sec. A few preganglionic parasympathetic fibers are unmyelinated. Acetylcholine is the neurotransmitter of most parasympathetic and sympathetic synapses and of presynaptic and postsynaptic parasympathetic neurons. The neurotransmitter of most postganglionic sympathetic neurons is norepinephrine (noradrenaline), although eccrine sweat glands are innervated by cholinergic postganglionic sympathetic neurons. Postganglionic axons are unmyelinated C fibers and small myelinated Aδ fibers. In adulthood, C fibers have a diameter of 0.25 to 1.35 μm, with conduction velocities between 0.5 and 2 m/sec, whereas Aδ fibers have diameters between 3 and 7 μm, with conduction velocities between 3 and 30 m/sec.

Autonomic involvement in neuropathies can affect the preganglionic autonomic neurons, postganglionic nerve bodies in sympathetic and parasympathetic ganglia, or postganglionic autonomic axons in peripheral nerves. Disorders of these systems are commonly classified according to the neurotransmitter of the affected postganglionic autonomic neuron: adrenergic (sympathetic), cholinergic (parasympathetic), or both (pandysautonomia).

Because postganglionic fibers are generally unmyelinated and are relatively inaccessible to electrical stimulation, standard methods of neurophysiologic testing are inadequate for assessment of autonomic function. Autonomic function is therefore more often assessed using a number of direct and indirect tests of sympathetic and parasympathetic function, each targeting end-organ responses to specific physiologic or pharmacologic stimuli.

Enteric Nervous System

The enteric nervous system functions as a separate division of the autonomic nervous system. The activity of gastrointestinal smooth muscle is modulated by extrinsic parasympathetic and sympathetic input, the intrinsic enteric nervous system, and locally produced neuropeptides that can act either as hormones or neurotransmitters. The excitatory postganglionic parasympathetic innervation to the gut originates in the vagus nerve and sacral segments S2-4. Postganglionic inhibitory sympathetic efferents to the

gastrointestinal system arise in the celiac, superior and inferior mesenteric ganglia and pass to the gut along the length of the corresponding arteries. The intrinsic enteric nervous system includes both the submucosal (Meissner's) plexus and the myenteric plexus sited between the outer (longitudinal) and inner (circular) layers of gut smooth muscles (Auerbach's plexus).[1]

Genitourinary Innervation

The detrusor muscle of the bladder is innervated by pelvic parasympathetic fibers arising from sacral segments S2-4 and passing through the pelvic plexus and nerves. The external sphincter of the bladder is also innervated by S2-4, through the pudendal nerves. The sympathetic nervous system supplies the bladder through projections from the sympathetic chain, although the significance of this in maintenance of continence is unclear.

Ontogenesis of the Autonomic Nervous System

Evolution of cardiovascular and thermoregulatory control in the fetus and infant are relatively well understood, with development of other autonomic systems being less well characterized. Catecholamines are present within the fetal adrenal medulla by 8 to 9 weeks gestational age, with reflex release being documented as early as 10 weeks.[2] Sympathetic function is relatively immature in early childhood, with most circulating catecholamines arising from the adrenal medulla rather than sympathetic innervation.

The cardiac parasympathetics are active from early in gestation, with a gradual fall in the baseline heart rate apparent from approximately 15 weeks of gestation to term. Vagal tone is relatively high in early childhood, which may explain why extreme bradycardia may occur in children after eyeball compression, sudden immersion in cold water, or the Valsalva maneuver.[3,4]

CLINICAL EVALUATION

Symptomatology

The clinical evaluation of a child with a suspected neuropathy should include inquiry as to symptoms referable to the autonomic system including orthostatic (postural) hypotension, sudomotor or secretomotor dysfunction, bladder or gastrointestinal involvement, and ophthalmic symptoms.

Orthostatic hypotension presents with dizziness, lightheadedness, near syncope, or syncope after standing. Some children are symptomatic only after precipitants such as hot baths, exercise, prolonged standing, or meals.[5] Syncope is relatively common in childhood and adolescence. At least 15% of children experience a syncopal episode before the end of the 2nd decade. Most of these are vasovagal in nature,[6,7] and in most cases a demonstrable trigger can be identified.[8] Paroxysmal hypertension and arrhythmias are occasionally seen in acute autonomic neuropathies and may be symptomatic if they cause significant impairment of cardiac output.

Sudomotor symptoms are investigated by asking the child or the parents whether they sweat on a hot day or after exercise. Autonomic dysfunction may manifest in the form of hypohidrosis or hyperhidrosis or localized abnormalities of sweat production such as gustatory sweating. Secretomotor function can be assessed by inquiry as to dry eyes, dry mouth, or impaired saliva production.

Gastrointestinal dysmotility in the autonomic neuropathies causes anorexia, early satiety, bloating, nausea, and vomiting. Diarrhea may alternate with constipation. Episodic vomiting is characteristic of familial dysautonomia, which can also be associated with pharyngeal incoordination. Weight loss may be prominent in children with gastroparesis.

Urinary retention, occasionally preceded by frequent micturition or incontinence, is seen in children with parasympathetic failure affecting the bladder. Nocturia and urinary frequency are also occasionally seen in the autonomic neuropathies. Sexual dysfunction is less frequently complained of in childhood but may manifest in the form of erectile or ejaculatory failure and retrograde ejaculation.

Children with impaired pupillary accommodation may complain of photophobia in bright sunlight, poor night vision, or difficulty focusing on near objects.

Postganglionic sympathetic dysfunction may be associated with small-fiber sensory dysfunction, resulting in paresthesia and lancinating pain of the extremities as well as anhidrosis or hyperhidrosis.

Clinical Evaluation of Autonomic Function

Blood Pressure and Heart Rate

Blood pressure and heart rate are best measured with an appropriately sized cuff (1) in the supine position after 5 to 10 minutes of rest and (2) after standing for 3 to 5 minutes. If orthostatic hypotension is suspected but not detected, the child is asked to perform light exercise, such as 10 squats, before rechecking the blood pressure. Orthostasis is a symptomatic reduction in systolic blood pressure greater than 20 mmHg on standing, with a concomitant drop in diastolic blood pressure greater than 10 mm Hg or a mean arterial blood pressure drop greater than 20 mm Hg, within 3 minutes of assuming the upright position.[9] Blood pressure recording should be repeated if abnormal.

Orthostatic hypotension reflects sympathetic dysfunction (adrenergic failure). On assumption of an upright posture, failure of normal splanchnic and lower extremity vasoconstriction causes dependent pooling of blood, decreased venous return, and a fall in cardiac output and systemic blood pressure. In children with adrenergic failure, there is no associated reflex tachycardia with orthostatic hypotension. In contrast, if reflex tachycardia is present, orthostatic falls in blood pressure may be secondary to hypovolemia or deconditioning.

Sudomotor Function

Dryness of the skin, whether global or regional, is clinically assessed by gently stroking the skin with the examiner's finger pads. Excessive sweating with blotching of the skin may be seen in children with acquired or familial dysautonomia.

Ophthalmic Function

Pupillary shape, size, and response to light and accommodation should be examined. Poorly reactive or unreactive (tonic) pupils are assessed by maintaining a strong light stimulus to the pupil for 1 minute. Corneal hypoesthesia and alacrima are common in children with familial dysautonomia. Ptosis may be seen in Horner's syndrome. Involuntary tear production in response to stimulation of the taste buds is termed a *gustolacrimal reflex* ("crocodile tears") and can occur unilaterally after facial nerve reinnervation, likely secondary to ephaptic transmission.

Vasomotor and Trophic Functions

Vasomotor and trophic changes to the extremities and nail beds are important clues to the presence of distal sympathetic or toxic neuropathies.

LABORATORY EVALUATION OF AUTONOMIC FUNCTION

Although clinical assessment may raise the possibility of autonomic involvement in neuropathic processes, laboratory evaluation is commonly required to confirm the location, distribution, and severity of autonomic dysfunction. Autonomic function is assessed using tests of sympathetic and parasympathetic responses to a range of physiologic or pharmacologic stimuli, each test reflecting function of a complex reflex arc. A range of investigations is required to adequately assess all aspects of autonomic function (Box 34-1). These investigations are quantitative, noninvasive procedures, which are of known sensitivity and specificity in adulthood.[10] Normal values are generally less well-established in childhood.

BOX 34-1
TESTS OF AUTONOMIC FUNCTION

Sympathetic Sudomotor
Quantitative sudomotor axon reflex testing
Thermoregulatory sweat test
Sympathetic skin response

Sympathetic Vasomotor
Beat-to-beat blood pressure responses to the Valsalva
    maneuver
Heart rate and blood pressure responses to
    head-up tilt
Pressor responses

Parasympathetic
Heart rate response to Valsalva maneuver
    (Valsalva ratio)
Heart rate response to standing (30:15 ratio)
Heart rate response to deep breathing
R-R interval variation

Autonomic function testing may be confounded by a number of variables, many of which can be controlled in childhood. Testing should be performed in a laboratory with experience in testing of children, preferably one with established age-appropriate norms for each investigation. Children should not be tested when acutely unwell or distressed. Where possible, all medications with potential effects on sympathetic or parasympathetic function should be discontinued at least 48 hours prior to testing. This includes diuretics, opioids, caffeine, and nicotine in addition to anticholinergic, sympathomimetic, and parasympathomimetic medications.

Quantitative Sudomotor Axon Reflex Test

Sweating, or sudomotor function, can be assessed by assessment of sweating patterns and quantity after elevation of body temperature, or by injection or local iontophoresis of cholinergic agents. Sudomotor function varies with temperature, age, and gender. Women produce approximately half the sweat volume of men.[10] At birth the body has a full complement of active sweat glands, which regress with increasing age.

The quantitative sudomotor axon reflex test (QSART) evaluates the function of postganglionic sympathetic cholinergic sudomotor fibers. In the QSART, iontophoresed acetylcholine activates sudomotor sympathetic C fibers,

which conduct antidromically to a branch point. These action potentials then reverse down a neighboring fiber, flowing orthodromically to the nerve terminal and causing release of acetylcholine to muscarinic receptors in sweat glands and activation of sweating. Sweat is captured in multicompartment cells and quantified using a sudorometer. Several sites are routinely tested—most commonly proximal foot, distal leg, proximal leg, and medial forearm.[11] Hyperhidrosis is common in the early stages of diabetic neuropathy,[12] distal hypohidrosis or anhidrosis being seen in neuropathies with significant postganglionic sudomotor dysfunction. Figure 34-1 shows normal QSART potentials recorded from a 9-year-old boy.

Thermoregulatory and Other Sweat Tests

The thermoregulatory sweat test (TST) measures sweat production after exposure to controlled heat produced by infrared lights in conditions of regulated humidity. Prior to heating, patients are painted with cornstarch, sodium carbonate, and alizarin red, a mixture that changes color when moistened by sweat. The central temperature is monitored by a thermal probe in the patient's mouth, skin probes simultaneously measuring the surface temperature. When the body temperature is elevated by 1°C or to more than 38°C, the patient is removed from the heating cabinet, and with the use of digital photography, the percentage of body demonstrating a normal sweat pattern is determined by a pixel count. The TST reflects both preganglionic and postganglionic sympathetic function and is complementary to the QSART in differentiating preganglionic versus postganglionic disorders. The TST reliably demonstrates both hyperhidrosis and anhidrosis in patients with autonomic neuropathies.[13]

Hyperhidrosis may be idiopathic or related to autonomic hyperreflexia. Patterns of hypohidrosis or anhidrosis may give insight into the underlying pathologic process. Distal changes are seen in the peripheral neuropathies, focal changes with peripheral nerve lesions, segmental loss after spinal cord injuries or sympathectomies, and global changes with diffuse disorders such as progressive autonomic failure or multisystem atrophy. The high activity level of young children can create technical difficulties with performance of TSTs. Figures 34-2 and 34-3 show normal and abnormal TSTs recorded from children.

Sudomotor function can also be quantified by iontophoresis of 2 mA of pilocarpine, for 5 minutes, to a 1 cm^2 area over the dorsum of the foot, and measurement of sweat production after taking a Silastic imprint of the tested area of skin. Electron microscopic examination of this Silastic imprint enables measurement of the number, size, and volume of the sweat beads produced. In the

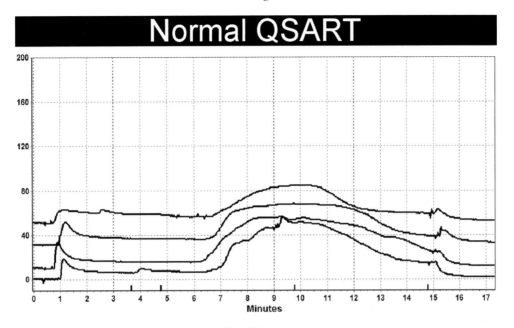

FIGURE 34–1

Normal quantitative sudomotor axon reflex test (QSART). These tracings demonstrate the sudomotor axon reflex in a 9-year-old boy in response to 1 mA of constant current applied for 5 minutes through each of four iontophoresis capsules. The locations of the recordings are (from top to bottom) *forearm, proximal leg, distal leg, and foot.*

Silastic imprint test, iontophoresed pilocarpine directly stimulates sweat glands rather than mediating an axon reflex. The Silastic imprint test may therefore be diagnostic even when the QSART response is absent.[14]

Sympathetic Skin Response

The sympathetic skin response (SSR) reflects changes in skin resistance in response to arousal stimuli such as electrical stimulation, deep inspiration, cough, and startle. The SSR measures sympathetic sudomotor function and can be recorded over the palm or sole, with reference electrodes placed over the dorsum of the hand or foot.[15] Responses are of variable amplitude and latency, and normal values are not well established in childhood, but asymmetric or absent responses may be significant in patients with sympathetic sudomotor or vasomotor dysfunction.[16,17] One weakness of this technique is that the response habituates quickly, and repeated attempts to elicit the response can cause it to attenuate.

Beat-to-Beat Blood Pressure and Heart Rate Responses to the Valsalva Maneuver

In the Valsalva maneuver children are asked to inhale deeply, then exhale forcibly into a mouthpiece connected to a manometer, maintaining an expiratory pressure of 40 mm Hg for 15 to 20 seconds while the blood pressure and heart rate are continuously monitored. Testing should be repeated until two similar responses are obtained. Four phases of the Valsalva response are recognized,[18] and they are demonstrated in Figure 34-4:

- Phase I: Expiration causes mechanical compression of the aorta and a rise in abdominal, thoracic, and blood pressure. The increased blood pressure causes a reflex increase in vagal tone, usually causing a decreased heart rate.
- Phase II: Continued expiration against resistance further increases the intrathoracic pressure, impeding venous return, decreasing stroke volume, and causing a fall in the blood pressure (early phase II [II$_e$]), which triggers reflex tachycardia and vasoconstriction mediated by increased sympathetic outflow and decreased parasympathetic activity, causing a recovery in the blood pressure (late phase II [II$_l$]). The phase II$_l$ is a sensitive marker of adrenergic cardiovascular function.
- Phase III: Expiration is completed. The intrathoracic pressure falls, causing the pulmonary venous capacitance to increase and leading to a fall in venous return, a fall in the blood pressure, and an increased heart rate.
- Phase IV: Venous return recovers, increasing cardiac output. Because of persisting increased systemic adrenergic cardiovascular activity, there is a rebound overshoot in systemic blood pressure over baseline, causing reflex, vagally mediated bradycardia.

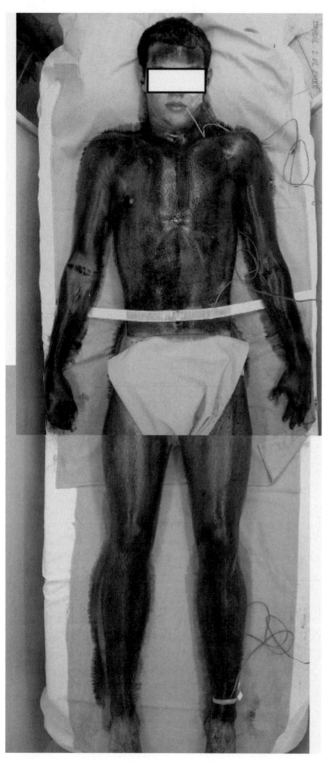

FIGURE 34–2
Normal thermoregulatory sweat test in a 16-year-old boy.

Phases I and III reflect mechanical changes in blood vessel capacitance, phases II_1 and IV_1 reflecting the effect of baroreceptor activation and resultant sympathetic and parasympathetic outflow. Autonomic neuropathies cause characteristic changes in the physiologic responses to the Valsalva maneuver. Sympathetic nervous system dysfunction causes failure of peripheral vasoconstriction in phase II_1, causing failure of blood pressure recovery in phase II_1 and absence of the normal blood pressure overshoot and reflex bradycardia in phase IV. Abnormal parasympathetic nervous system function results in decreased vagal tone and loss of the usual relative bradycardia following phase IV.

The *Valsalva ratio* (VR) is the ratio of the longest R-R interval during phase IV to that of the shortest R-R interval of phase II and can be used as a marker of cardiovagal function. Alternatively, the VR can be calculated by dividing tachycardia during phase II_1 by the reflex bradycardia following phase IV (within 30 seconds of phase III). The VR diminishes minimally with increasing age.[10] Other factors altering the VR include gender, positioning of the subject, expiratory pressure, duration of effort, inspiratory volume, volume status, and medications.[10] Normal values have been described in children older than 7 years of age.[19]

Heart Rate and Blood Pressure Responses to Active Standing and Head-Up Tilt

Orthostatic hypotension is the cardinal symptom of adrenergic dysfunction. Many children, especially those with vasovagal syncope, have normal baseline physical examinations, and on routine clinical testing no abnormalities will be identified. Provocative testing is often necessary to demonstrate a tendency to orthostatic hypotension, which can be identified and quantified either on active standing or on prolonged head-up tilt from a supine to erect position. Active standing is perhaps more physiologic and requires less equipment but can be difficult for children with neuromuscular disorders.

The standard laboratory test for orthostatic hypotension is the head-up tilt test, which uses a table with a supportive footboard and an electric motor controlling positioning of the patient at variable angulation. After a resting period (10 to 30 minutes) in the supine position patients are brought upright, usually to an angle of 60, 70, or 80 degrees (although an angle of 90 degrees might seem more physiologic, an excessive false-positive rate is often obtained at this elevation). Over the following 10 to 45 minutes the electrocardiogram and blood pressure are continuously monitored, the latter by finger plethysmography or arterial tonometry. In some laboratories infusions of isoproterenol are used as a provocative agent.

With active standing the fastest heart rate (shortest R-R interval) usually occurs around the 15th heartbeat, followed

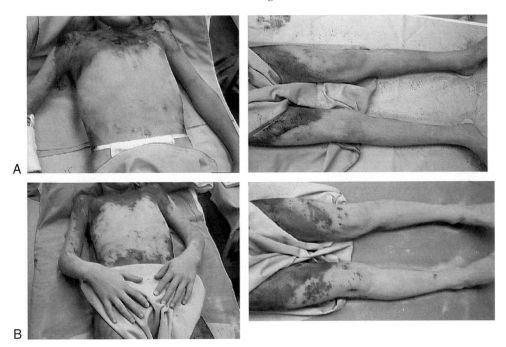

FIGURE 34–3

A, Abnormal thermoregulatory sweat test (TST) demonstrating anhidrosis over much of the trunk and distal extremities in a 7-year-old boy with an acquired inflammatory sensory and autonomic neuropathy. This child experienced severe distal neuropathic pain, gastrointestinal dysmotility, and blood pressure instability with slow clinical recovery over 3 to 4 months. B, A follow-up TST 1 year later demonstrated persistently decreased sweating over the trunk and distal extremities.

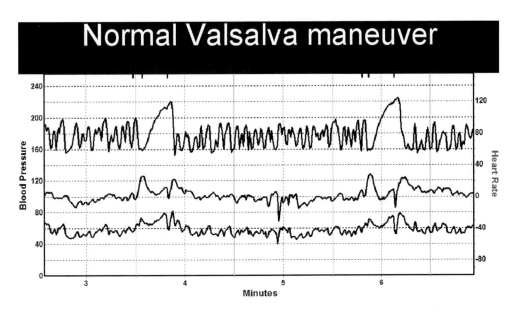

FIGURE 34–4

Valsalva maneuver. This figure demonstrates response to two Valsalva maneuvers performed several minutes apart by an 8-year-old boy. The upper tracing displays the heart rate. The lower two tracings demonstrate systolic and diastolic blood pressures. At the top of the figure, two narrowly spaced hatch marks indicate onset of the Valsalva maneuver. The single hatch mark 15 seconds later indicates completion of the maneuver. The Valsalva ratio (VR) is calculated by dividing the maximum heart rate generated by the Valsalva maneuver by the lowest heart rate occurring within 30 seconds of that peak heart rate. Here, the VR is approximately 2.

by maximal slowing around the time of the 30th heartbeat (longest R-R interval). The ratio of the longest-to-shortest R-R interval (30:15 ratio) should be greater than 1. If there is no change in heart rate on active standing, as is the case with vagal (parasympathetic) dysfunction, the 30:15 ratio is 1 or less.

The normal response to the head-up tilt test is a mild tachycardia, of the order of a 10- to 20- beats/min increase in the heart rate. The systolic blood pressure remains stable, the diastolic and mean blood pressures increasing slightly. Abnormal responses include vasovagal syncope, a dysautonomic response, and orthostatic intolerance.

Children with vasovagal syncope usually tolerate the first few minutes after tilting or active standing without difficulty. Five to 30 minutes after tilting, however, affected children develop nausea, sweatiness, and dizziness. Simultaneously there is an initial slow fall in the blood pressure, followed by an abrupt fall in blood pressure and heart rate, which may culminate in asystole, loss of consciousness, and, as a release phenomenon, muscular movements resembling a seizure.[20] A similar clinical phenomenon associated with cerebral hypoperfusion without systemic hypotension— cerebral syncope—has recently been described in childhood.[21] The pathogenesis of vasovagal syncope remains poorly understood. Physiologically inappropriate vagally mediated bradycardia and vasodilation may arise because of ventricular hypercontractility, although this theory is not universally accepted.[22]

Children with true orthostatic hypotension experience a fall in systolic blood pressure of more than 20 mm Hg on standing, with a concomitant drop in diastolic blood pressure of more than 10 mm Hg, within 3 minutes of assuming the upright position.[9] Concomitant failure of compensatory tachycardia is seen in patients with generalized (sympathetic and parasympathetic) autonomic dysfunction. In children with sparing of cardiac adrenergic innervation, the heart rate response is preserved. Mild adrenergic impairment may be associated with excessive blood pressure oscillations, an excessive reduction (>50%) in pulse pressure, an excessive (>30 beats/min) increment in heart rate, or a transient decrease in systolic blood pressure.

Children with severe cyanotic breath-holding spells demonstrate a decrease in diastolic blood pressure, without an increase in systolic blood pressure, on assuming upright posture. These children also demonstrate a significantly lower 30:15 ratio than controls.[23]

In adults, postural orthostatic tachycardia syndrome (POTS) characteristically results in an increase in the heart rate of at least 30 beats/min (to a rate > 130 beats/min), within 10 minutes of the head-up tilt, and without a significant decline in blood pressure. Diagnostic difficulty arises in children and adolescents when they become symptomatic during a tilt test with stable blood pressure and a greater than 30 beats/min increase in heart rate that still does not reach the proscribed 130 beats/min heart rate. For example, adolescents with resting heart rates of 52 beats/min can become symptomatic during a tilt test, more than doubling their heart rate to 120 beats/min, and still not meet the adult POTS criteria of a heart rate greater than 130 beats/min. Additional normative data need to be collected for children and adolescents to more reliably ascribe significance to observed changes.

In normal adult subjects, tilt testing results in positive responses in 0 to 65% of patients, depending on the protocol used. False-positive responses are obtained in 40% to 60% of children, possibly because of a heightened anxiety response to placement of an intravenous line prior to testing.[24-27] Sensitivity may be improved by use of a protocol employing a head-up tilt of no more than 70 degrees for 10 minutes or less.[27]

Heart Rate Response to Deep Breathing

Heart rate variation with the respiratory cycle, the phenomenon of *sinus arrhythmia*, is mediated by vagal efferent outflow. The heart rate usually increases with inspiration and decreases with expiration. The heart rate response to deep breathing (HR_{DB}) decreases with increasing age and is affected by the rate and depth of inspiration, but it is an accurate noninvasive gauge of parasympathetic cardiovagal function.[10] Patients are asked to breathe quietly for 5 minutes, then to breathe deeply once every 10 seconds for 1 minute. Changes in heart rate are most commonly measured in the form of changes in the R-R interval and are maximal at a breathing rate of 5 or 6 breaths/min (Fig. 34-5).[10] The standard deviation and the mean square of the successive difference of the R-R intervals are calculated for the period of deep breathing. The expiratory-to-inspiratory ratio is calculated for the period of deep breathing by dividing the longest R-R intervals during expiration (slowest heart rate [$R-R_{max}$]) by the shortest R-R intervals during inspiration (maximal heart rate [$R-R_{min}$]). The cycle is repeated and the values for three cycles of deep breathing are averaged. Positioning of the patient may alter the HR_{DB} and should be standardized. Other variables that may alter the HR_{DB} include salicylate medications and obesity. Compliance and effort are important. Normal values for HR_{DB} in children down to 5 years of age have been published but are based on small numbers of subjects.[19]

Children with pallid breath-holding spells have been shown to have less respiratory sinus arrhythmia than age-matched patients with cyanotic breath-holding spells or age-matched controls.[23]

An alternative measure of cardiovagal function is the 24-hour study of normal variation in heart rate variability,

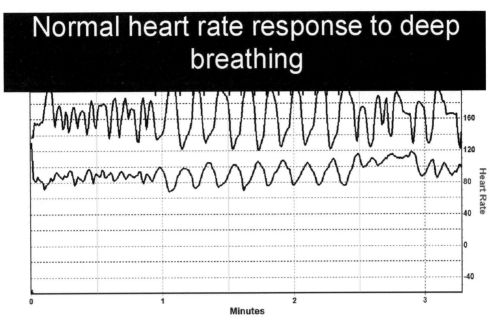

FIGURE 34–5

Heart rate response to deep breathing. This figure demonstrates a normal heart rate response to deep breathing in a 9-year-old girl. The upper trace monitors respiration (the rate can be calculated from the horizontal axis, which is labeled in minutes). The lower trace displays heart rate. The heart rate increases with inspiration and decreases with expiration.

recorded via ambulatory electrocardiographic (Holter) monitoring.[28] A number of indices of heart rate (R-R interval) variation are analyzed in the time domain, whereas commercially available programs are used to transform beat-beat fluctuations to the frequency domain by fast-Fourier transformation. Short-term oscillations in heart rate are transformed into a power spectrum, which is then broken down into frequency regions of interest. High-frequency bands (0.15 to 0.40 Hz) of the spectrum are thought to reflect parasympathetic (vagal) influences on the sinus node and can be heavily influenced by respiration.[29] Low-frequency bands (0.02 to 0.15 Hz) reflect both cholinergic and adrenergic activity.

Delayed maturation of cardiovagal function has been implicated in sudden infant death syndrome.[30,31] A loss of normal heart rate variability may be a sensitive marker of early cardiac autonomic neuropathy in childhood diabetes mellitus.[32] Heart rate variability was noted to normalize (increase) during sleep in patients with severe cyanotic breath-holding spells treated with supplemental iron.[33]

Quantitative Sensory Testing

Quantitative sensory testing (QST) objectively assesses and quantifies sensory function in patients at risk or with symptoms of neuropathy. QST determines the detection threshold of sensory stimuli and may be used to selectively test a number of discrete neuroanatomic pathways. The devices used administer increasingly or decreasingly strong calibrated physical (vibratory or thermal) or electrical stimuli.[34-36] Alternative methods require that patients report an increasingly strong stimulus, cease to detect a decreasingly strong stimulus (the method of limits), or identify whether or not a stimulus is felt (the method of levels).

This testing can be time consuming, and results with forced-choice algorithms may be affected by boredom or questions of secondary gain. Use of a 4, 2, 1 stepping algorithm with null stimuli may provide a more accurate estimate of sensory thresholds.[37] Measured sensory thresholds are also affected by the methods of testing, with normative standards varying between different devices. Quantitative testing of vibratory detection thresholds can be undertaken in children as young as 3 years of age, while thermal threshold detection can be performed from the age of 6 years. A number of recent studies have established normal values for cold and warm sensation and vibration detection thresholds in childhood.[38-40]

Analysis of Intraepidermal Nerve Fiber Density

The epidermis is abundantly innervated by nerve fibers originating from the dorsal root ganglia. These fibers are presumed to represent the terminal of C, and possibly Aδ, pain receptors. These can be defined by staining of skin (obtained by punch biopsy or suction blisters) with methylene blue or silver or by immunostaining for axonal markers. The punch skin biopsy has recently been established as a means of quantification of C and Aδ fibers within the skin. Intraepidermal nerve fiber density (IENFD) is significantly reduced, in a length-dependent fashion, in adults with small-fiber sensory neuropathies.[41] Nerve fiber loss correlates with abnormalities on clinical examination, neurophysiologic tests,[42] and QST.[35] This approach is less invasive, less laborious, and possibly more accurate than the alternative method of electron microscopic analysis of the small myelinated and unmyelinated fiber populations on sural nerve biopsy.[43]

IENFD analysis is technically challenging, however, and is best done in a center with expertise in this technique. Whether IENFD measurement will become an integral diagnostic tool in routine clinical practice remains to be determined. At this time, there is little collective experience of the use of IENFD in young children.

Intradermal Histamine Testing

The intradermal injection of histamine usually results in a phenomenon known as the *triple response*. The components of this response include (1) appearance, within a few seconds, of a localized erythematous reaction extending for several millimeters around the area of the injection, (2) a brighter flush, or "flare" developing over a slightly larger area (≈1 cm) over the next 10 to 20 seconds, and (3) a raised wheal, in the same area as the original erythematous area, developing over the next 1 to 2 minutes. Phase 1 is caused by the direct vasodilatory effect of histamine, phase 2 by histamine-induced stimulation of an axon reflex mediated by polymodal C-receptors causing further vasodilation, and phase 3 by local histamine-induced edema. Histamine is commonly available as a parenteral preparation of histamine phosphate.[44]

Testing is usually performed on the forearm, using 0.1 mL of 0.05 mg/cc histamine phosphate.[45] Intradermal histamine is commonly used as the "control" during intradermal allergy testing. The intradermal histamine test is used primarily in assessment of suspected hereditary sensory and autonomic neuropathies (HSANs), wherein abnormalities of the axon reflex cause failure of the flare response to histamine injection.

Pressor Responses

Isometric exercise, cold stimuli, and mental stress all cause increased sympathetic vasoconstrictor activity and, hence, increased blood pressure. Testing of these "pressor" responses reflects sympathetic nervous system function.

TABLE 34-1. TESTS OF PUPILLARY FUNCTION

Function	Autonomic System Tested
Pupillary response to light and accommodation	Parasympathetic
Pupillary pharmacologic tests	
0.125% Pilocarpine	Parasympathetic
2% Isonephrine, 4% cocaine	Postganglionic sympathetic
1% Omatropine	Sympathetic

Compliance with these tests is, however, difficult to achieve in young children. In adolescents, testing methods and normal values are no different than those used in the adult population.[46]

Assessment of Pupillary Responses

A combination of pharmacologic and infrared methods allows for the assessment of pupillary reflexes (Table 34-1). This can be of use in assessment of a variety of autonomic neuropathies.[47] In recent years the increasing availability of computer-based infrared video instruments has enabled convenient, quick, and noninvasive measurement of pupillometry in the clinical setting.[48]

Pupillometry is most frequently used for monitoring of parasympathetic pupillary function in children with diabetes mellitus. Impaired pupillary adaptation to darkness is common in patients with longstanding or poorly controlled diabetes mellitus. Pupillary parasympathetic dysfunction occurs before involvement of pupillary sympathetic innervation and appears to precede involvement of the cardiovascular system in diabetic autonomic neuropathy.[49] Loss of normal pupillary reflexes is seen in as many as 14% of children with adolescent diabetes[49] and is linked to both duration of disease and poor diabetic control.[50-52]

Other uses of pupillometry include differentiation of Horner's syndrome from physiologic anisocoria and quantification of relative afferent pupillary defects.

Assessment of Gastrointestinal Motility

Abnormalities of gastrointestinal motility can be investigated with a variety of anatomic and functional studies. In cases of suspected dysmotility, an early priority is the exclusion of mechanical gastrointestinal obstruction by radiography and videocinefluoroscopy, barium studies, and endoscopy.

Manometric studies are the most frequently used and best validated tests of gut motility.[53-55] Fasting and postprandial manometry can be used to identify abnormalities of esophageal, gastric, small bowel, and colonic motility[56] and can differentiate between neuropathic and myopathic causes of intestinal pseudo-obstruction.[57]

Other investigations to be considered include radionuclide scintigraphy, a noninvasive measure of gastric emptying.[54] This test requires ingestion of a meal labeled with radionuclides, with determination either of the percentage of the meal retained, or emptied, after a set period, or the time required for emptying 50% of the meal. Normal ranges are affected by age, obesity, and menstrual cycle.[58] The technique has been used to evaluate gastrointestinal motility in children with functional dyspepsia,[59] but normative data from age-matched children do not exist and are not likely to be collected from asymptomatic children due to ethical concerns. Radioactive tracers incorporated into standardized meals can be used to scintigraphically monitor small intestine and colonic transit times in adults,[60] whereas an intravenous radioactive tracer excreted into bile and delivered to the duodenum (Tc-HIDA) has also been used to evaluate small bowel transit time in adults.[61] These methods are not well established in pediatric practice.

A gastric emptying test using measurement of breath $^{13}CO_2$ after ingestion of radiolabeled foodstuffs has been correlated to scintigraphic gastric emptying times in adults.[62-64] The same concerns about lack of normative data in children are pertinent, although this method has been successfully used to measure orocecal transit times in childhood.[65] Three-dimensional single-photon emission computed tomography (SPECT) scanning before and after a liquid meal labeled with technetium pertechnetate can provide information on fasting and postprandial gastric volumes, assessing gastric "accommodation."[66] This technique has been used to evaluate symptomatic children and adolescents.

Ultrasonography and electrogastrography are also useful in some cases. Ultrasonography is used for real-time evaluation of gastric wall motion and emptying, but interpretation of findings is somewhat subjective and requires significant expertise. Electrogastrography records electrical activity of gastric muscle via leads placed on the abdominal wall. The normal 3 cycle/min gastric contraction rhythm, tachygastrias (3.6 to 9.9 cycle/min) and bradygastrias (1.0 to 2.4 cycle/min) can be recorded in a noninvasive and reproducible fashion.[58]

Assessment of Genitourinary Function

Bladder function studies[67] are of use in specific situations in clinical pediatrics. Investigations that can be used to evaluate the micturition reflex include assessment of postvoid residual volume, urodynamic studies, intravenous pyelography, renal ultrasonography, urethral sphincter electromyography (EMG), and cystourethrography.

Sexual function may be assessed in older children by means of penile plethysmography and intracavernosal papaverine injections. Normal values for pudendal somatosensory evoked potentials produced with electrical stimulation of the dorsal nerve of the penis or clitoris have been reported in children between 3 and 13 years of age.[68] Mechanical stimulation also can be used, and may be better tolerated, in eliciting the bulbocavernosus reflex and pudendal somatosensory evoked potentials in boys.[69] These techniques have been used to evaluate the pathophysiology of primary nocturnal enuresis.[70] In practice these investigations are rarely indicated in childhood.

CLASSIFICATION OF AUTONOMIC NEUROPATHIES

Acute Autonomic Neuropathies

Guillain-Barré Syndrome (Acute Inflammatory Demyelinating Polyradiculoneuropathy)

Autonomic involvement is common in children with Guillain-Barré syndrome (GBS). Vasomotor symptoms with peripheral vasoconstriction and episodes of excessive sweating are seen in as many as 50% of these patients.[71] Constipation develops in approximately 40% of children and may be associated with an adynamic ileus.[72] Urinary symptoms are usually transient, with retention and/or incontinence developing in 10% of patients.[73-75]

Although a life-threatening dysautonomia is rare in children with GBS, when it does develop this usually occurs in the acute phase of the disease and tends to correlate with the severity of somatic involvement.[76] GBS has also been associated with a supraventricular tachycardia or bradycardia that may cause wide fluctuations in blood pressure with alternating hypertension and hypotension.[72,76] Heart block and asystole are also described. Autonomic testing may reveal abnormalities of tests of cardiovagal, sudomotor, vasomotor, and adrenergic function in children with GBS.[72,76,77]

Symptomatic autonomic instability in children with GBS necessitates close supervision in an intensive care setting with careful monitoring of heart rate and blood pressure.[78] An adequate blood volume should be maintained because there may be extreme sensitivity to volume depletion. Antihypertensive medications should be avoided where possible in patients with alternating paroxysmal hypertension and hypotension because of the risk of supersensitivity to these agents. Sustained severe hypertension may be treated with a combined alpha- and beta-adrenergic blocker. Constipation should be anticipated and treated aggressively. Adynamic ileus is an uncommon complication of GBS but warrants monitoring.[79]

Other Acute Autonomic Neuropathies of Childhood

Although it is rare to find other examples of acute dysautonomia during childhood, restricted forms of autonomic

TABLE 34–2. CLASSIFICATION OF PEDIATRIC AUTONOMIC NEUROPATHIES

Acute and Subacute Autonomic Neuropathies	*Chronic Autonomic Neuropathies*
Pandysautonomias	*Pandysautonomias*
Immune mediated	Hereditary neuropathies
Guillain-Barré syndrome	Hereditary sensory and
Idiopathic autonomic	autonomic neuropathies
(pandysautonomia)	Fabry's disease
Drug induced	Nerve growth factor
Cisplatinum	deficiency (?)
Vincristine	Hereditary motor and
Vacor	sensory neuropathies°
Amiodarone	Friedreich's ataxia°
Toxins	Chronic small-fiber
Heavy metals	neuropathies
Acrylamide	Diabetes
Organic solvents°	Idiopathic pure autonomic
Postoperative	failure
Regional sympathectomy	
Postvagotomy	
Postorgan transplantation	
Traumatic	
Spinal cord injury	
Inborn errors of metabolism	
Porphyria	
Cholinergic dysautonomia	*Pure adrenergic neuropathies*
Botulism	Chronic idiopathic anhidrosis
Acute cholinergic neuropathy	Lambert-Eaton myasthenic
	syndrome
	Adies' syndrome
	Chagas' disease
	Pure cholinergic neuropathies
	Dopamine beta-hydroxylase
	deficiency
	Disorders of reduced
	* orthostatic tolerance*
	Postural orthostatic
	tachycardia syndrome

°Autonomic dysfunction not clinically prominent.

neuropathy are occasionally described (Table 34-2).[81-87] These include the syndromes of acute idiopathic autoimmune neuropathy (IAN) (also known as acute pandysautonomia) and acute cholinergic neuropathy. Postural orthostatic tachycardia syndrome (POTS) can also be of acute or subacute onset.

An autoimmune basis for these syndromes is suggested by four factors. First, there is a frequent association with a preceding viral infection.[81,82,85,88] Second, autoantibodies to ganglionic acetylcholine receptors are now identified.[89] Third, well-documented responsiveness to immunomodulatory therapies is now recorded.[90,91] Finally, postmortem studies in some cases have identified inflammatory infiltrates in autonomic and sensory ganglia.[90,92]

Acute Idiopathic Autoimmune Neuropathy. This commonly involves symptoms both of sympathetic (orthostatic hypotension and anhidrosis) and parasympathetic failure (constipation or diarrhea, dry eyes, dry mouth, and disturbance of bladder function). Neurologic examination in IAN demonstrates orthostatic hypotension, a fixed heart rate, and tonic pupils. Muscle strength, muscle stretch reflexes, and sensation are generally normal, although mild distal sensory deficits may occur.

Nerve conduction studies are generally normal in IAN, although minor abnormalities are occasionally identified.[85] The TST demonstrates widespread anhidrosis. The QSART is also markedly abnormal, indicating postganglionic sudomotor sympathetic failure. There is a loss of normal heart rate variability and a reduction in phase II of the Valsalva maneuver. Sural nerve biopsy in IAN may be normal or may reveal varying degrees of axonal degeneration and myelin remodeling, whereas skin biopsy may show involvement of epidermal C fibers.[85]

Acute Cholinergic Neuropathies. In contrast with other autonomic polyneuropathies, here the abnormalities are limited to the postganglionic cholinergic neuron.[83,84] Children with pure cholinergic failure present with alacrima, blurred vision, xerostomia, dysphagia, anhidrosis, constipation, and urinary retention. Abnormalities of gastrointestinal motility dominate the clinical picture in some cases. Involvement of postganglionic sympathetic sudomotor fibers causes loss of sweating and a tendency to hyperthermia. Physical examination may reveal an elevated body temperature, dry skin, dilated and unresponsive pupils, tachycardia, abdominal distention, and decreased bowel sounds. Prior to the onset of cholinergic failure a transient phase of increased cholinergic activity may result in a brief period of increased salivation, sweating, and diarrhea.

Autonomic studies demonstrate a loss of heart rate variability to the Valsalva and other maneuvers, although a baseline tachycardia may be exacerbated by maneuvers that increase sympathetic tone. The TST and QSART are markedly abnormal. The pupils are exquisitely sensitive to cholinomimetics.

Therapy. Hyperthermia should be avoided. Supportive treatment of orthostatic hypotension and bowel and bladder symptoms is important. Orthostatic symptoms are managed with aggressive hydration, increased salt intake, and elevation of the head of the bed.[93] Parenteral nutrition may be required, whereas cholinergic medications such as bethanechol may improve bowel and bladder function. Pilocarpine eye drops and artificial tears relieve ocular symptoms. Artificial saliva may also relieve discomfort. Medications used for orthostatic hypotension include midodrine and fludrocortisone. Adults with IAN have responded to treatment with corticosteroids[90] and intravenous immunoglobulin.[91,94,95]

Outcome. IAN and acute cholinergic neuropathy are generally monophasic illnesses. In most affected children, recovery of function is delayed and incomplete.[81,82,85,86,88]

Postural Orthostatic Tachycardia Syndrome

Clinical Introduction. POTS is a heterogeneous entity that is primarily characterized by orthostatic tachycardia. The cardinal feature is upright tachycardia that is variably associated with hypotension and supine tachycardia. With standing, there is a heart rate increment of at least 30 beats/min, usually to more than 120 beats/min, which is associated with lightheadedness, palpitations, tremulousness, anxiety, and nausea. Symptoms may be episodic or cyclical, but many patients experience daily symptoms. Most cases occur in young women between the ages of 20 and 50 years,[96] but POTS is now increasingly recognized in childhood.[97] Orthostatic tachycardia is also identified in adolescent chronic fatigue syndrome.[98]

Pathogenesis. This is variable and poorly understood for POTS. Some patients appear to have a reduced plasma volume; others have poor vasomotor tone due to adrenergic denervation resulting in alpha$_1$-adrenergic hypersensitivity; and still others have venous pooling in the splanchnic system and lower extremities. A decreased beta$_1$-adrenergic sensitivity is another postulated mechanism. In a single family POTS has been linked to abnormal function of the norepinephrine reuptake transporter protein.[99]

Neurophysiologic Testing. Approximately 50% of patients with POTS show abnormalities on autonomic testing. These include distal sudomotor failure on the QSART and TST as well as excessive HR$_{DB}$ variability. There is increased beat-to-beat blood pressure variability on the Valsalva maneuver, with an exaggerated phase II$_e$ and reduced or absent phase II$_l$. Phase IV may be normal or may be excessively large. The HR response to tilt is abnormal, with excessive tachycardia on tilt-up. As discussed earlier, the limits to normal increment in HR with head-up tilt are less well established in youth. The situation is diagnostically compounded by the relative resting bradycardia noted in healthy, fit children and adolescents.

Patients with excessive venous pooling have a reduction in pulse pressure. Some patients have a hypertensive response. In contrast to children with neurogenic orthostatic hypotension, patients with neuropathic POTS have stable blood pressure on head-up tilting and no evidence of generalized autonomic failure. The differential diagnosis of POTS also includes deconditioning, hypovolemia, prolonged bed rest, medication effect, and anxiety disorders.

Management of POTS. This includes adequate hydration, a high-salt diet, and elevation of the head of the bed.[22,100] Patients with excessive venous pooling may benefit from support stockings or treatment with midodrine, whereas those with beta-receptor supersensitivity can be treated with low-dose beta-blockers. The prognosis of POTS appears to be generally favorable.[101]

Porphyria

Clinical Introduction. The hepatic porphyrias are occasionally seen in adolescence.[102] Autonomic dysfunction, usually manifesting as autonomic hyperactivity, is frequent in acute intermittent porphyria and may also occur in variegate porphyria. Clinical features include persistent tachycardia, abdominal pain, nausea and vomiting, severe constipation, diarrhea, bladder distention, hyperhidrosis, and hypohidrosis. Painless vomiting may occur, in association with hypertension and tachycardia. Sudden death is reported during exacerbations of porphyria, possibly as a result of cardiac arrhythmias.

Neurophysiologic Investigations. Autonomic studies demonstrate abnormal sympathetic and parasympathetic function related to involvement of the vagus nerve and sympathetic ganglia.[103,104]

Management. This particularly includes avoidance of porphyrogenic drugs and supportive treatment of acute attacks.[105]

Toxic Autonomic Neuropathies

Toxic neuropathy may result from single doses or chronic exposure to neuropathic agents. A number of medications, industrial agents, and heavy metals have been related to the development of autonomic neuropathies (Table 34-3).[106]

TABLE 34–3. TOXIC AUTONOMIC NEUROPATHIES

Toxic Agent	Autonomic Symptomatology
Cisplatinum	Orthostatic hypotension, secretomotor failure, paralytic ileus
Vincristine	Orthostatic hypotension, constipation, abdominal pain, ileus and urinary retention, abnormal cardiovascular responses
Vacor	Postural hypotension, gastrointestinal dysfunction[220]
Arsenic	Hypohidrosis or hyperhidrosis
Mercury	Tachycardia, hypertension, acrodynia, and excessive sweating[221]
Thallium	Tachycardia, hypertension, and loss of sweating[222,223]
Organophosphates	Cholinergic crisis sweating, miosis, abdominal cramps, diarrhea, muscle cramps and fasciculations, mental confusion, and coma[222]
Jimsonweed poisoning	Constipation, abdominal pain, ileus and urinary retention, abnormal cardiovascular responses
Glue sniffing	Sudomotor failure, vasomotor instability, postural hypotension, and erectile failure[224]

Botulism

Clinical Introduction. Botulism presents with ptosis, blurred vision, ophthalmoplegia, and bulbar weakness, with progression in a few cases to generalized neuromuscular paralysis. Cholinergic failure in this disorder results in anhidrosis, dry eyes and mouth, pupillary dilation, paralytic ileus, and urinary retention.[107] Postural hypotension is less common.[108] Botulism type B may be more frequently associated with significant cholinergic neuropathy.

Altered autonomic function is also common in infantile botulism, in which *Clostridium botulinum* spores multiply within the intestine, producing additional botulinum toxin. Affected infants present with skeletal, respiratory, and bulbar weakness accompanied by tachyarrhythmias, decreased pupillary responses, and ileus (see Chapter 35).[109]

Neurophysiologic Testing. Nerve conduction studies in botulism show reduced compound muscle action potential (CMAP) amplitudes, with facilitation after exercise and rapid repetitive motor nerve stimulation with prolonged post-tetanic facilitation. Single-fiber EMG may reflect a neuromuscular transmission defect with both blocking and increased jitter.[110]

Autonomic testing reveals abnormal cardiovagal function and orthostatic hypotension.[108] Adrenergic function recovers before parasympathetic function, which in turn tends to improve before the resolution of neuromuscular blockade.

Treatment. This is mainly supportive. Administration of botulinum antitoxin is not warranted in infantile botulism because of the risk of anaphylaxis. Human botulinum immunoglobulin may be of benefit when given early in the disease course.[111]

Childhood Breath-holding

Clinical Introduction. Breath-holding spells of early childhood are involuntary stereotyped behavioral episodes most commonly seen in infancy, during which period they may affect as many as 5% of all children.[112] Usually precipitated by an emotional trigger such as fright, anger, or pain, breath-holding spells begin with active or full expiration, often with crying, followed within 10 to 15 seconds by a noiseless phase with a skin color change to pallor or cyanosis. If the episode continues, the child may experience a change in muscle tone—to limpness or opisthotonus, with loss of consciousness, possibly associated with clonic jerks and/or urinary incontinence. The episode terminates with an inspiratory gasp followed by the return of normal respiration, with or without a phase of drowsiness. Breath-holding spells may be "pallid," "cyanotic," or mixed.

Pathophysiology. *Pallid breath-holding spells* are associated with severe bradycardia or asystole that is attributed to parasympathetic vagally mediated cardiorespiratory inhibition.[113,114] Parasympathetic hypersensitivity in pallid breath-holders, and in a subset of cyanotic breath-holders, has been repeatedly demonstrated in studies reporting exaggerated responses to ocular compression.[112]

Cyanotic breath-holding spells are associated with oxygen desaturation during prolonged apnea, which may also be vagally mediated. Detailed autonomic testing of cyanotic breath-holders has demonstrated a tendency to increased pulse pressure (primarily due to decreased diastolic blood pressure) on upright standing, with an increase in the tachycardia seen on rising from the supine position. Children with cyanotic breath-holding spells may have an excessive immediate sympathetic response to stressors, which may be opposed by a concomitant tendency to parasympathetic hyperactivity.[23]

Differential diagnosis of breath-holding spells includes the long QT syndrome and other arrhythmias, seizures, orthostatic syncope, familial dysautonomia, and brainstem dysfunction related to tumors or malformations.

Therapy. A number of studies have demonstrated a link between iron deficiency anemia and breath-holding spells. Breath-holding spells are more common in infants with anemia, with or without iron deficiency, and in such cases may respond to dietary iron supplementation.[33,115-118] Treatment with iron supplementation, piracetam or tetrabenazine may be effective but is not usually required.

CHRONIC AUTONOMIC NEUROPATHIES

Hereditary Autonomic Neuropathies of Childhood

Hereditary autonomic neuropathies of childhood are individually uncommon in childhood but represent an important class of pediatric polyneuropathies. All except HSAN-1 are autosomal recessive disorders of migration and maturation of neural crest cells. There are three major clinical syndromes of HSAN:

1. HSAN with predominant lower extremity involvement, commonly manifesting in the 2nd or 3rd decade of life (HSAN-1)

2. HSAN with early presentation and generalized involvement (HSAN-2 to HSAN-5)

3. Spinocerebellar degeneration

The various forms of HSAN can be differentiated by the clinical history, physical examination, and standard neurophysiologic and autonomic testing. In addition, all (with the possible exception of HSAN-5) are associated with absence of the axon flare on intradermal histamine testing.

Hereditary Sensory and Autonomic Neuropathy Type 1

Clinical Introduction. HSAN-1 most commonly presents in adulthood but is occasionally seen in childhood. Affected individuals have slowly progressive loss of lower extremity pain and temperature sensation, with associated distal weakness, hyporeflexia, and anhidrosis. Pes cavus and other foot deformities may be present from childhood. The upper limbs are usually spared. Sensory loss causes recurrent foot infections, plantar ulcers, and osteomyelitis. Pain is frequent and may be lancinating. Distal symmetric muscle wasting and weakness may progress to significant disability.[119]

Genetics. This disorder is inherited in an autosomal dominant fashion and is caused in some kindreds by mutations in the serine palmitoyltransferase (*SPTLC1*) gene on chromosome 9q22.[120,121] Linkage to the HSAN-1 locus has been excluded in several kindreds, suggesting genetic heterogeneity in this disorder.[122]

Neurophysiology. Sensory and motor NCVs may be decreased, CMAP amplitudes are usually decreased, and sensory nerve action potential (SNAP) responses may be absent. Sensory thresholds are increased.

Pathologic studies of peripheral nerves reveal the severe loss of all sizes of myelinated and unmyelinated fibers as well as additional degeneration of the dorsal root ganglia.[123]

Hereditary Sensory and Autonomic Neuropathy Type 2

Clinical Introduction. HSAN-2 (congenital insensitivity to pain) is an autosomal recessive disorder presenting in infancy or early childhood with severe distal sensory loss. Affected children may develop a mutilating acropathy with ulcers and painless fractures of the feet and hands. There is generalized areflexia with distal anhidrosis. The pupils may be tonic, and there may be gastrointestinal dysmotility, episodic fever, and recurrent apnea.

Electrophysiologic studies demonstrate mild slowing of motor nerve conduction with absent SNAPs. Impaired sensory perception results in elevated vibratory and thermal perception thresholds.

Pathology. Sural nerve biopsy demonstrates marked loss of myelinated fibers and normal or increased numbers of unmyelinated fibers. As yet, no causative genetic mutation has been identified for HSAN-2.[124]

Hereditary Sensory and Autonomic Neuropathy Type 3

Clinical Introduction. Typical clinical features of HSAN-3 (familial dysautonomia, Riley-Day syndrome) include labile blood pressure, dysphagia, vomiting crises, pain insensitivity, and vasomotor instability. Sweating is preserved and, at times, even excessive. Affected children have an absence of overflow tears with emotional crying, and developmental delay is common, although intelligence is usually normal. Examination reveals hypotonia, areflexia, alacrima, and a pale, smooth tongue because of absence of the fungiform papillae. The corneal reflexes are absent. Corneal hypesthesia may result in ulceration and scarring.

Genetics. Familial dysautonomia is a recessively inherited disorder caused by mutations in an IkappaB kinase complex-associated protein[125] and associated with abnormal development and survival of peripheral autonomic and sensory neurons.

Neurophysiology and Related Studies. Adrenergic dysfunction in affected children is reflected in resting and orthostatic hypotension, which may be severe. Parasympathetic involvement may manifest with loss of heart rate variability and arrhythmias.[126] QST shows increased thresholds for pain, temperature, and vibration perception. No axon flare is seen after intradermal injection of histamine in HSAN-3. Instillation of dilute metacholine or pilocarpine into the conjunctiva causes pupillary miosis, reflecting hypersensitivity to cholinomimetics.

Other abnormal investigations include increased urinary excretion of homovanillic acid, with reduction of plasma dopamine beta-hydroxylase. In contrast to HSAN-4, however, the SSR is preserved.[17]

Pathology. There is a reduction in the number and size of sympathetic and parasympathetic ganglia, loss of sympathetic neurons from the intermediolateral columns, and marked depletion of unmyelinated fibers on sural nerve biopsy.[127]

Treatment. This is mainly preventive, supportive, and symptomatic. Death commonly results from aspiration pneumonitis or arrhythmias.

Hereditary Sensory and Autonomic Neuropathy Type 4

Clinical Introduction. Cardinal features of HSAN-4 (congenital insensitivity to pain with anhidrosis) include episodic high fevers, insensitivity to pain, and anhidrosis.[128] Affected children are usually mildly mentally retarded. Muscle strength and the muscle stretch reflexes are preserved, but loss of deep sensation may result in self-mutilating behavior and neuropathic fractures of the extremities.

Genetics. HSAN-4 is an autosomal recessive disorder linked to mutations in the gene for the tyrosine kinase receptor for nerve growth factor (*TRKA*).[129]

Neurophysiology. Standard studies are normal. Anhidrosis and dermal hyperkeratosis result in absence of the SSR or lack of sweat output during QSART. Insensitivity to pain is demonstrated on the QST.[124] Intradermal histamine injection induces a wheal but not a flare.[17,130,131]

Neuropathologic examination reveals absence of first-order afferent sensory neurons,[128] whereas nerve biopsy demonstrates loss of unmyelinated nerve fibers.[131,132]

Conventional assessment of skin biopsies in HSAN-4 may show normal or decreased numbers of intradermal nerve fibers.[131,133]

Hereditary Sensory and Autonomic Neuropathy Type 5

Clinical Introduction. Only three patients with HSAN-5 (congenital sensitivity to pain with partial anhidrosis) have been reported. Affected children have a congenital sensory neuropathy with selective loss of pain perception in the extremities.[45,134] Sensation of touch, vibration, and proprioception are preserved. Sweating is normal, as is cognition. HSAN-5 has significant clinical overlap with HSAN-4 and may be allelic with this condition.[135] The classification of these disorders is in evolution, with no firm agreement as to distinguishing clinical or histopathologic findings.[136-138]

Diagnostic Studies. Electrodiagnostic evaluations are normal. Cardiovascular autonomic studies may be mildly abnormal for age. The histamine flare response is variably abnormal.

Pathology. Sural nerve biopsy reveals a selective reduction of small myelinated fibers with a possible modest reduction in the number of small unmyelinated fibers.[45,134]

Dopamine Beta-Hydroxylase Deficiency

Clinical Introduction. A small number of patients are reported with this autosomal recessive disorder, which was first recognized in the late 1980s. The biochemical defect consists of isolated deficiency of dopamine beta-hydroxylase, the enzyme that converts dopamine into noradrenaline. Although most cases have been diagnosed in adulthood, symptoms have typically dated to early infancy or childhood. Typically patients present with postural hypotension and recurrent syncope that are commonly worsened by exercise. In some instances this disorder has contributed to delayed achievement of motor milestones. Physical examination may reveal bilateral ptosis and postural hypotension.[5]

Investigations. There is severe orthostasis with loss of sympathetic vasoconstrictor activity but preservation of parasympathetic function with dopamine beta-hydroxylase deficiency. Plasma epinephrine and norepinephrine levels are undetectable, but the plasma dopamine level is markedly elevated.[139]

Therapy. Dihydroxyphenylserine is usually highly effective for orthostasis in dopamine beta-hydroxylase deficiency.

Dopa Decarboxylase Deficiency

Clinical Introduction. This uncommon autosomal recessive disorder causes hypotonia and abnormal limb and eye movements. Autonomic crises, with paroxysmal sweating and intermittent hypothermia, are reported in most affected children. Cardiac and peripheral sympathetic responses may be absent or diminished on provocative testing.[140]

Biochemistry. The underlying defect leads to a deficiency of catecholamines and 5-hydroxytryptamine.

Treatment. These patients may respond to dietary supplementation with dopamine receptor agonists such as bromocriptine, tranylcypromine, and pyridoxine.

Nerve Growth Factor Deficiency

There is a single report of a 30-year-old woman with longstanding dizziness and orthostatic hypotension who was found, on investigation, to have a reduced skin axon-reflex flare response and selective impairment of adrenergic sympathetic function. Her plasma noradrenaline, adrenaline, dopamine, and dopamine beta-hydroxylase levels were undetectable.

Skin biopsy specimens showed loss of tyrosine hydroxylase and neuropeptide Y (markers of adrenergic sympathetic fibers) and of substance P and calcitonin gene-related peptide (sensory neuropeptides). A sural nerve biopsy specimen showed severe depletion of unmyelinated fibers. Nerve growth factor deficiency was confirmed on specific assay.[141]

Nerve growth factor deficiency has not as yet been reported in childhood; however, based on the long-term history of this initial case, one may need to consider this possibility in the differential diagnosis of childhood and adolescent orthostasis.

Fabry's Disease

Clinical Introduction. Fabry's disease is a rare X-linked disorder caused by deficiency of alpha-galactosidase A. Onset is typically in childhood or adolescence. The clinical hallmarks of Fabry's disease include attacks of neuropathic pain, angiokeratomas of skin, and progressive kidney disease. Other complications include renal failure, cardiac conduction disturbances, and stroke.

Investigations. Nerve conduction studies in Fabry's disease may be normal or mildly abnormal.[142,143] Preferential small-fiber involvement is indicated by the early elevation of skin cold and heat-pain detection thresholds and by loss of amplitude of SSRs in affected men.[144] Nerve biopsy demonstrates loss of small myelinated fibers,[145] whereas postmortem studies show a sensory ganglionopathy.[142]

Therapy. Two recent studies demonstrated efficacy of enzyme replacement in Fabry's disease.[146,147]

Acquired Chronic Autonomic Neuropathies of Childhood

Diabetic Neuropathy

Autonomic neuropathy in diabetes mellitus likely results from metabolic derangement due to hyperglycemia, accumulation of toxic products, and deficiency of neurotrophic growth factors, in addition to nerve ischemia related to decreased perfusion.[148] A proportion of patients with diabetic autonomic neuropathy have autoantibodies to autonomic nervous tissue structures, but it is unclear whether this is a primary or secondary phenomenon.

A number of studies have demonstrated evidence of subclinical autonomic neuropathy in adolescents with diabetes.[50,52,149-157] Cardiac manifestations of diabetic autonomic neuropathy include resting tachycardia, reduced heart rate variability, and loss of the normal circadian rhythm of blood pressure and heart rate.[32,157] Gastrointestinal involvement causes gastroparesis, enteropathy, gallbladder atony, and colonic hypomotility. Genitourinary complications of diabetes, and erectile dysfunction, are uncommon in pediatric practice.

Other findings include loss of normal pupillary reflexes.[50,51] Pupillary function tests may be more sensitive and reproducible than tests of heart rate variability and appear to correlate better with duration of diabetes mellitus and glycemic control.[52] Loss of heart rate and diurnal blood pressure variation occurs somewhat later in the disease course.[158]

Overt autonomic dysfunction is rare in pediatric diabetes. Identification of early autonomic dysfunction, however, enables stratification of children at high risk of microvascular and macrovascular complications of diabetes, in whom aggressive metabolic control may alter long-term outcome.[159]

Distal Small-Fiber Neuropathy

Distal small-fiber neuropathy (DSFN) is characterized by distal dysesthesia and postganglionic sympathetic dysfunction, occurring in the absence of significant somatic neuropathy. Sympathetic dysfunction manifests with vasomotor and sudomotor changes.[43] Small-fiber neuropathy is rare in childhood, most cases relating to systemic disorders such as HSAN and Fabry's disease. The incidence of DSFN in disorders such as childhood diabetes mellitus is uncertain. Idiopathic small-fiber neuropathy is extremely uncommon in childhood.[160]

The neurologic examination in idiopathic DSFN is usually unremarkable, as are standard EMG and nerve conduction studies. The QSART or TST are abnormal in about 80% of adults with DSFN, with the diagnostic yield being enhanced if multiple recording sites are used.[161] The sensitivity and specificity of these tests in childhood, however, are poorly established. Skin punch biopsy may demonstrate decreased density of intraepidermal C and Aδ fibers.[160]

Pure Cholinergic Neuropathies

Chronic Idiopathic Anhidrosis. This uncommon disorder is characterized by acquired total, subtotal, or segmental anhidrosis, in the absence of generalized adrenergic and cardiovagal failure. Affected patients are heat intolerant, becoming hot, flushed, dizzy, dyspneic, and weak after exercise or when the ambient temperature is high. Distal vasomotor changes and pupillary abnormalities may be present.

Chronic idiopathic anhidrosis probably comprises a heterogeneous group of disorders with restricted autonomic failure. The differential diagnosis includes acquired anhidrosis related to medications such as zonisamide and topiramate.[162,163]

Affected children have widespread anhidrosis on the TST, usually because of postganglionic impairment.[164] Other tests of autonomic function are normal. Pathologic studies are limited, but eccrine sweat glands may contain inflammatory cell infiltrates.[165]

Most patients have a stable disease course, few progressing to diffuse adrenergic failure. Treatment is focused on the avoidance of heat stress and use of environmental control measures such as cooling vests or air conditioning. Anecdotal reports of improvement with high-dose corticosteroids suggest a possible immune-mediated mechanism in some patients.[165]

Lambert-Eaton Myasthenic Syndrome

Lambert-Eaton myasthenic syndrome (LEMS) is rarely diagnosed in childhood. Common LEMS symptoms include weakness and dry eyes and mouth, whereas examination may reveal ptosis, transient diplopia, proximal weakness, and areflexia. Although many cases of adult LEMS are associated with an underlying neoplasm, particularly small cell lung carcinoma,[166] younger patients generally present with LEMS as part of a more general autoimmune tendency.[167-169]

Adie's Syndrome

A "tonic" pupil is large and reacts poorly, or not at all, to direct illumination with a bright light. An Adie's pupil is tonically dilated because of a postganglionic parasympathetic lesion of the ciliary ganglion.[170] *Adie's syndrome* refers to the combination of a tonic pupil with areflexia and decreased vibration sense, whereas the combination of a tonic pupil with hyporeflexia and segmental anhidrosis is known as *Ross' syndrome*.[171] In childhood, Adie's pupils may be unilateral or bilateral and may develop in isolation or in association with more widespread neurologic or autonomic abnormalities.[171-173]

Denervation hypersensitivity of the tonic pupil is demonstrated by pupillary constriction to subthreshold concentrations of parasympathomimetic agents, such as pilocarpine 0.125% or methacholine 2.5%.

Horner's Syndrome

Horner's syndrome results from disruption of the sympathetic innervation to the eye anywhere along its three-neuron circuit.[174]

Pigmentation of the iris depends on the distribution of melanocytic cells on the anterior border and within the stroma of the iris. The migration of these melanocytic cells into the iris late in gestation and after birth is modulated by the sympathetic nervous system.[175] Iris color is not fully developed until the 12th to 16th month of life.[176]

Congenital Horner's syndromes are therefore associated with heterochromia irides (asymmetry of iris color due to failure to acquire pigment in the iris on the affected side).[177] Congenital Horner's syndrome frequently occurs in association with a brachial plexus lesion incurred during the birth process.

Childhood Horner's syndrome has been described in congenital varicella,[178] birth trauma,[176] vascular lesions of the internal carotid or subclavian arteries,[179] and tumors of the neck and mediastinum including neuroblastoma,[180] ganglioneuroma,[181] and neurilemmoma.[182]

Pharmacologic testing of pupils in infants may be difficult to evaluate[183] or may yield false localizing information.[184,185]

Abnormalities of Gastrointestinal Innervation

Achalasia. This is typically characterized by absent peristalsis of the lower esophageal body and failure of relaxation of the lower esophageal sphincter due to postganglionic denervation of esophageal smooth muscle. Pathologically these changes are associated with inflammatory reactions in and around the myenteric nerves.[186] Achalasia may be congenital or acquired and usually presents with vomiting or dysphagia.

The investigation of choice for achalasia is esophageal manometry, which demonstrates failure of esophageal peristalsis, incomplete lower esophageal relaxation, a high-pressure lower esophageal sphincter, and raised intra-esophageal pressure. Treatment options include nifedipine, botulinum toxin injections, balloon dilation, or surgical myotomy.[56]

Gastroparesis. In gastroparesis, gastric hypomotility or antroduodenal incoordination causes impaired emptying of gastric contents into the duodenum in the absence of a mechanical obstruction. Pediatric causes of gastroparesis include prematurity, viral infection,[187] medications, and electrolyte imbalances.[56] Gastroparesis may also occur in association with diabetic neuropathy, myotonic dystrophy,[188] and Duchenne's muscular dystrophy.[189]

Diagnosis is by gastric emptying scan (radioscintigraphy), antroduodenal manometry, gastric ultrasound, or electrogastrography.[190] Erythromycin and other prokinetic agents may increase motility of the gastric antrum, which may also be improved by better metabolic control in diabetic children.[191]

Chronic Intestinal Pseudo-obstruction

Chronic intestinal pseudo-obstruction (CIP) due to impaired gut motility without mechanical obstruction is seen in association with a variety of neuropathic, myopathic, and systemic disorders.[192] CIP may be congenital or acquired, primary or secondary to a variety of conditions. More

generalized signs of autonomic dysfunction are seen in as many as 30% of patients with all forms of CIP.[193]

Congenital neuropathic forms result from failure of normal migration and/or differentiation of enteric neurons.[194] A proportion of patients have demonstrable intestinal neuronal dysplasia, with hyperplasia of Auerbach's and Meissner's plexuses and abnormally distributed gut neural elements. A familial X-linked recessive syndrome of CIP with malrotation and pyloric hypertrophy presents in the neonatal period.[195] An idiopathic form is also seen in childhood. Dominant and recessive forms of CIP are recognized. About a third of affected neonates have associated genitourinary dysfunction.[192]

Myopathic CIP is seen in infants with the megacystis-microcolon-intestinal hypoperistalsis syndrome and in gastrointestinal alpha$_2$-actin deficiency. The visceral myopathies are associated with vacuolar degeneration and progressive fibrosis of intestinal smooth muscle.[196] Dominant and X-linked visceral myopathies are recognized.

In a few children, CIP is associated with a sensorimotor neuropathy, ptosis, and/or external ophthalmoparesis,[197-199] with or without associated autonomic and urinary tract symptoms.[192,193]

Some (but not all) of these patients have demonstrable underlying disorders of mitochondrial function such as mitochondrial neurogastrointestinal encephalomyopathy (MNGIE).[200,201] MNGIE is an autosomal recessive disorder associated with multiple deletions and depletion of mitochondrial DNA from skeletal muscles and is caused by mutations in the gene for thymidine phosphorylase. Additional findings in affected children may include leukoencephalopathy, lactic acidosis, and abnormal electrocardiography.[202]

A subset of children with gastrointestinal dysmotility presenting within the neonatal period (documented during childhood with abnormal gastric emptying scans and antroduodenal manometry) has been shown to have abnormalities of the mitochondrial electron transport chain enzymes without meeting the criteria for MNGIE.[203]

Acquired forms of CIP may relate to viral myenteric neuritis caused by cytomegalovirus, herpes simplex virus, or Epstein-Barr virus[192,204] or to enteric myositis.[205] Alternating diarrhea and intestinal pseudo-obstruction are also occasionally seen in childhood dermatomyositis, myotonic dystrophy,[188,192] and Duchenne's muscular dystrophy.[192,206,207]

Diagnosis is by manometry, scintigraphy, and histopathology.[53,55,192,208,209] Colonic manometry may differentiate between primarily myopathic and neuropathic processes in children with acquired CIP.[54] Affected children may require jejunal or parenteral feeds in addition to treatment with prokinetic agents and management of bacterial overgrowth.

Hirschsprung's Disease. Hirschsprung's disease (aganglionic megacolon, HSCR) is caused by a congenital deficiency of the ganglion cells of the distal large bowel. The aganglionic segment, which commences at the internal anal sphincter and extends for a variable distance proximally, is tonically contracted. HSCR presents soon after birth with constipation and abdominal distention due to absence of parasympathetic ganglion cells from the intramural myenteric and submucosal plexuses of the distal colon. HSCR results from failure of normal craniocaudal migration of neurenteric ganglion cells from the neural crest to the distal part of the gut during weeks 5 to 12 of gestation. Seventy percent of HSCR cases are isolated, 12% related to chromosomal abnormalities, and 18% associated with other congenital abnormalities with or without other syndromal features.[210]

Other neurocristopathies variably associated with HSCR include the congenital central hypoventilation syndrome (Ondine's curse),[211] Riley-Day syndrome,[210] and congenital neuroblastoma.[173] A proportion of children with HSCR have findings of more generalized dysautonomia.[173,212,213] As many as 73% of affected infants with neurocristopathies have evidence of congenital Horner's syndrome or other pupillary abnormalities.[214]

HSCR is diagnosed on anorectal manometry and suction rectal biopsy demonstration of colonic aganglioniosis.[210] Treatment is by surgical resection of the aganglionic segment.

Functional Abdominal Pain. Generalized dysfunction of autonomic function (with relative preservation of parasympathetic function) has been documented in seven of eight children with "functional" abdominal pain investigated with thorough autonomic laboratory evaluations. These findings suggest that apparently idiopathic abdominal pain may be due in some cases to unmodulated peristalsis secondary to unopposed parasympathetic effect on bowel function.[215]

Abnormalities of Genitourinary Function

Bladder dysfunction is an uncommon manifestation of autonomic neuropathy in childhood but may be seen in association with the HSANs, mitochondrial cytopathies, diabetes mellitus, and acquired dysautonomias. As many as 10% of children with GBS have bladder symptoms, which usually manifest after the onset of peripheral weakness and which tend to parallel the severity of somatic involvement.[73-75]

Urinary retention may also be seen in acute dysautonomia.[216] Overflow incontinence may be seen in the mitochondrial syndrome of MNGIE.[217] Diabetic cystopathy is uncommon in pediatric practice, although adolescents with longstanding diabetes may have subclinical loss of bladder sensation and impairment of bladder emptying.[218]

REFERENCES

1. Camilleri M, Bharucha AE: Gastrointestinal dysfunction in neurologic disease. Semin Neurol 1996;16:203-216.
2. Shifferli PY, Caldeyro-Barcia R: Effects of atropine and beta-adrenergic drugs on the heart rate of the human fetus. *In* Boreus LO (ed): Fetal Pharmacology. New York, Raven Press, 1973, pp 259-275.
3. Miyazoe H, Harada Y, Yamasaki S, Tsuji Y: Clinical study on accentuated antagonism in the regulation of heart rate in children. Jpn Heart J 1998;39:481-487.
4. Gastaut H, Broughton R, De Leo G: Syncopal attacks compulsively self-induced by the Valsalva maneouvre in children with mental retardation. Electroencephalogr Clin Neurophysiol 1982;Suppl 35:323-329.
5. Mathias CJ, Bannister RB, Cortelli P, et al: Clinical, autonomic and therapeutic observations in two siblings with postural hypotension and sympathetic failure due to an inability to synthesize noradrenaline from dopamine because of a deficiency of dopamine beta hydroxylase. Q J Med 1990;75:617-633.
6. Ruckman RN: Cardiac causes of syncope. Pediatr Rev 1987;9:101-108.
7. Scott WA: Evaluating the child with syncope. Pediatr Annu 1991;20:350-359.
8. Ganzeboom KS, Colman N, Reitsma JB, et al: Prevalence and triggers of syncope in medical students. Am J Cardiol 2003;91:1006-1008, A8.
9. Consensus Committee of the American Autonomic Society and the American Academy of Neurology: Consensus statement on the definition of orthostatic hypotension, pure autonomic failure, and multiple system atrophy. Neurology 1996;46:1470.
10. Low PA: Laboratory evaluation of autonomic function. *In* Low PA (ed): Clinical Autonomic Disorders: Evaluation and Management, 2nd ed. Philadelphia, Lippincott-Raven, 1997, pp 179-208.
11. Low PA, Caskey PE, Tuck RR, et al: Quantitative sudomotor axon reflex test in normal and neuropathic subjects. Ann Neurol 1983;14:573-580.
12. Hoeldtke RD, Bryner KD, Horvath GG, et al: Redistribution of sudomotor responses is an early sign of sympathetic dysfunction in type 1 diabetes. Diabetes 2001;50:436-443.
13. Fealey RD, Low PA, Thomas JE: Thermoregulatory sweating abnormalities in diabetes mellitus. Mayo Clin Proc 1989;64:617-628.
14. Kennedy WR, Navarro X: Sympathetic sudomotor function in diabetic neuropathy. Arch Neurol 1989;46:1182-1186.
15. Hoeldtke RD, Davis KM, Hshieh PB, et al: Autonomic surface potential analysis: Assessment of reproducibility and sensitivity. Muscle Nerve 1992;15:926-931.
16. Shahani BT, Halperin JJ, Boulu P, Cohen J: Sympathetic skin response: A method of assessing unmyelinated axon dysfunction in peripheral neuropathies. J Neurol Neurosurg Psychiatry 1984;47:536-542.

17. Hilz MJ, Stemper B, Axelrod FB: Sympathetic skin response differentiates hereditary sensory autonomic neuropathies III and IV. Neurology 1999;52:1652-1657.

18. Benarroch EE, Opfer-Gehrking TL, Low PA: Use of the photoplethysmographic technique to analyze the Valsalva maneuver in normal man. Muscle Nerve 1991;14:1165-1172.

19. Ingall TJ, McLeod JG, O'Brien PC: The effect of ageing on the autonomic nervous system function. Aust N Z J Med 1990;20:570-577.

20. Driscoll DJ, Jacobsen SJ, Porter CJ, Wollan PC: Syncope in children and adolescents. J Am Coll Cardiol 1997;29:1039-1045.

21. Rodriguez-Nunez A, Fernandez-Cebrian S, Perez-Munuzuri A, et al: Cerebral syncope in children. J Pediatr 2000;136:542-544.

22. Stewart JM: Orthostatic intolerance in pediatrics. J Pediatr 2002;140:404-411.

23. Di Mario FJ Jr, Burleson JA: Autonomic nervous system function in severe breath-holding spells. Pediatr Neurol 1993;9:268-274.

24. Fouad FM, Sitthisook S, Vanerio G, et al: Sensitivity and specificity of the tilt table test in young patients with unexplained syncope. Pacing Clin Electrophysiol 1993;16:394-400.

25. Berkowitz JB, Auld D, Hulse JE, Campbell RM: Tilt table evaluation for control pediatric patients: Comparison with symptomatic patients. Clin Cardiol 1995;18:521-525.

26. de Jong-de Vos van Steenwijk CC, Wieling W, Johannes JM, et al: Incidence and hemodynamic characteristics of near-fainting in healthy 6- to 16-year old subjects. J Am Coll Cardiol 1995;25:1615-1621.

27. Lewis DA, Zlotocha J, Henke L, Dhala A: Specificity of head-up tilt testing in adolescents: Effect of various degrees of tilt challenge in normal control subjects. J Am Coll Cardiol 1997;30:1057-1060.

28. Massin M, von Bernuth G: Normal ranges of heart rate variability during infancy and childhood. Pediatr Cardiol 1997;18:297-302.

29. Lishner M, Akselrod S, Avi VM, et al: Spectral analysis of heart rate fluctuations: A noninvasive, sensitive method for the early diagnosis of autonomic neuropathy in diabetes mellitus. J Auton Nerv Syst 1987;19:119-125.

30. Antila KJ, Valimaki IA, Makela M, et al: Heart rate variability in infants subsequently suffering sudden infant death syndrome (SIDS). Early Hum Dev 1990;22:57-72.

31. Gordon D, Southall DP, Kelly DH, et al: Analysis of heart rate and respiratory patterns in sudden infant death syndrome victims and control infants. Pediatr Res 1986;20:680-684.

32. Massin MM, Derkenne B, Tallsund M, et al: Cardiac autonomic dysfunction in diabetic children. Diabetes Care 1999;22:1845-1850.

33. Orii KE, Kato Z, Osamu F, et al: Changes of autonomic nervous system function in patients with breath-holding spells treated with iron. J Child Neurol 2002;17:337-340.

34. Dyck PJ, Karnes JL, O'Brien PC, Zimmerman IR: Detection thresholds of cutaneous sensation in humans. In Dyck PJ, Thomas PK, Griffin JW, et al (eds): Peripheral Neuropathy, 3rd ed. Philadelphia, WB Saunders, 1993, pp 706-728.

35. Shy ME, Frohman EM, So YT, et al: Therapeutics and Technology Assessment Subcommittee of the American Academy of Neurology. Quantitative sensory testing: Report of the Therapeutics and Technology Assessment Subcommittee of the American Academy of Neurology. Neurology 2003;60:898-904.

36. Burns TM, Taly A, O'Brien PC, Dyck PJ: Clinical versus quantitative vibration assessment: Improving clinical performance. J Periph Nerv System 2002;7:112-117.

37. Dyck PJ, O'Brien PC, Kosanke JL, et al: A 4, 2, and 1 stepping algorithm for quick and accurate estimation of cutaneous sensation threshold. Neurology 1993;43:1508-1512.

38. Hilz MJ, Stemper B, Schweibold G, et al: Quantitative thermal perception testing in 225 children and juveniles. J Clin Neurophysiol 1998;15:529-534.

39. Hilz MJ, Axelrod FB, Hermann K, et al: Normative values of vibratory perception in 530 children, juveniles, and adults aged 3-79 years. J Neurol Sci 1998;159:219-225.

40. Meier PM, Berde CB, DiCanzio J, et al: Quantitative assessment of cutaneous thermal and vibration sensation and thermal pain detection thresholds in healthy children and adolescents. Muscle Nerve 2001;24:1339-1345.

41. Holland NR, Stocks A, Hauer P, et al: Intraepidermal nerve fiber density in patients with painful sensory neuropathy. Neurology 1997;48:708-711.

42. Herrmann DN, Griffin JW, Hauer P, et al: Epidermal nerve fiber density and sural nerve morphometry in peripheral neuropathies. Neurology 1999;53:1634-1640.

43. Holland NR, Crawford TO, Hauer P, et al: Small-fiber sensory neuropathies: Clinical course and neuropathology of idiopathic cases. Ann Neurol 1998;44:47-59.

44. Garrison JC: Histamine, bradykinin, 5-hydroxytryptamine, and their antagonists. In Gilman AG, Rall TW, Nies AS, Taylor P: Goodman and Gilman's The Pharmacological Basis of Therapeutics, 8th ed, Vol I. New York, Pergamon Press, 1991, pp 575-599.

45. Low PA, Burke WJ, McLeod JG: Congenital sensory neuropathy with selective loss of small myelinated fibers. Ann Neurol 1978;3:179-182.

46. Kelsey RM, Patterson SM, Barnard M, Alpert BS: Consistency of hemodynamic responses to cold stress in adolescents. Hypertension 2000;36:1013-1017.

47. Kawasaki A, Kardon RH: Disorders of the pupil. Ophthalmol Clin North Am 2001;14:149-168.

48. Wilhelm H, Wilhelm B: Clinical applications of pupillography. J Neuroophthalmol 2003;23:42-49.

49. Karavanaki K, Baum JD: Coexistence of impaired indices of autonomic neuropathy and diabetic nephropathy in a cohort of children with type 1 diabetes mellitus. J Pediatr Endocrinol Metab 2003;16:79-90.

50. Clarke CF, Piesowicz AT, Spathis GS: Pupillary size in children and adolescents with type 1 diabetes. Diabet Med 1989;6:780-783.

51. Karavanaki K, Davies AG, Hunt LP, et al: Pupil size in diabetes. Arch Dis Child 1994;71:511-515.

52. Schwingshandl J, Simpson JM, Donaghue K, et al: Pupillary abnormalities in type I diabetes occurring during adolescence: Comparisons with cardiovascular reflexes. Diabetes Care 1993;16:630-633.

53. Hyman PE: Chronic intestinal pseudo-obstruction in childhood: progress in diagnosis and treatment. Scand J Gastroenterol Suppl 1995; 213:39-46.

54. Di Lorenzo C, Flores AF, Reddy SN, et al: Colonic manometry in children with chronic intestinal pseudo-obstruction. Gut 1993;34:803-807.

55. Cucchiara S, Annese V, Minella R, et al: Antroduodenojejunal manometry in the diagnosis of chronic idiopathic intestinal pseudoobstruction in children. J Pediatr Gastroenterol Nutr 1994;18:294-395.

56. Hussain SZ, Di Lorenzo C: Motility disorders. Diagnosis and treatment for the pediatric patient. Pediatr Clin North Am 2002;49:27-51.

57. Parkman HP, Harris AD, Krevsky B, et al: Gastroduodenal motility and dysmotility: An update on techniques available for evaluation. Am J Gastroenterol 1995;90:869-892.

58. Koch KL: Diabetic gastropathy: Gastric neuromuscular dysfunction in diabetes mellitus: A review of symptoms, pathophysiology, and treatment. Dig Dis Sci 1999;44:1061-1075.

59. Chitkara DK, Delgado-Aros S, Bredenoord AJ, et al: Functional dyspepsia, upper gastrointestinal symptoms and transit in children. J Pediatr 2003;143:609-613.

60. Graff J, Brinch K, Madsen JL: Gastrointestinal mean transit times in young and middle-aged healthy subjects. Clin Physiol 2000;21:253-259.

61. Gryback P, Jacobsson H, Blomquist L, et al: Scintigraphy of the small intestine: A simplified standard for study of transit with reference to normal values. Eur J Nucl Med Mol Imaging 2002;29:39-45.

62. Ghoos YF, Maes BD, Geypens BJ, et al: Measurement of gastric emptying rate of solids by means of a carbon-labeled octanoic acid breath test. Gastroenterology 1993;104:1640-1647.

63. Lee JS, Camilleri M, Zinsmeister AR, et al: A valid, accurate, office-based non-radioactive test for gastric emptying of solids. Gut 2000;46:768-773.

64. Viramontes BE, Kim DY, Camilleri M, et al: Validation of a stable isotope gastric emptying test for normal, accelerated or delayed stomach emptying. Neurogastroenterol Motil 2001;13:567-574.

65. Van Den Driessche M, Van Malderen N, Geypens B, et al: Lactose-[^{13}C]ureide breath test: A new, noninvasive technique to determine orocecal transit time in children. J Pediatr Gastroenterol Nutr 2000;31:433-438.

66. Liau SS, Camilleri M, Kim DY, et al: Pharmacological modulation of human gastric volumes demonstrated non-invasively using SPECT imaging. Neurogastroenterol Mot 2001;13:533-542.

67. Fowler CJ: Neurological disorders of micturition and their treatment. Brain 1999;122:1213-1231.

68. Perretti A, Savanelli A, Balbi P, De Bernardo G: Pudendal nerve somatosensory evoked potentials in pediatrics: Maturation aspects. Electroencephalogr Clin Neurophysiol 1997;104:383-388.

69. Podnar S, Vodusek DB, Trsiner B, Rodi Z: A method of uroneurophysiological investigation in children. Electroencephalogr Clin Neurophysiol 1997;104:389-392.

70. Podnar S, Trsinar B, Vodusek DB: Neurophysiological study of primary nocturnal enuresis. Neurourol Urodyn 1999;18:93-98.

71. Billard C, Ponsot G, Lyon G, Arthuis M: Acute polyradiculoneuritis in children: Clinical and developmental aspects—prognostic factors apropos of 100 cases. Arch Franc Pediatr 1979;36:149-161.

72. Low PA, McLeod JG: The autonomic neuropathies. *In* Low PA (ed): Clinical Autonomic Disorders: Evaluation and Management. Boston, Little, Brown, 1993, pp 395-421.

73. Wheeler JS Jr, Siroky MB, Pavlakis A, Krane RJ: The urodynamic aspects of the Guillain-Barré syndrome. J Urol 1984;131:917-919.

74. Kogan BA, Solomon MH, Diokno AC: Urinary retention secondary to Landry-Guillain-Barré syndrome. J Urol 1981;126:643-644.

75. Truax BT: Autonomic disturbances in Guillain-Barré syndrome. Neurology 1984;4:462-468.

76. Tuck RR, McLeod JG: Autonomic dysfunction in Guillain-Barré syndrome. J Neurol Neurosurg Psychiatry 1981;44:983-990.

77. Persson A, Solders G: R-R variations in Guillain-Barré syndrome: A test of autonomic dysfunction. Acta Neurol Scand 1983;67:294-300.

78. Ropper AH: Acute autonomic emergencies and autonomic storm. *In* Low PA (ed): Clinical Autonomic Disorders: Evaluation and Management. Boston, Little, Brown, 1993, pp 747-760.

79. Burns TM, Lawn NC, Low PA, et al: Adynamic ileus in severe Guillain-Barré syndrome. Muscle Nerve 2001;24:963-965.

80. Young RR, Asbury AK, Corbett JL, Adams RD: Pure pan-dysautonomia with recovery: Description and discussion of diagnostic criteria. Brain 1975;98:613-636.

81. Neville BG, Sladen GE: Acute autonomic neuropathy following primary herpes simplex infection. J Neurol Neurosurg Psychiatry 1984;47:648-650.

82. Yahr MD, Frontera AT: Acute autonomic neuropathy: Its occurrence in infectious mononucleosis. Arch Neurol 1975;32:132-133.

83. Inamdar S, Easton LB, Lester G: Acquired postganglionic cholinergic dysautonomia: Case report and review of the literature. Pediatrics 1982;70:976-978.

84. Hopkins IJ, Shield LK, Harris M: Subacute cholinergic dysautonomia in childhood. Clin Exp Neurol 1981;17:147-151.

85. Suarez GA, Fealey RD, Camilleri M, Low PA: Idiopathic autonomic neuropathy: Clinical, neurophysiologic, and follow-up studies on 27 patients. Neurology 1994;44:1675-1682.

86. Colan RV, Snead OC III, Oh SJ, Kashlan MB: Acute autonomic and sensory neuropathy. Ann Neurol 1980;8:441-444.

87. Dune X, Lee WT, Shen YZ: Postmeningoencephalitic dysautonomia: Report of one case. Pediatr Neurol 2002;26:161-163.

88. Hart RG, Kanter MC: Acute autonomic neuropathy: Two cases and a clinical review. Arch Intern Med 1990;150:2373-2376.

89. Vernino S, Low PA, Fealey RD, et al: Autoantibodies to ganglionic acetylcholine receptors in autoimmune autonomic neuropathies. N Engl J Med 2000;343:847-855.

90. Stoll G, Thomas C, Reiners K, et al: Encephalo-myelo-radiculo-ganglionitis presenting as pandysautonomia. Neurology 1991;41:723-726.

91. Smit AA, Vermeulen M, Koelman JH, Wieling W: Unusual recovery from acute panautonomic neuropathy after immunoglobulin therapy. Mayo Clin Proc 1997;72:333-335.

92. Taubner RW, Salanova V: Acute dysautonomia and polyneuropathy. Arch Neurol 1984;41:1100-1101.

93. Low PA: Neurogenic orthostatic hypotension. *In* Johnson RT, Griffin JW (eds): Current Therapy in Neurologic Disease, 4th ed. St. Louis, Mosby-Year Book, 1993, pp 21-26.

94. Mericle RA, Triggs WJ: Treatment of acute pandysautonomia with intravenous immunoglobulin. J Neurol Neurosurg Psychiatry 1997;62:529-531.

95. Heafield MT, Gammage MD, Nightingale S, Williams AC: Idiopathic dysautonomia treated with intravenous gamma globulin. Lancet 1996;347:28-29.

96. Schondorf R, Low PA: Idiopathic postural orthostatic tachycardia syndrome: An attenuated form of acute pandysautonomia? Neurology 1993;43:132-137.

97. Stewart JM, Gewitz MH, Weldon A, Munoz J: Patterns of orthostatic intolerance: The orthostatic tachycardia syndrome and adolescent chronic fatigue. J Pediatr 1999;135:218-225.

98. Rowe PC, Bou-Holaigah I, Kan JS, Calkins H: Is neurally mediated hypotension an unrecognised cause of chronic fatigue? Lancet 1995;345:623-624.

99. Shannon JR, Flattem NL, Jordan J, et al: Orthostatic intolerance and tachycardia associated with norepinephrine-transporter deficiency. N Engl J Med 2000;342:541-549.

100. Low PA, Opfer-Gehrking TL, Textor SC, et al: Postural tachycardia syndrome (POTS). Neurology 1995;45(Suppl 5):S19-S25.

101. Stewart JM, Gewitz MH, Weldon A, Munoz J: Patterns of orthostatic intolerance: the orthostatic tachycardia syndrome and adolescent chronic fatigue. J Pediatr 1999;135:218-225.

102. Elder GH: Hepatic porphyrias in children. J Inherit Metab Dis 1997;20:237-246.

103. Fagius J, Wallin BG: Long-term variability and reproducibility of resting human muscle nerve sympathetic activity at rest, as reassessed after a decade. Clin Auton Res 1993;3:201-205.

104. Stewart PM, Hensley WJ: An acute attack of variegate porphyria complicated by severe autonomic neuropathy. Aust N Z J Med 1981;11:82-83.

105. Elder GH, Hift RJ: Treatment of acute porphyria. Hosp Med 2001;62:422-425.

106. Suarez GA: Autonomic neuropathies. *In* Jones HR, De Vivo DC, Darras BT (eds): Neuromuscular Disorders of Infancy, Childhood, and Adolescence: A Clinician's Approach. Philadelphia, Butterworth Heinemann Health 2003, pp 529-545.

107. Clay SA, Ramseyer JC, Fishman LS, Sedgwick RP: Acute infantile motor unit disorder: Infantile botulism? Arch Neurol 1977;34:236-243.

108. Vita G, Girlanda P, Puglisi RM, et al: Cardiovascular-reflex testing and single-fiber electromyography in botulism: A longitudinal study. Arch Neurol 1987;44:202-206.

109. Long SS: Infant botulism. Indian J Pediatr 1986;53:141-143.

110. Chaudhry V, Crawford TO: Stimulation single-fiber EMG in infant botulism. Muscle Nerve 1999;22:1698-1703.

111. Arnon SS: Infantile botulism. *In* Feigen RD, Cherry JD (eds): Textbook of Pediatric Infectious Diseases, 4th ed. Philadelphia, WB Saunders, 1998, pp 1570-1577.

112. Di Mario FJ Jr: Breath-holding spells in childhood. Am J Dis Child 1992;146:125-131.

113. Stephenson JB: Reflex anoxic seizures ("white breath-holding"): Nonepileptic vagal attacks. Arch Dis Child 1978;53:193-200.

114. DiMario FJ Jr, Chee CM, Berman PH: Pallid breath-holding spells: Evaluation of the autonomic nervous system. Clin Pediatr 1990;29:17-24.

115. Mocan H, Yildiran A, Orhan F, Erduran E: Breath holding spells in 91 children and response to treatment with iron. Arch Dis Child 1999;81:261-262.

116. Bhatia MS, Singhal PK, Dhar NK, et al: Breath holding spells: an analysis of 50 cases. Indian Pediatr 1990;27:1073-1079.

117. Dauod AS, Batieha A, al-Sheyyab M, et al: Effectiveness of iron therapy on breath-holding spells. J Pediatr. 1997;130:547-550.

118. Tam DA, Rash FC: Breath-holding spells in a patient with transient erythroblastopenia of childhood. J Pediatr 1997;130:651-653.

119. Auer-Grumbach M, De Jonghe P, Verhoeven K, et al: Autosomal dominant inherited neuropathies with prominent sensory loss and mutilations: A review. Arch Neurol 2003;60:329-334.

120. Bejaoui K, Wu C, Scheffler MD, et al: *SPTLC1* is mutated in hereditary sensory neuropathy, type 1. Nat Genet 2001;27:261-262.

121. Dawkins JL, Hulme DJ, Brahmbhatt SB, et al: Mutations in *SPTLC1*, encoding serine palmitoyltransferase long-chain base subunit-1, cause hereditary sensory neuropathy type I. Nat Genet 2001;27:309-312.

122. Auer-Grumbach M, Wagner K, Timmerman V, et al: Ulcero-mutilating neuropathy in an Austrian kinship without linkage to hereditary motor and sensory neuropathy IIB and hereditary sensory neuropathy I loci. Neurology 2000;54:45-52.

123. Dyck PJ: Neuronal atrophy and degeneration predominantly affecting peripheral sensory and autonomic neurons. *In* Dyck PJ, Thomas PK, Griffin JW, et al (eds): Peripheral Neuropathy, 3rd ed. Philadelphia, WB Saunders, 1993, pp 1065-1093.

124. Hilz MJ: Assessment and evaluation of hereditary sensory and autonomic neuropathies with autonomic and neurophysiological examinations. Clin Auton Res 2002;12(Suppl 1):I33-I43.

125. Anderson SA, Coli R, Daly IW, et al: Familial dysautonomia is caused by mutations of the *IKAP* gene. Am J Hum Genet 2001;68:753-758.

126. Axelrod FB, Putman D, Berlin D, Rutkowski M: Electrocardiographic measures and heart rate variability in patients with familial dysautonomia. Cardiology 1997;88:133-140.

127. Aguayo AJ, Nair CP, Bray GM: Peripheral nerve abnormalities in the Riley-Day syndrome: Findings in a sural nerve biopsy. Arch Neurol 1971;24:106-116.

128. Swanson AG, Buchan GC, Alvord EC Jr: Anatomic changes in congenital insensitivity to pain: Absence of small primary sensory neurons in ganglia, roots and Lissauer's tract. Arch Neurol 1965;12:12-18.

129. Indo Y, Tsuruta M, Hayashida Y, et al: Mutations in the TRKA/NGF receptor gene in patients with congenital insensitivity to pain with anhidrosis. Nat Genet 1996;13:485-488.

130. Shorer Z, Moses SW, Hershkovitz E, et al: Neurophysiologic studies in congenital insensitivity to pain with anhidrosis. Pediatr Neurol 2001;25:397-400.

131. Nolano M, Crisci C, Santoro L, et al: Absent innervation of skin and sweat glands in congenital insensitivity to pain with anhidrosis. Clin Neurophysiol 2000;111:1596-1601.

132. Itoh Y, Yagishita S, Nakajima S, et al: Congenital insensitivity to pain with anhidrosis: Morphological and morphometrical studies on the skin and peripheral nerves. Neuropediatrics 1986;17:103-110.

133. Verze L, Viglietti-Panzica C, Plumari L, et al: Cutaneous innervation in hereditary sensory and autonomic neuropathy type IV. Neurology 2000;55:126-128.

134. Donaghy M, Hakin RN, Bamford JM, et al: Hereditary sensory neuropathy with neurotrophic keratitis: Description of an autosomal recessive disorder with a selective reduction of small myelinated nerve fibres and a discussion of the classification of the hereditary sensory neuropathies. Brain 1987;110:563-583.

135. Houlden H, King RH, Hashemi-Nejad A, et al: A novel TRK A (NTRK1) mutation associated with hereditary sensory and autonomic neuropathy type V. Ann Neurol 2001;49:521-525.

136. Toscano E, Simonati A, Indo Y, Andria G: No mutation in the TRKA (NTRK1) gene encoding a receptor tyrosine kinase for nerve growth factor in a patient with hereditary sensory and autonomic neuropathy type V. Ann Neurol 2002;52:224-227.

137. Klein CJ, Sinnreich M. Dyck PJ: Indifference rather than insensitivity to pain. Ann Neurol 2003:53:417-418.

138. Toscano E, Simonati A, Indo Y, Andria G: No mutation in the TRKA (NTRK1) gene encoding a receptor tyrosine kinase for nerve growth factor in a patient with hereditary sensory and autonomic neuropathy type V. Ann Neurol 2002;52:224-227.

139. Man in't Veld AJ, Boomsma F, van den Meiracker AH, Schalekamp MA: Effect of unnatural noradrenaline precursor on sympathetic control and orthostatic hypotension in dopamine-beta-hydroxylase deficiency. Lancet 1987;21:1172-1175.

140. Swoboda KJ, Saul JP, McKenna CE, et al: Aromatic L-amino acid decarboxylase deficiency: Overview of clinical features and outcomes. Ann Neurol 2003;54(Suppl 6):S49-S55.

141. Anand P, Rudge P, Mathias CJ, et al: New autonomic and sensory neuropathy with loss of adrenergic sympathetic function and sensory neuropeptides. Lancet 1991;337:1253-1254.

142. Ohnishi A, Dyck PJ: Loss of small peripheral sensory neurons in Fabry disease. Arch Neurol 1974;31:120-127.

143. Sheth KJ, Swick HM: Peripheral nerve conduction in Fabry disease. Ann Neurol 1980;7:319-323.

144. Dutsch M, Marthol H, Stemper B, et al: Small-fiber dysfunction predominates in Fabry neuropathy. J Clin Neurophysiol 2002;19:575-586.

145. Kocen RS, Thomas PK: Peripheral nerve involvement in Fabry's disease. Arch Neurol 1970;22:81-88.

146. Eng CM, Guffon N, Wilcox WR, et al, and the International Collaborative Fabry Disease Study Group: Safety and efficacy of recombinant human alpha-galactosidase A: Replacement therapy in Fabry's disease. N Engl J Med 2001;345:9-16.

147. Schiffmann R, Kopp JB, Austin HA, et al: Enzyme replacement therapy in Fabry disease. JAMA 2001;285:2743-2749.

148. Dyck PJ: Nerve growth factor and diabetic neuropathy. Lancet 1996;348:1044-1045.

149. Aman J, Eriksson E, Lideen J: Autonomic nerve function in children and adolescents with insulin-dependent diabetes mellitus. Clin Physiol 1991;11:537-543.

150. Clarke CF, Eason M, Reilly A, et al: Autonomic nerve function in adolescents with type 1 diabetes mellitus: Relationship to microalbuminuria. Diabet Med 1999;16:550-554.

151. Sundkvist G, Almer L, Lilja B: Respiratory influence on heart rate in diabetes mellitus. BMJ 1979;1:924-925.

152. Mitchell EA, Wealthall SR, Elliott RB: Diabetic autonomic neuropathy in children: Immediate heart-rate response to standing. Aust Paediatr J 1983;19:175-177.

153. Young RJ, Ewing DJ, Clarke BF: Nerve function and metabolic control in teenage diabetics. Diabetes 1983;32:142-147.

154. Ringel RE, Chalew SA, Armour KA, et al: Cardiovascular reflex abnormalities in children and adolescents with diabetes mellitus. Diabetes Care 1993;16:734-741.

155. Donaghue KC, Fung AT, Fairchild JM, et al: Prospective assessment of autonomic and peripheral nerve function in adolescents with diabetes. Diabet Med 1996;13:65-71.

156. Verrotti A, Chiarelli F, Blasetti A, Morgese G: Autonomic neuropathy in diabetic children. J Paediatr Child Health 1995;31:545-548.

157. Barkai L, Madacsy L: Cardiovascular autonomic dysfunction in diabetes mellitus. Arch Dis Child 1995;73:515-518.

158. Madacsy L, Yasar A, Tulassay T, et al: Association of relative nocturnal hypertension and autonomic neuropathy in insulin-dependent diabetic children. Acta Biomed Ateneo Parmense 1995;66:111-118.

159. Oduwole A, Marcon M, Bril V, Ehrlich RM: Transient autonomic neuropathy in an adolescent with insulin-dependent diabetes mellitus. J Pediatr Endocrinol Metab 1995;8:195-197.

160. Wakamoto H, Hirai A, Manabe K, Hayashi M: Idiopathic small-fiber sensory neuropathy in childhood: A diagnosis based on objective findings on punch skin biopsy specimens. J Pediatr 1999;135:257-260.

161. Stewart JD, Low PA, Fealey RD: Distal small-fiber neuropathy: Results of tests of sweating and autonomic cardiovascular reflexes. Muscle Nerve 1992;15:661-665.

162. Arcas J, Ferrer T, Roche MC, et al: Hypohidrosis related to the administration of topiramate to children. Epilepsia 2001;42:1363-1365.

163. Okumura A, Hayakawa F, Kuno K, Watanabe K: Oligohidrosis caused by zonisamide. No To Hattatsu 1996;28:44-47.

164. Low PA, Zimmerman BR, Dyck PJ: Comparison of distal sympathetic with vagal function in diabetic neuropathy. Muscle Nerve 1986;9:592-596.

165. Ando Y, Fujii S, Sakashita N, et al: Acquired idiopathic generalized anhidrosis: Clinical manifestations and histochemical studies. J Neurol Sci 1995;132:80-83.

166. Shapira Y, Cividalli G, Szabo G, et al: A myasthenic syndrome in childhood leukemia. Dev Med Child Neurol 1974;16:668-671.

167. Tsao CY, Mendell JR, Friemer ML, Kissel JT: Lambert-Eaton myasthenic syndrome in children. J Child Neurol 2002;17:74-76.

168. Sanders DB: Lambert-Eaton myasthenic syndrome: Diagnosis and treatment. Ann N Y Acad Sci 2003;998:500-508.

169. Hoffman WH, Helman SW, Sekul E, et al: Lambert-Eaton myasthenic syndrome in a child with an autoimmune phenotype. Am J Med Genet 2003:199:77-80.

170. Harriman DGF, Garland HG: The pathology of Adie's syndrome. Brain 1968;91:401-418.

171. Shin RK, Galetta SL, Ting TY, et al: Ross syndrome plus: Beyond Horner, Holmes-Adie, and harlequin. Neurology 2000;55:1841-1846.

172. Ryan MM, Grattan-Smith PJ, Procopis PG, et al: Childhood chronic inflammatory demyelinating polyneuropathy: Clinical course and long-term outcome. Neuromusc Disord 2000;10:398-406.

173. Lambert SR, Yang LL, Stone C: Tonic pupil associated with congenital neuroblastoma, Hirschsprung disease, and central hypoventilation syndrome. Am J Ophthalmol 2000;130:238-240.

174. Kardon RH, Denison CE, Brown CK, Thompson HS: Critical evaluation of the cocaine test in the diagnosis of Horner's syndrome. Arch Ophthalmol 1990;108:384-387.

175. McCartney ACE, Riordan-Eva P, Howes RC, Spalton DJ: Horner's syndrome: An electron microscopic study of a human iris. Br J Ophthalmol 1992;76:746-749.

176. Giles CL, Henderson DA: Horner's syndrome: An analysis of 216 cases. Am J Ophthalmol 1958;46:289-301.

177. Cross SA: Evaluation of pupillary and lacrimal function. *In* Low PA (ed): Clinical Autonomic Disorders, 2nd ed. Philadelphia, Lippincott-Raven, 1997, pp 259-268.

178. Lambert SR, Taylor D, Kriss A, et al: Ocular manifestations of congenital varicella syndrome. Arch Ophthalmol 1989;107:52-56.

179. Sauer C, Levinsohn MW: Horner's syndrome in childhood. Neurology 1976;26:216-220.

180. Jaffe N, Cassady JR, Filler RM, et al: Heterochromasia and Horner's syndrome associated with cervical and mediastinal neuroblastoma. J Pediatr 1975;87:75-77.

181. McRae D, Shaw A: Ganglioneuroma, heterochromia iridis, and Horner's syndrome. J Paediatr Surg 1979;14:612-614.

182. Sayed AK, Miller BA, Lack EE, et al: Heterochromia iridis and Horner's syndrome due to paravertebral neurilemmoma. J Surg Oncol 1983;22:15-16.

183. Maloney WF, Younge BR, Moyer NJ: Evaluation of the causes and accuracy of pharmacologic localisation in Horner's syndrome. Am J Ophthalmol 1980;90:394-402.

184. Weinstein JM, Zweifel TJ, Thompson HS: Congenital Horner's syndrome. Arch Ophthalmol 1980;98:1074-1078.

185. Woodruff G, Buncic JR, Morin JD: Horner's syndrome in children. J Pediatr Ophthalmol Strabismus 1988;25:40-44.

186. Aggestrup S, Uddman R, Sundler F, et al: Lack of vasoactive intestinal polypeptide nerves in esophageal achalasia. Gastroenterology 1983;84:924-927.

187. Sigurdsson L, Flores A, Putnam PE, et al: Postviral gastroparesis: Presentation, treatment, and outcome. J Pediatr 1997;131:751-754.

188. Bodensteiner JB, Grunow JE: Gastroparesis in neonatal myotonic dystrophy. Muscle Nerve 1984;7:486-487.

189. Chung BC, Park HJ, Yoon SB, et al: Acute gastroparesis in Duchenne's muscular dystrophy. Yonsei Med J 1998;39:175-179.

190. Cucchiara S, Franzese A, Salvia G, et al: Gastric emptying delay and gastric electrical derangement in IDDM. Diabetes Care 1998;21:438-443.

191. White NH, Waltman SR, Krupin T, Santiago JV: Reversal of neuropathic and gastrointestinal complications related to diabetes mellitus in adolescents with improved metabolic control. J Pediatr 1981;99:41-45.

192. Faure C, Goulet O, Ategbo S, et al: Chronic intestinal pseudo-obstruction syndrome: Clinical analysis, outcome, and prognosis in 105 children. French-Speaking Group of Pediatric Gastroenterology. Dig Dis Sci 1999;44:953-959.

193. Bharucha AE, Camilleri M, Low PA, Zinsmeister AR: Autonomic dysfunction in gastrointestinal motility disorders. Gut 1993;34:397-401.

194. Navarro J, Sonsino E, Boige N, et al: Visceral neuropathies responsible for chronic intestinal pseudo-obstruction syndrome in pediatric practice: Analysis of 26 cases. J Pediatr Gastroenterol Nutr 1990;11:179-195.

195. Auricchio A, Brancolini V, Casari G, et al: The locus for a novel syndromic form of neuronal intestinal pseudo-obstruction maps to Xq28. Am J Hum Genet 1996;58:743-748.

196. Puri P, Lake BD, Gorman F, et al: Megacystis-microcolon-intestinal hypoperistalsis syndrome: A visceral myopathy. J Pediatr Surg 1983;18:64-69.

197. Steiner I, Steinberg A, Argov Z, et al: Familial progressive neuronal disease and chronic idiopathic intestinal pseudo-obstruction. Neurology 1987;37:1046-1050.

198. Ionasescu V, Thompson SH, Ionasescu R, et al: Inherited ophthalmoplegia with intestinal pseudo-obstruction. J Neurol Sci 1983;59:215-228.

199. Amato AA, Jackson CE, Ridings LW, Barohn RJ: Childhood-onset oculopharyngodistal myopathy with chronic intestinal pseudo-obstruction. Muscle Nerve 1995;18:842-847.

200. Hirano M, Silvestri G, Blake DM, et al: Mitochondrial neurogastrointestinal encephalomyopathy (MNGIE): Clinical, biochemical, and genetic features of an autosomal recessive mitochondrial disorder. Neurology 1994;44:721-727.

201. Li V, Hostein J, Romero NB, et al: Chronic intestinal pseudo-obstruction with myopathy and ophthalmoplegia: A muscular biochemical study of a mitochondrial disorder. Dig Dis Sci 1992;37:456-463.

202. Nishino I, Spinazzola A, Papadimitriou A, et al: Mitochondrial neurogastrointestinal encephalomyopathy: An autosomal recessive disorder due to thymidine phosphorylase mutations. Ann Neurol 2000;47:792-800.

203. Chitkara DK, Nurko S, Shoffner JM, et al: Abnormalities in gastrointestinal motility are associated with diseases of oxidative phosphorylation in children. Am J Gastroenterol 2003;98:871-877.

204. Vassallo M, Camilleri M, Caron BL, Low PA: Gastrointestinal motor dysfunction in acquired selective cholinergic dysautonomia associated with infectious mononucleosis. Gastroenterology 1991;100:252-258.

205. Ginies JL, Francois H, Joseph MG, et al: A curable cause of chronic idiopathic intestinal pseudo-obstruction in children: Idiopathic myositis of the small intestine. J Pediatr Gastroenterol Nutr 1996;23:426-429.

206. Leon SH, Schuffler MD, Kettler M, Rohrmann CA: Chronic intestinal pseudoobstruction as a complication of Duchenne's muscular dystrophy. Gastroenterology 1986;90:455-459.

207. Staiano A, Del Giudice E, Romano A, et al: Upper gastrointestinal tract motility in children with progressive muscular dystrophy. J Pediatr 1992;121:720-724.

208. Boige N, Faure C, Cargill G, et al: Manometrical evaluation in visceral neuropathies in children. J Pediatr Gastroenterol Nutr 1994;19:71-77.

209. Vanderwinden JM, Rumessen JJ, Liu H, et al: Interstitial cells of Cajal in human colon and in Hirschsprung's disease. Gastroenterology 1996;111:901-910.

210. Amiel J, Lyonnet S: Hirschsprung disease, associated syndromes, and genetics: A review. J Med Genet 2001;38:729-739.

211. Verloes A, Elmer C, Lacombe D, et al: Ondine-Hirschsprung syndrome (Haddad syndrome): Further delineation in two cases and review of the literature. Eur J Pediatr 1993;152:75-77.

212. Sagel SD, Cohen H, Townsend SF: Neonatal Hirschsprung disease, dysautonomia, and central hypoventilation. Obstet Gynecol 1999;93:834-836.

213. Staiano A, Santoro L, De Marco R, et al: Autonomic dysfunction in children with Hirschsprung's disease. Dig Dis Sci 1999;44:960-965.

214. Goldberg DS, Ludwig IH: Congenital central hypoventilation syndrome: Ocular findings in 37 children. J Pediatr Ophthalmol Strabismus 1996;33:175-180.

215. Chelimsky G, Boyle JT, Tusing L, Chelimsky TC: Autonomic abnormalities in children with functional abdominal pain: Coincidence or etiology? J Pediatr Gastroenterol Nutr 2001;33:47-53.

216. Kirby RS, Fowler CJ, Gosling JA, Bannister R: Bladder dysfunction in distal autonomic neuropathy of acute onset. J Neurol Neurosurg Psychiatry 1985;48:762-767.

217. Bardosi A, Creutzfeldt W, DiMauro S, et al: Myo-, neuro-, gastrointestinal encephalopathy (MNGIE syndrome) due to partial deficiency of cytochrome C oxidase: A new mitochondrial multisystem disorder. Acta Neuropathol 1987;74:248-258.

218. Gort E, Guell R, Valls O: Diagnosis of urinary bladder disorders in diabetic children. Acta Diabetol Lat 1984;21:153-160.

219. Johnson D, Kubic P, Levitt C: Accidental ingestion of Vacor rodenticide: The systems and sequelae in a 25-month-old child. Am J Dis Child 1980;134:161-164.

220. Warkany J, Hubbard DM: Mercury in urine of children with acrodynia. Lancet 1948;1:829-830.

221. Bahiga LM, Kotb NA, El-Dessoukey EA: Neurological syndromes produced by some toxic metals encountered industrially or environmentally. Z Ernahrungswiss 1978;17:84-88.

222. Rangel-Guerra R, Martinez HR, Villarreal HJ: Thallium poisoning: Experience with 50 patients. Gac Med Mex 1990;126:487-494.

223. Devathasan G, Low D, Teoh PC, et al: Complications of chronic glue (toluene) abuse in adolescents. Aust N Z J Med 1984;14:39-43.

SUGGESTED READINGS

Assessment: Clinical autonomic testing report of the Therapeutics and Technology Assessment Subcommittee of the American Academy of Neurology. Neurology 1996;46:873-880.

Di Mario FJ Jr, Bauer L, Baxter D: Respiratory sinus arrhythmia in children with severe cyanotic and pallid breath-holding spells. J Child Neurol 1998;13:440-442.

Dyck PJ, Kennel AJ, Magal IV, Kraybill EN: A Virginia kinship with hereditary sensory neuropathy, peroneal muscular atrophy, and pes cavus. Mayo Clin Proc 1965;40:685-694.

Hyman PE: Chronic intestinal pseudo-obstruction in childhood: Progress in diagnosis and treatment. Scand J Gastroenterol Suppl 1995;213:39-46.

Indo Y: Genetics of congenital insensitivity to pain with anhidrosis (CIPA) or hereditary sensory and autonomic neuropathy type IV: Clinical, biological, and molecular aspects of mutations in TRKA (*NTRK1*) gene encoding the receptor tyrosine kinase for nerve growth factor. Clin Auton Res 2002:12(Suppl 1):I20-I32.

Mackler B, Person R, Miller LR, et al: Iron deficiency in the rat: Biochemical studies of brain metabolism. Pediatr Res 1978;12:217-220.

Robertson D, Goldberg MR, Onrot J, et al: Isolated failure of autonomic noradrenergic neurotransmission: Evidence for impaired beta-hydroxylation of dopamine. N Engl J Med 1986;314:1494-1497.

Voorhess ML, Stuart MJ, Stockman JA, Oski FA: Iron deficiency anemia and increased urinary norepinephrine excretion. J Pediatr 1975;86:542-547.

35

Neuromuscular Transmission Defects

P. IAN ANDREWS AND DONALD B. SANDERS

THE NEUROMUSCULAR JUNCTION

Anatomy

The neuromuscular junction (NMJ) is the connection between peripheral motor nerve axon and skeletal muscle, that is, the nerve-muscle synapse (see reviews elsewhere[1-3]). Each motor neuron innervates many skeletal muscle fibers, but, with few exceptions, each human muscle fiber is innervated by a single axon.[4,5] In mammalian extraocular muscles (EOMs), 20% of fibers have multiple innervation.[6] The motor axons divide into multiple, fine branches, which lead to NMJs on each muscle fiber. Each branch terminates in a small swelling, known as the *terminal bouton*, which lies over a specialized region of the muscle fiber membrane, the end plate. The proximal side of the bouton is capped by the distal tip of the accompanying Schwann cell. Within the terminal bouton are vesicles of neurotransmitter acetylcholine (ACh), choline acetyltransferase (for synthesis of ACh), mitochondria (which provide energy for synthesis and release of ACh), transmembrane voltage-gated calcium channels (VGCCs), and the multiple cellular mechanisms required for regulated release of ACh into the synaptic cleft.

The synaptic cleft, the space between the presynaptic terminal bouton and the postsynaptic motor end plate, is approximately 50 to 100 nm wide (wider than the 15- to 30-nm synaptic clefts in the central nervous system [CNS]). Within this cleft, bathed in extracellular fluid, are the basement membrane, composed of collagen, glycoproteins and other extracellular matrix proteins, and the enzyme acetylcholinesterase (AChE), anchored by a collagen tail to the basal lamina adjacent to the end plate.

The postsynaptic membrane beneath each terminal bouton is thickened and deeply folded. The region of the terminal bouton from which ACh is released, the active zone, is directly opposite the tips of junctional folds of the postsynaptic membrane. The outer third of these folds are densely lined by ionotropic receptors for ACh (AChR)—more than 10,000 AChRs/μm^2. Deeper within the junctional folds are voltage-gated Na^+ channels.

Also located at the postsynaptic muscle membrane, near the AChR, are the muscle-specific tyrosine kinase (MuSK) and the receptor-associated synaptic protein, rapsyn (Fig. 35-1). During development, agrin is released from the motor nerve to interact with MuSK. This is then phosphorylated, leading to phosphorylation of rapsyn and clustering of AChRs on the postsynaptic muscle surface. MuSK is essential for development of the NMJ, although its role in mature muscle is not specifically defined.[7]

Molecular Biology of the AChR

The AChR is a ligand-gated ion channel. It is composed of specific combinations of five subunits, α, β, δ, and γ or ϵ, which are encoded by specific genes (Fig. 35-2). Adult AChRs are composed of two α subunits and one each of the β, δ, and ϵ subunits. Fetal (and denervated) AChRs are composed of two α subunits and one each of the β, δ, and γ subunits. The fetal form is present in early gestation. The adult form makes its appearance at 14 weeks' gestation. Cross-over between the fetal and adult forms is activity

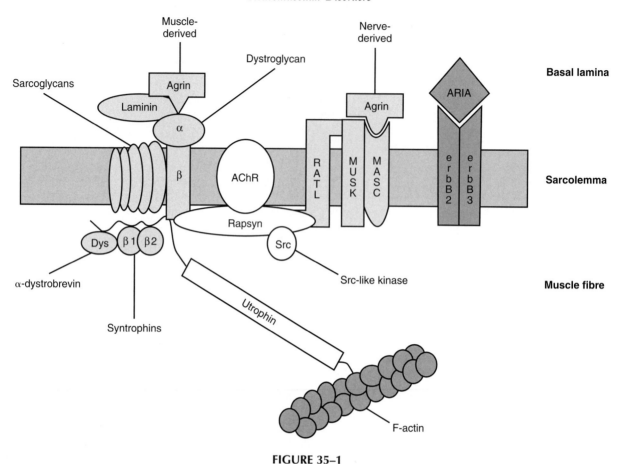

FIGURE 35–1

Molecular organization of the postsynaptic apparatus, showing some of the identified and hypothetical proteins in the postsynaptic neuromuscular junction membrane. (From Liyanage Y, Hoch W, Beeson D, Vincent A: The agrin/muscle-specific kinase pathway: New targets for autoimmune and genetic disorders at the neuromuscular junction. Muscle Nerve 2002;25:4-16.)

dependent[8] and mostly complete by 33 weeks' gestation in humans.[9,10] The subunits form a barrel-like structure that traverses the muscle membrane. The central pore allows regulated flux of cations, mostly Na^+ and K^+, after binding of ACh to the receptor. The pore opens (activates) when two ACh molecules attach to specific binding regions at the interfaces between one α and the γ and the other α and the δ subunits in fetal and denervated muscle and at the interfaces between one α and the ϵ and the other α and the δ subunits in adult muscle.

Mutations in different domains of the different subunits influence function of the AChR by altering the kinetics or affinity of ACh binding to the receptor or by altering kinetics of channel opening and closure. For example, slow-channel myasthenic syndromes are caused by various AChR mutations that increase the response to ACh and result in prolonged channel activation. Fast-channel syndromes are caused by mutations that reduce the response to ACh, resulting in abnormally brief openings of the channel and reduced synaptic cation flux. Mutations in AChR subunit genes, pre-

dominantly the ϵ subunit, also influence the formation of AChRs and may result in deficiency of AChRs at the end plate. Similarly, mutations in genes encoding proteins that regulate expression, localization, or concentration of AChRs in the postsynaptic membrane may influence the receptor. For example, mutation or microdeletion of the N-box promoter of the AChR ϵ subunit gene[11] and mutations in rapsyn[12] result in deficiency of AChRs at the end plate.

Adult AChRs at the NMJ turn over at a very slow rate, with a half-life of more than 10 days. Fetal AChRs turn over more quickly, due to internalization and degradation—their half-life is about 10 hours and constant synthesis is required for replacement of AChRs.

Embryology

The development of the mammalian NMJ is well reviewed elsewhere.[2,13] Motor neurons innervating the NMJ arise from multipotential progenitors in the ventral neural tube. Schwann cells are derivatives of the neural crest, which

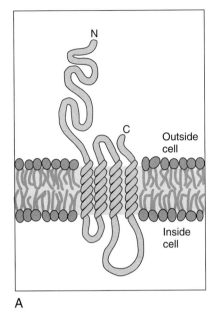
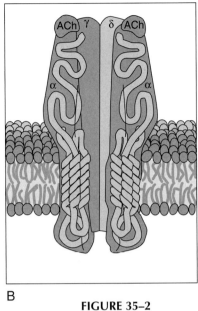
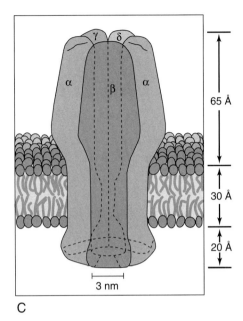

A   B   C

FIGURE 35–2

The structure of the acetylcholine (ACh) receptor. A, Each receptor subunit crosses the membrane four times. B and C, Five such subunits come together to form a complex structure that surrounds a central pore. ACh attachment points are indicated in B. (A-C, From Purves D, Augustine GJ, Fitzpatrick D, et al: Neuroscience. Sunderland, MA, Sinauer Associates, 1997.)

arises from the dorsal margin of the neural tube. Muscle fibers are derived from mesodermal cells, which migrate to peripheral sites, differentiate into myoblasts, and then align in "straps" and fuse to form myotubes. Prior to formation of the NMJ, the primitive myotubes express fetal AChRs diffusely over their surface. Nerve-muscle contact begins as the motor axon's growth cone reaches the newly formed myotube. Such contacts are loosely aggregated in the human fetus by 9 weeks' gestation. In these earliest synapses, the terminal boutons contain few presynaptic vesicles but are capable of rudimentary transmission.[14]

Presynaptic morphologic changes are virtually complete by the 10th week. The complicated structure of the postsynaptic membrane forms more slowly but is well established by 20 weeks' gestation.[14] Aggregation of the AChRs in the outer third of postjunctional membranes is carefully ordered and regulated.[2,7,15-17] Initiation of clustering of AChRs early in embryogenesis is dependent on MuSK and rapsyn and is independent of neural input. Agrin, a glycoprotein secreted into the basal lamina mostly from motor nerve terminals, induces and maintains further clustering of AChRs, rapsyn, sodium channels and other postsynaptic proteins in the postjunctional membrane. This process also utilizes MuSK, which phosphorylates AChRs and enhances their interaction with cytoskeletal components of the NMJ. Neuregulin (formerly known as *ARIA*) is also released from motor nerve terminals. It stimulates expression of AChR genes in specific muscle fiber nuclei that underlie the postsynaptic membrane to stimulate local synthesis of AChRs. In contrast, AChRs away from the NMJ are pruned via a

cascade of signals (initiated by action potentials [APs]) culminating in down-regulation of expression of AChR genes in muscle fiber nuclei away from the NMJ.

The primitive NMJ is initially innervated by multiple axons, but terminal branches segregate and withdraw to leave a single axon overlying each convoluted postsynaptic membrane. This process of "synapse elimination" is activity dependent. This developmental process is recapitulated following denervation injury to adult muscle fibers. Reinnervation begins with transient polyneural reinnervation and expression of the fetal AChRs, followed by synapse elimination.

Although maturation of the postsynaptic membrane is well established by 20 weeks' gestation, the surface area, complexity of junctional folds, and density of AChRs in the postsynaptic membrane continue to develop at least until term.[9] The synaptic concentration of AChE also increases through gestation and infancy. In parallel with morphologic changes, function matures during late gestation and infancy. For example, the NMJ of infants of 34 to 37 weeks' gestation have less reserve and are less able to sustain fast, repetitive activation than the NMJs in term infants, which, in turn, have less reserve than the adult NMJ.[18]

Neuromuscular Transmission

Features of neuromuscular transmission (NMT) are well reviewed in Reichardt and Kelly,[19] Engel,[20] and Elmqvist.[21] Spontaneous release of individual synaptic vesicles into the synapse (defined as one "quantum" of ACh, containing

5000 to 10,000 molecules of ACh) occurs continuously at the NMJ. Each quantum produces a miniature end plate potential, approximately 1 mV in amplitude. These miniature depolarizations are insufficient to activate neighboring voltage-gated sodium channels and, therefore, insufficient to initiate muscle contraction.

Propagation of an AP along the α-motor axon brings electrical depolarization to the terminal region of the axon. This depolarization opens VGCCs in the presynaptic bouton with consequent local influx of Ca^{2+} ions. This triggers fusion of many ACh-containing synaptic vesicles (typically 60 to 100) to the presynaptic membrane and release of ACh into the synaptic cleft. The amount of ACh released by a nerve AP is known as its *quantal content*. The released ACh diffuses across the synaptic cleft and binds reversibly to postsynaptic AChRs. Binding of ACh opens the channel within the receptor and permits rapid flux of cations, mostly Na^+, through the postsynaptic membrane, resulting in local depolarization—the end plate potential. This change in potential rapidly activates voltage-gated sodium channels deeper in the junctional folds, with further influx of Na^+ and launching of the muscle AP, which spreads along the muscle fiber to initiate muscle contraction. The enzyme AChE, highly concentrated in the synaptic cleft, rapidly hydrolyses ACh to terminate its effect.

The normal nerve AP generates an end plate potential of about 40 mV. This is considerably more than the 7- to 20-mV threshold required to activate the voltage-gated sodium channels and initiate muscle contraction. This excess or reserve in the system is the "safety factor" of NMT and ensures that each nerve impulse induces muscle contraction. The magnitude of the safety factor is relatively reduced in infants compared with children and adults. If a nerve impulse fails to induce a suprathreshold end plate depolarization, muscle contraction will not occur; that is, NMT is an "all or none" phenomenon. Failure of the nerve AP to generate a muscle AP is known as "blocking." Weakness is manifest when a significant proportion of NMJs is blocked.

All disorders of NMT are characterized by compromise of the safety factor. Processes that reduce the safety factor and produce muscle weakness include reduced synthesis, storage, or release of ACh; reduced activity of AChE in the synaptic cleft; and abnormal function of the postsynaptic complex.

In normal muscle, repetitive 2 to 5/sec activation of the nerve depletes immediately available presynaptic ACh stores within four or five stimuli. Because of the safety margin at normal NMJs, however, the released ACh still exceeds the threshold required for muscle contraction, and muscle APs normally result from all nerve depolarizations. When NMT is impaired, the threshold may not be achieved by all nerve activations, and muscle APs do not

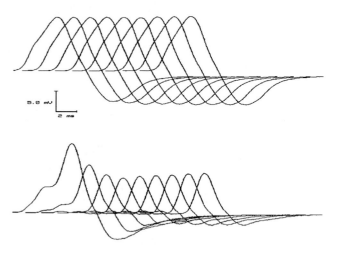

FIGURE 35–3

Compound muscle action potentials (CMAPs) elicited by repetitive motor nerve stimulation at 3/sec in a hand muscle: Normal (top) and myasthenia gravis (bottom). With optimum recording electrode placement, the CMAP waveform departs sharply from the baseline and is monophasic. In myasthenia gravis, the decrement begins with the second response of the train, is maximum at the fourth or fifth response, and resolves thereafter, giving a characteristic U-shaped or "saddle-shaped" train envelope. (Courtesy of D. B. Sanders, Duke University, Durham, North Carolina.)

occur with later nerve depolarizations in a series. This physiologic sequence forms the basis for the decremental response with repetitive nerve stimulation characteristic of many disorders of the NMJ (Fig. 35-3.)

Each nerve depolarization releases Ca^{2+} ions into the periterminal space, which increases the local concentration of calcium for 100 to 200 milliseconds. If another depolarization occurs during this time, the higher calcium concentration increases the number of ACh quanta released. In conditions of impaired NMT, this greater ACh release may briefly improve synaptic transmission, a phenomenon called *facilitation*. Marked facilitation after activation is characteristic of presynaptic blockade. Following the period of facilitation, the amplitude of end plate potentials falls, reducing the margin of safety for NMT (post-tetanic or postactivation exhaustion) for up to 10 minutes (Fig. 35-4).

ELECTRODIAGNOSTIC STUDIES RELEVANT TO INFANTS AND CHILDREN WITH DISORDERS OF NEUROMUSCULAR TRANSMISSION

The main electrodiagnostic techniques applied to children with disorders of NMT include nerve conduction studies (NCSs), repetitive motor nerve stimulation (RMNS)

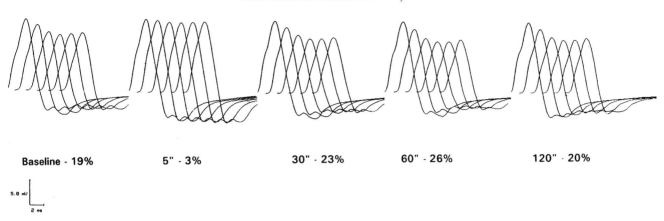

Baseline - 19%   5" - 3%   30" - 23%   60" - 26%   120" - 20%

FIGURE 35-4

Repetitive motor nerve stimulation studies with 3/sec stimulation in a hand muscle of a patient with myasthenia gravis, before and at indicated intervals after maximum voluntary contraction of the muscle. The percentage decrement of the fourth response of each train is noted. There is an initial 19% decrement, which virtually disappears immediately after activation, becomes maximum at 1 minute, and returns to the baseline value at 2 minutes. (Courtesy of D. B. Sanders, Duke University, Durham, North Carolina.)

studies, conventional needle electromyography (EMG), and single-fiber electromyography (SF-EMG). These studies are performed relatively infrequently in infants and children. They are often painful, and the small size of infants, especially preterm infants, makes them technically difficult. Patient cooperation with testing is often limited or short lived. Maintaining temperature is particularly important, since the core temperature of small infants quickly falls outside the confines of their neonatal incubator, which may adversely affect performance and interpretation of studies. Oftentimes, studies crucial for diagnosis, prognosis, and therapy are performed in the neonatal or pediatric intensive care unit (ICU) settings. Such studies are necessarily performed around tubes, intravenous (IV) lines, and restraints and in the presence of mechanical ventilation, medications, and multiple electrical devices. All these conspire to make the performance and interpretation of such studies challenging. Therefore, it is crucial that we thoughtfully and thoroughly evaluate clinical information before testing, to be certain that the studies are indicated and to plan the procedure. A suggested protocol for electrophysiologic testing of infants and children with suspected disorders of NMT is shown in Box 35-1.

Practical Considerations

Performance and interpretation of these tests require that the patient remain still during the procedure. Some testing also requires active patient cooperation, such as voluntary muscle contraction. RMNS and SF-EMG tests, the cornerstones of electrodiagnostic tests for disorders of NMT, are particularly demanding of stillness and cooperation. In practice, infants and young children usually

---

BOX 35-1
SUGGESTED PROTOCOL FOR ELECTROPHYSIOLOGIC ASSESSMENT OF NEONATES AND CHILDREN WITH SUSPECTED DISORDERS OF NEUROMUSCULAR TRANSMISSION

1. Motor and sensory nerve conduction studies and needle EMG in one symptomatic limb
2. A single supramaximal stimulus to identify potential repetitive CMAPs (see text) in two distal muscles
3. Baseline RMNS at 3 to 5 seconds, in two distal muscles
4. If step 3 produces no decrement, tetanizing stimulation at 50 Hz for 10 seconds, followed by 3 to 5/sec stimulation every 30 seconds until CMAP amplitude returns to baseline
5. If step 4 evokes an abnormal decrement, consider treatment with cholinesterase inhibitor and repeat step 4
6. If RMNS is normal, consider single-fiber EMG with volitional activation or axonal stimulation (see text)

CMAP, compound muscle action potential; RMNS, repetitive motor nerve stimulation.

need sedation to facilitate electrodiagnostic testing. Guidelines for premedication and sedation relevant to these patients are provided in the American Academy of

Pediatrics Guidelines for Monitoring Infants and Children after Sedation.[22,23] These tests are frequently performed on patients who are floppy and weak, in whom bulbar and respiratory function and reserve are limited. Such patients are at risk of dangerous respiratory compromise during sedation. Furthermore, treatment with cholinesterase inhibitors (e.g., edrophonium [Tensilon]) may induce acute bronchorrhea and salivation, adding further danger to an already compromised patient. Therefore, preadministration or coadministration of atropine or ready availability of atropine is required if cholinesterase inhibitors are to be used during testing. Similarly, following the procedure, these children may be "groggy," increasing the potential for falls. An experienced team, well-practiced in handling sedated children, prepared for pediatric resuscitation, providing monitoring on a one-to-one basis is required to facilitate electrodiagnostic testing in infants and children.

For outpatients who require sedation, we assess respiratory and bulbar function and potential drug interactions before the procedure. Protocols for sedation vary among institutions. We commonly use a combination of chloral hydrate (30 mg/kg for infants of 3 to 12 months, and 50 mg/kg after 12 months, to a maximum of 1 gm), pethidine (0.5 to 1 mg/kg/dose IV or 1.5 to 2 mg/kg/dose intramuscularly [IM] in children older than 3 months, to a maximum of 75 mg), and droperidol (0.05 mg/kg IM for infants 6 to 12 months of age, and 0.1 to 0.2 mg/kg IM after 12 months). The potential reversibility of pethidine and droperidol with naloxone makes this combination relatively safe, provided caution is applied.

In young infants and in the ICU setting, where the patient's ventilation is often controlled and patients are quite immobile, we commonly use midazolam (oral: 0.5 mg/kg initially and then 0.25 mg/kg if not sedated, to a maximum of 15 mg; nasal: 0.3 mg/kg to a maximum of 5 mg; IV: 0.1 mg/kg bolus titrated as required, often to about 0.3 mg/kg/dose, and repeated as required through the procedure). If necessary, midazolam can be rapidly reversed with flumazenil.

Some recommend general anesthesia, typically using midazolam and nitrous oxide, or propofol, with or without a short-acting narcotic agent for pain relief. None of these agents compromise NMJ function, and their short half-lives permit rapid recovery from sedation, minimizing the postanesthetic risk. Since these patients are often being investigated for undiagnosed neuromuscular disease, anesthetics that may precipitate neuroleptic malignant syndrome, especially halogenated inhalation agents such as halothane, should be avoided. Neuromuscular blocking agents must also be avoided. Patients in the ICU setting are often treated with multiple drugs, some of which may compromise function of the NMJ and confound diagnostic testing. Box 35-2 lists drugs that may fall into this category

---

BOX 35-2
DRUGS THAT MAY CAUSE INCREASED WEAKNESS IN DISORDERS OF NEUROMUSCULAR TRANSMISSION

1. Alpha-interferon, botulinum toxin, and D-penicillamine should be avoided in myasthenic patients.
2. The following drugs produce worsening of myasthenic weakness in most patients who receive them. Use with caution, and monitor the patient for exacerbation of myasthenic symptoms.
   Succinylcholine, D-tubocurarine, or other neuromuscular-blocking agents
   Quinine, quinidine, and procainamide
   Aminoglycoside antibiotics, particularly gentamicin, kanamycin, neomycin, and streptomycin
   Beta blockers (systemic and ocular preparations): propranolol, timolol maleate eyedrops
   Calcium-channel blockers
   Magnesium salts (including laxatives and antacids with high Mg^{2+} concentrations)
   Iodinated contrast agents
3. Many other drugs are reported to exacerbate the weakness in some patients with myasthenia gravis. All patients with myasthenia gravis should be observed for increased weakness whenever a new medication is started.*

° An up-to-date reference document for such adverse interactions is maintained on the Web site of the Myasthenia Gravis Foundation of America (*http://www.myasthenia.org/drugs/reference.htm*).

---

and should be discontinued prior to testing. If possible, electrical interference from machinery surrounding patients in the ICU should be reduced. Transport of the patient to the EMG laboratory may avoid such interference in some settings.

Older children, 6 or 8 years of age and older, may tolerate and cooperate with electrodiagnostic testing without sedation. The parents' encouragement and support is often crucial in obtaining the child's cooperation. The parents' help may be enlisted by clear explanation of the need for and methodology of the procedure. Simple, honest descriptions of the procedure to the child, and a calm, positive manner in the examiner facilitate patient cooperation and trust. However, high stimulation rates during RMNS are distressing, and SF-EMG, especially of facial and orbital muscles, requires considerable patient cooperation. Movement artifact needs to be avoided, or at least recognized, because it may falsely simulate a positive RMNS test. Therefore, complex studies of NMT may not be feasible without sedation, even in otherwise cooperative children. This decision frequently can be made only in the actual testing situation.

Nerve Conduction Studies

NCSs in infants and children are discussed in Chapter 6. Sensory and motor nerve conduction velocities (NCVs), distal latencies, and F-wave minimal latencies are typically normal in disorders of the NMJ.

The stimulus intensity required to elicit maximal compound muscle action potential (CMAP) amplitude is determined using a stimulus of 0.05-millisecond duration and increasing the stimulus intensity until there is a plateau of response, in that further increase in stimulus intensity produces no further increase in CMAP amplitude. The stimulus intensity is then increased by another 20% to 25%. This is the supramaximal stimulus. The experienced electromyographer minimizes discomfort by using the fewest necessary stimuli to determine the supramaximal stimulus. In presynaptic and more severe postsynaptic disorders of the NMJ, the CMAP amplitude is often reduced.

To enhance identification of the rare but important finding of repetitive CMAPs (R-CMAPs), responses to single supramaximal stimuli should be observed before RMNS is begun (see later).

Repetitive Motor Nerve Stimulation

Children and Adolescents

Many children older than 8 to 10 years of age can be examined using the same RMNS technique as adults, with appropriate adjustments for limb size. In our experience, children older than age 8 years can usually cooperate adequately without sedation. Shorter limb length requires great attention to stimulus artifacts. Stimulating electrodes with a shorter interelectrode distance (1.25 to 2 cm) should be used in infants and small children, but standard recording disk electrodes are suitable.

Choice of nerves for stimulation depends on the localization of symptoms. A muscle weakened by most disorders of NMT should reveal an abnormal decremental response to RMNS. Important potential exceptions include some congenital myasthenic syndromes (CMSs) and botulism (see later). Percutaneous stimulation at distal sites, recording over small distal muscles is often best tolerated and provides most reliable data, since the limb can be immobilized with an arm or leg board. Often the distribution of weakness, however, requires proximal muscle testing. For instance, the child with primarily bulbar weakness due to autoimmune myasthenia gravis may have normal RMNS of a peripheral nerve such as the ulnar or median. If this

occurs, then one needs to test a more proximal muscle, such as the trapezius or facial muscles. Muscle surface temperature should be maintained above 34°C in hand or foot muscles. Preparation of the skin with alcohol or mild abrasion improves conductance and reduces the required stimulus intensity. Submaximal stimulation and unnoticed movement of stimulating or recording electrodes may give false-positive results. Near-nerve needle stimulation, such as to musculocutaneous or femoral nerves, may facilitate supramaximal stimulation with relatively little discomfort. Anticholinesterase and other NMJ-modifying drugs should be avoided for 24 hours, if safe to do so. A reproducible decrement in testing of at least two nerves is desirable to confirm a disorder of NMT.

Slow RMNS is performed at 2 to 5/sec. Five to 10 supramaximal stimuli are applied. When NMT is impaired, the greatest proportional decrement occurs between the first and second responses, but the absolute decrement is maximal by the fourth or fifth response and frequently repairs by the seventh to tenth response. A reproducible decrement of more than 10% between the first and the lowest of the first five responses is abnormal. This finding indicates a disorder of NMT and is consistent with either presynaptic or postsynaptic dysfunction. Since the CMAP represents the sum of all individual muscle fiber APs, transmission across a significant proportion of individual NMJs must fail for the test to be abnormal. Therefore, RMNS is relatively insensitive to impaired NMT.

Slow RMNS following 10 to 60 seconds of activation by isometric exercise or high-frequency nerve stimulation (10 to 50/sec) may reveal abnormalities not identified in the resting muscle and thus enhance the diagnostic sensitivity of the test. When NMT is impaired, such activation increases CMAP amplitude or decreases the decrement for 1 to 2 minutes, followed by 2 to 10 minutes of enhanced decrement. In mildly affected muscles with most disorders of the NMJ, resting RMNS responses may be normal, but repeat administration of slow RMNS each minute after activation may unmask the deficit after a couple of minutes. In moderately involved muscles an abnormal decrement at rest is often repaired by activation and worsens again within minutes. In muscles with severe weakness due to a postsynaptic NMT abnormality, the baseline CMAP amplitude may be slightly reduced, a decrement is observed with slow RMNS, and transient facilitation may be noted after activation.

Rapid RMNS is particularly useful in patients with suspected presynaptic disorders, such as the Lambert-Eaton-like CMS, botulism and Lambert-Eaton myasthenic syndrome (LEMS) (see later). Hand or foot muscles are more likely than proximal muscles to show typical abnormalities in these conditions. Supramaximal stimulation at 20 to 50/sec is applied for 2 to 10 seconds in the infant and younger child. This is quite painful and is therefore often performed under anesthesia. In the normal NMJ such stimulation may briefly deplete the immediately available pool of ACh-containing vesicles, but the normal safety factor maintains NMT and CMAP amplitudes. In some presynaptic disorders, reduced release of ACh reduces the CMAP amplitude. Rapid RMNS increases extracellular Ca^{2+} concentration at the presynaptic nerve terminal, increasing ACh release, which then exceeds threshold for many previously blocked NMJs, and augments muscle contraction. This is reflected by a marked incremental response in CMAP amplitudes with rapid RMNS. Ten seconds of maximal voluntary contraction has a similar effect.

Administration of edrophonium IV or neostigmine, 0.15 mg/kg to a maximum of 2 mg subcutaneously, transiently repairs the decremental responses in most disorders of the NMJ. Important exceptions are congenital AChE deficiency, slow-channel myasthenic syndromes, and botulism.

Neonates

Transmission across the NMJ matures during gestation and infancy. Unfortunately, normative data regarding RMNS in preterm and term infants are limited. In general, infants display less reserve in NMT than older children and adults, characterized by reduced facilitation and reduced and delayed recovery following tetanizing stimulation.

One study of 17 normal neonates, born at 34 to 42 weeks' gestation, aged 1 day to 6 weeks, measured CMAP amplitudes before, during, and after 15-second epochs of repetitive nerve stimulation at 1, 2, 5, 10, 20, and 50/sec.[18] No decrement or facilitation was observed during or after 1 or 2/sec stimulation. One of the 17 infants showed a decrement of 19% during 5/sec stimulation, and this infant and one other showed a 14% transient decrement after the train. None showed a decrement during or after 10/sec stimulation. Twelve showed decremental responses (13% to 38%) during and six showed transient decremental responses (15% to 35%) after 20/sec stimulation. All showed decremental responses (17% to 84%) during and 13 showed transient decremental responses (10% to 120%) after 50/sec stimulation. Twelve showed post-tetanic exhaustion for 10 seconds to 10 minutes after 50/sec stimulation. In general, decrement and post-tetanic exhaustion were more common in preterm than term infants. One infant showed 14% facilitation of CMAP amplitude after a train of 1/sec stimulation. Four showed facilitation (11% to 19%) during 5/sec stimulation, akin to that seen on Lambert-Eaton syndrome.[24] None showed facilitation during or after higher stimulus rates.

Another study measured RMNS in ulnar nerve–hypothenar muscles in three normal term infants, using supramaximal 3/sec stimulation for 10 seconds and 10 and 50/sec stimulation for 5 seconds.[25] Decrements of 10% to 20% were observed during 3/sec stimulation (maximal between 4 and 8 seconds). No decrements were observed during faster stimulation. One infant showed 30% increment of CMAP amplitude during 50/sec stimulation; otherwise, increments with 10 and 50/sec stimulation varied from 2% to 15%. Following 3/sec stimulation, single stimuli produced CMAP amplitudes of within 10% of initial amplitudes. Following 10 and 50/sec stimulation, single stimuli produced CMAP amplitudes that varied from 80% to 105% of initial amplitudes.

In infants, RMNS is usually performed on median, ulnar, or peroneal nerves, although proximal nerves and muscles can be studied. Care needs to be taken to maintain skin temperature over distal muscles greater than 34°C. The limb is immobilized with appropriate restraints. Surface electrodes are secured by tape. The stimulating electrode should be as close as possible to the nerve and at least 4 cm from the recording electrodes. The stimulus intensity required to elicit maximal CMAP amplitude is normally less than for adults. Preparation of the skin with alcohol or mild abrasion improves conductance and reduces required stimulus intensity and stimulus artifacts.

Decrementing responses in infants must be interpreted in light of the findings in normal neonates described earlier. Decrements greater than 20% in two muscles can be taken as evidence of abnormal NMT. Lesser decrements greater than 10% should be interpreted with caution. Application of 1 to 5-sec trains of 20 to 50/sec stimulation permits identification of "postexercise" facilitation or decrement. Facilitation of more than 120% is abnormal for infants.[26]

Electromyography

EMG is discussed in Chapter 6. Conventional EMG is often normal in disorders of the NMJ, but three patterns of abnormality are recognized. These include short-duration, low-amplitude polyphasic motor unit APs (MUAPs) due to physiologic blocking of NMT during voluntary activation; unstable MUAPs; and (rarely) fibrillation potentials due to persistent transmission block with effective denervation of individual muscle fibers.

Single-Fiber EMG

SF-EMG selectively assesses transmission at individual NMJs and is the most sensitive method for identifying defective NMT in vivo.[27,28] SF-EMG is technically demanding and requires considerable expertise to be reliable. Recordings are made with a concentric needle electrode that contains a shielded central wire of 25-μm diameter that is exposed through a side port 3 mm from the needle tip. The small recording surface selectively registers activity from muscle fibers close to the electrode (300 μm compared to 1 cm with conventional concentric EMG needle

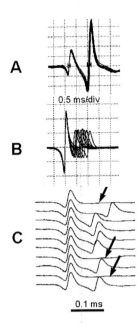

FIGURE 35–5

Single-fiber EMG recordings during voluntary activation. A, Ten superimposed discharges of a pair of potentials with normal jitter. B, Ten superimposed discharges of a pair of potentials with increased jitter. C, Ten consecutive discharges of a pair of potentials in which the second potential intermittently blocks (arrows). (A-C, From Sanders DB: Electrophysiologic study of disorders of neuromuscular transmission. In Aminoff MJ [ed]: Electrodiagnosis in Clinical Neurology. New York, Churchill Livingstone, 1999, pp 303-321.)

electrodes). A 500-Hz low-frequency filter further increases recording selectivity by reducing signals from more distant muscle fibers. This permits identification of APs from single muscle fibers. The latency between nerve activation and muscle fiber depolarization varies normally because of the quantal nature of synaptic transmission. This variability is the neuromuscular jitter. Jitter is inversely, but nonlinearly, related to the safety margin of the NMJ.[29] When NMT is sufficiently impaired, nerve impulses fail to elicit muscle APs and SF-EMG demonstrates intermittent impulse blocking (Fig. 35-5). When blocking occurs in many end plates in a muscle, there is clinical weakness. Jitter varies among different end plates in a muscle and from muscle to muscle. In diseases of abnormal NMT, jitter may be increased in muscles that are clinically normal and that show no decrement to RMNS.

SF-EMG jitter analysis can be performed during nerve stimulation or volitional muscle contraction. For the latter, the patient must activate and maintain a relatively constant firing rate of the tested motor units. The former requires only that the muscle be relaxed and is used for uncooperative patients, under sedation if necessary. Nerve twigs are stimulated repetitively with a monopolar needle electrode, using very low-intensity rectangular pulses. In both techniques, the SF-EMG needle is positioned within the muscle to record single muscle fiber APs of at least 200 μV amplitude. With voluntary activation, jitter is measured between APs from pairs of muscle fibers innervated by branches of the same axon. With stimulation, jitter is measured between the stimulus and APs from individual muscle fibers. Jitter is calculated as the mean difference between consecutive interpotential intervals (MCD) recorded during voluntary activation. With the stimulation technique, the MCD calculation uses the latency from stimulus to AP. Blocking is expressed as the percentage of AP pairs (with voluntary activation) or single APs (with nerve stimulation) in which any nerve depolarizations fail to produce muscle APs.

In myasthenia gravis, blocking occurs only when jitter values are highly abnormal. The degree of impairment varies within the muscle, and jitter must be measured in an adequate sample of end plates. Normal jitter varies among muscles, and normative values for jitter measured during volition are available for many muscles and for children older than 10 years of age.[30,31] For younger ages, especially term or preterm infants, normal jitter values must be assumed to be higher, and results should be interpreted accordingly.

The MCD value measured during axonal stimulation is less than that measured during voluntary activation of the same muscle since the jitter measured during axonal stimulation comes from only single end plates. Reference values for jitter during axonal stimulation have been determined for the extensor digitorum communis and orbicularis oculi muscles.[27,32] For other muscles, the normative values for stimulation jitter can be obtained by multiplying the normative values for voluntary activation by a conversion factor of 0.8. MCD values of 4 microseconds or less obtained during stimulation SF-EMG indicate that the muscle fiber is being directly stimulated; these values should not be used for assessment of NMT.

Jitter is greatest in weak muscles but may be abnormal even in muscles not judged to be clinically affected. Normal jitter in a weak muscle excludes a disorder of NMT as the cause of weakness. SF-EMG accurately identifies disordered NMT but may not necessarily distinguish between various pathogeneses. In general, however, jitter that is greater with higher rates of nerve activation indicates postsynaptic dysfunction (e.g., autoimmune myasthenia gravis), and jitter that is less with higher rates of stimulation indicates diminished presynaptic release of ACh (e.g., infantile botulism, LEMS). Because of its great sensitivity, SF-EMG may demonstrate abnormal jitter in other nerve or muscle disorders, including anterior horn cell disease, peripheral neuropathies, and myopathies.

BOX 35-3
DISORDERS OF NEUROMUSCULAR TRANSMISSION IN INFANCY AND CHILDHOOD

Prenatal or Neonatal Onset
Most congenital myasthenic syndromes (see text)
Transient neonatal myasthenia gravis
Hypermagnesemia

Onset in Later Infancy or Childhood
Some congenital myasthenic syndromes (see text)
Botulism
Autoimmune myasthenia gravis
Lambert-Eaton myasthenic syndrome
Toxins

Disorders of Neuromuscular Transmission

A relatively small number of uncommon disorders disrupt NMT during infancy and childhood (Box 35-3 and Table 35-1). In general, diagnosis depends on a high index of suspicion. The dominant clinical feature is weakness, which is often fatigable. This section briefly details the pathophysiology, clinical and laboratory features, and diagnosis of neonatal, infantile, and childhood syndromes of abnormal NMT. We focus on electrodiagnostic techniques relevant to these patients and highlight electrophysiologic features of these disorders, which often confirm a disorder of NMT and may offer clues to the specific diagnosis. Table 35-2 and Figure 35-6 summarize clinical features that help distinguish among the main differential diagnoses relevant to neonatal disorders of NMT.

Congenital Myasthenic Syndromes

The CMSs comprise a heterogeneous and growing group of uncommon disorders. They are caused by genetic defects of the NMJ, which reduce the safety margin and compromise the function of the NMJ. Syndromes are classified according to site of the defect (presynaptic, synaptic, and postsynaptic), when these can be determined; some syndromes are not well classified. Some mutations are "private" to each kinship, in which case mutation testing can be extremely difficult, whereas some mutations are common in different kinships. For example, a specific mutation in the AChR ε subunit is common in CMS with deficiency of AChRs at the end plate in patients of southeastern European or Gypsy descent but uncommon in patients of German descent.[33,34] It seems likely that more defects will be identified. Much of the work establishing the clinical,

electrophysiologic, pathologic, and genetic features of CMS has come from the group at the Mayo Clinic. Their recent review of the topic is comprehensive and useful.[35]

Clinical Features

Patients affected with CMS may have mild symptoms or severe, life-threatening disease. In the absence of a similarly affected family member, a high index of suspicion is required to make the diagnosis, especially given the limitations of clinical examination in the newborn period.

Most children affected with CMS, irrespective of the specific syndrome, have similar clinical features. Most have problems from birth, although presentation may be delayed because of the nonspecific nature and mildness of symptoms in some individuals. Patients with slow-channel syndromes and limb-girdle myasthenia, however, characteristically present in childhood or adolescence. Prenatal weakness may be manifest as reduced fetal movements, polyhydramnios, and arthrogryposis. Generalized weakness and hypotonia are common. Ptosis and strabismus may occur but are uncommon in some syndromes (notably end plate choline acetyltransferase deficiency, also known as *CMS with episodic apnea*; Lambert-Eaton-like CMS; and familial limb-girdle myasthenia). Weakness is typically exacerbated with crying or feeding during infancy and may be improved by sleep. Feeding difficulties and intermittent or persistent respiratory insufficiency are common and potentially life threatening. Motor development is often delayed. Fluctuating and fatigable weakness of extraocular, bulbar, trunk, and limb muscles may be demonstrable in toddlers and children. Scoliosis and lumbar lordosis, exaggerated by prolonged standing, may be noted.

Clinical manifestations of some syndromes are distinctive, and their recognition may facilitate precise diagnosis, as discussed in the following:

1. Recurrent, sudden bulbar weakness, dyspnea and apnea following fever, vomiting or excitement, or without precipitant, may occur in *choline acetyltransferase deficiency* (also known as *CMS with episodic apnea* and often reported as "familial infantile myasthenia.") Some patients manifest neonatal weakness and respiratory failure, which improves with age. Some seem well at birth. Episodic apnea begins during infancy or early childhood and may have a fatal outcome. Most patients are normal or only mildly weak between episodes.

2. Patients with congenital end plate AChE deficiency characteristically have slow and limited pupillary responses to light.[36,37]

3. Patients with slow-channel syndromes present in childhood or adolescence and typically show selective weakness of cervical and wrist and finger extensor muscles.

4. A rare CMS is associated with epidermolysis bullosa, a progressive myopathy and elevated serum creatine kinase

TABLE 35–1. CLINICAL FEATURES OF NEONATAL DISORDERS OF NEUROMUSCULAR TRANSMISSION AND MAJOR DIFFERENTIAL DIAGNOSES

Clinical Feature	CMS	TNMG	Botulism	SMA	Cervical Cord Injury	Myopathy	Central
Family history of similar problems	Often; most are autosomal recessive	Almost always	No	Usually autosomal recessive inheritance	No	Often; various inheritance patterns	Some are acquired Some have various inheritance patterns
Fetal hypokinesis (e.g., arthrogryposis, polyhydramnios, pulmonary hypoplasia)	Some syndromes	May occur, especially in asymptomatic mothers with antifetal AChR Abs	No	Rare	Usually cord injury occurs at delivery, but rarely may occur in utero; may cause hypokinesis	Some syndromes	Some syndromes
Alert and responsive	Yes	Yes	Yes	Yes	Yes, unless secondary asphyxia	Yes	No
Feeding difficulties	If severe	If severe	Common	Uncommon initially, more common as disease progresses.	Common, secondary to respiratory failure	Uncommon	Common
Respiratory difficulties	If severe	If severe	Common	Uncommon initially, common as disease progresses	Respiratory failure	Uncommon	If severe
Pupillary reactions	Normal, except for congenital end plate acetylcholinesterase deficiency	Normal	May have normal or impaired responses	Normal	Normal, may have Horner's syndrome	Normal	Usually normal
Ptosis and ophthalmoplegia	Some syndromes°	Yes, although less common than acquired MG	Frequent ptosis	No	No, but may have Horner's syndrome	Some syndromes†	No
Weakness	Yes	Yes	Yes	Yes	Yes	Yes	No
Reflexes	Normal	Normal	Normal or reduced	Absent	Initially absent	Normal or reduced	Normal or increased
Sensation	Normal	Normal	Normal	Normal	Absent or reduced below lesion	Normal	Normal, but blunted responses
Serum creatine kinase	Normal	Normal	Normal	May be mildly elevated	Usually normal; may be elevated with asphyxia	Elevated in some syndromes	May be elevated with asphyxia
Distinctive features	See text	See text	See text	Tongue and peripheral fasciculations	Usually acute onset at birth	Many syndromes have distinct clinical features	Many syndromes have distinct clinical features

° Ptosis and ophthalmoplegia are variable in several CMSs and may not be obvious in the neonatal period. CMSs that may manifest early-onset ptosis and ophthalmoplegia include paucity of synaptic vesicles, congenital end plate acetylcholinesterase deficiency; primary AChR deficiency, slow-channel syndromes, and fast-channel syndromes. Ptosis may be seen in childhood or adolescence in choline acetyltransferase deficiency (although eye movements may be spared and examination is often normal between crises in less severely affected children).

† Congenital myopathies associated with ptosis and ophthalmoplegia include myotubular myopathy, centronuclear myopathy, multicore–minicore myopathy, nemaline myopathy, congenital fiber-type disproportion, reducing body myopathy, congenital myopathy with type 1 fibers, minimal change myopathy, desmin myopathy, and congenital myotonic dystrophy.

CMS, congenital myasthenic syndrome; TNMG, transient neonatal myasthenia gravis; SMA, spinal muscular atrophy; AChR Ab, acetylcholine receptor antibody; MG, myasthenia gravis.

TABLE 35–2. ELECTROPHYSIOLOGIC FEATURES OF CONGENITAL MYASTHENIC SYNDROMES

Site of Defect	Disorder	Slow RMNS	Rapid RMNS	SF-EMG	Other Distinctive Features
Presynaptic	Choline acetyltransferase deficiency	Decrement in clinically weak muscles. Decrement only after prolonged stimulation between crises or in nonweak muscles	No facilitation	Increased jitter and blocking, progressively worse during prolonged activity	Decrement and jitter induced by prolonged activation repairs slowly, over 15-30 min
	Paucity of synaptic vesicles	Decrement	No facilitation	Increased jitter and blocking	
	Lambert-Eaton-like CMS	Decrement	Facilitation	Increased jitter and blocking	Low-amplitude CMAP
Synaptic	Congenital end plate AChE deficiency	Decrement, not repaired by AChE therapy	Decrement, not repaired by AChE therapy	Increased jitter and blocking	Repetitive CMAPs, not enhanced by cholinesterase inhibitors
Postsynaptic	Slow-channel CMS	Decrement, not repaired by AChE therapy	Decrement worsens at faster rates of RMNS	Increased jitter and blocking	Repetitive CMAPS, enhanced by cholinesterase inhibitors
	Fast-channel syndromes	Decrement	No decrement	Increased jitter and blocking	
	Primary AChR deficiency with or without minor kinetic abnormality	Decrement	Decrement may be partly repaired, and facilitation may be apparent	Increased jitter and blocking	
	CMS with rapsyn deficiency	Variable decrement	??	Increased jitter and blocking	Decrement with RMNS may be revealed after exercise
	CMS with plectin deficiency	Decrement	Decrement	Increased jitter and blocking	Myopathic features on EMG
Incompletely characterized syndromes	Familial limb-girdle myasthenia	Decrement	Early repair and late fall of with prolonged 10-Hz RMNS	Increased jitter and blocking	Myopathic features on EMG

RMNS, repetitive motor nerve stimulation; SF-EMG, single-fiber electromyogram; CMS, congenital myasthenic syndrome; CMAP, compound muscle action potential; AChR, acetylcholine receptor; AChE, acetylcholinesterase.

due to plectin deficiency.[38] Plectin is a filament-linking protein concentrated at the postsynaptic membrane at the NMJ, and deficiency produces a postsynaptic myasthenic pattern. Other features are related to absence of plectin from the sarcolemma, Z-disks in skeletal muscle, intercalated disks in cardiac muscle, and desmosomes in skin.

5. A syndrome of congenital myasthenia associated with elongated face, high-arched palate, mandibular prognathism, malocclusion, and particular weakness of facial and masticatory muscles has been reported among consanguineous Iraqi and Iranian Jews has been recently associated with rapsyn mutations.[39]

6. McQuillen and others since have reported families with fatigable limb-girdle weakness with myasthenic and myopathic features beginning in teenage years.[40]

Some slow-channel CMSs are inherited in an autosomal dominant fashion (or as a sporadic mutation), due to gain-of-function mutations. Slow-channel CMS may also be inherited as an autosomal recessive disorder with variable penetrance.[41] Other CMS show autosomal recessive inheritance, due to loss-of-function mutations. Therefore, some, but not all, probands will have similarly affected relatives. Despite autosomal dominant and recessive patterns of inheritance in the recognized syndromes, males are more

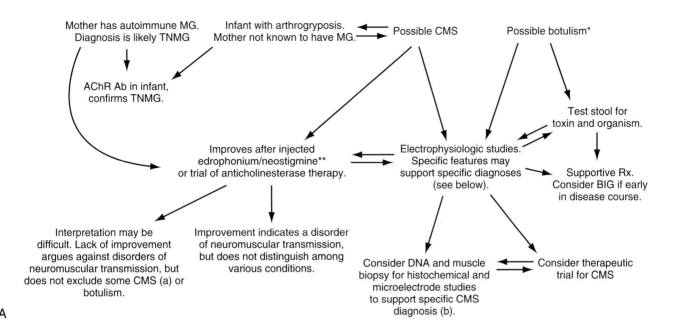

A

Procedure	Disorders of NMJ	Differential diagnoses
Sensory and motor nerve conduction studies	Normal velocities. CMAP amplitude may be reduced in severe NMJ dysfunction.	Slowed velocities in peripheral nerve disease. Reduced CMAP amplitudes in some myopathies.
Repetitive CMAPs	Consistent with congenital end-plate acetylcholinesterase deficiency and slow channel CMS.	Exogenous anticholinesterase.
Slow RMNS (0.5-3 stimuli/sec)	Decrement in most CMS (c) and TNMG; common in botulism	Normal, recognizing limited reserve in neonates, esp. preterm neonates.
Rapid RMNS (20-50 stimuli/sec)	Decrement in some CMS (d), increment in some CMS (e), neither decrement or increment in Fast Channel syndromes. Variable response in TNMG. Increment in botulism.	Normal, recognizing limited reserve in neonates.
Conventional EMG	Variable MUAPs. CMS with myopathy (and myopathic EMG) often presents in later childhood.	Abnormal in SMA, peripheral nerve disease and myopathies.
SFEMG	Increased jitter and blocking in all disorders of neuromuscular transmission.	Abnormal jitter in SMA, some peripheral neuropathies and myopathies.

B

FIGURE 35–6

Disorders of neuromuscular transmission (NMT) in infancy. A, A diagnostic approach to disorders of NMT in infancy. This algorithm offers an approach to assessment of infants with suspected disorders of NMT. It follows on from Table 35-1, which summarizes clinical features that help distinguish among disorders of NMT and the major differential diagnoses pertinent to infants. Specific information is also provided in the text. B, Electrodiagnostic testing for disorders of NMT and pertinent differential diagnoses. The following notes correspond to the letters in parentheses shown in the figure: (a) CMSs not responsive to anticholinesterases include end plate acetylcholinesterase deficiency, slow-channel CMS, and CMS with plectin deficiency; (b) CMSs that require DNA analysis for specific diagnosis include paucity of synaptic vesicles, fast-channel syndromes, primary AChR deficiency, and CMS with rapsyn deficiency; (c) CMSs that show decrement with slow RMNS include choline acetyltransferase deficiency (in weak muscles), paucity of synaptic vesicles, Lambert-Eaton-like CMS, end plate acetylcholinesterase deficiency, slow-channel CMS, fast-channel syndromes, primary AChR deficiency, and CMS with rapsyn deficiency; (d) CMSs that may show a decrement with rapid RMNS include choline acetyltransferase deficiency (prolonged stimulation may be required), end plate acetylcholinesterase deficiency, slow-channel CMS, primary AChR deficiency, and CMS with rapsyn deficiency; and (e) Lambert-Eaton-like CMS may show an increment with rapid RMNS.

CMS, congenital myasthenic syndrome; TNMG, transient neonatal myasthenia gravis; CNS, central nervous system; SMA, spinal muscular atrophy; AChR Ab, acetylcholine receptor antibody; BIG, botulinum immune globulin; RMNS, repetitive motor nerve stimulation; CMAP, compound muscle action potential; MG, myasthenia gravis; NMJ, neuromuscular junction; MUAP, motor unit action potential; SF-EMG, single-fiber EMG.

*Symptoms not present from birth, prior constipation, other clinical clues (see text).

**Prior injection of atropine reduces risk of respiratory compromise from bronchorrhea and excessive salivation.

commonly affected than females.[42] A family history of multiple deaths in infancy, stillbirths, or spontaneous abortions is a nonspecific but potentially important diagnostic clue.

Diagnosis

Potential differential diagnoses include transient neonatal myasthenia gravis (TNMG), infantile botulism, spinal muscular atrophy, cervical cord lesions, congenital myotonic dystrophy, congenital myopathies, Möbius syndrome, and the long list of causes of central neonatal hypotonia (such as brain malformation, Prader-Willi syndrome, and perinatal asphyxia). Table 35-2 and Figure 35-6 describe features that help distinguish among disorders with neonatal weakness and hypotonia. See also Chapters 20, 21, 22, 25, and 28, which discuss relevant differential diagnoses in detail.

Electrophysiologic Features

Electrodiagnostic studies are often helpful in evaluating patients with potential CMS. These studies can identify disordered NMT, thereby localizing the defect. They may also serve to exclude other disorders with similar clinical features. Some CMSs have distinctive electrophysiologic features that facilitate specific diagnoses. Table 35-2 summarizes the electrophysiologic features of CMS. These studies are often technically challenging, and relevant norms for preterm and term infants are limited (see Chapters 6 and 7); therefore, thoughtful selection of candidates for such studies is important.

Nerve Conduction Studies. NCVs are normal. Most syndromes also have normal CMAPs. CMAP amplitude may be reduced in Lambert-Eaton-like CMS and in severely affected patients with other CMS. In end plate AChE deficiency and slow-channel syndromes, R-CMAPs are seen after single supramaximal stimuli, due to abnormal prolongation of the end plate potential (Fig. 35-7). These distinctive discharges may not emerge until after the first few months of life.[43] In most cases the CMAP is followed within 5 to 8 milliseconds by a single, smaller R-CMAP (see Fig. 35-7). During low-frequency RMNS, consecutive R-CMAPs are smaller than the preceding ones (Fig. 35-8; see also Fig. 35-7), even at rates as low as 0.5/sec, and they may become unapparent after the first three or four stimuli. Exercise also abolishes the R-CMAPs, and they can easily be missed unless single stimuli are delivered at 5 to 10-second intervals in well-rested muscle. R-CMAPs can be difficult to see when the CMAP waveform is broad (see Fig. 35-8).[44]

Because cholinesterase inhibitors can produce R-CMAPs, it may be necessary to discontinue these medications for several hours before testing for R-CMAPs. Cholinesterase inhibitors cause an increase in the number and size of R-CMAPs in slow-channel myasthenic syndrome but have no effect in congenital end plate AChE deficiency.[45] This difference can be used to distinguish these conditions.

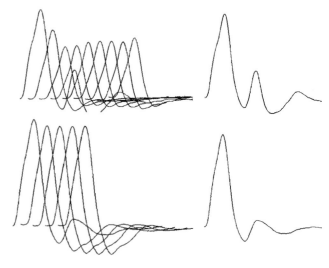

FIGURE 35–7

Repetitive motor nerve stimulation at 3/sec in a hand muscle of a patient with congenital end plate acetylcholinesterase deficiency, performed before (top) and immediately after (bottom) maximum voluntary contraction for 30 seconds. The initial response in each train is shown at right: the CMAP decrement and the size of the R-CMAP are less after activation. CMAP, compound muscle action potential; R-CMAP, repetitive CMAP. (Courtesy of D. B. Sanders, Duke University, Durham, North Carolina.)

Repetitive Motor Nerve Stimulation. In most forms of CMS, RMNS findings are identical to acquired myasthenia gravis. Slow RMNS in symptomatic regions produces a decrement greater than 10%. Higher rates of stimulation may produce a rate-dependent decrement, and exercise may partly or completely repair the decrement. AChE also repairs the decremental response to repetitive nerve stimulation in most CMS, the exceptions being end plate AChE deficiency and slow-channel CMS.

CMSs that have specific features on RMNS include the following:

1. Between crises and in mildly affected children with choline acetyltransferase deficiency, there is a decremental response to RMNS in weak muscles. In strong muscles a decremental response may be seen only after sustained voluntary muscle activity or prolonged nerve stimulation. This can be demonstrated by stimulating at 3 to 5/sec for 5 minutes, then delivering brief trains at the same stimulation rate (Fig. 35-9). The amplitude of the CMAP begins to fall progressively after 2 to 3 minutes of continuous stimulation. The subsequent brief trains demonstrate a decrement, which becomes less and may disappear after 20 to 30 minutes and which can be corrected by edrophonium. The progressive abnormality of NMT during sustained activity that characterizes this condition also can be demonstrated by measuring the jitter with SF-EMG during continuous axonal stimulation

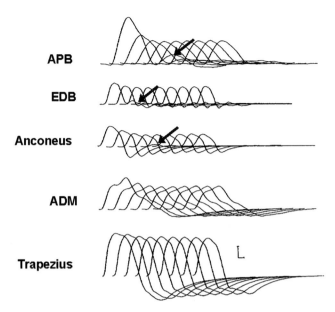

FIGURE 35–8

Repetitive motor nerve stimulation studies at 3/sec in five muscles of a patient with slow-channel congenital myasthenic syndrome. Repetitive compound muscle action potentials (R-CMAPs) are clearly visible in the abductor pollicis brevis (APB), extensor digitorum brevis (EDB) and anconeus (arrows). R-CMAPs were not obvious in the adductor digiti minimi (ADM) or trapezius, although there is a suspicious "shoulder" on the falling phase of the ADM CMAP. (From Bedlack RS, Bertorini TE, Sanders DB: Hidden afterdischarges in slow channel congenital myasthenic syndrome. J Clin Neuromusc Dis 2000;1:186-189.)

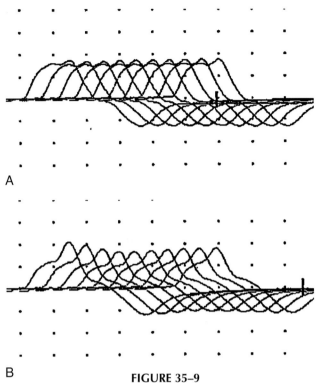

FIGURE 35–9

Repetitive motor nerve stimulation studies with 3/sec stimulation in hypothenar muscles of an 18-year-old woman with congenital choline acetyltransferase deficiency (congenital myasthenic syndrome with episodic apnea) before (A—no decrement) and after (B—30% decrement) continuous 3/sec stimulation for 5 minutes. (A and B, From Sanders DB: Electrophysiologic study of disorders of neuromuscular transmission. In Aminoff MJ [ed]: Electrodiagnosis in Clinical Neurology. New York, Churchill Livingstone, 1999, pp 303-321.)

(Fig. 35-10). The process is attributed to slow or decreased resynthesis of ACh or vesicular refilling.

2. CMAP amplitudes increase from a low baseline with brief tetanic stimulation (facilitation) in Lambert-Eaton-like CMS.

3. High-frequency repetitive nerve stimulation does not produce a decrement in fast-channel syndromes.

Conventional EMG. Standard concentric needle EMG shows normal insertional activity and MUAPs that vary in amplitude and waveform configuration. Fibrillation potentials and other abnormal spontaneous activity are seen in CMS associated with myopathy with plectin deficiency.[35] Complex, polyphasic MUAPs may be seen in CMS with myopathy and end plate dysfunction, notably slow-channel CMS and familial limb-girdle myasthenia.[40]

SF-EMG. All CMS syndromes show increased jitter with SF-EMG, as in acquired myasthenia gravis. In choline acetyltransferase deficiency, jitter may be normal in some end plates at rest and become progressively greater, with blocking, during continuous low-frequency stimulation (see Fig. 35-10).

Other Investigations

By definition, all patients with CMS have an inherited defect of NMT. Unlike autoimmune myasthenia, these patients do not have elevated AChR or MuSK autoantibodies or immune-mediated injury of the AChR, and they do not respond to immunotherapies. The specific gene defects underlying some syndromes are known. Therefore, DNA testing for candidate mutations is feasible in a growing proportion of these patients.

Sophisticated morphologic and microelectrode studies of muscle biopsy specimens, such as detailed cytochemical and structural examination for AChRs and AChE in the end plate, electron microscopy, microelectrode recordings, and patch-clamp recordings of currents passing through single AChR channels, are frequently required for precise diagnosis. Such studies are available only in a few centers.

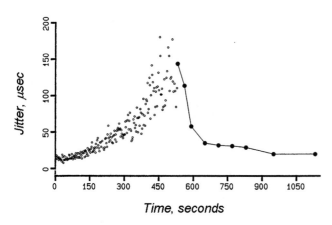

FIGURE 35–10

Jitter measured in a single end plate during and after prolonged axonal stimulation in the same patient as Figure 35-8. Each open circle represents the jitter in 50 consecutive responses during continuous 10/sec stimulation. Filled circles and solid line indicate jitter in 50 consecutive responses during intermittent 10/sec stimulation. (From Sanders DB: Diseases associated with disorders of neuromuscular transmission. In Brown WF, Bolton CF, Aminoff MJ (eds): Neuromuscular Function and Disease. Philadelphia, WB Saunders, 2002, pp 1345-1353.)

Treatment

Therapy for the genetic defects underlying CMS is not currently possible. Unlike therapy for autoimmune myasthenia gravis, there is no role for immune modulation in CMS. Nevertheless, NMT may be enhanced in some CMS, with resolution or diminution of symptoms. Progress in understanding of the underlying pathophysiology permits rational application of potential therapies. Table 35-3 details therapeutic options for the different syndromes. Responses are often only partial. Most syndromes are rare and often only small numbers of patients have been treated.

Longer-acting cholinesterase inhibitors (neostigmine and pyridostigmine) are often given as a trial, either diagnostically or therapeutically if a CMS is strongly suspected. As with autoimmune myasthenia gravis, many, but not all, patients with various CMS respond to cholinesterase inhibitors. Patients with end plate AChE deficiency have exaggerated muscarinic side effects with neostigmine and pyridostigmine. 3,4-Diaminopyridine (3,4-DAP) increases transmitter release at synapses. It blocks voltage-sensitive potassium channels, which enhances calcium entry into the presynaptic neuron, stimulating fusion of synaptic vesicles with the presynaptic membrane and facilitating transmitter release. It crosses the blood-brain barrier poorly, so the major site of action is the NMJ. It is useful in many forms of

TABLE 35–3. RESPONSE TO THERAPY AMONG CONGENITAL MYASTHENIC SYNDROMES

Site of Defect	Disorder	Clinical Response	Distinctive Features
Presynaptic	Choline acetyltransferase deficiency	Improved with cholinesterase inhibitors 3,4-DAP may be beneficial	Episodic crises; improves with age
	Paucity of synaptic vesicles	Improved with cholinesterase inhibitors	
	Lambert-Eaton-like CMS	Improved with guanidine[176] and 3,4-DAP[42]	Response to RMNS improved with guanidine and 3,4-DAP
Synaptic	Congenital end plate AChE deficiency	No effective therapy; possible role for atracurium[177]	Enhanced muscarinic side effects with cholinesterase inhibitors; repetitive CMAPs not enhanced by cholinesterase inhibitors
Postsynaptic	Slow-channel CMS	Improved with quinidine and fluoxetine[48,49]	Repetitive CMAPs enhanced by cholinesterase inhibitors; 3,4-DAP contraindicated
	Fast-channel syndromes	Improved with combination of cholinesterase inhibitors and 3,4-DAP	
	Primary AChR deficiency with or without minor kinetic abnormality	Often improved with cholinesterase inhibitors; 3,4-DAP may be beneficial	
	CMS with rapsyn deficiency	Improved with combination of cholinesterase inhibitors and 3,4-DAP	
	CMS with plectin deficiency	Improved with 3,4-DAP	
Incompletely characterized syndromes	Familial limb-girdle myasthenia	Improved with cholinesterase inhibitors and 3,4-DAP	

CMS, congenital myasthenic syndrome; AChE, acetylcholinesterase; AChR, acetylcholine receptor; DAP, diaminopyridine; RMNS, repetitive motor nerve stimulation; CMAP, compound muscle action potential.

CMS as well as autoimmune myasthenia gravis and autoimmune Lambert-Eaton syndrome.[46,47] Quinidine sulfate[48] and fluoxetine[49] normalize the prolonged opening episodes of mutant AChRs expressed in human embryonic kidney cell culture and have been used in patients with slow-channel CMS. Ephedrine has also been used in some patients with CMS when other treatments were not effective.[50]

Transient Neonatal Myasthenia Gravis

TNMG is a rare experiment of nature that underscores many aspects of the immunopathology of myasthenia gravis. During pregnancy, circulating maternal IgG antibodies normally cross the placenta to enter the fetal circulation, especially during the second half of gestation. Thus, pathogenic autoantibodies in the circulation of mothers with autoimmune myasthenia gravis may cross the placenta to enter the fetal circulation and interfere with the normal AChR function of the fetus. Clearance of these autoantibodies from the neonate may take up to 5 months after birth.

Virtually all infants of seropositive mothers have elevated circulating AChR antibodies, yet only about 10% to 20% manifest significant symptoms of TNMG.[51-53] Once an affected mother delivers an infant with TNMG, it is likely that her subsequent infants will be similarly affected.[52,54] TNMG has mostly been reported among infants of seropositive mothers, but it has been reported in infants of seronegative mothers, whose affected infants often have respiratory compromise.[54-60] There is no correlation between disease severity in mothers and their infants. There is only a poor correlation between maternal AChR antibody titers and disease severity in the infants, but, for each baby, falling AChR antibody titers correlate with clinical improvement. Accumulating evidence suggests that maternal autoantibodies directed against the fetal AChR (rather than the main immunogenic region of the adult AChR) are linked with fetal muscle weakness with in utero hypokinesis and arthrogryposis.[61-65] The observation that the first infant of an affected mother is often spared but subsequent infants are affected suggests that the mother may become immunized to fetal AChRs.[65] Some mothers with autoantibodies directed specifically against fetal AChR antigens may themselves be asymptomatic, which makes diagnosis difficult.[63]

Clinical Manifestations

Symptoms of muscle weakness due to transplacental passage of maternal pathogenic autoantibodies may occasionally be manifest by the fetus in utero. These include arthrogryposis, weak fetal movements, polyhydramnios (due to poor fetal swallowing), pulmonary hypoplasia (due to reduced fetal respiratory movements), hydrops fetalis, and stillbirth. Most infants manifest symptoms a few hours after birth, but symptoms may be delayed for up to 3 days. The main features are variably severe hypotonia, generalized weakness, facial diplegia, poor sucking, weak cry, intermittent cyanosis (especially during feeds), respiratory weakness, and respiratory failure. Ptosis and external ophthalmoplegia occur but often are not so marked as in autoimmune myasthenia gravis. Mental state, tendon jerks, bladder and bowel function, and sensation are preserved. Symptoms are transient, typically lasting about 3 weeks, but may extend for 3 months.[66] Once symptoms resolve, they do not reappear, although one report describes a patient with TNMG who later developed autoimmune myasthenia gravis.[67]

Diagnosis

In the mother already diagnosed with autoimmune myasthenia gravis, suspicion of TNMG in the affected infant is relatively simple. TNMG, however, may occur in infants of mothers with minimal symptoms, and, as previously mentioned, recurrent fetal disease, especially arthrogryposis, may be seen in infants of asymptomatic mothers with autoantibodies directed against the fetal form of the AChR. Potential differential diagnoses include CMS, infantile botulism, spinal muscular atrophy, cervical cord lesions, congenital myotonic dystrophy, congenital myopathies, Möbius syndrome, and the long list of causes of central neonatal hypotonia (such as brain malformation, Prader-Willi syndrome, and perinatal asphyxia). Table 35-1 and Figure 35-6 describe features that help distinguish among disorders with neonatal weakness and hypotonia. See also Chapter 26, that discusses relevant differential diagnoses in detail.

Detection of AChR antibodies in the mother and child is supportive of the diagnosis, although seronegative mothers have delivered affected infants. Transient improvement following injection of edrophonium or the longer-acting neostigmine supports a diagnosis of TNMG. However, it may be hard to assess the response in an intubated and ventilated neonate, not all affected infants respond (especially infants with arthrogryposis), and a response does not distinguish TNMG from some forms of CMS. In addition, affected neonates may be compromised by secondary asphyxia, which can confound diagnostic endeavors.

Electrophysiologic Features

Electrodiagnostic studies are rarely necessary but become important in infants of asymptomatic mothers and in those with equivocal response to edrophonium or other anticholinesterase inhibitors (Table 35-4).

Nerve Conduction Studies. NCVs and CMAPs are normal.

Repetitive Motor Nerve Stimulation. Low-frequency RMNS typically shows an abnormal decremental response.[52] It has been suggested that RMNS before and after administration of anticholinesterase improves accuracy of the diagnosis and may offer quantitative assessment of neuro-

TABLE 35–4. ELECTROPHYSIOLOGIC FEATURES OF MAJOR ACQUIRED CHILDHOOD MYASTHENIC SYNDROMES

Site of Defect	Disorder	Slow RMNS	Rapid RMNS	SF-EMG
Presynaptic	Infantile botulism	Inconsistent, usually modest decrement[85]	Modest incremental facilitation (50-100%) with 50/sec stimulation	Increased jitter and blocking, which decreases as stimulation frequency increases
	Lambert-Eaton myasthenic syndrome	Decrement	Marked (>200%) incremental facilitation	Increased jitter and blocking, which decreases as stimulation frequency increases
Postsynaptic	TNMG	Decrement	No data	Increased jitter and blocking, which increases as stimulation frequency increases
	Autoimmune MG	Decrement	Decrement may repair or improve	Increased jitter and blocking, which increases as stimulation frequency increases

RMNS, repetitive motor nerve stimulation; SF-EMG, single-fiber electromyogram; TNMG, transient neonatal myasthenia gravis; MG, myasthenia gravis.

muscular function and response to therapy.[52] Brief tetanic stimulation may transiently correct the defect in NMT (post-tetanic facilitation) and is followed by post-tetanic exhaustion.[68] With sustained rapid RMNS (10 to 50/sec), significant decrement may be seen throughout the stimulus train.[25] These results must be interpreted in light of the decremental responses that occur in normal neonates. One report describes abnormal RMNS of a 28-day-old term infant with arthrogryposis secondary to maternal autoimmune myasthenia gravis: Stimulation at 5/sec produced a decrement of 31% and at 30/sec of 88%.[62]

Conventional EMG. EMGs have rarely been reported with TNMG. A single infant with arthrogryposis and TNMG had a normal EMG.[69]

SF-EMG. To our knowledge, there are no reports of SF-EMG in patients with TNMG.

Therapy

Maternal AChR antibodies no longer enter the infant via the placenta after birth. Although breast milk does contain these antibodies, there is no evidence that they are active in human neonates, and there is no consensus against breast-feeding by myasthenic mothers. Newborn levels of AChR antibody fall progressively and the disease resolves spontaneously after several weeks. Supportive treatment is given until weakness disappears. Severely affected infants may require ventilatory support and nasogastric feeding. Pyridostigmine or neostigmine may be helpful. Exchange transfusion[70] and IV immunoglobulin (IVIg)[71] have been used with good effect. When intrauterine movement is reduced, and arthrogryposis is suspected, prenatal treatment of the mother with repeated plasma exchange (PEX) and corticosteroids may be considered to reduce maternal AChR antibody titers.[72]

Infantile Botulism

Clostridium botulinum is an obligatory anaerobic, gram-positive, spore-forming rod. Spores are ubiquitous in soil, agricultural products, and household dust. They have a particular propensity to multiply in the large intestine of infants younger than 5 months of age. The spores are excluded from the gut in exclusively breast-fed infants. Supplementation with contaminated foods may result in colonization, and honey has been implicated as the source in 16% to 32% of cases.[73,74] Minute quantities of the powerful botulinum toxin are absorbed through the colon and circulate to produce the systemic, paralytic disease *infantile botulism*. Infrequently, epidemics of paralysis may occur after ingestion of food containing the preformed toxin (now largely alleviated by modern food processing). Paralysis may also be induced by toxin released from wounds colonized by *C. botulinum*.

Multiple subspecies of *Clostridium* produce specific botulinum toxins, designated A through G. Toxins A and B are usually associated with infantile botulism. The toxin is composed of a heavy chain linked to a light chain. The heavy chain binds to specific gangliosides at the axon terminus of cholinergic motor neurons.[75] Once internalised by endosomic uptake, the light chain is cleaved and migrates from the endosome to the local cytoplasm. The light chains of each specific toxin target and inactivate specific proteins (SNAP 25, VAMP, syntaxin) involved in synaptic vesicle docking or exocytosis.[76-80] This prevents release of ACh from the presynaptic terminal, so that during the period of toxicity, the muscle is at least partly denervated. The lack of synaptic transmission reinstitutes the fetal pattern of unclustered AChRs. Following new synthesis and transport of new SNAP-25, VAMP or syntaxin, transmission across the NMJ is re-established and the adult morphology of the postsynaptic membrane is re-established.

Clinical Features

Median age of onset is 10 weeks; 95% of patients have onset before 6 months of age. Presentation may be as early as 1 week of age.[81] Severity and tempo of the disease are highly variable but can be catastrophic and rapid. Onset of weakness is usually subacute, often with late, precipitous deterioration. Days or months of constipation typically precede weakness. Parents report reduced spontaneous movements, lethargy, and poor feeding. Unlike food-borne botulism, infantile botulism does not occur in "epidemics." The disease is not spread by fecal-oral contamination from infected patients.

Examination typically shows mid size or large pupils with reduced or sluggish responses to light, reduced extraocular movements and ptosis, immobile face, drooling with reduced gag reflex, and weak cry. Ventilation may be compromised by bulbar and respiratory muscle weakness. One study, for instance, reported the need for mechanical ventilation in six of nine hospitalized infants.[82] Neck muscles are particularly weak, and the babies are diffusely hypotonic and weak. Tendon reflexes may be normal, reduced, or absent. Autonomic dysfunction, urinary retention, and the syndrome of inappropriate antidiuretic hormone secretion are reported.[83] Sensorium and sensation are normal. Patients are afebrile. Symptoms may be exacerbated by medications that interfere with NMJ function (see Box 35-2).

The most important consequence of the disease is respiratory failure due to weakness of bulbar and respiratory muscles. This may occur rapidly and is often quiet and undramatic. Crying, positioning for lumbar puncture, and sedative medications may provoke respiratory collapse. Careful observation is required, and patients should be mechanically ventilated if respiration is compromised.

Diagnosis

Initial diagnostic considerations often include sepsis and metabolic disease. In the typical case, given a high index of suspicion, the clinical features are quite distinctive. This often allows a presumptive diagnosis (without precluding consideration of important differentials requiring immediate treatment). Potential differential diagnoses include CMS; autoimmune myasthenia gravis (in older patients); Guillain-Barré syndrome; infections of the anterior horn cell (polio or other enteroviruses); various myopathies, especially those associated with ptosis and EOM weakness; venoms and toxins; brainstem tumors; and brainstem encephalitis (either infectious or postinfectious). Table 35-1 and Figure 35-6 detail features that help distinguish infantile botulism from some of these differential diagnoses.

In the appropriate clinical setting, electrodiagnostic studies (see later) confirm clinical suspicions in a timely manner. Some, but not all, affected infants respond to edro-phonium. (For details regarding edrophonium testing, see the later section on autoimmune myasthenia gravis.) Such a response indicates a disorder of NMT but does not distinguish among the various pathogeneses. Both the organism and the toxin can be recovered from stool specimens in most cases, although concomitant constipation means a gentle enema may be required to collect stool. Repeated samples may be required, which is feasible since the stool may yield toxin and organisms for up to 1 month.[84] The serum may occasionally be positive for toxin.[84]

Electrophysiologic Features

Gutierrez and associates proposed a protocol for electrophysiologic evaluation and diagnosis of infantile botulism (Box 35-4).[26] See also Table 35-4 for a summary of electrodiagnostic features.

Nerve Conduction Studies. Almost all infants with botulism have normal NCVs, distal latencies, and sensory nerve APs.[26,85] CMAPs are typically reduced in amplitude with short duration.

Repetitive Motor Nerve Stimulation. RMNS is crucial for accurate and rapid diagnosis of the presynaptic failure of NMT seen in infantile botulism. Because high

---

BOX 35-4
DIAGNOSIS IN INFANTILE BOTULISM

Proposed Electrodiagnostic Tests for Suspected Infantile Botulism[26]
1. Motor and sensory nerve conduction velocities in one arm and one leg
2. 2/sec RMNS in two distal muscles
3. Supramaximal single-nerve stimulation followed by 50/sec tetanization for 10 seconds and immediately thereafter by single-nerve stimuli at 30-second intervals until amplitude of CMAPs returns to baseline

Diagnostic Features Necessary for Electrodiagnosis of Infantile Botulism[26]
1. CMAPs of decreased amplitude in at least two muscles
2. Tetanic and post-tetanic facilitation defined by CMAP amplitude increased more than 120% from baseline
3. Post-tetanic facilitation lasting more than 120 seconds (often several minutes) and no post-tetanic exhaustion

CMAP, compound muscle action potential; RMNS, repetitive motor nerve stimulation.

stimulation rates are required, it is important to secure surface electrodes carefully. It has been suggested that 10 seconds of 50/sec stimulation is the best way to elicit the post-tetanic facilitation typical of infantile botulism.[26] It is important to be aware that volitional activity during the test may induce unsolicited, transient increment of CMAP amplitude in "baseline" measurements and produce a false-negative study.

Low-frequency stimulation (2 to 5/sec) produces variable responses—one study, for example, reported a decrement in 14 (56%) of 25 affected infants.[26] The characteristic and important finding is incrementally increasing CMAP amplitude with stimulation at 20 to 50/sec. Cornblath and colleagues showed that 23 (92%) of 25 had incremental responses which varied from 23 to 313% (mean 73%).[85] They identified incremental responses in 19 of 23 babies using 20/sec stimulation and in another 4 using 50/sec stimulation. RMNS tests tend to give normal results early in the clinical course or if disease is not too severe. Repeated studies or studies of multiple muscles improve the diagnostic yield. Other important electrodiagnostic clues are the prolonged period of post-tetanic facilitation (up to 21 minutes in one infant) and the absence of post-tetanic exhaustion.[86,87] The limitations of NMT testing in the normal immature neonatal NMJ must be considered in interpreting the results of RMNS in this age group (see Chapters 6 and 7).

Conventional EMG. EMG often shows frequent, brief, low-amplitude polyphasic MUAPs, and fibrillation and positive sharp wave potentials, consistent with the functional denervation produced by impaired ACh release.

SF-EMG. Stimulated SF-EMG may give the best electrodiagnostic information in these infants. Sedation or anesthesia is usually required. In four infants with typical RMNS features, stimulated SF-EMG of intrinsic hand muscles revealed abnormal jitter, which improved (i.e., decreased) with increasing rates of stimulation.[88] This response is similar to that in LEMS and is consistent with a presynaptic defect of NMT. It differs from autoimmune myasthenia gravis and other postsynaptic disorders, which show increasing jitter with increasing rates of stimulation. This technique may be more sensitive than RMNS in identifying the presynaptic defect of infantile botulism.[81,88]

Therapy

Infant botulism is a chronic process, and treatment is predominantly symptomatic. Human-derived botulinum immunoglobulin reduces severity and duration, if given within the first 3 days after admission to the hospital.[89] Mechanical ventilation is commonly indicated, and infants who require this support often need it for months. Enteral feeding is commonly indicated. Relief of constipation and urinary retention may be required. Antibiotics have no proven value, and gentamicin or other drugs affecting the

NMJ should be avoided. Infants may relapse during convalescence,[90] but long-term outcome is good.

Autoimmune Myasthenia Gravis

Autoimmune myasthenia gravis, known as *juvenile myasthenia gravis* when it occurs in children, is an antibody-mediated process targeting the postsynaptic component of the NMJ in skeletal muscle. The principal target is the AChR. A specific section of the extracellular domain of the alpha subunit is the main immunogenic region, although the autoimmune process is often directed against multiple targets (epitope spreading). Conventional testing identifies autoantibodies directed against the AChR in most, but not all, patients with autoimmune myasthenia gravis. About 80% of affected adults and adolescents, and about 50% of affected young children have detectable AChR antibodies, so-called seropositive patients.[91,92] Affected patients without detectable AChR antibodies are described as seronegative. Recent evidence indicates that about 50% of seronegative patients (mostly adults so far) with generalized disease have circulating autoantibodies directed against MuSK.[93-95]

Binding of autoantibodies to the AChR accelerates degradation of the AChR, blocks the ACh binding sites of the receptors, and induces local deposition of complement, including the membrane attack complement complex. This immune-mediated injury reduces the number of functional AChRs with subsequent disruption of normal NMT. This results in muscle weakness, the severity of which parallels the reduction in AChRs. MuSK autoantibodies induce disordered clustering of AChRs at the NMJ; however, initial studies have not demonstrated loss of MuSK or AChR at the end plate to explain the abnormal NMT or weakness in MuSK-positive myasthenia gravis.[96] The role of these antibodies is not yet clear. Neuromuscular fatigue, another characteristic clinical feature of autoimmune myasthenia gravis, is related to the additive effects of the normal reduction of ACh release during repeated nerve stimulation and the reduced number and function of the immunologically injured AChRs.[97]

Although autoantibodies directed against the AChR and neighboring postsynaptic proteins mediate clinical disease and T cells are not found at the affected NMJ, it is clear that the cell-mediated immune system plays a crucial role in the disorder. Nonspecific components of the immune response, such as complement, cytokines, and macrophages, are also involved in the inflammatory injury to the NMJ.

Conventional light microscopic studies are usually unrevealing in myasthenia gravis and thus are used mainly to exclude other diseases of nerve or muscle. Small accumulations of lymphoid cells ("lymphorrhages") are occasionally seen in peripheral muscle but are not specific for myasthenia gravis. Ultrastructural studies demonstrate reduction in the nerve terminal area and simplification of the postsynaptic membrane.[35] Special studies of AChR concentration demonstrate that the number of receptors is decreased at the NMJ in acquired myasthenia gravis.[98] IgG deposits are found on the postsynaptic membrane, as are complement deposits, which are also found in the synaptic clefts.[35,99] Studies such as these are important in advancing our understanding of the disease but have limited use in the clinical diagnosis of myasthenia gravis.

Clinical Features

Autoimmune myasthenia gravis rarely begins before 1 year of age. Fluctuating and fatigable weakness are the hallmarks of the disease. Symptoms are least apparent on awakening and become more obvious through the day. Frequent daytime naps may mask symptoms in infants. Onset and exacerbation of symptoms often follow febrile illnesses. Symptoms may also begin or be exacerbated after insect bites. Accurate assessment of strength and fatigability may be difficult in young children.

Weakness is most frequently manifest in the EOMs. Ptosis, strabismus, and diplopia affect almost 90% of children with autoimmune myasthenia gravis.[100] Fatigable ptosis and ophthalmoplegia may be unilateral or bilateral, with considerable variability over time. Involved muscles may differ from eye to eye, without conforming to neurogenic patterns of involvement. Bulbar weakness affects approximately 75% of patients[101] and may present with slow chewing and swallowing, drooling, weak or nasal voice, or poor pronunciation. Facial weakness may produce a characteristic flattened or horizontal smile. Limb muscles may also manifest weakness, most obvious as fatigability and an inability to run, climb stairs, or keep up with peers. Proximal weakness is most common. Systemic weakness may also involve the diaphragm and other muscles of respiration and may be sufficiently severe to cause respiratory failure ("myasthenic crisis"). The combination of bulbar weakness and weakness of respiratory musculature is of particular concern and requires specific recognition and assessment. Mental state, pupillary responses, tendon jerks, bladder and bowel function, and sensation are preserved.

Weakness remains limited to EOMs in about 10% to 15% of children and adolescents, so-called ocular myasthenia.[101-103] This pattern is common among patients with prepubertal onset[103,104] and Japanese[105] and Chinese patients.[106] Most patients manifest maximum disease severity within 1 year of disease onset. For instance, about 80% of patients who progress from ocular to generalized myasthenia do so within 1 year after onset of symptoms, and only 6% do so after 3 years.[107]

Thymoma occurs in about 15% of adults with myasthenia gravis but is rare in children and adolescents. For instance, only 5 of 248 patients with juvenile myasthenia gravis, all older than 14 years at diagnosis, had thymoma.[103,104] Other coincident autoimmune disorders are well recognized with myasthenia gravis, most commonly juvenile diabetes mellitus, thyroid disease, and juvenile rheumatoid arthritis.

Electrophysiologic Features

Electrodiagnostic features are summarized in Table 35-4.

Nerve Conduction Studies. Motor and sensory NCS are normal. R-CMAPs with single supramaximal stimuli are not observed, except with excessive administration of cholinesterase inhibitors.

Repetitive Motor Nerve Stimulation. RMNS is applied to nerves supplying clinically affected muscles. Distal muscles are more easily and reliably tested, but a decrement is seen more often in proximal or facial muscles. A decrement more than 10% with low-frequency RMNS in two nerves is required to confirm a disorder of NMT. Such an abnormal response does not distinguish autoimmune myasthenia gravis from other disorders of the NMJ. Severely affected muscles may show marked facilitation of CMAP amplitudes immediately following tetanic stimulation.

Conventional EMG. In experienced hands, conventional needle EMG may demonstrate MUAPs with a varying waveform, indicating abnormal NMT. CMAPs are usually normal, but amplitude and duration may be reduced, similarly to myopathy, in severely affected muscles.

SF-EMG. SF-EMG measurement of jitter is the most sensitive method to detect abnormal NMT in vivo but does not distinguish between autoimmune myasthenia gravis and CMS. This test can be especially useful, however, when the diagnosis of myasthenia cannot be confirmed by other means. Jitter measurements can be made during voluntary muscle activation in cooperative children as young as 8 years of age.[108] In children who cannot cooperate fully, jitter can be measured with axonal stimulation under sedation. Because these procedures require considerable expertise and are painful, they have a lesser role in diagnosis and management in children than in adults with myasthenia gravis. Referral to a unit experienced in pediatric electrophysiologic testing may be prudent in such cases.

Differential Diagnoses

The various CMSs are the most important differential diagnostic consideration, especially in young children and infants.[103,104] Figure 35-11 outlines features that help distinguish between these disorders. Most CMS syndromes present at birth, so questioning to evaluate weakness in the neonatal period is crucial in distinguishing CMS from acquired, autoimmune myasthenia gravis. Two forms of CMS—slow-channel syndrome and limb-girdle myasthenia—may present later in childhood or

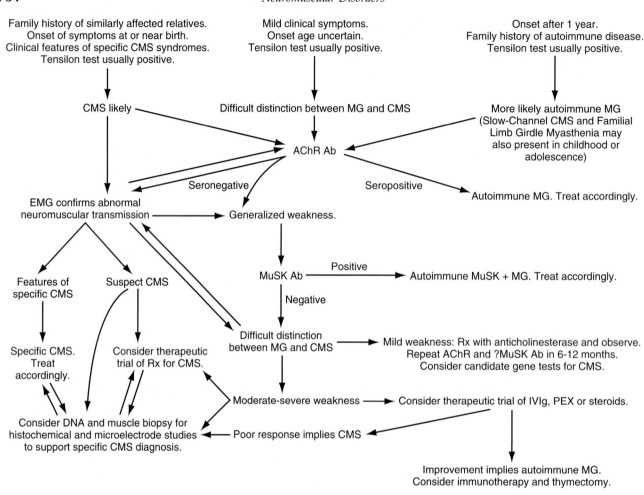

FIGURE 35–11

Algorithm for distinguishing autoimmune myasthenia gravis (MG) from congenital myasthenic syndromes (CMSs).
AChR Ab, acetylcholine receptor antibody; MuSK, muscle-specific tyrosine kinase; IVIg, intravenous immunoglobulin; PEX,
plasma exchange.

adolescence and remain important differential diagnoses in older children and adolescents. Other disorders of NMT of childhood that may mimic autoimmune myasthenia gravis include botulism and autoimmune-mediated LEMS. Various myopathies, especially those associated with ptosis and EOM weakness, venoms and toxins (including tick paralysis) are relevant differential diagnoses, as are brainstem tumors, brainstem encephalitis (either infectious or postinfectious), Guillain-Barré syndrome (especially the Miller-Fisher variant), mass lesions near the orbit, cavernous sinus, or sella turcica, diphtheria, and Fazio-Londe disease (progressive bulbar paralysis of childhood). Remote paraneoplastic effects of neuroblastoma[71] and conversion reaction also need consideration in the differential diagnosis.

Diagnosis

The most important factor in arriving at the correct diagnosis is a high index of clinical suspicion. A therapeutic challenge with edrophonium, a short-acting cholinesterase inhibitor, is a useful aid for the diagnosis of autoimmune myasthenia gravis. If there is clear improvement in weak muscles following administration, the test is considered positive. The transient response and the induced behavioral distress can make interpretation of the test difficult. Atropine needs to be available for resuscitation, especially in children with respiratory distress in whom edrophonium-induced bronchorrhea may be dangerous. Not all patients with autoimmune myasthenia gravis display a convincingly positive response to edrophonium. For instance, one study reported that 8% of children failed to respond.[109] Improvement after edrophonium may also occur in denervating diseases and rarely in some myopathies.[110-112] Occasional reports describe inconsistent positive responses to edrophonium in adult patients with diseases not associated with abnormal NMT.[113] Neostigmine also inhibits AChE and may be administered IM or subcutaneously as a diagnostic test. Improvement begins in 10 to 15 minutes and lasts 1 to 4 hours. This prolonged action enables better observation of the response. The same side effects and precautions apply as for edrophonium testing, and the longer duration of action increases the risk of cholinergic worsening.

Antibodies that bind to the AChR are detected by coprecipitation of the patient's serum IgG with human skeletal muscle AChR. A positive assay for these binding antibodies in the appropriate clinical context is diagnostic of autoimmune myasthenia gravis. Many patients, especially young children, with autoimmune myasthenia gravis, however, do not have elevated AChR autoantibodies. (Thirty-six percent to 50% of prepubertal patients, 18% to 32% of peripubertal patients, and < 9% of postpubertal adolescents with acquired myasthenia gravis are seronegative.[91,103,104,114]) This high prevalence of seronegative myasthenia gravis in young children increases the difficulty of making the important distinction between seronegative autoimmune myasthenia gravis and CMS. Repeated AChR antibody measurements may demonstrate conversion from seronegative to seropositive, confirming a diagnosis of autoimmune myasthenia gravis over time. Assays for modulating or blocking antibodies have not enhanced detection of AChR antibodies in children who are seronegative for the conventional AChR binding antibody assay.[92,103] Recently, autoantibodies to MuSK have been demonstrated in about 50% of patients with generalized, seronegative autoimmune myasthenia gravis, including some young children.[93-95] Patients with purely ocular disease seem not to have detectable MuSK antibodies. In only one report have MuSK antibodies been found in patients with elevated AChR antibodies or thymoma.[115]

As outlined earlier, readily available tests may not distinguish between autoimmune myasthenia gravis and CMS in young seronegative children with suspected autoimmune myasthenia gravis (see Fig. 35-11). In such patients, with moderate to severe weakness that is not adequately controlled by anticholinesterase medications, a trial of PEX or IVIg should be considered. Definite improvement supports a diagnosis of autoimmune myasthenia gravis. For mildly affected, young children, a noninvasive distinction between seronegative, autoimmune myasthenia gravis and CMS may not be possible. In such cases, the benefit of a potential diagnosis must be weighed against the invasiveness and logistical demands of muscle biopsy and special studies to demonstrate the characteristic findings of CMS, versus

the risk-benefit ratio of chronic immunosuppression or thymectomy if the diagnosis is not autoimmune myasthenia gravis. The growing number of diagnostic DNA tests for CMS may partly alleviate this management dilemma.

Therapy

Therapeutic strategies for autoimmune myasthenia gravis in children are similar to those in adults. Four categories of treatment are currently employed: anticholinesterase medications, short-term immunomodulation (PEX, IVIg, and pulsed IV methylprednisolone), thymectomy, and long-term immunosuppression (e.g., corticosteroids, azathioprine, and cyclosporine). The decision to offer any treatment implies that the expected benefits outweigh the expected risks and that the family understands the concepts involved. Increasingly, we aim for cure, complete resolution of signs and symptoms, or sufficient improvement to enable a full and active lifestyle. Although autoimmune myasthenia gravis is one of the best characterized human autoimmune disorders, there is much to learn about the mechanisms that initiate and sustain the process to optimize treatment.

Interpretation of the effect of thymectomy in childhood myasthenia gravis needs to be guarded.[102,109,116] Studies of thymectomy in myasthenic children and adolescents suggest that the procedure is generally effective, producing complete remission in 11% to 75% of patients and improvement in 57% to 95%.[117,118] These uncontrolled studies suggest that thymectomy within the first 12 months of onset of symptoms is more effective than delayed thymectomy. The role of thymectomy for children and adolescents with purely ocular weakness is not well defined. More information is required to develop a consensus on the exact role and timing of thymectomy in the very young patients. Published reports have not described deleterious clinical consequences of thymectomy for young patients, although follow-up has often been limited.[103,117,118]

Treatment of patients with seronegative myasthenia gravis is traditionally similar to that of patients with elevated AChR antibodies, including PEX, IVIg, and immunosuppression. The role of thymectomy in seronegative children and adolescents has not been specifically addressed. Although most reports suggest that thymectomy is often beneficial in seronegative patients,[97,119,120] some have suggested less benefit among seronegative than seropositive patients.[121,122] None of the few reported seronegative myasthenia gravis patients with circulating anti-MuSK antibodies who have undergone thymectomy have shown benefit from the procedure,[93,95] and the role of thymectomy in these patients is still uncertain. Clinical and epidemiologic studies that address these concerns may modify standard practice and facilitate more specific therapy in the future. These observations may have particular relevance to prepubertal patients, who have the highest frequency of seronegative disease.

Lambert-Eaton Myasthenic Syndrome

LEMS is a rare antibody-mediated disorder of the NMJ. Presynaptic VGCC terminals of the NMJ and postganglionic autonomic synapses are the targets of the autoimmune process. The pathophysiologic mechanism is not completely understood, but recent evidence suggests that LEMS autoantibodies bind, cross-link, and down-regulate the number of P/Q-type VGCCs rather than blocking their function.[123,124] The consequence is reduced nerve-evoked neurotransmitter release at these sites, which causes the end plate potential to fall below the threshold required for activation of the voltage-gated sodium channels within the postsynaptic folds. This results in weakness and autonomic dysfunction. One recent study reported 17 (15%) of 110 patients diagnosed with LEMS on clinical and electrophysiologic grounds did not have detectable anti-P/Q-type VGCC antibodies.[125] In passive transfer experiments, sera from "seronegative" and "seropositive" patients produced comparable reduction of quantal content of end plate potentials, implying a similar antibody-mediated process.[125]

LEMS is most commonly seen in adults, typically after 40 years of age. A small number of pediatric cases are reported, all older than 7 years at onset,[126-131] and children and adolescents make up a small proportion of larger series.[125,132,133] LEMS is often a paraneoplastic disorder. Approximately 50% of patients have cancer at onset of the disease or within 4 years of disease onset. Small-cell lung cancer is the most commonly associated malignancy in adults. Leukemia and Burkitt's lymphoma have been associated in childhood cases. Approximately 20% of patients, including a few children, have one or more other autoimmune diseases, including autoimmune myasthenia gravis, pernicious anemia, systemic lupus erythematosus, autoimmune thyroid disease, celiac disease, insulin-dependent diabetes, vitiligo, Sjögren's disease, rheumatoid arthritis, and immune-mediated glomerulonephritis.[133]

Clinical Features

Gradual onset of weakness over months is the major symptom, although rapid deterioration associated with aggressive malignancy may occur. Proximal muscles are predominantly affected, especially the thighs and legs. Weak muscles may be painful. The weakness identified by examination often seems milder than symptoms suggest. Ptosis, diplopia, and/or bulbar weakness is present in about 50%, but, unlike autoimmune myasthenia gravis, purely ocular weakness is rare.[133,134] In some patients, strength improves immediately after exercise (facilitation) but becomes less with sustained activity. Respiratory muscles

may be weak, although respiratory failure due to weakness is rare. Tendon jerks are usually reduced or absent but may be elicited immediately following 10 seconds of voluntary contraction. Most patients have a dry mouth, which may precede weakness. Pupillary dysfunction and constipation are also common, and specific autonomic testing is usually abnormal, even in the absence of symptoms.[135]

Electrophysiologic Features

Patients with LEMS have characteristic electrophysiologic findings. Diagnosis in childhood requires a high index of suspicion and a diagnostic protocol that includes assessment of responses to voluntary muscle contraction and/or tetanic stimulation. Details in the following sections rest predominantly on observations in adults but are consistent with the few reports of children with LEMS. Table 35-4 summarizes electrodiagnostic findings.

Nerve Conduction Studies. Routine motor and sensory NCS are normal. Baseline CMAP amplitudes are usually reduced, often less than 10% of normal. R-CMAPs with a single supramaximal stimulus are not observed.

As described earlier, activation of the nerve enhances calcium influx into the distal nerve terminal and augments ACh release. This physiologic response transiently corrects the presynaptic defect of LEMS. Demonstration of this phenomenon is a crucial part of the electrodiagnosis of LEMS. This can be done most simply by measuring the CMAP at rest and immediately after the patient voluntarily maximally contracts the tested muscle for 10 seconds (Fig. 35-12). A supramaximal stimulus should be delivered as soon as possible (<5 seconds) after relaxation. The ampli-

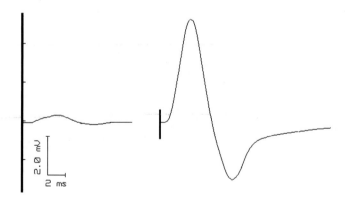

FIGURE 35–12

Compound muscle action potentials recorded from a hand muscle in a patient with Lambert-Eaton myasthenic syndrome, before (left) and after (right) maximum voluntary contraction of the muscle for 10 seconds. (From Sanders DB: Electrophysiologic study of disorders of neuromuscular transmission. In Aminoff MJ [ed]: Electrodiagnosis in Clinical Neurology. New York, Churchill Livingstone, 1999, pp 303-321.)

tude of the postactivation CMAP is compared to that of the rested state. Most patients with LEMS show more than 100% facilitation in a hand or foot muscle tested in this fashion. The duration of the CMAP should be measured to ensure it is not shortened, producing "pseudofacilitation."

Repetitive Motor Nerve Stimulation. RMNS is applied to nerves supplying clinically affected muscles. Distal muscles are more easily and reliably tested and are always more abnormal than proximal muscles in LEMS.[136] A decrement of more than 10% is seen during slow RMNS in 98% of patients[132] and is similar to the abnormal responses seen in autoimmune myasthenia gravis. Typically, the decrement disappears, or is much less, immediately after a brief period of vigorous voluntary contraction, which usually shows more than 100% facilitation of the initial train response compared with the resting state.

Rapid RMNS at 20 to 50/sec applied for 5 to 10 seconds typically produces an initial decrement, followed by a marked facilitation (Fig. 35-13). Facilitation greater than 50% in any muscle is suggestive of LEMS but may also be seen in autoimmune myasthenia gravis. Facilitation of

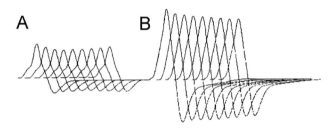

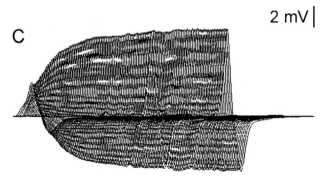

2 mV

FIGURE 35–13

Repetitive motor nerve stimulation studies in the abductor digiti minimi muscle of a patient with Lambert-Eaton myasthenic syndrome, with 3/sec stimulation at baseline (A) and immediately after maximum voluntary contraction of the muscle for 10 seconds (B). C, Intratetanic facilitation of 153% during 20/sec stimulation for 10 seconds. (A-C, From Sanders DB: Diseases associated with disorders of neuromuscular transmission. In Brown WF, Bolton CF, Aminoff MJ [eds]: Neuromuscular Function and Disease. Philadelphia, WB Saunders, 2002, pp 1345-1353.)

more than 100% in all muscles tested or more than 400% in any individual muscle is almost diagnostic of LEMS. If facilitation is less than 50% in all muscles tested, the patient may still have LEMS, especially if weakness has been present only for a short time.

When LEMS is mild, electrophysiologic findings may resemble those of autoimmune myasthenia gravis, with normal CMAP amplitudes, a decremental response with slow RMNS, and little facilitation. One helpful distinguishing feature, however, is that electrophysiologic findings are frequently less severe than clinical findings would suggest in patients with autoimmune myasthenia gravis, but the opposite applies to patients with LEMS.

Conventional EMG. In experienced hands, conventional needle EMG demonstrates unstable MUAPs that vary in waveform with muscle contraction, indicating abnormal NMT (Fig. 35-14).

SF-EMG. SF-EMG measurement of jitter is markedly increased and frequently out of proportion to the degree of clinical weakness. Impulse blocking is frequent. Increasing the stimulation rate from 2 to 15/sec decreases jitter and blocking. Although this inverse relationship between rate of stimulation and degree of jitter and blocking is typical of LEMS, this pattern is not seen in all end plates or in all patients with LEMS. Furthermore, this pattern may occasionally be seen in autoimmune myasthenia gravis.[137,138]

Diagnosis

LEMS is uncommon in childhood and adolescence. Co-occurrence with lymphoproliferative disorders and autoimmune diseases is well recognized. In such patients, cachexia and systemic malaise may seem to account for symptoms, thereby obscuring diagnosis. A high index of suspicion is required. Electrodiagnostic studies are characteristic but require particular attention to responses to voluntary muscle contraction or tetanic stimulation. In the appropriate clinical context, noninvasive diagnosis is possible by identification of elevated circulating levels of P/Q-type VGCC antibodies. These autoantibodies are elevated in 85% of adults with LEMS, but little data exist regarding their frequency in childhood LEMS. Immunotherapy reduces titers; therefore, testing needs to be performed prior to such therapy. Low titers of these antibodies are also found in disorders with elevated levels of IgG, such as systemic lupus erythematosus and rheumatoid arthritis.

Autoimmune myasthenia gravis is an important differential diagnosis, but the insidious onset of predominantly proximal weakness and limited ocular and bulbar involvement often make myopathy an initial consideration. Other potential differential diagnoses include slow-channel myasthenic syndrome, familial limb-girdle myasthenia, acquired botulism, autonomic and peripheral neuropathies, arthritis (when pain is prominent), and conversion disorder.

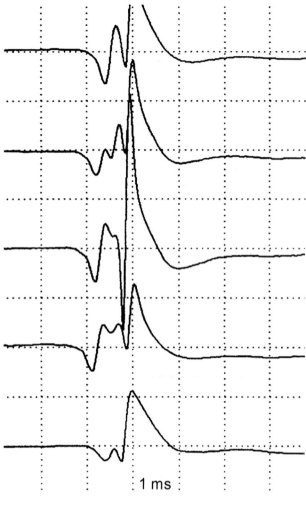

FIGURE 35–14

"Unstable" motor unit action potentials (MUAPs) recorded with a concentric needle electrode in a patient with myasthenia gravis. MUAP shape variation is due to intermittent blocking of individual single muscle fiber action potentials. (From Sanders DB: Diseases associated with disorders of neuromuscular transmission. In Brown WF, Bolton CF, Aminoff MJ [eds]: Neuromuscular Function and Disease. Philadelphia, WB Saunders, 2002, pp 1345-1353.)

Therapy

Because LEMS is frequently a paraneoplastic disorder, diagnosis requires diligent search for an underlying malignancy. Lymphoproliferative disorders seem most common in pediatric patients. Other autoimmune disorders should also be sought. Since onset of LEMS may precede other disorders, these associated diseases need to be considered beyond the initial assessment. Treatment of the underlying malignancy may ameliorate LEMS symptoms. Drugs that may compromise NMT need to be avoided (see Table 35-2).

Cholinesterase inhibitors are often ineffective but may improve strength and dry mouth in mildly affected pa-

tients. Guanidine hydrochloride inhibits uptake of calcium by subcellular organelles, thereby increasing calcium concentration in the cytoplasm and facilitating neurotransmitter release. Strength and autonomic symptoms are improved with cautious escalation of dose to about 30 mg/kg/day. Side effects may be serious and are more common at higher doses. Coadministration of cholinesterase inhibitors augments effects and permits dose reduction. 3,4-DAP improves strength and autonomic function in most patients.[139,140] The optimal dose varies from 15 to 50 mg/day. Coadministration of cholinesterase inhibitors usually augments the therapeutic effect and permits use of a lower dose of 3,4-DAP.[139]

In mildly affected patients, these symptomatic treatments may be sufficient. In more severely affected patients, immunotherapy is often indicated, recognizing that symptoms may not be completely controlled. Prednisone, azathioprine, cyclosporine, other immunosuppressive agents, IVIg, and PEX have been used with benefit.

Disorders of Neuromuscular Transmission Caused by Drugs and Toxins

Many drugs and chemicals may interfere with NMT.[141,142] NMJ dysfunction secondary to botulinum toxin is described earlier. A few other relevant examples are detailed in subsequent sections. Table 35-2 lists drugs that may adversely affect NMT and should be avoided, or used with caution, in patients with disorders of the NMJ. A common theme among patients with drug-induced NMJ dysfunction is the multifactorial nature of the process. For example, postoperative respiratory depression is a frequent presentation, since these patients typically have neuromuscular blockade during the operation and fail to recover as quickly as expected because of coadministered drugs or underlying disorders that interfere with NMT. Similarly, administration of aminoglycoside antibiotics often precipitates significant weakness in patients treated with other drugs or who have underlying disorders that interfere with NMT.

Neonatal Hypermagnesemia

Magnesium is essential for activation of multiple enzymes and preservation of the macromolecular structure of DNA, RNA, and ribosomes. About 60% of body stores are in bone, about 40% is intracellular, and about 1% is extracellular. One third of serum magnesium is bound to protein, mostly albumin, and levels of free magnesium are influenced by pH and protein concentration. The ionized fraction is believed to be the physiologically active component of the circulating pool. Excess magnesium reduces release of presynaptic ACh in the NMJ and sympathetic synapses, at least partly via blockade of Ca^{2+} entry into the presynaptic bouton.[143] Exogenous calcium partly corrects the reduction of ACh release induced by hypermagnesemia.[144] Hypermagnesemia also disturbs NMT by reducing end plate sensitivity to applied ACh.[144]

Maternal preeclampsia is often treated with high doses of magnesium sulfate. Magnesium readily crosses the placenta. Maternal and fetal levels equilibrate over about 2 hours, and fetal levels exceed maternal levels after 24 hours,[145] so levels of magnesium are elevated in infants born to mothers treated with high doses. Other potential causes of hypermagnesemia include ingestion of magnesium-containing cathartics, milk-alkali syndrome, acute oliguria with ketosis, neoplasms with skeletal involvement, hypothyroidism, viral hepatitis, tissue damage, and lithium therapy.[146] Magnesium levels are usually sufficiently high to produce neuromuscular symptoms only among patients with excessive exogenous administration of magnesium.[146]

The typical infant with neonatal hypermagnesemia presents soon after birth with variably severe CNS depression, hypotonia, weakness, reduced tendon reflexes, and progressive abdominal distention.[147,148] Symptoms and signs in the infant that parallel serum magnesium levels and levels higher than 7.0 mmol/L may be fatal (Table 35-5). Hypermagnesemia is often associated with hypocalcemia.[145,146,148,149] Symptoms are usually temporary until excess magnesium is spontaneously excreted by the neonatal kidney over 24 to 48 hours.[145] Magnesium may also be removed by dialysis or exchange transfusion.[146,150] Raising serum calcium levels results in rapid improvement in strength.[144,147]

Hypermagnesemia does not influence NCVs. Studies of one hypermagnesemic adult[151] and eclamptic women before and after administration of magnesium sulfate[149] show that hypermagnesemia is associated with low CMAP amplitudes at rest; variable decrement with 2/sec stimulation; considerable facilitation (≈50% increment in CMAP amplitude) with 20/sec RMNS; and variable, often lesser, facilitation after

TABLE 35–5. SERUM MAGNESIUM LEVELS AND CLINICAL MANIFESTATIONS

Serum Mg, mmol/L	Symptoms
1.5-4.5	Cutaneous flushing, nausea, hypotension, vomiting
2.0-5.0	ECG changes, decreased deep tendon reflexes, CNS depression, bradycardia, drowsiness, unsteadiness, diaphoresis
>4.5	Respiratory depression, unresponsiveness
>5.0	Absent deep tendon reflexes, voluntary muscle paralysis
>7.0	Asystole, cardiac arrest

CNS, central nervous system; ECG, electrocardiogram.
Adapted from Huey CG, Chan K-M, Wong ET, et al: Los Angeles County–University of Southern California Medical Center Clinical Pathology Case Conference: Extreme hypermagnesemia in a neonate. Clin Chem 1995;41:615-618.

exercise. These findings are similar to those exhibited by patients with LEMS, who also have reduced ACh release due to reduced Ca^{2+} entry to the presynaptic terminal (see earlier).

In the clinical setting of a hypermagnesemic infant born to a mother treated with magnesium sulfate, electrodiagnostic studies are not usually required, since symptoms are usually transient and diagnosis rests on clinical suspicion and measurement of serum magnesium. The few reports of electrophysiologic testing in hypermagnesemic neonates show significant decrement with 2/sec stimulation[148,152] but neither decrement nor facilitation with 50 and 100/sec RMNS.[148] This pattern is also seen in LEMS.

Venoms

Venoms contain multiple pharmacologically active components, many of which exert effects at the NMJ. The pathophysiology of many of these toxins is well summarized elsewhere.[153-155] Toxins may bind to specific targets, such as presynaptic calcium channels (e.g., toxin from the funnel web spider, *Agelenopsis aperta*[156]), potassium channels, or the AChR (e.g., venoms of snakes from the families Elapidae [cobras, coral snakes, mambas, and kraits] and Hydrophilidae [sea snakes]), and some effects may be due to nonspecific binding. Some toxins interfere with NMT at multiple sites. Some venoms contain phospholipase A_2, which interferes with release of ACh from presynaptic terminals.[157] The exact pathophysiologic mechanism of many toxins remains unclear. Some toxins are temperature sensitive; for instance, fish toxins are typically inactivated by heat (e.g., immersion in hot water).[153]

Electrodiagnostic studies are reported infrequently, and observations vary according to the different toxins. An example of a presynaptic toxin is the venom of the Papuan taipan (*Oxyuranus scutellatus canni*). Local pain and lymphadenopathy and consumptive coagulopathy occur within hours of the bite.[158] Myasthenic symptoms, including ptosis, external ophthalmoplegia, bulbar weakness, and weakness of respiratory and peripheral musculature, progress over the next hours. Electrodiagnostic tests have been reported in 3 patients.[158] NCVs were normal. CMAP amplitudes were reduced. RMNS at 3 Hz produced subtle decrement at rest (6% to 13%). Following voluntary contraction or 10 seconds of supramaximal 20-Hz stimulation, the amplitude of the initial potential in a train was greater than the initial CMAP at rest (120% to 170%), but the subsequent decrement was much greater (53% to 75%). This complex postactivation effect lasted up to 30 minutes. SF-EMG revealed markedly increased jitter and blocking. Edrophonium 10 mg IV did not alter these electrophysiologic features. The authors hypothesized a presynaptic block due to severe depletion of available ACh vesicles. These observations are concordant with the pathophysiology of taipoxin, the purified venom of the Australian taipan, which is characterized by a gradual reduction to complete absence of ACh release from presynaptic terminals.[158,159] Ultrastructural studies show indentations like empty vesicles frozen in a state of fusion with the presynaptic membrane and absence of ACh vesicles from the nerve terminal, as if formation and recycling of vesicles have been arrested.[159,160]

Other toxins produce postsynaptic dysfunction. For example, one of several toxins from the Taiwan krait (*Bungarus multicinctus*) is alpha-bungarotoxin, which binds specifically to the AChR and is used in identification of the AChR. Krait venom also contains presynaptic toxins, including phospholipase A₂, and this presynaptic block likely explains the lack of benefit with edrophonium.[161,162] Venom from the cobra acts postsynaptically, and patients present with variably severe myasthenic weakness.[163] One paper reported excessive decrement with 5-Hz RMNS, which normalized with edrophonium 10 mg IV.[161]

Organophosphate Poisoning

Organophosphates are organic derivatives of phosphoric acid. They may be absorbed through the skin, ingested, or inhaled. They were developed during World War II as highly toxic nerve gases. They remain in common use throughout the world as pesticides. Accidental and suicide-intended poisonings are well reported. Organophosphates inhibit carboxyl esterase enzymes, including AChE. AChE has two binding sites for its substrate, ACh. Organophosphates bind to one of these sites, the esteratic site, preventing attachment and subsequent degradation of ACh. Although initially reversible, the binding between organophosphates and AChE becomes irreversible, a process known as "aging."[164]

Three overlapping clinical syndromes are reported following ingestion.[165-170] An acute cholinergic crisis due to irreversible inhibition of ACh in central and peripheral nicotinic and muscarinic synapses develops over hours after exposure. It is characterized by variably severe miosis, rhinorrhea, excessive salivation, dyspnea, bronchoconstriction, bradycardia, vomiting, urinary and fecal incontinence, variably severe CNS dysfunction (including coma and delirium), muscle fasciculation, and depolarizing paralysis (type 1 paralysis). This acute illness is often fatal or associated with anoxic brain injury, unless the patient is resuscitated and ventilation maintained. As or after the cholinergic crisis resolves, an "intermediate syndrome" associated with persistent AChE inhibition may follow (see later). A delayed, distal, sensory-motor neuropathy, and occasional CNS axonal loss[169] may occur 1 to 5 weeks after poisoning, at least partly attributed to interference with neuropathy target esterase.[171,172]

The intermediate syndrome occurs in 41% to 68% of patients with acute organophosphate poisoning.[166,170] It is more likely to occur with severe poisoning and severe acute cholinergic crisis, than with less severe poisoning; and specific organophosphates seem more or less prone to induce the syndrome.[166,170] The intermediate syndrome begins as the cholinergic crisis resolves, oftentimes with an intervening symptom-free period of 1 to 4 days.[165-167,170] It usually persists for a week or two but may last up to 38 days.[166] Prolonged inhibition of red blood cell membrane AChE, reducing function to less then 10% of normal, parallels symptoms.[166,170] The prolonged inhibition of AChE is attributed to persistence of the toxins and redistribution of toxins with high-lipid solubility from fat stores.[166] Direct muscle injury has also been implicated in the pathogenesis of the weakness.[170] Symptoms are mostly related to the degree of disordered NMT. Dysphagia, hoarseness of voice, ptosis, external ophthalmoplegia, and weakness of neck flexors occur first and are quickly followed by proximal weakness and respiratory failure, then diffuse weakness and areflexia. Bouts of muscarinic dysfunction (as experienced in the acute cholinergic crisis) may recur during the intermediate syndrome. Recovery occurs in a specific order: cranial nerve dysfunction recovers first, followed by neck flexors, followed by respiratory and proximal musculature.[165-167,170]

Studies in experimental animals revealed excessive decrement with RMNS at 20/sec and increased jitter and blocking with SF-EMG in a dose-dependent manner.[173] Healthy human volunteers exposed to low doses of sarin vapor, an organophosphate, showed a reduction of red blood cell AChE activity to about 60% of normal.[174] Serial SF-EMG studies showed excessive jitter and occasional blocking, in the absence of clinical signs of neuromuscular dysfunction.

Electrophysiologic studies of distal limb muscles in humans with the intermediate syndrome show normal NCVs.[165-167] They reveal a continuum of abnormalities between the acute cholinergic crisis and the intermediate syndrome. Early in the disease course R-CMAPS may be induced by supramaximal nerve stimulation. In the first few days of the intermediate syndrome, several patterns are reported: (1) excessive decrement with low frequency stimulation (1 to 3/sec) and normal responses to rapid RMNS; (2) excessive decrement with intermediate rates of RMNS (10 to 20/sec) and normal responses with slow rates of stimulation (2/sec) or very rapid stimulation (50/sec); or (3) normal responses to slow RMNS, but marked decrement with rapid RMNS (20 to 50/sec), without post-tetanic facilitation. After the first few days of the intermediate syndrome, a decrement-increment response with rapid RMNS (20 to 50/sec) or isolated increments (up to 220%) with 10 to 20 cycle/sec RMNS are reported. Conventional EMG is normal. These findings have generally been interpreted as indicative of both presynaptic and (predominantly) postsynaptic dysfunction.

Treatment of acute poisoning begins with removal of the patient from the contaminated area and removal of contaminated clothing.[175] Following ingestion, intragastric activated charcoal may reduce adsorption. Supportive measures, including mechanical ventilation, are crucial. Atropine should be administered to control muscarinic effects and may need to be readministered frequently for several days. Pralidoxime is an oxime that reactivates cholinesterases. It is useful in controlling nicotinic symptoms and may also need to be administered repeatedly for several days. Neither drug is particularly helpful for CNS symptoms. Presuming vital functions are maintained with supportive care, full recovery is often possible, although long-lasting central and peripheral axonal injury is also recognized.[169,172]

REFERENCES

1. Salpeter MM, Loring RH: Nicotinic acetylcholine receptors in vertebrate muscle: Properties, distribution, and neural control. Progr Neurobiol 1985;25:297-325.
2. Sanes JR, Lichtman JW: Development of the vertebrate neuromuscular junction. Annu Rev Neurosci 1999;22:389-442.
3. Kandel ER, Siegelbaum SA: Signalling at the nerve-muscle synapse: Directly gated transmission. *In* Kandel ER, Schwartz JH, Jessel TM (eds): Principles of Neural Science. New York, McGraw-Hill, 2000, pp 187-206.
4. Lateva ZC, McGill KC, Johanson EM: Electrophysiological evidence of adult human skeletal muscle fibers with multiple endplates and polyneuronal innervation. J Physiol 2002;544:549-565.
5. McComas AJ, Kereshi S, Manzano GM: Multiple innervation of human muscle fibers. J Neurol Sci 1984;64:55-64.
6. Kaminski HJ, Ruff RL: Ocular muscle involvement by myasthenia gravis. Ann Neurol 1997;41:419-420.
7. Liyanage Y, Hoch W, Beeson D, Vincent A: The agrin/muscle-specific kinase pathway: New targets for autoimmune and genetic disorders at the neuromuscular junction. Muscle Nerve 2002;25:4-16.
8. Missias AC, Chu GC, Klocke BJ, et al: Maturation of the acetylcholine receptor in skeletal muscle: Regulation of the gamma-to-epsilon switch. Dev Biol 1996;179:223-238.
9. Hesselmans LFGM, Jennekens FGI, van den Ord CJM, et al: A light and electron microscopical study of B-50 (GAP-43) in human intramuscular nerve and neuromuscular junctions during development. J Neurol Sci 1989;89:301-311.
10. Mishina M, Takai T, Imoto K, et al: Molecular distinction between fetal and adult forms of muscle acetylcholine receptor. Nature 1986;321:406-411.
11. Abicht A, Lochmuller H: What's in the serum of seronegative MG and LEMS? MuSK et al: Neurology 2002;59:1672-1673.
12. Ohno K, Engel AG, Shen XM, et al: Rapsyn mutations in humans cause endplate acetylcholine receptor deficiency and myasthenic syndrome. Am J Hum Genet 2002;70:875-885.
13. DeLepeyriere O, Henderson CE: Motoneuron differentiation, survival, and synaptogenesis. Curr Opinion Genet Devel 1997;7:642-650.
14. Fidzianska A: Human ontogenesis: II. Development of the human neuromuscular junction. J Neuropathol Exp Neurol 1980;39:606-615.
15. Lin W, Burgess R, Dominguez B, et al: Distinct roles of nerve and muscle in postsynaptic differentiation of the neuromuscular synapse. Nature 2001;410:1057-1064.
16. Borges LS, Ferns M: Agrin-induced phosphorylation of the acetylcholine receptor regulates cytoskeletal anchoring and clustering. J Cell Biol 2001;153:1-12.
17. Sanes JR, Jessel TM: The formation and regeneration of synapses. *In* Kandel ER, Schwartz JH, Jessel TM (eds): Principles of Neural Science. New York, McGraw-Hill, 2000, pp 1087-1114.
18. Koenigsberger MR, Patten B, Lovelace RE: Studies of neuromuscular function in the newborn: I. A comparison of myoneural function in the full term and premature infant. Neuropaediatrie 1973;4:350-361.
19. Reichardt LF, Kelly RB: A molecular description of nerve terminal function. Annu Rev Biochem 1983;52:871-926.
20. Engel AG: The neuromuscular junction. *In* Engel AG, Banker BQ (eds): Myology. New York, McGraw-Hill, 1986, pp 209-254.
21. Elmqvist D: Neuromuscular transmission with special reference to myasthenia gravis. Acta Physiol Scand 1965;64:249.
22. Committee on Drugs: Guidelines for monitoring and management of pediatric patients during and after sedation for diagnostic and therapeutic procedures [Addendum]. Pediatrics 2002;110:836-838.
23. Committee on Drugs: Guidelines for monitoring and management of pediatric patients during and after sedation for diagnostic and therapeutic procedures. Pediatrics 1992;89:1110-1115.
24. Lambert EH, Eaton LM, Rooke ED: Defect of neuromuscular conduction associated with malignant neoplasms. Am J Physiol 1956;187:612-613.
25. Wise GA, McQuillen MP: Transient neonatal myasthenia. Arch Neurol 1970;22:556-565.
26. Gutierrez AR, Bodensteiner J, Gutmann L: Electrodiagnosis of infantile botulism. J Child Neurol 1994;9:362-365.
27. Stålberg E, Trontelj JV: Single-Fiber Electromyography: Studies in Healthy and Diseased Muscle, 2nd ed. New York, Raven Press, 1994.
28. Sanders DB: Single-fiber EMG in myasthenia gravis. *In* Kimura J, Shibasaki H (eds): Recent Advances in Clinical Neurophysiology. Amsterdam, Elsevier, 1996, pp 288-291.
29. Lin T-S, Cheng KS: Characterization of the relationship between motor end-plate jitter and the safety factor. Muscle Nerve 1998;21:628-636.

30. Bromberg MB, Scott DM: Single-fiber EMG reference values: Reformatted in tabular form. Muscle Nerve 1994;17:820-821.

31. Gilchrist JM, Ad hoc Committee: Single-fiber EMG reference values: A collaborative effort. Muscle Nerve 1992;15:151-161.

32. Trontelj JV, Khuraibet A, Mihelin M: The jitter in stimulated orbicularis oculi muscle: Technique and normal values. J Neurol Neurosurg Psychiatry 1988;51:814-819.

33. Abicht A, Stucka R, Karcagi V, et al: A common mutation (epsilon1267delG) in congenital myasthenic patients of Gypsy ethnic origin. Neurology 1999;53:1564-1569.

34. Engel AG: 73rd ENMC International Workshop: Congenital myasthenic syndromes. Neuromuscul Dis 2001;11:315-321.

35. Engel AG, Ohno K, Harper CM: Congenital myasthenic syndromes. *In* Jones HR, De Vivo DC, Darras BT (eds): Neuromuscular Disorders of Infancy, Childhood, and Adolescence: A Clinician's Approach. Philadelphia, Butterworth Heinemann Health 2003, pp 555-574.

36. Hutchinson DO, Walls TJ, Nakano S, et al: Congenital endplate acetylcholinesterase deficiency. Brain 1993;116:633-653.

37. Shapira YA, Sadeh ME, Bergtraum MP, et al: Three novel *COLQ* mutations and variation of phenotypic expressivity due to G240X. Neurology 2002;58:603-609.

38. Banwell BL, Russel J, Fukudome T, et al: Myopathy, myasthenic syndrome, and epidermolysis bullosa simplex due to plectin deficiency. J Neuropathol Exp Neurol 1999;58:832-846.

39. Goldhammer Y, Blatt I, Sadeh M, Goodman RM: Congenital myasthenia associated with facial malformation in Iraqi and Iranian Jews. Brain 1990;113:1291-1306.

40. McQuillen MP: Familial limb-girdle myasthenia. Brain 1966;89:121-132.

41. Croxen R, Hatton C, Shelley C, et al: Recessive inheritance and variable penetrance of slow-channel congenital myasthenic syndromes. Neurology 2002;59:162-168.

42. Vincent A, Newsom-Davis J, Wray D, et al: Clinical and experimental observations in patients with congenital myasthenic syndromes. Ann N Y Acad Sci 1992;681:451-460.

43. Hutchinson DO, Engel AG, Walls TJ, et al: The spectrum of congenital end-plate acetylcholinesterase deficiency. Ann N Y Acad Sci 1993;681:469-486.

44. Bedlack RS, Bertorini TE, Sanders DB: Hidden afterdischarges in slow channel congenital myasthenic syndrome. J Clin Neuromusc Dis 2000;1:186-189.

45. Harper CM: Congenital myasthenic syndromes. *In* Brown WF, Bolton CF, Aminoff MJ (eds): Neuromuscular Function and Disease. Philadelphia, WB Saunders, 2002, pp 1687-1695.

46. Harper CM, Engel AG: Treatment of 31 congenital myasthenic syndrome patients with 3,4-diaminopyridine [Abstract]. Neurology 2000;54(Suppl 3):A395.

47. Anlar B, Varli K, Ozdirim E, Ertan M:3,4-diaminopyridine in childhood myasthenia: Double-blind, placebo-controlled trial. J Child Neurol 1996;11:458-461.

48. Harper CM, Engel AG: Quinidine sulfate therapy for the slow-channel congenital myasthenic syndrome. Ann Neurol 1998;43:480-484.

49. Harper CM, Fukudome T, Engel AG: Treatment of slow-channel congenital myasthenic syndrome with fluoxetine. Neurology 2003;60:1710-1713.

50. Felice KJ, Relva GM: Ephedrine in the treatment of congenital myasthenic syndrome. Muscle Nerve 1996;19:799-800.

51. Namba T, Brown SB, Grob D: Neonatal myasthenia gravis: A report of two cases and review of the literature. Pediatrics 1970;45:488-504.

52. Papazian O: Transient neonatal myasthenia gravis. J Child Neurol 1992;7:135-141.

53. Volpe JJ: Neuromuscular disorders: Levels above the lower motor neuron to the neuromuscular junction. *In* Volpe JJ (ed): Neurology of the Newborn. Philadelphia, WB Saunders, 1995, pp 606-633.

54. Morel E, Eymard B, Vernet-der Garabedian B, et al: Neonatal myasthenia gravis: A new clinical and immunologic appraisal on 30 cases. Neurology 1988;38:138-142.

55. Gardnerova M, Eymard B, Morel E, et al: The fetal/adult acetylcholine receptor antibody ratio in mothers with myasthenia gravis as a marker for the transfer of the disease to the newborn. Neurology 1997;48:50-54.

56. Vernet-der Garabedian B, Eymard B, Bach JF, Morel E: Alpha-bungarotoxin blocking antibodies in neonatal myasthenia gravis: Frequency and selectivity. J Neuroimmunol 1989;21:41-47.

57. Vernet-der Garabedian B, Lacokova M, Eymard B, et al: Association of neonatal myasthenia gravis with antibodies against the fetal acetylcholine receptor. J Clin Invest 1994;94:555-559.

58. Tzartos SJ, Efthimiadis A, Morel E, et al: Neonatal myasthenia gravis: Antigenic specificities of antibodies in sera from mothers and their infants. Clin Exp Immunol 1990;80:376-380.

59. Heckmatt JZ, Placzek M, Thompson AH: An unusual case of neonatal myasthenia. J Child Neurol 1987;2:63-66.

60. Mier AK, Havard CW: Diaphragmatic myasthenia in mother and child. Postgrad Med J 1985;61:725-727.

61. Stoll C, Ehret-Mentre MC, Treisser A, Tranchant C: Prenatal diagnosis of congenital myasthenia with arthrogryposis in a myasthenic mother. Prenat Diagn 1991;11:17-22.

62. Dinger J, Prager B: Arthrogryposis multiplex in a newborn of a myasthenic mother—case report and literature. Neuromuscul Dis 1993;3:335-339.

63. Vincent A, Newland C, Brueton L, et al: Arthrogryposis multiplex congenita with maternal autoantibodies specific for a fetal antigen. Lancet 1995;346:24-25.

64. Riemersma S, Vincent A, Beeson D, et al: Association of arthrogryposis multiplex congenita with maternal antibodies inhibiting fetal acetylcholine receptor function. J Clin Invest 1996;98:2358-2363.

65. Matthews I, Sims G, Ledwidge S, et al: Antibodies to acetylcholine receptor in parous women with myasthenia:

Evidence for immunization by fetal antigen. Lab Invest 2002;82:1407-1417.

66. Desmedt JE, Borenstein S: Time course of neonatal myasthenia gravis and unsuspectedly long duration of neuromuscular block in distal muscles. N Engl J Med 1977;296:633.

67. Teng P, Osserman KE: Studies in myasthenia gravis: Neonatal and juvenile types. J Mt Sinai Hosp 1956;23:711-727.

68. Branch CE, Swift TR, Dyken PR: Prolonged neonatal myasthenia gravis: Electrophysiological studies. Ann Neurol 1978;3:416-418.

69. Barnes PRJ, Kanabar DJ, Brueton L, et al: Recurrent congenital arthrogryposis leading to a diagnosis of myasthenia gravis in an initially asymptomatic mother. Neuromuscul Disord 1995;5:59-65.

70. Donat JFG, Donat JR, Lennon VA: Exchange transfusion in neonatal myasthenia gravis. Neurology 1981;31:911-912.

71. Bassan H, Muhlbaur B, Tomer A, Spirer Z: High-dose intravenous immunoglobulin in transient neonatal myasthenia gravis. Pediatr Neurol 1998;18:181-183.

72. Carr SR, Gilchrist JM, Abuelo DN, Clark D: Treatment of antenatal myasthenia gravis. Obstet Gynecol 1991;78:485-489.

73. Spika JS, Shaffer N, Hargrett-Bean N, et al: Risk factors for infant botulism in the United States. Am J Dis Child 1989;143:828-832.

74. Arnon SS, Midura TF, Damus K, et al: Honey and other environmental risk factors for infantile botulism. J Pediatr 1979;94:331-338.

75. Black JD, Dolly JO: Interaction of ^{125}I-labeled botulinum neurotoxins with nerve terminals: I. Ultrastructural autoradiographic localization and quantitation of distinct membrane acceptors for types A and B on motor nerve. J Cell Biol 1986;103:521-534.

76. Schiavo G, Benfenati F, Poulain B, et al: Tetanus and botulinum-B neurotoxins block neurotransmitter release by proteolytic cleavage of synaptobrevin. Nature 1992;359:832-835.

77. Blasi J, Chapman ER, Link E, et al: Botulinum neurotoxin A selectively cleaves the synaptic protein SNAP-25. Nature 1993;365:160-163.

78. Blasi J, Chapman ER, Yamasaki S, et al: Botulinum neurotoxin C1 blocks neurotransmitter release by means of cleaving HPC-1/syntaxin. EMBO J 1993;12:4821-4828.

79. Huttner WB: Snappy excitotoxins. Nature 1993;365:104-105.

80. Schiavo G, Rossetto O, Catsicas S, et al: Identification of the nerve terminal targets of botulinum neurotoxins serotypes A, D, and E. J Biol Chem 1993;268:23784-23787.

81. Crawford TO: Infantile botulism. *In* Jones HR, De Vivo DC, Darras BT (eds): Neuromuscular Disorders of Infancy, Childhood, and Adolescence: A Clinician's Approach. Philadelphia, Butterworth Heinemann Health 2003, pp 547-554.

82. Thompson JA, Glasgow LA, Warpinski JR, Olson C: Infant botulism: Clinical spectrum and epidemiology. Pediatrics 1980;66:936-942.

83. Long SS: Botulism in infancy. Pediatr Infect Dis J 1984;3:266-271.

84. Hathaway CL, McCroskey LM: Examination of feces and serum for diagnosis of infant botulism in 336 patients. J Clin Microbiol 1987;25:2334-2338.

85. Cornblath DR, Sladky JT, Sumner AJ: Clinical electrophysiology of infantile botulism. Muscle Nerve 1983;6:448-452.

86. Fakadej AV, Gutmann L: Prolongation of post-tetanic facilitation in infant botulism. Muscle Nerve 1982;5:727-729.

87. Sheth RD, Lotz BP, Hecox KE, Waclawik AJ: Infantile botulism: Pitfalls in electrodiagnosis. J Child Neurol 1999;14:156-158.

88. Chaudhry V, Crawford TO: Stimulation single-fiber EMG in infant botulism. Muscle Nerve 1999;22:1698-1703.

89. Arnon SS: Infantile botulism. *In* Feigin RD, Cherry JD (eds): Textbook of Pediatric Infectious Diseases. Philadelphia, WB Saunders, 1998, pp 1570-1577.

90. Glauser TA, Maguire HC, Sladky JT: Relapse of infantile botulism. Ann Neurol 1990;28:187-189.

91. Andrews PI, Massey JM, Sanders DB: Acetylcholine receptor antibodies in juvenile myasthenia gravis. Neurology 1993;43:977-982.

92. Sanders DB, Andrews PI, Howard JF Jr, Massey JM: Seronegative myasthenia gravis. Neurology 1997;48(Suppl 5):S40-S51.

93. Sanders DB, el-Salem K, Massey JM, et al: Clinical aspects of MuSK antibody positive seronegative myasthenia gravis (SNMG). Neurology 2003;60:1978-1980.

94. Scuderi F, Marino M, Colonna L, et al: Anti-P110 autoantibodies identify a subtype of "seronegative" myasthenia gravis with prominent oculobulbar involvement. Lab Invest 2002;82:1139-1146.

95. Hoch W, McConville J, Helms S, et al: Auto-antibodies to the receptor tyrosine kinase MuSK in patients with myasthenia gravis without acetylcholine receptor antibodies. Nature Medicine 2001;7:365-368.

96. Selcen D, Fukuda T, Shen XM, Engel AG: Are MuSK antibodies the primary cause of myasthenic symptoms? Neurology 2004;62:1945-1950.

97. Drachman DB: Medical Progress: Myasthenia gravis. N Engl J Med 1994;330:1797-1810.

98. Fambrough DM, Devreotes PN, Gardner JM, Card DJ: The life history of acetylcholine receptors. Progr Brain Res 1979;49:325-334.

99. Engel AG, Sahashi K, Lambert EH, Howard FM: The ultrastructural localization of the acetylcholine receptor, immunoglobulin G and the third and ninth complement components at the motor end-plate and their implications for the pathogenesis of myasthenia gravis. *In* Aguayo AJ, Karpati G (eds): Current Topics in Nerve and Muscle Research. Amsterdam, Excerpta Medica, 1979, pp 111-122.

100. Brodsky MC, Baker RS, Hamed LM: Pediatric Neuro-ophthalmology. New York, Springer, 1996.

101. Rodriguez M, Gomez MR, Howard FM Jr, Taylor WF: Myasthenia gravis in children: Long-term follow-up. Ann Neurol 1983;13:504-510.

102. Linder A, Schalke B, Toyka KV: Outcome in juvenile-onset myasthenia gravis: A retrospective study with long-term follow-up of 79 patients. J Neurol 1997;244:515-520.

103. Evoli A, Batocchi AP, Bartoccioni E, et al: Juvenile myasthenia gravis with prepubertal onset. Neuromuscul Dis 1998;8:561-567.

104. Andrews PI, Massey JM, Howard FM Jr, Sanders DB: Race, sex, and puberty influence onset, severity, and outcome in juvenile myasthenia gravis. Neurology 1994;44:1208-1214.

105. Fukuyama Y, Suzuki M, Segawa M: Studies on myasthenia gravis in childhood. Paediatr Univ Tokyo 1970;18:57-68.

106. Wong V, Hawkins BR, Yu YL: Myasthenia gravis in Hong Kong Chinese: II. Paediatric disease. Acta Neurol Scand 1992;86:68-72.

107. Grob D, Arsura EL, Brunner NG, Namba T: The course of myasthenia gravis and therapies affecting outcome. Ann N Y Acad Sci 1987;505:472-499.

108. Sanders DB, Stålberg EV: AAEM Minimonograph #25: Single-fiber electromyography. Muscle Nerve 1996;19:1069-1083.

109. Afifi AK, Bell WE: Tests for juvenile myasthenia gravis: Comparative diagnostic yield and prediction of outcome. J Child Neurol 1993;8:403-411.

110. Oh SJ, Cho HK: Edrophonium responsiveness not necessarily diagnostic of myasthenia gravis. Muscle Nerve 1990;13:187-191.

111. Rosenberg ML: Spasm of the near reflex mimicking myasthenia gravis. J Clin Neuro-Ophthalmol 1986;6:106-108.

112. Dirr LY, Donofrio PD, Patton JF, Troost BT: A false-positive edrophonium test in a patient with a brainstem glioma. Neurology 1989;39:865-867.

113. Okamoto K, Ito J, Tokiguchi S, Furusawa T: Atropy of bilateral extraocular muscles—CT and clinical features of seven patients. J Neuro-Ophthalmol 1996;16:286-288.

114. Snead OC, Benton JW, Dwyer D, et al: Juvenile myasthenia gravis. Neurology 1980;30:732-739.

115. Ohta K, Shigemoto K, Kubo S, et al: MuSK antibodies in AChR AB-seropositive MG vs AChR Ab-seronegative MG. Neurology 2004;62:2132-2133.

116. Adams C, Theodorescu D, Murphy EG, Shandling B: Thymectomy in juvenile myasthenia gravis. J Child Neurol 1990;5:215-218.

117. Seybold ME: Thymectomy in childhood myasthenia gravis. Ann N Y Acad Sci 1998;841:731-741.

118. Andrews PI: A treatment algorithm for autoimmune myasthenia gravis in childhood. Ann N Y Acad Sci 1998;841:789-802.

119. Frist WH, Thirumalai S, Doehring CB: Thymectomy for the myasthenia gravis patient: Factors influencing outcome. Ann Thorac Surg 1994;57:334-338.

120. Blossom GB, Ernstoff RM, Howells GA, et al: Thymectomy for myasthenia gravis. Arch Surg 1993;128:855-862.

121. Verma PK, Oger JJ: Seronegative generalized myasthenia gravis: Low frequency of thymic pathology. Neurology 1992;42:586-589.

122. Evoli A, Batocchi AP, Lo Monaco M, et al: Clinical heterogeneity of seronegative myasthenia gravis. Neuromuscul Dis 1996;6:155-161.

123. Magnelli V, Grassi C, Parlatore E, et al: Down-regulation of non-L-, non-N-type (Q-like) Ca^{2+} channels by Lambert-Eaton myasthenic syndrome (LEMS) antibodies in rat insulinoma RINm5F cells. FEBS Lett 1996;387:47-52.

124. Pinto A, Iwasa K, Newland C, et al: The action of Lambert-Eaton myasthenic syndrome immunoglobulin G on cloned human voltage-gated calcium channels. Muscle Nerve 2002;25:715-724.

125. Nakao YK, Motomura M, Fukudome T, et al: Seronegative Lambert-Eaton myasthenic syndrome: Study of 110 Japanese patients. Neurology 2002;59:1773-1775.

126. Dahl DS, Sato S: Unusual myasthenic state in a teen-age boy. Neurology 1974;24:897-901.

127. Brown JC, Johns RJ: Diagnostic difficulties encountered in the myasthenic syndrome sometimes associated with carcinoma. J Neurol Neurosurg Psychiatry 1974;37:1214-1224.

128. Chelmicka-Schorr E, Bernstein LP, Zurbrugg EB, Huttenlocher PR: Eaton-Lambert syndrome in a 9-year-old girl. Arch Neurol 1979;36:572-574.

129. Argov Z, Shapira Y, Averbuch-Heller L, Wirguin I: Lambert-Eaton myasthenic syndrome (LEMS) in association with lymphoproliferative disorders. Muscle Nerve 1995;18:715-719.

130. Shapira Y, Cividalli G, Szabo G, et al: A myasthenic syndrome in childhood leukemia. Dev Med Child Neurol 1974;16:668-671.

131. Tsao C-Y, Mendell JR, Freiner ML, Kissel JT: Lambert-Eaton myasthenic syndrome in children. J Child Neurol 2002;17:74-76.

132. Tim RW, Massey JM, Sanders DB: Lambert-Eaton myasthenic syndrome (LEMS): Clinical and electrodiagnostic features and response to therapy in 59 patients. Ann N Y Acad Sci 1998;841:823-826.

133. Wirtz PW, Sotodeh M, Nijnuis M, et al: Difference in distribution of muscle weakness between myasthenia gravis and the Lambert-Eaton myasthenic syndrome. J Neurol Neurosurg Psychiatry 2002;73:766-768.

134. Wirtz PW, Smallegange TM, Wintzen AR, Verschuuren JJ: Differences in clinical features between the Lambert-Eaton myasthenic syndrome with and without cancer: An analysis of 227 published cases. Clin Neurol Neurosurg 2002;104:359-363.

135. Khurana RK: Paraneoplastic autonomic dysfunction. *In* Low PA (ed): Clinical Autonomic Disorders. Boston, Little, Brown, 1993, pp 506-511.

136. Tim RW, Massey JM, Sanders DB: Lambert-Eaton myasthenic syndrome: Electrodiagnostic findings and response to treatment. Neurology 2000;54:2176-2178.

137. Trontelj JV, Stålberg E: Single motor end-plates in myasthenia gravis and LEMS at different firing rates. Muscle Nerve 1991;14:226-232.

138. Sanders DB: The effect of firing rate on neuromuscular jitter in Lambert-Eaton myasthenic syndrome. Muscle Nerve 1992;15:256-258.

139. Sanders DB, Massey JM, Sanders LL, Edwards LJ: A randomized trial of 3,4-diaminopyridine in Lambert-Eaton myasthenic syndrome. Neurology 2000;54:603-607.

140. McEvoy KM, Windebank AJ, Daube JR, Low PA: 3,4-Diaminopyridine in the treatment of Lambert-Eaton myasthenic syndrome. N Engl J Med 1989;321:1567-1571.

141. Argov Z, Mastaglia FL: Disorders of neuromuscular transmission caused by drugs. N Engl J Med 1979;301:409-413.

142. Howard JF Jr: Adverse drug effects on neuromuscular transmission. Semin Neurol 1990;10:89-102.

143. Ravin R, Parnas H, Spira ME, Parnas I: Partial uncoupling of neurotransmitter release from [Ca^{2+}] by membrane hyperpolarization. J Neurophysiol 1999;81:3044-3053.

144. Del Castillo J, Engbark L: The nature of the neuromuscular block produced by magnesium. J Physiol 1954;124:370-384.

145. Lipsitz PJ: The clinical and biochemical effects of excess magnesium in the newborn. Pediatrics 1971;47:501-509.

146. Huey CG, Chan K-M, Wong ET, et al: Los Angeles County–University of Southern California Medical Center Clinical Pathology Case Conference: Extreme hypermagnesemia in a neonate. Clin Chem 1995;41:615-618.

147. Lipsitz PJ, English IC: Hypermagnesemia in the newborn infant. Pediatrics 1967;40:856-862.

148. Rasch DK, Huber PA, Richardson CJ, et al: Neurobehavioral effects of neonatal hypermagnesemia. J Pediatr 1982;100:272-276.

149. Ramanathan J, Sibai BM, Pillai R, Angel JJ: Neuromuscular transmission studies in pre-eclamptic women receiving magnesium sulfate. Am J Obstet Gynecol 1988;158:40-46.

150. Engel RR, Elin RJ: Hypermagnesemia from birth asphyxia. J Pediatr 1970;77:631-637.

151. Swift TR: Weakness from magnesium containing cathartics. Muscle Nerve 1979;2:295-298.

152. L'Hommedieu CS, Huber PA, Rasch DK: Potentiation of magnesium-induced neuromuscular weakness by gentamicin. Crit Care Med 1983;11:55-56.

153. Church JE, Hodgson WC: The pharmacologic activity of fish venoms. Toxicon 2002;40:1083-1093.

154. Hodgson WC, Wickramaratna A: Animal toxins of Asia and Australia: In vitro neuromuscular activity of snake venoms. Clin Exp Pharmacol Physiol 2002;29:807-814.

155. Geh S-L, Vincent A, Rang S, et al: Identification of phospholipase A$_2$ and neurotoxic activities in the venom of the New Guinea small-eyed snake (*Micropechis ikaheka*). Toxicon 1997;35:101-109.

156. Uchitel OD, Protti DA, Sanchez V, et al: P-type voltage-dependent calcium channel mediates presynaptic calcium influx and transmitter release in mammalian synapses. Proc Natl Acad Sci 1992;89:3330-3333.

157. Swift TR: Disorders of neuromuscular transmission other than myasthenia gravis. Muscle Nerve 1981;4:334-353.

158. Connolly S, Trevett AJ, Nwokolo NC, et al: Neuromuscular effects of Papuan taipan snake venom. Ann Neurol 1995;38:916-920.

159. Kamenskaya M, Thesleff S: The neuromuscular blocking action of an isolated toxin from the elapid (*Oxyuranus scutellatus*). Acta Physiol Scand 1974;90:716-724.

160. Fohlman J, Eaker D, Karlsson E, Thesleff S: Taipoxin, an extremely potent presynaptic neurotoxin from the venom of the Australian snake Taipan (*Oxyuranus scutellatus*). Eur J Biochem 1976;68:457-469.

161. Watt G, Theakston RDG, Hayes CG, et al: Positive response to edrophonium in patients with neurotoxic envenoming by cobras (*Naja philippinensis*). N Engl J Med 1986;315:1444-1448.

162. Sanmuganathan PS: Myasthenic syndrome of snake envenomation: A clinical and neurophysiological study. Postgrad Med 1998;74:596-599.

163. Su C, Chang CC, Lee CY: Pharmacological properties of the neurotoxin of cobra venom. *In* Russell FE, Saunders PR (eds): Animal Toxins. Oxford, Pergamon Press, 1967, pp 259-267.

164. Ehrich M: Organophosphates. *In* Wexler P (ed): Encyclopedia of Toxicology. San Diego, Academic Press, 2002, pp 467-471.

165. Senanayake N, Karalliedde L: Neurotoxic effects of organophosphorus insecticides: An intermediate syndrome. N Engl J Med 1987;316:761-763.

166. De Bleecker J, Van Den Neucker K, Colardyn F: Intermediate syndrome in organophosphorus poisoning: A prospective study. Crit Care Med 1993;21:1706-1711.

167. He F, Xu H, Qin F, et al: Intermediate myasthenia syndrome following acute organophosphates poisoning—an analysis of 21 cases. Hum Exp Toxicol 1998;17:40-45.

168. Moretto A, Lotti M: Poisoning by organophosphorus insecticides and sensory neuropathy. J Neurol Neurosurg Psychiatry 1998;64:463-468.

169. Chuang C-C, Lin TS, Tsai MC: Delayed neuropathy and myelopathy after organophosphate intoxication. N Engl J Med 2002;347:1119-1121.

170. John M, Oomen A, Zachariah A: Muscle injury in organophosphorous poisoning and its role in the development of the intermediate syndrome. Neurotoxicology 2003;24:43-53.

171. Johnson MK: Target for initiation of delayed neurotoxicity by organophosphorus esters: Biochemical studies and toxicological applications. Rev Biochem Toxicol 1982;4:141-212.

172. Sevim S, Aktekin M, Dogu O, et al: Late-onset polyneuropathy due to organophosphate (DDVP) intoxication. Can J Neurol Sci 2003;30:75-78.

173. Yang D, Tao L, He F: Electroneurophysiologic studies in rats of acute dimethoate poisoning. Toxicol Lett 1999;107:249-254.

174. Baker DJ, Sedgwick EM: Single-fibre electromyographic changes in man after organophosphate exposure. Hum Exp Toxicol 1996;15:369-375.

175. Linden CH, Lovejoy FHJ: Poisoning and drug overdosage. *In* Fauci AS, Braunwald E, Isselbacher KJ, et al (eds): Harrison's Principles of Internal Medicine. New York, McGraw-Hill, 1998, pp 2523-2543.

176. Bady B, Chauplannaz G, Carrier H: Congenital Lambert-Eaton myasthenic syndrome. J Neurol Neurosurg Psychiatry 1987;50:476-478.

177. Breningstall GN, Kurachek SC, Fugate JH, Engel AG: Treatment of congenital endplate acetylcholinesterase deficiency by neuromuscular blockade. J Child Neurol 1996;11:345-346.

36

Muscle Disorders in Children: Neurophysiologic Contributions To Diagnosis and Management

Nancy L. Kuntz

Diagnosis of muscle disorders in children requires an assessment of clinical history, physical examination, and laboratory test data. More specifically, diagnostic considerations comprise the following:
- Clinical history, including presenting symptoms and family history
- Physical findings
- Blood tests, including muscle enzymes, serum biochemical tests, and inflammatory markers
- Exercise testing
- Molecular genetics testing
- Imaging, including ultrasonography (US), magnetic resonance imaging (MRI), and magnetic resonance spectroscopy (MRS)
- Muscle biopsy, including immunohistochemistry, electron microscopy, and biochemical analyses
- Neurophysiologic testing, including nerve conduction studies (NCS) and electromyography (EMG)

NCS and EMG offer valuable insight into the physiology of the motor unit and are important tools in the diagnosis of neuromuscular disorders in infants, children, and adolescents. However, the goal is to reach an accurate diagnosis as directly as possible with the least potential discomfort and risk to the child.

Optimal diagnosis of muscle disorders does not always require NCS or needle EMG. There are a number of reasons for this, including the following:

- Neurophysiologic techniques are not as accurate at diagnosing myopathic disorders in childhood as they are for diagnosing neuropathic disorders.[1-4]
- Less-invasive techniques such as US scans of muscle have been successfully used for screening in cases of suspected neuromuscular disease.[5,6]
- Diagnosis of certain clinically suspected muscle disorders can be confirmed by newly developed techniques including DNA testing,[7] MRI of muscle,[8,9] and MRS.[10]
- A significant percentage of young children (35%) experience extreme behavioral distress when undergoing NCS and/or EMG.[11] Although conscious sedation can be used to minimize physical discomfort and emotional distress, this adds a degree of potential morbidity and increases the time requirement and cost of the procedure.

However, neurophysiologic techniques provide a unique insight into the physiology of the motor unit, including the functional status of disordered muscle. This chapter discusses the potential contribution of neurophysiologic techniques to the diagnosis of disorders of muscle function.

Pathologic changes in childhood muscle disorders can include loss of muscle fibers, fiber necrosis with associated denervation, alteration in membrane excitability or ability to utilize available substrates to produce energy, or changes in excitation-contraction coupling. This altered muscle physiology produces changes in NCS and needle EMG

BOX 36-1
CLASSIFICATION OF MYOPATHIES IN CHILDREN

Hereditary
Congenital myopathies
Muscular dystrophies
Channelopathies
   Chloride channelopathies
   Calcium channelopathies
   Sodium channelopathies
Metabolic myopathies
   Disorders of glycogen metabolism
   Disorders of lipid metabolism
   Disorders of nucleotide metabolism
   Disorders of mitochondrial energy metabolism

Acquired
Inflammatory myopathies
Toxic myopathies
Myopathies associated with endocrine or systemic
   disorders

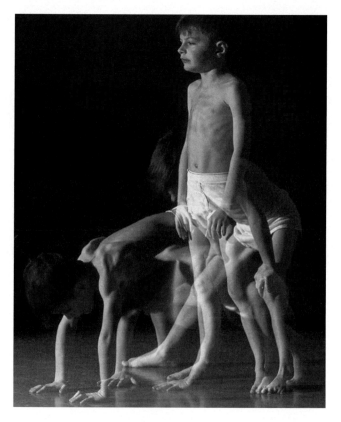

FIGURE 36–1
"Gower's sign," or using the arms to push off the thighs to stand up from the floor, is a sensitive clinical sign of proximal lower extremity weakness.

findings. For example, severe loss of muscle can lead to low compound muscle action potential (CMAP) amplitudes on NCS. The presence of fewer muscle fibers in each motor unit potential (MUP) produces shorter duration, low-amplitude MUPs. Rapid recruitment occurs when less mechanical force is produced with activation of each MUP.[12] There are circumstances when these data will refine the differential diagnosis and other circumstances in which this information may be used to provide prognostic information or monitor response to therapy.[13]

Box 36-1 contains a simple classification of muscle disorders in children. An encyclopedic discussion of diagnostic considerations in muscle disorders in children is beyond the scope of this chapter. A number of excellent references are available for this purpose.[14-20] Figure 36-1 demonstrates, by time-lapse photography, the Gower's phenomenon, in which children with proximal lower extremity weakness use upper extremity support on the thigh to stand up from a crouch. This clinical phenomenon identifies proximal lower extremity weakness sensitively but is nonspecific, emphasizing the need for additional diagnostic efforts. This chapter provides an overview of diagnostic considerations relating to muscle disorders in children, with particular emphasis on the potential contribution of neurophysiologic techniques.

CONGENITAL MYOPATHIES

Congenital myopathies are a group of relatively less common, inherited myopathies with a variety of characteristic histologic profiles. Box 36-2 contains a listing of the most commonly occurring congenital myopathies. In these disorders, hypotonia and weakness are associated with relatively preserved muscle stretch reflexes and normal sensation. The clinical spectrum is quite variable. Among those with the most severe clinical courses are infants with X-linked myotubular myopathy who have decreased intrauterine movements and a difficult delivery followed by respiratory insufficiency and dysphagia that frequently limit survival. At the milder end of the clinical spectrum are a number of these disorders in which adolescents (or even adults) present with mild hypotonia and proximal/facial weakness sometimes associated with respiratory weakness or skeletal deformities. Traditionally considered nonprogressive, clinical strength has been noted to decline in association with growth, weight gain, and skeletal deformities including progressive scoliosis. Diagnosing congenital

BOX 36-2
CONGENITAL MYOPATHIES

Bethlem myopathy
Cap disease
Central core disease
Centronuclear myopathy
Congenital fiber size disproportion
Desmin storage myopathy
Fingerprint body myopathy
Multicore/minicore disease
Myopathy with lysis of type 1 fibers
Myopathy with tubular aggregates
Myotubular myopathy
Nemaline myopathy
Reducing body myopathy
Sarcotubular myopathy
Spheroid body myopathy
Trilaminar myopathy
Zebra body myopathy

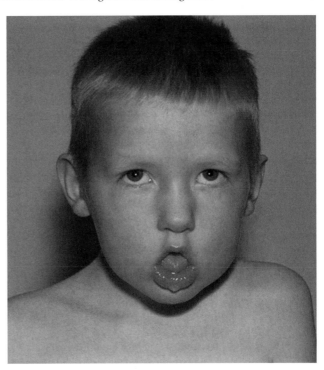

FIGURE 36–2
Facial weakness is a sensitive but nonspecific clinical finding in children with congenital myopathy.

myopathies is important because of the genetic implications for the family and because of the prognostic implications for the individual child who may be at increased risk of malignant hyperthermia in response to anesthetic agents. Figure 36-2 demonstrates the facial weakness observed in a young boy with nemaline myopathy.

Genetic linkage studies are providing a new perspective on the congenital myopathies. For example, nemaline myopathy has been shown to link to at least three different regions on chromosomes with different target proteins having been identified: nebulin,[21] alpha-actin,[22] and tropomysin.[23] Clinicogenetic correlation has led to the separation of centronuclear/myotubular myopathy into two separate disorders, with centronuclear being reserved for an autosomal recessive disorder associated with a milder phenotype and myotubular myopathy used for the X-linked recessive severe phenotype described earlier.

When specific gene mutations are identified for each of the congenital myopathies, DNA testing will likely become the preferred method of diagnosis. In the interim, muscle biopsy with clinical and pedigree correlation is the standard. Muscle US can be used as a tool to identify appropriately involved muscles for biopsy. The Neuromuscular Clinic at Hammersmith Hospital has been exploring the use of muscle US for diagnosis of neuromuscular disorders since 1980. A prospective study involving 222 consecutively evaluated new children referred to the pediatric muscle clinic demonstrated nonspecific abnormalities in 4 (57%)

of the 7 children with congenital myopathies.[24] The Royal Hospital for Sick Children in Glasgow reported their experience evaluating 100 children with suspected neuromuscular disease. They reported that the sensitivity of US in detecting neuromuscular disease was 78% with a 91% specificity. US was more reliable in children older than 3 years of age where the sensitivity was 81% and the specificity was 96%. The sensitivity for detecting nonspecific abnormalities in children with biopsy-confirmed congenital myopathies was 70%.[6] Clinicians at Istanbul University recently evaluated use of muscle US and EMG for evaluation of floppy infants. US and EMG were diagnostically equivalent and showed complete concordance with eventual pathologic or molecular genetics diagnoses. Of the 41 infants, the following 39 diagnoses were reached: 16 neurogenic disease, 6 myopathic disorders, and 17 central disorders. Two of the 41 infants remained undiagnosed after muscle US, EMG, and muscle/nerve biopsy.[5] The sensitivity and specificity of muscle US appear to be as high or higher than those of needle EMG, suggesting that muscle US may emerge as an important screening and diagnostic technique in pediatric neuromuscular disease. For example, a characteristic pattern of muscle involvement on MRI of thigh muscle (involvement of the peripheral region of the vastus lateralis and hamstring muscles with relative sparing of the central portions of these muscles) has recently been described in three generations of patients from one family with Bethlem myopathy. This diagnosis can be confirmed by molecular genetic analysis of the *COL6* gene.[25]

Concordance between neurophysiologic testing and muscle biopsy results for infants and children with congenital myopathies has varied between 10% and 50% in different laboratories.[1,3,4] In addition to small MUPs that are excessively polyphasic and recruit rapidly, abnormal spontaneous activity can be seen during needle EMG of congenital myopathies. Needle EMG in children with myotubular myopathy[26] and spheroid body myopathy[27] can demonstrate fibrillation potentials and occasional myotonic discharges. Fibrillation potentials have also been described in nemaline myopathy,[28] congenital fiber-type disproportion myopathy,[29] and desmin storage myopathy.[30] This emphasizes the importance of disciplining oneself to evaluate MUPs as well as spontaneous activity during each study and to avoid reflexively assuming that neurogenic disorders are the cause of fibrillation potentials.

MUSCULAR DYSTROPHIES

Muscular dystrophy (MD) refers to a type of inherited muscle disorder characterized by progressive weakness and muscle necrosis. During the past decade understanding of the pathophysiology of this group of disorders has increased and been associated with a parallel increase in the availability of relevant diagnostic tools. Eventually, all forms of MD may be diagnosed by molecular genetic analysis of the underlying gene defect. Categorization according to these gene defects will be straightforward, although significant phenotypic variation is being observed within specific gene defects. Box 36-3 outlines forms of MD that are most frequent in infants and children. Underlying gene defect and protein abnormalities have not been defined for all forms of

MD; therefore, current classifications also use clinical phenotypes (e.g., limb-girdle muscular dystrophy [LGMD], congenital muscular dystrophy [CMD]).

Clinical presentation, family history, and level of muscle enzymes can be used to make certain presumptive diagnoses that lead directly to DNA testing without performing neurophysiologic testing or muscle biopsy.[7] For example, 4- or 5-year-old boys with large calves, a tendency to toe-walk, a mildly waddling gait, and markedly elevated serum creatine kinase (CK) have a presumptive diagnosis of Duchenne's MD type of dystrophinopathy. Figure 36-3 demonstrates the prominent hypertrophy of calf muscles that is suggestive of Duchenne's MD in young boys. In most of these children, a DNA deletion test can confirm the diagnosis. However, there are more generic clinical presentations of MD such as a floppy infant with arthrogryposis or an older child with slowly progressive proximal weakness and mildly elevated serum CK. In these circumstances, the differential diagnoses are too broad to proceed directly to DNA analysis. These infants or children would benefit from neurophysiologic testing to refine their respective differential diagnoses: central hypotonia versus disorder of the motor unit for the floppy infant or muscle disorder versus neurogenic process for an older child with indeterminate proximal weakness. Awareness of the neurophysiologic findings in these various disorders prepares for the most efficient diagnostic evaluation.

Dystrophinopathies

In early stages of Duchenne- and Becker-type dystrophinopathies, NCSs are normal and needle EMG demonstrates normal to mildly increased insertional activity with sparse fibrillation potentials. MUPs are of short duration, low amplitude and rapidly recruiting with an increased proportion of polyphasic potentials. As this type of dystrophy progresses with muscle necrosis, attempts at repair and subsequent fibrosis, increased numbers of fibrillation potentials, and polyphasic MUP with satellite potentials are noted. Eventually, reduced recruitment of MUPs is noted.[31] A clinically milder spectrum of dystrophinopathies has been recognized including X-linked isolated cardiomyopathies, phenotypic presentation of myalgia and exercise intolerance, as well as hyperCKemia. Neurophysiologic studies of peripheral nerve and skeletal muscle (NCS and EMG) are frequently normal in these patients.

Congenital Muscular Dystrophies

CMDs are a heterogeneous group of disorders with congenital onset of progressive weakness associated with a dystrophic muscle biopsy. The central nervous system is involved in a number of forms of CMD. Arthrogryposis and

---

BOX 36-3
MUSCULAR DYSTROPHIES IN
INFANTS AND CHILDREN

Dystrophinopathies
Congenital muscular dystrophies
Facioscapulohumeral dystrophy
Emery-Dreifuss muscular dystrophy
Limb-girdle muscular dystrophies
Myotonic dystrophy
Proximal myotonic myopathy

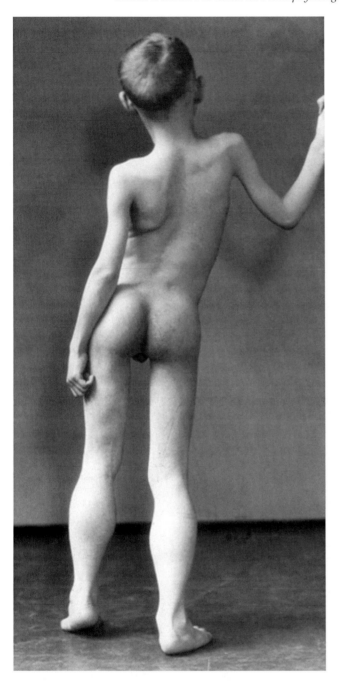

FIGURE 36–3

Disproportionate hypertrophy of calf muscles is a clinical finding in boys with Duchenne's muscular dystrophy.

peripheral neuropathy have been described in CMD.[14] There are currently nine forms of CMD that have been linked to a genetic defect and multiple additional clinical syndromes for which the genetic defect is being sought.[32] Muscle biopsies demonstrate nonspecific dystrophic changes. Real-time US of muscle demonstrated abnormali-

ties in 86% of 14 infants and children with CMD.[24] In CMDs showing little clinical progression and associated with normal or mildly elevated serum CK, NCSs are normal and needle EMG shows normal spontaneous activity with nonspecific MUP changes consistent with a myopathy.[33,34] A demyelinating peripheral neuropathy[35] and central conduction slowing in somatosensory evoked potentials have been described in merosin-deficient CMD.[36] Imaging, neurophysiologic testing, and standard muscle histology do not readily differentiate the various forms of CMD. Pattern of clinical involvement, muscle immunohistochemistry, and molecular genetic studies provide the most definitive diagnosis of CMD.[14]

Facioscapulohumeral Dystrophy

Facioscapulohumeral dystrophy (FSHD) is an autosomal dominant disorder with onset in childhood of slowly progressive weakness of selected muscles. Because of the mild and slowly progressive nature of the weakness, it is not uncommon for individuals to first seek medical attention during adult life. Extraocular, bulbar, respiratory, and cardiac muscles are usually not affected. A deletion creating a 4q35 DNA "short fragment" has been described in individuals with FSHD. This short fragment is not present in individuals with scapuloperoneal MD, which clarifies that this is a separate disorder.[14] Neurophysiologic findings parallel the stage of muscle breakdown. In early or mild FSHD, NCS are normal and needle EMG demonstrates short, low-amplitude polyphasic MUPs that recruit rapidly. Sparse fibrillation potentials are present in muscles with ongoing fiber necrosis.[37]

Limb-Girdle Muscular Dystrophies

LGMDs are a heterogeneous group of disorders with progressive weakness involving primarily the shoulder and hip girdles. Somewhat less than two thirds of individuals with this phenotype have an identifiable gene defect with the rest waiting to be clarified through further research. There are more than a dozen disorders with separate protein defects that have been identified including deficiencies of various forms of sarcoglycans, dystroglycan, calpain-3, dysferlin, caveolin, and others.[14,38] Neurophysiologic findings and muscle imaging studies can assist diagnostically by improving on clinical ability to specify the pattern of muscle involvement. For example, MRI scanning can demonstrate greater involvement of posterior thigh muscles with sparing of hip abductors suggestive of calpainopathy.[39] However, the current role of neurophysiologic testing is to differentiate LGMD from neurogenic disorders such as spinal muscular atrophy that may present with a similar phenotype.

Emery-Dreifuss Muscular Dystrophy

Emery-Dreifuss muscular dystrophy (EDMD) is an X-linked recessive disorder with progressive proximal weakness notable for onset of joint contractures early in the clinical course and for the presence of cardiac conduction defects. Needle EMG demonstrates fibrillation potentials in some patients and short-duration, low-amplitude, polyphasic MUPs that recruit rapidly.[40] A rare autosomal dominant form of EDMD has been described.[14] Definitive diagnosis is made by immunohistochemical staining for emerin in muscle or skin biopsies or by deletion analysis.

Myotonic Dystrophy

Myotonic dystrophy (MyD) is an autosomal dominant multisystem disorder that involves skeletal and heart muscle and is associated with cataracts, premature balding, and endocrine abnormalities. MyD is caused by an unstable trinucleotide repeat on chromosome 19. The clinical severity correlates with the number of repeats; therefore, infants with congenital onset demonstrate the largest number of repeats.[41] DNA testing is the preferred method for diagnosing MyD. However, neurophysiologic examinations are performed on patients in whom MyD is not yet suspected: for example, family members unaware of or in denial of their MyD who are being evaluated for neuromuscular complaints or floppy infants who may present with congenital MyD prior to diagnosis in their mother.

Recognition of the characteristic neurophysiologic profile is valuable. In older children and young adults with MyD, NCSs are normal with the exception that a transient decrement in CMAP amplitude may occur in response to repetitive stimulation or brief (10-second) exercise. The reduced CMAP amplitude returns to normal in less than 2 minutes after brief exercise.[42] There are several reports of fibrillation potentials and/or myotonic discharges noted in infants with a congenital form of MyD.[10,43-45] One report noted that in the youngest infants, the fibrillation potentials were most prominent and the myotonic discharges least well defined.[43] Figure 36-4 demonstrates the abnormal spontaneous activity recorded in infants with congenital MyD. Abnormal spontaneous activity was not universally observed in infants with congenital MyD.[46] MUPs were reported as either normal or possessing mildly short duration and low amplitude.

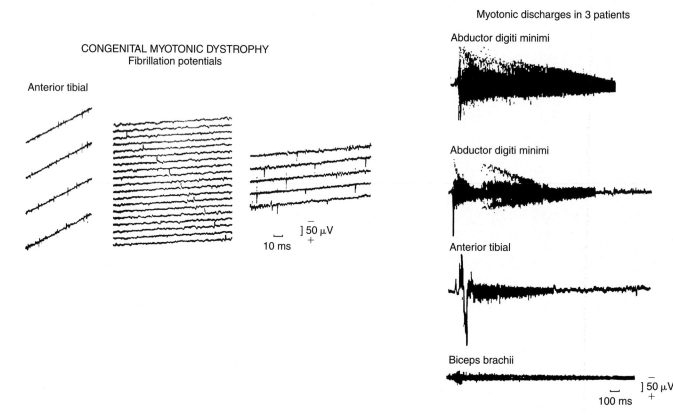

FIGURE 36–4

Abnormal spontaneous activity on needle EMG; both fibrillation potentials (left) and myotonic discharges (right), from several infants with congenital myotonic dystrophy are shown.

CONGENITAL MYOTONIC DYSTROPHY
Motor unit potentials

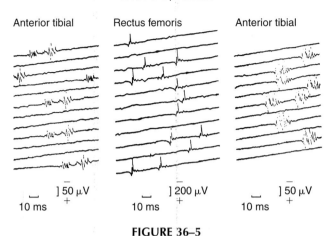

FIGURE 36–5

Low-amplitude, excessively polyphasic voluntary motor unit potentials from several infants with congenital myotonic dystrophy are displayed. These findings can be present in other muscle disorders as well.

Figure 36-5 demonstrates a number of low-amplitude, polyphasic MUPs recorded in an infant with congenital MyD. Careful prospective studies have not been performed to determine the age at which children with MyD first demonstrate myotonia and dystrophic MUP changes on needle EMG. Abnormal spontaneous activity is not observed during infancy in childhood-onset MyD. One child had classic MyD confirmed clinically and electromyographically at 7 years of age after a normal needle EMG was documented in the newborn period (personal observation). Clinical and EMG myotonia has been described in an 18-month-old child with noncongenital MyD. Clinical myotonia is demonstrable before 5 years of age in only 12% of children known to have MyD. When sought, clinical myotonia is present in most MyD children by 10 years of age. Myotonic discharges on needle EMG are easier to elicit than clinical myotonia.[47] Myotonic discharges are not present in all muscles in any individual with MyD, and the intensity has been described to vary directly with the degree of individual muscle weakness.[48]

Proximal Myotonic Myopathy

Proximal myotonic myopathy (PROMM) is an autosomal dominant disorder characterized by progressive, proximal weakness and myotonia. Clinical onset is most frequent during adult years; however, childhood onset has been observed. Cataracts and cardiac arrhythmias are associated clinical findings.[41] In contrast to MyD, PROMM lacks involvement of facial, respiratory, and distal muscles. PROMM has been linked to chromosome 3q, and patients lack the excess CTG repeats seen in MyD.[14] Needle EMG is useful to demonstrate myotonic discharges when they are not clinically apparent and to differentiate this disorder from phenotypically similar spinal muscular atrophy. In PROMM, myotonic discharges can be sparse throughout muscles. Brief runs of very high frequency spontaneous discharges (180 to 240 Hz) have been described.[49]

Over the past decade, muscle imaging techniques such as US and MRI have been used both to screen for muscle involvement as well as to identify selective involvement of muscles to aid in the diagnosis of dystrophies. For example, US evaluation of the degree of involvement of the soleus muscle differentiates between X-linked and autosomal dominant forms of EDMD better than clinical assessment.[50] US imaging has also been used to direct muscle biopsy to selectively involved muscles.[51] In summary, neurophysiologic techniques are not the primary tool for diagnosing suspected MD. However, neurophysiologic testing has an important role in excluding neurogenic disorders when the clinical presentation is more generic. Furthermore, findings on needle EMG reflect ongoing pathophysiology and can therefore differentiate between the MyDs and other myotonic disorders.

CHANNELOPATHIES

Channelopathies are a group of muscle disorders characterized by delayed relaxation and/or episodic weakness. Recent research has identified dysfunction of various sarcolemmal ion channels as the underlying defect. Table 36-1

TABLE 36–1. CHANNELOPATHIES: CLINICAL FINDINGS

Abnormal Ion Channel	Disorder	Pattern of Inheritance	Episodic Weakness	Clinical Myotonia
Chloride	Myotonia congenita	AD	No	Yes
Calcium	Hypokalemic periodic paralysis	AD	Yes	No
Sodium	Potassium-sensitive periodic paralysis	AD	Yes	Yes
	Paramyotonia congenita	AD	No	Yes
	Myotonia fluctuans	AD	No	Varies

AD, autosomal dominant.

TABLE 36–2. CHANNELOPATHIES: ELECTRODIAGNOSTIC FINDINGS

Abnormal Ion Channel	Disorder	CMAP Amplitude		Insertional Activity				Motor Unit Potentials	
		Resting	Attack	Resting	Attack	Exercise	Cold	Voluntary Movement	During Paralysis
Chloride	Myotonia congenita	NL	—	Short MyD	—	↑	±↑	NL°	—
Calcium	Hypokalemic periodic paralysis	NL	↓	NL	—			NL	Decreased recruitment
								Myop†	Electrical silence
Sodium	Potassium-sensitive periodic paralysis	NL	↓	Long MyD	↑	↓	↑	NL	Same
	Paramyotonia congenita	NL	↓	Long MyD	↑	↓		NL	Same
	Myotonia fluctuans	NL	—	Variable	—	↓	±	NL	—

° MUPs can be difficult to isolate because of the profuse myotonic discharges.
† Small polyphasic MUP recruiting rapidly late in course if patients develop fixed weakness.
NL, normal; MyD, myotonic discharges; MUP, motor unit potential.

lists the primary characteristics of each of these relatively uncommon disorders. In some circumstances, classic clinical presentation and positive family history make diagnosis of myotonia congenita (MC), paramyotonia congenita (PC), or a form of periodic paralysis straightforward. However, in uncooperative young patients with myotonia or in children with a history of episodic weakness who are asymptomatic at presentation, diagnosis can be more challenging. Neurophysiologic techniques including NCS, repetitive stimulation, prolonged exercise testing, and needle EMG are helpful in reaching a definitive diagnosis. Table 36-2 outlines the results of neurophysiologic testing in these disorders. The change in CMAP amplitude after prolonged exercise in several channelopathies is demonstrated in Figure 36-6.

Chloride Channelopathy: Myotonia Congenita

Myotonia consists of delayed relaxation of muscle contraction. Neurophysiologically, repetitive discharges of biphasic spike potentials that wax and wane in amplitude and frequency are observed. Most nondystrophic myotonic disorders present during childhood. Myotonia is the primary symptom of the several forms of MC. These disorders have been linked to dysfunction of the skeletal muscle chloride channel whose DNA coding exists on the long arm of chromosome 7. Clinical myotonia decreases the speed and coordination of movements and in this disorder affects facial, bulbar, and extremity muscles producing symptoms such as eyelid lag, choking, and stumbling. Children with this disorder have well-developed muscle bulk, which is more difficult to appreciate in infants and toddlers until their "baby fat" is lost. Weakness is not present in the autosomal dominant form of this disorder and is a minor feature in the autosomal recessive form.[41]

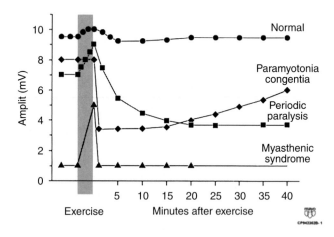

FIGURE 36–6

Compound muscle action potential amplitudes monitored before, during 5 minutes of exercise, and for the next 30 to 60 minutes can demonstrate characteristic changes in channelopathies such as paramyotonia and forms of periodic paralysis. Findings in a normal control and in a subject with myasthenic syndrome are displayed for comparison.

Myotonic discharges and normal MUPs on needle EMG have been documented as early as 2 weeks of age in an infant from a family with known MC.[52] Neurophysiologic findings are similar in both genetic forms of MC. NCSs are normal for age. Brief periods (10 seconds) of exercise or repetitive stimulation can decrease evoked CMAP amplitudes that then revert to normal with a brief period (<1 minute) of rest. Needle EMG demonstrates brief-duration myotonic discharges that become more prominent with cooling of the muscle and less prominent with exercise.[53] Muscle biopsy is either normal or shows only minor nonspecific changes. DNA mutation analysis for confirmation of diagnosis is available.

Calcium Channelopathy: Hypokalemic Periodic Paralysis

Hypokalemic periodic paralysis (hypo-KPP) is an autosomal dominant disorder that is characterized by episodes of muscle weakness most prominently affecting limb muscles. Clinical onset typically occurs during the 2nd decade of life, although children do develop symptoms at younger ages. Episodes of weakness in hypo-KPP are precipitated by rest after exercise or high carbohydrate and salt intake. The weakness can last anywhere from several hours in a mild attack to longer than 24 hours. This disorder has been linked to abnormalities in the skeletal muscle calcium channel whose gene is located on the long arm of chromosome 1. Between attacks, NCS and needle EMG are normal. During attacks of weakness, the affected muscles demonstrate proportionately decreased CMAP amplitudes. Needle EMG demonstrates decreased insertional activity and reduced recruitment of voluntarily activated MUPs in weak muscles. MUPs are of normal configuration.[54]

However, diagnostic testing is frequently conducted when children are asymptomatic. An exercise protocol has been devised that monitors the CMAP amplitude at rest, during 2 to 5 minutes of vigorous exercise, and for 40 minutes after exercise. More than 70% of patients with periodic paralysis demonstrate CMAP amplitude changes outside the normal range on this prolonged exercise test (> 50% decrease in CMAP amplitude, primarily during the first 20 minutes postexercise) (see Fig. 36-1). A greater decrease of postexercise facilitation in CMAP amplitude is also usually observed.[55] Children and adults with hypo-KPP who have repeated attacks of weakness can develop fixed, proximal weakness and demonstrate small, polyphasic MUPs that recruit rapidly on needle EMG.[56]

Sodium Channelopathy

Potassium-Sensitive Periodic Paralysis

Potassium-sensitive periodic paralysis (PSPP) is an autosomal dominant disorder that has historically been referred to as *hyperkalemic periodic paralysis*. However, serum potassium level is not always elevated during attacks of weakness. Administration of oral potassium precipitates or worsens this disorder, which is increasingly felt to include most of the rare cases previously referred to as *normokalemic periodic paralysis*. This is one of the clinical disorders linked to abnormalities of skeletal muscle sodium ion channels whose gene resides on the long arm of chromosome 17. Attacks of weakness tend to be shorter (minutes to several hours) and are more likely to involve cranial-innervated and respiratory muscles than in hypo-KPP. Clinical onset of symptoms in PSPP is usually in the 1st decade of life. Clinical myotonia can be observed but is mild. Typical precipitants of clinical attacks include fasting or rest after exercise.

Between attacks of weakness, needle EMG can demonstrate increased insertional activity, myotonic discharges, and complex repetitive discharges. In PSPP, myotonic discharges noted on needle EMG tend to be of longer duration than in MC. This clinical and electrical myotonia often worsens with exercise (paradoxical myotonia).[19] During the onset of weakness, insertional activity progressively decreases in parallel to the decrease in recruitment of voluntarily activated MUPs.[57] Except for the presence of abnormal insertional activity on needle EMG, the neurophysiologic findings on NCS, exercise testing, and needle EMG are similar to those seen in hypo-KPP.

Paramyotonia Congenita

PC is an autosomal dominant disorder characterized by clinically significant paradoxical myotonia that is worsened by exposure to cold and/or repeated contraction. Clinical findings are present from birth and tend to be most prominent in facial, bulbar, and upper extremity muscles. Some affected families have episodic weakness, particularly in response to prolonged exercise or exposure to cold. PC is associated with mutations in the same alpha subunit of the skeletal muscle sodium channel as occurs in PSPP.[19]

NCS are normal at rest. Brief periods (10 seconds) of exercise produce a prompt and significant fall in CMAP amplitude that recovers to normal values slowly over 15 to 90 minutes (see Fig. 36-1), Repetitive stimulation can produce a decrement in CMAP amplitude.[58] Needle EMG demonstrates myotonic discharges with a longer duration than in MC. Myotonic discharges initially increase with exercise and cooling; however, with prolonged exposure, the myotonic discharges decrease in association with reduced recruitment of MUPs. If exposure is long enough, weakness in association with electrical silence on needle EMG is noted.[59]

Myotonia Fluctuans

Myotonia fluctuans is an autosomal dominant disorder that is characterized by potassium-sensitive myotonia that does not worsen with exposure to cold nor demonstrate episodes of weakness. The clinical severity of myotonia fluctuans varies widely over time in the same patient but tends to decrease with exercise. Clinical onset is during infancy. Myotonic discharges can be demonstrated by needle EMG at times when clinical myotonia is not evident. Myotonia fluctuans is clinically similar to "acetazolamide-responsive MC," which also links to the gene coding for the alpha subunit of the skeletal muscle sodium channel.[60]

METABOLIC MYOPATHIES

All of the hereditary metabolic myopathies involve dysfunction of some aspect of muscle energy metabolism, that is, disorders of glycogen metabolism, disorders of lipid metabolism, disorders of nucleotide metabolism, and disorders of mitochondrial energy generation. The clinical presentation varies widely, from hypotonic, significantly weak infants to infants or children with fixed proximal muscle weakness to normally functioning older children who experience muscle cramps or myoglobinuria with exercise. The one unifying symptom in metabolic myopathies is episodic worsening of symptoms or crises during periods of physiologic stress with overexertion or intercurrent illness.

Disorders of Glycogen Metabolism

Glycogen breakdown produces glucose, which serves as the major source of fuel for energy production in muscle during exercise, particularly during a high-intensity regimen. There are a number of well-characterized disorders of glycogen metabolism. Abnormalities in muscle-specific isoforms of enzymes involved in glycogen metabolism explain the greater involvement of skeletal muscle in many of these disorders. However, cardiac muscle, liver, and erythrocytes can also be involved. When disorders of muscle glycogen metabolism are suspected, usual diagnostic approaches include exercise testing, phosphorus magnetic resonance spectography (P-MRS), and muscle biopsy with special histochemical staining.

In disorders of muscle glycogen metabolism, prolonged exercise or the forearm ischemic exercise test can produce a clinical contracture of muscle that is electrically silent.[61] Physiologic tests of muscle response to exercise play an important role in diagnosing metabolic muscle disorders. The forearm ischemic exercise test is a useful physiologic test of the glycolytic metabolism in muscle. A normal increase in lactate in response to exercise excludes disorders of glycolysis. Use of this test in children is limited by the discomfort created by exercise under conditions of muscle ischemia. Bruno and colleagues[62] at the Gaslini Children's Hospital Muscle Service in Genoa, Italy, described results from a "semi-ischemic exercise test" in 30 children between 7 and 16 years of age referred to their clinic. Modification in this testing procedure involved inflating the sphygmomanometer cuff to the level of, but not above, mean arterial pressure. All children older than 9 years of age were able to exercise for the prescribed 1 minute and raised their plasma ammonia concentrations 5- to 10-fold above baseline. The only children who experienced any discomfort (but no muscle contracture) were two children whose lactate levels did not increase with exercise and whose muscle biopsies subsequently demonstrated abnormalities of myophosphorylase and phosphofructokinase, respectively. In all other children older than 9 years of age, the lactate levels increased 2.6-fold above baseline.[62] Adult patients with glycolytic muscle disorders demonstrated similar results to forearm exer-

cise testing whether ischemia was produced or not.[61,63] Cycle ergometry has been used to produce aerobic exercise for physiologic testing. With this technique, abnormalities are detected in muscle disorders that impair oxidative metabolism such as mitochondrial myopathies, myophosphorylase deficiency, and phosphofructokinase deficiency.[20]

Muscle US demonstrated nonspecific abnormalities in fewer than half of the children studied with metabolic muscle disorders.[6,24] In adults, P-MRS of exercising muscle has assisted in clarifying the physiology of some metabolic muscle disorders. It can differentiate between disorders of glycogenolysis (phosphorylase deficiency) and glycolysis (blocks at or distal to phosphofructokinase) by whether glycolytic intermediate metabolites accumulate.

Among disorders of glycogen metabolism, acid maltase deficiency (type II glycogenosis) and debrancher enzyme deficiency (type III glycogenosis) demonstrate the most abnormal insertional and spontaneous activity on needle EMG. The degree of increased insertional activity and amount of spontaneous activity (fibrillation potentials, myotonic discharges, complex repetitive discharges) observed is greater in affected infants than in children who present at an older age.[64] Fibrillation potentials and myotonic discharges have been noted along with small polyphasic MUPs in weak muscles in patients with phosphofructokinase deficiency.[65] An infant who succumbed at 13 weeks with severe hypotonia and weakness was discovered at autopsy to have muscle phosphorylase deficiency. Needle EMG had demonstrated diffuse fibrillation potentials with an increased percentage of polyphasic MUPs.[66] However, most types of metabolic myopathies have either normal or mildly small MUPs noted on needle EMG.

Disorders of Lipid Metabolism

Free fatty acids are used to fuel muscle activity during fasting and prolonged exercise. Unlike the glycogenoses, disorders of lipid metabolism are caused by generalized (rather than muscle-specific) enzyme deficiencies. The clinical severity of these disorders appears to be related to the completeness of the enzyme deficiency.[67] Individuals with higher levels of residual enzyme activity tend to have symptoms limited to skeletal muscles such as exercise-induced cramps, exercise intolerance, or myoglobinuria. Those individuals with little residual enzyme activity generally have symptoms indicating involvement of multiple organs including heart and liver as well as skeletal muscle.[20] There are more than two dozen different enzyme deficiencies creating disorders of fatty acid oxidation that have been identified and characterized over the past several decades. These disorders can be divided into disorders of fatty acid transport into mitochondria and disorders of intramitochondrial beta oxidation. All of these disorders are relatively uncommon.

Needle EMG usually demonstrates normal MUPs. However, small, polyphasic, rapidly recruited MUPs and occasional fibrillation potentials have been reported in some of these disorders.[68] Cui and colleagues[69] at the Peking Union Medical College Hospital described EMG findings in 18 patients with lipid storage myopathy and described abnormal spontaneous activity in 14% of patients with various forms of lipid storage myopathy. All patients demonstrated short-duration MUPs, and 46% had an increased proportion of polyphasic potentials. They documented a lower incidence of abnormal spontaneous activity in patients with lipid storage myopathy as compared to patients with inflammatory muscle disease.[69] Forearm exercise tests show normal lactate and ammonia responses in patients with disorders of lipid metabolism. During episodes of metabolic decompensation, diagnosis of fatty acid oxidation disorders can be made by looking at the pattern of metabolites in serum and urine. Confirmation of the disorder can be made through genetic testing for several disorders including carnitine palmitoyltransferase II deficiency and medium-chain acyl-coenzyme A dehydrogenase deficiency or through enzyme assay on muscle or fibroblast cultures for the other disorders.[20,70]

Disorders of Nucleotide Metabolism

Myoadenylate deaminase deficiency is a metabolic alteration of uncertain clinical significance since it is found in 1% to 2% of all people, including asymptomatic top athletes.[71] During exercise testing, individuals with myoadenylate deaminase deficiency demonstrate a normal rise in plasma lactate with a flat plasma ammonia curve.

Disorders of Mitochondrial Energy Generation

Mitochondria contain the intracellular machinery necessary for conversion of carbohydrates, lipids, and protein into usable energy via aerobic metabolism. The proteins necessary for these biochemical pathways are genetically coded by DNA located in both the cell nucleus (nuclear DNA [nDNA]) as well as mitochondrial DNA (mtDNA). Although each cell has only two copies of nDNA, each has large numbers of mtDNA, and the proportion of mtDNA possessing a mutation varies between cells, between different organs in the same individual, and between individuals. This phenomenon is termed *heteroplasmy* and is part of the basis for the clinical variability in mitochondrial encephalomyopathies.[72] Abnormal mitochondrial energy generation can be caused by defects in mtDNA, defects in nDNA coding for mitochondrial proteins, or defects in nDNA control over mtDNA replication.[18] Organs such as skeletal and heart muscle, liver, kidney, and brain with active

metabolisms are more susceptible to dysfunction. Multiple clinical phenotypes have been described and include symptoms referable to the central and peripheral nervous systems, heart, skeletal muscle, liver, bone marrow, gastrointestinal tract, kidney, and endocrine system. A detailed delineation of the numerous syndromic presentations of mitochondrial disease that involve muscle such as myoclonic epilepsy with ragged-red fibers and progressive external ophthalmoplegia are beyond the scope of this chapter, but excellent references are available.[73]

Needle EMG either demonstrates normal MUPs or mild changes consisting of small, polyphasic rapidly recruiting MUPs. NCS sometimes demonstrate presence of a peripheral neuropathy that can be part of the phenotype. Diagnosis is usually made through a combination of clinical pattern of involvement; family history; search for other organ involvement (electrocardiogram, complete blood count, calcium, phosphorus, liver function tests, renal function tests, lactate, pyruvate); MRI head scan; and cerebrospinal fluid (protein, lactate and pyruvate). Definitive diagnosis frequently requires muscle biopsy for standard histology, electron microscopy, or biochemical testing of enzyme activity. Increasingly, molecular genetic studies are available to confirm the diagnosis of mitochondrial encephalomyopathies.[18]

P-MRS has been used to objectively assess response to treatment trials in mitochondrial myopathies.[10] The noninvasive nature of P-MRS makes it ideal for monitoring oxidative metabolism in muscle both for screening patients with exercise intolerance and for monitoring treatment trials. The technique requires cooperation with an exercise protocol that, as always, presents a challenge in infants and young children. There is currently limited experience using this technique in children.

INFLAMMATORY MYOPATHIES

Inflammatory myopathies in children nearly always present as dermatomyositis in which there is a vasculitis affecting both skin and muscle. Diagnosis is made in the presence of a pathognomonic rash involving malar, periorbital, and extensor surfaces of the limbs in combination with proximal muscle weakness and muscle pain. Figure 36-7 demonstrates that the skin changes in young children with dermatomyositis can be subtle, as a periorbital rash in a young boy with dermatomyositis is shown. Laboratory findings include elevation of muscle enzymes and inflammatory markers, needle EMG changes of myopathy with or without fibrillation potentials, and muscle biopsy changes demonstrating vasculitis, necrosis, or inflammatory infiltrate. Each individual patient does not present with all defining abnormalities. In a review of 131 cases of polymyositis in

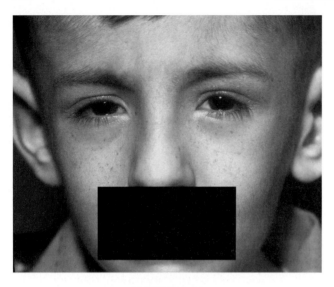

FIGURE 36–7
The periorbital rash seen in this young boy with dermatomyositis is subtle and nondiagnostic. Neurophysiologic testing can be useful when clinical findings are indeterminate in children with inflammatory myopathies.

Newcastle upon Tyne, United Kingdom, different diagnostic criteria were met by varying proportions of patients: proximal weakness (92%), elevated CK (64%), abnormal needle EMG (89%), and abnormal muscle biopsy (83%). However, the abnormalities were "classic" or independently diagnostic of inflammatory myopathy in only 45% of the EMGs and 65% of the muscle biopsies.[74] Only 20% of the patients in this series were children or adolescents.

A description of 105 children with juvenile dermatomyositis cared for at the Hospital for Sick Children in Toronto, Canada, indicated that electromyography was abnormal in 86 of 104 patients in whom it had been performed.[75] Neurophysiologic testing on 22 children with inflammatory myopathy evaluated at our institution demonstrated short-duration, low-amplitude MUPs with rapid recruitment and an increased proportion of polyphasic MUPs in all children studied. Approximately three fourths of the children without prior treatment and one half of the children with some prior treatment demonstrated fibrillation potentials on needle EMG. Two untreated patients had complex repetitive discharges. The degree of abnormal spontaneous activity was proportional to the degree of muscle weakness and elevation of serum muscle enzymes more than the duration of symptoms. None of the children had abnormal insertional activity or fibrillation potentials limited to paraspinal muscles.[76] Polymyositis is extremely rare in children and has primarily been observed in infants.[77]

MRI has been used to identify focal involvement of muscles in patchy processes such as inflammatory myopathy and has been useful in directing diagnostic muscle biop-

sies to the affected areas.[78] Short tau inversion recovery (STIR) MRI pulse sequences of the proximal thigh and buttocks of 26 children with dermatomyositis demonstrated edema in skin, subcutaneous tissue, fascia, or muscle in 50% to 85% of the children. These changes were noted to vary directly with disease activity in several children followed over time. Edema was present in the subcutaneous tissue (25%) and muscle (38%) of 8 children who had STIR MRI performed but who were determined on follow-up to not have dermatomyositis. Eventual diagnoses for these children included other connective tissue disease, carrier of Duchenne's MD, no defined musculoskeletal disorder, and juvenile polymyositis. Five children with dermatomyositis, who were noted to have subcutaneous edema on STIR MRI, developed clinically apparent calcinosis at the same location within 9 months.[79] Therefore, although abnormalities on STIR MRI are not pathognomonic for dermatomyositis, changes indicating edema would appear to correlate with disease activity and be potentially useful in monitoring efficacy of treatment.

Noninvasive P-MRS has been used to characterize metabolic abnormalities in the muscles of 13 children with dermatomyositis. Changes observed during rest, two graded levels of exercise, and postexercise recovery indicated defective oxidative phosphorylation in the mitochondria of muscles demonstrating inflammation on MRI sequences. MRS findings were normal in 2 children who had responded quickly and dramatically to previous steroid treatment and whose muscles did not demonstrate inflammation on MRI sequences. Authors suggest that quantitative, noninvasive P-MRS data are useful for evaluating patients and optimizing treatment in dermatomyositis. Of the 13 children with dermatomyositis in this series reported by rheumatologists, only 1 child had undergone muscle biopsy and only 1 child had undergone a diagnostic needle EMG. The other 11 children were believed to have clinical presentations pathognomonic for dermatomyositis.[80]

MRI has proven useful in diagnosing and assessing the location and extent of abscesses in muscle. A hyperintense signal on T2-weighted and STIR sequences as well as a hyperintense rim on T1-weighted images that enhanced after gadolinium administration has been noted.[81] Clinicians so frequently omit portions of the classical diagnostic evaluation for juvenile dermatomyositis (muscle enzymes, EMG, and muscle biopsy) that several groups have considered changing the diagnostic criteria in children.[75]

TOXIC MYOPATHIES

Various prescription medications as well as over-the-counter drugs and drugs of abuse are capable of damaging or causing dysfunction of skeletal muscle. Table 36-3 contains a chart relating type of neurophysiologic

TABLE 36–3. AGENTS WITH POTENTIAL FOR SKELETAL MUSCLE TOXICITY IN CHILDREN

Pathology	Agents	NCS Changes	Needle EMG Changes	References
Necrotizing myopathy	Cyclosporine, tacrolimus, labetalol, propofol, alcohol	Normal	Increased insertional activity; fibrillation potentials; small, polyphasic MUPs recruiting rapidly; proportional to weakness	27, 82, 83
Autophagic lysosomal myopathy	Chloroquine, hydroxychloroquine, amiodarone	Axonal sensorimotor peripheral neuropathy	Same as necrotizing myopathy (chloroquine—rare myotonic discharges)	84, 85
Antimicrotubular myopathy	Vincristine	Axonal sensorimotor peripheral neuropathy	Same as necrotizing myopathy	86
Mitochondrial myopathy	Zidovudine	Normal	Some patients have increased insertional activity and small, rapidly recruiting polyphasic MUPs	87
Inflammatory myopathy	L-Tryptophan, D-penicillamine, cimetidine, L-dopa, phenytoin, lamotrigine	Normal ± low CMAP amplitude	Same as necrotizing myopathy	88, 89
Myofibrillar myopathy	Emetine		Same as necrotizing myopathy	90
Steroid myopathy	Corticosteroids	Normal	Normal	91
Acute quadriplegic myopathy	Corticosteroids, neuromuscular blocking agents, and sepsis	Low CMAP amplitudes	± Fibrillation potentials, positive sharp waves; decreased recruitment early → small, rapidly recruiting polyphasic MUPs	92
Type 2 muscle fiber atrophy (neuromyopathy)	Omeprazole	Axonal sensorimotor peripheral neuropathy	Small, rapidly recruiting, polyphasic MUPs	93

MUP, motor unit potential; CMAP, compound muscle action potential; NCS, nerve conduction study.

abnormalities with the medications and other agents that have been reported to injure muscle in children. For example, zidovudine can cause a myopathy demonstrating ragged-red fibers on muscle biopsy. Zidovudine, a nucleoside analog, is believed to cause a depletion of mtDNA by being incorporated during its replication.[18]

ENDOCRINE- RELATED MYOPATHIES

Abnormalities of calcium homeostasis, adrenal function, thyroid function, or pituitary function have been clinically associated with hypotonia and muscle weakness.[52] Usually, the muscle symptoms are mild and less noticeable than other features such as changes in growth or development. NCS are usually normal. Needle EMG can demonstrate normal MUPs or show nonspecific MUP changes such as an excess of low-amplitude, short-duration, polyphasic MUPs that recruit rapidly.

SUMMARY

Neurophysiologic techniques are an important part of the diagnostic repertoire for neuromuscular disorders in infants and children. These techniques are important in the following:

- Establishing the primary diagnosis of disorders of anterior horn cell, peripheral nerve, and neuromuscular junction
- Characterizing the underlying pathophysiology of disorders when the phenotypic presentation is generic
- Screening hypotonic infants to help differentiate between central and peripheral causes and provide more focus for further diagnostic testing
- Evaluating skeletal muscle channelopathies with the characteristic abnormalities in response to NCS, repetitive stimulation, prolonged exercise testing, and needle EMG

Currently, US and MRI imaging of muscle are able to provide the same degree of concordance with muscle biopsy as NCS and needle EMG in the diagnosis of primary myopathies in infants and children. Since the former techniques are less invasive, neurophysiologic techniques will likely play a secondary role when primary muscle disorders, other than channelopathies, are suspected. However, infants and children frequently present with clinically indistinct problems, and neurophysiologic testing is useful at those times. Finally, new applications of current techniques and future development of technology may create new roles for neurophysiologic techniques in children. There are potential roles for neurophysiologic techniques in monitoring response to treatment in anticipated treatment trials in childhood neuromuscular disorders. It is also possible that further advances in motor unit quantitation, requiring less time and active patient cooperation, may improve the sensitivity and specificity of neurophysiologic techniques for muscle disorders in children.[94]

REFERENCES

1. David WS, Jones HR Jr: Electromyography and biopsy correlation with suggested protocol for evaluation of the floppy infant. Muscle Nerve 1994;17:424-431.
2. Jones HR Jr: EMG evaluation of the floppy infant: Differential diagnosis and technical aspects. Muscle Nerve 1990;13:338-347.
3. Packer RJ, Brown MJ, Berman PH: The diagnostic value of electromyography in infantile hypotonia. Am J Dis Child 1982;136:1057-1059.
4. Russell JW, Afifi AK, Ross MA: Predictive value of electromyography in diagnosis and prognosis of the hypotonic infant. J Child Neurol 1992;7:387-392.
5. Aydinli N, Baslo B, Caliskan M, et al: Muscle ultrasonography and electromyography correlation for evaluation of floppy infants. Brain Dev 2003;25:22-24.
6. Zuberi SM, Matta N, Nawaz S, et al: Muscle ultrasound in the assessment of suspected neuromuscular disease in childhood. Neuromuscul Disord 1999;9:203-207.
7. Darras BT, Jones HR Jr: Diagnosis of pediatric neuromuscular disorders in the era of DNA analysis. Pediatr Neurol 2000;23:289-300.
8. Chan WP, Liu GC: MR imaging of primary skeletal muscle diseases in children. AJR Am J Roentgenol 2002;179:1989-1997.
9. Mercuri E, Pichiecchio A, Counsell S, et al: A short protocol for muscle MRI in children with muscular dystrophies. Eur J Paediatr Neurol 2002;6:305-307.
10. Argov Z, Lofberg M, Arnold DL: Insights into muscle diseases gained by phosphorus magnetic resonance imaging. Muscle Nerve 2000;23:1316-1334.
11. Hays RM, Hackworth SR, Speltz ML, Weinstein P: Exploration of variables related to children's behavioral distress during electrodiagnosis. Arch Phys Med Rehabil 1992;73:1160-1162.
12. Harper CM Jr: Myopathies. *In* Jones HR Jr, Bolton CF, Harper CM Jr (eds): Pediatric Clinical Electromyography. Philadelphia, Lippincott-Raven, 1996, pp 387-443.
13. Sandstedt PER, Henriksson KG, Larsson LE: Quantitative electromyography in polymyositis and dermatomyositis: A long-term study. Acta Neurol Scand 1982;65:110-121.
14. Bertorini TE, Igarashi M: Muscular dystrophies. *In* Pourmand R (ed): Neuromuscular Diseases: Expert Clinicians' Views. Philadelphia, Butterworth Heinemann, 2001, pp 227-284.
15. Dubowitz V: Muscle Disorders in Childhood, 2nd ed. London, WB Saunders, Ltd, 1995.
16. Engel AE, Franzini-Armstrong C: Myology, 2nd ed. New York, McGraw-Hill, 1994.
17. Goebel HH, Muller J, Gillen HW, Merritt AD: Autosomal dominant spheroid body myopathy. Muscle Nerve 1978;1:14-26.
18. Hirano M, Nishino I, DiMauro S: Mitochondrial myopathies. *In* Pourmand R (ed): Neuromuscular Diseases: Expert Clinicians' Views. Philadelphia, Butterworth Heinemann, 2001, pp 411-437.
19. Riggs JE: Skeletal muscle channelopathies. *In* Pourmand R (ed): Neuromuscular Diseases: Expert Clinicians' Views. Philadelphia, Butterworth Heinemann, 2001, pp 381-392.
20. Vissing J, Haller RG: Metabolic myopathies. *In* Pourmand R (ed): Neuromuscular Diseases: Expert Clinicians' Views. Philadelphia, Butterworth Heinemann, 2001, pp 393-410.
21. Pelin K, Hilpela P, Donner K, et al: Mutations in the nebulin gene associated with autosomal recessive nemaline myopathy. Proc Natl Acad Sci U S A 1999;6:2305-2310.
22. Nowak KJ, Wattanasirichaigoon D, Goebel HH, et al: Mutations in the skeletal muscle alpha-actin gene in patients with actin myopathy and nemaline myopathy. Nat Genet 1999;23:208-212.
23. Laing NG, Wilton SD, Akkari PA, et al: A mutation in the alpha tropomyosin gene *TPM3* associated with autosomal dominant nemaline myopathy. Nat Genet 1995;9:75-79.
24. Heckmatt JZ, Dubowitz V: Real-time ultrasound imaging of muscles. Muscle Nerve 1988;11:56-65.
25. Mercuri E, Cini C, Counsell S, et al: Muscle MRI findings in a three-generation family affected by Bethlem myopathy. Eur J Paediatr Neurol 2002;6:309-314.
26. Hawkes CH, Absolon MJ: Myotubular myopathy associated with cataract and electrical myotonia. J Neurol Neurosurg Psychiatry 1975;38:761-764.
27. Hanna JP, Ramundo ML: Rhabdomyolysis and hypoxia associated with prolonged propofol infusion in children. Neurology 1988;50:301-303.
28. Shy GM, Engel WK, Somers JE, Wanko T: Nemaline myopathy: A new congenital myopathy. Brain 1963;86:793-810.
29. Cavanagh NPC, Lake BD, McMeniman P: Congenital fiber type disproportion myopathy: A histological diagnosis with an uncertain clinical outlook. Arch Dis Child 1979;54:735-743.
30. Edstrom L, Thornell LE, Eriksson A: A new type of hereditary distal myopathy with characteristic sarcoplasmic bodies and intermediate (skeletin) filaments. J Neurol Sci 1980;47:171-190.
31. Kugelberg E: Electromyography in muscular dystrophies: Differentiation between dystrophies and chronic lower motor neuron lesions. J Neurol Neurosurg Psychiatry 1949;12:129-136.
32. Muntoni F, Bertini E, Bonnemann C, et al: 98th ENMC International Workshop on Congenital Muscular Dystrophy (CMD), 7th Workshop of the International Consortium on CMD, 2nd Workshop of the MYO CLUSTER project GENRE, October 26-28, 2001,

Naarden, The Netherlands. Neuromuscul Disord 2002;12:889-896.

33. Banker B: The congenital muscular dystrophies. *In* Engel AG, Franzini-Armstrong C (eds): Myology, 2nd ed. New York, McGraw-Hill, 1994, pp 1188-1191.

34. Jones HR Jr: Evaluation of the floppy infant. *In* Jones HR Jr, Bolton CF, Harper CM Jr (eds): Pediatric Clinical Electromyography. Philadelphia, Lippincott-Raven, 1996, pp 37-104.

35. Shorer Z, Philpot J, Muntoni F, et al: Demyelinating peripheral neuropathy in merosin-deficient congenital muscular dystrophy. J Child Neurol 1995;10:472-475.

36. Mercuri E, Muntoni F, Berardinelli A, et al: Somatosensory and visual evoked potentials in congenital muscular dystrophy: Correlation with MRI changes and muscle merosin status. Neuropediatrics 1995;26:3-7.

37. Tawil R, Figlewicz DA, Griggs RC, Weiffenbach B: Facioscapulohumeral dystrophy: A distinct regional myopathy with a novel molecular pathogenesis. FSH Consortium. Ann Neurol 1998;43:279-282.

38. Bushby KM: Diagnostic criteria for the limb-girdle muscular dystrophies: Report of the ENMC Consortium on Limb-Girdle Dystrophies. Neuromuscul Disord 1995;5:71-74.

39. Pollitt C, Anderson LV, Pogue R, et al: The phenotype of calpainopathy: Diagnosis based on a multidisciplinary approach. Neuromuscul Disord 2001;11:287-296.

40. Merlini L, Granata C, Dominici P, Bonfiglioli S: Emery-Dreifuss muscular dystrophy: Report of five cases in a family and review of the literature. Muscle Nerve 1986;9:481-485.

41. Moxley RT III: Myotonic Disorders in childhood: Diagnosis and treatment. J Child Neurol 1997;12:116-129.

42. Aminoff MJ, Layzer RB, Satya-Murti S, Faden AI: The declining electrical response of muscle to repetitive nerve stimulation in myotonia. Neurology 1977;27:812-816.

43. Kuntz NL, Daube JR: Electrophysiology of congenital myotonic dystrophy. EEG Clin Neurophysiol 1983;56:S20.

44. Swift TR, Ignacio OJ, Dyken PR: Neonatal dystrophia myotonica: Electrophysiologic studies. Am J Dis Child 1975;129:734-737.

45. Young RSK, Ganz DL, Zalneraitis EL, Krishnamoorthy KS: Dysmaturation in infants of mothers with myotonic dystrophy. Arch Neurol 1981;38:716-719.

46. Aicardi J, Conti D, Gontieres F: [Neonatal forms of Steinert's mytonic dystrophy.] J Neurol Sci 1974;22:149-164.

47. Harper PS: Myotonic dystrophy. Major Probl Neurol 1979;9:170-209.

48. Streib EW, Sun SF: Distribution of electrical myotonia in myotonic muscular dystrophy. Ann Neurol 1983;14:80-82.

49. Ricker K, Koch MC, Lehmann-Horn F, et al: Proximal myotonic myopathy: Clinical features of a multisystem disorder similar to myotonic dystrophy. Arch Neurol 1995;52:25-31.

50. Mercuri E, Counsell S, Allsop J, et al: Selective muscle involvement on magnetic resonance imaging in autosomal dominant Emery-Dreifuss muscular dystrophy. Neuropediatrics 2002;33:10-14.

51. Heckmatt JZ, Dubowitz V: Diagnostic advantage of needle muscle biopsy and ultrasound imaging in the detection of focal pathology in a girl with limb girdle dystrophy. Muscle Nerve 1985;8:705-709.

52. Harel S, Chui LA, Shapira Y: Myotonia congenita (Thomsen's Disease): Early diagnosis in infancy. Acta Paediatr Scand 1979;68:225-227.

53. Nielsen VK, Friis ML, Johnson T: Electromyographic distinction between paramyotonia congenita and myotonia congenita: Effect of cold. Neurology 1982;32:827-832.

54. Engel AG, Lambert EH, Rosevear JW, Tauxe WN: Clinical and electromyographic studies in a patient with primary hypokalemic periodic paralysis. Am J Med 1965;38:626-640.

55. McManis PG, Lambert EH, Daube JR: Exercise test in periodic paralysis. Muscle Nerve 1986;9:704-710.

56. Dyken M, Zeman W, Rusche T: Hypokalemic periodic paralysis: Children with permanent myopathic weakness. Neurology 1969;19:691-699.

57. Buchthal F, Engback L, Gamstorp I: Paresis and hyperexcitability in adynamia episodica hereditaria. Neurology 1958;8:347-351.

58. Burke D, Skuse NF, Lethlean AK: An analysis of myotonia in paramyotonia congenita. J Neurol Neurosurg Psychiatry 1974;37:900-906.

59. Subramony SH, Malhorta CP, Mishra SK: Distinguishing paramyotonia congenita and myotonia congenita by electromyography. Muscle Nerve 1983;6:374-379.

60. Ricker K, Moxley RT, Heine R, Lehmann-Horn F: Myotonia fluctuans: A third type of muscle sodium channel disease. Arch Neurol 1994;51:1095-1102.

61. Kazemi-Esfarjani P, Skomorowska E, Jensen TD: No need for ischemia in the forearm exercise test for McArdle's disease. Neurology 2000;54(Suppl 3):A332.

62. Bruno C, Bado M, Minetti C, Cordone G: Forearm semi-ischemic exercise test in pediatric patients. J Child Neurol 1998;13:288-290.

63. Kissel JT, Beam W, Bresolin N, et al: Physiologic assessment of phosphoglycerate mutase deficiency: Incremental exercise tests. Neurology 1985;35:828-833.

64. Engel AG, Gomez MR, Seybold ME, Lambert E: The spectrum and diagnosis of acid maltase deficiency. Neurology 1973;23:95-106.

65. DiMauro S, Tsujino S: Nonlysosomal glucogenoses. *In* Engel AG, Franzini-Armstrong C (eds): Myology, 2nd ed. New York, McGraw-Hill, 1994, pp 1554-1576.

66. DiMauro S, Hartlage PL: Fatal infantile form of muscle phosphorylase deficiency. Neurology 1978;28:1124-1129.

67. DiDonato S: Disorders of lipid metabolism affecting skeletal muscle: Carnitine deficiency syndromes, defects in catabolic pathway, and Chanarin disease. *In* Engel AG, Franzini-Armstrong C (eds): Myology, 2nd ed. New York, McGraw-Hill, 1994, pp 1587-1609.

68. Engel AG, Angelini C: Carnitine deficiency of human skeletal muscle with associated lipid storage myopathy: A new syndrome. Science 1973;179:899-902.

69. Cui L, Tang X, Zhang Q, et al: EMG study in the diagnosis

and differential diagnosis of lipid storage myopathy. Chin Med Sci J 1998;13:42-44.

70. Bank WJ, DiMauro S, Bonilla E, et al: A disorder of muscle lipid metabolism and myoglobinuria: Absence of carnitine palmityl transferase. N Engl J Med 1975;292:443-440.

71. Verzijl HTFM, van Engelen BGM, Luyten JA, et al: Genetic characteristics of myoadenylate deaminase deficiency. Ann Neurol 1998;44:140-143.

72. Schon EA, Bonilla E, DiMauro S: Mitochondrial DNA mutations and pathogenesis. J Bioenerg Biomembr 1997;29:131-149.

73. Hirano M, DiMauro S: Clinical features of mitochondrial myopathies and encephalomyopathies. *In* Lane R (ed): Handbook of Muscle Disease. New York, Marcel Dekker, 1996, pp 479-503.

74. DeVere R, Bradley WG: Polymyositis: Its presentation, morbidity and mortality. Brain 1975;98:637-666.

75. Ramanan AV, Feldman BM: Clinical features and outcomes of juvenile dermatomyositis and other childhood-onset myositis syndromes. Rheum Dis Clin North Am 2002;28:833-857.

76. Kuntz NL: Electrophysiology of childhood inflammatory myopathy. Muscle Nerve 1983;6:536-537.

77. Thompson CE: Infantile myositis. Dev Med Child Neurol 1982;24:307-313.

78. Kaufman LD, Gruber BL, Gerstman DP, Kaell AT: Preliminary observations on the role of magnetic resonance imaging for polymyositis and dermatomyositis. Ann Rheum Dis 1987;46:569-572.

79. Kimball AB, Summers RM, Turner M, et al: Magnetic resonance imaging detection of occult skin and subcutaneous abnormalities in juvenile dermatomyositis. Arthritis Rheum 2000;43:1866-1873.

80. Park JH, Niermann KJ, Ryder NM, et al: Muscle abnormalities in juvenile dermatomyositis patients. Arthritis Rheum 2000;43:2359-2367.

81. Soler R, Rodriguez E, Aguilera C, Fernandez R: Magnetic resonance imaging of pyomyositis in 43 cases. Eur J Radiol 2000;35:59-64.

82. Campellone JV, Lacomis D, Kramer DJ, et al: Acute myopathy after liver transplantation. Neurology 1998;50:46-53.

83. Willis JK, Tilton AH, Harkin JC, Boineau FG: Reversible myopathy due to labetalol. Pediatr Neurol 1990;6:275-276.

84. Stein M, Bell MJ, Ang LC: Hydroxychloroquine neuromyotoxicity. J Rheum 2000;27:2927-2931.

85. Wasay M, Wolfe GI, Herrold JM, et al: Chloroquine myopathy and neuropathy with elevated CSF protein. Neurology 1998;51:1226-1227.

86. Bradley WG, Lassman LP, Pearce GW, Walton JN: The neuropathy of vincristine in man: Clinical electrophysiological and pathological studies. J Neurol Sci 1970;10:107-131.

87. Dalakas MC, Illa I, Pezeshkpour GH, et al: Mitochondrial myopathy caused by long-term zidovudine therapy. N Engl J Med 1990;322:1098-1105.

88. Dimachkie MM, Vriesendorp FJ, Heck KA: Phenytoin-induced dermatomyositis: Case report and literature review. J Child Neurol 1998;13:577-580.

89. Schaub JE, Williamson PJ, Barnes EW, Trewby PN: Multisystem toxicity with lamotrigine. Lancet 1994;344:481.

90. Mateer JE, Farrell BJ, Chou SS, Gutmann L: Reversible ipecac myopathy. Arch Neurol 1985;42:188-190.

91. Rothstein JM, Delitto A, Sinacore DR, Rose SJ: Muscle function in rheumatic disease patients treated with corticosteroids. Muscle Nerve 1983;6:128-135.

92. Lacomis D, Giulani MJ, Van Cott A, Kramer DJ: Acute myopathy of intensive care: Clinical, electromyographic, and pathological aspects. Ann Neurol 1996;40:645-654.

93. Faucheux JM, Tourneize P, Viguier A, et al: Neuromyopathy secondary to omeprazole treatment. Muscle Nerve 1998;21:261-262.

94. Nandedkar SD, Sanders DB, Stalberg EV: Automatic analysis of the electromyographic interference pattern: II. Findings in control subjects and in some neuromuscular diseases. Muscle Nerve 1986;9:491-500.

37

Neuromuscular Problems of the Critically Ill Neonate, Child, and Adolescent

Basil T. Darras, Charles F. Bolton, and H. Royden Jones, Jr.

OVERVIEW

Clinical Setting

Three clinical sets of acute neuromuscular disorders occasionally confront the pediatric intensivist and/or the pediatric neurologist. Many of these are primary disorders of the motor unit that present acutely and may require urgent admission to a neurologic intensive care unit (ICU). Because of the variable presentations of sometimes similar disorders, as well as some illnesses that are particularly unique to babies and toddlers, in comparison to older children, we have thought it best to discuss these various processes apropos to these two respective age groups.[1,2] Although this creates somewhat artificial categories, we find this provides a practical format for evaluating an acutely paralyzed child. The third category relates to acute motor unit disorders developing in a child hospitalized with an acute systemic illness that requires intensive care management. It is the combination of the systemic illness and its therapy per se that predisposes the child to these various relatively uncommon acute motor unit disorders.

There is a rather unique differential diagnosis specific to both newborns and toddlers. These disorders present either at birth or shortly thereafter with lesions at each level of the peripheral motor unit. Typical examples seen at or shortly after birth include Werdnig-Hoffman disease, neonatal congenital polyneuropathies, an intrauterine onset of Guillain-Barré syndrome (GBS), and infantile-onset

myotonic dystrophy or glycogen storage myopathies. Within the first 3 to 6 months of life, and rarely as late as up to 1 year of age, previously healthy infants may develop infantile botulism, other unique genetically determined congenital neuromuscular transmission disorders, and, rarely, postvaccine poliomyelitis. Clinical examination is difficult due to the small size of young children, the confined space, the endotracheal tubes, the vascular lines, and the splints and bandages applied to the parts of the body.

The older child and adolescent are predisposed to certain peripheral motor unit disorders that require critical care management, similar to the adult patient. These primarily include GBS and autoimmune myasthenia gravis (MG). Both disorders have an increasing incidence among older children. However, when GBS and MG affect children, both may vary significantly from their traditional presentation. The pseudoencephalopathic form of GBS is a good example. Additionally, some uncommon entities, such as tick paralysis, always deserve careful consideration in the differential diagnosis of an acutely paretic child. The neuromuscular complications of extended intubation and sepsis affecting either the muscle cell or peripheral nerve also occur in children.

Careful review of the clinical records by the primary physician, or someone as junior as an astute intern, or the nondiagnostic results of an imaging study often lead the clinicians to pursue further testing. The differential diagnosis of these various motor unit disorders is also significantly aided by utilizing clinical neurophysiology techniques,

763

particularly nerve conduction studies (NCSs) and electromyography (EMG)[3] or electroencephalography (EEG), and cerebrospinal fluid (CSF) analysis. These studies provide the clinician an objective means to appropriately assign a specific pathoanatomic or neurophysiologic site for the child's illness.

There is an interesting but relatively uncommon set of neuromuscular disorders that develop in a child predominantly as a phenomena secondary to either sepsis or status asthmaticus. These processes may independently affect each primary portion of the peripheral motor unit from the anterior horn cell, to the peripheral nerve, neuromuscular junction (NMJ), or muscle fiber per se. Thus, in comparison to the other disorders discussed in this chapter wherein a primary individual motor unit disorder presents in an acute fashion requiring intensive care management, this set of illnesses is usually serious but self-limited and somehow secondary to a toxic process related to the underlying illness.

Infantile Nerve Conduction Studies and EMG

When studying infants and toddlers, both the pediatric neurologist and the clinical neurophysiologist must familiarize themselves with the maturational norms for NCSs and needle EMG. Accurate clinical correlations depend on making interpretations utilizing these evolutionary set parameters that proceed over the first 3 years of life. If one does not consider these changes, it is possible to inappropriately conclude that an infant has a motor unit disease when indeed the findings are normal for age.

During early childhood, the process of peripheral myelination is an ongoing one. NCS parameters are only one half as fast in newborns as the "adult" values that are usually first attained by age 3 years.[4] In addition, the responsiveness of the NMJ is also immature during infancy. Presently, this is still a difficult and poorly defined area at this age. Few, if any, well-defined repetitive motor nerve stimulation (RMNS) normative standards are defined for NMJ evaluation in newborns and young infants with recognized techniques.[4] This sometimes makes it difficult to provide clear-cut definitions of abnormality in this young age group when evaluating some possible infantile neuromuscular transmission defects (NMTDs).

Similarly, there is an established maturation process related to the definition of motor unit potential (MUP) size among different age groups.[4] Needle EMG is the most accurate means to differentiate lesions at the anterior horn cell level from a primary myopathic process. With the former there is a marked diminution in the number of firing motor units; characteristically, these MUPs are also more rapidly recruited and may often be of higher amplitude

and longer duration, not unlike the findings in adult motor neuron diseases. In contrast, the MUPs characteristic of myopathies are typically smaller and recruited in increased numbers. However, the distinction between normal and myopathic is often more difficult to make in infants and toddlers because normally their MUPs are more diminutive than those found in older children. It is also more challenging to get some infants to activate their muscles long enough to appreciate the classic increased activation and early recruitment of large numbers of low-amplitude, short-duration MUPs seen in a typical myopathy.

In addition, one must not rely primarily on the presence of abnormalities with needle insertion. Fibrillation potentials and positive waves are nonspecific findings that have no potential localizing value. These are found in many infantile lesions affecting all pathoanatomic levels of the motor unit, including processes affecting the anterior horn cell (spinal cord injury, spinal muscular atrophy [SMA], poliomyelitis), polyneuropathies, NMJ defects (infantile botulism), and a number of myopathies.[1,2,4,5]

One always needs to consider whether any clinical evidence is present suggesting that possibly some infectious or metabolic process is superimposed on a previously unsuspected mild case of one of the various motor unit disorders that may present as a floppy infant.[2] In that instance, the acute "stress" may have temporarily led to the mild or subtle decomposition of the underlying motor unit function. In fact, some of the more acute neuromuscular lesions discussed earlier may not be operative. In this instance, once the inciting mechanism is corrected, the infant will return to baseline.

Respiratory Considerations

ICUs in children's hospitals are supporting children who require endotracheal intubation and ventilatory support, intravenous infusions, and sophisticated monitoring devices. A significant number have disorders of the nervous system, particularly those involving the brainstem, high cervical spinal cord, peripheral nerve, NMJ, and muscle. EMG studies of children in the ICU are valuable for localizing the site of nervous system dysfunction to the brain, peripheral nerve, NMJ, and muscle.

Phrenic nerve conduction and needle EMG of the diaphragm are of particular value in pinpointing the site of dysfunction in the neuromuscular respiratory system. In recent years, Bolton has performed these studies with increasing frequency for the evaluation of infants and older children with unexplained limb weakness, hypotonia, and difficulty in weaning from the ventilator (Table 37-1). The results were valuable in establishing a diagnosis and in following the course of the illness. No complications occurred.[6]

TABLE 37-1. NEUROPHYSIOLOGIC TESTS IN THE PEDIATRIC ICU

Conditions	Site of Dysfunction	Test	References
Severe encephalopathy	Brain	Electroencephalography (EEG) Somatosensory evoked potential Brainstem auditory evoked potential	Picton et al, 1999[94]
Neurologic respiratory insufficiency	Brain, spinal cord, phrenic nerves, neuromuscular junction, diaphragm	Transcranial and cervical magnetic stimulation	Zifko et al, 1996[95]
		Phrenic nerve somatosensory evoked potential Phrenic nerve conduction Repetitive phrenic nerve stimulation Needle EMG of the diaphragm Automated interference pattern analysis of the diaphragm Power spectral analysis of the diaphragm	Zifko et al, 1995[96] Chen et al, 1995[97] Zifko et al, 1997[98] Bolton et al, 1992[99] Collins et al, 1997[100] Chen et al, 1996[101]
Polyneuropathies	Peripheral nerves	Motor and sensory nerve conduction, needle EMG	Bolton et al, 1986[69]
Neuromuscular transmission defects	Neuromuscular junction	Repetitive limb nerve stimulation	Kimura, 1989[102]
		Stimulated single-fiber EMG	Schwartz et al, 1997[103]
Myopathies	Skeletal muscle	Motor and sensory nerve conduction, needle EMG Direct muscle stimulation	Bolton et al, 1986[69] Rich et al, 1997[77]
Other tests		Measurement of muscle force and "sound"	Bolton et al, 1989[104]

ICU, intensive care unit.

Technical Considerations and General Approach

Clinical neurophysiologists are often concerned that technical problems prevent effective studies in the pediatric ICU. However, with attention to certain details, all studies normally performed in the adult ICU can be performed in the pediatric ICU (see Table 37-1). The clinical examination is difficult due to the small size of young children, the confined space of an incubator, the endotracheal tubes, the vascular lines, and the splints and bandages applied to parts of the body.

EMG studies can be readily performed in the pediatric ICU using a portable EMG. Newer instruments with improved hardware and software have greatly reduced the incidence of artifact. Physicians in the pediatric ICU must be consulted regarding the child's clinical status to determine what tests can be safely performed, considering the child's condition and the necessity for maintenance of treatment and monitoring devices. To remove the possibility of 60 cycle/sec artifact, all devices attached to the patient that are not absolutely necessary should be unplugged from the wall.

During the procedure of applying surface electrodes or in stimulating peripheral nerves, residents, fellows, or the attending nurse need to assist, if necessary, in the proper positioning of the infant, adjusting the position of endotracheal tubes and vascular lines.

Sedation should be given under the direction of the intensivist as to dosage and timing, especially to avoid the pain of RMNS when there is a question of an NMTD or during needle EMG yet permitting the evaluation of voluntary muscle activity. Although the application of an electrical stimulus near an intravascular line, whose destination is the heart, is of theoretical concern in regard to induction of arrhythmias or asystole, Bolton and colleagues have often stimulated at these sites in adults and children and have never had such a complication. Opinion from cardiology experts indicates the electrical stimuli are too small to cause such a complication.

Septic patients frequently have elevation in body temperature, which may spuriously decrease latencies and amplitudes of the compound muscle action potential (CMAP). Hence, limb-skin surface temperatures should be routinely recorded.

When applying electrodes, it may be necessary to splint the limb to avoid excessive movement, which may loosen electrode contact. When performing needle EMG, short-needle electrodes are best as the underlying nerve, muscle, and bone may be near the skin surface. Evaluation of the chest wall with needle EMG, where underlying muscle, including the diaphragm, may be very near the skin surface, the needle should be advanced through the tissues carefully, constantly monitoring the presence or absence of insertional activity to make sure that one is always in muscle.

When performing needle EMG of the diaphragm, it may be necessary to briefly discontinue intermittent mandatory ventilation to observe the type of voluntary respirations, as reflected in electrical activity from the diaphragm during inspiration. During this time, the child should be kept on enough pressure support to supply oxygen, and the child's condition should be monitored by observing the heart rate, respiration, and blood gases. Mechanical ventilation should be immediately resumed if the child appears to be in respiratory or cardiac distress.

When needle EMG of the diaphragm is performed, the heart rate and respirations should be closely watched. If the infant seems in distress, the chest wall should be auscultated to determine if there are decreased breath sounds on the side that the procedure was performed. In the event of possible pneumothorax, an emergency chest radiograph should be performed. We have not yet had this complication in children and have had only two instances in the 400 procedures that we have performed in adults (C.F.B.). Adults who appear to be at risk from this rare complication are those with asthma and who are on a ventilator. Presumably, children in similar situations are also at risk.

ACUTE INFANTILE NEUROMUSCULAR CRISES

Babies may present during the neonatal period with floppy infant syndrome or, acutely, with a flaccid paralysis after being healthy during the first few months of their life.[4] Some newborns, presenting primarily with an acute respiratory compromise during the immediate neonatal period, are concomitantly observed to be hypotonic, sometimes to the degree of being identified as a floppy baby. A variety of congenital or developmental lesions at any level of the peripheral motor unit from motor neuron to muscle cell per se may lead to this picture. There is a different subset of disorders for newborns and infants, as discussed here, in comparison to the older child reviewed later.

Rarely during the first year of life a small group of previously healthy infants unexpectedly develop a precipitous neuromuscular crisis. Specific clinical mechanisms that require consideration in this instance include a previously unrecognized SMA, GBS, infantile botulism, familial MG now recognized to be secondary to an end plate deficiency of choline acetyltransferase, or, rarely, postvaccine poliomyelitis and, potentially, as in adults, West Nile virus.

Anterior Horn Cell

Spinal Muscular Atrophy

The Werdnig-Hoffmann form of spinal muscular atrophy (SMA-1) is one of the most common causes of floppy infant syndrome. It is the primary example of a classic anterior horn cell disorder of infancy.[1,2] Usually, these infants either present as a floppy baby or with failure to develop early motor milestones between 1 and 3 months of age. Most are easily recognized early because of their typical clinical presentation as a floppy baby with an alert facies, absent muscle stretch reflexes, and fasciculations of their tongue. This diagnosis is usually made by a combination of EMG and genetic DNA analysis.[2] Occasionally, however, parents and pediatricians have not recognized a relatively subtle clinical presentation until an acute illness leads to hospitalization. Eventually a respiratory distress develops, such as with an acute bronchiolitis. This requires neonatal ICU monitoring, When the infant cannot be weaned, neurologic consultation and eventually EMG are performed, leading to the diagnosis.

Babies who have SMA demonstrate a typical constellation of EMG findings. These include low-amplitude CMAPs, normal motor conduction velocities (MCVs), and distal latencies (DLs), as well as intact sensory nerve action potentials (SNAPs). Needle EMG primarily demonstrates a marked decrease in the number of MUPs. Many of these MUPs are larger than normal and fire at increased rates. These are associated with widespread active denervation, characterized by many fibrillation potentials and positive waves.

In babies with SMA-1 wherein respiratory muscles are affected sufficiently to require mechanical ventilation, electrophysiologic studies may be valuable when the diagnosis of the neuromuscular condition is still in doubt. In addition to the traditional EMG signs affecting limb muscles, studies of the respiratory system may help establish motor neuron disease as the reason for the respiratory insufficiency rather than potential cardiac or pulmonary causes. Here, phrenic NCSs should reveal near-normal latencies but reduced CMAP amplitudes from the diaphragm.

On needle EMG, it may be difficult to detect fibrillation potentials and positive sharp waves, but the number of MUPs with each inspiration should be reduced. With a more chronic SMA in the rare circumstances when children have been placed on ventilators, diaphragm needle EMG may reveal little evidence of fibrillation and positive sharp waves, simply large MUPs in decreased numbers due to denervation and collateral reinnervation.

DNA analysis for the 5q11-13 mutation of the survival motor neuron gene (*SMN*) is the appropriate means to make the diagnosis. Occasionally, with babies requiring ICU monitoring and treatment, the clinician may need to make a more rapid diagnosis. This is one of the primary indications for using EMG in the setting of SMA-1. It provides information allowing for appropriate clinical management as well as parental counseling.

Acute Postimmunization Poliomyelitis

Acute postimmunization poliomyelitis is an even more unusual form of anterior horn cell disease; however, an acute vaccine-associated poliomyelitis deserves mention in the differential diagnosis of any infant or child with an acute weakness.[7] One must be alert to the potential for West Nile virus to affect the adult motor neuron[8] and thus potentially also that in a child. One of the authors (H.R.J.) has personally been aware of three cases of acute flaccid infantile paralysis, secondary to live vaccine-related immunization poliomyelitis, that occurred within just a few years during the mid 1990s.[7,9,10] An acute febrile illness preceded a progressive asymmetric extremity weakness, head lag, irritability, and lethargy at age 3 to 4 months, 1 month subsequent to receiving type 3 polio immunization. CSF findings included a cellular pleocytosis with 100 to 580 white blood cells, protein values between 82 and 143 mg/dL, and glucose of 49 mg/dL in one.[7] EMG demonstrated classic electrophysiologic evidence of an acute asymmetric anterior horn cell disorder.

Current Centers for Disease Control and Prevention guidelines require that the initial immunization protocol use the Salk killed vaccine as the primary immunization method for all children.[11] It is thought that this new infantile immunization protocol will also make postvaccination-related poliomyelitis of historic interest in North America. However, this rare complication needs to be always considered in any immigrant baby arriving from economically underdeveloped countries that are still using the live vaccine.

Peripheral Nerve

Some congenital hypomyelinating polyneuropathies present in the newborn period with a clinical phenotype similar to SMA-1, Werdnig-Hoffman disease (i.e., as a floppy baby with a frog-leg posture and tongue fasciculations). These infants may be so ill that they require intensivist support.[2] In contradistinction to SMA-1, these babies have distinct EMG findings characterized by very slow MCVs, with low-amplitude, sometimes dispersed CMAPs, and, most important, absent SNAPs. When the CMAPs are dispersed, the possible diagnosis of a primarily acquired demyelinating polyneuropathy is of foremost consideration and not SMA-1. At Children's Hospital Boston (CHB), 6% of 111 floppy babies evaluated in our EMG laboratory had a peripheral neuropathy.[1,2] These neuropathies were more common among arthrogrypotic infants implying an early fetal involvement.[1] The absence

of SNAPs is the most important EMG clue suggesting that the baby has one of these rare neonatal polyneuropathies. The nerve pathologies included primary axonal, demyelinating, and widespread neuronal degeneration.[12]

Rarely, GBS occurs in newborns and should be included in the differential diagnosis of neonatal flaccid paralysis.[13-15] In one instance a baby with GBS presented soon after birth.[13] The mother had another autoimmune disease, chronic ulcerative colitis. During the 30th week of pregnancy she noted that her fetus was significantly less active.[13] This baby was quadriparetic when delivered at 37 weeks. Neurologic examination at 3 days of age demonstrated severe leg and moderate proximal arm weakness and generalized absence of muscle stretch reflexes. The CSF protein was normal (38 mg/dL). However, motor NCS demonstrated profound motor NCV slowing (3 to 15 m/sec), with conduction block and temporal dispersion in many nerves. Needle EMG revealed active denervation in many muscles. No specific treatment was provided; his recovery was gradual and complete by age 1 year.[13]

Another pregnant mother developed severe GBS herself during the 29th week.[14] She became tetraplegic and was still respirator dependent when her baby was born at 38 weeks. Although initially appearing healthy, her baby became hypotonic, with marked respiratory distress and feeding problems 12 days postpartum; his CSF protein was 243 mg/dL. An EMG was typical for GBS. Both the mother and child had IgG antibodies positive for recent cytomegalovirus infection. Intravenous immunoglobulin therapy led to a complete resolution within 2 weeks.[14] One presumes his GBS developed in utero.[14] GBS also occurred in yet another pregnant woman. Although this baby had poor spontaneous ventilation at delivery and required brief intubation during the next 5 days of observation, no other signs of GBS developed.[15] Nevertheless, this infant and mother both had high antibody titers to human peripheral nerve myelin glycolipids.[15]

Even without any recognized intrauterine complications, GBS may develop as early as 3 weeks of age. Previously healthy babies may present with an acute, rapidly progressive and often severe hypotonia, with possible respiratory distress and feeding difficulties.[16] Additionally chronic inflammatory demyelinating polyneuropathy subsequently developed in one infant who experienced an acute GBS at age 7 weeks.[17]

An EMG is the essential diagnostic means to differentiate GBS from other acute floppy infant syndromes.[16] Absent SNAPs, profound motor conduction slowing, and dispersed CMAPs are the quintessential EMG clues. In the previously noted CHB EMG review of 111 floppy babies, only one of the six infants with a polyneuropathy had EMG findings commensurate with GBS.[1]

Although tick paralysis mimics acute GBS in children, we are unaware of an infantile case. Nonetheless, any baby with an acute onset of generalized muscle weakness needs to be searched for a tick, particularly in the scalp.[18]

Neuromuscular Junction

Maternal Related

Of the various NMJ disorders occasionally encountered among newborns, transient neonatal MG is the most easily recognized and probably most common. Typically, 15% to 20% of infants born to mothers with autoimmune MG develop myasthenic symptoms.[19,20] Another even less common NMJ disorder occurs at birth when a baby's mother has developed eclampsia, necessitating treatment with magnesium sulfate. This cation potentially predisposes the infant to development of an acute presynaptic NMJ disorder.[21,22] Neither neonatal maternal MG or magnesium induced NMTDs often leads to a request for an EMG. Although we have seen neither entity in more than 26 years at CHB, one needs to keep the possibility of same in the differential diagnosis of any acutely ill newborn floppy infant.

Congenital Myasthenic Syndromes (CMSs)

A number of rare congenital myasthenic syndromes occur during infancy (see Chapter 35). Their specific pathophysiologic site varies among the presynaptic NMJ, the synapse, or the postsynaptic NMJ. An end plate deficiency of choline acetyltransferase is a congenital myasthenic syndrome that predisposes the baby to an acute-onset NMJ disorder. Typically, these babies have recurrent episodic apnea. In contrast, it is unusual for other congenital myasthenic syndrome forms to have such an acute presentation.

Infantile Botulism

The clinical presentation of infantile botulism is usually stereotyped. Typically, a previously healthy infant, between ages 10 days and 6 months, has the acute onset of hypotonia, generalized weakness, poor feeding, dysphagia, and constipation.[23-29] Infantile botulism may also present with unexplained acute respiratory distress in babies younger than 6 months of age. When this is severe it may require ventilatory support. Therefore, one must keep this diagnosis at the forefront with any previously healthy baby who becomes acutely hypotonic and sometimes even respiratory compromised. It is possible that infantile botulism is more common than is currently recognized.

EMG is the most useful early diagnostic tool because bacteriologic confirmation requires a few weeks. Sensory NCSs are normal. However, motor conduction studies reveal markedly reduced amplitudes of CMAPs with little change in latency. Needle EMG showed abnormal spontaneous activity, remarkably low-amplitude and short-duration fibrillation potentials in half the infants. The number of MUPs

firing on attempted voluntary contraction may be remarkably reduced, low amplitude, and polyphasic.

Most babies with infantile botulism have clear-cut evidence of an NMTD (Chapter 35). Low-rate RMNS, at 2 to 5 Hz, may demonstrate a decremental response.[30] The primary EMG technique for diagnosing infantile botulism is more rapid RMNS rates of 20 to 50 Hz.[30] A post-tetanic facilitation varying between 23% and 313%, with a mean of 73%, was documented in 23 of 25 babies.[30] A longer period of post-tetanic facilitation was also observed.[31] One may not always be able to confirm a diagnosis of infantile botulism with EMG because not all cases have a documented facilitation with RMNS.[30,32] However, in most instances of infantile botulism, babies have a typical EMG diagnostic triad[33] that includes (1) low-amplitude CMAPs (beware of normal maturation standards for age); (2) post-tetanic facilitation; and (3) absence of post-tetanic exhaustion.[32]

Muscle

Congenital myopathies typically present as a floppy infant syndrome, but most babies are not sick enough to require neonatal ICU monitoring. In addition, myopathies do not typically cause acute infantile flaccid paralysis and/or respiratory distress. However, occasionally we are asked to see a baby in the neonatal ICU who is found to have a primary myopathy.

Certain myopathies, particularly congenital muscular dystrophy and congenital myopathies, may be severe enough to require endotracheal intubation and ventilatory support. To determine if the respiratory system is affected and is the main reason for respiratory insufficiency, in contrast to primary cardiac and pulmonary causes, phrenic nerve conduction and needle EMG of the chest wall muscles and diaphragm are often of assistance.

Children with myopathies have phrenic NCSs demonstrating low-amplitude diaphragm CMAPs but normal latencies. Needle EMG variably demonstrates fibrillation potentials and positive sharp waves, or in the case of myotonic dystrophy, myotonia, within chest wall muscles and diaphragm.

Myotonic dystrophy is one of the few dystrophies that presents as a severely floppy infant. Babies with congenital myotonic dystrophy may have severe generalized hypotonia requiring intubation at birth because of their associated respiratory compromise. Sometimes, the diagnosis is suspected clinically by their classic facies with "tenting" of the mouth that appears like an upside down letter "V." Most of all infants with muscular dystrophy have a family history of myotonic dystrophy; however it is often unrecognized in the parent, usually the mother who has a milder form. Clinical clues to a minor maternal presence include a history of premature cataract removal or mild subclinical myotonia and/or distal weakness on clinical examination.

When confronted with the typical clinical phenotype, DNA testing is 98% to 99% accurate in both infants with myotonia dystrophy as well as their symptomatic or asymptomatic mothers. Myotonia detectable by EMG may be present in the hypotonic newborn infant, as early as age 5 days, although it sometimes is not always evident this early.[34,35] Occasionally profuse fibrillations are the most predominant finding. Here one needs to carefully search for the myotonia. Sometimes a maternal EMG detects previously unsuspected myotonia.[2] If this does occur, a subsequent follow-up EMG in the infant, in the face of a negative initial one, is not needed; a DNA test quickly establishes the diagnosis. In the past, however, EMG testing had been able to detect later onset myotonia in some of these infants.[35]

Metabolic Myopathy: Phosphofructokinase Deficiency

Rarely, metabolic myopathies present in neonates with severe hypotonia and respiratory weakness in the period. We evaluated one floppy baby @ CHB with arthrogryposis multiplex congenita (AgMC) whose EMG was distinctly abnormal with a profusion of myopathic MUPs. Biopsy led to a diagnosis of phosphofructokinase deficiency.[36] Another fatal case, later proven to be muscle phosphorylase deficiency, presented at age 4 weeks with feeding difficulties, tiring easily, and severe respiratory distress. This infant had a rapidly progressive course, becoming hypotonic with generalized weakness.[5]

Although his EMG demonstrated myopathic MUPs, the abundant concomitant fibrillation potentials were wrongly interpreted as "consistent with spinal muscular atrophy."[5] Such instances emphasize the importance of careful attention, by the electromyographer, to the motor unit profile and not the insertional finding per se. In fact the motor units in this case were typically myopathic in this baby with muscle phosphorylase deficiency similar to our case of phosphofructokinase deficiency.[36]

Respiratory Dysfunction

Spinal Cord

If the high cervical spinal cord is damaged, endotracheal intubation and ventilation may be required. Conditions that may induce this are trauma at birth, compression by neoplasm, hemorrhage or infection, or acute transverse myelitis. Motor and sensory conduction studies of limb nerves will be normal. Since the phrenic nerves arise from C3, C4, and C5 segments, CMAP amplitudes from the diaphragm may be considerably reduced or absent, although latencies relatively preserved. Needle EMG will show decreased or absent numbers of MUPs. Muscles innervated by high cervical seg-

ments that are involved will show fibrillation potentials and positive sharp waves after 2 weeks. To further confirm the localization, needle EMG of the cervical paraspinal muscles and of shoulder muscles supplied predominantly by C4 (i.e., upper border of the trapezius and levator scapulae) should also show evidence of denervation.

In lower cervical spinal cord lesions, often due to traumatic hyperextension injuries of the neck resulting in quadriplegia, respiratory difficulty is due to upper motor neuron weakness of chest wall muscles. Thus, phrenic NCSs and needle EMG of the diaphragm will be normal. However, there will be a relative lack of firing of MUPs from chest wall muscles and fibrillation potentials and positive sharp waves will not be present.

Phrenic Neuropathy

The phrenic nerve may be traumatized by surgery, during delivery, or other mechanisms. Phrenic nerve conduction reveals reduced amplitudes. Standard nerve conduction and needle EMG of upper limbs help further localize the lesion. The brachial plexus may be damaged at delivery to produce Erb's palsy (upper plexus) or Klumpke's paralysis (lower plexus).

Polyneuropathies and Respiratory Compromise

GBS either demyelinating or axonal forms sometimes require ventilation in an ICU when they lead to quadriplegia and difficulty in breathing. In regard to the respiratory system, phrenic NCSs reveal prolongation of latencies and reduction or dispersion of the diaphragm CMAP. On needle EMG of the diaphragm, there is decreased recruitment of MUPs with each inspiration. Axonal polyneuropathies do not affect phrenic nerve conduction latency, but the diaphragm CMAP is reduced or absent. There are abundant fibrillation potentials and positive sharp waves on needle EMG of the diaphragm, while the number of MUPs recruited with each inspiration is reduced or absent.

Critical Illness Myopathy or Polyneuropathy

Typically these disorders develop after admission to the ICU, usually as a complication of the systemic inflammatory response syndrome (sepsis). This is either a primary axonal degeneration of peripheral nerve fibers, or a toxic myopathy with consequent difficulty in weaning from the ventilator. This appears to be a much less frequent occurrence in pediatric, as opposed to adult, ICU. The reader is referred to a more detailed description of the critical illness neuromuscular disorders discussed later in this chapter.

Autonomic Nervous System

The sympathetic skin response can be successfully recorded from both the hand and foot in response to a loud clap; the usual method of electrical stimulation of a peripheral nerve may not always be effective in the environment of the pediatric ICU. The cardiac R-R interval also can be measured. Such studies may be of value in assessing the autonomic nervous system.

ACUTE NEUROMUSCULAR CRISES IN THE OLDER CHILD

Anterior Horn Cell

Since the inception of our EMG laboratory in 1979 at CHB, we are unaware of any acute poliomyelitis, beyond infancy. Unfortunately, one needs to always consider this possibility, as some parents still decline to have their children appropriately immunized. Additionally, with increasing air travel and children being adopted, immigrating, or visiting worldwide, one always needs to consider the possibility of poliomyelitis in countries with less than ideal immunization standards. As there is an increasing incidence of West Nile infection, with its proclivity to affect motor neurons, we need to always investigate this possibility in any child presenting with an acute asymmetric multiple extremity flaccid weakness or a monoparesis and lacking sensory findings.[8] Rarely, we have seen a few instances of subacute polio in children coming from those nations where standard immunization is not routinely available. These kids generally present with a monoparesis sometimes with the question of a mononeuropathy or a plexopathy.

EMG findings include diminished CMAP amplitudes, no more than minimal decrease in MCV, normal distal motor latencies, and normal SNAPs. On needle EMG there is a relatively marked diminution in the number of active MUPs with these tending to fire more rapidly than normal. Abnormal insertional activity, characterized by runs and trains of positive waves and fibrillation potentials, is evident by 10 to 14 days.

Peripheral Nerve

GBS is the most common cause for an acute generalized paralysis in the older child.[37] When confronted with any child having acute flaccid paralysis GBS, an acute myelopathy from either a spinal cord tumor or transverse myelitis and tick paralysis are the three most important entities in the differentiation from the GBS. A few other rare etiologies require consideration in the evaluation of acute pediatric polyneuropathies. These include various toxins, such as tick paralysis, buckthorn wild cherry, and organophosphate pesticide poisoning[38]; heavy metals, glue or gasoline sniffing; the rare circumstance of a child with sometimes unsuspected Charcot-Marie-Tooth type 1 receiving vincristine[39,40]; infectious diseases such as diphtheria; and metabolic errors including porphyria, Leigh's disease, and hypokalemia or potentially hyperkalemia from Addison's disease.

Transverse myelitis or spinal cord tumor can have a relative rapid evolution of increasing weakness, numbness, concomitant areflexia, and sometimes most importantly problems with urination. Babinski signs may not appear at first. The sphincter difficulty, although sometimes present early on in the course of GBS, generally clears within the first 24 hours with GBS. EMG can be confusing as one of the earliest EMG signs of GBS is the prolongation or loss of F waves. If a cord tumor involves the anterior horn cells at a level of L5-S1 or C6-C8, F waves appropriate to peripheral nerves having their origin at these levels will be abnormal. Rather than awaiting the clinical profile to evolve, the wise thing is to obtain a magnetic resonance imaging (MRI) early whenever one has the slightest degree of hint of a primary spinal cord lesion.

Acute tick paralysis always needs consideration in the differential diagnosis of GBS or MG, particularly among children from the preschool ages and older.[18,41-45] Tick paralysis is an often unsuspected and unidentified disorder. The precise site of this biologic toxin is not yet defined. Each child with acute flaccid paralysis requires careful inspection of the scalp to exclude this unusual diagnosis. Early presence of pupillary involvement is a particularly helpful clue,[18] allowing the clinician to differentiate tick paralysis from GBS or MG. Total ophthalmoplegia may occur and many have some degree of extraocular muscle paresis occasionally mimicking the Miller-Fisher GBS variant.

Most likely the site of action is at the distal axonal terminal or possibly at the NMJ. Experimental data have suggested that tick paralysis is related to the presynaptic NMJ causing decreased acetylcholine release.[46] Typical EMG findings in tick paralysis include diminished CMAP amplitudes with preserved MCVs, motor DLs, and SNAPs.[18,44,45] These findings are similar to acute motor axonal neuropathy or even some early demyelinating forms of GBS. The reduced CMAP improved dramatically after the tick was removed.[44,45] In some children the early appearance of fibrillation potentials, as soon as 24 to 48 hours, may lead to diagnostic confusion if one does not pay close attention to the total constellation of neurophysiologic findings.[44,45]

Rarely, a child with GBS will develop fixed dilated pupils and other bulbar findings. Both diphtheria and botulism are diagnostic considerations with this clinical set particularly when there is predominant bulbar involvement.[47] MG or poliomyelitis also enters into this differential diagnosis, but in these instances the pupillary responses are preserved.

Severe pain mimicking a meningoencephalopathic process was the initial emergency department presentation in some children who later were identified as having GBS @CHB.[48] Initially they all were so irritable and difficult to examine that they received either a brain computed tomography or MRI scan, and when normal and anticipating an infection, these were followed by CSF examination. The finding of an albuminocytologic dissociation led to neurologic consultation and subsequently an EMG that helped confirm this diagnosis.

Our two most common EMG findings in GBS included a reduced CMAP in 83%, with absent or prolonged long latency waves in 81%.[37] Primary signs of demyelination, including conduction block, temporal dispersion, or MCV slowing, occurred in 70% to 74% of our children; in contrast, findings usually implying a significant axonal component characterized by low-amplitude mean distal CMAP of less than 20% of normal occurred in 22%. SNAPs were abnormal in 70% but not necessarily the same nerves as affected on motor conduction studies.[39] Although isolated absence of F waves may be an early sign of GBS in a number of children,[39] if the child has had an acute onset of leg weakness, areflexia, and back pain, a diagnosis of transverse myelitis or even a surgically remediable tumor always requires consideration. Although EMG is generally normal in this setting, if segmental anterior horn cells are affected, both the CMAPs and F waves may be abnormal. This leads to neurophysiologic mimicking of the typical early GBS findings.

Neuromuscular Junction Disorders in the Toddler and Older Child

Any child presenting with extraocular muscle weakness manifested by diplopia, ptosis, bulbar, and generalized weakness must be considered as most likely having an NMTD. These children often require hospitalization, sometimes in an intensive care setting. When autoimmune MG occurs in the pediatric age group, it is typically quite similar to its presentation in adults varying from an acute bulbar respiratory crisis requiring intensive care, or failure to wean from a respirator, to a more ingravescent course.

This applies to children of any age, even in toddlers, as we have experienced in one 15-month-old child. The youngest child with non-neonatal autoimmune MG that we are aware of was 9 months old.[49] Although most autoimmune MG children present with ptosis and/or diplopia,[50] we occasionally see other clinical settings, some of which require urgent intensive care management. For instance we evaluated one teenager being followed by an otolaryngologist for progressive but variable speech

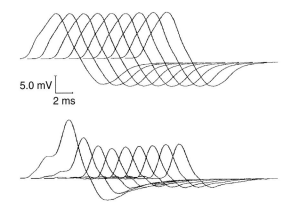

FIGURE 37–1

Compound muscle action potentials (CMAPs) elicited by repetitive motor nerve stimulation at 3/sec in a hand muscle: normal (top) and myasthenia gravis (bottom). With optimum recording electrode placement, the CMAP waveform departs sharply from the baseline and is monophasic. In myasthenia gravis, the decrement begins with the second response of the train, is maximum at the fourth or fifth response, and resolves thereafter, giving a characteristic "U-shaped" or "saddle-shaped" train envelope. (Courtesy of D. B. Sanders, Duke University, Durham, North Carolina.)

difficulties when she suddenly developed severe dysphagia and increasing respiratory distress.

The appropriate EMG evaluation and neurophysiologic findings are detailed in Chapter 35. EMG provides an excellent means to demonstrate the presence of an NMTD by identifying the presence of a decrement to RMNS (Fig. 37-1). This is particularly germane in the acutely ill child or adolescent with a typical clinical picture and in whom one needs to begin therapy and cannot wait for antibody study results.

These adolescents generally respond to acute immunomodulatory therapy and more prolonged chronic immunotherapy as well as thymectomy (see Chapter 35).[51]

Muscle

Channelopathies

Some of the various channelopathies, particularly hyperkalemic and hypokalemic periodic paralysis, always warrant consideration in the differential diagnosis of acute GBS. As these are autosomal dominant sodium or calcium channelopathies, there is usually a well-documented family history. Clinically the episodes of paralysis are relatively short-lived on most occasions. Routine NCS findings are normal; however, prolonged periods of exercise with EMG monitoring can evoke a diminution in CMAP amplitudes.[3] Needle EMG often demonstrates significant myotonic-like discharges with the hyperkalemic variant (see Chapter 36).

TABLE 37–2. DIFFERENTIATING FEATURES OF CRITICAL ILLNESS NEUROMUSCULAR DISORDERS

Features	Acute Quadriplegic/ Necrotizing Myopathy	Hopkins' Syndrome	Critical Illness Polyneuropathy
Age group	Children, adolescents	Young children	Elderly (rarely in children)
Risk factors	NMBAs and/or steroids	Status asthmaticus	Multiorgan failure/sepsis
Timing	Variable	<2 wk	>2 wk
Clinical findings	Purely motor		Sensory and motor
Limbs affected	Quadriparesis	Monoparesis	Quadriparesis
Pain	Muscular tenderness	Mild	Unusual
Reflexes	↓	Normal in unaffected limbs	Absent or ↓
Recovery	Good (slow, complete); may be rapid	Poor	Good (slow, complete); may be incomplete
Creatine kinase	Normal to ↑↑↑°	Normal	Less than twice upper normal value
Nerve conduction studies	Normal SNAPs; ↓↓ CMAPs	Normal SNAPs	↓ SNAP and CMAP amplitudes
Electromyography	Myopathic	Localized neuropathic	Neuropathic
Muscle excitability	Absent or ↓↓	Normal	Normal
Spinal fluid	Not reported	Pleocytosis	Normal
Muscle biopsy	Type II atrophy; myosin loss	Not reported	Grouped atrophy; axonal loss

° Normal to mildly increased in acute quadriplegic myopathy; significantly increased in acute necrotizing myopathy.
  NMBA, neuromuscular blocking agent; SNAP, sensory nerve action potential; CMAP, compound muscle action potential.

We do call attention to Moxley's case illustration[52] of an 18-month-old child with a previously unrecognized sodium channel myotonia who presented with respiratory stridor and increasing difficulty breathing, secondary to an acute bronchiolitis. She had trouble opening her eyes that was worsened with crying, as was her stridor. This child had somewhat elevated serum potassium levels presumably secondary to her increased respiratory effort. These findings were all compatible with a form of paradoxical myotonia. This clinical combination exacerbated her underlying sodium channelopathy with vocal cord myotonia and led to ever increasing respiratory stridor. EMG performed on this child showed generalized myotonia.

Dermatomyositis

Occasionally one may witness the acute onset of dermatomyositis in the pediatric age group. More commonly, this illness slowly evolves and does not require evaluation in the acute care setting.

PRIMARY CRITICAL ILLNESS NEUROMUSCULAR DISORDERS

Occasionally an acute, severe generalized weakness, often mimicking a hospital-acquired GBS, develops in children during the course of a critical illness. Typically such kids have an overwhelming sepsis or status asthmaticus. These syndromes may affect each level of the peripheral motor unit, that is, anterior horn cell (Hopkins' syndrome), peripheral nerve (critical illness polyneuropathy [CIP]), NMJ (persistent neuromuscular blockade), and muscle cell per se (acute quadriplegic myopathy [AQM] or acute

necrotizing myopathy of intensive care). In children a myopathic mechanism usually predominates. Their neurologic presentation is typically one of a failure to wean from the respirator.[53-56]

EMG is particularly valuable for assessing the precise anatomic site for these various entities. Additional scientific advances in EMG, especially diaphragmatic EMG and phrenic nerve stimulation, have further broadened the indications for pediatric EMG particularly in the critical care setting. An additional diagnostic value of EMG occurs when primary motor unit disorders have a clinical presentation mimicking various disorders of the central nervous system, such as pseudoencephalopathic GBS.[48] The primary disorders are outlined in the following sections.

Segmental Anterior Horn Cell Disease

Segmental anterior horn cell disease (Hopkins' syndrome) is a poliomyelitis-like illness that occurs following status asthmaticus and primarily in childhood. It is characterized by rapidly progressive and permanent monoplegia or diplegia (Table 37-2).[57-66] The etiology remains unknown. Despite its resemblance to poliomyelitis, all 27 reported patients were appropriately immunized against polio (Table 37-3). Other possible etiologies included enteroviruses and herpes simplex virus (HSV)-1. CSF culture in one 7-year-old child with Hopkins' syndrome demonstrated primary HSV-1 infection, supporting the viral hypothesis.[67,68] An outbreak indistinguishable from Hopkins' syndrome was due to an epidemic of enterovirus 71[67]; however, these children did not have acute asthma. Since all patients with Hopkins' syndrome recently received steroids, the possibility of an immunologically mediated mechanism, perhaps an underlying im-

TABLE 37–3. FEATURES OF 27 CHILDREN WITH HOPKINS' SYNDROME*

Feature	Outcome
Age of onset	13 mo-11 yr
Sex, male/female	19/8
Immunization (polio)	27/27
Days to pareses after asthma	1-11
Spinal fluid protein (mild elevation)	6/13 reported
Spinal fluid pleocytosis	13/13 reported
Denervation on EMG	17/17 reported
Slowed conduction velocities	4/15
Virus isolation	
Enteroviruses	5/22
HSV-1 (spinal fluid)	1/22
Permanent paralysis	27/27
Monoplegia	21
Diplegia	4
Hemiplegia	2

* Data derived from cases reported in the literature.[58-65]

  HSV, herpes simplex virus.

  Adapted from Sheth RD, Bolton CF: Neuromuscular complications of sepsis in children. J Child Neurol 1995;10:346-352.

munodeficiency and/or steroid-mediated susceptibility of patients to invasion of the anterior horn cells by a virus, is also postulated.[65]

EMG is typical of a segmental anterior horn cell disease; this is characterized by a decrease in the number of MUPs, normal MCVs, potentially low-amplitude CMAPs, and normal sensory studies. Cervical spine MRI in Hopkins' syndrome revealed swelling and edema in the region of the clinically involved segments.[63,68] Not surprisingly, surgical exploration of the brachial plexus was unremarkable in one instance.[61]

Critical Illness Polyneuropathy

Initially described by Bolton and associates in 1984,[54] CIP, associated with sepsis and multiorgan failure, has sensorimotor axonal characteristics. This is primarily a distal axonopathy, and its pathogenesis remains uncertain. It is possible that humoral and cellular processes result in disturbed or lack of vascular autoregulation with increased microvascular permeability, endoneural edema, and capillary occlusion.[54,69]

The onset of the neuropathy is difficult to recognize because of the frequently associated encephalopathy, the severity of the underlying illness, and the use of neuromuscular blocking agents (NMBAs) in conjunction with ventilatory support (see Table 37-2). It is usually noted when the patient cannot be weaned from the mechanical ventilator.

Clinical findings in CIP include distally predominant extremity weakness and loss of muscle stretch reflexes. Sensory loss is difficult to demonstrate but is sometimes detectable when patients can cooperate for a neurologic examination. The presence of significant cranial neuropathies should suggest another pathophysiologic process because these nerves are rarely involved in CIP.

EMG demonstrates an axonal neuropathy.[69,70] NCSs demonstrate reduced amplitude of both motor and sensory responses. Significant nerve conduction slowing or blocks do not occur with CIP and, if present, suggest other diagnostic possibilities, particularly GBS. Phrenic NCSs show either reduced or absent responses.[71] Needle EMG in extremity musculature, as well as the diaphragm, demonstrates neurogenic MUPs, fibrillation potentials, and positive sharp waves.[69] Serum CK levels are usually normal or mildly elevated. Neuropathologic studies show motor sensory axonal degeneration without significant inflammation or demyelination.[69]

The differential diagnosis here includes acute GBS, porphyria, botulism, myasthenic crisis, prolonged neuromuscular blockade, and critical illness myopathy.[70] Recovery may be slow and incomplete.

Persistent Neuromuscular Blockade

Persistent neuromuscular blockade follows the discontinuation of NMBAs that unexplicably continue to have a pharmacologic effect. This results in prolonged weakness and inability to wean from the ventilator. It occurs more frequently in children who have impaired renal or hepatic function. Persistent neuromuscular blockade is seen with all NMBAs, including pancuronium, vecuronium, and atracurium.[72-74] Serum creatine kinase (CK) levels are usually normal.

RMNS demonstrates a decremental response of the CMAP, identifying the NMJ as the primary anatomic site of this physiologic abnormality. Rarely, no motor response is obtained in the child with severe prolonged blockade or in those with AQM.

Typically, children with persistent neuromuscular blockade have weakness that lasts for only a few days and should not persist for more than a week once the NMBAs are discontinued. If the weakness persists beyond 7 days, other conditions such as AQM need consideration. Thus the EMG studies must be repeated if the weakness persists, particularly in instances where no motor responses are present on initial evaluation. Normal motor conduction studies with a concomitant decrement on RMNS support the diagnosis of prolonged blockade. In contrast, the presence of persistently reduced or absent motor responses is compatible with the possible diagnosis of AQM.[74,75]

Acute Quadriplegic Myopathy

AQM is also known as *critical illness myopathy*, *critical care myopathy*, *acute myopathy*, and *acute myopathy with selective loss of myosin filaments*.[70,76] Asthma is the most common predisposing condition. This is typically in conjunction with the use of intravenous corticosteroids, nondepolarizing NMBAs, and aminoglycosides.[75] However, AQM is also described in patients with sepsis who were not treated with either NMBAs or corticosteroids.[77-79] Other predisposing conditions for AQM include pneumonia, organ transplantation (e.g., heart, liver, lung),[80] hepatic failure, and acidosis.[70] One recent study from Toronto noted that 8 (57%) of the 14 critically ill children with muscle weakness were solid-organ or bone marrow transplant recipients.[81] This study aimed to establish the incidence of muscle weakness in children admitted to a pediatric ICU for longer than 24 hours. Fourteen (1.7%) of 830 children had generalized muscle weakness and most had received NMBAs, corticosteroids, or aminoglycoside antibodies. In most patients with AQM, the CK level is normal or mildly elevated.[77,82,83] Nevertheless, in a small number of patients, CK levels may be significantly elevated.

Most patients with AQM are severely affected, having significant weakness or even paralysis, as well as inability to be weaned from the ventilator. In contrast, a few patients may have only mild weakness. Extraocular movements are usually preserved, sensation is intact, and muscle stretch reflexes are decreased proportionate to the decrease in strength. If the child exhibits facial grimacing in response to rigorous painful stimulation of the distal extremities, implying intact sensory pathways, a myopathic mechanism for the quadriparesis needs to be suspected; nonetheless, the differentiation cannot usually be made clinically. In a series of 8 adults with AQM, biopsy demonstrated loss of thick myofilaments EMG.[84]

Among seven children who underwent NCS, the overall electrodiagnostic studies were myopathic in four, normal in two, showed compressive neuropathies in one, and a mild demyelinative polyneuropathy in another patient.[81] NCSs in AQM are usually normal except for diminished CMAP amplitudes.[75,77]

In four of the five children who had an EMG performed, the study showed myopathic findings, and in the fifth it was normal. Needle EMG often records early recruited low-amplitude, short-duration motor units as well as fibrillation potentials.[85] In one of our CHB adolescents with asthma, the extreme severity of the changes near the muscle surface, including many complex repetitive discharges, mimicked the findings seen in primary dermatomyositis. However, other children may be unable to activate their muscles due to an associated encephalopathy or inability to generate any voluntary activity.

The resulting lack of clear EMG findings, combined with the fact that either CIP or AQM may occur in septic patients who have not received corticosteroids or NMBAs, combined with the coexistence of these two syndromes in certain patients, sometimes make their differentiation

extremely difficult. The presence of normal SNAPs and small CMAPs suggests AQM, but small or absent SNAPs indicative of CIP do not necessarily exclude AQM.

Muscle biopsy shows loss of myosin adenosine triphosphatase staining that can be localized or be maximal in the center (corelike) of the myofibers; electron microscopy shows loss of myosin-thick filaments.[81-84] There is relative sparing of actin filaments and Z disks (Fig. 37-2). Light microscopy commonly shows small, angulated, atrophic predominantly type II fibers, with basophilic staining of the cytoplasm with hematoxylin and eosin staining. Most corelike lesions are seen in type I fibers.[84] Necrosis of myofibers is usually mild, but in some cases it can be quite severe. Muscle biopsy demonstrating now these classic pathologic findings is diagnostic of AQM. However, this procedure does not always provide a definitive differentiation between AQM and CIP. This is because the characteristic loss of myosin is seen in only a fraction of patients with AQM.[86] Also, the finding of low-amplitude CMAPs is not diagnostic of a polyneuropathy and may indicate AQM.[84] Significant conduction slowing or conduction blocks are not consistent with either CIP or AQM but rather a demyelinating polyneuropathy.

Although myopathic MUPs having an early recruitment pattern are indicative of a myopathic process, *myopathic potentials* may also occur with prolonged neuromuscular blockade from the use of nondepolarizing NMBAs; thus, standard 2-Hz RMNS is required as part of the electrophysiologic evaluation of these patients.[70]

When the child is very weak or the EMG findings are hard to interpret, direct muscle stimulation is employed to study muscle membrane excitability; the latter is normal in patients with CIP and reduced or absent in patients with AQM. Muscle is reported to be electrically inexcitable in AQM.[77,87] Therefore, in patients with AQM, direct muscle stimulation does not lead to action potentials. The membrane excitability does return with clinical recovery of patients.

Although rapid recovery is sometimes observed, the usual clinical course for AQM is slow (weeks or months) and may be incomplete.[56,88] In a study of five children with critical illness neuromuscular disease, both children with critical illness myopathy recovered completely within 3 weeks and 6 months.[89]

AQM is probably a disorder of protein turnover in muscle. Increased activation of specific proteases such as calpain, a calcium-activated protease, has been found in muscle of patients with AQM. This may be crucial in the pathogenesis of this disorder (Fig. 37-3).[78] These patients demonstrate significant overexpression of caspases, calpain, cathepsin B, and ubiquitin with numerous apoptotic nuclei within the muscle fibers.[90] Proteolytic proteases are also pathogenetically important in AQM; these stimulate apop-

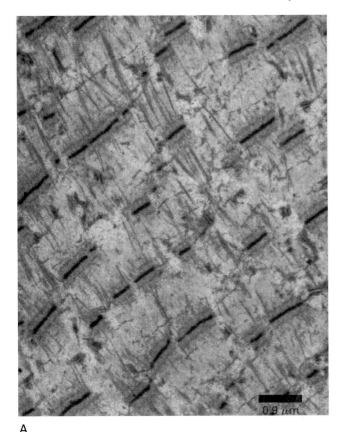

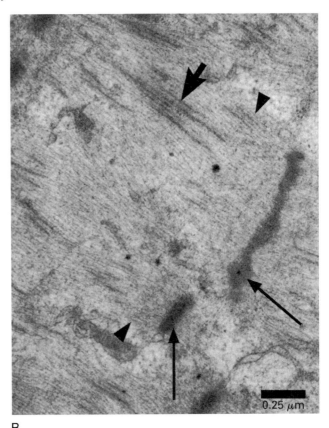

A   B

FIGURE 37–2

Electron micrographs showing loss of thick filaments and myofibrillar disorganization (A) and remaining thick (myosin) filaments (short arrow), thin (actin) filaments (arrowheads), and Z bands (long arrows) (B). Note the relative sparing of Z disks and actin filaments. A, original magnification, × 11,000; B, original magnification, × 40,500. (A and B, From Scully RE, Mark EJ, McNeely WF, et al: Case 11-1997: Case records of the Massachusetts General Hospital. N Engl J Med 1997;336:1079-1088.)

tosis. However, it is not yet clear why the thick filaments are preferentially involved.[90]

Corticosteroids, and other conditions such as sepsis, also stimulate muscle catabolism, which is further amplified by muscle inactivity initially related to neuromuscular blockade and later to lack of membrane excitability (see Fig. 37-3). Sepsis per se and renal or respiratory failure are often associated with significant acidosis. This in turn may also lead to high cytokine levels with their own catabolic effect on muscle. This usually persists despite treatment of sepsis and/or withdrawal of corticosteroids and NMBAs. Thus, it is possible that the ensuing paralysis subsequent to lack of membrane excitability prevents muscle from switching to an anabolic state. Therefore, AQM recovery is usually a slow process.[91]

Acute Necrotizing Myopathy of Intensive Care

Acute necrotizing myopathies of intensive care most typically are associated with severe pulmonary disorders, severe sepsis, or subsequent to organ transplants. Most patients have received high-dose intravenous corticosteroids in conjunction with low to moderate doses of NMBAs. Patients with acute necrotizing myopathy of intensive care have muscle biopsy demonstrating panfascicular muscle fiber necrosis, suggesting that acute necrotizing myopathy may be a severe form of AQM.

This pathology contrasts with the multiple pyogenic abscesses typical for pyomyositis, a condition of septic patients endemic to the tropics. This rare disorder is usually associated with significant CK elevation, myoglobinuria, and myopathic EMG findings.[92]

In contrast serum CK levels are sometimes, but not uniformly, markedly elevated with AQM. Rarely an associated myoglobinemia occurs that may lead to acute renal failure.[85,92] The CK level per se is not a very helpful tool for making the differentiation between a myopathic or neuropathic lesion. Only 3 of 14 patients with critical illness myopathy of the AQM variety had an elevated

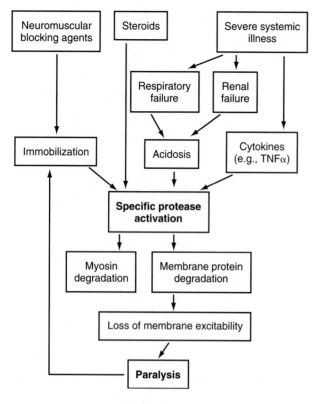

FIGURE 37–3

Risk factors for the development of acute quadriplegic or necrotizing myopathy. TNF, tumor necrosis factor. (Modified from Salviati L, Laverda AM, Zancan L, et al: Acute quadriplegic myopathy in a 17-month-old boy. J Child Neurol 2000;15:63-66.)

CK with a maximal value being a very mild 331 U/L.[56] EMG may exclude a polyneuropathy and often demonstrates a myopathy; however, in certain cases the EMG findings are challenging and difficult to interpret. The muscle biopsy is necessary to define the typical primary loss of thick skeletal muscle filaments.

CONCLUSIONS

When infants develop an acute flaccid paralysis, there is a clinical differential diagnosis somewhat dissimilar to that considered in the older child. In newborns and during the first 6 months of life, certain unusual syndromes require careful consideration.[93] Infantile botulism is a good example. We question whether this illness may be more common than currently recognized. This is particularly relevant among infants with acute indeterminate respiratory distress. GBS is another example of a possibly under-recognized or not-considered illness in the evaluation of

the floppy infant syndrome, particularly so with those babies who may have had an intrauterine onset. At times the clinical presentation of some acute pediatric motor unit disorders, such as GBS, mimics central nervous system lesions including various encephalopathies, even brain death, or acute myelopathies such as transverse myelitis or spinal cord tumors. MRI provides an important diagnostic tool for making this differentiation.

EMG is for defining the presence of a number of peripheral motor unit lesions. Pediatric neurologic and intensive care colleagues need to be encouraged to increase their utilization of EMG in some of these ICU settings. This is especially true when the initial clinical suspicions are not supported by the various investigations. The important finding that infantile botulism or a severe form of axonal GBS can clinically mimic brain death always needs top consideration in the emergency department and the ICU. An EEG may provide the important information of relatively spared brain function and thus lead to consideration of the importance of EMG to define these severe ICU-associated anterior horn cell disorders, peripheral neuropathies, NMTDs, or myopathies.

REFERENCES

1. David WS, Jones HR Jr: Electromyography and biopsy correlation with suggested protocol for evaluation of the floppy infant. Muscle Nerve 1994;17:424-430.
2. Jones HR Jr: Evaluation of the floppy infant. *In* Jones HR Jr, Bolton CF, Harper CM (eds): Pediatric Clinical Electromyography. Philadelphia, Lippincott-Raven, 1996, pp 37-104.
3. Jones HR Jr, Bolton CF, Harper CM (eds): Pediatric Clinical Electromyography. Philadelphia, Lippincott-Raven, 1996, p 487.
4. Jones HR Jr, Harmon RL, Bolton CF, et al: An approach to pediatric electromyography. *In* Jones HR Jr, Bolton CF, Harper CM (eds): Pediatric Clinical Electromyography. Philadelphia, Lippincott-Raven, 1996, pp 1-36.
5. DiMauro S, Hartlage P: Fatal infantile form of muscle phosphorylase deficiency. Neurology 1978;28:1124-1129.
6. Bolton CF, Zifko U, Bird SJ: Clinical neurophysiology in the intensive care unit. Suppl Clin Neurophysiol 2000;53:29-37.
7. David WS, Doyle JJ: Acute infantile weakness: A case of vaccine-associated poliomyelitis. Muscle Nerve 1997;20:747-749.
8. Al-Shekhlee A, Katirji B: Electrodiagnostic features of acute paralytic poliomyelitis associated with West Nile virus infection. Muscle Nerve 2004;29:376-380.
9. Beausoleil JL, Nordgren RE, Modlin JF: Vaccine-associated paralytic poliomyelitis. J Child Neurol 1994;9:334-335.

10. Goldstein J: Infantile poliomyelitis in a recently immunized baby seen at Yale, personal communication, 1995.

11. Recommendations of the Advisory Committee on Immunization Practices: Revised recommendations for routine poliomyelitis vaccination. MMWR Morb Mortal Wkly Rep 1999;48:590.

12. Gabreels-Festen A, Gabreels F: Congenital and early infantile neuropathies. *In* Jones HR Jr, De Vivo DC, Darras BT (eds): Neuromuscular Disorders of Infancy, Childhood, and Adolescence: A Clinician's Approach. Philadelphia, Butterworth Heinemann Health, 2003, pp 361-389.

13. Jackson AH, Baquis GD, Shah BL: Congenital Guillain-Barré syndrome. J Child Neurol 1996;11:407-410.

14. Luijckx GJ, Vles J, de Baets M, et al: Guillain-Barré syndrome in mother and newborn child. Lancet 1997;349:27.

15. Rolfs A, Bolik A: Guillain-Barré syndrome in pregnancy: Reflections on immunopathogenesis. Acta Neurol Scand 1994;89:400-402.

16. Jones HR Jr: Childhood Guillain-Barré syndrome: Clinical presentation, diagnosis, and therapy. J Child Neurol 1996;11:4-12.

17. Pasternak JF, Fulling K, Nelson J, et al: An infant with chronic, relapsing polyneuropathy responsive to steroids. Dev Med Child Neurol 1982;24:504-524.

18. Grattan-Smith PJ, Morris JG, Johnston HM, et al: Clinical and neurophysiological features of tick paralysis. Brain 1997;120:1975-1987.

19. Lefvert AK, Osterman PO: Newborn infants to myasthenic mothers: A clinical study and an investigation of acetylcholine receptor antibodies in 17 children. Neurology 1983;33:133-138.

20. Papazian O: Transient neonatal myasthenia gravis. J Child Neurol 1992;7:135-141.

21. Lipsitz PJ: The clinical and biochemical effects of excess magnesium in the newborn. Pediatrics 1971;47:501-509.

22. Sokal MM, Koenigsberger MR, Rose JS, et al: Neonatal hypermagnesemia and the meconium-plug syndrome. N Engl J Med 1972;286:823-825.

23. Pickett J, Berg B, Chaplin E, et al: Syndrome of botulism in infancy: Clinical and electrophysiologic study. N Engl J Med 1976;295:770-772.

24. Clay SA, Ramseyer JC, Fishman LS, et al: Acute infantile motor unit disorder: Infantile botulism? Arch Neurol 1977;34:236-243.

25. Hoffman RE, Pincomb BJ, Skeels MR: Type F infant botulism. Am J Dis Child 1982;136:270-271.

26. Schwartz RH, Eng G: Infant botulism: Exacerbation by aminoglycosides. Am J Dis Child 1982;136:952.

27. Thompson JA, Glasgow LA, Warpinski JR, et al: Infant botulism: Clinical spectrum and epidemiology. Pediatrics 1980;66:936-942.

28. Shukla AY, Marsh W, Green JB, et al: Neonatal botulism [Abstract]. Neurology 1991;41(Suppl 1):202.

29. Donley DK, Knight P, Tenorio G, et al: A patient with infant botulism, improving with edrophonium [Abstract]. Muscle Nerve 1991;41:201.

30. Cornblath DR, Sladky JT, Sumner AJ: Clinical electrophysiology of infantile botulism. Muscle Nerve 1983;6:448-452.

31. Fakadej AV, Gutmann L: Prolongation of post-tetanic facilitation in infant botulism. Muscle Nerve 1982;5:727-729.

32. Sheth RD, Lotz BP, Hecox KE, et al: Infantile botulism: Pitfalls in electrodiagnosis. J Child Neurol 1999;14:156-158.

33. Gutierrez AR, Bodensteiner J, Gutmann L: Electrodiagnosis of infantile botulism. J Child Neurol 1994;9:362-365.

34. Swift TR, Ignacio OJ, Dyken PR: Neonatal dystrophia myotonica: Electrophysiologic studies. Am J Dis Child 1975;129:734-737.

35. Kuntz NL, Daube JR: Electrophysiology of Congenital Myotonic Dystrophy. Rochester, MN, AAEE Course E, American Association of Electromyography and Electrodiagnosis, 1984.

36. Swoboda KJ, Specht L, Jones HR Jr, et al: Infantile phosphofructokinase deficiency with arthrogryposis: Clinical benefit of a ketogenic diet. J Pediatr 1997;131:932-934.

37. Bradshaw DY, Jones HR Jr: Guillain-Barré syndrome in children: Clinical course, electrodiagnosis, and prognosis. Muscle Nerve 1992;15:500-506.

38. Dirik E, Uysal KM: Organophosphate-induced delayed polyneuropathy [Abstract]. Pediatr Neurol 1994;11:111.

39. Jones HR Jr: Guillain-Barré syndrome: Perspectives with infants and children. Semin Pediatr Neurol 2000;7:91-102.

40. Graf WD, Chance PF, Lensch MW, et al: Severe vincristine neuropathy in Charcot-Marie-Tooth disease type 1A. Cancer 1996;77:1356-1362.

41. Haller JS, Fabara JA: Tick paralysis: Case report with emphasis on neurological toxicity. Am J Dis Child 1972;124:915-917.

42. Donat JR, Donat JF: Tick paralysis with persistent weakness and electromyographic abnormalities. Arch Neurol 1981;38:59-61.

43. Kincaid JC: Tick bite paralysis. Semin Neurol 1990;10:32-34.

44. Swift TR, Ignacio OJ: Tick paralysis: electrophysiologic studies. Neurology 1975;25:1130-1133.

45. Cherington M, Synder RD: Tick paralysis: Neurophysiologic studies. N Engl J Med 1968;278:95-97.

46. Cooper BJ, Spence I: Temperature-dependent inhibition of evoked acetylcholine release in tick paralysis. Nature 1976;263:693-695.

47. Bakshi N, Maselli RA, Gospe SM Jr, et al: Fulminant demyelinating neuropathy mimicking cerebral death. Muscle Nerve 1997;20:1595-1597.

48. Bradshaw DY, Jones HR Jr: Pseudomeningoencephalitic presentation of pediatric Guillain-Barré syndrome. J Child Neurol 2001;16:505-508.

49. Geh VS, Bradbury JA: Ocular myasthenia presenting in an 11-month-old boy. Eye 1998;12:319-320.

50. Mullaney P, Vajsar J, Smith R, et al: The natural history and ophthalmic involvement in childhood myasthenia gravis at the Hospital for Sick Children. Ophthalmology 2000;107:504-510.

51. Andrews PI: A treatment algorithm for autoimmune myasthenia gravis in childhood. Ann N Y Acad Sci 1998;841:789-802.

52. Moxley RT III: Channelopathies affecting skeletal muscle: Myotonic disorders including myotonic dystrophy and periodic paralysis. *In* Jones HR Jr, De Vivo DC, Darras BT (eds): Neuromuscular Disorders of Infancy, Childhood, and Adolescence: A Clinician's Approach. Philadelphia, Butterworth Heinemann Health, 2003, pp 783-812.

53. Sheth RD, Pryse-Phillips WE, Riggs JE, et al: Critical illness neuromuscular disease in children manifested as ventilatory dependence. J Pediatr 1995;126:259-261.

54. Bolton CF, Gilbert JJ, Hahn AF, et al: Polyneuropathy in critically ill patients. J Neurol Neurosurg Psychiatry 1984;47:1223-1231.

55. Goulden KJ, Dooley JM, Peters S, et al: Critical illness polyneuropathy: A reversible cause of paralysis in asthmatic children [Abstract]. Ann Neurol 1989;26:451.

56. Lacomis D, Zochodne DW, Bird SJ: Critical illness myopathy. Muscle Nerve 2000;23:1785-1788.

57. Hopkins IJ, Shield LK: Poliomyelitis-like illness associated with asthma in childhood [Letter]. Lancet 1974;1:760.

58. Shapiro GG, Chapman JT, Pierson WE, et al: Poliomyelitis-like illness after acute asthma. J Pediatr 1979;94:767-768.

59. Blomquist HK, Bjorksten B: Poliomyelitis-like illness associated with asthma. Arch Dis Child 1980;55:61-63.

60. Manson JI, Thong YH: Immunological abnormalities in the syndrome of poliomyelitis-like illness associated with acute bronchial asthma (Hopkin's syndrome). Arch Dis Child 1980;55:26-32.

61. Nihei K, Naitoh H, Ikeda K: Poliomyelitis-like syndrome following asthmatic attack (Hopkins syndrome). Pediatr Neurol 1987;3:166-168.

62. Shahar EM, Hwang PA, Niesen CE, et al: Poliomyelitis-like paralysis during recovery from acute bronchial asthma: Possible etiology and risk factors. Pediatrics 1991;88:276-279.

63. Wakamoto H, Morimoto T, Nagao H, et al: MRI in poliomyelitis-like syndrome. Pediatr Radiol 1992;22:533-534.

64. Batley R, Johnson EW: Asthmatic amyotrophy: Three cases. Am J Phys Med Rehabil 1991;70:332-334.

65. Sheth RD, Bolton CF: Neuromuscular complications of sepsis in children. J Child Neurol 1995;10:346-352.

66. Liedholm LJ, Eeg-Olofsson O, Ekenberg BE, et al: Acute postasthmatic amyotrophy (Hopkins' syndrome). Muscle Nerve 1994;17:769-772.

67. Hayward JC, Gillespie SM, Kaplan KM, et al: Outbreak of poliomyelitis-like paralysis associated with enterovirus 71. Pediatr Infect Dis J 1989;8:611-616.

68. Kyllerman MG, Herner S, Bergstrom TB, et al: PCR diagnosis of primary herpesvirus type I in poliomyelitis-like paralysis and respiratory tract disease. Pediatr Neurol 1993;9:227-229.

69. Bolton CF, Laverty DA, Brown JD, et al: Critically ill polyneuropathy: Electrophysiological studies and differentiation from Guillain-Barré syndrome. J Neurol Neurosurg Psychiatry 1986;49:563-573.

70. Gutmann L: Critical illness neuropathy and myopathy. Arch Neurol 1999;56:527-528.

71. Hart DE, Rojas LA, Rosario JA, et al: Childhood Guillain-Barré syndrome in Paraguay, 1990 to 1991. Ann Neurol 1994;36:859-863.

72. O'Connor M, Russell WJ: Muscle strength following anaesthesia with atracurium and pancuronium. Anaesth Intensive Care 1988;16:255-259.

73. Partridge BL, Abrams JH, Bazemore C, et al: Prolonged neuromuscular blockade after long-term infusion of vecuronium bromide in the intensive care unit. Crit Care Med 1990;18:1177-1179.

74. Segredo V, Caldwell JE, Matthay MA, et al: Persistent paralysis in critically ill patients after long-term administration of vecuronium. N Engl J Med 1992;327:524-528.

75. Bird SJ, Rich MM: Neuromuscular complications of critical illness. Neurologist 2000;6:2-11.

76. MacFarlane IA, Rosenthal FD: Severe myopathy after status asthmaticus. Lancet 1977;2:615.

77. Rich MM, Bird SJ, Raps EC, et al: Direct muscle stimulation in acute quadriplegic myopathy. Muscle Nerve 1997;20:665-673.

78. Showalter CJ, Engel AG: Acute quadriplegic myopathy: Analysis of myosin isoforms and evidence for calpain-mediated proteolysis. Muscle Nerve 1997;20:316-322.

79. Latronico N, Fenzi F, Recupero D, et al: Critical illness myopathy and neuropathy. Lancet 1996;347:1579-1582.

80. Perea M, Picon M, Miro O, et al: Acute quadriplegic myopathy with loss of thick (myosin) filaments following heart transplantation. J Heart Lung Transplant 2001;20:1136-1141.

81. Banwell BL, Mildner RJ, Hassall AC, et al: Muscle weakness in critically ill children. Neurology 2003;61:1779-1782.

82. Lacomis D, Petrella JT, Giuliani MJ: Causes of neuromuscular weakness in the intensive care unit: A study of ninety-two patients. Muscle Nerve 1998;21:610-617.

83. Lacomis D, Giuliani MJ, Van Cott A, et al: Acute myopathy of intensive care: Clinical, electromyographic, and pathological aspects. Ann Neurol 1996;40:645-654.

84. Sander HW, Golden M, Danon MJ: Quadriplegic areflexic ICU illness: Selective thick filament loss and normal nerve histology. Muscle Nerve 2002;26:499-505.

85. Zochodne DW, Ramsay DA, Saly V, et al: Acute necrotizing myopathy of intensive care: Electrophysiological studies. Muscle Nerve 1994;17:285-292.

86. Primavera A, Abbruzzese M: Case 11-1997: Critical-illness myopathy. N Engl J Med 1997;337:862-863.

87. Rich MM, Teener JW, Raps EC, et al: Muscle is electrically inexcitable in acute quadriplegic myopathy. Neurology 1996;46:731-736.

88. Salviati L, Laverda AM, Zancan L, et al: Acute quadriplegic myopathy in a 17-month-old boy. J Child Neurol 2000;15:63-66.

89. Tabarki B, Coffinieres A, Van Den Bergh P, et al: Critical illness neuromuscular disease: Clinical, electrophysiological, and prognostic aspects. Arch Dis Child 2002;86:103-107.

90. Di Giovanni S, Mirabella M, D'Amico A, et al: Apoptotic features accompany acute quadriplegic myopathy. Neurology 2000;55:854-858.

91. Ruff RL: Why do ICU patients become paralyzed? Ann Neurol 1998;43:154-155.

92. Lannigan R, Austin TW, Vestrup J: Myositis and rhabdomyolysis due to *Staphylococcus aureus* septicemia. J Infect Dis 1984;150:784.

93. Jones HR Jr, Darras BT: Acute care pediatric electromyography. Muscle Nerve 2000;23(Suppl):S53-S62.

94. Picton TW, Taylor MJ, Durieux-Smith A: Brainstem auditory evoked potentials in infants and children. *In* Aminoff MJ (ed): Electrodiagnosis in Clinical Neurology, 4th ed. Philadelphia, Churchill-Livingstone, 1999, pp 485-511.

95. Zifko U, Remtulla H, Power K, et al: Transcortical and cervical magnetic stimulation with recording of the diaphragm. Muscle Nerve 1996;19:614-620.

96. Zifko UA, Young BG, Remtulla H, et al: Somatosensory evoked potentials of the phrenic nerve. Muscle Nerve 1995;18:1487-1489.

97. Chen R, Collins S, Remtulla H, et al: Phrenic nerve conduction study in normal subjects. Muscle Nerve 1995;18:330-335.

98. Zifko U, Nicolle MW, Remtulla H, et al: Repetitive phrenic nerve stimulation study in normal subjects. J Clin Neurophysiol 1997;14:235-241.

99. Bolton CF, Grand'Maison F, Parkes A, et al: Needle electromyography of the diaphragm. Muscle Nerve 1992;15:678-681.

100. Collins SJ, Chen RE, Remtulla H, et al: Novel measurement for automated interference pattern analysis of the diaphragm. Muscle Nerve 1997;20:1038-1040.

101. Chen R, Collins SJ, Remtulla H, et al: Needle EMG of the human diaphragm: Power spectral analysis in normal subjects. Muscle Nerve 1996;19:324-330.

102. Kimura J: Techniques of repetitive stimulation. *In* Kimura J (ed): Electrodiagnosis in Diseases of Nerve and Muscle: Principles and Practice, 2nd ed. Philadelphia, FA Davis, 1989, pp 257-278.

103. Schwartz J, Planek J, Briegel I, et al: Single fiber electromyography, nerve conduction studies, and conventional electromyography in patients with critical illness polyneuropathy: Evidence for a lesion of terminal axons. Muscle Nerve 1997;20:696-701.

104. Bolton CF, Parkes A, Thompson TR, et al: Recording sound from human skeletal muscle: Technical and physiological aspects. Muscle Nerve 1989;12:126-134.

38

The Interrelation of DNA Analysis with Clinical Neurophysiology in the Diagnosis of Chronic Neuromuscular Disorder of Childhood

BASIL T. DARRAS AND H. ROYDEN JONES, JR.

The rapidly evolving genetic discoveries vis-à-vis the molecular pathogenesis of many neuromuscular disorders have led to a major diagnostic expansion and sometimes a concomitant reclassification of these various pathophysiologic entities, especially those having a slowly ingravescent, chronic clinical presentation with symmetric and proximal muscle weakness. An increasing number of more chronic pediatric motor unit disorders are now diagnosable using a number of genetic DNA and neuroimmunologic modalities. These particularly include well-known myopathies such as Duchenne's dystrophy, as well as the spinal muscular atrophies (SMAs), increasingly some of the polyneuropathies; lastly, one can anticipate similar modalities for diagnosing the rare congenital neuromuscular transmission disorders (NMTDs). The current diagnostic approaches to the more common childhood neuromuscular diseases are discussed in the chapter, emphasizing the importance of newer nonneurophysiologic diagnostic techniques that in some instances make electromyography (EMG) unnecessary.

Our current laboratory diagnostic approach to more common pediatric neuromuscular disorders seen at Children's Hospital Boston (CHB) emphasizes the importance of DNA analyses. These many genetic tests currently available, are defined relative to the appropriate timing of pediatric nerve conduction studies (NCSs), needle EMG, as well as muscle biopsy. Certain major genetic discoveries now provide the primary means for diagnosis. This particularly includes dystrophin assessment for Duchenne's (DMD) or Becker's muscular dystrophy (BMD) and often survival motor neuron (SMN) DNA analysis, when there is a significant clinical suspicion of an SMA.[1] DNA testing via polymerase chain reaction (PCR)/Southern blot assay is one of the primary studies. Similarly standard muscle biopsy is enhanced by using immunohistochemistry and Western blot assay with antibodies against various muscle proteins. Therefore, an EMG is no longer used in the evaluation of a young boy with a Duchenne/Becker phenotype. Similarly these are much less commonly required to diagnose SMA, although there are clinical settings wherein the concomitant use of both studies is warranted.

Currently we still use EMG for the initial evaluation of certain polyneuropathies. For those children having a suspected hereditary neuropathy, such as the Charcot-Marie-Tooth (CMT) phenotype, EMG is the preferred initial study to identify whether the primary pathophysiologic mechanism is demyelinating, such as in CMT-1a, where DNA analysis is available, or axonal, where few specific genetic defects are identified. This is also particularly relevant in babies where genetic analysis has failed to confirm a diagnosis (as in suspected SMA) and the infant may have a congenital polyneuropathy, or more likely a myopathy where a muscle biopsy is necessary for diagnosis. EMG is almost essential for diagnosis of Guillain-Barré syndrome (GBS) or chronic inflammatory demyelinating poly-neuropathy (CIDP). Similarly with certain pediatric NMTDs, particularly infantile botulism, EMG is the primary means for early diagnosis, although stool culture may eventually provide a specific diagnosis. When the diagnosis of myasthenia gravis (MG) is not of the essence, anti-acetylcholine receptor antibody testing is the most accurate means in both infants and children. These studies allow one to confirm the presumed clinical diagnosis accurately and less invasively than standard NCS/EMG. However, repetitive motor nerve stimulation (RMNS) is still an effective means to confirm a clinical diagnosis of MG or, as noted, with infantile botulism. Engel anticipates that specific DNA testing will soon become available to provide a diagnostic means for some of the various con-genital NMTDs.[2] The role of magnetic resonance imaging (MRI) for the evaluation of inflammatory myopathies rather than muscle biopsy or EMG is still being evaluated.

Although genetic DNA testing is highly effective, it has added another level of complexity to an already complex diagnostic field (Table 38-1). As a consequence this has left a number of neurologists uncertain about the indications for invasive procedures, especially EMG; this is par-ticularly relevant in the practice of child neurology. This chapter reviews the state of the art for selecting the appropriate studies in a child presenting with a chronic neuromuscular disorder. It is always important to consider the entire motor unit when evaluating any child with proximal weakness; therefore, this chapter is organized in a traditional anatomic fashion, looking at each major division of the peripheral motor unit from the motor neuron to the skeletal muscle cell.

ANTERIOR HORN CELL

SMA Werdnig-Hoffman disease (SMA-1) and SMA-2 typically present as a floppy baby either close to birth or by 6 to 12 months of age. In most infants with SMA-1 or SMA-2, the clinical presentation is stereotyped and the diagnosis can easily be confirmed by DNA analysis. This therefore obviates the need for an EMG and/or muscle biopsy. Both SMA-1 and SMA-2, as well as SMA-3, share the same genetic defect on chromosome 5q11-13. The PCR test looks for deletion of exons 7 and 8 of the *SMN* gene on chromosome 5q11-13.[1] In each of the three SMA phenotypes, this clinically available DNA test is the diag-nostic tool of choice as outlined in detail in Chapter 30.

Sometimes, although clinically seemingly apparent, an SMA diagnosis needs to be confirmed rapidly because the

infant is in distress and decisions surrounding the need for early diagnosis and thus issues of ongoing respiratory support are raised by our colleagues. Generally when this occurs with infants, it is in the setting of a failure to wean after an episode of bronchiolitis and for the first time it is recognized that the baby is very hypotonic.

Because EMG is also very accurate for making an SMA diagnosis,[3] we are still asked to perform an EMG in some of these hypotonic infants pending the DNA results. EMG also provides supportive diagnostic value in this setting. When this study defines a primary motor neuron disorder, such results provide the infant's clinician with a preliminary and accurate test, which, in combination with DNA testing, will reassure parents that two accurate tests have con-firmed the sad prognosis that an SMA diagnosis implies.

Finally, in the atypical cases of hypotonic infants, when DNA testing has not confirmed the presumed clinical diag-nosis of SMA, an EMG is performed to establish where in the peripheral motor unit the responsible lesion has occurred (Table 38-1). The EMG findings are well delin-eated in typical SMA. Classically the major finding is a marked diminution in the number of motor unit potentials (MUPs) recruited. These MUPs typically have a longer duration and occasionally a higher amplitude than normal. Concomitantly one finds profuse fibrillation potentials. No other disorders in this age group have these EMG characteristics unless the baby has had the rare infantile poliomyelitis, and here the findings are usually rather asymmetric in contrast to the more symmetric results in SMA. To date we are unaware of EMG findings in West Nile virus infections of children, although the adult counterparts are similar to those of poliomyelitis.[4]

Muscle biopsy is usually not needed. During the last 8 years, we have performed only a single muscle biopsy in a floppy infant with a typical SMA-like EMG and twice-negative DNA testing; the muscle biopsy showed typical small- and large-group atrophy, supporting the diagnosis of SMA. This baby might have had a nonchromosome 5 SMA or a mutation(s) in the *SMN* gene not detectable with the currently used PCR-based methodology.

With the older child or adolescent one may delineate the findings of SMA-3 in the EMG laboratory when inves-tigating a youngster with an indeterminate proximal weak-ness. In contrast to the babies with SMA-1 and SMA-2, Kugelberg-Welander disease (SMA-3) presents between ages 2 and 14 years with proximal weakness and modest creatine phosphokinase (CPK) elevation (<1000 IU/L). However, occasionally these children present to the EMG laboratory prior to having made the diagnosis of SMA. Here the findings are more chronic, and although the motor unit changes are similar to those of SMA-1 and SMA-2, one does not find the signs of active denervation.

Thus EMG continues to prove of value in some clinical

TABLE 38–1. RECOMMENDED APPROACH TO CHILDHOOD NEUROMUSCULAR DISORDERS

	Diagnostic Test or Procedure		
Suspected Clinical Diagnosis	*First Option*	*Second Option*	*Third Option*
Duchenne/Becker MD	DNA	MBx	
LGMDs	DNA°	MBx	EMG/NCS†
Congenital muscular dystrophies	MBx	DNA	EMG/NCS†
Emery-Dreifuss MD	DNA	MBx	EMG/NCS†
FSH MD	DNA	MBx	EMG/NCS‡
MyD	DNA	EMG/NCS	
Periodic paralysis/myotonias	DNA	EMG/NCS	
Metabolic	MBx	DNA	EMG/NCS‡
Congenital myopathies	MBx	DNA§	EMG/NCS¶¶
DM/PM	MRI	MBx	EMG/NCS‡
Indeterminate proximal weakness	EMG/NCS	RMNS	MBx/DNA
SMA	DNA	EMG/NCS	MBx¶
CIDP	EMG/NCS	CSF	NBx
CMT phenotypes	EMG/NCS	DNA	
Neuromuscular transmission disorders	EMG/NCS	RMNS	Antibodies/DNA°°

° To exclude DMD/BMD (if positive).
† In atypical, sporadic cases with low CK values.
§ If available.
¶ If EMG/NCS consistent with SMA but DNA test is negative.
¶¶ In certain cases, EMG/NCS may be the first option.
°° For congenital myasthenic syndromes.
‡ Optional.
DNA, DNA/genetic testing; MBx, muscle biopsy; NBx, nerve biopsy; EMG, electromyography; NCS, nerve conduction study; MRI, magnetic resonance imaging; RMNS, repetitive motor nerve stimulation; MD, muscular dystrophy; LGMD, limb-girdle muscular dystrophy; FSH, facioscapulohumeral; MyD, myotonic dystrophy; DM/PM, dermatomyositis/polymyositis; SMA, spinal muscular atrophy; CIDP, chronic inflammatory demyelinating polyneuropathy; GBS, Guillain-Barré syndrome; AIDP, acute inflammatory demyelinating polyneuropathy; CSF, cerebrospinal fluid; CMTs, Charcot-Marie-Tooth phenotypes (hereditary motor and sensory neuropathies); DMD, Duchenne's muscular dystrophy; BMD, Becker's muscular dystrophy.
Modified from Darras BT, Jones HR Jr: Diagnosis of pediatric neuromuscular disorders in the era of DNA analysis. Pediatr Neurol 2000;23:289-300.

settings wherein SMA enters the differential diagnosis. DNA testing is indeed the study of choice here; however, EMG maintains its diagnostic value, although in a more supplementary fashion, today.

PERIPHERAL NERVE

Chronic Inflammatory Demyelinating Polyneuropathy

Occasionally a child with CIDP presents with a slowly evolving painless proximal and/or distal weakness that is often initially thought to be compatible with a dystrophy or other myopathy. In contrast with most primary myopathies, however, the muscle stretch reflexes are usually diminished or absent. This neurologic finding is the best clinical clue to the diagnosis of CIDP in a child with slowly evolving proximal weakness, particularly one having normal serum creatine kinase (CK) values. In CIDP, the cerebrospinal fluid is usually acellular and the cerebrospinal fluid protein is significantly elevated in about 90% of the cases. There appears to be little additional diagnostic value from performing a sural nerve biopsy in children with CIDP.[5]

An EMG is the primary testing modality leading to a diagnosis of CIDP. It is important to perform with the slightest consideration because often this diagnosis may not be clinically suspected. Typically, NCS performed in children with this inflammatory demyelinating polyneuropathy, as well as GBS, demonstrate pronounced slowing of conduction velocity. Normally motor NCSs are 50 to 70 m/sec in healthy children 3 years of age and older versus 15 to 35 m/sec in those affected with either CIDP or GBS. Additionally, distal latencies are usually prolonged, and the compound muscle action potentials (CMAPs) are dispersed, sometimes associated with evidence of conduction block, prolongation of latencies of F and H waves, or absent F waves. These EMG/NCS findings are often asymmetric in distribution. These findings are quite distinct and serve to differentiate these inflammatory neuropathies from a myopathy (Fig 38-1). It is important to recognize CIDP because this polyneuropathy usually responds well to treatment with intravenous immunoglobulin and/or corticosteroids.

Hereditary Motor Sensory Polyneuropathies

Currently, most hereditary motor sensory neuropathies are classified genetically. In a substantial number of children,

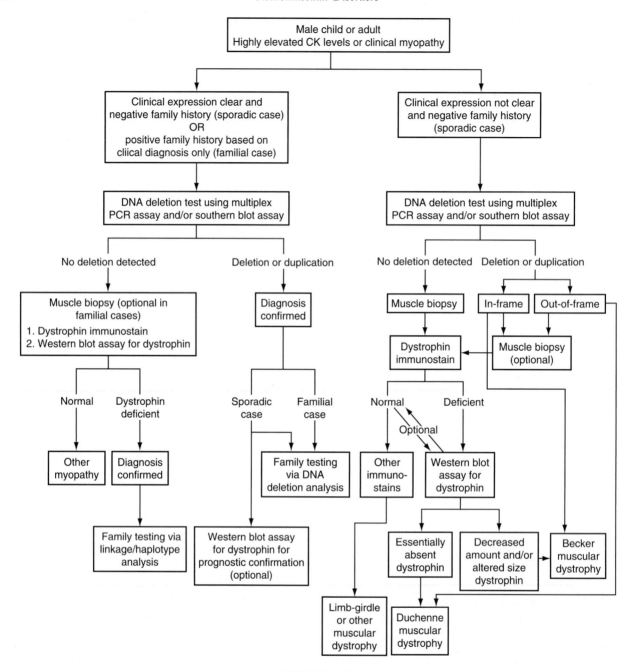

FIGURE 38–1

Algorithm for molecular diagnosis of Duchenne's and Becker's muscular dystrophy. The diagnosis can be confirmed in most patients by DNA deletion analysis; a muscle biopsy is optional if the in-frame, out-of-frame status of the deletion is known and also in familial cases. CK, creatine kinase; PCR, polymerase chain reaction. (From Darras BT, Menache CC, Kunkel LM: Dystrophinopathies. In Jones HR Jr, De Vivo DC, Darras BT [eds]: Neuromuscular Disorders of Infancy, Childhood, and Adolescence: A Clinician's Approach. Philadelphia, Butterworth Heinemann Health, 2003, pp 649-699.)

one has available DNA testing. CMT-1 is a demyelinating polyneuropathy inherited as an autosomal dominant disorder. The main subtypes of CMT-1 are CMT-1A (chromosome 17p11-12, *PMP22* gene duplication), CMT-1B (chromosome 1q22-23, *Po* gene), CMT-1C (unknown chromosome and causal gene), and CMT-X1 (chromosome Xq13, *connexin 32* gene). CMT-2 (hereditary motor sensory neuropathy type 2) is an axonal form of neuropathy with five known genetic subtypes but unknown genes. There are autosomal dominant and autosomal recessive forms of CMT-3 (Dejerine-Sottas disease); some of the autosomal dominant cases are related to mutations in the *PMP22* (CMT-1A) and *Po* (CMT-1B) genes.

Currently it is primarily the demyelinating CMT-1A, CMT-1B, and CMT-X1 subtypes and a proportion of CMT-3 cases that can be tested genetically. Only a few of the uncommon axonal forms (CMT-2) have any precise DNA testing available. Therefore, given the substantial expense of the genetic tests and the reliability of EMG in classifying the disease as either a demyelinating or axonal variant, we prefer to confirm the diagnosis of CMT-1a first by classifying it by EMG. We then proceed with genetic testing if the electrophysiologic findings support the diagnosis of a demyelinative form of CMT (see Table 38-1). In axonal CMT disease the genetic testing may be negative in many cases because commercially available DNA tests for the most common axonal types are not yet available.

NEUROMUSCULAR TRANSMISSION DEFECTS

One has to always be aware of the syndrome of infantile botulism, a presynaptic defect of neuromuscular transmission. This illness typically affects infants between ages 10 days and 6 months. The presentation is one of acute generalized hypotonia, difficulty in eating, and constipation. Infantile botulism also needs consideration in any infant up to 6 months old presenting with unexplained respiratory distress. In its most severe state, the presentation may be acute and require ventilatory support. Bacteriologic confirmation requires a few weeks; however, confirmation of the diagnosis of infantile botulism can be made in a few days by a direct in vivo assay of botulinum toxin from the stool. EMG and NCS are the most useful early diagnostic tools. Most babies with infantile botulism have clear-cut evidence of an NMTD. The primary EMG/NCS abnormalities with infantile botulism are low-amplitude CMAPs with at least a 25% and often greater than 100% post-tetanic facilitation.

Congenital myasthenic syndromes can be classified according to the site of the defect, that is, presynaptic, synaptic, postsynaptic, and mixed.[2] These usually present during infancy with generalized hypotonia and fluctuating weakness, weak cry and suck, respiratory distress, apnea, and feeding difficulties. During late infancy and childhood, fluctuating ptosis, ophthalmoparesis, and abnormal fatigability with exertion are typical presentations. The tests for anti-acetylcholine receptor antibodies are negative. The diagnosis is based on clinical history and examination, family history (if present), EMG findings, edrophonium (Tensilon) test, and the clinical response to acetylcholinesterase inhibitors. The results of edrophonium testing are positive in most types

of congenital myasthenic syndromes, except in acetylcholinesterase deficiency and in the classic slow-channel syndrome. During motor NCS, these latter two disorders characteristically demonstrate repetitive CMAPs after a single stimulus. In most children in addition to detailed EMG studies, in vitro microphysiologic, ultrastructural, and histochemical studies of intercostal muscle biopsies are required to establish these various diagnoses.

The child with acquired MG may present with acute generalized weakness, bulbar weakness, and/or ocular findings (ptosis, ophthalmoparesis) (see Chapter 35). The NMTD is at a postsynaptic location. In children MG most often occurs in the juvenile age group, but occasionally MG may begin in the preschool child. The youngest child we have seen was 15 months old. Isolated proximal weakness is rarely a primary presenting feature of MG.

Although Lambert-Eaton myasthenic syndrome (LEMS) is extremely uncommon in childhood, a few well-documented cases of this presynaptic NMTD are documented.[6-8] Two presented with isolated proximal muscle weakness and were initially not clinically thought to have LEMS. However, careful EMG demonstrated not only a decremental defect in NMT at rest, but with exercise or high-frequency repetitive stimulation, the classic and diagnostic finding of a greater than 200% facilitation of the CMAP is observed. Because LEMS responds to corticosteroid therapy, it is important to use an EMG to identify the rare child whose proximal weakness may represent the presenting symptom of this almost unique pediatric defect in neuromuscular transmission.

MYOPATHIES

Myopathy is a term that covers the entire spectrum of primary disorders of skeletal muscle. Infants typically present with generalized weakness and/or hypotonia, with or without suppression of muscle stretch reflexes, and quite uncommonly with respiratory and feeding difficulties, mild dysmorphology, and/or contractures. Older children have a more varied presentation with a primary proximal, distal, generalized, or focal weakness. Concomitant fatigability, periodic paralysis, myotonia, intermittent weakness with or without muscle aches, or myoglobinuria are common accompaniments.

Until the mid-1980s, it was typical for a child with a suspected myopathy usually to have had a tripartite laboratory investigation sequentially, including (1) serum enzymes (e.g., CPK, aldolase), (2) EMG, and (3) muscle biopsy. The EMG was usually performed prior to proceeding with a muscle biopsy. At that time, although we appreciated that muscular dystrophies are genetically determined conditions, with well-established modes of inheritance, their precise chromosomal localization and the specific affected genes were just beginning to be identified. Subsequently, specific clinically available DNA tests have been isolated in rapid succession beginning with the dystrophin gene.[9] During recent decades, more and more genes have been identified with the concomitant development of specific DNA testing modalities.[10] Therefore, both EMG and muscle biopsy are infrequently used, particularly in the evaluation of any infant or child presenting with the typical phenotype of Duchenne's or Becker's dystrophy. Instead, a simple dystrophin algorithm is now available. When one is unable to successfully identify a precise myopathy with today's many standard DNA studies, as outlined in the subsequent portions of this chapter, additional motor unit loci differential diagnostic considerations are considered. Many, including SMA, CIDP, CMT, and the rare NMJ disorders, still require an EMG for appropriate diagnosis as outlined earlier in this chapter. Although SMA is also now diagnosable by DNA testing, it is occasionally not clinically suspected until an EMG is actually performed.

Duchenne's and Becker's Muscular Dystrophies

Recognizing that the Duchenne gene was on the X chromosome, a linkage was identified between a polymorphic DNA marker (known as RC8) and the *DMD* gene in 1983. This was one of the first genes to be linked to a restriction fragment length polymorphism. Since the DNA marker was in the middle of the short arm of the X chromosome, in a position referred to as *Xp21*, the gene for DMD was mapped within that area. Similarly the *BMD* gene was also mapped to the same locus, suggesting that *DMD* and *BMD* were either closely linked to each other or possibly allelic. A few years later, in 1986, the *DMD-BMD* gene was isolated by Kunkel's group at CHB,[9] and within another year the protein product, named *dystrophin*, was characterized.[9] Further basic research introduced Southern and Western blot methodology and later the PCR as new tools for diagnosis of these two most common dystrophinopathies, DMD and BMD.[10-12]

When "molecular" DNA methods for the diagnosis of dystrophinopathies became available, pediatric EMG was no longer necessary in the evaluation of children with possible DMD/BMD. Some pediatric neurologists recommend an EMG for the so-called atypical phenotypes. However, atypical presentations of DMD/BMD are extremely rare.[13] Children with probable DMD/BMD usually present with proximal weakness, lordosis, and pseudohypertrophy of the calves and with markedly elevated serum CPK levels (in the thousands). In this clinical setting, as shown in the proposed algorithm (see Fig. 38-1), we initially perform a DNA deletion test and in some instances, but not always, a muscle

biopsy (see Table 38-1). A deletion is detected in about 65% of males with DMD and 80% of males with BMD and confirms the diagnosis.[14] Intragenic duplications account for about 6% of cases[10,15]; in the remaining children the molecular lesions leading to DMD or BMD are point mutations or splicing errors, which are not detectable with the currently used PCR and/or Southern blot techniques. Analysis of nondeletion mutations is available only on a research basis. Many believe that a muscle biopsy is not needed if the PCR DNA test is positive for a deletion, especially if the in-frame/out-of-frame status of the deletion is known[16]; also, a muscle biopsy is optional in familial cases and in patients with an obvious phenotype.[10] When the DNA analysis is negative in a child with probable dystrophinopathy and negative family history, one then will need to proceed to a muscle biopsy; the tissue can be immunostained specifically for the presence or absence of dystrophin[17] and be used for dystrophin quantitation via Western blot analysis (see Fig. 38-1).

Patients with DMD have less than 5% of the normal quantity of dystrophin. Patients with dystrophin levels between 5% and 20% of normal, regardless of protein size, seem to develop an intermediate phenotype (mild DMD or severe BMD).[18] Children and adolescents with mild to moderate BMD usually have levels above 20%; in 80% of BMD cases the dystrophin protein molecule is decreased in size (truncated). EMG may still be necessary for patients with probable BMD whose CPK values are less than 1000 IU/L to differentiate from neuropathic causes of proximal weakness (e.g., SMA-3 or other rare denervating conditions) with mild to moderate elevations in CPK levels (usually < 1000 IU/L).

Limb-Girdle Muscular Dystrophies

Limb-girdle muscular dystrophies (LGMDs) may be either autosomal recessive or autosomal dominant (Table 38-2).[19] Most autosomal recessive cases have earlier onset, rapid progression, and relatively high CPK values. Children with autosomal recessive LGMDs may be clinically indistinguishable from those with DMD or BMD. However, in contrast with DMD, cognitive function is normal in patients with these dystrophies (e.g., sarcoglycanopathies). If the CPK is more than 1000 IU/L in a child with a myopathic phenotype, thus making other nonmyopathic motor unit disorders less likely (e.g., SMA), we next proceed to a dystrophin DNA test (see Table 38-1); given that this test is positive in 65% to 80% but not all DMD/BMD cases, a dystrophinopathy is not excluded.

Muscle biopsy is the next appropriate diagnostic procedure. Immunohistochemistry, with antibodies against sarcoglycans, dystrophin, dystroglycans, and merosin, may then provide a means for a specific biopsy diagnosis (e.g. alpha-sarcoglycanopathy), but this is not invariable. If the biopsy

TABLE 38–2. LIMB-GIRDLE MUSCULAR DYSTROPHIES

Gene	Gene Location	Protein	Type of Heredity
LGMD-1A	5q31	Myotilin	AD
LGMD-1B	1q11-q21	Lamin A/C	AD
LGMD-1C	3p25	Caveolin-3	AD
LGMD-1D	6q23	?	AD
LGMD-1E	7q	?	AD
LGMD-2A	15q15	Calpain-3	AR
LGMD-2B	2p13	Dysferlin	AR
LGMD-2C	13q12	γ-sarcoglycan	AR
LGMD-2D	17q12	α-sarcoglycan	AR
LGMD-2E	4q12	β-sarcoglycan	AR
LGMD-2F	5q33-q34	δ-sarcoglycan	AR
LGMD-2G	17q11-q12	Telethonin	AR
LGMD-2H	9q31-q34.1	TRIM32	AR
LGMD-2I	19q13.3	FKRP	AR
LGMD-2J	2q31	Titin	AR

LGMD, limb-girdle muscular dystrophy; AD, autosomal dominant; AR, autosomal recessive; FKRP, fukutin-related protein; TRIM32, tripartite motif-containing protein.
Modified from Darras BT, Jones HR Jr: Diagnosis of pediatric neuromuscular disorders in the era of DNA analysis. Pediatr Neurol 2000;23:289-300.

suggests a myopathic process but DNA testing and immunohistochemistry for all of the just-mentioned proteins is normal, then certain less common testing may need to be pursued in selected research laboratories. Currently these include calpain-3 (LGMD-2A),[20] dysferlin (LGMD-2B),[21,22] telethonin (LGMD-2G),[23] TRIM32 (LGMD-2H),[24] fukutin-related protein (LGMD-2I),[25] and titin (LGMD-2J).[26]

The autosomal dominant LGMD patients usually have a later age at onset and a more ingravescent clinical progression. The CPK values in these individuals may not be as significantly elevated. However, in LGMD-1C, related to caveolin mutations,[27] CPK values are elevated 4-fold to 25-fold, and the clinical onset of this form of LGMD may begin in childhood. When such is clinically suspected, DNA testing for caveolin mutations is currently available only in the research setting.[28] Some sporadic dominant cases, and even autosomal recessive ones with modest CPK elevation, may be clinically indistinguishable from SMA-3, the Kugelberg-Welander form. Because SMA-3 may also have a modest CPK elevation (<1000 IU/L), an EMG is particularly useful in this setting for differentiating a neurogenic from a myopathic process. This offers the means to decide whether to proceed with DNA testing for SMA or a muscle biopsy for a potential myopathy (see Table 38-1).

Congenital Muscular Dystrophies

Infants with congenital muscular dystrophy (CMD) present in the newborn period as floppy babies, often with arthrogryposis, clinically not unlike infants with a severe

---

BOX 38-1
CLASSIFICATION OF CONGENITAL MUSCULAR DYSTROPHIES (CMD)*

1. Classical CMD
2. Merosin-deficient CMD
   a. Primary merosin deficiency
   b. Secondary merosin deficiency
3. Merosin-positive CMD
   a. Classic CMD without distinguishing features
   b. Rigid spine syndrome
   c. CMD with distal hyperextensibility (Ullrich type)
   d. CMD with mental retardation or sensory abnormalities
4. CMD with central nervous system abnormalities
   a. Fukuyama's CMD
   b. Muscle-eye-brain disease
   c. Walker-Warburg syndrome

* See Table 38-3 for genetic loci based on the categories in this list.
From Jones K, North K: Congenital muscular dystrophies. *In* Jones HR Jr, De Vivo DC, Darras BT (eds): Neuromuscular Disorders of Infancy, Childhood, and Adolescence: A Clinician's Approach. Philadelphia, Butterworth Heinemann Health, 2003, pp 633-647.

congenital myopathy. However in contrast with the congenital myopathies, some but not all of these uncommon CMD babies have variably elevated serum CK levels. The classification of CMDs is shown in Box 38-1. To date, a laminin-alpha2 (merosin)[29,30] (in the chromosome 6q22 form of CMD), fukutin (in Fukuyama's CMD),[31,32] and other genetic defects are delineated in a substantial subset of these patients (Table 38-3). Box 38-2 shows a recent biochemical classification of CMDs. Unfortunately, commercial DNA testing for merosin, fukutin, or other gene mutations is not available at the moment.

Therefore EMG is still performed in this subset. The MUPs are of short duration and low amplitude, and usually there are no abnormalities on insertion. As with the various congenital myopathies, the diagnosis is made by muscle biopsy, which shows widespread dystrophic changes. Merosin-negative cases shows no merosin in the sarcolemma of the muscle fibers with muscle immunostaining using antimerosin antibodies. In the CMDs with structural central nervous system anomalies, and also muscular dystrophy, congenital (MDC)-1C and MDC-1D, immunostaining with anti-alpha-dystroglycan monoclonal antibodies (VIA4-1) has evolved into a useful diagnostic marker.

TABLE 38–3. GENETIC LOCI FOR CONGENITAL MUSCULAR DYSTROPHIES (CMD) IDENTIFIED TO DATE

Disease*	Mode of Inheritance	Gene Location	Symbol (Gene Product)
1. Classic CMD			
a. Primary merosin deficiency (MDC1A)	AR	6q2	LAMA2 (laminin-alpha2 chain of merosin)
b. Secondary merosin deficiency (MDC1B)	AR	1q42	?
c. Secondary merosin deficiency (MDC1C)	AR	19q13.3	FKRP (fukutin-related protein)
d. Merosin (+): Rigid spine syndrome	AR	1p35-36	RSMD1 (selenoprotein N)
e. Merosin (+): Ullrich muscular dystrophy	AR	21q22.3	COL6 A$\frac{1}{2}$ (collagen VI-alpha $\frac{1}{2}$ chain)
	AR	2q37	COL6A3 (collagen VI-alpha3 chain)
2. CMD with CNS abnormalities			
a. Fukuyama CMD	AR	9q31-33	FCMD (fukutin)
b. Muscle-eye-brain disease	AR	1p32-p34	POMGnT1 (glycosyltransferase)
c. Walker-Warburg syndrome	AR	9q34.1	POMT1 (mannosyltransferase)

* See Box 38-1 for a summary of the classification of CMD as detailed in this column.
  AR, autosomal recessive; CMD, congenital muscular dystrophy; CNS, central nervous system.
  Modified from Jones K, North K: Congenital muscular dystrophies. *In* Jones HR Jr, De Vivo DC, Darras BT (eds): Neuromuscular Disorders of Infancy, Childhood, and Adolescence: A Clinician's Approach. Philadelphia, Butterworth Heinemann Health, 2003, pp 633-647.

BOX 38-2
BIOCHEMICAL CLASSIFICATION OF CONGENITAL MUSCULAR DYSTROPHIES (CMDs)

Conditions affecting the endoplasmic reticulum
  SEPN1 (RSMD1)
Conditions involving the extracellular matrix
  Laminin alpha-2 (MDC-1A)
  Integrin alpha-7 (CMD)
  Collagen VI (Ullrich syndrome)
Conditions affecting the glycosylation of proteins
  Fukutin (FCMD)
  FKRP (MDC-1C)
  Large (MDC-1D)
  POMT1 (WWS)
  POMGnT1 (MEB)

SEPN1, selenoprotein N1; RSMD1, rigid spine syndrome 1; MDC, muscular dystrophy, congenital; CMD, congenital muscular dystrophy; FCMD, Fukuyama's congenital muscular dystrophy; FKRP, fukutin-related protein; WWS, Walker-Warburg syndrome; MEB, muscle-eye-brain disease.

Emery-Dreifuss Muscular Dystrophy

Emery-Dreifuss muscular dystrophy (EDMD) is an X-linked recessive (chromosome Xq28), autosomal dominant, or autosomal recessive condition (chromosome 1q21) with onset in late childhood or adult life.[33-37] EDMD is characterized by humeroperoneal distribution of muscle weakness typically associated with fixed contractures (particularly at the elbows, neck), cardiac arrhythmias, and slowly progressive clinical course. Mutations in the *emerin* (Xq28)[37] and *lamin A/C* genes (1q21)[34,38] are responsible for the EDMD form of muscular dystrophy. In the X-linked variety of EDMD, DNA testing for *emerin* gene mutations is now clinically available. Therefore, EMG is not required when this type of dystrophy is suspected and the appropriate DNA test is positive.

EMG may confirm the myopathic nature of the process in both the autosomal and X-linked sporadic cases of EDMD where there are relatively low CPK values and negative family history. Recently, DNA testing for the *lamin A/C* gene mutations has become commercially available also. Therefore, muscle biopsy in EDMD is unnecessary if the mutation analysis is positive for an *emerin* or *lamin A/C* mutation. However, a muscle biopsy can provide further evidence for the diagnosis of X-linked EDMD by demonstrating (via immunohistochemistry) an absence of nuclear immunostaining for *emerin* (see Table 38-1). Furthermore, as with EMG, a muscle biopsy may confirm the myopathic nature of the process in atypical, sporadic cases or in rare cases without detectable mutations.

Facioscapulohumeral Dystrophy

Facioscapulohumeral (FSH) dystrophy is an autosomal dominant type with a distinct phenotype.[39,40] As of this date, the precise genetic defect in this major form of FSH dystrophy has yet to be identified. However, the diagnosis in FSH dystrophy can be suspected and/or easily made clinically in most patients with this disorder. Typically, these children have prominent facial as well as scapulohumeral muscle weakness. Paradoxical to other dystrophies a striking asymmetry of muscle involvement is a typical feature of FSH dystrophy.

The occurrence of this phenotype quite often leads to diagnostic consideration of a mononeuropathy or plexopathy by clinicians not familiar with the asymmetric presentation of FSH dystrophy, who may order an EMG/NCS for a suspected focal neuropathic process. Instead, the EMG often demonstrates the presence of many low-amplitude, short-duration MUPs consistent with a myopathy. Concomitant neuropathic EMG findings may be related to secondary nerve injuries from stretching of the brachial plexus or to focal compression neuropathies affecting the proximal sciatic nerve or branches of the radial, median, or ulnar nerves; there are no reports describing the pathology of these neuropathies.

A commercial DNA test is now available for FSH muscular dystrophy (see Table 38-1)[41]; most patients with classic FSH for whom detailed molecular studies have been done there is a chromosomal rearrangement within the subtelomere of chromosome 4q (4q35).[42] A tandem array of 3.3 kb repeated DNA elements (D4Z4) is deleted in patients with FSH dystrophy (Fig. 38-2).[43] In the general population, the number of repeat units varies from 11 to more than 100; in patients with FSH dystrophy, an allele of

1-10 residual units is observed because of the deletion of an integral number of these units.[44] This new diagnostic test is positive in 93% of typical FSH dystrophy cases.[45] Nonetheless, the exact gene defect is not known yet; thus, the sensitivity of the genetic test for atypical cases remains uncertain.[46] In typical cases, we see no value in performing a muscle biopsy.

Myotonic Muscular Dystrophy

Clinical myotonia is defined as delayed muscle relaxation or involuntary stiffness accompanied by the finding of myotonic discharges on needle EMG. The myotonic dystrophy (MyD) phenotype is usually obvious in older children and adults with the typical temporalis, masseter, and sternocleidomastoid muscle wasting, lending to the hatchet-like appearance of the face, distal weakness, and, in the older MyD individual, frontal balding.[47] The MyD gene (myotonin protein kinase or myotonin) is located on the long arm of chromosome 19; the mutation is an abnormal expansion of the trinucleotide repeat (CTG)n in the 3′ noncoding region of the *myotonin* gene.[48,49] When MyD is

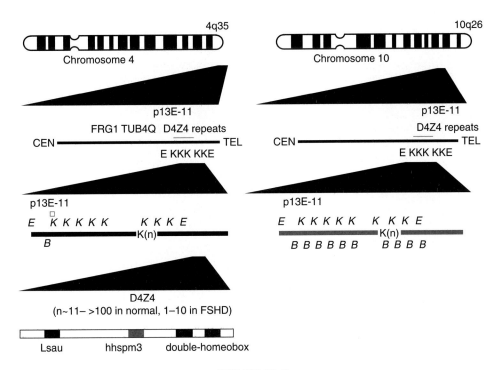

FIGURE 38–2

Diagrammatic representation of the hierarchical genetic organization of the telomeric regions of chromosomes 4q and 10q. In patients with facioscapulohumeral dystrophy, there are less than 10 copies of the D4Z4 repeat on chromosome 4, whereas in normal individuals there are approximately 11 to 100 copies. The presence of a restriction site for BlnI in the 10q repeats allows these two chromosomal repeats to be differentiated. B, BlnI; E, EcoRI; K, KpnI restriction sites. CEN, centromere; TEL, telomere. (From Orrell RW, Darras BT, Griggs RC: Facioscapulohumeral dystrophy, scapuloperoneal syndromes, and distal myopathies. In Jones HR Jr, De Vivo DC, Darras BT [eds]: Neuromuscular Disorders of Infancy, Childhood, and Adolescence: A Clinician's Approach. Philadelphia, Butterworth Heinemann Health, 2003, pp 701-716.)

suspected clinically, DNA testing (see Table 38-1) is 98% to 99% accurate.[50]

Infants with congenital MyD present with severe hypotonia, poor feeding, facial weakness, leading to an unusual "tenting" of the mouth, and club feet and sometimes with associated severe respiratory and feeding difficulties. Typically these MyD infants have mothers affected by MyD. On occasion, when we perform an EMG in a floppy infant, the presentation of MyD in the mother is atypical and, therefore, her diagnosis has not been previously suspected. Some clinical clues to the maternal diagnosis may include premature cataract surgery, some mild neck flexor or distal muscle weakness, or actual clinical myotonia that the mother thought was normal for her.

When one performs an EMG in a MyD neonate, the myotonic discharges may be somewhat atypical, being less prevalent or persistent. In some MyD infants the EMG-recorded myotonia has a higher discharge frequency than in the adult forms of this disorder (see Chapter 36). Myotonic discharges may not even appear in some infants for several months or years; thus, an EMG may be normal in a floppy infant with MyD. If the EMG is normal in the infant and the mother has suspicious signs for MyD, an EMG in the mother is optional, but if it shows myotonia, this can quickly support the diagnosis and the need for a DNA test in her; if the DNA test is positive in the mother, blood should be drawn from her floppy infant for DNA analysis. In contrast, if the mother had MyD diagnosed previous to her pregnancy by clinical, EMG, and/or genetic studies, DNA testing[51,52] is indicated in the infant prior to EMG. If the MyD diagnosis in this floppy infant is confirmed by DNA testing, EMG is not necessary.

Other Myotonic Disorders, Including Periodic Paralysis

Myotonia is not specific for MyD; it occurs clinically and electrophysiologically in other genetically determined disorders including myotonia congenita, both Thomsen's and Becker's forms, paramyotonia congenita, myotonia fluctuans, and hyperkalemic periodic paralyses.[53] Myotonic discharges are also observed during the EMG of the rare child with centronuclear myopathy, acid maltase deficiency, and some nongenetic entities including dermatomyositis/polymyositis, hypothyroid myopathy, and in rare patients (usually adults) receiving lipid-lowering drugs.

Genetic testing has identified a host of channelopathies affecting the sodium (paramyotonia congenita, hyperkalemic periodic paralysis, myotonia fluctuans), calcium (hypokalemic periodic paralysis), and chloride (autosomal dominant myotonia congenita of Thomsen, autosomal recessive myotonia congenita of Becker) channels.[54] DNA laboratory analyses of these most common mutations within

the sodium, calcium, or chloride channel genes are currently available. If the clinical setting is compatible with one of these diagnoses, we usually initiate DNA testing first, which, if positive, will confirm the diagnosis (see Table 38-1). However, despite the availability of DNA tests for these various myotonic disorders or the periodic paralyses, novel or rare, so-called private mutations cannot be detected in all cases.[53] In the absence of a family history, or a characteristic clinical presentation, an EMG is often useful in confirming the presence of myotonia in some of these disorders, namely myotonia congenita, paramyotonia congenita, myotonia fluctuans, and hyperkalemic periodic paralysis. This finding supports the need for DNA analysis.

Metabolic Myopathies

The metabolic myopathies are a group of muscle disorders resulting from failed energy production related primarily to defects in glycogen, lipid, or mitochondrial metabolism. Typically these individuals present with either dynamic symptoms such as exercise intolerance, myalgias, or myoglobinuria and/or static symptoms, primarily fixed muscle weakness.

Except for the rare circumstance, where we serendipitously uncover a newborn with glycogen storage disease, usually presenting as generalized infantile hypotonia and sometimes with arthrogryposis, we do not routinely perform EMG in children with suspected metabolic myopathies. The detection of myotonic discharges in children with an otherwise myopathic EMG may be useful in suspecting the rare infantile and/or juvenile cases of acid maltase deficiency. In most metabolic myopathies, however, a muscle biopsy for light microscopy, electron microscopy, immunohistochemistry, and biochemistry remains the mainstay of the laboratory investigation.[55] Currently DNA testing is increasingly available in a few enzymatic defects, such as phosphorylase deficiency (see Table 38-1).[56]

Congenital Myopathies

The term *congenital myopathies* refers to a group of genetically determined, slowly progressive or nonprogressive muscle disorders usually presenting at birth. Typically these present with generalized infantile hypotonia, the so-called floppy baby syndrome, with or without feeding or respiratory difficulties, and sometimes various dysmorphic features. To date, a few specific gene abnormalities have been characterized for some of the congenital myopathies (e.g., centronuclear,[57,58] nemaline rod,[59-62] and central core)[63-65]; however, DNA testing is not commercially available for all of them yet.

Muscle biopsy has been the definitive diagnostic tool over the past 3 decades; these demonstrate distinctive features.

In possible congenital myopathies, especially in the floppy infant with normal or very mildly elevated CK levels, we continue to order and perform EMGs prior to performing a muscle biopsy (see Table 38-1). The EMG can be normal or show myopathic findings with low-amplitude CMAPs and small polyphasic, rapidly recruited MUPs. The definition of so-called myopathic MUPs is particularly challenging in this age group because the normal infant's MUPs are relatively small. Thus, one is more likely to have difficulty defining a myopathic process in these infants than a neurogenic process.

Fibrillation potentials are most likely to be identified in centronuclear (myotubular) myopathy but are also seen in many other myopathies, including other congenital ones.[66] The presence of abnormal spontaneous activity may lead to diagnostic errors, especially if misinterpreted as a neuropathic sign.[3] It is the MUP per se that is the EMG key to differentiating between a neurogenic and myopathic disorder.[3]

On occasion in this setting, one unexpectedly finds slow motor NCS, and absent sensory nerve action potentials, compatible with a congenital polyneuropathy or even CIDP. However, in most other instances, a muscle biopsy is still required to make a specific histologic diagnosis. We anticipate that eventually DNA testing will be more widely applicable to the investigation of the floppy infant increasingly replacing the need for EMG with evaluation of myopathies.

Inflammatory Myopathies

Inflammatory myopathies are immunologically mediated disorders that are not genetically determined. However, unless the presentation is absolutely typical with the classic dermatologic changes, most of our children presenting with proximal weakness without a typical skin rash, or with normal muscle enzymes, undergo EMG and/or muscle biopsy to confirm the diagnosis (see Table 38-1) because they may mimic a number of the genetically determined myopathies. In some instances, however, if the presentation is classic for childhood dermatomyositis, an MRI can demonstrate areas of muscle inflammation and, unlike muscle biopsy, can assess large areas of muscle tissue, thus avoiding problems with sampling errors of proximal muscles.[67] This is further defined in Chapter 36.

OVERVIEW AND CONCLUSIONS

EMG stills serves as an extension of the neurologic examination. It continues to be a useful tool for the evaluation of both the floppy infant and an older child with muscle weakness for two primary reasons. First, EMG is particularly sensitive to the detection of an abnormality of the peripheral motor unit, providing the clinician a means to help distinguish between central nervous system versus peripheral motor unit hypotonia or weakness. Second, when there is an initial consideration of a peripheral mechanism, an EMG provides a reliable means to define the presence of a neuronopathy, or a peripheral neuropathy (see Table 38-1). Often these findings may help the clinician determine the need for DNA analysis and/or a muscle biopsy.

Multiple maturational changes need to be accounted for and/or technical difficulties that may be encountered during the performance of pediatric EMG. This is particularly true with the varied norms for NCSs during ages 0 to 3 years, as well as the size of normal MUPs on needle EMG.[68,69]

One needs to utilize these norms to avoid overcalling the presence of myopathic potentials. When dealing with the issue of a myopathy in floppy infants, a positive correlation between EMG and myopathic muscle biopsies has ranged between 10% and 76%.[66] Even experienced pediatric electromyographers sometimes encounter difficulty distinguishing the normally low amplitude, short duration MUPs of a neonate from those MUPs classically identified in a structural myopathy.[3,69] Therefore, it is important to emphasize that a normal EMG does not exclude a myopathy, particularly of the congenital type.

The electrodiagnostic evaluation of NMTDs in infancy and early childhood, particularly congenital lesions, is often more difficult. There are no well-defined norms for the newborn infants' immature neuromuscular junction when they require RMNS (see Chapter 35).[70] This is an area where eventually DNA testing will be especially useful for defining these extremely uncommon congenital NMTDs. However, with NMTDs such as infantile botulism[71] or MG (see Chapter 35) one can find a significant value for the utility of EMG for making a rapid clinical neurophysiologic diagnosis.

With the increased availability of specific DNA testing allowing precise diagnosis of a number of myopathies, as outlined earlier, one might speculate that there is less need for pediatric EMG/NCS at a large referral hospital such as CHB. In fact, there is not; many EMG/NCSs are still ordered. The proportion of patients with genetically determined myopathies seen in a pediatric neuromuscular clinic is rather small. As shown in Figure 38-3, no significant decrease in the number of EMGs performed yearly (mean annual number, 146; range, 97 to 174) occurred in the EMG laboratory at our hospital during the so-called molecular era. It is estimated that approximately 20% of cases of infantile hypotonia are produced by disease of the peripheral motor unit. However, in the remaining 80% the central origin of the hypotonia and/or weakness is not always obvious, and some EMGs are performed to determine whether the infant has a peripheral process and

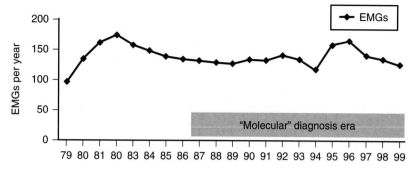

FIGURE 38–3

Number of EMGs performed yearly in the EMG laboratory at Children's Hospital Boston during a 20-year period (1979 to 1999). No significant decrease in the number of EMGs has occurred during the "molecular" diagnosis era.

also to distinguish myopathies from disorders of the motor neuron, peripheral nerve, and neuromuscular junction.

Therefore, EMGs and NCSs continue to have an important role in the evaluation of many children referred to our neuromuscular service at CHB. Overall, our EMG laboratory continues to perform approximately 130 to 160 EMGs per year (see Fig. 38-3). The slight diminution in numbers of evaluations for myopathies, that are much more elegantly identified by DNA testing, is made up by the recognition of the ever-increasing value of EMG in new settings, particularly in the critical care units.[72]

REFERENCES

1. Crawford TO: Spinal muscular atrophies. *In* Jones HR, De Vivo DC, Darras BT (eds): Neuromuscular Disorders of Infancy, Childhood, and Adolescence: A Clinician's Approach. Philadelphia, Butterworth Heinemann Health, 2003, pp 145-166.
2. Engel AG, Ohno K, Harper CM: Congenital myasthenic syndromes. *In* Jones HR, De Vivo DC, Darras BT (eds): Neuromuscular Disorders of Infancy, Childhood, and Adolescence: A Clinician's Approach. Philadelphia, Butterworth Heinemann Health, 2003, pp 555-574.
3. David WS, Jones HR Jr: Electromyography and biopsy correlation with suggested protocol for evaluation of the floppy infant. Muscle Nerve 1994;17:424-430.
4. Al-Shekhlee A, Katirji B: Electrodiagnostic features of acute paralytic poliomyelitis associated with West Nile virus infection. Muscle Nerve 2004;29:376-380.
5. Burns TM, Dyck PJ, Darras BT, Jones HR: Chronic inflammatory demyelinating polyradiculoneuropathy. *In* Jones HR, De Vivo DC, Darras BT (eds): Neuromuscular Disorders of Infancy, Childhood, and Adolescence: A Clinician's Approach. Philadelphia, Butterworth Heinemann Health, 2003, pp 445-468.
6. Chelmicka-Schorr E, Bernstein LP, Zubrugg EB, Huttenlocher PR: Eaton-Lambert syndrome in 9-year-old girl. Arch Neurol 1979;36:572-574.
7. Streib EW, Rothner AD: Eaton-Lambert myasthenic syndrome: Long-term treatment of three patients with prednisone. Ann Neurol 1981;10:448-453.
8. Tsao CY, Mendell JR, Friemer ML, Kissel JT: Lambert-Eaton myasthenic syndrome. J Child Neurol 2002;17:74-76.
9. Hoffman EP, Brown RJ, Kunkel LM: Dystrophin: The protein product of the Duchenne muscular dystrophy locus. Cell 1987;51: 919-928.
10. Darras BT: Molecular genetics of Duchenne and Becker muscular dystrophy. J Pediatr 1990;117:1-15.
11. Darras BT, Harper JF, Francke U: Prenatal diagnosis and detection of carriers with DNA probes in Duchenne's muscular dystrophy. N Engl J Med 1987;316:985-992.
12. Darras BT, Koenig M, Kunkel LM, Francke U: Direct method for prenatal diagnosis and carrier detection in Duchenne/Becker muscular dystrophy using the entire dystrophin cDNA. Am J Med Genet 1988;29:713-726.
13. Darras BT, Jones HR: Diagnosis of neuromuscular disorders in the era of DNA analysis: The role of pediatric electromyography. Pediatr Neurol 2000;23:289-300.
14. Den Dunnen JT, Grootscholten PM, Bakker E, et al: Topography of the Duchenne muscular dystrophy (DMD) gene: FIGE and cDNA analysis of 194 cases reveals 115 deletions and 13 duplications. Am J Hum Genet 1989;45:835-847.
15. Hu XY, Ray PN, Murphy EG, et al: Duplicational mutation at the Duchenne muscular dystrophy locus: Its frequency, distribution, origin, and phenotype genotype correlation. Am J Hum Genet 1990;46:682-695.
16. Monaco AP, Bertelson CJ, Liechti-Gallati S, et al: An explanation for the phenotypic differences between patients bearing partial deletions of the DMD locus. Genomics 1988;2:90-95.
17. Arahata K, Ishiura S, Ishiguro T, et al: Immunostaining of skeletal and cardiac muscle surface membrane with antibody against Duchenne muscular dystrophy peptide. Nature 1988;333;861-863.
18. Hoffman EP, Kunkel LM, Angelini C, et al: Improved diagnosis of Becker muscular dystrophy by dystrophin testing. Neurology 1989;39:1011-1017.
19. Bonnemann CG, McNally EM, Kunkel LU: Beyond dystrophin: Current progress in the muscular dystrophies. Curr Opin Pediatr 1996;8:569-582.
20. Richard I, Broux O, Allamand V, et al: Mutations in the proteolytic enzyme calpain 3 cause limb-girdle muscular dystrophy type 2A. Cell 1995;81:27-40.
21. Bittner RE, Anderson LV, Burkhardt E, et al: Dysferlin

deletion in SJL mice (SJL-Dysf) defines a natural model for limb girdle muscular dystrophy 2B [Letter]. Nat Genet 1999;23:141-142.

22. Matsuda C, Aoki M, Hayashi YK, et al: Dysferlin is a surface membrane-associated protein that is absent in Miyoshi myopathy. Neurology 1999;53:1119-1122.

23. Moreira ES, Wiltshire TJ, Faulkner G, et al: Limb-girdle muscular dystrophy type 2G is caused by mutations in the gene encoding the sarcomeric protein telethonin. Nat Genet 2000;24:163-166.

24. Frosk P, Weiler T, Nylen E, et al: Limb-girdle muscular dystrophy type 2H associated with mutation in TRIM32, a putative E3-ubiquitin-ligase gene. Am J Hum Genet 2002;70:663-672.

25. Driss A, Noguchi S, Amouri R, et al: Fukutin-related protein gene mutated in the original kindred limb-girdle MD 2I. Neurology 2003;60:1341-1344.

26. Hackman JP, Vihola AK, Udd AB: The role of titin in muscular disorders. Ann Med 2003;35:434-441.

27. Minetti C, Sotgia F, Bruno C, et al: Mutations in the caveolin-3 gene cause autosomal dominant limb-girdle muscular dystrophy. Nat Genet 1998;18:365-368.

28. McNally EM, de Sa Moreira E, Duggan DJ, et al: Caveolin-3 in muscular dystrophy. Hum Mol Genet 1998;7:871-877.

29. Tome FM, Evangelista T, Leclerc A, et al: Congenital muscular dystrophy with merosin deficiency. C R Acad Sci: III. 1994;317:351-357.

30. Helbling-Leclerc A, Zhang X, Topaloglu H, et al: Mutations in the laminin alpha 2-chain gene *(LAMA2)* cause merosin-deficient congenital muscular dystrophy. Nat Genet 1995;11:216-218.

31. Toda T, Segawa M, Nomura Y, et al: Localization of a gene for Fukuyama-type congenital muscular dystrophy to chromosome 9q31-33. Nat Genet 1993;5:283-286.

32. Kobayashi K, Nakahori Y, Miyake M, et al: An ancient retrotransposal insertion causes Fukuyama-type congenital muscular dystrophy. Nature 1998;394:388-392.

33. Hopkins LC, Jackson JA, Elsas LJ: Emery-Dreifuss humeralperoneal muscular dystrophy; an X-linked myopathy with unusual contractures and bradycardia. Ann Neurol 1981;10:230-237.

34. Di Barletta MR, Ricci E, Galluzzi G, et al: Different mutations in the *LMNA* gene cause autosomal dominant and autosomal recessive Emery-Dreifuss muscular dystrophy. Am J Hum Genet 2000;66:1407-1412.

35. Rowland LP, Fetell M, Olarte M, et al: Emery-Dreifuss muscular dystrophy. Ann Neurol 1979;5:111-117.

36. Yates JR, Warner JP, Smith JA, et al: Emery-Dreifuss muscular dystrophy: Linkage to markers in distal Xq28. J Med Genet 1993;30:108-111.

37. Bione S, Maestrini E, Rivella S, et al: Identification of a novel X-linked gene responsible for Emery-Dreifuss muscular dystrophy. Nat Genet 1994;8:323-327.

38. Bonne G, Di Barletta MR, Varnous S, et al: Mutations in the gene encoding lamin A/C cause autosomal dominant Emery-Dreifuss muscular dystrophy. Nat Genet 1999;21:285-288.

39. Munsat TL, Piper D, Cancilla P, Mednick J: Inflammatory myopathy with facioscapulohumeral distribution. Neurology 1972;22:335-347.

40. Taylor DA, Carroll JE, Smith ME, et al: Facioscapulohumeral dystrophy associated with hearing loss and Coats syndrome. Ann Neurol 1982;12:395-398.

41. Kohler J, Rohrig D, Bathke KD, Koch MC: Evaluation of the facioscapulohumeral dystrophy phenotype in correlation to the occurrence of 4q35 and 10q26 fragments. Clin Genet 1999;55:88-94.

42. Griggs RC, Tawil R, Storvick D, et al: Genetics of facioscapulohumeral muscular dystrophy: New mutations in sporadic cases. Neurology 1993;43:2369-2372.

43. Hewitt JE, Lyle R, Clark LN, et al: Analysis of the tandem repeat locus D4Z4 associated with facioscapulohumeral muscular dystrophy. Hum Mol Genet 1994;3:1287-1295.

44. Tawil R, Figlewicz DA, Griggs RC, Weiffenbach B: Facioscapulohumeral dystrophy: A distinct regional myopathy with a novel molecular pathogenesis. FSH Consortium. Ann Neurol 1998;43:279-282.

45. Ricci E, Galluzzi G, Deidda G, et al: Progress in the molecular diagnosis of facioscapulohumeral muscular dystrophy and correlation between the number of KpnI repeats at the 4q35 locus and clinical phenotype. Ann Neurol 1999;45:751-757.

46. Vitelli F, Villanova M, Malandrini A, et al: Inheritance of a 38-kb fragment in apparently sporadic facioscapulohumeral muscular dystrophy. Muscle Nerve 1999;22:1437-1441.

47. Harper PS: Myotonic dystrophy—the clinical picture. *In* Myotonic Dystrophy. London, WB Saunders, 1989, pp 13-36.

48. Aslanidis C, Jansen G, Amemiya C, et al: Cloning of the essential myotonic dystrophy region and mapping of the putative defect. Nature 1992;355:548-551.

49. Brook JD, McCurrach ME, Harley HG, et al: Molecular basis of myotonic dystrophy: Expansion of a trinucleotide (CTG) repeat at the 3′ end of a transcript encoding a protein kinase family member. Cell 1992;68:799-808.

50. Harley HG, Rundle SA, Reardon W: Unstable DNA sequence in myotonic dystrophy. Lancet 1992;339:1125-1128.

51. Brunner HG, Nillesen W, van Oost BA: Presymptomatic diagnosis of myotonic dystrophy. J Med Genet 1992;29:780-784.

52. Suthers GK, Huson SM, Davies KE: Instability versus predictability: The molecular diagnosis of myotonic dystrophy. J Med Genet 1992;29:761-765.

53. Moxley RT III: Channelopathies affecting skeletal muscle in childhood: Myotonic disorders including myotonic dystrophy and periodic paralysis. *In* Jones HR, De Vivo DC, Darras BT (eds): Neuromuscular Disorders of Infancy, Childhood, and Adolescence: A Clinician's Approach. Philadelphia, Butterworth Heinemann Health, 2003, pp 783-812.

54. Moxley RT III: Carrell-Krusen Symposium Invited Lecture-1997. Myotonic disorders in childhood: Diagnosis and treatment. J Child Neurol 1997;12:116-129.

55. Darras BT, Friedman NR: Metabolic myopathies: A clinical approach: I. Pediatr Neurol 2000;22:87-97.

56. Darras BT, Friedman NR: Metabolic myopathies: A clinical approach: II. Pediatr Neurol 2000;22:171-181.

57. Thomas NST, Sarfarazi M, Roberts K, et al: X-linked myotubular myopathy (MTM1) evidence for linkage to Xq28 DNA marker loci. J Med Genet 1990;27:284-287.

58. Laporte J, Hu LJ, Kretz C, et al: A gene mutated in X-linked myotubular myopathy defines a new putative tyrosine phosphatase family conserved in yeast. Nat Genet 1996;13:175-182.

59. Laing NG, Majda BT, Akkari PA, et al: Assignment of a gene *(NEMI)* for autosomal dominant nemaline myopathy to chromosome I. Am J Hum Genet 1992;50:576-583.

60. Laing NG, Wilton SD, Akkari PA, et al: A mutation in the alpha tropomyosin gene *TPM3* associated with autosomal dominant nemaline myopathy. Nat Genet 1995;9:75-79.

61. Nowak KJ, Wattanasirichaigoon D, Goebel HH, et al: Mutations in the skeletal muscle alpha-actin gene in patients with actin myopathy and nemaline myopathy. Nat Genet 1999;23:208-212.

62. Pelin K, Hilpela P, Donner K, et al: Mutations in the nebulin gene associated with autosomal recessive nemaline myopathy. Proc Natl Acad Sci U S A 1999;96:2305-2310.

63. Haan EA, Freemantle CJ, McCure JA: Assignment of the gene for central core disease to chromosome 19. Hum Genet 1990;86:187.

64. Quane KA, Healy JM, Keating KE, et al: Mutations in the ryanodine receptor gene in central core disease and malignant hyperthermia. Nat Genet 1993;5:51-55.

65. Lynch PJ, Tong J, Lehane M, et al: A mutation in the transmembrane/luminal domain of the ryanodine receptor is associated with abnormal Ca²⁺ release channel function and severe central core disease. Proc Natl Acad Sci U S A 1999;96:4164-4169.

66. Jones HR Jr: EMG evaluation of the floppy infant: Differential diagnosis and technical aspects. Muscle Nerve 1990;13:338-347.

67. Miller LC, Tucker LB, Schaller JG: Dermatomyositis and polymyositis. *In* Burg FD, Ingelfinger JR, Wald ER, Polin RA (eds): Gellis and Kagan's Current Pediatric Therapy. Philadelphia, WB Saunders, 1996, pp 386-387.

68. Feinstein B, Lindegard B, Nyman E, Wohlfart G: Morphologic studies of motor units in normal human muscles. Acta Anat (Basel) 1955;23:127-142.

69. Jones HR Jr: Electromyographic evaluation of the floppy infant: Myotonia dystrophica. *In* Jones HR Jr, Bolton CF, Harper CM Jr (eds): Pediatric Clinical Electromyography. Philadelphia, Lippincott-Raven, 1996, pp 88-89.

70. Cornblath DR, Sladky JT, Sumner AJ: Clinical electrophysiology of infantile botulism. Muscle Nerve 1983;6:448-452.

71. Jones HR, Darras B: Acute care pediatric electromyography. Muscle Nerve 2000;23:S53-S62.

SUGGESTED READINGS

Bischoff C, Stålberg E, Falck B, Edebol Eeg-Olofsson K: Reference values of motor unit action potentials obtained with multi-MUAP analysis. Muscle Nerve 1994;17:842-851.

Bradshaw DY, Jones HR: Guillain-Barré syndrome in children: Clinical course, electrodiagnosis, and prognosis. Muscle Nerve 1992;15:500-506.

Bradshaw DY, Jones HR: Pseudoencephalopathic presentation of pediatric Guillain-Barré syndrome. J Child Neurol 2001;16:505-508.

Bruno C, Hayes AP, Di Mauro S: Glycogen storage diseases of muscle. *In* Jones HR, De Vivo DC, Darras BT (eds): Neuromuscular Disorders of Infancy, Childhood, and Adolescence: A Clinician's Approach. Philadelphia, Butterworth Heinemann Health, 2003, pp 813-832.

Committee on Drugs: Guidelines for monitoring and management of pediatric patients during and after sedation for diagnostic and therapeutic procedures. Pediatrics 1992;89:1110-1115.

Cornelio F, Bresolin N, DiMauro S: Congenital myopathy due to phosphorylase deficiency. Neurology 1983;33:1383-1385.

Daube JR: The description of motor unit potentials in electromyography. Neurology 1978;28:623-625.

Daube JR: Needle examination in electromyography: American Association of Electromyography and Electrodiagnosis. Rochester, MN, Mayo Clinic, 1979.

de Carmo RJ: Motor unit action potential parameters in human newborn infants. Arch Neurol 1960;3:136-140.

Dyck PJ, Lais AC, Ohta M, et al: Chronic inflammatory polyradiculoneuropathy. Mayo Clin Proc 1975;50:621-637.

Eng GD: Electrodiagnosis. *In* Molnar GE (ed): Pediatric Rehabilitation, 2nd ed. Baltimore, Williams & Wilkins, 1992, pp 143-165.

Engel AG, Gomez MR, Seybold ME, Lambert EH: The spectrum and diagnosis of acid maltase deficiency. Neurology 1973;23:95-106.

Griffin JW, Sheikh K, Li CY: Acute axonal motor neuropathy. *In* Jones HR, De Vivo DC, Darras BT (eds): Neuromuscular Disorders of Infancy, Childhood, and Adolescence: A Clinician's Approach. Philadelphia, Butterworth Heinemann Health, 2003, pp 425-432.

Jones HR: Guillain-Barré syndrome: Perspectives with infants and children. Semin Pediatr Neurol 2000;7:91-102.

Jones HR, Harmon RL, Bolton CF, Harper CM: An approach to pediatric electromyography. *In* Jones HR, Bolton CF, Harper CM: Pediatric Clinical Electromyography. Philadelphia, Lippincott-Raven, 1996, pp 1-36.

Jones HR, Miller RG, Turk MA, Wilbourn AJ: The pediatric EMG examination: General considerations [Panel Discussion]. AAEE Course A. Myopathies, floppy infant, and electrodiagnostic studies in children: Tenth Annual Continuing Education Course. Rochester, MN, American Association of Electromyography and Electrodiagnosis, 1987, pp 39-46.

McManis P, Lambert EH, Daube JR: The exercise test in periodic paralysis. Muscle Nerve 1986;9:704-710.

Pachman LM: Juvenile dermatomyositis and other inflammatory myopathies. *In* Jones HR, De Vivo DC, Darras BT (eds): Neuromuscular Disorders of Infancy, Childhood, and Adolescence: A Clinician's Approach. Philadelphia, Butterworth Heinemann Health, 2003, pp 901-937.

Sacco G, Buchthal F, Rosenfalck P: Motor unit potentials at different ages. Arch Neurol 1962;6:366-373.

Samaha FJ, Quinlan JG: Dystrophinopathies: Classification and complications. J Child Neurol 1996;11:13-20.

Simmons Z, Wald JJ, Albers JW: Chronic inflammatory demyelinating polyradiculoneuropathy in children: I. Presentation, electrodiagnostic studies, and initial clinical course, with comparison to adults. Muscle Nerve 1997;20:1008-1015.

Sladky JT, Brown MJ, Berman PH: Chronic inflammatory demyelinating polyneuropathy of infancy: A corticosteroid-responsive disorder. Ann Neurol 1986;20:76-81.

Sonoo M, Stålberg E: The ability of MUP parameters to discriminate between normal and neurogenic MUPs in concentric EMG: Analysis of the MUP "thickness" and the proposal of "size index." Electroencephalogr Clin Neurophysiol 1993;89:291-303.

Stålberg E, Bischoff C, Falck B: Outliers, a way to detect abnormality in quantitative EMG. Muscle Nerve 1994;17:392-399.

Stålberg E, Nandedkar SD, Sanders B, Falck B: Quantitative motor unit potential analysis. J Clin Neurophysiol 1996;13:410-422.

Swoboda K, Specht L, Jones HR, et al: Infantile phosphofructokinase deficiency with arthrogryposis: Clinical benefit using a ketogenic diet. Pediatrics 1997;131:932-934.

Turk MA: Pediatric electrodiagnosis. Phys Med Rehabil 1989;3:791-808.

Turk MA: Pediatric electromyography. *In* AAEE Course E: Pediatric EMG: Seventh Annual Continuing Education Course. Rochester, MN, American Association of Electromyography and Electrodiagnosis, 1984, pp 7-8.

Willison RG: Analysis of electrical activity in healthy and dystrophic muscle in man. J Neurol Neurosurg Psychiatry 1964;27:386-394.

IV

Other Neurophysiologic Techniques

39

Magnetoencephalography

JAMES W. WHELESS, EDUARDO M. CASTILLO, AND ANDREW C. PAPANICOLAOU

HISTORY

Hans Christian Oersted discovered in the early 19th century that electric currents generated magnetic fields, with the direction of the magnetic field described by the simple right-hand rule. The right-hand rule states that when the thumb of the right hand is pointed in the direction of current flow, the fingers curl in the direction of the associated magnetic field. This is as true for bioelectric currents, such as those flowing within neurons, as it is for currents in power lines. Biomagnetic fields directly reflect electrophysiologic events of the brain, and they pass through the tissues of the body without distortion. Thus, their measurement and characterization can provide new insight into human physiology and the working of the brain. Neuromagnetism is the study of magnetic signals generated by currents arising from ion movements in the nerve cells of the peripheral or central nervous system. The measurement of magnetic fields produced by intracranial currents is the proper subject of magnetoencephalography (MEG), which has developed into an important functional imaging technique.

The first concrete step toward the goal of measuring biomagnetic signals and localizing their source was taken in the early 1960s when magnetic signals produced by current sources in the human heart were recorded.[1] This was a critical step because it demonstrated the feasibility of such a recording in spite of the fact that heart signals are about a million-fold weaker than the magnetic field of the earth and that these measurements were undertaken with instruments that, from their present perspective, may be considered quite crude. However, magnetic fields in the brain could not

be easily measured until the development of the superconducting quantum interference device (SQUID). The second significant step was taken in 1970 when Cohen and associates described the use of the SQUID inside a magnetically shielded room to improve the quality of the magnetic signals from the heart.[2] This opened the door to the development of equipment to record signals from the human brain. The third milestone occurred 2 years later when Cohen made the first successful measurements of magnetic fields generated by intracranial currents, the same ones that give rise to the electroencephalogram (EEG), thus launching the technique of MEG.[3] Identification of the origin of such neuromagnetic signals was successfully attempted soon after and continues to be the central theme of MEG investigations. It was hypothesized that extracranial measurement of intracranial magnetic fields would make an important contribution to the study of epilepsy and noninvasive functional mapping. The genesis of the magnetic field is linked to two distinct neuronal activities: (1) action potential currents and (2) postsynaptic currents. Both activities are related to the exchange of sodium and potassium ions.

Stimuli, whether somatosensory, visual, auditory, or linguistic, evoke brain activity soon after they impinge on sensory receptors. One basic aspect of such activity is the intracellular flow of ions, which generate electric currents and magnetic fields. Traditionally, intracranial currents associated with ongoing cerebral activity, specific brain responses to sensory stimuli, and activities specific to preparation and execution of movement have been recorded noninvasively from the scalp as time-varying voltages. EEG, the study of spontaneous brain electrical activity and sensory and

TABLE 39–1. COMPARISON OF MEG AND EEG

Criteria	EEG	MEG
Origin (for both)	Fluctuations of membrane potential of the dendritic tree of cortical neurons	
Signal measured	Electrical potential change (extracellular current)	Magnetic fields (intracellular current)
Dipole orientation recorded	Radial >> tangential (radial = top of cortical gyri)	Tangential to scalp surface (in sulci)
Field spread by volume conduction	Yes	No
Used for functional mapping	No	Yes
Use in epilepsy (localization)	Interictal, ictal	Interictal

motor event-related potentials or evoked potentials, is based on the correspondence between intracranial currents and the result of voltages on the scalp. On the basis of this correspondence, it has been possible to address a variety of questions regarding the nature of normal and pathologic brain processes, since many such processes are reflected in the morphology of voltage variations on the surface of the head.

Among those issues that cannot be addressed satisfactorily using surface voltage measurements is the precise location of the sources of the currents that give rise to specific aspects or components of the voltage waveforms, whether these are particular evoked potential components or epileptic spikes seen on the EEG record.[4] One factor that complicates precise localization of intracranial current sources on the basis of EEG records is volume conduction. If, for instance, one wants to localize the source of current evoked by a visual stimulus, one has to contend with the fact that this is the primary current, originating in a cluster of cells in the visual cortex, that has given rise to extracellular secondary currents, which spread through the conducting volume of the head surface onto the scalp and are thus recorded as voltages. This effect is unavoidable since the cluster of cells from which the primary currents originated is inevitably embedded in surrounding tissue such as other neurons and glial cells, cerebrospinal fluid, meninges, skull, and scalp. Each of these tissues has a different conductivity value, and their geometric arrangement is quite irregular. The irregularity of these conductors results in sufficient distortion of the volume currents that translate the primary currents to the scalp to render precise location of the intracranial source extremely problematic. It is mainly this difficulty that MEG can overcome by virtue of the following specific advantages of magnetic recordings (Table 39-1).[4]

INSTRUMENTATION AND TECHNIQUE OF MEG/MAGNETIC SOURCE IMAGE

MEG entails the extracranial detection of brain magnetic fields by use of biomagnetometry. Electric currents, which produce the voltages on the scalp that serve as the basis for EEG, also produce magnetic fields. MEG records the mag-

netic flux associated with electrical currents in activated sets of neurons.[*] It allows tracking of brain activity in real time, but unlike evoked (electrical) potentials, the sources of this activity can be accurately estimated because they are not distorted by differences in conductivity among the brain, skull, and scalp. Deduction of the sources from the measured magnetic field distribution is simple, and both spatial and temporal aspects of the activity can be determined with remarkable accuracy (0.1 to 1 cm and 1 millisecond, respectively).[4-6] Several algorithms for source modeling of the MEG data have been proposed.[4,5] The most widely used source model is the equivalent current dipole. The estimated source location (i.e., the activated brain region) is identified using the following procedure: Three fudicial points are defined on the subject's head surface. Usually they are clear anatomic landmarks such as the two preauricular points and the nasion. These three points define the coordinate system that includes the brain and the position of the magnetometers relative to it. The line between the preauricular points defines the y-axis of the coordinate system. The line between the nasion and the midpoint of the y-axis and perpendicular to it defines the x-axis and the line perpendicular to the x-y plane, passing through the intersection of the x- and y-axes, defines the z-axis of the coordinate system. Usually, lipid markers (e.g., vitamin E pills) are attached to these three fudicial points, and a structural magnetic resonance imaging (MRI) scan is taken, either before or after the MEG recording session. The position of the markers is visible on the MRI scans. Therefore, the relative position of all brain structures with respect to the position of the source of activity is known. The locations of these activity sources are estimated and projected onto the structural images of the brain (MRI), creating the magnetic source image (MSI), which displays the activated brain regions (Fig. 39-1).

The biomagnetic fields detected by MEG are extremely small compared to the earth's magnetic field; at times the neuronal noise may be as much as 10,000 times the neuronal magnetic field being monitored. Detection of the small magnetic field requires both a magnetically shielded room and the use of sophisticated instrumentation involving superconducting technology (Fig. 39-2). (Both a SQUID and bio-

---

[*]A detailed description of whole-head MEG can be found in Reference 4.

Spike

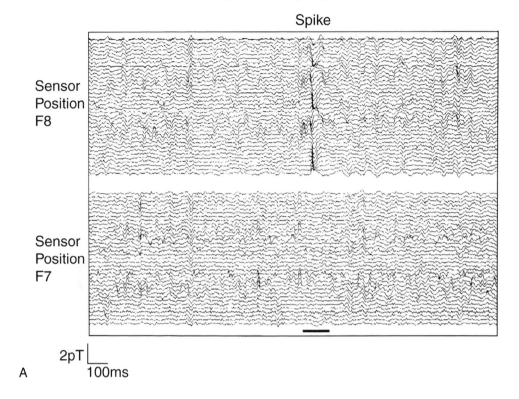

Sensor Position F8

Sensor Position F7

2pT ⌊
A   100ms

Superior

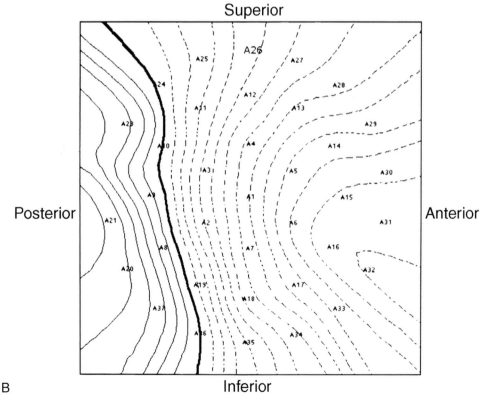

Posterior   Anterior

B

Inferior

FIGURE 39–1

A, MEG waveforms recorded from symmetric, homotopic channel positions centered over an F8 spike (above). The MEG waveforms for each probe are ordered according to the number of each sensor coil in the detector array. The displayed time begins—2 seconds before the spike and continues for 1.5 seconds after the spike. B, An isocontour MEG map of the magnetic field for the F8 probe position at the latency corresponding to the peak of the spike. The pattern shows a typical dipolar pattern suitable for modeling the source as a single equivalent current dipole.

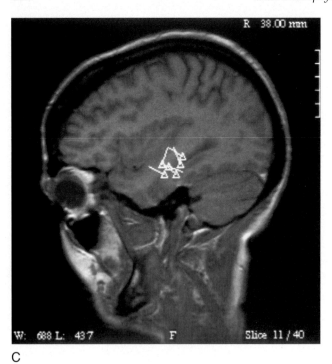

C

FIGURE 39–1—Cont'd

C, *Representative source localization of individual interictal spikes overlaid on corresponding sagittal T1-weighted MR image creating the MSI.*

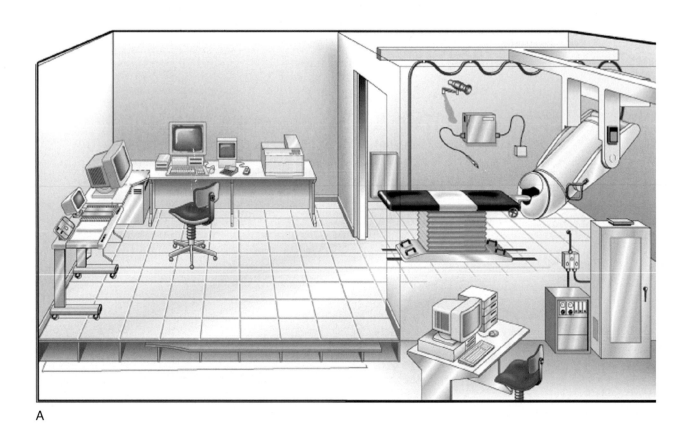

A

FIGURE 39–2

A, *Typical room design for the whole-head MEG system.*

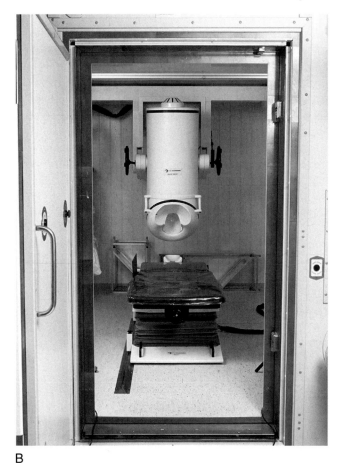

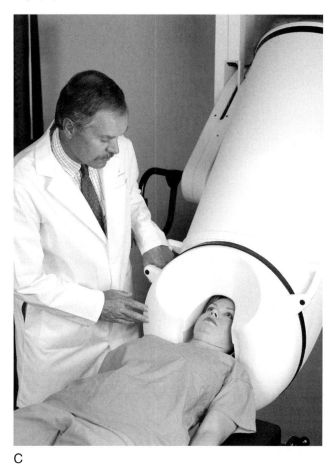

FIGURE 39–2—Cont'd

B, *Magnetically shielded room with whole-head MEG and Dewar flask (upper cylinder).* C, *Patient in whole-head MEG.*

magnetometer are utilized.) A biomagnetometer consists of niobium detection coils immersed in liquid helium contained within a Dewar flask. A SQUID acts as a magnetic-field-to-voltage converter for the detection coils of the biomagnetometer, which are positioned close to the scalp surface. The weak neuronal magnetic fields are monitored by the biomagnetometer and then displayed as a contour map of magnetic fields. The contour map is an image of the magnetic field amplitudes that emanate from the neuronal source located in a sulcus or fissure. The X, Y, and Z coordinates of the source are identified in reference to three points designated prior to the acquisition of the MEG data. Once these three points have been identified on the corresponding MRI, it is possible to calculate X, Y, and Z coordinates and superimpose the MEG location on the MRI, creating the MSI.

Repetitive application of a given stimulus results in repeated evocation of the same electrical currents and magnetic fields. MEG consists of (1) recording magnetic flux on the head surface associated with electrical currents in acti-

vated neuronal aggregates (modeled as equivalent current dipoles); (2) estimating the location of such sets, referred to as *activity sources* or *event-related fields* (ERFs); and (3) projecting the ERFs onto an MRI of the brain to identify and envision the activated brain regions (MSI).[4] In most laboratories, all MSI recordings are made with a multichannel neuromagnetometer consisting of more than 100 magnetometers arranged to cover the entire head.

FUNCTIONAL MAPPING WITH MEG

MSI can be performed after somatosensory, auditory, or visual stimuli and the corresponding evoked potential is detected and mapped onto an MRI, allowing noninvasive determination of eloquent primary sensory cortices.[5] Williamson and Kaufman estimated that 100,000 to 1 million neurons could be simultaneously involved in the generation of a magnetic evoked response.[6] With recurring presentations of stimuli, these signals can be recorded as ERFs on the head surface. ERFs, similar to evoked potentials, are waveforms that represent temporal variations in brain activity time-locked to the presentation of stimuli. Some of the waveforms are noted to occur consistently across different experimental conditions and are known as components. There are two basic components: (1) early, extending up to 150 to 200 milliseconds following stimulus onset; and (2) late, lasting several hundred milliseconds after stimulus onset. Early components of the ERF waveform reflect activation of the primary sensory cortex.[7-17] Late components have been shown to reflect activation of the association cortex.[18-23] It is by estimation of the regions that contribute to systematic variations in late portions of the ERF waveform that delineation of the outline of the brain circuits responsible for cognitive and linguistic function can be accom-

plished. The typical recording session, during which the participant must remain still, rarely exceeds 10 minutes for each task, making it possible both to repeat measurements to establish the reliability of results and to test the young and restless. ERFs can be reliably elicited by experimentally controlled events, such as the presentation of auditory,[9-12] visual,[8] or tactile stimuli,[13-17] as well as during engagement in cognitive tasks.[19-23] Castillo and associates recently validated a new experimental paradigm for simultaneous sensory and motor mapping using MEG recordings.[24] They delivered pneumatically driven mechanical taps to the distal index finger by a balloon diaphragm and asked the subjects to respond with full hand extension if they felt a pressure pulse. They were able to reliably localize primary and secondary sensory cortices, premotor cortices, and primary motor cortex (Fig. 39-3). The interplay between sensory and motor

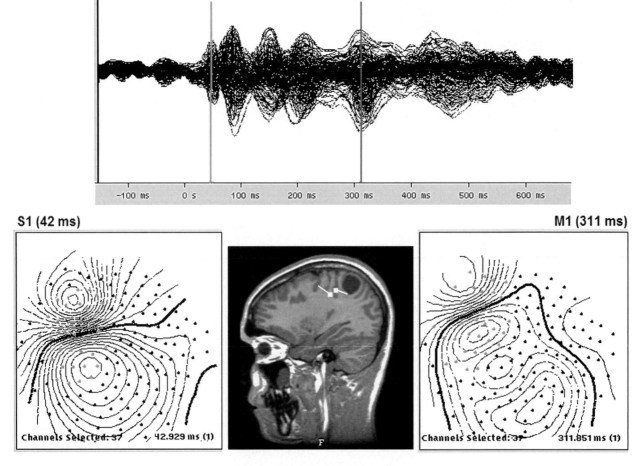

FIGURE 39–3

Averaged waveform, isofield magnetic maps (corresponding to S1 and M1 responses), and coregistration of S1 (primary sensory cortex) and M1 (primary motor cortex) estimated sources onto patients MRI (sagittal view). The MSI shows the proximity of the estimated sensory and motor sources to a 3-cm septated cyst in the left parietal lobe involving the gray matter and underlying white matter. The patient had infrequent complex partial seizures characterized by right arm numbness and decreased level of awareness.

cortex was readily observed in real time using MEG recordings in the content of a cued motor task.

Brain functions studied by MEG allow tracking of neural activation with the millisecond time scale relevant for cortical dynamics. MEG is the only noninvasive technology that has this capability. MSI has been validated and established for all primary sensory modalities, depending on the nature of the stimulus used (Fig. 39-4). The location of MEG-derived sources of brain activity can be compared with the result of invasive (presurgical or intraoperative) localization procedures. These studies have reported excellent agreement between the two sets of observations suggesting that

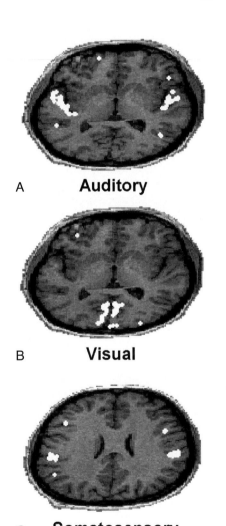

A 　**Auditory**

B 　**Visual**

C 　**Somatosensory**

FIGURE 39–4

Source localization of primary auditory cortex (A), visual (B), and somatosensory cortices (C), with MEG. Note that the equivalent current dipole (ECD) clusters obtained with responses prior to 150 milliseconds activate primary auditory, visual, and somatosensory cortices. Other ECDs seen represent later responses.

it is indeed feasible to estimate the location of the intracranial generators of the ERFs with a high degree of precision in realistic situations.[25-29] Comparisons between preoperative MEG mapping and intraoperative electrocortical stimulation have demonstrated a correlation of 4 to 10 mm between the MEG sources and the electrocortical stimulation localization.[5,26-29] Such information makes the spatial relationship between a cortical lesion and motor or sensory cortex more evident. MSI results facilitate risk-to-benefit assessment of proposed surgery, the process of informed consent, and decisions regarding the operative approach.

To take advantage of these unique properties, MEG is used increasingly in mapping functional brain areas in patients that are undergoing surgery for the resection of tumors, arteriovenous malformations, and epileptogenic tissue.[28,30-32] Currently, functional mapping performed by MEG is predominantly used to assess primary sensory cortices. Often, however, resection of areas associated with more complex brain functions such as those involved in comprehension of language is necessary.

Until recently, localization of functional cortex relied on invasive techniques.[29,33,34] For MEG to be able to provide information that can be used in surgical planning, it is important to establish its capacity to reveal the location of brain areas that show activity uniquely related to certain key language functions. Among the issues that MSI is called to address, identification of brain regions mediating language has always been the most urgently sought. Advance knowledge of the language-specific zones can facilitate surgical planning and reduce morbidity associated with resection of eloquent cortex, especially in cases of epilepsy surgery.

Using two recognition memory tasks for words (one auditory and one visual), Breier and Simos and their coworkers validated the ability of MEG to localize areas associated with receptive language function.[35-40] The average time to complete and validate these tasks was 10 to 20 minutes in cooperative children, adolescents, and adults. Three main results emerged from these initial trials. First, activity sources computed during the initial 150 to 200 milliseconds of the ERF waveform were consistently localized in the vicinity of modality-specific cortices, depending on the task. In the word task, most sources were localized in temporal-parietal areas during later portions of the waveform.[40] Second, activity sources computed within corresponding time periods in the two different word tasks were localized to the same brain areas. As such, MEG is modality independent in patients with intact reading skills (i.e., the same area was localized with either an auditory or visual verbal task). Additionally, the test-retest reliability of anatomic locations was validated (Fig. 39-5).[35] The third result that emerged from these initial studies is the variability among people in the precise localization of language activity

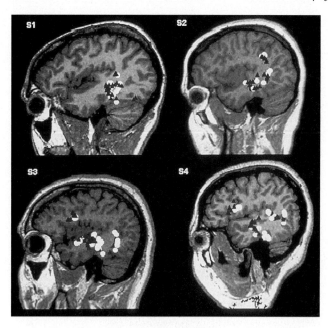

FIGURE 39–5

Examples of activity sources computed during late portions of the event-related fields (150 milliseconds after stimulus onset or later) in four representative subjects. Clusters of sources spanning 1.5 cm in the medial-lateral direction were superimposed on a single sagittal scan from the left hemisphere. The white circles represent sources found in the context of the first session of the word recognition task, whereas the triangles indicate sources found during the second session. Note the spatial overlap of sources in the temporal as well as in the frontal lobe (the latter in subjects S3 and S4 only). When possible, sources in the inferior and basal temporal cortices are also shown.

sources. This is likely the result of interindividual variability in the functional organization of cortical areas. This was a critically important finding when addressing individual patients and considering neurosurgical procedures near eloquent language cortex.

The reliability and validity of MSI data for the purpose of lateralization and localization of cortical areas active during the processing of linguistic material were verified by comparing the degree of concordance between MSI and the Wada procedure or electrical stimulation mapping.[41-46*] In eighty-five consecutive patients an excellent agreement has been found between MSI and Wada language laterality scores (Table 39-2).[46] Noninvasive lateralization of language function using a methodology such as MSI has a number of advantages, including elimination of health risk, potential

* See References 43 and 44 for detailed descriptions of the MEG filters, settings, and analysis used during the language task.

TABLE 39–2. HEMISPHERE DOMINANCE FOR LANGUAGE: MEG VERSUS WADA*

Wada	MEG		
	Left	*Bilateral*	*Right*
Left	57	7	0
Bilateral	2	15	1
Right	0	1	2

° N = 85.
Wada, intracarotid amobarbital test.
From Papanicolaou AC, Simos PG, Castillo EM, et al:
Magnetoencephalography: A non-invasive alternative to the Wada procedure.
J Neurosurg 2004;100:867-876.

for test-retest reliability studies, and ability to use a number of different tasks of extended duration. In addition, the problems inherent in the Wada procedure, including potential overanesthetization or underanesthetization and anomalous distribution of anesthetic due to cross-flow or atypical vascularization are eliminated. Furthermore, although the Wada procedure provides only data regarding lateralization of language function, MSI is capable of providing data regarding precise intrahemispheric localization of areas involved in language function (Fig. 39-6),[43,44] and these data have been shown to be valid in comparison with electrocortical stimulation. To date, in more than 40 consecutive patients, perfect agreement was found between MSI-based noninvasive mapping of receptive language-specific brain areas and intraoperative and extraoperative language mapping using direct electrocortical stimulation. The MSI mapping protocol provided correct localization even in patients with atypical language representation (Fig. 39-7).[45] In all of these atypical cases, MSI derived information was found to be extremely useful in surgical planning by (1) helping to determine the optimal extent of the craniotomy, (2) helping to assess surgical risk, and (3) helping to tailor the location and extent of the cortical resection. The accuracy of the localization procedure was apparently unaffected by the type and extent of pathologic conditions in the brain or the presence of preoperative language and cognitive deficits. This is particularly important in epilepsy surgery patients who have been shown to have a wider spatial distribution of language cortex, especially in patients with lower intelligence, poorer education, and worse verbal and memory skills.[48-50] Ojemann and colleagues' extensive intraoperative studies revealed no one posterior language site (Wernicke's area) that interrupted naming in more than 36% of patients tested, and less than 30% had no posterior sites whatsoever.[51] Schwartz and associates later verified this and noted no one posterior site disturbing language function in more than 40% of patients tested.[52] Based on this work documenting discrete localization of language function in individual patients, but substantial individual variability,

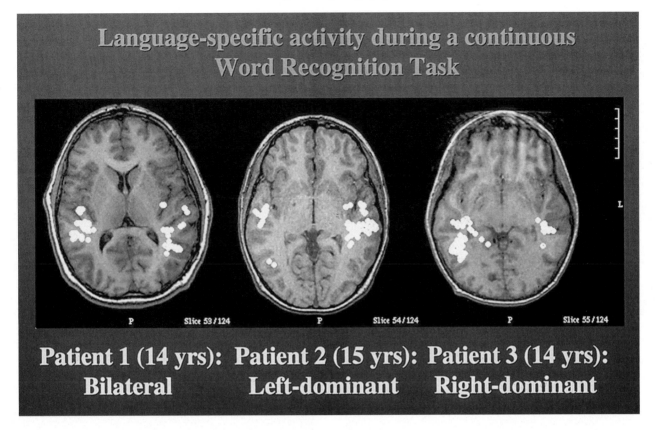

FIGURE 39–6

MSI coregistered scans for three representative patients showing, from left to right (the hemisphere on the right side of the figure is the left hemisphere), bilateral activity, predominantly left hemisphere activity, and predominantly right hemisphere activity during MSI testing of language function. These patients showed similar interhemispheric asymmetries in behavior during the intracarotid amobarbital procedure.

mapping for language localization has become an accepted part of resective surgical technique for epilepsy.

Finally, care should be taken to screen patients for the presence of a reading disability. Activation profiles in these individuals, in the context of reading tasks, can be dramatically different from those of normal, relatively skilled readers.

Another use of MEG is in describing the time course of neurophysiologic events associated with the presentation of external stimuli and/or engagement of the subject in an experimental task, which became possible by the excellent temporal resolution of MEG recordings (Fig. 39-8).[23,53] As a result, the range of questions to which MEG could help provide answers is not restricted to which brain areas become more active in response to an external event (as in the case of functional imaging techniques that rely on measurements of blood flow and metabolism) but also to the relative timing of the engagement of different brain areas (Table 39-3). Both temporal and spatial resolutions are critical to understand brain processing of cognitive functions (see discussion

of dyslexia later).[37,40,54,55] MEG is the only imaging technology that provides this information.

IDENTIFICATION OF LANGUAGE-SPECIFIC BRAIN ACTIVITY IN DYSLEXIA USING MEG

Dyslexia is a specific disability in learning to read that often persists into adulthood when early interventions are inadequate. Developmental reading disability (dyslexia) affects a significant portion of otherwise normal children (estimates of between 4% and 17% of the school-age population in North America).* One of the hallmark manifestations of this disorder is a persistent difficulty with phonologic pro-

---

* See Reference 56 for a review by Habib for discussion of the neuropathologic, electrophysiologic, and in vivo imaging modalities previously studied in patients with dyslexia.

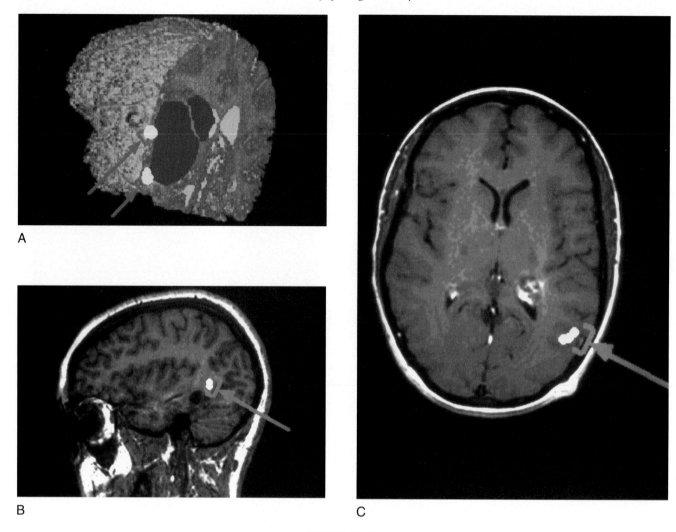

FIGURE 39–7

A, A 25-year-old male with recent onset of partial seizures. Three-dimensional rendering of MRI shows a large left temporal tumor (pathology: pleomorphic xanthoastrocytoma). Two distinct receptive speech areas are identified by MEG (circles) and confirmed by operative mapping (brackets). Corticectomy was performed between the two areas. B, A 16-year-old female with recent onset of partial seizures. Sagittal T1-weighted MRI shows left inferior temporal cystic lesion (pathology: well-differentiated oligodendroglioma). MEG (circles) and operative mapping (bracket) reveal receptive language area immediately superior and posterior to the lesion, allowing a complete surgical resection. C, A 32-year-old female with episodes of decreased speech fluency. Axial T1-weighted MRI reveals a cavernous malformation in the atrium of the left lateral ventricle. MEG (circles) and operative mapping (bracket) reveal atypical location of receptive speech (posterior to usual location). The lesion was approached posterior to the receptive speech area.

cessing, which leads to difficulty with word recognition skills, particularly phonologic decoding.* Although phonologic decoding is by definition required for reading out loud, it is also believed to be critically involved in silent reading of real words by skilled readers. Cortical regions that are specifical-

ly involved in phonologic decoding have been identified by MSI.[41,47] Children with persistent dyslexia face significant socioeconomic challenges in our current information (and language)-based society. As such, strategies that allow early identification of the neural basis of dyslexia and subsequent intervention programs are critically important to remediation of dyslexia. An understanding of dyslexia requires information of the time course of reading as well as anatomic information, and MEG is the only functional imaging method that can, at present, readily provide such data (Fig. 39-9).

---

* The process of phonologic decoding involves mapping of individual ortho-graphic segments onto the corresponding phonologic elements to arrive at a complete phonologic representation. This is used to read words that contain regular spelling to sound correspondences, such as "hint" and "alone."

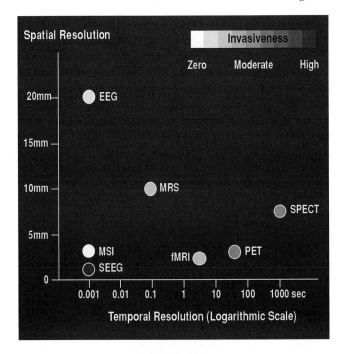

FIGURE 39–8

MEG compared to other functional imaging technologies on the basis of (1) invasiveness, (2) spatial resolution, and (3) temporal resolution.[4,5] PET, positron emission tomography; SPECT, single-photon emission computed tomography; SEEG, stereoencephalography; MRS, magnetic resonance spectroscopy; fMRI, functional magnetic resonance imaging.

TABLE 39–3. FUNCTIONAL IMAGING TECHNIQUES

Criteria	MEG	fMRI°
Noninvasive	+	+
Measures changes in local metabolic demand	–	+
Measures changes in intracellular electrical currents	+	–
High spatial resolution	+	+/–
High temporal resolution	+	–

°fMRI, functional magnetic resonance imaging.

Activation profiles of individuals with dyslexia are dramatically different, depending on whether they were presented with a visual or auditory word task (Fig. 39-10).[57,58] MSI has demonstrated the existence of a distinct spatiotemporal profile of brain activation associated with word and pseudoword reading that reliably differentiates between individual children with and without dyslexia. The validity of this procedure for obtaining spatiotemporal profiles of activation during complex cognitive tasks has been demonstrated in clinical studies in which MSI-derived maps showed excellent concordance when compared with invasive brain maps.[41-44] Localization of language-specific brain regions

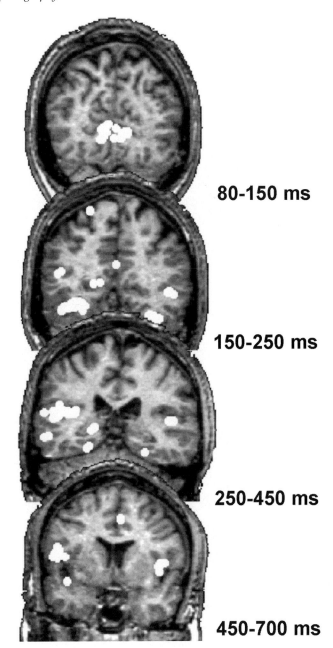

80-150 ms

150-250 ms

250-450 ms

450-700 ms

FIGURE 39–9

Series of coronal T1-weighted MR images showing the temporal course of activity during word reading, from mesial occipital (upper panel) to frontal areas (lower panel). (The left hemisphere is on the left side.) The spatiotemporal profile of neurophysiologic activity associated with the brain mechanism that supports reading features initial activation in the occipital visual areas (within the first 150 milliseconds after the onset of the printed stimulus), followed by activity in the occipitotemporal and basal temporal cortices (between 150 and 300 milliseconds, predominantly in the left hemisphere), and finally by activation of posterior superotemporal, inferoparietal, and inferofrontal regions (again, predominantly in the left hemisphere).

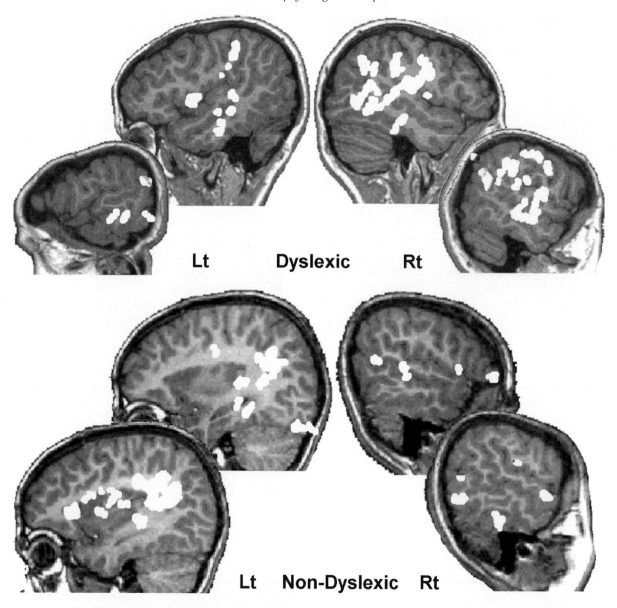

FIGURE 39–10

Reformatted sagittal T1-weighted MRI of a representative dyslexic and nondyslexic child during single word reading task.
Sources occurring between 100 and 300 milliseconds after visual stimulus onset were typically located in basal temporal cortices.
Temporoparietal (TMP) sources usually became active later, between 300 and 1200 milliseconds after stimulus onset. Note that dyslexic
children show homotopic (right TMP) activation during the visual word recognition task when compared with normal children.
Both groups show normal left TMP activation during the auditory word task (not shown). Lt, left; Rt, right.

may be altered in patients with dyslexia.[59-62] As a result, care should be taken to screen patients for the presence of a reading disability prior to a neurosurgical procedure.

The aberrant MEG profile in children with dyslexia features predominant activation of the right posterior superior temporal gyrus (STGp), and the right inferior parietal region (angular and supramarginal gyri). In contrast, most normal readers display predominant activation of the left STGp and the left inferior parietal region.[58] With respect to all other sources of activity, impaired and nonimpaired readers' MEG profiles are indistinguishable.

These differences appear to be specific to an important component of reading, namely phonologic processing, which is a major predictor of success in reading acquisition.[57,58]

Phonologic decoding is dependent on and disrupted by stimulation of the left STGp.[46,63] This area displays normal levels of activity during performance of simple word recognition tasks presented in the auditory modality. The discrepancy in the activation profiles between the auditory and the printed word processing tasks points to a functional disruption in the brain circuit that supports reading (i.e., difficulty converting print into sound [phonologic decoding]). MEG has been used to document a specific, aberrant activation profile in children with dyslexia, which became normal following successful remedial instruction (focusing on the development of phonologic processing and decoding skills) (Fig. 39-11).[64] This suggests that reading difficulties in many children represent a variation of normal development. Consistent with this is the recent demonstration of similar, aberrant MEG activation profiles in kindergarten children, who on the basis of their performance on tests of prereading skills, were found to be at risk for developing reading problems.[65]

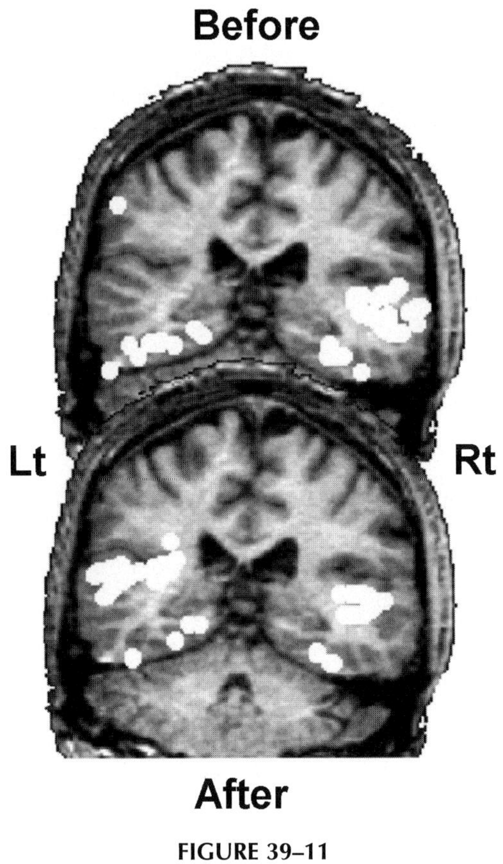

Before

Lt   **Rt**

After

FIGURE 39–11
Coronal T1-weighted MRI obtained during the single word reading task in a representative dyslexic child before and after intervention (80 hours of one-on-one phonics instruction) showing change from predominant activation of homotopic right temporoparietal areas to normal (left TMP) predominant activation as in nonimpaired readers. Lt, left; Rt, right.

The implications of these findings for education are clear: Instruction seems to play a significant role in the development of natural systems that are specialized for reading. MSI could serve as an objective evaluation tool to assess the efficacy of particular intervention strategies in children with dyslexia.

MEG IN EPILEPSY

In 1982, researchers at the University of California–Los Angeles first described the use of MEG to localize epileptiform discharges in human subjects, leading to the consideration of this technique for clinical use.[66]

MEG subsequently was investigated as a noninvasive method for localizing epileptic activity,[67-71] although technical limitations restricted its application until recently. Recent developments, particularly large-array sensors, have improved MEG localization of interictal epileptic spike sources and dramatically decreased the time needed to complete a study. (The typical duration of a MEG epilepsy study is now 30 to 60 minutes.[72-77]) The emergence of large-array, and now whole-head sensor arrays, has allowed MEG to be used in the preoperative assessment of patients for epilepsy surgery. A prospective, two-center study of 58 patients being evaluated for epilepsy surgery compared the ability of MEG, MRI, and video-EEG (V-EEG) to identify the resected epileptogenic zone, when referenced to surgical outcome.[32] MEG was second only to ictal intracranial V-EEG in predicting the epileptogenic zone for the entire group of patients who had an excellent surgical outcome. Overall, MEG localization was better than MRI, scalp V-EEG (interictal or ictal), and interictal intracranial V-EEG in spite of limitations of MEG. Patients were selected who demonstrated interictal spikes on previous routine and scalp V-EEG studies, resulting in a high rate of positive MEG studies. This study suggested MEG is helpful in evaluating patients for epilepsy surgery and has the advantage of allowing coregistration of the epileptic discharge and functional neocortex on a MSI image (Fig. 39-12). This would facilitate surgical planning (resection or intracranial electrode placement) by using a noninvasive technique. Since then, other centers have reported on their experience using whole-head MEG for the evaluation of epilepsy patients.[78-84] MEG appears to be especially useful for the study of patients with neocortical epilepsy (lesional or nonlesional) and helps guide the placement of subdural grid electrodes in patients with nonlesional epilepsy. MSIs provide data on the spatial relations of brain lesions, epileptogenic areas, and functional cortex. All of this information can be incorporated into a frameless, stereotaxic neuronavigational system allowing intraoperative identification of the corresponding brain regions. MEG can differentiate between patients with mesial and lateral temporal seizure

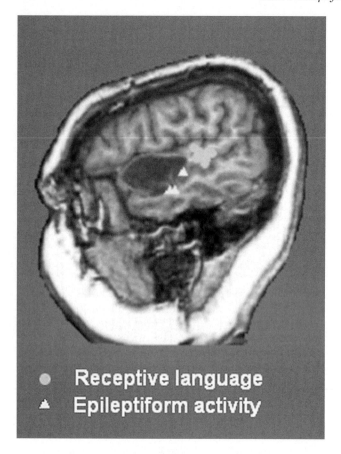

FIGURE 39–12

MSI obtained in an adolescent female with a left temporal cystic lesion documents the anatomic relationship of the lesion to the irritative zone (triangles) and receptive speech areas (circles). This noninvasive information was helpful in planning the surgical procedure and discussing the risk-to-benefit ratio with the family preoperatively. The findings were confirmed with subdural grid recordings; she had a left temporal lobectomy and is now seizure free, without language impairment.

onset (Fig. 39-13)[79,80] and provide prognostic information regarding surgical outcome in temporal lobe epilepsy.[80,85]

In conclusion, it appears that MEG provides complementary and confirmatory information in the work-up of epilepsy surgery candidates.[32,78] MEG is used in the diagnosis of epilepsy for two primary tasks: (1) localization of the area generating interictal spikes (irritative zone); and (2) functional mapping of cortical areas and demonstrating the relationship of these areas to the presumed area of seizure onset. MEG should improve the noninvasive evaluation of epilepsy patients and further reduce the need for invasive procedures. A major limitation of MEG has been the recording of seizures because long-term recordings cannot be performed on a routine basis.

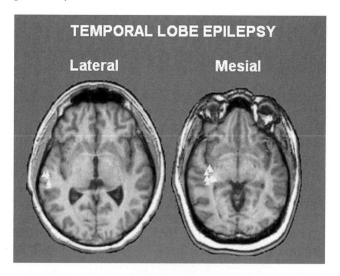

FIGURE 39–13

Axial MSI views (the right temporal lobe is on the left side) demonstrating the different dipole location (triangles) recorded in two patients, one with mesial temporal lobe syndrome and one with lateral neocortical temporal epilepsy.

EVALUATION OF CEREBRAL PLASTICITY AND FUNCTIONAL REORGANIZATION WITH MEG

MEG provides a view of the function of the brain, and its spatial resolution is sufficient to give indications of functional organization and reorganizational plasticity. Recent MEG studies suggest the functional organization of the auditory cortex is dynamic and modifiable over hours (short-term plasticity) and that early music training (before age 10 years) leads to an expansion in the cortical representation of complex harmonic sounds (long-term plasticity).[86] Subsequently, Breier and associates[16] reported an adolescent female with a large left hemisphere arteriovenous malformation in the frontoparietal region who underwent brain mapping of the somatosensory cortex using a whole-head neuromagnetometer. Results indicated the presence of two complete somatosensory maps in the unaffected, right hemisphere (Fig. 39-14). Papanicolaou and colleagues described the use of MEG in addressing the issue of brain reorganization for basic sensory and linguistic functions in a series of 10 children and young adults.[87,88] These patients presented with a wide variety of conditions, ranging from tumors and focal epilepsy to reading disability. In all cases, clear evidence of reorganization of the brain mechanisms of either somatosensory or linguistic functions or both was obtained, demonstrating the utility of MEG in studying, completely noninvasively, the issue of plasticity in the developing brain.

Obviously, functional reorganization does not occur in all cases. In fact, in which particular situations it may occur,

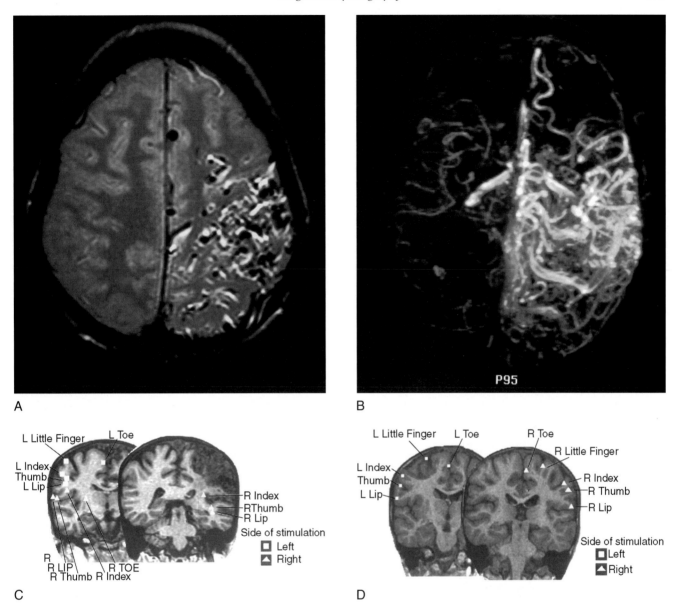

FIGURE 39–14

Axial (proton-density weighted) MRI (A) and MRA of the brain (B) demonstrating a large left cerebral arteriovenous malformation (the left cerebral hemisphere is on the right side, per radiologic convention). The MEG sources of somatosensory evoked magnetic responses for the patient (C) and a neurologically intact volunteer (D) are projected on a coronal slice through somatosensory cortex. The white squares represent sources activated by stimulation of areas on the left side of the body, whereas the triangles represent sources activated by stimulation of areas on the right side. The correspondence between areas stimulated and activated sources in the cortex is indicated. The volunteer has normal interhemispheric symmetry in somatotropic organization. The patient's intact right hemisphere contains the expected map of the contralateral (left) side of the body in the expected area. It also contains a complete map of the ipsilateral right body that is located inferiorly. In the left hemisphere, areas representing the right side of the body are found in inferior parietal and temporal lobes.

what specific factors precipitate it, and what factors determine its precise nature and extent all are open questions inviting investigation. Further detailed and direct study of the extent of functional reorganization and its nature under various circumstances is now feasible through MEG.

LIMITATIONS OF MEG

Although MEG provides a wealth of noninvasive information (delineation of eloquent cortex and irritative zone), there are some limitations to the current technology. Patients with metal implants (i.e., extensive dental fillings or braces, ventriculoperitoneal shunts, aneurysm clips, vagus nerve stimulator generators) in the head and chest area generate excess noise, interfering with the ability to obtain a reliable MEG study. Young children or noncooperative patients will not be able to perform cognitive tasks for assessment of language areas. Sleep, an activator of epileptiform abnormalities, may require artificial induction with chloral hydrate in some patients. If chloral hydrate sedation is not successful, propofol, in low doses, can be used with success in some patients. Patients requiring deeper levels of anesthesia to complete the MEG examination may not show any epileptic dipoles due to the anesthesia.

To date, only few studies addressed the question of the diagnostic yield of MEG because typically those patients who exhibited frequent interictal spikes on scalp EEG were referred for MEG recordings.[32,78,79] The diagnostic yield of MEG in patients without interictal spikes on scalp EEG is uncertain but probably very low for the detection of the irritative zone.[89] Whether MEG can detect if there is a single epileptogenic zone in patients with multifocal interictal epileptiform abnormalities is not known. Finally, ictal recordings are difficult to obtain on a routine basis. Seizures are usually accompanied by movement and asso-

ciated artifact, which can make MEG data difficult to interpret. The patient is required to stay in a fixed position over a prolonged period, so patients must have frequent seizures (multiple a day) to record one. This is usually possible only in simple partial seizures (epilepsia partialis continua) (Fig. 39-15) or frequent complex partial seizures that have little movement at the onset.[75,90-96]

CONCLUSIONS: CLINICAL USE OF MEG

The advent of whole-head MEG systems facilitated a major breakthrough for the MEG evaluation of functional cortex and epilepsy patients, allowing rapid recordings from the entire surface of the brain. MEG studies can now be performed on a routine basis as a clinical tool. MEG is indicated for (1) localization of the irritative zone in lesional and nonlesional epilepsy surgery patients, (2) functional mapping of eloquent cortex and demonstrating the relationship of these areas to the brain lesion or epileptogenic area, and (3) assessment of normal and abnormal language development and the impact of treatment strategies. In the future MEG may help with the understanding of normal develop-

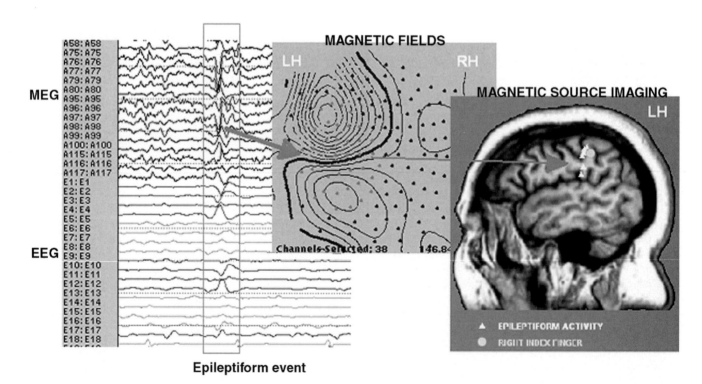

FIGURE 39–15

Ictal MEG recorded during right body (distal arm) epilepsia partialis continua reveals a clear, time-locked MEG dipole with each twitch. The EEG showed intermittent sharp activity that was not time locked. The MSI reveals overlap of the ictal events (triangles) over the right-hand area (squares).

ment and plasticity or functional reorganization after head injury or stroke.

Current MEG computerized software programs allow sampling of brain activity of 250 Hz, giving a temporal resolution of 4 milliseconds. The strength of MEG lies in the combination of rapid sampling and superior source localization. MEG is the only noninvasive method of brain imaging that has the capability of accurately tracking brain-specific functions, due to this high resolution. MEG studies can contribute to the understanding of cerebral activation sequences in healthy subjects or patients with neurologic diseases or special cognitive functions. This necessitates neurologists having an understanding of MEG and how to incorporate this new method of noninvasive brain mapping into their practice.

REFERENCES

1. Baule GM, McFee R: Detection of the magnetic field of the heart. J Appl Physics 1963;36:2066-2073.
2. Cohen D, Edelsack E, Zimmerman JE: Magnetocardiograms taken inside a shielded room with a super conducting point-contact magnetometer. Appl Physics Lett 1970;16:278-280.
3. Cohen D: Magnetoencephalography: Detection of the brain's electrical activity with a super conducting magnetometer. Science 1972;175:664-666.
4. Papanicolaou AC: Fundamentals of Functional Brain Imaging. Lisse, Netherlands, Swets & Zeitlinger, 1998.
5. Rowley HA, Roberts TPL: Functional localization by magnetoencephalography. Neuroimag Clin North Am 1995;5:695-710.
6. Williamson SJ, Kaufman L: Analysis of neuromagnetic signals. *In* Gevins AS, Remonds A (eds): Handbook of Electroencephalography in Clinical Neurophysiology, Vol 1. New York, Elsevier, 1987, pp 405-448.
7. Nakasato N, Kumabe T, Kanno A, et al: Neuromagnetic evaluation of cortical auditory function in patients with temporal lobe tumors. J Neurosurg 1997;86:610-618.
8. Seiki K, Nakasato N, Fujita S, et al: Neuromagnetic evidence that the P100 component of the pattern reversal visual evoked response originates in the bottom of the calcarine fissure. Electroencephalogr Clin Neurophysiol 1996;100:436-442.
9. Eulitz C, Diersch E, Pantev C, et al: Magnetic and electrical brain activity evoked by the processing of tone and vowel stimuli. J Neurosci 1995;15:2748-2755.
10. Papanicolaou AC, Baumann SB, Rogers RL, et al: Localization of auditory response sources using MEG and MRI. Arch Neurol 1990;47:33-37.
11. Papanicolaou AC, Rogers RL, Baumann SB, et al: Source localization of two evoked magnetic field components using two alternative procedures. Exp Brain Res 1999;80:44-48.
12. Zouridakis G, Simos PG, Papanicolaou AC: Multiple bilaterally asymmetric cortical sources account for the auditory N1m component. Brain Tomogr 1989;10:183-189.
13. Elbert T, Junghofer M, Schulz B, et al: The separation of overlapping neuromagnetic source in first and second somatosensory cortices. Brain Tomogr 1997;7:275-282.
14. Galen CC, Schwatz B, Rieke K, et al: Intrasubject variability and validity of somatosensory location using a large array biomagnetometer. Electroencephalogr Clin Neurophysiol 1994;90:145-156.
15. Hari R, Karthu J, Hamalainen M, et al: Functional organization of the human first and second somatosensory cortices: A neuromagnetic study. Eur J Neurosci 1993;5:724-734.
16. Breier JI, Simos PG, Wheless JW, et al: A magnetoencephalography study of cortical plasticity. Neurocase 1999;5:277-284.
17. Roberts TPL, Disbrow EA, Roberts HC, et al: Quantification and reproducibility of tracking cortical extent of activation by use of functional MR imaging and magnetoencephalography. AJNR Am J Neuroradiol 2000;21:1377-1387.
18. Rogers RL, Basile LF, Papanicolaou AC: Localization of the P3 sources using magnetoencephalography and magnetic resonance imaging. Electroencephalogr Clin Neurophysiol 1991;79:308-321.
19. Rogers RL, Basile LF, Papanicolaou AC, et al: Magnetoencephalography reveals two distinct sources associated with late positive evoked potentials during visual oddball task. Cereb Cortex 1993;3:163-169.
20. Simos PG, Basile LF, Papanicolaou AC: Source localization of the N400 response in a sentence-reading paradigm using evoked magnetic fields and magnetic resonance imaging. Brain Res 1997;762:29-39.
21. Basile LFH, Rogers RL, Bourbon WT, et al: Slow magnetic fields from human frontal cortex. Electroencephalogr Clin Neurophysiol 1994;90:157-165.
22. Kuriki S, Hirata Y, Fujimaki N, et al: Magnetoencephalographic study on the cerebral neural activities related to the processing of visually presented characters. Cognit Brain Res 1996;4:185-199.
23. Ioannides AA, Liu L, Theofilou D, et al: Real-time processing of affective and cognitive stimuli in the human brain extracted from MEG signals. Brain Topogr 2000;13:11-19.
24. Castillo EM, Simos PG, Wheless JW, et al: Integrating sensory and motor mapping in a comprehensive MEG protocol: Clinical validity and replicability. NeuroImage 2004;21:973-983.
25. Morioka T, Yamamoto T, Mizushima A, et al: Comparison of magnetoencephalography, functional MRI, and motor evoked potentials in the localization of the sensory motor cortex. Neurol Res 1995;17:361-367.
26. Hund M, Rezai AR, Kronberg E, et al: Magnetoencephalographic mapping: Basis of a new functional risk profile in the selection of patients with cortical brain lesions. Neurosurgery 1997;40:936-940.
27. Sutherling W, Crandall PH, Darcey TM, et al: The magnetic and electric fields agree with intracranial localizations of somatosensory cortex. Neurology 1988;38:1705-1714.

28. Orrison WW: Magnetic source imaging in stereotactic and functional neurosurgery. Stereotact Funct Neurosurg 1999;72:89-94.

29. Gallen CC, Sobel DF, Waltz T, et al: Noninvasive presurgical neuromagnetic mapping of sensory cortex. Neurosurgery 1993;32:260-268.

30. Rezai AR, Hund M, Kronberg E, et al: The interactive use of magnetoencephalography in stereotactic image-guided neurosurgery. Neurosurgery 1996;39:92-102.

31. Roberts T, Rowley H, Kucharczyk J: Applications for magnetic source imaging to presurgical brain mapping. Neuroimag Clin North Am 1995;5:251-266.

32. Wheless JW, Willmore LJ, Breier JI, et al: A comparison of magnetoencephalography, MRI, and V-EEG in patients evaluated for epilepsy surgery. Epilepsia 1999;40:931-941.

33. Lesser RP, Luders H, Morris HH, et al: Electrical stimulation of Wernicke's area interferes with comprehension. Neurology 1986;36:658-663.

34. Ojeman G, Ojeman J, Lettich E, et al: Cortical language localization in left, dominant hemisphere: An electrical stimulation mapping investigation in 117 patients. J Neurosurg 1989;7:316-326.

35. Breier JI, Panagiotis SG, Zouridakis G, et al: Lateralization of activity associated with language function using magnetoencephalography. J Clin Neurophysiol 2000;17:503-510.

36. Simos PG, Breier JI, Zouridakis G, et al: Identification of language specific brain activity using magnetoencephalography. J Clin Exp Neuropsychol 1998;20:706-722.

37. Breier JI, Simos PG, Zouridakis G, et al: Relative timing of neuronal activity in distinct temporal lobe areas during a recognition memory task for words. J Clin Exp Neuropsychol 1998;20:782-790.

38. Simos PG, Breier JI, Zouridakis G, et al: Assessment of functional cerebral laterality for language using magnetoencephalography. J Clin Neurophysiol 1998;15:364-372.

39. Breier JI, Simos PG, Zouridakis G, et al: Lateralization of cerebral activity in auditory verbal and non-verbal memory tasks using magnetoencephalography. Brain Topogr 1999;12:89-97.

40. Breier JI, Simos PG, Zouridakis G, et al: Temporal course of regional brain activation associated with phonologic decoding. J Clin Exp Neuropsychol 1999;21:465-476.

41. Breier JI, Simos PG, Wheless JW, et al: Language dominance in children as determined by magnetic source imaging and the intracarotid amobarbital procedure: A comparison. J Child Neurol 2001;16:124-130.

42. Breier JI, Simos PG, Zouridakis G, et al: Language dominance determined by magnetic source imaging: A comparison with the Wada procedure. Neurology 1999;53:938-945.

43. Simos PG, Papanicolaou AC, Breier JI, et al: Localization of language-specific cortex by using magnetic source imaging and electrical stimulation mapping. J Neurosurg 1999;91:787-796.

44. Papanicolaou AC, Simos PG, Breier JI, et al: Magnetoencephalographic mapping of the language-specific cortex. J Neurosurg 1999;90:85-93.

45. Simos PG, Breier JI, Maggio WW, et al: Atypical temporal lobe language representation: MEG and interoperative stimulation mapping correlation. Neuro Rep 1999;10:139-142.

46. Simos PG, Breier JI, Wheless JW, et al: Brain mechanisms for reading: The role of the superior temporal gyrus in word and pseudoword naming. Neuro Rep 2000;11:2443-2447.

47. Papanicolaou AC, Simos PG, Castillo EM, et al: Magnetoencephalography: A non-invasive alternative to the Wada procedure. J Neurosurg 2004;100:867-876.

48. Devinsky O, Perrine K, Hirsch J, et al: Relation of cortical language distribution and cognitive function in surgical epilepsy patients. Epilepsia 2000;41:400-404.

49. Devinsky O, Perrine K, Llinas R, et al: Anterior temporal language areas in patients with early onset of temporal lobe epilepsy. Ann Neurol 1993;34:727-732.

50. Perrine K: Future directions for functional mapping. Epilepsia 1994;35(Suppl 6):S90-S102.

51. Ojemann G, Ojemann J, Lettich E, Berger M: Cortical language localization in left, dominant hemisphere. J Neurosurg 1989;71:316-326.

52. Schwartz TH, Devinsky O, Doyle W, Perrine K: Function-specific high-probability "nodes" identified in posterior language cortex. Epilepsia 1999;40:575-583.

53. Salmelin R, Hari R, Lounasmaa OV, et al: Dynamics of brain activation during picture naming. Nature 1994;368:463-465.

54. Elbert T, Keil A: Imaging in the fourth dimension. Nature 2000;404:29-31.

55. Patel AD, Ballaban E: Temporal patterns of human cortical activity reflect tone sequence structure. Nature 2000;404:80-84.

56. Habib M: The neurological basis of developmental dyslexia: An overview and working hypothesis. Brain 2000;132:2373-2399.

57. Simos PG, Breier JI, Fletcher JM, et al: Cerebral mechanisms involved in word reading in dyslexic children: A magnetic source imaging approach. Cereb Cortex 2000;10:809-816.

58. Simos PG, Breier JI, Fletcher JM, et al: Brain activation profiles in dyslexic children during non-word reading: A magnetic source imaging study. Neurosci Lett 2000;290:61-65.

59. Pugh KR, Mencl WE, Jenner AR, et al: Functional neuroimaging studies of reading and reading disability (developmental dyslexia). Mental Retard Dev Disabil Res Rev 2000;6:207-213.

60. Salmelin R, Service E, Kiesila P, et al: Impaired visual word processing in dyslexia revealed with magnetoencephalography. Ann Neurol 1996;40:157-162.

61. Salmelin R, Helenius P, Service E: Neurophysiology of fluent and impaired reading: A magnetoencephalographic approach. J Clin Neurophysiol 2000;17:163-174.

62. Heim S, Eulitz C, Kaufmann J, et al: Atypical organization of the auditory cortex in dyslexia as revealed by MEG. Neuropsychologia 2000;38:1749-1759.

63. Simos PG, Breier JI, Fletcher JM, et al: Brain mechanisms for reading words and pseudowords: An integrated approach. Cerebr Cortex 2002;12:297-305.

64. Simos PG, Fletcher JM, Bergman E, et al: Dyslexia-specific brain activation profile becomes normal following successful remedial training. Neurology 2002;58:1203-1213.

65. Simos PG, Fletcher JM, Foorman BR, et al: Brain activation profiles during the early stages of reading acquisition. J Child Neurol 2002;17:159-163.

66. Barth DS, Sutherling W, Engel J, et al: Neuromagnetic localization of epileptiform spike activity in the human brain. Science 1982;218:891-894.

67. Barth DS, Sutherling W, Engel J, et al: Neuromagnetic evidence of spatially distributed sources underlying epileptiform spikes in the human brain. Science 1984;223:293-296.

68. Eisenberg HM, Papanicolaou AC, Baumann SB, et al: Magnetoencephalographic localization of interictal spike sources. J Neurosurg 1991;74;660-664.

69. Rose DF, Smith PD, Sato S: Magnetoencephalography and epilepsy research. Science 1987;238:329-335.

70. Sato S, Smith PD: Magnetoencephalography. J Clin Neurophysiol 1985;2:173-192.

71. Sutherling WW, Crandall PH, Cahan LD, et al: The magnetic field of epileptic spikes agrees with intracranial localizations in complex partial epilepsy. Neurology 1988;38:778-786.

72. Hari R, Ahonen A, Forss N, et al: Parietal epileptic mirror focus detected with a whole-head neuromagnetometer. Neuro Rep 1993;5:45-48.

73. Paetau R, Kajola M, Hari R: Magnetoencephalography in the study of epilepsy. Neurophysiol Clin North Am 1990;20:169-187.

74. Smith JR, Schwartz BJ, Galen C, et al: Utilization of multichannel magnetoencephalography in the guidance of ablative seizure surgery. J Epilepsy 1985;8:119-130.

75. Stefan H, Schneider S, Feistel H, et al: Ictal and interictal activity in partial epilepsy recorded with multichannel magnetoencephalography: Correlation of electroencephalography/electrocorticography, magnetic resonance imaging, and single photon emission computed tomography, and position emission tomography findings. Epilepsia 1992;33:874-887.

76. Tiihonen J, Hari R, Kajola M, et al: Localization of epileptic foci using a large-area magnetometer and functional brain anatomy. Ann Neurol 1990;27:283-290.

77. Stefan H, Schneider S, Abraham-Fuchs K, et al: Magnetic source localization in focal epilepsy. Brain 1990;113:1347-1359.

78. Ochi A, Otsubo H, Sharma R, et al: Comparison of electroencephalographic dipoles of interictal spikes from prolonged scalp video-electroencephalography and magnetoencephalographic dipoles from short-term recording in children with extratemporal lobe epilepsy. J Child Neurol 2001;16:661-667.

79. Baumgartner C, Pataraia E, Lindinger G, et al: Magnetoencephalography in focal epilepsy. Epilepsia 2000;41(Suppl 3):S39-S47.

80. Iwaski M, Nakasato N, Shamoto H, et al: Surgical implications of neuromagnetic spike localization in temporal lobe epilepsy. Epilepsia 2002;43:415-424.

81. Minassian BA, Otsubo H, Weiss S, et al: Magnetoencephalographic localization in pediatric epilepsy surgery: Comparison with invasive intracranial electroencephalography. Ann Neurol 1999;46:627-633.

82. Otsubo H, Ochi A, Elliott I, et al: MEG predicts epileptic zone in lesional extrahippocampal epilepsy: 12 pediatric surgery cases. Epilepsia 2001;42:1523-1530.

83. Stefan H, Hummel C, Hopfengartner R, et al: Magnetoencephalography in extratemporal epilepsy. J Clin Neurophysiol 2000;17:190-200.

84. King DW, Park YD, Smith JR, et al: Magnetoencephalography in neocortical epilepsy. *In* Williamson PD, Siegel AM, Roberts DW, et al (eds): Neocortical Epilepsies: Advances in Neurology. Philadelphia, Lippincott Williams & Wilkins, 2000, pp 415-423.

85. Ishibashi H, Simos PG, Castillo EM, et al: Detection and significance of focal, interictal, slow-wave activity visualized by magnetoencephalography for localization of a primary epileptogenic region. J Neurosurg 2002;96:724-730.

86. Pantev C, Lutkenhoner B: Magnetoencephalographic studies of functional organization and plasticity of the human auditory cortex. J Clin Neurophysiol 2000;17:130-142.

87. Papanicolaou AC, Simos PG, Breier JI, et al: Brain plasticity for sensory and linguistic functions: A functional imaging study using magnetoencephalography with children and young adults. J Child Neurol 2001;16:241-252.

88. Ishibashi H, Simos PG, Wheless JW, et al: Multimodality functional imaging evaluation in a patient with Rasmussen's encephalitis. Brain Dev 2002;24:239-244.

89. Pataraia E, Baumgartner C, Lindinger G, Deecke L: Magnetoencephalography in presurgical epilepsy evaluation. Neurosurg Rev 2002;25:141-159.

90. Ishibashi H, Morioka T, Shigeto H, et al: Three-dimensional localization of subclinical ictal activity by magnetoencephalography: Correlation with invasive monitoring. Surg Neurol 1998;50:157-163.

91. Shiraishi H, Watanabe Y, Watanabe M, et al: Interictal and ictal magnetoencephalographic study in patients with medial frontal lobe epilepsy. Epilepsia 2001;42:875-882.

92. Oishi M, Kameyama S, Morota N, et al: Fusiform gyrus epilepsy: The use of ictal magnetoencephalography [Case Report]. J Neurosurg 2002;97:200-204.

93. Tilz C, Hummel C, Kettenmann B, Stefan H: Ictal onset localization of epileptic seizures by magnetoencephalography. Acta Neurol Scand 2002;106:190-195.

94. Eliashiv DS, Elsas SM, Squires K, et al: Ictal magnetic source imaging as localizing tool in partial epilepsy. Neurology 2002;59:1600-1610.

95. Maggio V, Ng Y, Simos PG, et al: Correlation of ictal magnetoencephalography with ictal electroencephalographic recordings. Epilepsia 2002;43(Suppl 7):315.

96. Ishibashi H, Simos PG, Wheless JW, et al: Localization of ictal and interictal bursting epileptogenic activity in cortical dysplasia: Agreement of magnetoencephalography and electrocorticography. Neurol Res 2002;24:525-530.

40

Transcranial Magnetic Stimulation: An Overview

KARIN EDEBOL EEG-OLOFSSON

Magnetic stimulation through the skull of the human motor cortex was first reported in 1985 by Barker and coworkers.[1] Transcranial magnetic stimulation (TMS) is a noninvasive method used to assess motor pathway conduction, and TMS has become a widely used tool in research and clinical work in a large range of disorders.[2-13] TMS in children has been reported in varying disorders with motor involvement,[14-17] in the operating room, and has been reported in children with psychiatric diagnoses[18-21] and epilepsy.[22] However, the application of TMS has been somewhat limited in children, although the method offers unique possibilities to gain insight into the motor system.

BIOPHYSICS AND PHYSIOLOGY OF TMS

The Magnetic Stimulator

Magnetic stimulators mainly consist of two parts: (1) a system of high-voltage, high-current capacitors and (2) the inductor, which is the coil itself. As the capacitors discharge, a brief pulse of magnetic field (measured in tesla) is produced, causing rapid changes in the magnetic field within a millisecond. This leads to induction of electrical currents of 100- to 200-microsecond duration in biologic tissues nearby.[7,11,23-24] Nervous tissue is not excited by the magnetic field itself but by the induced current. The induced current flows in the opposite direction of the coil

current, in a plane parallel to the coil. This favors excitation of horizontally oriented cortical fibers in contrast with transcranial electrical stimulation (TES), which produces vertically oriented currents.[23,24] The higher the speed of change of the magnetic field, the higher is the strength of the induction current. The intensity of the magnetic field declines with distance from the coil. The induction current is proportional to the conductivity of the tissues; for example, neural tissue is easily excited, whereas in bone, fat, and skin only low-voltage currents are induced.[7,23]

Different types of magnetic coils have been designed. Large, round coils produce the strongest magnetic fields but do not give very focal stimulation owing to penetration to greater depth with distribution of magnetic fields through larger volumes of tissue. Smaller coils (e.g., "figure 8") give a weaker magnetic field but more focal stimulation. The induced currents at magnetic stimulation are concentrated below the center of the coil. In a large, round coil the maximum magnetic field is at the midpoint of the leading inner edge, and in a figure-8 coil it is under the bar of "8."[11,23,26] In clinical routine, a conventional large round coil is of good use, both for transcranial and motor root stimulation.

Stimulation of Neuronal Tissue

Magnetic stimulation excites the pyramidal tract cells of the motor cortex, the corticomotor neurons.[7,11,26,45] These cells are stimulated by transcranial magnet trans-synaptically or directly excited. In contrast, TES activates pyramidal cells in the depth of the brain, at the axon hillock, or at the first or second node of Ranvier. Thus, motor evoked potentials (MEPs) after TMS reflect the excitability state of the corticomotor neurons as well as the spinal motor neurons, whereas MEPs after TES depend on the excitability state of the spinal motor neurons only.

Recording of Magnetic Evoked Potentials

MEPs are mostly recorded from limb muscles, usually of the hand and lower limb. However, MEPs may also be recorded from muscles of the trunk or cranial nerves or elsewhere. At TMS, motor units (MUs) are recruited; the smallest are recruited first, and thereafter larger ones, in accordance with the size principle. Hand muscles have the lowest threshold stimulus since their cortical representational area is large, whereas muscles with a smaller representation in cortex, for example, proximal limb muscles, require a higher threshold stimulus to elicit MEPs.

TMS Parameters

In standard TMS investigations the motor threshold (MTh), MEP amplitude, MEP latency, and central motor conduction time (CMCT) are calculated. In addition to these, a calculation of the silent period (SP) as well as paired-pulse TMS can be carried out.

MTh is a function of both cortical and spinal mechanisms; that is, MTh reflects the excitability in the most excitable corticospinal neurons. MTh is increased by drugs such as carbamazepine and phenytoin that influence the sodium-channel function. MTh is the lowest TMS intensity that will give rise to an MEP of a minimum size of 50 to 100 μV at muscle rest and 100 to 200 μV at muscle activation. The MTh is about 25% lower at activation compared with muscle at rest. The MTh is also lower in distal muscles compared to proximal muscles. A high MTh is seen after a lesion on the corticospinal tract, such as after a stroke or spinal cord injury. A low MTh may be seen in conditions with increased corticospinal excitability, such as in untreated general idiopathic epilepsy, early in the course of amyotrophic lateral sclerosis, and in some psychiatric disorders.

MEP amplitude is usually calculated peak to peak (millivolt) and is usually expressed in percentage of maximal compound muscle action potential (CMAP) at electrical stimulation of the peripheral nerve to muscle. Thus,

$$MEP\% = obtained\ MEP \div maximal\ CMAP \times 100$$

MEP% is a measurement of the actual portion of spinal alpha motor neurons activated by TMS. The MEP amplitude

increases by increasing stimulus intensity.[18] The amplitude also increases at voluntary muscle activation due to increased activity in spinal motor neurons.[27] The MEP amplitude is also affected by the position of the coil.[6]

MEP% is lowered when there is an increased dispersion of multiple corticospinal discharges that leads to phase cancellation and in conditions with disturbed conduction in the corticospinal tract due to axonal (neuronal) loss, as well as in situations with severe decreased excitability in the corticospinal and/or spinal motor neurons. Some antiepileptic drugs may induce very high MThs.

MEP (corticomuscular) latency is measured from the stimulus artifact to the onset of motor response (in milliseconds). MEP latency varies with the distance to the muscle and thus is also related to the height of the investigated person.

CMCT is the corticomuscular latency minus the peripheral motor conduction time, which can be obtained by root stimulation or by using F-latency in the formula

$$(F + M - 1)/2$$

where F is the minimum F-latency and M is the distal motor latency.[28] The estimated time delay for antidromic activation of the spinal alpha motor neuron is 1 millisecond. The CMCT at root stimulation is 0.5 to 1.4 milliseconds longer for cervical roots compared with the F-method and 3.0 to 4.1 milliseconds longer for lumbosacral roots.

CMCT is 2 or 3 milliseconds shorter when a muscle is activated owing to a decreased need for temporal summation to reach a discharge threshold (especially in spinal alpha motor neurons) and facilitation of recruitment of larger and faster alpha motor neurons. Position of the coil affects the CMCT; the shortest CMCT is obtained when the coil is placed in optimal position,[29] the so-called hot spot in relation to the target muscle.

SP gives information about γ-amino-butyric acid (GABA)-mediated mechanisms controlling motor cortex excitability. TMS at voluntary contraction of the recording muscle gives an MEP followed by a pause of 200 to 300 milliseconds, the SP, before electromyographic (EMG) activity reappears. SP is measured from the end of the MEP to the restart of EMG activity. SP has a longer duration in the hand and forearm muscles compared to muscles of the upper arm. The duration of SP is correlated to the stimulus intensity.[12,30] The degree of voluntary activation is not important for the duration of SP. The cortical SP reflects the general degree of inhibitory mechanisms mainly within the sensorimotor loop. SP is increased in stroke with motor neglect. Decreased SP is seen in epilepsy, stroke, Parkinson's disease, "stiff man" syndrome, and tetanus. In cranial dystonia, SPs in facial muscles are shorter than in controls owing to hyperexcitability of the cortical inhibitory neurons.[31]

In *paired-pulse TMS* two TMS stimuli are given with variable intensity and different interstimulus intervals, and intracortical inhibition and excitation may be studied. If the interstimulus interval is short, MEP obtained after suprathreshold stimulation is inhibited by a previous conditioning of a subthreshold stimulus due to GABA-mediated intracortical inhibition.[13] A longer interstimulus interval gives, in contrast, a facilitation that is mediated by gluta-minergic receptors.[13] In the first case there is a short-latency intracortical inhibition that is GABA mediated, and in the second case there is a short-latency intracortical facilitation mediated by glutaminergic receptors. Thus, paired-pulse TMS may be used in research as well as in clinical disorders to study intracortical excitation and inhibition.

Repetitive TMS

Pascual-Leone and coworkers[32] first observed repetitive TMS (rTMS) in a train at 5 Hz and 120% MTh-induced MEPs that became successively larger. rTMS affects the corticospinal excitability also after the duration of the train. In one study, healthy subjects were given short trains of rTMS with 20 stimuli at 5, 10, and 20 Hz during relaxation of the target muscle. Cortical excitability, reflected by the size of MEP amplitude, was after a suprathreshold TMS pulse decreased for up to 1 second after the end of the rTMS. This post-train suppression was stronger after longer trains or higher frequencies of rTMS.[33] When the intensity of rTMS was increased, there was instead a post-train facilitation. The authors concluded that the effects seen after rTMS depend on frequency, intensity, and duration and that inhibition is reached by a smaller number of stimuli and with a relatively lower threshold compared to facilitation.[33] In one study, a subthreshold low-frequency rTMS stimulation (1 Hz) was given to subjects during 10 minutes, and MEPs were measured before and after the train.[34] The MEP amplitude was reduced by the train, and this effect lasted for about 10 minutes after the train was completed; that is, there was a depressed cortical excitability beyond the rTMS train.

TMS IN CHILDREN: SUBJECTIVE REACTIONS AND MATURATIONAL ASPECTS

How children perceive TMS was studied in normal children and children with attention-deficit hyperactivity disorder (ADHD).[35] Of the 38 children who were investigated with single-pulse TMS, 34 said that they would repeat the investigation. There are some children who find the investigation uncomfortable; however, most children consider it painless.

In healthy children, an early study[36] of TMS showed that during full muscular relaxation MEPs could be obtained in the upper extremity after the first year of life and in the lower extremity after the fourth year of life. CMCT was dependent on age (i.e., maturation), and adult values could not be obtained before the age of about 10 years. The maturational profile for the peripheral conduction was faster, whereas root stimulation (cervical and lumbar) reached adult values at about 3 years of age.

TMS has been used in studies on development of motor performance skills in children. Ten young school children aged 6 to 9 years were compared to 10 adults aged 22 to 26 years in a study of motor performance tasks that included finger tapping, ballistic movement, and diadochokinesis.[37] The central conduction time under facilitation (slight voluntary activation of the target muscle) and the postexcitatory SP were similar to those in adults. However, CMCT under relaxation of the target muscle and the MEP latency difference between relaxation and facilitation differed significantly between the children and adults (the children did not reach the same level of performance as the adults). These findings indicate that although children of early school age possess mature fast corticospinal pathways, the neuronal maturation and performance will undergo further maturation to reach adult levels. The same research group reported a study of 112 subjects aged 0.2 to 30 years where hand motor function and TMS were investigated.[25] CMCTs at relaxation and facilitation reached adult values at different times, reflecting maturation at cortical and spinal levels. A stable phase for CMCT and reaction time was reached during childhood, and the tract parameters related to motor speed and skill continued into adulthood. The findings indicated that the maturation of the fast corticospinal tract is completed first and the related motor performance is developed thereafter. In a recent report,[38] finger-tapping speed and mirror movements were studied in 43 healthy right-hand subjects aged 6 to 26 years, and TMS was performed with focal stimulation over the cortical hand areas. MEPs were recorded from left and right first dorsal interossei muscles. MTh and ipsilateral and contralateral SPs were measured. MEP thresholds of the right hemisphere were longer than those on the left in all subjects. With increasing age of the children, MEP thresholds decreased, ipsilateral SP duration increased, and ipsilateral SP latency decreased and these findings were closely related to acquisition of faster finger-tapping skills.

TMS SET-UP IN DAILY CLINICAL ROUTINE

Prior to magnetic stimulation, electrical stimulation of the ulnar nerve at the wrist and the deep peroneal nerve at the knee was performed to record muscle responses from the abductor digiti minimi and the tibialis anterior muscles, respectively. This was done to ensure the possibility of obtaining MEPs of the target muscle during magnetic stimulation.

Muscle responses are recorded by silver cup electrodes 10 mm in diameter. No specific preparation is needed for TMS. A magnetic stimulator (with a circular coil C-100 and a pulse width of 300 μsec biphasic) is used to elicit motor evoked potentials both by cortical stimulation (the coil is moved tangentially to the cortex for study of the upper limbs and is centered sagitally for the lower limbs) and root stimulation (the coil is centered over the C7 and L4 spinous processes to study the upper and lower limbs, respectively). The MEP recordings are done bilaterally with muscles at rest and during slight voluntary contraction for facilitation. During the procedure, the stimulation intensity is increased progressively and the coil is moved tangentially over the scalp until the maximum amplitude and the shortest latency of the response are obtained. CMCT is calculated by subtracting the peripheral conduction time with root stimulation from the total conduction time with cortical stimulation.[23,39]

Difficulty in eliciting lower limbs MEPs may occur not only in disease states but also in normal persons.[24] In children, there is in the clinical setting not seldom a lack of normative values both in cortical latency and CMCT. CMCT per se can be calculated according to the formula

$$CMCT \text{ (msec)} = MEP - [(F - MAP - 1)/2 + MAP]$$

where MEP refers to MEP latency, F to minimal F-wave latency, and MAP to distal motor latency on peripheral stimulation.[39]

CLINICAL APPLICATIONS OF MAGNETIC EVOKED POTENTIALS IN CHILDHOOD

TMS in Motor Function Evaluation

In disorders with symptoms and signs from the motor system, TMS has been used in pediatric patients. In one study TMS was carried out in children after treatment for childhood acute lymphoblastic leukemia.[40] Neurologic signs and symptoms were common after treatment: in 41% of 32 children the tendon reflexes were depressed, 63% had gross motor difficulties, and 34% had dysdiadochokinesia. Latencies of the motor evoked potentials were significantly prolonged along the entire motor nervous system in patients compared to an age-, sex-, and height-matched control group. The conduction delay within the peripheral nervous system (PNS) was related to the post-therapeutic interval

after administration of vincristine and the lesions within the central nervous system (CNS) to the number of injections of intrathecal methotrexate. The MEP amplitudes elicited by TMS showed a wider variation than in control children. No clear abnormalities were found, whereas magnetic stimulation of the PNS gave significantly lower amplitudes than in the healthy children. The authors found TMS to be a practical, painless, and objective method to study treatment-related toxicity both in the CNS and PNS.

In a case report, one 13-year-old child was followed up with TMS as well as somatosensory evoked potentials after transverse myelitis.[17] Four weeks after onset, MEP amplitudes were decreased and latencies prolonged. After 6 and 12 weeks the MEP amplitudes successively became higher and the latencies shorter, and these findings paralleled the clinical recovery.

In two children with multiple sclerosis, TMS showed a raised MTh in the upper limb in one of the children, and in the other child the MEP latency was increased and CCT prolonged to the right anterior tibial muscle.[14] Thus, TMS may well be one of the tools in the assessment of children with multiple sclerosis.

Rett's syndrome is a progressive encephalopathy affecting mainly girls, who lose fine motor ability and develop gross motor dysfunction with spastic pareses, mental retardation, and epilepsy. In a study of 31 persons aged 2 to 28 years, the results were compared to 112 healthy subjects aged 1 month to 35 years.[15] There was no difference in the peripheral conduction time between patients and controls, but the mean CMCT was shorter in the younger patients, especially in the youngest. These findings were interpreted as reflecting cortical and/or spinal hyperexcitability during the early stages of Rett's syndrome. In another report, three children were studied with TMS.[16] In the two youngest children, 4 and 6 years old, the CMCT was significantly shortened compared to age-matched healthy children. CMCT in a somewhat older child (11 years) was short but not significantly ($P = 0.06$). These findings confirm the shortening of CMCT in Rett's syndrome, implying a cortical hyperexcitability, with impaired function of the corticospinal tracts.

In a study on konzo (an acute, nonprogressive spastic paraparesis or quadriparesis affecting poor and undernourished populations in Central African countries), motor pathways were analyzed using TMS[41] in 15 children and adults living in the Democratic Republic of Congo. The muscle responses were recorded from hand and lower limb muscles. MEPs were either absent or showed prolonged CMCT in these patients.

Malnourished children in India have undergone TMS.[42,43] In one study 20 children aged 3 to 8 years were compared to 20 normal children.[42] MEPs were recorded from the abductor pollicis brevis and extensor digitorum brevis muscles.

TMS and root stimulation at the cervical and lumbar spine were performed. In malnourished children the cortical threshold was significantly increased, the CMCT was prolonged, and the MEP amplitude was decreased. These findings indicate asymptomatic involvement of the corticospinal pathways in malnutrition.

TMS in Child Psychiatry

In a study of children with psychiatric diagnoses it was found that in tic disorder a shortened cortical SP was noted, indicating deficient inhibitory mechanisms in the sensorimotor loop, whereas in ADHD a decreased intracortical inhibition was found that could indicate deficient inhibitory mechanisms within the motor cortex.[21] In children with a combination of the two disorders, a mixture of shortened cortical SP and reduced intracortical inhibition was found, providing evidence of additive affects at the level of motor system exitability.[20] The authors stated that "the decreased inhibitory mechanisms within the entire sensorimotor loop and especially the motor cortex may be essential neurobiological substrates of the deficient inhibitory motor control and regulation in the tic disorder and ADHD, respectively."[20] TMS was performed in a study on 21 children with tic disorder and 25 healthy controls aged 10 to 16 years.[19] The cortical SP was significantly shortened compared with healthy children but did not depend on tic localization. Intracortical inhibition and excitation did not differ between patients and controls, and the MTh was normal. The findings confirm earlier results from studies in adults with decreased motor control in the tic disorder. In a report on children with ADHD contralateral SP and transcallosally mediated ipsilateral SP were investigated. The ipsilateral SP latencies were significantly longer and their duration was shorter in the children with ADHD compared with healthy sex- and age-matched children, whereas the contralateral SP, MEP amplitude, and MTh were similar in both groups.[18] Ipsilateral SP latencies tended to decrease with age and the ipsilateral SP duration tended to increase. The shortened ipsilateral SP in the patient group could be explained by an imbalance between inhibitory and excitatory drives on the neuronal network between cortex layers III and V, and the longer latency possibly indicated a defective myelination of fast-conducting transcallosal fibers in ADHD.

rTMS is a novel treatment for varying psychiatric disorders undergoing trials with TMS.[44] In the motor cortex of patients with schizophrenia, for example, TMS has showed inhibitory deficits.[8]

TMS in Childhood Epilepsy

In CNS disorders such as epilepsy, prolonged cortical SP has been found after TMS in the generalized form.[9] In progressive myoclonic epilepsy, TMS has shown hyperexcitable cortical responses.[10]

TMS was performed in 13 children with benign childhood epilepsy with centrotemporal spikes, of whom 5 were untreated and 8 were treated with sodium valproate,[22] and in 10 age-matched controls. MEPs were recorded from the first dorsal interossei muscle at relaxation. MTh intensity was significantly higher in the treated group of children; a significant increase in threshold intensity was also observed in the untreated patients after starting valproate treatment. All other MEP parameters measured (CMCT, latency and duration of MEPs) showed no difference between controls and untreated and treated children.

TMS in Surgery

TMS is an excellent tool to monitor spinal surgery. In the past, somatosensory evoked potentials and direct stimulation of neural spinal tissue to muscles were used as neurophysiologic methods in spinal surgery; however, TMS has also been added to the list of methods for intraoperative monitoring in adults as well as in children.

REFERENCES

1. Barker AT, Jalinous R, Freeston IL: Noninvasive magnetic stimulation of the human motor cortex. Lancet 1975;1:1106-1107.
2. Abbruzzese G, Marchese R, Trompetto C: Motor cortical excitability in Huntington's disease. J Neurol Neurosurg Psychiatry 2000;68:120-121.
3. Abbruzzese G, Trompetto C: Clinical and research methods for evaluating cortical excitability. J Clin Neurophysiol 2002;19:307-321.
4. Berardelli A, Inghilleri M, Cruccu G, et al: Electrical and magnetic stimulation in patients with corticospinal damage due to stroke or motor neuron disease. Electroencephalogr Clin Neurophysiol 1991;81:389-396.
5. Currà A, Modugno N, Inghilleri M, et al: Transcranial magnetic stimulation techniques in clinical investigation. Neurology 2002;59:1851-1859.
6. Di Lazzaro V, Oliviero A, Profice P, et al: The diagnostic value of motor evoked potentials. Clin Neurophysiol 1999;110:1297-1307.
7. Dvořák J, Herdmann J, Vohánka S: Motor evoked potentials by means of magnetic stimulation in disorders of the spine. Methods Clin Neurophysiol 1992;3:45-64.
8. Fitzgerald PB, Brown TL, Daskalakis ZJ, Kulkarni J: A transcranial magnetic stimulation study of inhibitory deficits in the motor cortex in patients with schizophrenia. Psychiatry Res 2002;114:11-22.
9. Macdonell RA, King MA, Newton MR, et al: Prolonged cortical silent period after transcranial magnetic stimulation in generalized epilepsy. Neurology 2001;57:706-708.

10. Manganotti P, Tamburin S, Zanette G, Fiaschi A: Hyperexcitable cortical responses in progressive myoclonic epilepsy: A TMS study. Neurology 2001;57:1793-1799.

11. Terao Y, Ugawa Y: Basic mechanisms of TMS. J Clin Neurophysiol 2002;19:322-343.

12. Weber M, Eisen AA: Magnetic stimulation of the central and peripheral nervous systems. Muscle Nerve 2002;25:160-175.

13. Ziemann U, Hallett M: Basic neurophysiological studies with TMS. *In* George MS, Belmaker RH (eds): Transcranial Magnetic Stimulation in Neuropsychiatry. Washington, DC, American Psychiatry Press, 2000, pp 45-98.

14. Dan B, Christiaens F, Christophe C, Dachy B: Transcranial magnetic stimulation and other evoked potentials in pediatric multiple sclerosis. Pediatr Neurol 2000;22:136-138.

15. Heinen F, Petersen H, Fietzek U, et al: Transcranial magnetic stimulation in patients with Rett syndrome: Preliminary results. Eur Child Adolesc Psychiatry 1997;6(Suppl 1):61-63.

16. Nezu A, Kimura S, Takeshita S, Tanaka M: Characteristic response to transcranial magnetic stimulation in Rett syndrome. Electroencephalogr Clin Neurophysiol 1998;109:100-103.

17. Noguchi Y, Okubo O, Fuchigami T, et al: Motor-evoked potentials in a child recovering from transverse myelitis. Pediatr Neurol 2000;23:436-438.

18. Buchmann J, Wolters A, Haessler F, et al: Disturbed transcallosally mediated motor inhibition in children with attention deficit hyperactivity disorder (ADHD). Clin Neurophysiol 2003;114:2036-2042.

19. Moll GH, Wischer S, Heinrich H, et al: Deficient motor control in children with tic disorder: Evidence from transcranial magnetic stimulation. Neurosci Lett 1999;272:37-40.

20. Moll GH, Heinrich H, Rothenberger A: [Transcranial magnetic stimulation in child and adolescent psychiatry: Excitability of the motor system in tic disorders and/or attention deficit hyperactivity disorders] Z Kinder Jugendpsychiatr Psychother 2001;29:312-323.

21. Moll GH, Heinrich H, Trott GE, et al: Children with comorbid attention-deficit hyperactivity disorder and tic disorder: Evidence for additive inhibitory deficits within the motor system. Ann Neurol 2001;49:393-396.

22. Nezu A, Kimura S, Ohtsuki N, Tanaka M: Transcranial magnetic stimulation in benign childhood epilepsy with centro-temporal spikes. Brain Dev 1997;19:134-137.

23. Eisen A: Cortical and peripheral nerve magnetic stimulation. Methods Clin Neurophysiol 1992;3:65-84.

24. Eisen A, Shtybel W: AAEM Minomonograph No. 35: Clinical experience with transcranial magnetic stimulation. Muscle Nerve 1990;13:995-1011.

25. Fietzek UM, Heinen F, Berweck S, et al: Development of the corticospinal system and hand motor function: Central conduction times and motor performance tests. Dev Med Child Neurol 2000;42:220-227.

26. Rothwell JC: Techniques and mechanisms of action of transcranial stimulation of the human cortex. J Neurosci Methods 1997;74:113-122.

27. Hess CW, Mills KR, Murray NM: Magnetic stimulation of the human brain: Facilitation of motor responses by voluntary contraction of ipsilateral and contralateral muscles with additional observations on an amputee. Neurosci Lett 1986;71:235-240.

28. Robinson LR, Jantra R, MacLean IC: Central motor conduction times using transcranial stimulation and F-wave latencies. Muscle Nerve 1988;11:174-180.

29. Wilson SA, Lockwood RJ, Thickbroom GW, Mastaglia FL: The muscle silent period following transcranial magnetic cortical stimulation. J Neurol Sci 1993;114:216-222.

30. Cantello R, Gianelli M, Civardi C, Mutani R: Magnetic brain stimulation: the silent period after the motor evoked potential. Neurology 1992;42:1951-1959.

31. Currà A, Romaniello A, Berardelli A, et al: Shortened cortical silent period in facial muscle of patients with cranial dystonia. Neurology 2000;54:130-135.

32. Pascual-Leone A, Valls-Solé J, Wasserman EM, Hallett M: Responses to rapid-rate transcranial magnetic stimulation of the human motor cortex. Brain 1994;117:847-858.

33. Modugno N, Nakamura Y, Mackinnon CD, et al: Motor cortex excitability following short trains of repetitive magnetic stimuli. Exp Brain Res 2001;140:453-459.

34. Romero JR, Anschel D, Sparing R, et al: Subthreshold low-frequency repetitive transcranial magnetic stimulation selectively decreases facilitation in the motor cortex. Clin Neurophysiol 2002;113:101-107.

35. Garvey MA, Kaczynski KJ, Becker DA, Bartko JJ: Subjective reactions of children to single-pulse transcranial magnetic stimulation. J Child Neurol 2001;16:891-894.

36. Müller K, Hömberg V, Lenard HG: Magnetic stimulation of motor cortex and nerve roots in children: Maturation of corticomotor neuronal projections. Electroencephalogr Clin Neurophysiol 1991;81:63-70.

37. Heinen F, Fietzek UM, Berweck S, et al: Fast corticospinal system and motor performance in children—conduction precedes skill. Pediatr Neurol 1998;19:217-221.

38. Garvey MA, Ziemann U, Bartko JJ, et al: Cortical correlates of neuromotor development in healthy children. Clin Neurophysiol 2003;114:1662-1670.

39. Rossini PM, Pauri F: Central motor conduction time studies. Electroencephalogr Clin Neurophysiol Suppl 1999;51:199-211.

40. Harila-Saari AH, Huuskonen UE, Tolonen U, et al: Motor nervous pathway function is impaired after treatment in childhood acute lymphoblastic leukemia: A study with motor evoked potentials. Med Pediatr Oncol 2001;36:345-351.

41. Tshala-Katumbay D, Edebol Eeg-Olofsson K, Kazadi-Kayembe T, et al: Analysis of motor pathway involvement in konzo using transcranial electrical and magnetic stimulation. Muscle Nerve 2002;25:230-235.

42. Karak B, Misra S, Garg RK, Katiyar GP: A study of transcranial magnetic stimulation in older (>3 years) patients of malnutrition. Neurol India 1999;47:229-233.

43. Tamer SK, Misra S, Jaiswal S: Central motor conduction time in malnourished children. Arch Dis Child 1997;77:323-325.

44. Lin KL, Pascual-Leone A: Transcranial magnetic stimulation and its applications in children. Chang Gung Med J 2002;25:424-436.

45. Rossini PM, Berardelli A, Deuschl G, et al: Applications of magnetic cortical stimulation. The International Federation of Clinical Neurophysiology. Electroencephalogr Clin Neurophysiol 1999;52:171-185.

41

Sphincter Dysfunction

Karin Edebol Eeg-Olofsson

Anal sphincter dysfunction in children is not common; however, when it occurs, it often causes considerable distress in the concerned child. Neurophysiologic evaluation in anal sphincter dysfunction is indicated for severe constipation and anal incontinence.

Constipation of slight to moderate degree is not uncommon in otherwise healthy children. This kind of constipation responds effectively to medical treatment and/or behavioral modification in most cases.[1,2] Children with chronic constipation may have increased colonic transit time. In a study on 38 children aged 2 to 14 years, 50% had normal colonic transit time, whereas 37% had left colonic and rectosigmoid delays, and 13% had global delay; 64% of those with distal delay had also paradoxical anal contraction.[3] Children with motor disabilities often have constipation, and in children with myelomeningocele (MMC) this is due to dyssynergia of the pelvic floor causing both constipation and anal incontinence. In a Nordic study of 527 children with MMC, aged between 4 and 18 years, 412 had disturbed bowel control; that is, only 21% of the children could control the bowel function.[4,5] In children with moderate and severe cerebral palsy, constipation is a frequent problem owing to inactivity and it is enhanced by low intake of fluid. Severe constipation may also be seen in gluten enteropathy and in Hirschsprung's disease. Few healthy children have severe constipation; however, in those children who do, neurophysiologic evaluation may be quite useful to rule out or confirm sphincter spasm and dyssynergia in the external anal sphincter (EAS).

Anal incontinence may be due to congenital malformations, such as those occurring in VACTERL syndrome

consisting of widespread malformations (*v*ertebra, *a*nal, *c*ardiac, *t*rachea, *e*sophagus, *r*enal, *l*imbs). Spinal cord and plexus lesions are further rare causes of anal incontinence. Another rare cause of anal incontinence is sexual abuse of boys. As mentioned earlier, children with MMC often have a combination of anal incontinence and constipation. In most cases, anal incontinence leading to fecal soiling in children is functional and will sooner or later disappear spontaneously.[6]

INVESTIGATION OF CONSTIPATION

By analyzing the electromyographic (EMG) activity during squeeze and strain in the EAS, a strain-to-squeeze index can be measured. This gives information about an eventual paradoxical activation such as dyssynergia of the EAS, which normally should be silent or have little activity during strain. This investigation is of use in severe constipation and forms a basis for treatment with biofeedback or botulinum toxin. The youngest patient who has undergone this investigation was 7 years old, in my experience.

Method

After appropriate preparation with sedation and local anesthetics (see later), the child is placed in left lateral position. Hook electrodes are inserted bilaterally in the EAS, 3 to 4 mm from the midline to a depth of 5 to 8 mm. For the investigation a computerized EMG machine has been used, set on a sweep length of 200 milliseconds and amplitude setting of 0.1 to 0.2 mV, using the program for spontaneous activity where amplitude cursors are available.

The child is asked to relax, then squeeze maximally during some seconds and thereafter relax again; this is repeated three times. Then the child is asked to strain maximally for some seconds and thereafter relax; this is also repeated three times. The mean value in amplitude of three squeezes respectively of three strains can then be obtained and a strain-to-squeeze index calculated. An index of 50% or higher is regarded as significant pathology. It may lead to biofeedback treatment in older children and adults and a trial with botulinum toxin in children with severely disturbed bowel emptying.[7-9]

INVESTIGATION OF ANAL INCONTINENCE

In children older than 14 years of age, the same standard method is used as in adults, namely analysis of pudendal nerve distal latency with St. Mark's electrode, concentric needle EMG of EAS and sometimes the puborectalis muscle, and fiber density in EAS.[10] In young children there is so far no applicable electrode for pudendal nerve neurography. Fiber density in EAS is painful and should be avoided in younger children. Thus, concentric needle EMG of EAS is the method of choice. Needle EMG in EAS gives information about the presence of neurogenic changes in the muscle. The puborectalis muscle might also be difficult to investigate in adults and is usually excluded when investigating children to avoid unnecessary discomfort.

Method

After appropriate preparation with sedation and local anesthetics (see later), the child is placed in the left lateral position. EAS is reached by insertion 3 to 4 mm from the midline and at a depth of 3 to 5 mm. The investigation is done bilaterally, preferentially in the middle of the muscle corresponding to 3 and 9 o'clock. Since EAS normally is active also during sleep to maintain continence, motor unit potentials (MUPs) can be collected for quantitative analysis with little voluntary activation. However, most children are tense at this examination and squeeze, so it is not difficult to obtain enough MUPs (Fig. 41-1). For young children it may be quite difficult to undergo quantitative EMG of EAS even when the preparations have been good. In those children a semiquantitative technique can be applied. This method is quite fast and still reliable, although not as exact as quantitative EMG where the MUPs are averaged. Semiquantitative analysis implies picking up several MUPs as the child is squeezing maximally. The MUPs form an interference pattern and from this single MUPs are chosen

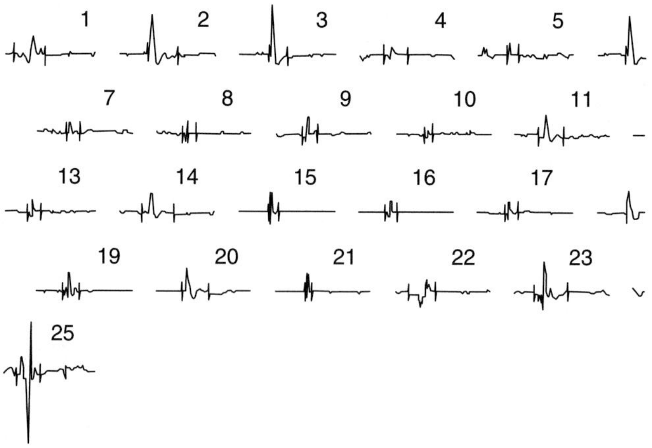

	MUP	Amp	Dur
Simple	1	367	11.2
MUPs (84%)	2	651	11.2
	3	830	7.6
	4	157	9.2
	5	304	4.6
	6	635	11.4
	7	167	5.2
	8	293	4.8
	9	323	6.2
	10	125	3.4
	11	360	9.2
	12	128	2.4
	13	235	5.0
	14	345	12.6
	15	443	4.2
	16	241	4.6
	17	258	5.2
	18	413	10.0
	20	414	10.6
	21	342	2.4
	22	401	9.6
	Mean	354	7.2
Polyphasic	19	331	6.8
MUPs (16%)	23	663	12.8
	24	813	17.0
	25	1650	9.0
	Mean	864	11.4
All	Mean	435	7.8
MUPs	rel.SD		

FIGURE 41–1

Quantitative EMG in a 3-year-old boy with skin-covered myelomeningocele and anal incontinence. The motor unit potentials (MUPs) are from the right external anal sphincter. Collection of 25 MUPs shows normal mean amplitude (435 μV) and duration (7.8 milliseconds). No neurogenic lesion was found.

and automatically measured (Fig. 41-2). The amplitude parameter is quite appropriate, but the duration of the MUPs is not exact with this method (Fig. 41-3). Approximately 20 collected MUPs are enough for both quantitative and semiquantitative EMG. It is difficult to get enough

Muscle	#	Amp				Dur				Area				Poly %
		uV	rel.SD	<min	>max	ms	rel.SD	<min	>max	uVms	rel.SD	<min	>max	
Right sphincter ani	23	459	-	-	-	9.9	-	-	-	825	-	-	-	9
Left sphincter ani	20	401	-	-	-	9.0	-	-	-	698	-	-	-	10

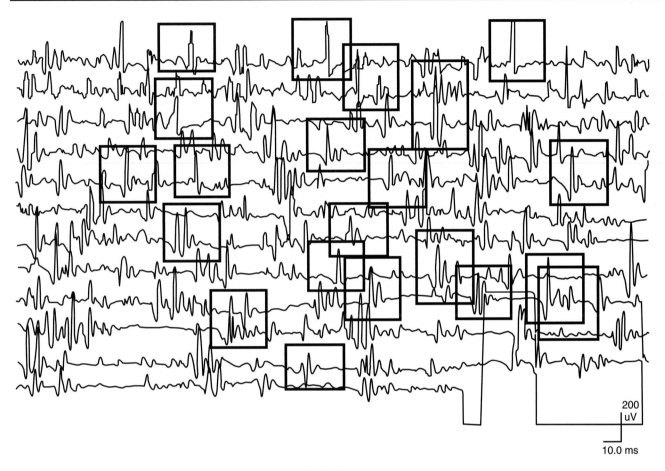

FIGURE 41–2

Semiquantitative EMG in a 10-year-old boy with anal incontinence. Collection of 23 MUPs from those recruited at squeeze shows normal findings (mean amplitude 459 μV). No neurogenic lesion was identified.

relaxation in the EAS to study spontaneous activity at rest, especially in children. Thus, EMG of EAS gives information about MUPs,[11] that is, whether they are normal, have reinnervation potentials as in inactive neurogenic changes, or are myopathic (rare).

PREPARATIONS FOR INVESTIGATIONS

Pain relief and sedation are important when performing needle EMG in the anal sphincter, because the area is highly sensitive to pain. Disregarding pain and anxiety in children when there are ways to alleviate and soothe would be unethical.

Prior to the examination, all children receive an application of EMLA cream (contains lidocaine and prilocaine) over the skin (and mucous membrane) covering the needle insertion area. EMLA cream is applied 1 hour before the examination. In the anal region the cream does not attach very well though, even when the creme is properly covered with the plastic film made for its use.

The children are also given midazolam (Dormicum), a benzodiazepine derivative with hypnotic effect. In the recommended dosage the child becomes drowsy. Even if the child is not optimally cooperating, it is usually not difficult to get him or her to squeeze (i.e., activate) the EAS. Midazolam is given after parental consent and can be administered in different ways (oral, rectal, nasal, intravenous). It provides an

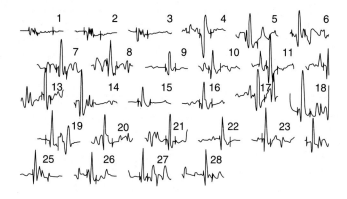

	MUP	Amp	Dur
Simple	4	1328	9.4
MUPs (68%)	6	1094	11.0
	7	1129	9.0
	8	1089	8.8
	9	709	8.2
	10	856	10.4
	11	1395	9.2
	15	596	10.8
	16	833	10.0
	17	1183	8.6
	18	1496	10.2
	20	1056	8.0
	21	1073	7.8
	22	1067	9.4
	23	1360	7.4
	24	1083	12.2
	26	1005	7.6
	27	1058	7.0
	28	1092	7.2
	Mean	1079	9.1
Polyphasic	1	243	19.6
MUPs (32%)	2	417	13.0
	3	377	9.0
	5	1065	8.8
	12	1376	11.2
	13	1187	7.4
	14	1452	14.2
	19	1125	10.8
	25	1068	12.6
	Mean	923	11.8
All	Mean	1029	10.0
MUPs	rel.SD		

FIGURE 41–3

Semiquantitative EMG in a 5{1/2}-year-old boy with anal incontinence due to VACTERL syndrome (see text). Collection of motor unit potentials (MUPs) was from the left external anal sphincter (EAS). MUPs numbered 1 to 28 have increased amplitudes (mean amplitude 1029 μV). The finding is consistent with an inactive neurogenic lesion of the EAS.

amnesia for the investigation, which is a positive side effect. After the administration of midazolam, the child is observed for at least 2 hours to recover fully from the sedation. Documentation should be provided for the dosage, method and time of administration, and the reaction to the drug.

PRACTICAL HINTS

EMG evaluation of the anal sphincter implies a somewhat more difficult situation compared to EMG of extremity muscles. The technique itself is the same, but the choice of muscle (EAS) presents a stressful situation for the child, the parents, and the clinician. Informing the parents that the investigation will cause pain despite measures to relieve pain and anxiety in the child is important, as is informing the child that the investigation may be somewhat difficult for him or her but it will be done fast. The examination should be performed in a quick, friendly, and confident way. The child will in almost all cases cry during the examination and will need soothing after it is completed. Evaluation for anal incontinence and constipation means two needle insertions (with standard concentric needle vs. hook electrodes), but the pain caused by the insertion is of short duration. Thus, despite discomfort in connection with the investigation, it is possible to carry out a neurophysiologic evaluation of sphincter dysfunction in children.

REFERENCES

1. Youssef NN, Di Lorenzo C: Treatment options for refractory childhood constipation. Curr Treat Options Gastroenterol 2002;5:377-387.
2. Loening-Baucke V: Encopresis. Curr Opin Pediatr 2002;14:570-575.
3. Gutierrez C, Marco A, Nogales A, Tebar R: Total and segmental colonic transit time and anorectal manometry in children with chronic idiopathic constipation. J Pediatr Gastroenterol Nutr 2002;35:31-38.
4. Lie HR, Lagergren J, Rasmussen F, et al: Bowel and bladder control of children with myelomeningocele: A Nordic study. Dev Med Child Neurol 1991;33:1053-1061.
5. Hagelsteen JH, Lagergren J, Lie HR, et al: Disability in children with myelomeningocele: A Nordic study. Acta Paediatr Scand 1989;78:721-727.
6. Rintala RJ: Fecal incontinence in anorectal malformations, neuropathy, and miscellaneous conditions. Semin Pediatr Surg 2002;11:75-82.
7. Karlbom U, Edebol Eeg-Olofsson K, Graf W, et al: Paradoxical puborectalis contraction is associated with impaired rectal evacuation. Int J Colorect Dis 1998;13:141-147.
8. Wald A: Slow transit constipation. Curr Treat Options Gastroenterol 2002;5:279-283.

9. Karlbom U, Hålldén M, Edebol Eeg-Olofsson K, et al: Results of biofeedback in constipated patients: A prospective study. Dis Colon Rectum 1997;40:1149-1155.

10. Österberg A, Graf W, Edebol Eeg-Olofsson K, et al: Results of neurophysiologic evaluation in fecal incontinence. Dis Colon Rectum 2000;43:1256-1261.

11. Podnar S, David B: Comparison of different quantitative EMG methods in the external anal sphincter muscle [Abstract]. Presented at the 11th International Congress of EMG and Clinical Neurophysiology, Prague, September 1999.

Index

Page numbers followed by the letter b refer to boxed material. Page numbers followed by the letter f refer to figures; those followed by the letter t refer to tables.